Fundamentals of Surgical Practice

Third Edition

Edited by

Andrew N. Kingsnorth MS, FRCS, FACS
Consultant Surgeon, Derriford Hospital and Honorary Professor of Surgery,
Peninsula College of Medicine and Dentistry, Plymouth, UK

Douglas M. Bowley FRCS [Gen Surg]
Consultant Surgeon, Heart of England NHS Foundation Trust and Senior Lecturer,
Academic Department of Military Surgery and Trauma,
Royal Centre for Defence Medicine, Birmingham, UK

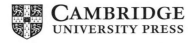

CAMBRIDGE
UNIVERSITY PRESS

CAMBRIDGE UNIVERSITY PRESS
Cambridge, New York, Melbourne, Madrid, Cape Town,
Singapore, São Paulo, Delhi, Tokyo, Mexico City

Cambridge University Press
The Edinburgh Building, Cambridge CB2 8RU, UK

Published in the United States of America by Cambridge University
Press, New York

www.cambridge.org
Information on this title: www.cambridge.org/9780521137225

First published by Greenwich Medical Media 1998
Second Edition published by Cambridge University Press 2006
Third Edition published 2011

Printed in the United Kingdom at the University Press, Cambridge

*A catalogue record for this publication is available from the British
Library*

Library of Congress Cataloguing in Publication data
Fundamentals of surgical practice / edited by Andrew N. Kingsnorth,
MS, FRCS, FACS, Consultant Surgeon, Derriford Hospital and
Honorary Professor of Surgery, Peninsula College of Medicine and
Dentistry, Plymouth, UK, Douglas M. Bowley, FRCS [Gen Surg],
Consultant Surgeon, Heart of England NHS Foundation Trust and
Senior Lecturer, Academic Department of Military Surgery and
Trauma, Royal Centre for Defence Medicine, Birmingham, UK. – Third
Edition.
    p. ; cm.
Includes bibliographical references and index.
ISBN 978-0-521-13722-5 (pbk.)
1. Surgery.   I. Kingsnorth, Andrew N., 1948– editor.
II. Bowley, Douglas M., editor.
[DNLM: 1. Surgical Procedures, Operative. WO 500]
RD32.F86   2011
617 – dc22   2010048439

ISBN 978-0-521-13722-5 Paperback

Contents

Contents

Contributors

Donald J. Adam
Consultant Surgeon, Heart of England NHS
Foundation Trust and Senior Lecturer, Department of
Vascular Surgery, Birmingham University,
Birmingham, UK

Matthew Bowles
Consultant Surgeon, Derriford Hospital, Plymouth,
UK

Douglas M. Bowley
Consultant Surgeon, Heart of England NHS
Foundation Trust, and Senior Lecturer, Academic
Department of Military Surgery and Trauma, Royal
Centre for Defence Medicine, Birmingham, UK

Tim Campbell Smith
Department of Colon and Rectal Surgery, University
College London Hospitals, London, UK

Peter Cant
Consultant Surgeon, Department of Surgery,
Derriford Hospital, Plymouth, UK

Martin W. Claridge
Specialist Registrar in Surgery, Birmingham
University Department of Vascular Surgery, Heart of
England NHS Foundation Trust, Birmingham, UK

Jon Clasper
Consultant Surgeon, Frimley Park NHS Foundation
Trust and Defence Professor of Trauma and
Orthopaedics, Academic Department of Military
Surgery and Trauma, Royal Centre for Defence
Medicine, Birmingham, UK

Jamie J. Coleman
Senior Lecturer, Department of Clinical
Pharmacology, College of Medical and Dental
Sciences, University of Birmingham, Birmingham,
UK

Mark G. Coleman
Consultant Surgeon, Department of Surgery,
Derriford Hospital, Plymouth, UK

Angela Cottrell
Department of Urology, Derriford Hospital,
Plymouth, UK

Nicholas J. Cowley
Specialist Registrar, Department of Anaesthesia,
University Hospitals Birmingham NHS Foundation
Trust, Birmingham, UK

Anthony R. Cox
Lecturer in Clinical Therapeutics, School of
Pharmacy, Aston University, Birmingham,
UK

Tania C.S. Cubison
Consultant Surgeon, Department of Burns,
Reconstruction and Plastic Surgery, Queen Victoria
Hospital, East Grinstead, East Sussex, UK, and Royal
Army Medical Corps, UK

Chris Cunningham
Colorectal Surgeon, Department of Colorectal
Surgery, John Radcliffe Hospital, Oxford, UK

Richard Cunningham
Consultant Microbiologist, Department of
Microbiology, Derriford Hospital, Plymouth,
UK

Ross Davenport
Trauma Research Fellow, Trauma Clinical Academic
Unit, Royal London Hospital, Whitechapel, London,
UK

Andrew Dickinson
Consultant Surgeon, Department of Urology,
Derriford Hospital, Plymouth, UK

Mark Duxbury
Clinical Scientist and Honorary Consultant Surgeon, University of Edinburgh, Royal Infirmary, Edinburgh, UK

John Evans
St. Mark's Hospital, Middlesex, UK

Deborah Harrington
Specialist Registrar, Department of Thoracic Surgery, Heart of England NHS Foundation Trust, Birmingham, UK

Steven D. Heys
Professor of Surgical Oncology and Consultant Surgeon, Deputy Head, Division of Applied Medicine, School of Medicine and Dentistry, University of Aberdeen, Aberdeen, UK

Riffatt Hussein
Education Fellow, Heart of England NHS Foundation Trust, Birmingham, UK

Anant Kamat
Consultant Surgeon, Department of Neurological Surgery, Derriford Hospital, Plymouth, UK

Robin H. Kennedy
Consultant Surgeon, Department of Colorectal Surgery, St. Mark's Hospital, Middlesex, UK

Walter W.K. King
Clinical Professor, Department of Surgery, Chinese University of Hong Kong and Centre Director, Plastic and Reconstructive Surgery Centre, Hong Kong Sanatorium and Hospital, Hong Kong

Andrew N. Kingsnorth
Consultant Surgeon, Derriford Hospital and Honorary Professor of Surgery, Peninsula College of Medicine and Dentistry, Plymouth, UK

Gerald Langman
Consultant Histopathologist, Heart of England NHS Foundation Trust, Birmingham, UK

Evangelos Mazaris
PhD Student, The West London Renal and Transplant Centre, Imperial College NHS Healthcare Trust, Hammersmith Hospital, London, UK

Chantal Meystre
Consultant, Palliative Care Physician, Heart of England NHS Foundation Trust and Medical Director, Marie Curie Hospice, Solihull, Birmingham, UK

Mark J. Midwinter
Consultant Surgeon, University Hospitals Birmingham NHS Foundation Trust and Defence Professor of Surgery, Royal Centre for Defence Medicine, Birmingham, UK

Angela L. Neville
Assistant Professor of Surgery, Harbor-UCLA Medical Center, Los Angeles, CA, USA

Arvind Pallan
Consultant Radiologist, Heart of England NHS Foundation Trust, Birmingham, UK

James Palmer
Consultant Surgeon, Department of Neurological Surgery, Derriford Hospital, Plymouth, UK

Vassilios Papalois
Consultant Transplant and General Surgeon, The West London Renal and Transplant Centre, Imperial College NHS Healthcare Trust, Hammersmith Hospital, London, UK

Rowan W. Parks
Consultant Surgeon, Edinburgh Royal Infirmary and Reader in Surgery, Department of Clinical and Surgical Sciences, University of Edinburgh, Edinburgh, UK

Michael A. Scott
Consultant Surgeon, Department of Surgery, Gloucestershire Royal Hospital, Gloucester, UK

Richard S. Steyn
Consultant Surgeon, Department of Thoracic Surgery, Heart of England NHS Foundation Trust, Birmingham, UK

Nigel Tai
Consultant Trauma and Vascular Surgeon, Trauma Clinical Academic Unit, Royal London Hospital and Senior Lecturer, Royal Centre for Defence Medicine, Birmingham, UK

Paul K.H. Tam

Chair Professor and Chief of Paediatric Surgery and Pro-Vice Chancellor and Vice-President (Research), The University of Hong Kong, Queen Mary Hospital, Hong Kong

Paris Tekkis

Consultant Colorectal Surgeon, Chelsea and Westminster Hospital and The Royal Marsden Hospital, London, UK

Jeffrey L. Tong

Consultant Anaesthetist, University Hospitals Birmingham NHS Foundation Trust, Department of Anaesthesia and Critical Care, Royal Centre for Defence Medicine, Birmingham, UK

Tim Wheatley

Consultant Surgeon, Department of Upper Gastrointestinal Surgery, Derriford Hospital, Plymouth, UK

Antonius B.M. Wilmink

Consultant Vascular Surgeon, Birmingham University Department of Vascular Surgery, Heart of England NHS Foundation Trust, Birmingham, UK

Alistair Windsor

Consultant Surgeon, Department of Colorectal Surgery, University College London Hospitals, London, UK

John K.S. Woo

Clinical Associate Professor, Chinese University of Hong Kong and Consultant, Department of Surgery, Prince of Wales Hospital, Hong Kong

Preface

The surgeon of today is witness to unprecedented change in the delivery of healthcare. Our populations are ageing and the available options for treatment are expanding. Surgeons are becoming increasingly specialist and patients in hospital are sicker than ever before. Pressures on trainees include a shorter working week and there is an emphasis on operating theatre efficiency, which reduces opportunity for supervised trainee operating. Add to this the increasing scrutiny of an individual surgeon's outcomes that can act to limit a trainee's exposure to operative experience. Traditional team structures of surgical firms and the apprentice-style training have been consigned to history.

Over recent years, the examination process in surgery has also changed and the Intercollegiate Surgical Curriculum Project now emphasizes the different domains of surgical practice, based on the Can-MEDS framework and underpinned by the principles of Good Medical Practice. As well as becoming a surgical expert, with the appropriate knowledge, clinical skills, technical skills and professional attitudes, a surgeon must develop skills as a Communicator, Collaborator, Manager, Health Advocate, Scholar and Professional. These are admirable goals and the examination system is indeed evolving to assess the full range of these qualities.

This new edition of Fundamentals of Surgical Practice is aimed at the surgeon in training preparing for the Intercollegiate MRCS Examination. The book follows the syllabus for the examination, which has been agreed by, and is common to, the Surgical Royal Colleges of Great Britain and Ireland. The syllabus integrates basic sciences, principles of surgery-in-general and important generic surgical topics. The authors are dedicated surgical educators and we hope this book will communicate some of our passion for surgery to you as much as we hope it helps you progress in your professional careers.

Andrew Kingsnorth and Douglas Bowley

Pharmacology and the safe prescribing of drugs

Jamie J. Coleman, Anthony R. Cox and Nicholas J. Cowley

Understanding the pharmacological principles and safe use of drugs is just as important in surgical practice as in any other medical specialty. With an ageing population with often multiple comorbidities and medications, as well as an expanding list of new pharmacological treatments, it is important that surgeons understand the implications of therapeutic drugs on their daily practice. The increasing emphasis on high quality and safe patient care demands that doctors are aware of preventable adverse drug reactions (ADRs) and interactions, try to minimize the potential for medication errors, and consider the benefits and harms of medicines in their patients. This chapter examines these aspects from the view of surgical practice and expands on the implications of some of the most common medical conditions and drug classes in the perioperative period.

The therapeutic care of surgical patients is obvious in many circumstances – for example, antibacterial prophylaxis, thromboprophylaxis, and postoperative analgesia. However, the careful examination of other drug therapies is often critical not only to the sustained treatment of the associated medical conditions but to the perioperative outcomes of patients undergoing surgery. The benefit–harm balance of many therapies may be fundamentally altered by the stress of an operation in one direction or the other; this is not a decision that should wait until the anaesthetist arrives for a preoperative assessment or one that should be left to junior medical or nursing staff on the ward. Think for example of the difference between the need to stop oral anticoagulants used for atrial fibrillation versus the abrupt cessation of long-term corticosteroids. The strategy for different patients, for different conditions, and for different drug treatments is, not surprisingly, varied. There are some basic rules for many circumstances and these should be considered carefully by

experienced surgical staff prior to any operative intervention. Whilst not possible in emergency situations, it is also wise to involve any other specialists who provide ongoing treatments in the discussion about elective, planned surgery well in advance. The general rule is that medications with withdrawal potential should be continued perioperatively, non-essential medications that increase surgical risk should be stopped before surgery, and clinical judgement should be exercised in other circumstances. Many hospitals also have policies or protocols relating to perioperative prescribing: prescribers should be familiar with these and follow them.

Medication history

An accurate medication history is essential for the safe prescribing of medication, and there is evidence that there is an unintentional variance between preadmission and on admission medicines of between 30%–70% across all types of hospital admissions. Failure to accurately resolve differences in the medication history across boundaries in clinical care, which is often referred to as medicines reconciliation, can lead to preventable adverse drug events. As a result of this, a technical patient safety solution for medicines reconciliation on hospital admissions was jointly issued by the National Institute for Health and Clinical Excellence (NICE) and the National Patients Safety Agency (NPSA) in 2007. In the surgical setting, knowledge of the patient's drugs and their comorbidities is essential so that the risk of perioperative decompensation can be determined.

The latest advice is that in order to properly reconcile a patient's medication history at least two sources of information about the drugs should be sought, with one source preferably being the patient themselves.

Fundamentals of Surgical Practice, Third Edition, ed. Andrew N. Kingsnorth and Douglas M. Bowley.
Published by Cambridge University Press. © Cambridge University Press 2011.

Table 1.1 CASES – a useful mnemonic to remember important aspects within a surgical history

	Surgical relevance
Contraception	Pregnancy in female patients Risk of venous thromboembolism
Anticoagulation	Risk of bleeding Need for decision about perioperative continuation or other management
Steroids	Requirement for steroids in surgery to prevent Addisonian crisis
Ethanol	Risk of alcohol withdrawal Interaction with anaesthetic
Smoking	Lung disease

The process should also involve a pharmacist, but this is not always possible. The overall process should ensure that important medicines aren't stopped inadvertently on admission and that new medicines are prescribed, with a complete knowledge of what a patient is already taking.

Taking a medication history is not always as simple as asking a patient what drugs they are on. Attempts to obtain accurate primary care records from the general practitioner should be made. However, patients can stop prescribed medicines without informing their general practitioner, or even tailor their own dosage (for example, to avoid a suspected adverse reaction). Focused questions should be asked to uncover information that will subsequently be useful in the patient's journey.

Elements of the medication history that are often missed are over-the-counter medicines; non-oral medicines (e.g. eyedrops, creams or inhalers); the oral contraceptive; complementary and alternative therapies (including potent herbal products that can interfere with cytochrome P450 enzymes, such as St John's Wort) and 'borderline substances' (e.g. vitamins, food supplements). Such substances should be specifically asked about, as many patients may not consider them medicines or will not volunteer them due to possible concerns that healthcare professionals will not approve of their use. In surgical practice there are some additional questions that are worth asking about which have been given the acronym CASES (see Table 1.1).

A further part of the medication history – which ties in with the past medical and surgical history – is prior drug exposure. While prior history of allergies from exposure to drugs (especially penicillin and related drugs) is commonly obtained, drug history taking also provides an important opportunity to explore any previous exposure to other agents used in the perioperative period (e.g. anaesthetic gases, analgesics). This information is useful if the patient has had prior adverse reactions to medicines, in which case a more extensive review of the history and previous medical notes may be required. The appropriate flagging and documentation of any intolerances or allergies is vitally important. For example, the prescription of a penicillin-related drug to a penicillin-allergic patient is deemed a 'never happen event' in the health service.

Adverse drug events

Adverse events in healthcare are an inevitable outcome of both acute and elective admissions – but are much less acceptable when considered to be preventable. Adverse drug reactions (ADRs) are defined as appreciably harmful or unpleasant reactions, resulting from an intervention related to the use of a medicinal product; adverse effects usually predict hazard from future administration and warrant prevention, or specific treatment, or alteration of the dosage regimen, or withdrawal of the product. ADRs are a common factor in hospital admissions, accounting in a large UK study for 6.5% of acute hospital admissions in whole or part (Pirmohamed *et al.* 2004). In most cases these ADRs were judged to be potentially or definitely avoidable. Whilst the majority of these events result in medical admissions, rather than surgical admissions, there are some notable drug-attributable symptoms that may masquerade as surgical emergencies. It is fairly common knowledge that angiotensin-converting enzyme (ACE) inhibitors have been associated with cases of pancreatitis, but much less commonly known that the same agents can cause intestinal angioedema and lead to repeated laparotomies for suspected peritonitis before the true diagnosis is made (Coleman 2007).

Adverse drug reactions and medication errors can also cloud an inpatient admission, leading to increased morbidity, increased length of stay, and occasionally more serious outcomes or death. Approximately 15% of inpatients will experience an ADR during hospital admission, although a lower proportion of surgical patients (12%) experience adverse drug reactions during their stay (Davies *et al.* 2009). The most commonly implicated drugs are: loop diuretics, opioids, compound analgesics (e.g. cocodamol), systemic

Table 1.2 Selected potential drug interactions with anaesthetics and neuromuscular blockers

Drug group	Interacting drug	Interaction
Anaesthetic agents	Alpha-blockers	Enhanced hypotensive effect
	Antipsychotics	Hypotension
	ACE inhibitors and angiotensin-II receptor antagonists	Severe hypotension. May need discontinuing 24 hours prior to surgery
	Adrenaline (epinephrine)	Risk of arrhythmias with volatile general anaesthetics
	Calcium channel blockers	Enhanced hypotensive effect (and AV delay with verapamil)
	Lithium	Enhance effects of muscle relaxants
	Methylphenidate	Risk of hypertension with volatile general anaesthetics
	Monoamine oxidase inhibitors (MAOIs)	British National Formulary advises should be stopped 2 weeks before surgery (risk of hypo- and hypertension). May be due to confounding by other drugs such as pethidine and ephedrine
	Tricyclic antidepressants	Increase risk of arrhythmias and hypotension during anaesthesia
Neuromuscular blockers	Anticonvulsants	Effects of competitive neuromuscular blockers are reduced and shortened with chronic use of phenytoin and carbamazepine
	Antibiotics: aminoglycosides, vancomycin, clindamycin and polymixins	Neuromuscular blockade prolonged and increased
	Digitalis glycosides (e.g. digoxin)	Risk of ventricular arrhythmias with suxamethonium
	Lithium	Effects of neuromuscular blockers enhanced

corticosteroids, inhaled beta-agonists, antibiotics (penicillins, cephalosporins and macrolides), oral anticoagulants and low molecular weight heparins. Again, as with drug-induced admissions, over half of ADRs emerging during a hospital stay are preventable.

Suspected ADRs can be reported to the Yellow Card scheme, which was started in 1964 in the wake of the thalidomide disaster. The scheme is a spontaneous reporting scheme – incidents are detected and reported by healthcare professionals. For new drugs and vaccines under intensive surveillance – identified by the inverted black triangle symbol in the British National Formulary – all suspected ADRs should be reported regardless of how trivial they may appear.

For established drugs and vaccines, only serious suspected reactions should be reported. Serious reports include disability, life-threatening or deadly reactions, and medically significant reactions, such as bleeding or congenital birth defects. Further guidance on ADR reporting is given in the *British National Formulary* and at the MHRA Yellow Card reporting website http://www.yellowcard.gov.uk.

Drug interactions

Drug interactions are an important cause of adverse drug reactions, with around 17% of adverse drug events related to interactions between drugs. One particular concern in the perioperative setting is the interaction between pre-existing medications and the potential drugs used in the operative setting (e.g. anaesthetic drugs, analgesics). Drug interactions can be broadly split into pharmacokinetic and pharmacodynamic interactions. Pharmacokinetic interactions are those influencing the absorption, distribution, metabolism and excretion of drugs. Pharmacodynamic interactions occur when the effects of one drug are influenced by the presence of a competitor drug at its specific receptor site, or by indirect effects. These can be antagonistic or additive or synergistic in nature.

Judging the importance of a particular drug interaction can be difficult. Evidence from clinical studies is generally lacking, and when available can be from pharmacokinetic/pharmacodynamic studies performed in small numbers of healthy young volunteers, who are not representative of the patient groups in which interactions may occur. Case reports and case series can therefore be important sources of information about interactions, although care must be taken due to the inherent limitations of such evidence in terms of causality. Information sources such as the British National Formulary and Stockley's Drug Interactions handbook provide useful summarized information for clinicians. Some interactions with drugs used in the operative setting are given in Table 1.2.

Medication errors

Medication errors have been defined as 'a failure in the treatment process that leads to, or has the potential to lead to, harm to the patient'. These can occur either because the wrong plan has been chosen (i.e. a contraindicated drug prescribed due to lack of knowledge), or because a good plan has been implemented poorly, preventing the intended outcome (i.e. poor handwriting on a prescription leading to the administration of the wrong drug).

Errors can be at the skill-based level (slips and lapses), the rule-based level (poorly chosen or inappropriate rules) and the knowledge-based level (application of knowledge to a novel situation). Errors have two broad categories: errors in the planning of an intentional act, known as mistakes; and errors in execution of an act, known as slips (acts of commission) and lapses (acts of omission).

Slips and lapses are unconscious acts or omissions and occur when a prescriber has the correct plan for treatment, but fails to carry it out accurately. An example might be picking the wrong drug strength from a computer list when prescribing. These are not amenable to training or threats.

Mistakes occur when error arises in an attempt to deal with a complex situation, through lack of knowledge, or the application of poor or inappropriate rules. An example would be an inadvertent overdose due to lack of knowledge of the use of a drug in renal failure.

Another subset are violations, which are defined as deliberate – but not always reprehensible – deviations from those practices deemed necessary to maintain the safe operation of a potentially hazardous system. In the context of prescribing, an example might be the taking of deliberate short-cuts in a badly designed electronic prescribing system.

Accurate information about patients and access to good information about drugs can mitigate some prescribing errors. Adherence to good principles of prescribing and hospital policies can also help reduce the opportunity for some medication errors. For example, writing micrograms in full rather than the abbreviation mcg can prevent confusion between micrograms (mcg) and milligrams (mg).

Distractions and momentary loss of attention will always have the potential to cause medication errors. Additionally, complex systems of care can contain so-called 'latent' errors within the system. These built-in failures, due to policies or custom and practice, do not cause harm until events conspire to allow an error to pass the normal defences.

Nil by mouth

Whether a patient can take food or fluids by mouth prior to surgery often seems to influence whether the patient will receive medications via the oral route. For adult elective surgery in healthy adults without gastrointestinal disease it is usual to restrict oral solids for 6 hours before surgery, with only water or clear fluids allowed up until 2 hours before surgery. In most instances therefore it is allowable to give routine medications with these clear fluids until 2 hours before the operation. If gastrointestinal problems are present preoperatively and certainly in operations where the patient is starved postoperatively, alternative methods of drug administration or medication strategies must be employed (for example converting to a parenteral preparation for a period of time). Many other processes will affect the absorption of oral medications during this period, including diminished blood flow to the gut, villous atrophy, mucosal ischaemia and diminished motility from postoperative ileus. Local guidelines or medicine information department or senior clinical/pharmacist advice may be required to ensure that the right dose for the medicine is used for the chosen route of administration. Staff administering the drugs should be clear which drugs are intended to be given on the day of operation and which are purposely omitted, otherwise the prescriber's intent may not be followed.

Discharge at home drugs

Ensuring that patients are discharged on the correct medication is an essential part of good surgical practice. It is tempting to only provide details about new medications relevant to the surgery, but unless this is obvious to other care providers there is a risk of failing to communicate essential information about the patient. This process also helps to ensure that the intended resumption of long-term medicines is not overlooked. When the patient leaves the hospital the provision of appropriate advice both to the patient and within the discharge letter is essential. Think of the example of a patient with a recent splenectomy; providing the correct advice will ensure that the general practitioner is aware that the oral penicillin has to be given for life as well as ensuring that the patient knows the precautions to be taken for the future. Another example would be providing the correct advice about the cessation of anti-anginal therapy but continuation of antiplatelet treatment following coronary artery bypass surgery – failure to get this right may lead to adverse outcomes for the patient. The surgical practitioner must ensure that the discharge at home drugs are clearly recorded on the discharge letter, particularly noting the reasons and intended length of course for new medications and the reasons for stopping previous at home medicines.

The next section of the chapter concentrates on specific diseases and drug classes known to be relevant for surgical patients in clinical practice. Specific information about individual drugs should always be sought from an up-to-date reference source such as the British National Formulary (BMJ 2009).

Analgesics

Analgesics for surgical patients may be divided into those serving to relieve chronic pain unrelated to any planned surgical intervention, chronic pain related to the condition being managed or acute pain related to a surgical intervention. Although the therapies used to manage each form of pain may overlap, it is important to understand why each analgesic is prescribed, in order to predict fluctuations in analgesic requirement in the perioperative period. For example, a patient may attend for elective cholecystectomy with a background of chronic intermittent abdominal pain, in addition to weight-related chronic back pain. He or she may already be taking a significant number of analgesics to control their pain. Without prior knowledge of the reasons for taking each analgesic and their doses, it would be difficult to plan their postoperative analgesic requirements. In particular, opiates are frequently under-dosed in the postoperative period in tolerant individuals. A patient maintained on a large dose of sustained-release morphine for chronic pain will not respond to a conventional acute dose perioperatively, and the dose will need to be individually tailored.

Routes of administration of analgesics

Different classes of opioid, or different routes of administration – for example the transcutaneous fentanyl patch – have differing pharmacokinetic profiles. Importantly, however, there is a class effect in which tolerance from one form of opioid will necessitate

Table 1.3 Opioid strength to achieve equivalence to 10 mg oral morphine

Opioid analgesic	Relative potency	Dose of drug
Morphine (oral)	1	10 mg
Codeine (oral)	0.1	100 mg
Tramadol	0.2	50 mg
IV/IM morphine	4	2.5 mg
IV/IM pethidine	0.3	30 mg
Oxycodone (oral)	2	5 mg
Buprenorphine (oral)	40	250 mcg
Fentanyl (oral)	75	130 mcg

increased dosing of all other drugs within the opioid family. There is no reason why a patient maintained on a fentanyl patch for chronic pain should not continue this through the perioperative period, with standard intermittent morphine prescription for breakthrough pain. Knowledge of the relative strength of one opioid compared to another is valuable in determining likely requirements for breakthough pain (see Table 1.3).

The choice of route of administration of an analgesic drug will be influenced by the type of surgery, and by the postoperative monitoring environment. Abdominal surgery may reduce the likelihood of enteral absorption of analgesics, and an alternative route of administration should be used until good absorption can be guaranteed. Care must be taken, particularly in patient groups with abnormal metabolism or excretion of drugs such as the elderly or those with acute or chronic renal impairment, not to allow accumulation of potent analgesics such as morphine with resultant respiratory depression and over-sedation. Patient-regulated analgesics such as 'as required' analgesics or patient-controlled analgesia (PCA) opiate infusions are inherently safer than using regular potent analgesics or infusions, particularly outside a high-dependency environment. PCA must not, however, be used as the exclusive form of analgesia, as this will result in fluctuating levels of pain, and in particular interfere with rest and sleep in the early postoperative period. Again, regular analgesia must be adjusted with knowledge of baseline requirements, and regularly reviewed in the postoperative period, titrated to the patient's pain. A useful method of titrating regular analgesic requirement is to review the 'as required' or PCA dose delivered over the preceding 24 hours, and to use this dose to guide the regular analgesic requirement over the following 24 hours.

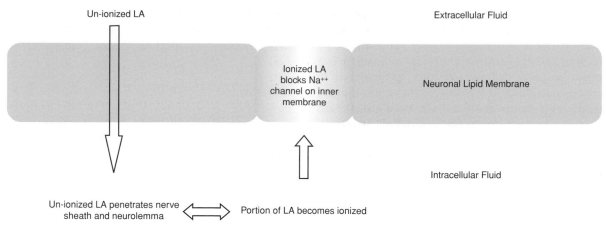

Figure 1.1 Diagram showing LA dissociation/neuronal penetration.

The World Health Organization (WHO) pain ladder

The WHO pain ladder provides a simple strategy to pain management on the basis that analgesics have different and synergistic modes of action (WHO 2009). Additionally, it is clear that analgesic drugs have adverse effects, and these are usually dose-dependent. With these two points in mind, the WHO pain ladder, originally devised for management of cancer-related pain, advises the initiation of simple analgesics such as paracetamol, followed by the addition (rather than replacement) of weak and then strong opiates. Nonsteroidal anti-inflammatory drugs (NSAIDs) are excellent forms of postoperative pain relief, again working synergistically with paracetamol and opiates. These drugs may be used regularly for short durations unless there are contraindications (e.g. peptic ulcer disease). They should be used with extreme caution in the elderly and those with renal impairment or heart failure, and where their antiplatelet function is undesirable. A single dose of diclofenac in a critically unwell postoperative patient could well render them anuric.

Drug dependence and perioperative analgesia

Patients with a background of illicit opiate drug abuse are likely to be tolerant to conventional doses of opiate analgesics. Postoperative analgesia is therefore often a problem in these patients. Clearly drug abusers feel pain just as the rest of us do, and it is not good practice to ignore their analgesic requirements. An effective strategy will include liberal use of non-opiate analgesics, and regional analgesia where possible. When opiates are required, it should be accepted that small doses may be ineffective, and an increase in dose should be prescribed with careful supervision and clear patient boundaries. The inpatient perioperative period is not the time to be attempting to wean the patient's opiate dependence, and attempting to do so will make the working environment strained. However, a degree of common-sense prescribing is also clearly required.

Local anaesthetics

As well as systemic administration of drugs, local anaesthetics provide a valuable form of pain relief in the perioperative period. Local anaesthetics work on nerve conduction locally, to prevent transmission of the pain impulse, specifically by blocking the neuronal Na^{2+} channels. Knowledge of their mechanism of action can help in their effective practical application. Local anaesthetics are all weak bases. They are fully ionized in an acidic solution at the point of injection, where upon entry into tissue at neutral pH they become only partially dissociated. Only the un-ionized portion of the drug is able to pass through the lipid membrane of a nerve to the internal surface where the Na^{2+} channel is accessed and blocked. It is for this reason that local anaesthetics penetrate infected tissue poorly; the acidic environment favours ionization of the local anaesthetic, and therefore poor penetration of the neuronal lipid membrane (Figure 1.1).

A surgeon will regularly infiltrate local anaesthetic, and therefore knowledge of the choice, dosing and toxicity is essential. There are recommended maximum doses of local anaesthetics which aim to avoid toxicity. Rather confusingly though, maximum doses for local anaesthetic drugs are published in milligrams, or milligrams per kilogram, whereas local anaesthetics are usually available as percentage solutions. For example a 1% solution of lidocaine (lignocaine) contains 1g (1000 mg) of lidocaine in 100 ml of solvent. Therefore, each millilitre of 1% lidocaine will contain 10 milligrams (1000/100 mg) of the active drug.

Local anaesthetic toxicity is caused by systemic absorption and relates specifically to peak serum concentrations of drug, and subsequent adverse central nervous system and cardiovascular effects. Peak serum concentration is not always directly proportional to the dose given, although the recommended dose maximums for each drug are a good guide. Peak serum concentration is related to the rate of systemic absorption of the drug in the tissue being infiltrated, which can depend on the vascularity of the site or concurrent administration of local vasoconstrictors. Infiltration of local anaesthetic with adrenaline into poorly vascularized lipomatous tissue, for example, will result in a very slow rate of systemic drug absorption, and ongoing metabolism of drug during this period will prevent a high peak concentration even with fairly high dosing. Conversely, a very small inadvertent intravascular injection, even within the recommended dose range, will lead to an immediate spike in serum concentration, and have the potential to cause cardiovascular collapse. The treatment of severe local anaesthetic toxicity is therefore a prerequisite for safe surgical practice. Seizures and cardiovascular collapse should be treated using standard resuscitation protocols (i.e. an airway, breathing, circulation algorithm). Cardiopulmonary resuscitation in the event of cardiorespiratory arrest may have to be prolonged to allow drug metabolism to less toxic levels and return of spontaneous cardiac output. More recently, however, protocols for administration of a lipid emulsion infusion (Intralipid®) have been developed (AAGBI 2007). The lipid emulsion preferentially absorbs the un-ionized local anaesthetic in a similar way to the lipid neuronal membrane, lowering serum concentrations and speeding recovery markedly.

Antibiotics

Antibiotics may be administered prophylactically to reduce the incidence of surgical site infections, or may be used to treat infection empirically or based on the results of isolated organisms from microbiological cultures. Choice of prophylactic or empirical antibiotic therapy should be guided by local microbial resistance patterns, and will differ from one geographical region to another and even from one specialty to another. There has been a drive to reduce excessive antibiotic administration in the perioperative period in order to reduce the incidence of resistant organisms, as well as inadvertent gut proliferation of organisms such as *Clostridium difficile*. When indicated, a single dose of prophylactic antibiotic, given at full treatment dose, should be administered within 30–60 minutes of skin incision. Generally speaking, this will be on arrival in theatre at the time of anaesthesia or during surgical site preparation. Whilst the majority of antibiotics may be administered as an intravenous bolus, there are a few notable exceptions, including vancomycin, ciprofloxacin and erythromycin, which must be delivered slowly in a diluted solution; this becomes relevant when antibiotics should be initiated prior to arrival in the theatre suite in order to achieve adequate serum concentrations at the initiation of surgery to minimize risk of infection.

Route of administration may also be best decided on with knowledge of each antibiotic's bioavailability. For example, the quinolones, such as ciprofloxacin, are absorbed so well orally that even in the presence of severe infection the intravenous route is only indicated if there is concern about the effectiveness of enteral absorption.

Use of prophylactic antibiotics for certain surgical procedures has been until recently recommended for groups of patients with structural cardiac lesions or prosthetic valves in order to prevent infective endocarditis. Although there is conflicting advice from one authority to another, it is now generally considered that the risk of infective endocarditis may be actually lower than the incidence of severe antibiotic-related complications from blanket antibiotic use. Currently the advice is to consider the risk on a case by case basis (NICE 2008).

When treating established infections, awareness of the differences in mechanism of action of antibiotics can have practical implications for patient management. For instance, aminoglycoside antibiotics such as gentamicin are most efficacious at peak serum concentrations – favouring large, once-daily, dosing regimens. Other antibiotics, such as the glycopeptides including vancomycin, work best when a serum concentration is steadily maintained, and are less effective if levels are allowed to dip. The site of infection may also dictate the choice of antibiotic. Although a microbiological sample may reveal that a bacterium is sensitive to a number of classes of antibiotic, it does not follow that each antibiotic will be equally as effective. For example, quinolones will penetrate lung parenchyma much more effectively than most penicillins (Honeybourne 1994).

Cardiovascular medications

Cardiovascular morbidity is present in many surgical patients and there are a large number of associated drug classes used to control hypertension, symptoms of heart failure or ischaemic heart disease, and to limit cardiovascular disease progression. A patient's usual medication should be noted, and only adjusted if there is a good clinical reason to do so. It is not acceptable for a patient with significant cardiovascular disease on multiple medications for disease control to have these drugs omitted because of admission to a surgical ward.

Hypertension

Perioperative cardiovascular instability is related to the degree of chronic uncontrolled hypertension. Medications used to control high blood pressure should be established weeks to months before attending for surgery. It is important to understand why hypertension needs to be controlled, in order to appreciate why the acute correction of blood pressure does not appreciably reduce perioperative cardiovascular risk. The chronic hypertensive patient will develop left ventricular hypertrophy, and so at times of surgical or postoperative stress the bulky myocardium will have an increased oxygen demand, but a reduced period of perfusion (occurring during diastole) and therefore an increased chance of perioperative myocardial ischaemia. The chronic hypertensive patient will also have a relatively high peripheral vascular resistance. This leads to significantly higher demands on the heart, which is pumping against high resistance, and a tendency towards cardiovascular lability in the perioperative period; particularly following the administration of vaso-active drugs such as general anaesthetic agents. It is vital that long term preoperative cardiovascular optimization has taken place, as these highlighted problems will persist until cardiovascular remodelling has taken place. In fact overzeal-

ous, rapid correction of blood pressure may actually worsen morbidity by reducing perfusion pressures to organs without sufficient time for end organs to compensate.

Beta-adrenoceptor blocking drugs

This drug class deserves a special mention with regards to the perioperative period. Beta-adrenoceptor blocking drugs (beta-blockers) are commonly prescribed for both hypertension and for ischaemic heart disease. When prescribed for ischaemic heart disease, they should not be abruptly discontinued, as the patient will be at higher risk of perioperative cardiovascular adverse events if stopped. Beta-blockers prevent peri- and postoperative tachycardia, thus increasing the time spent in diastole for good myocardial perfusion. Conversely, initiating beta-blockers in the perioperative period in those at high risk of cardiovascular events may not be the right thing to do. A recent Canadian trial has examined the evidence and concluded that reduced cardiovascular mortality is offset by an increased incidence of stroke in this group (POISE 2008). The ability to mount a tachycardic response to a state of hypovolaemia will be blunted in patients recently started on beta-blockers, and in a postoperative ward with infrequent monitoring this may be missed, leading to serious adverse events.

Angiotensin-converting enzyme (ACE) inhibitors

ACE inhibitors and angiotensin receptor blockers are potent drugs, with significant benefits in many patients with chronic cardiovascular disease. They have potent vasodilating properties, and there is some concern about their use immediately prior to anaesthesia. Certainly patients treated with ACE inhibitors may already fit into a high-risk category for general anaesthesia. The vasodilatation caused by general anaesthesia or neuraxial (spinal) blockade will act synergistically with ACE inhibitors and rarely may cause refractory hypotension during anaesthesia, which may be difficult to control with standard vasoconstrictors (Colson *et al.* 1999). This problem is usually manageable during the period of close monitoring at anaesthesia and rarely leads to patient harm. Protocols of discontinuing one cardiac medication but continuing another often lead to confusion and as a result the omission of all drugs preoperatively; this situation must be avoided by employing clear communication regarding these therapies. Some authorities advocate suspension of all cardiovascular drugs in certain cases where the risk of rebound hypotension is marked, such as situations where there are anticipated large perioperative fluid shifts or when the patient is maintained on multiple antihypertensive medications.

Statins

Statins (hydroxy methylglutaryl coenzyme A reductase inhibitors) are drugs commonly prescribed as primary prophylaxis in those at risk of cardiovascular disease, and for secondary prevention following a cardiac event. These drugs have traditionally been felt to be beneficial when taken long term as part of a cholesterol-lowering strategy. These drugs may have other beneficial properties including anti-inflammatory and vasodilatory functions and there is some evidence for improved outcome in surgical patients who are taking statins. The evidence does not currently favour routine perioperative statin initiation (Dunkelgrun *et al.* 2009); however, patients already taking these drugs should not have them stopped in the perioperative period if possible.

Antiplatelet agents

Many patients with cardiovascular comorbidities will be maintained on antiplatelet agents such as aspirin or clopidogrel, often in combination for their synergistic effect on platelet function. It is helpful to be aware of their mechanism of action, as this can aid good patient management and minimize disruption of these agents. Aspirin is an irreversible cyclooxygenase (COX) inhibitor, which, once bound, will prevent normal platelet function for the life of the platelet (approximately one week). Clearly there will be a gradual improvement in overall platelet function for every day that aspirin is discontinued, as new platelets replace old. Similarly, clopidogrel acts on platelets, irreversibly binding to platelet ADP receptors, and will act for the life of the platelet. Theoretically therefore a prolonged period of cessation of at least a week is required to reduce bleeding complications for both of these agents. However, evidence is less clear and individual practice varies. The decision to stop treatment is easy if the thrombotic risk is small and the risk of bleeding is overwhelming; but situations are rarely this clear cut. It is also vitally important to know the reason for the antiplatelet prescription, as the risks of discon-

tinuation for primary prophylaxis are not the same as for those patients on them following percutaneous coronary revascularization. Indeed, for this group, in particular those having had drug-eluting coronary stents inserted within the last year, discussion with a cardiologist is essential to weigh up the significant risk of stent occlusion associated with only a short period of drug cessation (Chassot *et al.* 2007).

A recent systematic review has suggested that aspirin use should not be stopped in the perioperative period unless the risk of bleeding exceeds the thrombotic risk from withholding the drug. With the exception of recent drug-eluting stent implantation, clopidogrel use should be stopped at least 5 days prior to most elective surgery (O'Riordan *et al.* 2009). The timing for restarting these drugs should be guided by a risk–benefit evaluation based on the consequences of postoperative haemorrhage versus the likelihood of adverse thrombotic events.

Anticoagulants and perioperative anticoagulation

Anticoagulant medication may be used in the community for treatment or prevention of thromboembolic disease, and for prevention of prosthetic heart valve thrombosis. Anticoagulants are also used widely during inpatient care for thromboprophylaxis. Warfarin is the most common anticoagulant used in the community. It is a far from ideal agent, requiring regular dose monitoring, with a variable genetic sensitivity to the drug, and numerous drug–drug and drug–food interactions. For those patients maintained on warfarin in the community there will need to be a management plan formulated prior to surgery not only to reduce the risk of perioperative bleeding but to minimize the risk of thromboembolism whilst off oral anticoagulants. Clearly, the management plan will be influenced by the indication for anticoagulation. Withholding warfarin that is being used for uncomplicated atrial fibrillation is associated with a relatively low stroke risk of around 1.5% per year. The importance of multidisciplinary liaison with haematology and cardiology must be emphasized for complicated patients. For example, a patient with a metal mitral valve and other cardiac risk factors will have a much higher risk of thrombotic complications than a patient with an uncomplicated bileaflet metal aortic valve. Therefore, it is appropriate to initiate some patients on heparin anticoagulation around the operative period, when discontinuing warfarin (Bonow *et al.* 2006).

Heparins exert their anticoagulant effect through inhibiting thrombin and activated factor X via actions on anti-thrombin. Heparins may be administered by intravenous infusion or by intermittent subcutaneous injection. Heparins may be divided into unfractionated heparin and low molecular weight (LMW) heparins. Unfractionated heparin has a number of advantages as a parenteral anticoagulant. When given as an intravenous infusion, it can be rapidly loaded to achieve therapeutic anticoagulation in a short period, and its half-life of around 1 hour allows complete correction of the coagulation profile following a short period of discontinuation of therapy. The level of anticoagulation can be easily assessed using activated clotting time (ACT) or activated partial thromboplastin time (aPTT), allowing dose manipulation using a dose-adjustment nomogram. A further advantage is the ability to reverse its action with the drug protamine, when more rapid correction of anticoagulation is required. Unfractionated heparin is used much less frequently than it was due to alternative options but it still has a place in therapy. The disadvantages include the need for a constant infusion via an accurate syringe driver, the occurrence of subtherapeutic levels during any period of disconnection or between syringe changes, and the drug's liability to swings in effect, leading to periods of potentially harmful under or over anticoagulation.

The low molecular weight heparins were designed to overcome many of the disadvantages of unfractionated heparin and achieve a reliable, steady level of anticoagulation with a relatively easy once or twice daily subcutaneous administration. The reduced binding to plasma proteins is responsible for the more predictable dose–response relationship and longer plasma half-life. The half-life of approximately 12 hours is significantly longer than that of unfractionated heparin, but shorter than oral anticoagulants such as warfarin. The LMW heparins also have reasonably predictable pharmacokinetics with weight-based drug calculation, thus allowing reasonably accurate anticoagulation without the need for monitoring in most patients. Unfortunately though in situations where monitoring is required, for example in pregnant or morbidly obese patients whose metabolism of the drug is not expected to be normal, routine coagulation screen will not guide therapy for LMW heparins and specialist testing of Factor Xa levels is required and is not widely avail-

able. Dose reductions for renal impairment are also advised.

Heparin-induced thrombocytopenia (HIT)

HIT is an immune-mediated reaction to heparin, in particular unfractionated heparins, leading to consumption of platelets usually occurring 1–2 weeks after initiating therapy, although sooner if there has been prior exposure to the drug. The condition results in severe thrombocytopaenia with bleeding complications and paradoxical thrombosis, unless the condition is recognized early and heparin is discontinued. Alternative short-acting anticoagulants are available, all with advantages and disadvantages, and specialist haematology advice should be sought prior to their use.

Respiratory medication

Patients with chronic respiratory disease may be maintained on regular inhaled bronchodilators or inhaled corticosteroids. Generally, these are continued perioperatively, although in certain situations conversion to a nebulized route of delivery may be more appropriate. General anaesthesia involves manipulation of a possible already irritable airway, and although inhaled anaesthetic agents have bronchodilator properties, significant bronchospasm may be precipitated by intubation of the airway. Unavoidable postoperative lung atelectasis may be more manifest in this group, and escalation to higher doses of nebulized bronchodilator may be appropriate. Nebulization of bronchodilators may be more appropriate if a postoperative patient has poor inspiratory effort, or if they are unable to comply with a reasonable inhalation technique.

Many patients will require perioperative supplemental oxygen, and this should not be withheld with the preconception that it will precipitate type 2 respiratory failure with hypercapnoea. Postoperative hypoventilation and hypoxia is a multifactorial phenomenon requiring careful patient examination to accurately diagnose. For instance, inadequate re-expansion of lungs may be secondary to pain, or occasionally due to excessive opiate administration. Patients with underlying lung disease are most susceptible to respiratory complications following surgery, and safe drug prescribing should focus on multimodal opiate-sparing analgesia. These patients benefit from regional techniques of pain control such as epidural analgesia more than any other group, in particular following high abdominal or thoracic incisions (Popping *et al.* 2008).

Renal medication

Patients with renal disease, in particular those approaching end-stage renal failure (ESRF), may require multiple drug treatments. These patients are likely to be suffering from associated comorbidities and may also be on medication for difficult-to-control hypertension; they may also have ischaemic or valvular heart disease, and are at a generalized higher risk of infection. They may require high doses of diuretic to maintain an adequate urine output, or may be oliguric/anuric if in established ESRF. The key to fluid management is to continue their usual diuretic medication, or fluid restriction, bearing in mind that there may be significant fluid shifts perioperatively which will require intermittent fluid bolus management.

Renally excreted drugs, in particular drugs from the opiate class, may be cautiously used in patients with renal failure. Regular opiate prescription should be avoided in severe renal impairment, and reliance on 'as required' analgesia or PCA is advisable. A common misconception is that loading doses should be reduced; this is not the case. A carefully titrated dose of morphine should be used until pain is controlled; subsequent requirements may be much lower if elimination is severely deranged.

Drugs used in endocrine disorders

Diabetes mellitus

Diabetic blood glucose control in the perioperative period frequently causes confusion amongst healthcare professionals and subsequently leads to suboptimal patient management. The traditional requirement of sliding-scale insulin for all diabetics undergoing any operation is outdated, leading to unnecessary interventions and increased patient risks without benefit. Fundamental to safe diabetes management is knowledge of what type of diabetes the patient has, and what operation they are going to undergo.

Type 2 diabetes

This form of diabetes is the commonest form in older adults and the elderly, stemming from insulin resistance. Patients are often overweight, and this may be worsened if they have been initiated on insulin therapy,

which is an anabolic hormone, encouraging fat deposition. Individuals will be maintained either on dietary control, oral medication or insulin therapy. In order to anticipate what is likely to happen to blood glucose following starvation for surgery or suspension of oral diabetes medication, an awareness of mechanisms of drug action is essential.

Biguanides

Metformin is the only biguanide licensed in the UK, and it has a multimodal method of action. It sensitizes cells to the action of insulin, so improving the effectiveness of circulating endogenous insulin: it also reduces gluconeogenesis, glycogenolysis and fatty acid oxidation. Patients on these drugs will not become hypoglycaemic, as they are producing and regulating their own insulin. Furthermore, if they are being starved for surgery, their blood glucose will tend towards normal over time. Historically, there has been concern about the development of severe lactic acidosis in the perioperative period if biguanide medications are not discontinued in advance. In supra-therapeutic levels, biguanides inhibit the mitochondrial respiratory pathway, causing anaerobic metabolism. It is likely that the problem has been somewhat overstated, and the drug may be continued in relatively minor surgery. It is, however, contraindicated in the presence of significant renal impairment, as the drug is likely to accumulate, and lactic acidosis is therefore more likely to develop. For this reason, during major surgery, particularly in patients with pre-existing renal dysfunction, metformin should be discontinued until the patient is fully recovered.

Other oral hypoglycaemic drugs

Sulphonylureas such as gliclazide increase endogenous insulin secretion, and so do have an inherent risk of precipitating hypoglycaemia if not discontinued in patients who are nil by mouth on the day of surgery. Longer-acting sulphonylureas such as glibenclamide are more likely to precipitate hypoglycaemia. Newer drugs such as the thiazolidinediones are less likely to precipitate hypoglycaemia, although the manufacturers still advise their discontinuation perioperatively.

Insulins

These may be divided into short-acting and longer-acting insulins. Doses are very variable from one individual to another, and may be very large in patients with significant insulin resistance. If usual doses are not discontinued during periods of starvation, there is a high risk of hypoglycaemia. Type 2 diabetics are less likely to become hyperglycaemic following insulin discontinuation than type 1 diabetics unless they have failure of pancreatic beta cell function; in type 2 diabetics periods of starvation will cause blood glucose levels to fall towards normal. Postoperative insulin requirements will be titrated to the individual; and prescription is dependent on postoperative course and expected resumption of a normal diet. It is important to bear in mind that insulin requirements also increase with the stress response to surgery. Unfortunately, a proportion of type 2 diabetics will over time fail to generate their own insulin, and these patients must be treated in a similar fashion to type 1 diabetics.

Type 1 diabetes

In contrast to type 2 diabetes, this disease is characterized by a lack of endogenous insulin secretion. Individuals are completely dependent on exogenous insulin to prevent ongoing glucose generation and glycogen breakdown. If these patients are starved preoperatively and have their insulin withheld, there is a risk of ongoing and worsening hyperglycaemia, and eventually ketoacidosis. Hyperglycaemia will precipitate diuresis and result in dehydration. These patients require close scrutiny perioperatively, although during minor or day-case surgery there may be relatively minimal disruption to the patient's normal insulin regime.

Insulin sliding scales

Intravenous insulin is most commonly administered via a syringe driver using a short-acting insulin infused at a rate based on the serum (or capillary) blood glucose, which is regularly monitored and adjusted. In order to smooth out swings in blood glucose, intravenous fluids are usually modified to those containing glucose when blood sugar is low. A degree of common sense must also be applied here, as large amounts of 5% dextrose can lead to hyponatraemia, and prolonged use of restrictive protocols without monitoring electrolytes can cause morbidity and mortality. Patients on high baseline levels of subcutaneous insulin are likely to require higher rates of infusion, and scales should be adjusted accordingly if blood glucose control is not being achieved. At-risk groups likely to benefit from sliding-scale insulin are those with likely prolonged

Table 1.4 Equivalent doses for corticosteroids compared to prednisolone (adapted from *British National Formulary* 2009)

Equivalent anti-inflammatory drug dose (British National Formulary)	
Prednisolone 10 mg is equivalent to	Betamethasone 1.5 mg Cortisone acetate 50 mg Deflazacort 12 mg Dexamethasone 1.5 mg Hydrocortisone 40 mg Methylprednisolone 8 mg Triamcinolone 8 mg

periods of starvation, those with no or unknown postoperative enteral absorption, those with labile blood sugars and type 1 diabetics. Tight glycaemic control perioperatively may also reduce the incidence of surgical infective complications.

Steroid therapy

Patients who are maintained on long-term corticosteroids should not have their medication discontinued perioperatively for two reasons. Firstly, the underlying condition being managed with steroids may flare following withdrawal, and secondly, the patient's hypothalamo-pituitary-adrenal (HPA) axis will be suppressed with maintenance doses of steroid equivalent greater than or equal to 10 mg prednisolone daily. Furthermore, it can take up to a year for the HPA axis to normalize following steroid courses of more than 2–4 weeks.

Steroid requirement may increase markedly during the stress of surgery, and this is directly related to the degree of surgical insult. Minor surgery requires no more than the intravenous equivalent of the patient's normal dose of oral steroid. Moderate or major surgery necessitates a short period of increased dosing, to simulate the natural surge following surgery, ideally via continuous intravenous infusion, although intermittent boluses of intravenous steroid are acceptable. Patients with HPA axis failure (for example due to Addison's disease) will not mount a stress response even if the maintenance dose of steroid is low, and will therefore of course require additional steroid (Marik and Varon 2008).

Care should be taken when converting one form of steroid to another, as relative potencies vary considerably (see Table 1.4). Additionally, not all steroid preparations act equally on the mineralocorticoid and corticosteroid axes; dexamethasone for instance has little mineralocorticoid activity, and will lead to inadequate mineralocorticoid function if used as a replacement

Table 1.5 Steroid treatment regimen for surgical patients (adapted from Nicholson *et al.* 1998)

Use the following steroid cover for patients who have received a regular daily dose of more than 10 mg prednisolone or equivalent in the last three months:	
Minor surgery	25 mg hydrocortisone at induction
Moderate surgery	Usual pre-op steroids +25 mg hydrocortisone at induction +100 mg hydrocortisone/day
Major surgery	Usual pre-op steroids +25 mg hydrocortisone at induction +100 mg hydrocortisone/day for 2–3 days. Resume normal oral therapy when gastrointestinal function has returned

for oral prednisolone – potentially resulting in Addisonian crisis. For this reason, hydrocortisone is usually used as an intravenous alternative to prednisolone; further information is given in Table 1.5.

Oestrogens and progestogens

Women of child-bearing age may be using one of many oestrogen or progestogen-based contraception methods. Postmenopausal women may be taking hormone replacement therapy (HRT). The risk of perioperative deep venous thrombosis or pulmonary embolus is slightly elevated whilst patients are taking these drugs. Minor surgery with early mobilization carries minimal risk to the patient, unlike the much higher risk of thromboembolism if the patient becomes pregnant following advice to discontinue their contraception. For this reason, most authorities would advocate continuation of hormone-based contraception unless a high risk of thromboembolism is identified. There is more controversy over HRT, as the risks of discontinuing the medication are lower, and the patients tend to rest in higher risk categories by virtue of age and other potential comorbidities. There is still no clear answer, with comparable rates of thromboembolism noted following orthopaedic surgery in those on or off HRT therapy if adequate thromboprophylaxis is given (Hurbanek *et al.* 2004).

Further reading

Bonow RO, Carabello BA, Kanu C *et al.* ACC/AHA 2006 guidelines for the management of patients with valvular heart disease: a report of the American College of Cardiology/American Heart Association Task Force on Practice Guidelines. *Circulation* 2006;**114**:e84–231.

British National Formulary 58. BMJ Publishing Group / Royal Pharmaceutical Publishing Group, 2009.

Calvey N, Williams N. *Principles and Practice of Pharmacology for Anaesthetists*. 5th edn. Blackwell, 2008.

Chassot PG, Delabays A, Spahn DR. Perioperative antiplatelet therapy: the case for continuing therapy in patients at risk of myocardial infarction. *Br J Anaesth* 2007;**99**(3):316–328.

Coleman JJ. Antihypertensive drugs. In Aronson JK (ed). *Side Effects of Drugs Annual 29*. Elsevier, 2007.

Colson P, Ryckwaert F, Coriat P. Renin angiotensin system antagonists and anesthesia. *Anesth Analg* 1999;**89**:1143–1155.

Davies EC, Green CF, Taylor S *et al.* Adverse drug reactions in hospital in-patients: a prospective analysis of 3695 patient-episodes. *PLoS ONE* 2009;**4**(2):e4439. doi:10.1371/journal.pone.0004439

Dunkelgrun M, Boersma E, Poldermans D *et al.* Dutch Echocardiographic Cardiac Risk Evaluation Applying Stress Echocardiography Study Group. Bisoprolol and fluvastatin for the reduction of perioperative cardiac mortality and myocardial infarction in intermediate-risk patients undergoing noncardiovascular surgery: a randomized controlled trial (DECREASE-IV). *Ann Surg* 2009;**249**(6):921–926.

Honeybourne D. Antibiotic penetration into lung tissue. *Thorax* 1994;**49**(2):104–106.

Hurbanek JG, Jaffer AK, Morra N, Karafa M, Brotman DJ. Postmenopausal hormone replacement and venous thromboembolism following hip and knee arthroplasty. *Thromb Haemost* 2004;**92**(2):337–343.

Marik PE, Varon J. Requirement of perioperative stress doses of corticosteroids: a systematic review of the literature. *Arch Surg* 2008;**143**:1222–1226.

National Institute for Health and Clinical Excellence (NICE). CG64 Prophylaxis against infective endocarditis. London, 2008.

Nicholson G, Burrin JM, Hall GM. Perioperative steroid supplementation. *Anaesthesia* 1998;**53**:1091–1104.

O'Riordan JM, Margey RJ, Blake G, O'Connell R. Antiplatelet agents in the perioperative period. *Arch Surg* 2009;**144**:69–76.

Pirmohamed M *et al.* Adverse drug reactions as cause of admission to hospital: prospective analysis of 18 820 patients. *BMJ* 2004;**329**(7456):15–19.

POISE Study Group. Effects of extended-release metoprolol succinate in patients undergoing non-cardiac surgery (POISE trial): a randomised controlled trial. *Lancet* 2008;**371**:1839–1847.

Popping DM, Elia N, Marret E *et al.* Protective effects of epidural analgesia on pulmonary complications after abdominal and thoracic surgery. A meta-analysis. *Arch Surg* 2008;**143**(10):990–999.

The Association of Anaesthetists of GB and Ireland (AAGBI). Guidelines for the management of severe local anaesthetic toxicity, 2007. Available at: http://www.aagbi.org/publications/guidelines.htm.

World Health Organization (2009) WHO pain ladder. Available at: http://www.who.int/cancer/palliative/painladder/en/ (accessed 03 January 2010).

Chapter

2

Fundamentals of general pathology

Gerald Langman

'Disease is life under abnormal conditions and pathology is physiology contending the obstacles.'
Rudolf Virchow

Pathology is the scientific study of disease and represents a bridge between basic science and clinical medicine. General pathology introduces the essential concepts of disease and forms the basis for the understanding of systematic pathology and ultimately clinical medicine. It is not the aim of this chapter to provide a detailed account of the pathological processes and underlying molecular events. These are well described in general pathology text books. The purpose is rather to introduce the basic ingredients of pathology so as to better understand, diagnose and treat a wide spectrum of diseases.

Cell injury and death

Cell injury represents the initial trigger in a cascade of biochemical events which eventually manifests as disease. Injury is defined as an alteration in cell structure or function resulting from some insult that exceeds the ability of the cell to compensate through normal physiological adaptive mechanisms. The outcome will depend on the type, duration and severity of the injury as well as the type of cell and its physiological state. Reversible cell injury occurs when the cell's highly evolved healing process is able to restore normal cell function when the stimulus is removed. When the injury is too extensive to permit reparative responses, the cell suffers irreversible damage and dies. This can take the form of either necrosis or apoptosis.

Causes of cell injury

Hypoxia: hypoxia is a pathological condition defined as an inadequate supply of oxygen delivered to the tissues. It is the most common cause of cellular injury and is divided into four types.

- Hypoxic hypoxia is either the result of cardiopulmonary failure in which the lungs are unable to efficiently transfer oxygen from the alveoli to the blood or a consequence of a decrease in the amount of breathable oxygen as encountered at high altitude.
- Anaemic hypoxia is seen when the total amount of haemoglobin is too small to supply the body's oxygen needs or when haemoglobin that is present is rendered non-functional. An example of the former is following severe bleeding and the latter is encountered with carbon monoxide poisoning.
- Stagnant hypoxia is when blood flow through the capillaries is insufficient to supply the tissues, such as following a thrombosis.
- Histotoxic hypoxia is when the cells of the body are unable to use the oxygen, such as following cyanide poisoning.

Physical agents: mechanical injury is the most common example and includes fractures, crush injuries, laceration and haemorrhage. Burns, frostbite, sudden changes in pressure (barotrauma), radiation and electric shock are other physical injuries which may be harmful to cells and tissues.

Chemical agents: these include simple chemicals such as glucose and salt in hypertonic solutions, while even water and oxygen, critical for the integrity and function of the cell, can cause damage in excess. Other agents include poisons, pollutants, insecticides, herbicides, carbon monoxide, asbestos, alcohol, narcotics and tobacco as well as the actions of therapeutic drugs.

Fundamentals of Surgical Practice, Third Edition, ed. Andrew N. Kingsnorth and Douglas M. Bowley.
Published by Cambridge University Press. © Cambridge University Press 2011.

Infectious agents: these range from infectious proteins called prions to large parasites and also include viruses, rickettsiae, bacteria and fungi. Injury can be mediated directly by the pathogen, by an immunological mediated response typically seen in tuberculosis or, as in the case of *Clostridium difficile*, indirectly by the actions of a toxin.

Immunological reaction: the immune system protects against foreign proteins; however, an exaggerated response results in allergy and anaphylaxis, while suppression renders the body vulnerable to infection. In autoimmune diseases endogenous antigens are targeted by the immune system.

Genetic derangements: these include not only inherited mutations which may lead to congenital malformations, abnormal proteins or inborn errors of metabolism but also acquired mutations of somatic cells, responsible for the development of cancers.

Nutritional disorders: these may be the result of deficiencies, excesses or lack of an appropriate balance of nutrients, causing disease such as malnutrition, vitamin deficiencies and obesity.

Targets of injury

The injury can either target a cell constituent, such as the cell membrane or genetic apparatus, or it can affect the function of the cell by impeding aerobic respiration or protein synthesis. This sets in motion a range of biochemical processes including the generation of oxygen free radicals, ATP depletion, defects in membrane permeability and loss of electrolyte homeostasis. Because many of these mechanisms are interrelated, it leads to wide-ranging secondary effects.

Morphological manifestations of cellular injury

Morphological changes become apparent only after the critical biochemical system has become deranged. There is also a delay before these changes manifest. They are first appreciated ultrastructurally, and subsequently at a microscopic level, before they are apparent grossly.

Cellular swelling: cellular swelling, also referred to as hydropic degeneration, is a common and reversible form of cell injury. It reflects the cells' inability to maintain homeostasis leading to an influx of water and extracellular ions. It is characterized by cytoplasmic vacuolization at a microscopic level and macroscopically by swelling and pallor of the involved organ.

Fatty change: fatty change is another reversible cell injury and targets cells dependent on or involved in fat metabolism. It most commonly affects the liver and reflects an imbalance between the amount of fat entering a cell and its rate of utilization.

Intracellular accumulation: intracellular accumulation of substances is either a consequence of cell injury, such as haemosiderin following haemorrhage, or, as in the case of amyloid deposition, may cause cellular dysfunction. Both excess of normal cellular constituents, such as lipid, glycogen and proteins, and abnormal exogenous and endogenous substances may accumulate in the cytoplasm of the cell.

Extracellular matrix alteration: changes in the extracellular environment may also be a consequence of cellular injury and death. The best example is calcification, which results when fatty acids and phosphate ions are released by the damaged cell and react with calcium ions, forming insoluble calcium salts.

Necrosis and apoptosis

Cell death is the end result of irreversible cell injury and morphologically is expressed as either necrosis or apoptosis.

Necrosis

Necrosis follows the breakdown of the cell membrane with release of cytoplasmic contents, including lysosomal enzymes, into the extracellular space. The subsequent degradative enzyme action and protein denaturation is responsible for the morphological changes encountered in necrosis. These changes include pyknosis (shrinkage), karyorrhexis (fragmentation) and karyolysis (dissolution) of the nucleus and eosinophilia (increased pink staining) of the cytoplasm. Necrotic cell death is associated with an intense inflammatory response. When this is absent, as seen when cell death occurs post mortem, the process is called autolysis.

Several morphological patterns of necrosis are recognized.

- Coagulative necrosis. This is the pattern of necrosis seen in all tissues, except the brain,

Table 2.1 Features which distinguish necrosis from apoptosis

	Necrosis	Apoptosis
Stimuli	Always pathological. Think of necrosis as cell 'homicide'.	A physiological regulated process but occasionally pathological. Think of apoptosis as cell 'suicide'.
Morphological features	Loss of membrane integrity. Begins with swelling of the cytoplasm and mitochondria. Ends with total cell lysis. Large areas of tissue.	No loss of membrane integrity. Begins with shrinkage of the cytoplasm and shrinkage of the nucleus. Ends with fragmentation of the cell into smaller bodies (apoptotic bodies). Single cells.
Biochemical features	No energy requirement (passive). Random digestion of DNA.	Energy (ATP) dependent process (active). Non-random fragmentation of DNA.
Tissue reaction	Inflammation with secondary injury to surrounding tissues.	No inflammation or tissue injury but phagocytosis of apoptotic bodies.

Table 2.2 Cardinal signs of inflammation

Sign	Mechanism
Redness	Vascular dilatation
Heat	Hyperaemia
Swelling	Fluid exudation
Pain	Pressure from the swelling Chemical mediators
Loss of function	Due to pain and swelling

following hypoxic cell death. There is denaturation and precipitation of cellular proteins with preservation of the outline of the cell.

- Colliquative necrosis. This results from enzymatic digestion of the cell following a bacterial infection and is due to lysosomal enzymes released by recruited white blood cells. Ischaemic injury to brain tissue also results in colliquative necrosis.
- Caseous necrosis. A change closely associated with tuberculosis, it refers to a type of tissue death in which all cellular outline is lost and tissue appears crumbly and cheese-like.
- Fat necrosis. Rather than a specific type of necrosis it is a descriptive term that follows trauma to adipose tissue or pancreatitis. The release of intracellular fat by the damaged adipocytes leads to a brisk inflammatory response with phagocytosis of the fat cells by neutrophils and macrophages. In pancreatitis there is destruction of fat cells due to the action of pancreatic lipase.
- Gangrene. This occurs when necrotic skin or mucosa is colonized by bacteria, usually anaerobes, which are only capable of attacking damaged tissue. The tissues are discoloured due to

the deposition of sulphides derived from haemoglobin and foul-smelling due to the action of enzymes with the release of hydrogen sulphide, a process termed putrefaction.

Apoptosis

Apoptosis is a coordinated and internally programmed process that mediates the death of cells in a variety of physiological and pathological events. As a part of the normal physiological process it eliminates unwanted, functionally abnormal or senescent (old and worn out) cells. Examples include embryogenesis, normal cell turnover, such as intestinal crypt epithelium, induction and maintenance of immune tolerance and endocrine-dependent tissue atrophy. However, apoptosis may also be induced by pathological processes such as viral infections and radiation.

Cells undergoing apoptosis show characteristic biochemical and morphological features. These include cell shrinkage, chromatin condensation and partition of the nucleus and cytoplasm into membrane-bound apoptotic bodies. These are then phagocytosed and digested by adjacent cells which, in contrast to necrosis, does not illicit an inflammatory reaction.

Inflammation

Inflammation is a physiological response of vascularized tissue to injury which serves to bring defence and healing. The stimuli include many of the endogenous and exogenous factors that result in tissue injury and death. It is mediated by chemical factors which, via vascular and cellular responses, are responsible for the cardinal signs (Table 2.2) that define inflammation.

Inflammation may be acute or chronic. Acute inflammation, a process which takes a few days, is characterized by increased blood flow, exudation and an influx of polymorphonuclear granulocytes, also known as leuokocytes, neutrophils or polymorphs.

In contrast, chronic inflammation may take weeks to months or even years to resolve and is not associated with any vascular changes. Mononuclear inflammatory cells, especially lymphocytes and macrophages, are the principal cell type and the end result is scarring.

Acute inflammation

Acute inflammation may be divided into three phases. First there is a vascular phase followed by a cellular phase and finally a phase of either resolution or suppuration. Each phase is orchestrated by several chemical mediators termed cytokines. These are either produced locally, predominantly by inflammatory cells, or derived from the plasma. Histamine, serotonin, interferon, prostaglandins and leukotrienes are examples of mediators produced at the site of inflammation, while kinins and factors of the complement, coagulation and fibrinolytic cascades are formed in the plasma. Other mediators include nitric oxide and oxygen radicals. The beneficial effects of acute inflammation are the dilution and inactivation of toxins, removal of dead tissue and foreign material and a fibrin barrier to the spread of infection.

Vascular phase

Following transient and brief vasoconstriction, mediated by a neuronal reflex, there is dilatation of the vessels followed by an increased flow of blood to the injured area. This process, which is accentuated by the opening of additional vascular channels, is termed active hyperaemia. This must be differentiated from passive hyperaemia, more commonly referred to as congestion, which refers to a relative stasis of blood within the tissue resulting in a rise in venous pressure.

Vasodilatation is accompanied by increased blood vessel permeability. Bradykinin and histamine lead to an immediate, transient increase in permeability through the walls of venules, while endothelial cell injury is followed by a delayed but persistent vascular permeability through both capillaries and venules. As a consequence there is leakage of fluid containing plasma proteins, particularly fibrinogen, into tissues, a process termed exudation. Exudate carries protein, fluid and cells from local blood vessels into the damaged area to mediate local defences.

Cellular phase

The two main cell types in acute inflammation are the neutrophil and the monocyte. The neutrophil is the defining cell of acute inflammation. It is distinguished by its lobulated nucleus and characterized by its ability to engulf and digest microorganisms and other small products. The neutrophil survives only a few hours after emigration. The monocyte is part of the mononuclear phagocyte system and is involved in phagocytosis as well as an immune accessory cell presenting antigens to lymphocytes for antibody synthesis. Monocytes, which migrate from the bloodstream to other tissues, differentiate into tissue-resident macrophages.

The cellular stage is heralded by the emigration of neutrophils from the blood into the injured tissue, a complex process involving vascular changes and chemotaxis (Figure 2.1). Damaged endothelium becomes sticky due to the expression of selectins on the cell surface and is followed by the 'capture' of leukocytes, termed margination. This process occurs in the venules where the slowing of blood flow, a result of increased blood viscosity due to leakage of plasma into the tissue, and loss of the axial stream increases the contact period between cells and the vessel walls. Margination is followed by adhesion between the inflammatory cells and endothelium and this is mediated by integrins.

The active amoeboid and energy-dependent movement of these marginated leucocytes through the vessel wall is termed emigration. This occurs through intercellular junctions which then reform once emigration is completed. Red blood cells may also escape into the extravascular space, a process termed diapedesis. In contrast to emigration, this is a passive process and dependent on hydrostatic pressure forcing the red blood cells out of the vessels.

Following extravasations, leukocytes emigrate in tissues toward the site of injury by a process called chemotaxis. This is mediated by endogenous chemical agents such as leukotrienes and by products of the complement system as well as endogenous factors such as bacterial products. There is a biphasic cellular response in acute inflammation with neutrophils appearing first in large numbers followed by a relative increase in monocytes. This is because neutrophils are more numerous in the blood and more motile than monocytes.

Phagocytosis refers to the process whereby particles, such as bacteria, are ingested and destroyed by neutrophils or macrophages. This is preceded by the coating of the target protein by specific IgG class antibodies and the C3 component of complement, termed

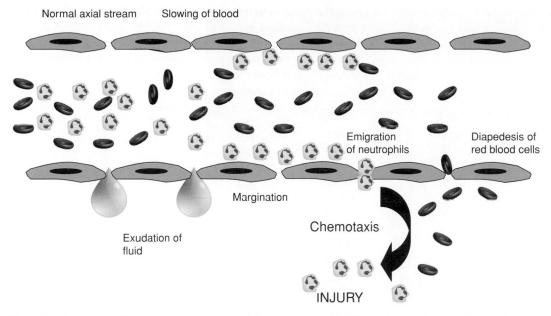

Normal axial stream   Slowing of blood

Emigration
of neutrophils

Diapedesis of
red blood cells

Margination

Chemotaxis

Exudation of
fluid

INJURY

Figure 2.1 Formation of the exudate in acute inflammation with leakage of fluid due to increased permeability, passive escape of red blood cells and steps in the emigration of neutrophils.

opsonification. Via specific receptors on the surface of the neutrophil or macrophage, the opsonized particle is then enveloped by cytoplasm and included in a phagocytic vacuole called a phagosome. Cytoplasmic lyzosomes fuse with the phagosome followed by enzymatic digestion of the particle, a process aided by a low pH inside the vacuole and hydrogen peroxide. Phagocytosis not only results in the destruction and removal of microorganisms but also the release of lysosomal enzymes into the tissues which helps digest and remove inflammatory debris.

The sequelae

1. Resolution: the restoration to normality requires no damage to the supporting structure. It is usually the result of mild inflammation due to chemical or physical insults or to infections which do not cause necrosis.
2. Suppuration: this is usually the result of a severe local injury with tissue necrosis caused by pyogenic organisms. The intense emigration of neutrophils produces an inflammatory exudate called 'pus' which contains dead tissue cells, dead and dying inflammatory cells, bacteria and a protein-rich fluid. When it occurs in solid tissue it forms an abscess.

3. Fibrosis: replacement by scar tissue occurs when the cells cannot regrow, such as following a myocardial infarction, or when the tissue architecture has been destroyed.
4. Chronic inflammation: this occurs when the damaging agent persists and results in continuing tissue destruction and attempts to heal by fibrous repair.
5. Local harmful effects: swelling associated with acutely inflamed tissues may disrupt important functions. This is a particular problem in the upper airways where the swollen larynx or epiglottis may occlude the airway. Swelling in the brain following trauma or infarction may cause further damage by local pressure necrosis and, if persistent, herniation. The exuberant and inappropriate inflammatory response seen following an allergic reaction potentiates the local effects of acute inflammation.

Chronic inflammation

Chronic inflammation is an inflammatory process that persists over an extended period. Central to the development of chronic inflammation is the persistence of the damaging agent with continuing tissue necrosis, organization and repair all occurring concurrently.

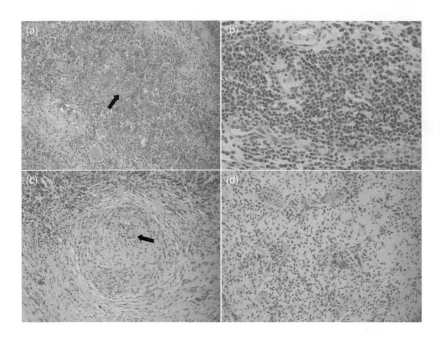

Figure 2.2 Morphological patterns of inflammation. (a) Acute inflammation with necrosis (arrow) surrounded by neutrophils and increased vascularity. (b) Chronic inflammation with lymphocytes and plasma cells. (c) A granuloma with a single giant cell (arrow). (d) Granulation tissue with a vascular proliferation and increased number of vessels in a loose connective tissue background.

Eradication or neutralization of the insult is required before tissue destruction abates and there is healing by fibrous intent. Whereas acute inflammation is 'vascular and phagocytic', chronic inflammation is 'immunological and fibrotic'.

Cell population

Mononuclear inflammatory cells, typically lymphocytes, plasma cells and macrophages, are the key effector cells in chronic inflammation and are involved in a tissue-based immune response to the damaging agent. In some types of chronic inflammation the fusion of macrophages creates multinucleated giant cells. Examples include foreign body giant cells in response to poorly digestible matter and Langhans' giant cells associated with granulomas.

Causes of chronic inflammation

Acute inflammation may progress to chronic inflammation when there are persistent or repeated attacks by the initiating agent or due to a failure to remove foreign material or poorly digestible necrotic tissue, such as bone.

Chronic inflammatory changes, however, may be there from the outset and this is seen in the setting of autoimmune diseases, foreign bodies or certain microorganisms. The microbiological infections are those with a low inherent pathogenicity but which incite an immunological response, such as mycobacteria.

Consequences of chronic inflammation

The continuing inflammation with tissue destruction and fibrosis may lead to:

Fistula formation: this is an abnormal connection between two epithelial lined organs. Examples include colovesical fistulas in diverticular disease and anorectal fistulas in Crohn's disease.

Sinus formation: tissue destruction leads to the formation of a chronically inflamed passage or tract, communicating with the skin.

Morphological patterns of inflammation

Both the causative agent and the tissue contribute to the type of inflammation. Recognizing this pattern can assist in identifying the cause of the disease (Figure 2.2).

Serous, fibrinous and suppurative inflammation

Serous, fibrinous and suppurative inflammation is the gross manifestation of the increased vascular permeability that accompanies inflammation. They differ in their cellular composition and protein content.

Serous inflammation represents the leakage of low molecular weight plasma components through minimally inflamed vessels. It often involves the serous lining of a body cavity, accompanied by copious effusion of non-viscous fluid, but is also seen in skin blisters.

Fibrinous inflammation occurs when there is a large increase in vascular permeability with outpouring of soluble protein components, most notably fibrin, though severely inflamed vessels. This commonly occurs on serous membranes where the extravasated fibrinogen is cleaved to form insoluble fibrin. Fibrinous adhesions may form when adjacent structures, such as loops of bowel, become stuck together by a loose fibrin matrix. The fibrin may be reabsorbed or organized with the deposition of scar tissue.

Suppurative inflammation is associated with exudation of neutrophils, in addition to plasma proteins, through inflamed vessel walls. This material, known as pus, may accumulate on the surface forming a purulent exudate or in serous cavities where it is termed an empyema. Alternatively an abscess may form when the pus is localized in a walled-off focus.

Granulation tissue

Fibrin deposits that remain moist and retain contact with a vascular supply undergo the process of fibrovascular organization. New vessels and fibroblasts extend into the fibrin, which is replaced by scar tissue, forming granulation tissue.

Ulcerative inflammation

This refers to the loss of surface epithelium, from any cause, with an inflammatory response in the underlying tissue. Extension of an ulcer through the wall of a hollow viscus is referred to as a perforation. This must be distinguished from penetration, where there is extension of the ulcer into a solid organ.

Granulomatous inflammation

This is a form of chronic inflammation characterized by the microscopic compact collection of epithelioid cells and giant cells, both representing altered macrophages, together with lymphocytes. Necrosis may be present. They are the result of a limited but diverse number of diseases, which include infections such as tuberculosis, foreign material and sarcoidosis.

Wounds and wound healing

Classification of wounds

A wound is an injury to the skin caused by mechanical force, and they are divided into open wounds, where the skin is either cut, torn or punctured, and closed wounds, where blunt trauma causes a contusion.

Open wounds are classified according to the nature of the injury which caused the wound. Incised wounds are caused by a sharp object such as a knife. This should not be confused with a laceration, which is an irregular tear-like wound caused by blunt trauma. An abrasion is a superficial wound where the epidermis is scraped off. Other types of open wounds include penetration, puncture and gunshot wounds.

Closed wounds are usually the result of blunt external injury. Contusions (bruises) arise due to damage to the tissues beneath the skin while a haematoma is the consequence of blood vessel injury which causes blood to collect under the skin. Crush injuries are caused by a large force applied over a long period of time.

Wound healing

Wound healing or repair occurs after there has been tissue destruction. The causes have been alluded to previously but the most common include infection, ischaemia and trauma. The repair process involves four sequential but overlapping phases: (1) haemostasis, (2) inflammation, (3) regeneration and (4) repair. This is an intricate and well-orchestrated process involving cellular constituents, stroma and an array of growth factors. The outcome is not uniform but depends on the type and extent of the injury and a host of endogenous and exogenous factors which govern repair.

Haemostasis

Following tissue injury, blood escapes from the vessels. The damaged endothelial lining of blood vessels exposes von Willebrand factor, which leads to platelet adhesion and aggregation. Activation of the clotting cascade follows with the formation of a fibrin plug, commonly known as a clot.

Inflammation

Once blood loss has been stopped, acute inflammation follows. Vasodilatation results in hyperaemia at the edges of the wound and within an hour neutrophils arrive. They phagocytize debris and bacteria and they also cleanse the wound by secreting proteases that break down damaged tissue. After two days the macrophage, attracted by growth factors released by platelets and other cells, becomes the predominant cell in the wound. In addition to engulfing bacteria and debriding damaged tissue by the release of proteases, they also secrete growth factors involved in regeneration.

Inflammation is important in preventing infection, removing debris and initiating the process of repair. However, if the inflammation persists, as seen with contaminated wounds, continuing tissue damage may delay healing. Cleansing and debridement of wounds is therefore paramount in their management.

Regeneration and repair

Repair of the wound requires fibrosis of the stromal tissue and re-epithelialization of the surface lining. The activity of both the fibroblast and the epithelial cell requires nutrients and oxygen and this is ensured by the proliferation of new vessels, a process called angiogenesis or neovascularization. This is driven by growth factors released by cells, notably macrophages and platelets, in a low-oxygen environment.

As the inflammation subsides, and concurrently with angiogenesis, fibroblasts begin to appear in the wound. They start to proliferate approximately 2–3 days after the injury and by the end of the first week they are the main cell type in the wound, laying down a collagen matrix. Platelet-derived growth factor and transforming growth factor-beta are important in the proliferation and migration of fibroblast as well as the production of the extracellular matrix. This combination of inflammatory cells, new blood vessels and collagen formation is termed granulation tissue.

Initially it is only the fibrin clot that is keeping the wound closed. The deposition of collagen provides greater strength to the wound and also provides the framework for the other cells involved in the reparative process to attach, grow and differentiate. Collagen is initially laid down perpendicular to the surface but after epithelialization realignment to the horizontal occurs. The wound strength is 10% of normal tissue after the first week and this increases to 50% by the end of the third month, eventually reaching 80% of the strength of normal tissue.

Epithelialization begins within the first 24 hours of wound injury via regenerating basal keratinocytes at the wound edges and dermal appendages. Migration of keratinocytes is stimulated by the loss of contact inhibition. This describes the process when a breach in a cell culture monolayer stimulates cell division until the breach is healed. The cells slide over each other as they migrate to cover the defect. They only move over viable tissue and therefore tunnel between the clot above and the viable tissue below. In open wounds granulation tissue is required for the cells to migrate across. Epithelial cells have the ability to phagocytize debris and via the secretion of plasminogen activator and metalloproteinases are able to digest the clot and damaged extracellular matrix as they migrate to cover the defect. Migration is complete once the cells from either end meet and new basement membrane is formed by proteins secreted by the keratinocytes.

Contraction commences approximately a week after wounding, when fibroblasts have differentiated into myofibroblasts. Myofibroblasts attach to each other as well as the extracellular matrix and wound edges. The actin fibres within the myofibroblast contract, pulling the edges of the wound together and decreasing the area for epithelial regrowth. As the myofibroblasts contract, fibroblasts lay down collagen to reinforce the wound.

Initially type I and III collagen is produced by fibroblasts. Whilst this joins the wound, it is of low tensile strength. During the maturation process, which may take over a year, type III collagen is gradually degraded and type I collagen is laid down in its place. Once disorganized, collagen fibres are rearranged, cross-linked, and aligned along tension lines. This change in fibre type and reorganization increases the tensile strength of the wound.

Healing by primary and secondary intention
Primary intention

This occurs when the edges of a cleanly incised wound are kept together. There is little tissue loss and, as a result, scarring is kept to a minimum. This is typically seen following a sutured surgical incision (Figure 2.3).

Secondary intention

When there is tissue loss or infection or when the edges of the wound are kept apart, there is healing by secondary intention. The healing differs from primary intention by the formation of granulation tissue and as a consequence there is a broader scar (Figure 2.3).

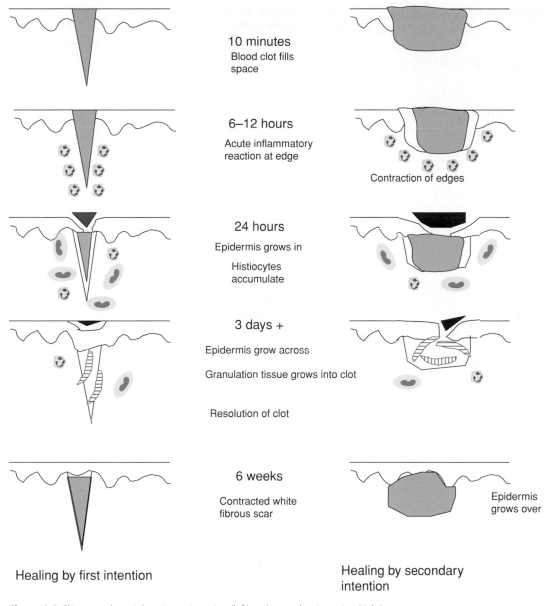

10 minutes

Blood clot fills space

6–12 hours

Acute inflammatory reaction at edge

Contraction of edges

24 hours

Epidermis grows in

Histiocytes accumulate

3 days +

Epidermis grow across

Granulation tissue grows into clot

Resolution of clot

6 weeks

Contracted white fibrous scar

Epidermis grows over

Healing by first intention

Healing by secondary intention

Figure 2.3 Skin wound repair by primary intention (left) and secondary intention (right).

Complications of wound healing

As described above, wound healing progresses in a predictable and timely fashion. Any endogenous or exogenous factor that disrupts the normal course of events may result in aberrant healing.

Complications include:

- Infection

- Pyogenic granuloma. This refers to excessive granulation tissue which may delay or prevent proper healing.
- Keloid formation. There is exuberant scar tissue, extending beyond the margins of the wound.
- Dehiscence. The edges of the wound separate, often the result of infection.
- Malignant change. A rare complication following chronic wounds.

Repair in bone

Bone fractures are usually the result of high force impact or stress. However, when the bone is weakened by medical conditions such as osteoporosis or cancer, trivial injury may cause the bone to break; these fractures are referred to as pathological fractures.

The basic healing processes are similar to those described in skin wounds, modified by the tissue reactions to bone. Immediately after a fracture there is haemorrhage due to damage of the blood vessels with haematoma formation. There is also necrosis of bone at the fracture site. Within the first week there is recruitment of inflammatory cells to the fracture site with phagocytosis of fibrin and red blood cells and removal of necrotic bone by osteoclasts. There is also granulation tissue formation with replacement of the blood clot by a matrix of collagen. A provisional callus of woven bone forms within the second to fourth week. The periosteal cells, found on the surface of bone, and some of the fibroblasts in the granulation tissue differentiate into osteoblasts and chondroblasts which lay down osteoid and cartilage respectively. This is followed by calcification of the osteoid tissue. A definite callus of lamellar bone is formed within four to 12 weeks. Osteoclasts remove cartilage and woven bone and the new bone is deposited in an orderly fashion around blood vessels. Within the ensuing months there is remodelling of the bone with reconstitution of the normal structure.

Complications of fracture

Immediate alignment and immobilization of the fractured bone is required to aid healing and prevent complications. These include:

- malalignment
- fibrous union; woven bone requires immobilization and, if not, there is incomplete replacement of fibrous tissue by provisional callus
- non-union; if there is interposition of soft tissue between the ends of bone, granulation tissue cannot close the gap
- delayed union; may be caused by poor blood supply, minimal adjacent soft tissue or fracture through a site devoid of periosteum.

Repair in the central nervous system

Neurons are permanent cells and cannot regenerate. Necrosis in the brain leads to phagocytosis by microglial cells, peripheral gliosis by astrocytes and liquification of the central necrotic area. The end result is a fluid-filled cavity. Unlike healing in other sites, collagen is not a feature.

General factors governing repair

Various local and systemic factors may retard wound healing.

Local factors

- Poor blood supply
- Presence of foreign material
- Excessive movement
- Poor apposition of wound edges
- Previous scar or irradiation
- Presence of infection.

Systemic factors

- Elderly
- Poor nutrition; vitamin C is required for collagen synthesis and zinc for the cross-linkage of collagen; deficiency results in defective collagen and wound strength is diminished
- Immunosuppression; steroid hormone treatment decreases the inflammatory response and decreases fibroblast proliferation.

Vascular disorders

Thrombosis

Normally blood within the vascular tree is kept within a fluid state. However, when the mechanisms that keep blood flowing are disrupted, a thrombus is formed. The pathological process whereby a solid or semisolid mass from the constituents of the blood is formed within the vascular system is termed thrombosis. This must be differentiated from haemostasis, which describes the physiological process whereby an injury to the blood vessel is repaired without interruption to the flow of blood.

Appearance of the thrombus

The thrombus is adherent to the wall of the vessel in which it was formed. They are composed predominantly of platelets and fibrin, with low red cell content, and as a result appear pale and friable. When they occur in fast-flowing blood, such as the aorta, they show parallel linear streaks termed lines of Zahn.

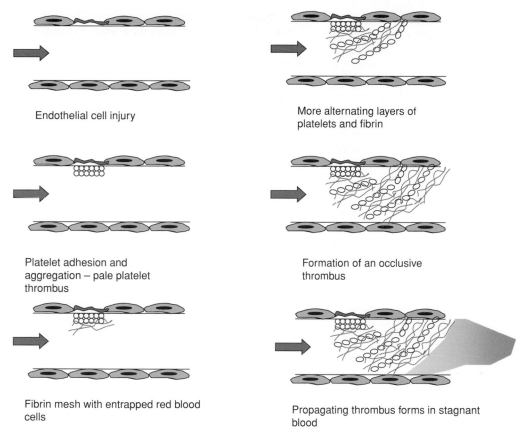

Endothelial cell injury

More alternating layers of platelets and fibrin

Platelet adhesion and aggregation – pale platelet thrombus

Formation of an occlusive thrombus

Fibrin mesh with entrapped red blood cells

Propagating thrombus forms in stagnant blood

Figure 2.4 Mechanism of thrombus formation.

These are produced by alternating layers of paler platelets, with some fibrin, separated by darker lines containing more red blood cells (Figure 2.4). However, these laminations are not as evident when the thrombus is formed in smaller arteries or veins where the blood flow is slower.

A thrombus must be differentiated from a clot, a solid mass which forms in blood which is not circulating. These have an even plum-red colour and, at post mortem, also have a surface yellow layer due to the slower sedimentation of white blood cells than red blood cells prior to clot formation.

Factors predisposing to thrombosis

Changes causing thrombosis may occur in one of three circumstances, referred to as Virchow's triad.

- Endothelial injury
- Alteration in the flow of blood
- Abnormalities in the composition of blood.

Injury to the endothelial lining is of particular importance in the formation of thrombi in the heart and arterial system. It is commonly seen on ulcerated atheromatous plaques in atherosclerosis and overlying a myocardial infarction. However, it is also encountered in mechanical and chemical damage as well as the result of inflammation or infection.

Turbulence, which disrupts the normal laminar flow of blood and causes further endothelial injury, contributes to thrombi in the arteries and heart. This is seen in the setting of atherosclerosis, aneurysm and cardiac conduction defects. Stasis is more important in thrombosis involving the slow-flowing venous circulation. Deep-vein thrombosis following long-haul air travel is a prime example.

Alteration in the composition of blood leading to thrombosis is termed hypercoagulability. This may either be the result of primary or secondary causes.

Primary hypercoagulability states are due to hereditary defects involving the coagulation pathways. These include Factor V Leiden, prothrombin mutation and protein C, protein S and antithrombin deficiencies. Secondary, or acquired, conditions are classified as either high risk or low risk. High-risk conditions include advanced malignancy and antiphospholipid antibodies, while tobacco smoking and the oral contraceptive tablet are classified as low-risk conditions. Advanced carcinomas of the pancreas or lung may produce procoagulant tumour products which create a hypercoagulable state; this is referred to as Trousseau's syndrome.

The fate of the thrombus

1. Propagation: a thrombus may extend in the direction of the heart. This means it is anterograde in veins or retrograde in arteries.
2. Resolution: this involves the break-up of the thrombus via the fibrinolytic pathway with restoration of the flow of blood. This is aided by thrombolytic drugs, which are most effective in the first few hours, before the fibrin meshwork is fully developed.
3. Organization and recanalization: this involves the ingrowth of endothelial cells, fibroblasts and smooth muscle cells into the thrombus. Capillary vessels coalesce and allow partial restoration of blood flow.
4. Embolization: portions of the thrombus or propagated clot may break off and form an embolus.

Embolism

Embolism is the migration of abnormal material, an embolus, via the blood stream and its impaction in a vessel.

Types of emboli

Emboli may be classified on the nature of the embolic material

- Thromboembolism – a fragment of a thrombus
- Cholesterol embolism – a portion of ulcerated atheromatous plaque
- Tumour embolism – embolism of fragments of tumour
- Fat embolism – embolism of fat and bone fragments following a fracture
- Air embolism – embolism of air or nitrogen bubbles

- Amniotic fluid embolism – amniotic fluid with fetal cells and hair enters the maternal circulation via the placental bed
- Septic embolism – embolism of pus containing bacteria
- Foreign body embolism – embolism of foreign material such as talc in intravenous drug abusers, or, more rarely, bullets that have entered the vascular system.

Consequences of emboli

The vast majority of emboli originate from thrombi (thromboembolism) and may involve either the venous or arterial circulation. Spread is in the direction of blood flow. Rarely paradoxical spread occurs when a venous embolus crosses to the arterial circulation via a cardiac septal defect.

Venous thromboemboli usually arise from the calf, leg or pelvic veins and impact in the lungs after passing through the right side of the heart; this forms a pulmonary embolism. The size of the embolus will determine not only where it will lodge, but also the effects thereof. Large pulmonary emboli impact in the pulmonary artery and bifurcation (saddle embolus) and cause sudden death or acute right heart failure. Blockage of medium- to small-sized pulmonary arteries may give rise to a wedge-shaped pulmonary infarct. As the lung has a dual blood supply, the infarct is haemorrhagic. When multiple small pulmonary emboli obliterate a large proportion of the pulmonary capillary bed, pulmonary hypertension ensues.

Systemic thromboemboli refer to the travel of emboli through the arterial circulation. Most originate from the mural thrombi in the left ventricle, overlying myocardial infarctions. They may also arise from atheromatous lesions in the aorta and its major branches, atrial thrombi or vegetations on the cardiac valve cusps. The major sites of embolization include the lower limbs, brain, spleen, kidney and mesentery, where the occlusion of the artery results in an infarct.

Ischaemia

Ischaemia is the result of impaired blood supply to an organ resulting in hypoxic damage to susceptible cells. A decrease in cardiac output in shock results in generalized and temporary ischaemia and the effect is felt in organs most susceptible to a low oxygen tension. This is in contrast to incomplete occlusion in an artery, which results in local and chronic effects.

Non-occlusive atheroma in the coronary and limb arteries results in angina pectoris and claudication respectively.

Infarction

An infarction is the process of tissue necrosis resulting from either arterial or venous occlusion of that tissue's blood supply; the area of dead tissue is termed an infarct.

Arterial occlusion is usually caused by a thrombus or embolus. In venous occlusion, the outflow of blood decreases and the associated increase in pressure prevents arterial inflow. Whilst venous occlusion may be the result of a thrombus, it is usually seen in the setting of external compression due to torsion, volvulus or strangulated hernia.

Infarcts are classified according to their colour, which is a reflection of their arterial supply, and presence or absence of bacterial contamination.

1. White/pale infarcts. These occur due to occlusion of arterial supply in organs with an end artery supply, such as the kidney, spleen and heart. Initially a small haemorrhagic area is seen due to the destruction of vessel walls in the necrotic area. Lysis of the erythrocytes occurs within 24–48 hours and the infarct becomes pale. The infarct is typically wedge-shaped with the apex towards the vascular occlusion and the base at the edge of the organ

2. Red/haemorrhagic infarcts. The macroscopic appearance is of markedly swollen necrotic tissue which is red due to the presence of numerous erythrocytes. It is seen in the following circumstances:

   · tissue with a dual blood supply (liver, lung)
   · tissue with a rich blood supply (small bowel)
   · re-perfusion of infarcted tissue
   · venous occlusion.

3. Septic infarcts. Bacterial contamination of an infarct is usually seen as a consequence of septic emboli or, in the case of small bowel infarcts, infection of the necrotic tissue by a proliferation of commensal organisms.

Aneurysm

An aneurysm is a localized abnormal dilatation of any vessel, including the heart, due to weakening of the vessel wall. This should be differentiated from the so-called 'false' aneurysm which is formed when blood leaking out of a vein or artery is contained next to the vessel by the surrounding tissue. In essence, a false aneurysm is actually a haematoma in communication with the vessel from which it arose.

Aneurysms may be described according to their shape. When there is circumferential involvement of the vessel, it is termed a fusiform aneurysm. A saccular aneurysm arises when only part of the circumference of the wall is involved; the aneurysm then communicates with the original lumen via an ostium.

Types of aneurysms

Atherosclerotic aneurysms

These are the commonest type of aneurysm with a predilection for the abdominal aorta as well as the iliac, femoral and popliteal arteries. The intimal-based plaque causes ischaemic-related damage and destruction of the media with thinning and weakening of the vessel wall.

Vasculitis and related aneurysms

Non-infective causes of vasculitis, such as polyarteritis nodosa and giant cell arteritis which involve medium to large arteries, may be associated with aneurysm formation.

Infection of an artery that significantly weakens its wall is termed a mycotic aneurysm. This is usually a consequence of a septic embolus in the setting of infective endocarditis. Tertiary syphilis was once the commonest cause of arterial aneurysms. Medial destruction of the wall is the result of narrowing of the small vessels in the adventitia (vasa vasora) by the surrounding inflammatory reaction. The ascending aorta, where the vasa vasora are most numerous, is preferentially involved.

Berry aneurysms

Berry aneurysms, a type of saccular aneurysm, are congenital in nature with weakness of the vessel wall. Weak and thinned parts of the cerebral circulation, especially the branch points in the circle of Willis, are particularly vulnerable. They are more common in the setting of hypertension where the increased pressure causes the vessel wall to bulge; rupture leads to subarachnoid haemorrhage.

Dissecting aortic aneurysms

A dissecting aneurysm is characterized by dissection of blood within the media of the aorta, splitting the

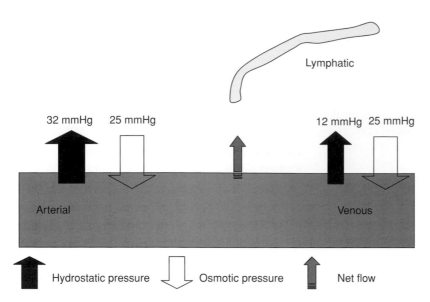

Figure 2.5 Factors involved in regulating the normal interchange of fluid.

lamina planes. This follows a tear into the intima and inner media which is usually sited in the ascending aorta. The dissection will narrow or occlude ostia of any aortic branch along its path and, occasionally, the blood may rupture back into the lumen of the aorta via a second tear. Aortic dissection is associated with hypertension and conditions where there is an abnormality of connective tissue which involves the aorta. Marfan's syndrome is such a condition where the weakening of the wall is due to loss of smooth muscle cells and elastin in the aortic media with replacement by mucopolysaccharide.

Cardiac aneurysms

This is seen after a transmural myocardial infarction where the weakened fibrotic myocardial wall bulges during systole.

Complication of aneurysms

- Pressure on adjacent structures
- Rupture with haemorrhage
- Occlusion of branches, either by direct pressure or mural thrombus formation
- Thromboembolism.

Oedema

Oedema is the accumulation of excess fluid in the intercellular tissue spaces or in one or more cavities of the body. Depending on the cause, oedema may be generalized or localized. Anasarca refers to severe and generalized oedema characterized by widespread swelling of the subcutaneous tissue. Accumulation of fluid within the serous lined cavities of the body is referred to as ascites, pleural effusion and pericardial effusion when it occurs within the peritoneal, pleural and pericardial cavities respectively.

Formation of oedema

Understanding the formation of oedema requires knowledge of the factors involved in regulating the normal interchange of fluid as proposed by Starling (Figure 2.5). Hydrostatic pressure at the arteriolar end of the capillary bed causes fluid to move out into the interstitial space. Protein molecules are too large to leave the vessel and the loss of intravascular fluid increases the plasma osmotic pressure. This acts to draw fluid from the interstitial space into the venular end of the capillary bed where the hydrostatic pressure is lower. Not all the interstitial fluid returns to the venules and the excess is drained by the lymphatic system. The rate of leakage of fluid is therefore determined by:

- an increase in hydrostatic pressure within the blood vessel
- a decrease in the oncotic pressure of the plasma
- an increase in vessel wall permeability
- an impairment in the flow of lymph
- retention of salt and water by the kidney.

Table 2.3 Classification of oedema

	Localized oedema	Generalized oedema
Increased hydrostatic pressure	Venous thrombosis External pressure on veins Cirrhosis (ascites)	Cardiac failure
Increased vascular permeability	Any cause of an acute inflammatory process	Hypoxia Bacterial toxins
Decreased plasma osmotic pressure	–	Loss of protein in the urine (nephrotic syndrome) or gut Reduced synthesis of protein by the liver (cirrhosis) Inadequate intake or absorption (malnutrition and malabsorption)
Retention of salt by the kidney	–	Reduced renal function Increased rennin-angiotensin-aldosterone secretion
Abnormality of lymphatics	Congenital absence of lymphatics Obstruction of lymphatics: Carcinoma Irradiation Surgical removal of lymphatics Filarial worms	–

Types of oedema fluid

When the oedema is the result of an inflammatory process, it is termed an exudate. The leakage of fluid, which is rich in protein, is due to increased vascular permeability. Typically the specific gravity is greater than 1.02, reflecting a protein concentration over 3 g/dl.

The fluid of a non-inflammatory oedema is called a transudate with a low protein level and a specific gravity below 1.02. This is due to changes in the variables regulating the movement of fluid other than increased vessel wall permeability.

Classification of oedema

Oedema can be localized or generalized. Increased hydrostatic pressure, depending on the cause, may result in either localized or generalized oedema. Inflammatory oedema is usually localized while a decrease in the osmotic pressure results in generalized body swelling (Table 2.3).

Disorders of growth, differentiation and morphogenesis

The size of a cell population may be altered by changing the rate of cell proliferation and differentiation on one hand and increasing or decreasing apoptosis on the other hand. Factors regulating this balance may result in disorders of growth, which include conditions that are either physiological or pathological in nature (Figure 2.6). Apart from neoplasia, which will be discussed in the next section, the adaptation remains subject to normal regulatory control mechanisms.

Failure of growth or maintenance of growth

Agenesis: this represents complete absence of an organ and its associated primordium (earliest recognizable stage) dating from embryonic development.

Aplasia: this is the absence of an organ or tissue due to lack of development of the primordium.

Hypoplasia: hyoplasia is the lack of development to the full mature size. It is a less severe form of aplasia.

Agenesis, aplasia and hypoplasia are usually congenital rather than acquired.

Atrophy: atrophy is the acquired shrinkage in the size of an organ or tissue due to reduction in the size of the cell. Occasionally the number of cells is also reduced. Causes of atrophy include poor nourishment, diminished blood supply, loss of hormonal stimulation, loss of nerve innervation, disuse or lack of exercise and ageing.

Most of the causes are pathological. However, atrophy may be physiological, as part of normal development, and includes shrinking and involution of the thymus in early childhood and the tonsils in adolescence.

Overgrowth with normal cell differentiation

Hyperplasia: hyperplasia is considered to be either a physiological or pathological response to a specific

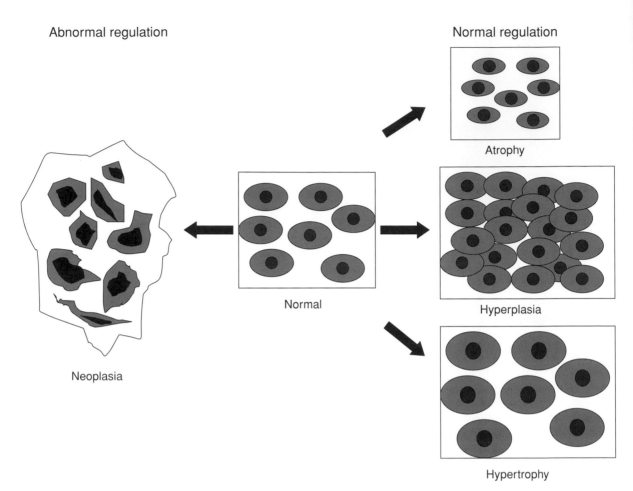

Figure 2.6 Common terminology relating to growth.

stimulus which results in an increase in the number of cells leading to an increase in the size of an organ. Only cells that undergo division, to replace those lost, are capable of undergoing hyperplasia.

Physiological hyperplasia is most frequently the result of hormonal stimulation. Examples include increase in the number of breast lobules prior to lactation and the enlargement of the uterus during pregnancy. Compensatory hyperplasia, in turn, refers to the growth of an organ when part of that organ is either removed or lost. This process, which is mediated by an array of growth factors, is seen when a portion of the liver is removed.

Pathological hyperplasia refers to the effect of an overproduction of hormones on target cells. Endometrial hyperplasia, for example, is due to the relative or absolute increase in oestrogen while androgen stimulation of the prostate gland leads to

benign prostatic hyperplasia. Unlike neoplasia (see later), the process is reversible if the hormonal stimulus is removed.

Hypertrophy: hypertrophy is the increase in the size of the organ or tissue due to increase in the size of the cell. It occurs in non-dividing cells, such as skeletal muscle, although cells capable of dividing may also be involved. Unlike hyperplasia, there is no increase in the number of cells. However, the two processes may occur together.

Hypertrophy is the result of increased functional demand and particularly affects muscular organs. Examples include increase in the skeletal muscle fibre cells in athletes, hypertrophy of the myocardium in hypertension and enlargement of the bladder muscle in urinary outflow obstruction. Hamartoma: a hamartoma is a congenital malformation due to the disorganized, haphazard overgrowth of tissue normally present at that site. Unlike a neoplasm, the growth is coordinated and occurs at the same rate as the surrounding tissue. Metaplasia: metaplasia is the reversible transformation of one type of differentiated tissue into another. This change is brought about by an abnormal stimulus which the original cell is not able to withstand. The new tissue, however, is more suited to this new environment. If the stimulus that caused metaplasia is removed or ceases, the tissue returns to its normal pattern of differentiation.

Metaplasia most commonly occurs in epithelial linings. It may involve mesenchymal tissue with the transformation of fibrous tissue to bone (osseous metaplasia) or cartilage (cartilagenous metaplasia). This is less clearly an adaptive response and frequently occurs following injury.

Metaplasia is not without consequences. Whilst the new cells are able to withstand the stresses that the epithelium is faced with, it is also accompanied by a loss of epithelial function. The metaplasia of the normal columnar pseudostratified ciliated epithelium in the bronchi to squamous epithelium in response to smoking is accompanied by the loss of mucus secretion, an important protective mechanism. A further undesirable response is the propensity for the metaplastic epithelium to undergo neoplastic transformation if the irritant is not removed.

Accumulations and depositions

Amyloid

Amyloid is an extracellular pathological fibrillar protein exhibiting a beta pleated sheet structure. Accumulation of this protein in various tissues and organs may lead to amyloidosis. Amyloid is inert and does not excite an inflammatory reaction.

Chemical composition

The essential component of amyloid is the protein fibril. Regardless of the type of amyloid, the polypeptide protein chains are arranged in a beta-pleated sheet configuration. The protein is also associated with other components, such as serum amyloid P component, a glycoprotein.

The chemical composition of the protein fibrils is related to the precursor protein, of which there are two main types:

- AL. The AL (amyloid light chain) type is composed of whole immunoglobulin light chains or fragments thereof. They are produced by plasma cells and their deposition is associated with monoclonal proliferations of these cells.
- AA. They consist of a polypeptide derived from a circulating precursor called SAA (serum amyloid associated) protein. SAA is an acute-phase protein which is synthesized in the liver and is normally present in trace amounts. AA amyloidosis is therefore associated with disorders that cause a sustained high level of SAA.

Other precursor proteins include:

- Transthyretin. This is present in some hereditary forms and also in the heart of elderly individuals (senile cardiac amyloidosis).
- Hormones. Localized amyloid deposits may be derived from calcitonin in medullary carcinomas of the thyroid.
- Beta-2-microglobulin. This is the precursor for amyloid seen in patients on long-term haemodialysis.
- Beta-2-amyloid protein. This constitutes the core of the plaques found in the brains of patients with Alzheimer's disease.

Classification

The classification is based on the fact that the different chemical types of amyloid occur in distinct clinical settings and these may occur in localized or systemic forms.

Immunocyte-derived systemic amyloidosis. Amyloid in this category is of the AL type and occurs in 15% of cases of myeloma and in 5% of benign monoclonal gammopathy. Less commonly AL amyloidosis may occur with B cell lymphomas. The protein is found in mesenchymal tissues such as the heart, kidneys, bowel, tongue and skin. Reactive systemic amyloidosis. The amyloid deposits in this category are of the AA type. This occurs in any condition capable of sustaining a prolonged acute-phase response such as chronic inflammatory conditions (rheumatoid arthritis) and chronic infections (tuberculosis). Because it is secondary to inflammatory conditions it is frequently referred to as secondary amyloidosis. Neoplastic diseases such as Hodgkin's disease and renal cell carcinomas are also capable of causing this type of amyloidosis. The protein is deposited in many parenchymal organs including the liver, spleen, kidneys and adrenals.

Localized amyloidosis. Senile amyloidosis, senile cerebral amyloidosis and endocrine amyloidosis result in the deposition of amyloid in a single organ.

Clinical effects

The presence of amyloid in the basement membrane of small blood vessels affects the transfer of nutrients, salts and water. The consequence depends on the organ involved. Cardiac involvement results in heart failure while deposition in the kidney causes the nephrotic syndrome or renal failure.

Diagnosis

Amyloid appears as pink amorphous deposits on conventional haematoxylin and eosin stained sections. Congo red stains amyloid a pale pink colour but also imparts an apple-green birefringence when examined by polarized light. Histological confirmation of the clinical diagnosis requires a biopsy of an involved organ or tissue.

Haemosiderosis and haemochromatosis

Most of the iron in the body is present in the red blood cells where it is bound to haemoglobin. When red blood cells are broken down the iron compounds are seen as haemosiderin granules in the macrophages. More widespread deposition of haemosiderin occurs in haemosiderosis and haemochromatosis.

Haemosiderosis. This is an iron overload disorder resulting from the accumulation of haemosiderin. It occurs in a localized form around areas of haemorrhage such as haematomas and haemorrhagic infarcts, while haemosiderin in the lung may reflect micro-haemorrhages that accompany heart failure. Generalized haemosiderosis is seen with repeated blood transfusions and haemolytic anaemia with haemosiderin present in the mononuclear phagocytes of the liver, bone marrow, spleen and lymph nodes. The pigment does not damage the parenchymal cells and organ function is not impaired.

Haemochromatosis. This is an inherited disease resulting from, in the majority of cases, a single amino acid change in the haemachromatosis gene

(HFE). This results in increased iron absorption from the small intestine and deposition of iron in parenchymal organs, notably the liver, myocardium, pancreas and skin. The iron is toxic to the cells and results in cirrhosis, heart failure and diabetes.

Calcification

Heterotopic calcification is the pathological deposition of calcium salts in tissues other than osteoid or enamel. Two main types are recognized: dystrophic and metastatic calcification. A third type is the deposition of calcium salts in calculi.

Dystrophic calcification

In this condition the serum levels of calcium and phosphate are normal but the tissue in which the calcification occurs is either dead or degenerate. This includes the necrotic tissue of previous infection or fat necrosis or degenerative tissue in atheroma plaques. Severe clinical effects may be associated with deposition in the cardiovascular system where calcification of the vessels may aggravate ischaemia and calcification in heart valves leads to rigidity and loss of function.

Metastatic calcification

This is the precipitation of calcium salts in apparently normal tissue as a result of generalized upset in calcium–phosphate metabolism. This is usually accompanied by hypercalcaemia with predilection for calcification in the kidney, lung, stomach, blood vessel walls and the cornea.

Causes of metastatic calcification include primary or secondary hyperparathyroidism, excessive calcium absorption from the gastrointestinal tract and conditions in which there is an excess of calcium mobilized from the bones such as immobilization and bone destruction by tumour.

Calculi

Calculi are masses of precipitated material, usually derived from secretions, which are deposited in the lumen or excretory ducts of the urinary bladder, biliary system, salivary gland, pancreas or prostate. Calcium is an important mineral in many stones.

Neoplasia

The classic definition of a neoplasm is an abnormal mass of tissue, the growth of which exceeds and is

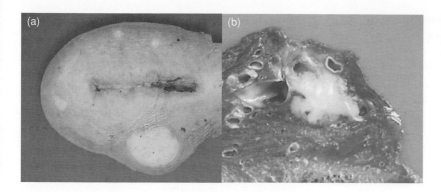

Figure 2.7 Circumscription of a benign leiomyoma in the wall of the uterus (a) compared to infiltrative squamous cell carcinoma arising from the lung (b).

uncoordinated with that of the normal tissues, and persists in the same excessive manner after cessation of the stimulus which evoked the change. However, this has been challenged with examples of neoplasms, such as Kaposi's sarcoma in HIV-positive patients and lymphomas in organ-transplant patients, shrinking when their immune status improves. Furthermore leukaemia and most forms of carcinoma *in situ* do not form mass lesions, while some neoplasms, such as naevi, are not progressive.

Neoplasms are clonal in that they are descended from a single progenitor cell. It may be more attractive to define neoplasms as clonal proliferations. Whilst this is frequently used in the diagnosis of lymphomas, the demonstration of clonality is not always possible and by no means practical for neoplasms involving solid organs.

The term 'tumour', frequently used synonomously with neoplasm, means swelling. Whilst most neoplasms are tumours, not all tumours are neoplasms.

Classification

Various histological and functional characteristics of tumours are used to separate them into three groups (1) those that are benign and have a favourable course, (2) pre-malignant lesions and (3) malignant tumours, frequently referred to as cancers, which, by definition, invade and metastasize. Benign tumours are not always harmless and if untreated may have compressive effects on adjacent organs or structures. A malignant tumour carries a more serious prognosis because of its defining characteristics. It may arise *de novo*, from a pre-existing benign tumour or from pre-malignant lesions. The latter refers to neoplasms which do not invade or destroy but, given enough time, will transform into a cancer.

- Benign tumours usually grow slowly compared to malignant tumours although there are exceptions. Histologically the proportion of cells seen to be in mitosis, the mitotic index, is used to describe the proliferation rate of the tumour. However, this does not reflect the growth rate of the tumour, which is dependent not only on the proportion of cells undergoing mitosis but also on the duration of the cell cycle and the rate of cell loss. Nevertheless it is useful when used in conjunction with other features.

- Benign tumours recapitulate the tissue from which they arise and are termed well differentiated. A squamous cell papilloma, for example, is lined by stratified squamous epithelium, identical in its composition to the normal epidermis. Malignant tumours may be well differentiated but are more often less well differentiated. In undifferentiated tumours it is not possible to determine their cell of origin.

- Pleomorphism describes the variation in cell size, shape and staining characteristics. This is frequently accompanied by a high nuclear to cytoplasmic ratio and is a typical finding in the cells of malignant tumours. Anaplasia refers to markedly pleomorphic cells such that the tissue or origin can no longer be determined.

- Benign tumours grow expansively, compressing the surrounding tissues, and are frequently encapsulated. The ability to infiltrate adjacent tissue, invade vessels and spread to distant sites are the major criteria of malignant tumours (Figure 2.7).

- Pre-malignant lesions are also referred to as intraepithelial neoplasia. There is abnormality of maturation and differentiation of an epithelial cell lining, a process termed dysplasia. When there is involvement of the full thickness of the epithelium it is referred to as severe dysplasia or carcinoma *in situ*. Until there is breach of the basement membrane separating the epithelium from the underlying stroma, there is no risk of metastatic spread.

Nomenclature

Tumour nomenclature conveys an indication of the tumour's derivation and frequently its behaviour. Benign tumours have the suffix -oma, which is preceded by an indication of the cell of origin. A papilloma is a benign tumour of either squamous or transitional epithelium while a lipoma is a benign tumour of adipose tissue. Malignant tumours use the suffix carcinoma if the tumour is of epithelial origin and sarcoma if it is derived from the mesoderm. A squamous cell carcinoma is a malignant tumour of squamous cells and a liposarcoma is a malignant tumour of adipose tissue. However, there are exceptions to these rules. A melanoma is not a benign tumour of melanocytes but a malignant tumour.

Table 2.4 provides a summary of neoplasms based on their tissue of origin and behaviour.

Spread of malignant tumours

Routes of spread

Direct spread

This refers not only to infiltrative spread through the organ of origin with direct extension into adjacent organs, but also to spread along the epithelial surface. This is seen in Paget's disease of the breast, where tumour permeates the epidermis of the nipple.

Lymphatic spread

Tumour invades lymphatic spaces. The cells may then break off and travel to lymph nodes where they colonize the peripheral sinus before replacing the entire node. Alternatively the tumour cells may grow inside lymphatics as a continuous cord of tumour. These thickened lymphatics may be visualized macroscopically and when extensive are termed lymphangitis carcinomatosis. Carcinomas, such as those involving the breast, colon, lung and stomach, frequently involve regional lymph nodes. In contrast, sarcomas spread

Table 2.4 Tumour nomenclature based on tissue of origin and behaviour

Tissue of origin	Benign	Malignant
Epithelium		
Squamous	Papilloma	Squamous cell carcinoma
Transitional	Papilloma	Transitional cell carcinoma
Glandular	Adenoma	Adenocarcinoma
Mesoderm		
Fibrous	Fibroma	Fibrosarcoma
Adipose	Lipoma	Liposarcoma
Vascular	Angioma	Angiosarcoma
Osseous	Osteoma	Osteosarcoma
Neuroectodermal	Carcinoid tumour	Small cell carcinoma
Melanocytic	Naevus	Melanoma
Lymphoreticular		Lymphomas
Trophoblast	Hydatidiform mole	Choriocarcinoma
Germ cells	Mature teratoma	Immature teratoma

by the blood stream and rarely involve the lymphatic route.

Blood spread

Tumour cells may infiltrate the walls of small vessels and then embolize to distant organs and set up bloodborne metastases. Spread occurs not only in the systemic circulation but also in the portal circulation and paravertebral venous plexus.

Trans-coelomic spread

A carcinoma which has reached the serosal surface in the peritoneal cavity can then disseminate to any other organ in the cavity. Cells which become dislodged from the main tumour are dispersed in the peritoneal fluid and can implant at other sites. This is particularly the case in ovarian tumours. Spreading of tumour cells by a similar mechanism may also occur in the pleural and pericardial cavities as well as in the subarachnoid space.

Mechanisms of metastasis

Metastatic spread refers to the spread of tumour from one site or organ to another non-adjacent site or organ. This occurs when a subpopulation of cells in a given malignant tumour acquires the necessary biological characteristics allowing it to disseminate. The process is complex and involves the production of proteolytic enzymes capable of degrading the surrounding extracellular matrix, increased motility of the tumour cells and decreased cellular adhesion. There is a great variability in the ability of tumours to metastasize. Osteosarcomas, for example, show micrometastases at the time of diagnosis, while intracranial tumours never spread outside the cranial cavity. Furthermore some organs, such as the liver, lungs, brain, kidneys, adrenal and bone, are frequently involved, while skeletal muscle and myocardium are rarely the site of metastatic deposits. This propensity for certain tumours to seed in particular organs is often referred to as the 'seed and soil' theory, whereby the microenvironment of the tissue provides the favourable conditions for the tumour cells to form a separate mass away from the primary tumour.

Laboratory diagnosis of neoplasms

Not all tumours are neoplastic. A mass in the lung may represent fibrosis, infection or cancer and a definitive diagnosis is critical for the further clinical management. Least-invasive procedures are preferred but, depending on the location of the tumour, this may not always be possible. The following methods are available to obtain tumour tissue for microscopic confirmation.

Cytology

Cytology involves the study and interpretation either of cells that have desquamated freely from epithelial surfaces or body cavities (exfoliative cytology) or of cells that have been forcibly removed from various tissues (fine needle aspiration cytology).

Biopsy

This involves a procedure in which a portion of the tumour is sampled and fixed in a suitable fixative prior to processing in the laboratory and histological assessment. The time taken from receipt of the specimen in the laboratory to a histological diagnosis depends on the size of the biopsy and complexity of the tumour. Most results will be available the next day. A range of techniques are used to acquire the tissue, including punch biopsy, tru-cut biopsy, open biopsy and endoscopic procedures. Access is problematic for deep-seated tumours which may require radiologically guided or operative methods to gain representative samples of tissue.

Clinical data are invaluable in the assessment of any biopsy. Prior radiotherapy may explain bizarre cytological features while history of a previous tumour

resection may prevent the erroneous diagnosis of a primary cancer. The histological interpretation of tumours is frequently supplemented by immunohistochemistry. This involves using a spectrum of monoclonal antibodies directly against cell components in order to determine the cell of origin (histogenesis) of the tumour. The demonstration of intermediate filaments in the cytoplasm of anaplastic cells confirms a diagnosis of carcinoma over melanoma or lymphoma.

Frozen section

Frozen sections are most frequently used in the operative setting when further surgical management is dependent on histological assessment. This may be to confirm a cancer or to assess margins of excision. Fresh tissue is frozen by liquid nitrogen, cut on a microtome and stained prior to examination under the microscope. The procedure usually takes 10 minutes. Once the diagnosis has been made, the tissue is thawed, fixed and processed. The quality of the prepared tissue sections is not optimal and occasionally the diagnosis has to be deferred till wax-embedded tissue sections are available.

Grading and staging

Grade

The tumour grade is a histological measure of the extent to which cancer cells are similar in appearance and function to healthy cells of the same tissue type. This is also referred to as differentiation and relates to the clinical behaviour of the tumour. The better-differentiated tumours have the most favourable outcome, while the poorly differentiated tumours follow a more aggressive course. For many tumours the grade is a subjective measurement with poor inter-observer variability. However, certain tumours have specific grading systems based on defined histological criteria such as mitotic activity, degree of anaplasia and architectural growth pattern. Examples include the Bloom-Richardson score for breast carcinomas and the Gleason score for prostate carcinomas.

Stage

The stage of a tumour is the extent of involvement based on pathological, radiological and clinical parameters. Whereas the grade of a tumour may be determined on a biopsy, a pathological stage requires careful examination of the resected specimen for criteria such as tumour location, size, extent of spread, lymph node involvement and metastatic spread. The TNM system is the most commonly used staging system and is based on the extent of the tumour (T), lymph node involvement (N), and the presence of metastasis (M). A number is added to each letter to indicate the size or extent of the tumour and the extent of spread. Most cancers are then staged from 0 to 4 using a combination of the TNM score.

Both grade and stage are used together to plan further treatment, estimate prognosis and determine eligibility for clinical trials.

Systemic effects and paraneoplastic syndromes

In addition to local effects, neoplasms, especially malignant tumours, may have additional systemic effects. These include anaemia, fever, cachexia and the production of hormones by tumours involving endocrine organs.

The paraneoplastic syndromes are a constellation of symptoms which are the consequence of the cancer but not due to their local or distant spread. The symptoms are mediated by humoral factors (hormones and cytokines) excreted by tumour cells or by an immune response against the tumour. Hormones elaborated by differentiated tumours involving endocrine organs are not included. The paraneoplastic syndromes result in symptoms involving predominantly the endocrine, neurological, mucocutaneous and haematological systems. Examples include ectopic ACTH causing Cushing's syndrome in small cell lung carcinomas and cerebellar degeneration in breast carcinomas.

Principles of cancer screening

Cancer screening involves testing asymptomatic individuals in order to diagnose the early stage of disease, which must be amenable to therapeutic intervention and management, in the hope of reducing mortality and suffering.

For a cancer to be suitable for screening the following criteria need to be satisfied:

- the cancer should be a significant burden in the community
- the cancer should have a precursor or early stage
- the screening test should be acceptable for the population, inexpensive and relatively accurate
- effective treatment is available for the detected disease.

Examples of successful screening programmes include the cervical smear for detecting cervical intraepithelial neoplasia and faecal occult blood for identifying colonic polyps or early cancers.

Carcinogenesis

The process of conversion of normal cells to a malignant tumour is called carcinogenesis and agents which cause this are termed carcinogens. The integrity of a tissue or organ depends on a tightly regulated balance between cell proliferation and programmed cell death. Cancer is essentially a disease in which there is uncontrolled tissue growth and carcinogenesis describes an alteration of the genes that control the balance between cell proliferation and cell death.

Proto-oncogenes and oncogenes

Proto-oncogenes are genes that are involved in promoting cell growth and are critical for growth, repair and homeostasis. These include genes that encode for growth factors and growth factor receptors and those that are intracytoplasmic signal-transducing proteins and nuclear regulatory proteins.

Transformation of the proto-oncogenes to oncogenes is brought about by either (1) changes in the structure of the gene or (2) disregulation of gene expression with increased production of a structurally normal product. Mutations, which include point mutations, deletions, and insertions within the coding sequence of the gene, alter the function or stability of its protein product. There are various mechanisms whereby the regulation of the gene may be affected. Increased copy numbers of the gene itself lead to overexpression of their products. Chromosomal translocations bring a transcriptionally active gene close to a proto-oncogene with similar effects. An additional mechanism involves the regulation of gene expression through chemical, non-mutational changes in DNA structure, a process called epigenetics. DNA methylation of a proto-oncogene suppresses its expression. Loss of that methylation can induce aberrant expression of the gene which may lead to cancer.

Tumour suppressor genes

Tumour suppressor genes encode for proteins which either have a dampening or repressive effect on the regulation of the cell cycle or promote apoptosis. They are transcriptional factors which are activated by cellular stresses, such as hypoxia, or DNA damage. Their function is to halt the cell cycle so that DNA repair can take place. A mutation that damages either the tumour suppressor gene or the signal that controls its expression may interfere with DNA repair and cause mutations to accumulate in the cell. Some of these mutations may lead to cancers; p53, encoded by the TP53 gene, is a well-known tumour suppressor protein. Mutations that affect the DNA repair genes are also strongly associated with high cancer risks.

Genes that regulate cell death

Both oncogenes and tumour suppressor genes ultimately have an effect on cell proliferation. However, genes that prevent apoptosis are also important in maintaining the equilibrium between cell proliferation and cell death. The anti-apoptotic Bcl-2 protein, a product of the Bcl-2 gene, is overexpressed in follicular B-cell lymphomas that carry the t(14;18) translocation. This places the Bcl-2 gene next to the transcriptionally active immunoglobulin heavy chain locus, leading to the transcription of excessively high levels of Bcl-2.

Mutations

A mutation caused by a carcinogen needs to affect a gene involved in regulating the balance between cell proliferation and cell death before it can cause a tumour. Even then the development of a tumour requires 'multiple hits' whereby a stepwise accumulation of genetic alterations in these critical genes is required before the normal cell transforms into a cancer cell.

There are two copies of each gene in a cell, one from each parent. Each copy is termed an allele. Oncogenes are dominant in that they represent gain-of-function mutations. This means that a mutation in just one copy of a particular proto-oncogene is enough to make that gene a true oncogene. In contrast tumour suppressor genes are recessive as they contain loss-of-function mutations. Mutations need to occur in both copies of the gene to render that gene non-functional.

Hereditary cancer syndromes involve tumour suppressor genes where the offspring inherits a normal copy from one parent and a defective copy from the other. The mutation, which is present in all the cells of the body (germ line mutation), lies dormant and it is only when the other allele is mutated that the cancer phenotype manifests; this is referred to as the Knudson two-hit hypothesis. Examples include the APC gene in

adenomatous polyposis coli and Rb gene mutations in retinoblastoma.

Carcinogenic agents

Chemical carcinogens

Most chemical carcinogens require metabolic activation before they react with the DNA of the cell. This causes irreversible but undetectable DNA damage to the cell and requires a second non-carcinogenic agent, a promoter, to produce the tumour. There are many examples of chemical carcinogens and these include polycyclic hydrocarbons which are metabolically activated by the cytochrome P450 system. They are produced in the combustion of tobacco and may well play a part in the causation of smoking-related cancers. Aromatic amines and azo dyes, implicated in bladder cancer, and nitrosamines which may cause gastrointestinal cancers are other examples.

Physical carcinogens

Since the early days of radiotherapy it has been known that irradiation can cause skin and other cancers. Following the dropping of the atomic bombs on Japan there was a marked increase in the incidence of acute leukaemia with an average latent period of 6 years. This was followed years later by a rising incidence in many solid organ tumours. The effect of radiation at a cellular level is either acute cell death or mutation.

The increased risk of skin tumours in fair-skinned people exposed to long-term ultraviolet radiation is well known. The radiation produces pyrimidine dimers which damage the phosphodiester backbone of the DNA molecule. Patients with xeroderma pigmentosum, an autosomal recessive condition in which there is defective DNA repair, have a very high incidence of cancers in sun-exposed skin. The molecular basis of these tumours rests on the inability to repair ultraviolet-light-induced DNA damage.

Asbestos fibres are carcinogenic on account of their physical rather than chemical properties. There is a very strong correlation between asbestos exposure, particularly crocidolite asbestos, and mesothelioma. Long latency periods, typically many decades, are the rule rather than the exception.

Viral carcinogenesis

Both DNA and RNA viruses have been shown to be capable of transforming normal cells in tissue culture. Whilst the presence of a virus or its nucleic acid in a tumour does not prove the virus is the causative agent, there is sufficient evidence to indicate that viruses are oncogenic in a number of human tumours.

DNA viruses

For these viruses to be oncogenic, their DNA needs to be integrated into the host cell genome. Viral genes are transcribed and the cell is said to be transformed. Human papillomavirus is associated with cervical cancers, Epstein-Barr virus with Burkitt's lymphoma and hepatitis B virus with hepatocellular carcinoma.

RNA viruses

RNA oncogenic viruses, termed retroviruses, require that their RNA genome be copied to DNA prior to integration in the host cell. It does so by means of an enzyme called reverse transcriptase with subsequent integration of the DNA into the host genome. RNA viruses which cause tumours are human T-cell lymphotropic virus 1 (HTLV-1) which causes adult T-cell leukaemia and HTLV-2, which is implicated in hairy cell leukaemia.

Surgical immunology

Immunoglobulins and their function

Immunoglobulins are glycoproteins which are produced by plasma cells in response to an antigen. They have a four-chain structure as their basic unit composed of two identical light chains and two identical heavy chains. Each chain is composed of a variable and constant region, based on the variability of their amino acid sequence. The chains are held together by disulphide bonds forming a Y-shaped structure. The arms of the Y, or the Fab region, contain two identical fragments each composed of the light chain, variable heavy chain and the first domain of the constant heavy chain. It is involved in antigen binding. The remainder of the molecule, or the Fc region, is made up of the second and third domain of the constant heavy chain.

Immunoglobulins are divided into five different classes based on differences in the amino acid sequences in the constant region of the heavy chains. These include IgG, IgM, IgA, IgD and IgE. All immunoglobulins within a given class will have very similar heavy chain constant regions. Immunoglobulins can also be classified by the type of light chain that they have. Light chain types are based on differences

in the amino acid sequence in the constant region and include kappa and lambda light chains.

The general function of immunoglobulins is the binding of antigens. It is the variable regions of the light and heavy chains which bind to specific antigenic determinants. This triggers a variety of effector functions, mediated by the Fc portion of the immunoglobulin, which include activation of the complement system and binding to various cell types. This binding can activate the cell to perform functions such as phagocytosis.

Cytokines

Cytokines are signalling molecules, or mediators, involved in the induction and regulation of the immune response. They are secreted by specific cells of the immune system and have their effect on neighbouring cells. This is termed autocrine or paracrine signalling depending on whether the same type of cell or different cells are targeted. Apart from mediating natural immunity, cytokines also play a role in regulating lymphocyte growth, activation and differentiation, activation of inflammatory cells and stimulation of haematopoiesis. Cytokines encompass a large and diverse family of polypeptides and include interleukins and interferons.

The complement cascade

The complement system comprises a group of proteins in the blood which 'complements' the cells of the immune system in elimination of pathogens and foreign cells from the body. It is part of the innate immune system that is a generalized non-adaptable response activated in an antigen non-specific manner.

There are three separate activation triggers which activate three pathways. Antigen–antibody complexes activate the classical pathway, bacterial cell surface activates the alternative pathway and mannose-binding lectin activates the lectin pathway. Circulating inactive precursor proteins are cleaved into their active forms to initiate an amplifying cascade of further cleavages. Common to all three pathways is the cleavage of C3 by the enzyme C3 convertases. The most dramatic effect is the activation of the membrane attack complex which results in lysis of cells or microbes. Complement-derived factors perform the other major functions. C3b binds to the surface of cells, enhancing phagocytosis; in this role it acts as an opsonin. C5a is an important chemotactic protein, helping recruit inflammatory cells, while both C3a and C5a have anaphylatoxin activity, directly triggering histamine release from mast cells as well as increasing vascular permeability and smooth muscle contraction.

Hypersensitivity reactions

The immune system is a powerful weapon that protects against disease by identifying and destroying pathogens and even tumour cells. However, in some individuals the reaction to an antigen is inappropriate and excessive and when pathological changes occur the patient is said to be hypersensitive.

Hypersensitivity reactions are divided into four types based on the mechanisms involved and the time taken for the reaction.

Type I hypersensitivity: anaphylaxis

Following sensitization to an allergen, antibody, primarily IgE, is bound to mast cells and basophils. After a second exposure, the allergen binds to the IgE molecule on the mast cell and basophils, triggering degranulation. Histamine is the most abundant and fastest-acting of the contents released and leads to smooth muscle contraction of blood vessels and bronchi as well as increased vascular permeability. This may lead to bronchospasm, oedema and hypotension.

Type II hypersensitivity: cytotoxic reaction

Type II hypersensitivity reactions are mediated by antibodies binding to antigenic determinants intrinsic to the cell membrane or foreign antigens adsorbed on the cell surface. Subsequent cell damage is the result of complement-dependent reactions or antibody-dependent cell-mediated cytotoxicity. In the complement-dependent pathway (examples of which include transfusion reactions and erythroblastosis fetalis) binding of the antibody to the cell surface leads to activation of the complement cascade. This may result in lysis of the cell by generation of a membrane attack complex or enhanced phagocytosis by the binding of C3b fragment to the cell surface (opsonization). In antibody-dependent cell-mediated cytotoxicity, the binding of low concentrations of antibody to the target cells results in cell lysis by a variety of nonsensitized cells. These cells, which include NK (natural killer) cells, recognize the bound antibody via Fc receptors on their cell surface.

Type III hypersensitivity: immune-complex deposition

This hypersensitivity reaction is mediated by soluble antigen–antibody immune complexes. The reaction may be systemic as seen with serum sickness, or localized to individual organs such as the skin in Arthus reaction or the kidney in lupus nephritis. The antigen may be exogenous (bacterial, viral, parasitic or foreign proteins) or endogenous. Endogenous antigens are self components to which the body produces antibodies.

Antigen–antibody results in tissue damage through activation of complement and recruitment of neutrophils. The degree of damage depends on the ratio of soluble antigen to that of antibody. Equal amounts of antigen and antibody result in complexes precipitating at the site where they are formed with a localized and mild reaction. In contrast when there is a large antigen excess, the complexes become soluble and circulate, causing systemic reactions.

Type IV hypersensitivity: delayed or cell-mediated

Type IV hypersensitivity is the clinically observable outcome of a cell-mediated immune reaction in the tissues of a sensitized individual. Cell-mediated immunity refers to the immune response of T-lymphocytes and macrophages rather than B-lymphocytes and antibodies.

T-cells are activated by antigens that are typically cell bound. A macrophage, which has previously engulfed the foreign cell, presents the antigen to specific T-lymphocytes. These T-lymphocytes are either CD4+ helper or CD8+ cytotoxic cells. The CD8+ cells are directly cytotoxic while the CD4+ cells secrete cytokines which activate cytotoxic T cells and recruit and activate monocytes and macrophages.

Type IV hypersensitivity reactions are involved in the pathogenesis of granulomas due to infections and foreign antigens and contact sensitivity.

Diseases mediated by immunological mechanisms

This encompasses a group of conditions referred to as autoimmune diseases in which structural and/or functional damage is produced by the action of antibodies or immunological competent cells against normal body components.

The spectrum of disease can be divided into those that are systemic and are not confined to any organ (systemic lupus erythematosis, rheumatoid arthritis) and those that affect a single organ (pernicious anaemia, Graves' disease).

Rheumatoid arthritis

Rheumatoid arthritis is a common systemic disease, invariably affecting the joints, associated with a variety of immunological abnormalities involving both the cellular and humoral immune systems. Most patients have an auto-antibody, rheumatoid factor, directly against autologous immunoglobulin. The articular lesion is characterized by chronic inflammation and proliferation of the synovium which gradually erodes the cartilage. Extra-articular features include subcutaneous rheumatoid nodules, vasculitis, serositis and lymphadenopathy.

Pernicious anaemia

In pernicious anaemia there is autoimmune destruction of the gastric parietal cells leading to loss of intrinsic factor and failure of acid production. The absorption of vitamin B12 is dependent on intrinsic factor and the loss thereof leads to deficiency of this vitamin and megaloblastic anaemia. Pathologically pernicious anaemia is characterized by atrophic gastritis affecting the body of the stomach.

Graves' disease

Graves' disease or thyroiditis is the commonest cause of thyrotoxicosis and is the result of an auto-antibody directed against the thyroid epithelial cells. This auto-antibody, known as long-acting thyroid stimulator, mimics the stimulatory action of thyroid stimulating hormone.

Immunodeficiency

Immunodeficiency occurs when the immune system is less active than normal, resulting in recurring and life-threatening infections. Immunodeficiency can be the result of either a genetic disease, such as severe combined immunodeficiency, pharmaceuticals or an infection.

Transplantation

Transplantation is the transfer of cells, tissues or organs between genetically similar individuals (allograft). The outcome depends on the closeness of the transplantation antigens between the donor and the recipient and the success of immunosuppressive measures to prevent rejection.

The HLA system

The surface of all cells expresses determinants which are recognized as foreign by the immune system of other individuals. The most important antigen in organ transplantation is the human leukocyte antigen (HLA) system, so called because it was first discovered on leukocytes. The genetic control of the protein is on chromosome 6, extending over four loci (A–D). Multiple alternative forms of the gene are present at each locus and the gene product on the cell surface is therefore extremely variable. Closeness of the HLA match is a major factor favouring prolonged graft survival.

Pathology of rejection

The cellular (T-cell mediated) immune response is more important than the humoral (antibody mediated) immune response in the pathogenesis of organ rejection. The humoral type targets the vasculature. The antidonor antibodies are either present before transplantation or develop during transplantation.

Hyperacute rejection is caused by pre-formed antibodies. Rejection occurs within minutes to hours following revascularization of the graft with the development of immune-complex-mediated thrombi and fibrinoid necrosis of the vessels. Acute rejection occurs a few weeks to months after transplantation and has both cellular and humoral components. Chronic rejection is seen after months or years and presents with a slow decline in organ function. It is usually the result of healing of repeated attacks of acute rejection.

Graft-versus-host disease is peculiar to bone marrow transplantation in which the grafted immunocompetent cells recognize the host as foreign and mount an immunological attack.

Further reading

Finlayson C, Newell B. *Pathology at a Glance*. 1st edn. Wiley-Blackwell, 2009.

Kumar V, Abbas, Fausto N, Aster J. *Robbins and Cotran Pathological Basis of Disease*. 8th edn. Elsevier, 2009.

Lakhani S, Dilly S, Finlayson C, Dogan A. *Basic Pathology*. 3rd edn. Arnold, 2003.

Reid R, Roberts F. *Pathology Illustrated*. 6th edn. Elsevier Churchill Livingstone, 2005.

Underwood J, Cross S. *General and Systematic Pathology*. 5th edn. Elsevier Churchill Livingstone, 2009.

Fundamentals of surgical microbiology

Richard Cunningham

Bacteriology for surgeons

Microbiology testing is increasingly automated with same-day PCR tests for organisms such as MRSA and *C. difficile* now widely available. Despite these advances, the pus and tissue samples of most interest to surgeons take at least two days to produce full culture and sensitivity results. There is good evidence that appropriate early antibiotics reduces morbidity in septic shock, and 8 hours delay is associated with an approximately 10-fold increase in mortality. Treatment of severe surgical infections therefore requires an empirical choice of antibiotics, based on knowledge of local flora and resistance rates. If the sample is sent immediately for microscopy, the regimen can be amended on day one if necessary. A basic knowledge of bacterial taxonomy will enable the surgical trainee to understand why different antibiotics are required in different situations, and to refine empirical therapy as supplementary results become available.

The Gram stain

First devised in 1844, this staining technique is still fundamental to bacteriology today. It allows prediction of the cause of infection within minutes, and at minimal cost. Laboratories base subsequent biochemical identification and susceptibility testing on the initial Gram stain of the surgical sample, so it is crucial that samples are collected carefully, and transported promptly. The categories of organisms differentiated by the Gram stain of particular relevance to surgical practice are described below:

Gram-positive cocci (GPC)

These have a thick peptidoglycan cell wall, so retain the purple crystal violet/iodine complex. Individual organisms are rounded, and form clumps, e.g. *Staphylococcus aureus*, pairs, e.g. *Enterococcus faecalis*, or chains, e.g. Group A Streptococcus.

Staphylococci

The crucial distinction within this group is between the coagulase-positive species *Staphylococcus aureus*, which is a virulent surgical pathogen, and the many species of coagulase-negative staphylococci, e.g. *S. epidermidis*, which are only of importance when infecting prosthetic joints or cannulae. *S. aureus* is further defined by the presence of antibiotic resistance (e.g. MRSA) or production of specific toxins (e.g. Panton-Valentine Leucocidin, PVL).

Streptococci

The taxonomy of this group is complex, and is mainly based on the type of haemolysis seen on blood agar and the presence of cell wall antigens.

Alpha haemolytic streptococci cause a greenish discolouration of blood agar, and are generally of low virulence. This group includes numerous species which are common causes of endocarditis.

Beta haemolytic streptococci cause complete haemolysis around their colonies, and produce a number of potent exotoxins. They are grouped using carbohydrate antigens on the cell wall into Lancefield groups A, B, C, F and G. Group A (also known as *S. pyogenes*) is highly virulent, and a major cause of surgical site infection.

Group D streptococci (enterococci) are now reclassified into a separate genus, and are mainly relevant in abdominal and urological surgery. They are generally of low virulence, but as they are inherently resistant to cephalosporins may cause problems on units where these are widely prescribed.

Fundamentals of Surgical Practice, Third Edition, ed. Andrew N. Kingsnorth and Douglas M. Bowley.
Published by Cambridge University Press. © Cambridge University Press 2011.

Gram-positive bacilli (GPB)

Aerobic Gram-positive bacilli such as Corynebacteria (also known as Diphtheroids) are of limited surgical importance, though they may cause infection of intravenous cannulae and ventricular shunts. Anaerobic Gram-positive bacilli include the Clostridia, which are major causes of gas gangrene (*C. perfringens*) and colitis (*C. difficile*).

Gram-negative bacilli (GNB)

Aerobic Gram-negative bacilli include enterobacteriaceae such as *Escherichia coli*, *Klebsiella* and *Proteus* spp. These are normal bowel flora, and may cause intra-abdominal sepsis, urinary tract infection and postoperative pneumonia. Hospital-acquired GNB such as *Enterobacter cloacae* and *Serratia* spp. are often multi-resistant. The above organisms derive their energy by fermenting carbohydrates, but others such as *Pseudomonas aeruginosa* use oxidative metabolism instead. They tend to be opportunistic, nosocomial pathogens and again are often multi-resistant.

Anaerobic GNB include *Bacteroides* and *Fusobacteria*. *Bacteroides fragilis* is a major cause of intra-abdominal abscesses. It is usually found as part of a mixed infection, and drainage and metronidazole are the main treatments. *Fusobacterium necrophorum* is the cause of Lemierre's syndrome, a persistent systemic infection following septic thrombophlebitis of the internal jugular vein.

Disinfection and sterilization

Disinfection

Disinfection is a physical process applied to the skin, environment or medical devices to kill most microorganisms and render the object or planned procedure 'safe'. It does not guarantee complete killing of microorganisms, and many viruses and bacterial spores are unaffected by standard disinfection methods. For example, hand washing with soap and water is essential during outbreaks of gastroenteritis as alcohol hand gels have no effect on *C. difficile* spores and norovirus particles.

Disinfectants do not penetrate the skin or external surfaces, and are inactivated to some extent by dirt, so preliminary cleaning is essential. The most potent disinfectants such as concentrated hypochlorite are too toxic for use on skin.

Aqueous or alcoholic chlorhexidine solution is the preferred skin disinfectant for most purposes. It is rapidly active against bacteria which cause surgical site infection, allergic reactions are rare, and the chlorhexidine component has some residual effect after evaporation of the carrier liquid. As with all alcoholic solutions, pooling of excess liquid can be hazardous if diathermy is used.

Hypochlorite solutions at various concentrations are the most widely used environmental disinfectants in hospital practice, particularly for 'deep cleaning' during outbreaks. Their main limitation is the corrosive effect after repeated use, which causes pitting of metal and vinyl surfaces. This makes the surface impossible to clean and significantly shortens the usable life of the item.

Commercial systems are now available which can fill an entire ward and all its equipment with a fog of hydrogen peroxide, which when activated remotely is very effective at inactivating microorganisms. The compounds are highly toxic while in use, so a limitation of these systems is the requirement to empty and completely seal the ward for the duration of the procedure. They have the advantage that bedside lockers, computers, soft furnishings, etc. are not damaged by the process and so can be disinfected *in situ*.

Sterilization

Sterilization kills all microorganisms including spores and viruses. Conventional sterilization cycles do not reliably inactivate prions. Prior to sterilization by heat, ionizing radiation or chemicals, instruments must be thoroughly cleaned. Modern practice is to centralize these processes in a single large department, as this makes quality control of the complex processes much simpler. Concerns about iatrogenic transmission of spongiform encephalopathy have led to increased regulation of traceability of surgical instruments, which is only practical on an industrial scale, often shared across more than one hospital site.

Autoclaving or high-pressure steam sterilization is the most widely used method for processing large numbers of surgical instruments. Chemical sterilization is used for heat-labile instruments such as endoscopes. It is inherently more difficult to control, and is reliant on adequate cleaning before the sterilization process. Some of the chemicals used are toxic and need occupational health monitoring of staff who are potentially exposed. If logistics and availability of instruments allow, it is generally preferable for these processes to be centralized rather than being carried out on a small scale by clinical staff.

Nosocomial infections

MRSA

Strains of methicillin-resistant *Staphylococcus aureus* have been associated with hospital-acquired infection (HAI) since the early 1960s. The current generation of epidemic strains have been circulating in the UK since the 1980s, and since 2005 highly virulent community-acquired strains have become a major problem in the USA. Public and political anxiety about this organism has led to fundamental changes in the regulation of infection control, with mandatory screening of all elective admissions in England since 2009, and emergency admissions from 2011.

Microbiology of MRSA

The MRSA cell wall contains an abnormal penicillin-binding protein coded by the *mecA* gene. This confers resistance to all penicillin and cephalosporin antibiotics (apart from a currently unlicensed cephalosporin called ceftibiprole). Other resistance mechanisms are frequently associated, including variable resistance to macrolides, clindamycin, quinolones, rifampicin, trimethoprim and gentamicin.

Laboratory diagnosis can be by conventional culture or PCR. Culture and susceptibility testing from a standard swab takes at least 2 days, or longer if highly sensitive liquid culture is used. This is the most cost-effective method for routine preoperative screening, where sensitivity and low cost is more important than speed of detection.

PCR testing is technically more difficult, and significantly more expensive. It is most effective when a same-day result is useful, e.g. screening before urgent surgery, or on admission to a critical care unit. Highly automated systems are now available which allow near patient testing within 1 hour, though these are even more expensive than laboratory-based tests. Another drawback of PCR tests is that they will detect strains which carry an incomplete *mecA* gene. These have probably descended from true MRSA strains but have subsequently reverted to methicillin susceptibility.

Epidemiology of MRSA

MRSA HAI has been highly prevalent in the UK and southern European countries since the 1980s. The Netherlands and Scandinavian countries have historically had much lower rates; this reflects conservative antibiotic use, uncrowded wards, and an expectation from patients that healthcare workers should routinely wash their hands before any patient contact. Screening and isolation of patients repatriated from high-prevalence countries has allowed the Netherlands in particular to maintain an impressively low level of MRSA, though this is threatened in recent years by community-acquired MRSA as a consequence of antibiotic use in intensive pig farms.

In contrast, by 2003 in the UK over 40% of *S. aureus* bacteraemia was caused by MRSA. The issue became so politically charged that infection control became a government priority, alongside waiting times and financial targets. Multiple interventions of variable scientific merit were introduced and heavily performance-managed by the Department of Health. Some such as easy availability of alcohol hand gel and improved care of central lines are universally accepted as effective. Others such as the 'bare below the elbows' campaign and universal screening are more controversial. Aspects of these initiatives have undeniably been very successful, with MRSA bacteraemia in England falling from 600 cases per month in 2006 to 200 per month in 2009. MRSA bacteraemia has a mortality of up to 25%.

Community-acquired MRSA is an emerging problem in the USA. This has been driven by a single strain (USA-300) which produces a toxin called Panton-Valentine Leucocidin (PVL). This toxin is rapidly cidal to polymorphs and patients typically present with severe, persistent cutaneous abscesses. Fulminant, haemorrhagic pneumonia is a rare but often fatal presentation, even in previously fit young people. USA-300 can also cause the same range of surgical infections as any other *S. aureus* strain, though generally more severely. These strains have not yet become widely established in the UK, though this is unlikely to continue indefinitely.

Treatment of MRSA

The range of antibiotics active against most MRSA strains has expanded substantially in recent years; however, the new agents are costly and glycopeptides (vancomycin and teicoplanin) remain the mainstay of treatment. Glycopeptides are effective in bacteraemia if given in appropriate doses, but penetrate poorly into abscesses, consolidated lung or infected bone. They are significantly less active than flucloxacillin against sensitive *S. aureus* strains, and response to treatment is often slow. They can be combined with a second, better-penetrating agent such as oral rifampicin for deep-seated infection. If this is done it is crucial to stop both antibiotics at the same time, as rifampicin monotherapy induces resistance within days. Combination therapy of vancomycin with gentamicin is potentially nephrotoxic; teicoplanin is a safer option in this setting. Vancomycin levels require close attention to timing of both dosing and sample collection; ideally trough levels should be maintained between 15 and 20 mg/l.

Newer MRSA active antibiotics include linezolid, tigecycline and daptomycin. Linezolid has the advantage of oral administration, and despite its high cost may be useful as an alternative to inpatient treatment. The main toxicity is a relatively high incidence of bone marrow suppression, which requires FBC monitoring weekly while it is being administered. Tigecycline is also active against anaerobes and many Gram negatives, so may be a useful monotherapy for mixed MRSA and bowel flora infections. Daptomycin is a once-daily IV antibiotic licensed for complex skin and soft tissue infections. Its main toxicities are nausea and rarely myositis. Creatinine kinase should be measured weekly while on daptomycin.

Most MRSA strains are susceptible to oral agents such as doxycycline, erythromycin, fusidic acid and trimethoprim. These agents, used singly or in combination, are adequate for most minor infections; the choice of agents depends on local susceptibility patterns.

MRSA infection control

Mandatory screening of patients admitted to NHS hospitals means that MRSA will become increasingly rare on surgical wards. Newly identified carriers should be started on a topical decolonization regimen, typically daily washes with triclosan or chlorhexidine, and concurrent nasal mupirocin ointment for 5 days. This will eliminate carriage in up to 40% of cases under ideal conditions, but recolonization from the environment, family members or the patient's own bowel flora is common. The number of viable organisms on the patient's skin is significantly reduced by the regimen, so it is a useful measure perioperatively, even if ulti-

mately unsuccessful. It is not helpful to delay surgery awaiting negative screens, as recolonization may occur while these are being processed. A better approach is to start decolonization 1–2 days before surgery, and supplement the usual operative prophylaxis with an MRSA active agent such as 400 mg teicoplanin, given IV at induction of anaesthesia.

As the prevalence of MRSA decreases, and when patients are proven to be negative on admission, clusters of incident cases are increasingly apparent. When epidemiologically linked cases occur, staff screening may be necessary to detect asymptomatic carriers. These should be decolonized as described above; systemic antibiotics are also sometimes necessary to eradicate throat and bowel carriage. Dermatitis is a recognized cause of refractory MRSA carriage, and may sometimes be exacerbated by skin disinfectants. MRSA-colonized healthcare workers suffer significant stress and anxiety, and should be managed confidentially by occupational health services, with input from the infection control team and other relevant specialists.

Clostridium difficile-associated diarrhoea (CDAD)

Clostridium difficile

This *spore-forming anaerobe* has become a major cause of morbidity and mortality across the developed world. The incidence has increased sharply since 2000, though coordinated control measures including mandatory reporting of cases has had some success at reducing numbers of new cases in the UK.

Microbiology of *C. difficile*

Ingested *C. difficile* spores or vegetative organisms rarely become established in the gastrointestinal tract of healthy people; innate defences include gastric acid, mucosal antibodies and, most importantly, a normal bowel flora. Not all strains are toxigenic, and there is some evidence that carriage of non-toxigenic strains may be protective. Most toxigenic strains produce two toxins, A and B. These cause an intense inflammatory response in the colon, with a wide spectrum of illness ranging from mild self-limiting diarrhoea to toxic megacolon and death. Diagnosis has traditionally been based on toxin detection in stool samples, commonly by enzyme immunoassay (EIA). It has recently been shown that these tests have very poor specificity and sensitivity, and should ideally be confirmed either by looking for the specific cytopathic effect of toxin on cell cultures, or more rapidly by PCR. Another EIA-based test looks for a *C. difficile* specific form of glutamate dehydrogenase (GDH). This test cannot differentiate toxigenic and non-toxigenic strains, so again is not adequate when used alone. Epidemic strains can be distinguished by molecular typing methods; this is increasingly important as hypervirulent strains such as 027 have been identified in recent years. This strain produces higher amounts of toxin, is associated with severe disease, higher mortality, and may respond less well to metronidazole than other strains.

Epidemiology of CDAD

Traditionally regarded as a hospital pathogen, community-acquired infections are increasingly recognized. These are often not associated with prior antibiotic use, and the mechanism of transmission and pathogenesis is still uncertain.

Hospital-acquired CDAD is strongly associated with increasing age and use of broad-spectrum antibiotics. The strongest association is with overuse of cephalosporins, clindamycin and quinolones, but the associated antibiotics change over time, and in different locations. Surgeons should use their local antibiotic policy as this will be tailored to their local *C. difficile* strains and resistance patterns.

An association between CDAD and use of proton pump inhibitors was first described in 2003, and subsequently confirmed in multiple studies and meta-analysis.

Spores are relatively resistant to gastric acid, and it may be that suppressing gastric acidity increases the risk of CDAD by allowing acid-susceptible vegetative cells to survive transit through the stomach. PPI use approximately doubles the risk of CDAD, which is a significant issue given the widespread, often inappropriate use of PPIs in the general population.

It should be noted that *C. difficile* spores are resistant to alcohol, so conventional soap and water hand-washing is essential when dealing with infected patients.

Treatment of CDAD

Mild cases will usually resolve after withdrawal of the offending antibiotic, but moderate and severe cases require specific treatment. Oral metronidazole is effective within 72 hours in most moderate cases,

Table 3.1 Features of severe *Clostridium difficile* diarrhoea

Temperature >38.5°C
Hypotension
White cell count >15 × 10^9/l
Serum albumin <25 mg/l
Serum creatinine >50% above baseline
Ileus
Colonic dilatation on CT scan or abdominal X-ray

and should be continued for 10 days. Severe cases, which are defined in Table 3.1, should be treated with oral vancomycin, as this has a more rapid effect than metronidazole. Intravenous vancomycin does not penetrate the gut lumen, and has no role. Recurrence of symptoms is very common, and can be due to both relapse of the same strain and reinfection with a new one. In one study PPI use increased the risk of CDAD relapse four fold. Numerous regimens, including pulsed antibiotics, tapered antibiotics, IV immunoglobulin, and even administration of donor faeces, have been tried. None has a good evidence base, and expert advice should be sought if a patient relapses more than once. Toxic megacolon is a serious complication of CDAD, with a mortality of over 35%. It is often preceded by a reduction in the frequency of diarrhoea, and patients suspected of having this complication must be monitored closely. Early colectomy may be life saving.

Antibiotic use

Prophylaxis

Appropriate use of perioperative antibiotic prophylaxis has had a dramatic effect on the incidence of surgical site infection. Consideration of its use before skin incision has been incorporated into the WHO Surgical Safety Checklist. When implemented properly, the beneficial effect far exceeds that obtained from technologies such as laminar air flow, at much lower cost. Unfortunately many misconceptions exist, particularly about duration of treatment. The prophylactic regimens used in Plymouth in 2010 are summarized in Table 3.2, but units should develop their own policies, informed by local resistance rates. General principles include the following:

- Prophylactic antibiotics must be at therapeutic levels in the blood before the first incision; this is best achieved by administration at induction of anaesthesia. Preoperative prophylaxis is essential because even the most expert surgical incision

Table 3.2 Plymouth Hospitals' surgical antibiotic prophylaxis guidelines

Procedure	Antibiotic
Cardiac	Flucloxacillin + gentamicin Teicoplanin + gentamicin if penicillin-allergic
Gastrointestinal	Co-amoxiclav Cefuroxime + metronidazole if penicillin-allergic
Vascular	Co-amoxiclav Cefuroxime + metronidazole if penicillin-allergic
Lower limb amputation	As above + penicillin/metronidazole for 5 days
Gynaecological	Co-amoxiclav Cefuroxime + metronidazole if penicillin-allergic
Termination of pregnancy	Metronidazole single dose, doxycycline for 7 days
Neurosurgery	Cephradine Co-amoxiclav or add metronidazole if sinuses/mucosa involved
General orthopaedic	Cephradine
Fractured neck of femur	Teicoplanin + gentamicin (given separately)
Plastic	Flucloxacillin Cephradine if penicillin-allergic
Breast reconstruction/implants	Co-amoxiclav Cephradine + metronidazole if penicillin-allergic
Urology	TURP single-dose gentamicin
Prostatic biopsy	Single-dose levofloxacin

causes microscopic haematomas deep within the wound. If skin organisms have been inoculated into these, postoperative antibiotics will not penetrate in time to prevent bacterial multiplication.

- Appropriate spectrum antibiotics to cover likely infecting organisms should be used. In practice, simple agents such as co-amoxiclav or cephalosporin and metronidazole combinations are effective for most purposes. They may not be adequate when a patient is known or suspected of carrying multi-resistant organisms such as MRSA or ESBL (extended spectrum beta lactamase producers). Such patients can usually be protected by single doses of teicoplanin, meropenem or gentamicin, in addition to the usual agents. They should be discussed with the microbiologist

before going to theatre, as the additional antibiotics required may not be readily available in the anaesthetic room.

- There is very little evidence that more than a single dose of prophylactic antibiotics adds to the therapeutic effect. An exception is when surgery is prolonged beyond 3 hours or there is significant blood loss, in which case intraoperative doses should be given. In settings where postoperative infection is catastrophic, such as in vascular and orthopaedic implant surgery, use of up to 24 hours prophylaxis is not unreasonable.

- Endocarditis prophylaxis in patients with prosthetic or damaged valves is often provided by the standard regimens used; again such cases should be discussed early with the microbiologist.

Therapy

Table 3.3 summarizes the policy for empirical antibiotic use in Plymouth Hospitals NHS Trust in 2010. This may not be appropriate in other locations and should be amended in light of local resistance patterns and flora. General principles to remember include the following:

- All UK hospitals must now have an antibiotic prescribing group, including a specialist antibiotic pharmacist, microbiologist and relevant clinicians.

- Always collect appropriate cultures before starting or changing an antibiotic, as even an inadequate choice or dosage may be enough to prevent positive cultures.

- Always document the agent, route of administration and suspected infection in the case notes. Remember the impact on the patient's bacterial flora may last months or years, and this information will influence future antibiotic choices.

- Use the narrowest spectrum possible, taking into account the severity of the infection. For example, oral trimethoprim is adequate for most cases of simple cystitis, even with a resistance rate of 20%, as little harm will result from having to change agents when culture results are available. On the other hand, ventilator-associated pneumonia can be rapidly fatal, so a broad-spectrum combination such as piperacillin-tazobactam and vancomycin is justifiable pending culture results.

Table 3.3 Summary of Plymouth Hospitals' empirical antibiotic guidelines

Suspected septicaemia		
Source	**Initial empirical therapy**	**Oral switch**
IV cannula	Flucloxacillin* + gentamicin (review gentamicin at 24 hours)	Flucloxacillin
Urinary tract	Trimethoprim + gentamicin (review gentamicin at 24 hours)	Trimethoprim
Neutropenia	Piperacillin/tazobactam – consider gentamicin in clinically unstable. Refer to unit protocol	n/a
Other	Amoxicillin + gentamicin + metronidazole	Co-amoxiclav
* Substitute vancomycin iv if colonized with MRSA		
Add vancomycin to all PNEUMONIA regimens if previously MRSA colonized and when treating empirically. Screen for MRSA before starting antibiotics and stop if negative		
Asthma	Antibiotics not indicated	
Infective exacerbation COPD	Doxycycline	

Community-acquired pneumonia
  Non-severe
  Severe
	Amoxicillin + doxycycline
	Levofloxacin if penicillin-allergic
	Co-amoxiclav + doxycycline
	Levofloxacin if penicillin allergic	

Hospital-acquired pneumonia	Within 5 days of admission treat as for community-acquired disease More than 5 days after admission IV Pipericillin/tazobactam and cover for MRSA with po Doxycycline OR IV Vancomycin till proven negative Non-severe allergy to penicillin replace pipericillin/tazobactam with meropenem Severe allergy to penicillin replace pipericillin/tazobactam with levofloxacin	
For severe infections consult with a medical microbiologist, especially those conditions marked with φ		
Clostridium difficile colitis	Metronidazole po or in severe disease Vancomycin po for 10 days	
Limb cellulitis	Flucloxacillin	
Facial cellulitis	Co-amoxiclav	
Diabetic foot infection deep to the fascial layers	Co-amoxiclav Where oral treatment is preferred consider clindamycin + levofloxacin after discussion with a microbiologist	
Uncomplicated UTI	Trimethoprim	
φBacterial meningitis	Ceftriaxone (plus amoxicillin if at risk of listeria)	
φIntracranial infection	Ceftriaxone + metronidazole	
φSeptic arthritis, osteomyelitis	Flucloxacillin + gentamicin (review gentamicin at 24 hours) or sodium fusidate po if known staphylococcal infection	
φPelvic inflammatory disease	Co-amoxiclav + doxycycline Consider stat IM/IV ceftriaxone if infection with gonococcus likely	

- Only use parenteral antibiotics when oral absorption is impaired, or immediate high blood levels are required. Some antibiotics such as quinolones, rifampicin and linezolid produce the same blood levels when given orally as IV, avoiding the discomfort and risks of intravenous cannulation. As a minimum, intravenous antibiotics should be reviewed daily and switched to oral as early as possible.
- Home administration of intravenous antibiotics requires significant resources to implement safely and can usually be avoided with appropriate oral therapy.

Viral infections of relevance to surgery

Blood-borne viruses and surgery

Blood-borne viruses (BBV), particularly HIV, hepatitis B (HBV) and hepatitis C (HCV), are a rare but significant hazard of surgical practice. Not only may they cause serious illness to surgeons who acquire them occupationally, chronic carriage may bring a surgical career to a premature end. Restrictions on healthcare workers who carry BBV are under constant review; the latest recommendations are available on the UK Department of Health website. The following is general guidance on avoiding infection with, or transmission of, these agents.

Surgery on BBV carriers

The prevalence of these viruses varies enormously in different ethnic and social groups and, generally, universal preoperative screening is not performed. This is because of the practical difficulty of obtaining informed consent, the issue of false negatives and, more frequently, false positives, and use of universal precautions whether the patient is a BBV carrier or not. Patients with risk factors for BBV carriage should be encouraged to consent to testing, and all surgical trainees should be comfortable with carrying out the appropriate level of pre-test counselling in various situations. The overall risk of HIV transmission from a needle stick injury from an intravenous drug user in the UK is very approximately 1 in 15 000; however for hepatitis C it is around 1 in 70, reflecting the higher prevalence of hepatitis C in this population.

Exposure-prone procedures (EPP)

These are defined as procedures where injury to the worker may result in exposure of the patient's open tissues to their blood. This includes procedures where the worker's gloved hands may be in contact with sharp instruments, needle tips or sharp tissues (spicules of bone or teeth) inside a patient's open body cavity, wound or confined anatomical space where the hands or fingertips may not be completely visible at all times. Examples and more detailed guidance is available on the UK Department of Health website.

Vaccination against blood-borne viruses

All surgeons carrying out EPP should be immunized against HBV, and have their antibody response confirmed. Following a case where a carrier surgeon submitted another person's blood sample for analysis, this must now be performed by the hospital Occupational Health Department. Current guidance is that those who generate an anti-HBs level greater than 100 IU should have a single booster dose 5 years later. Further immunization of those whose level is between 10 IU and 100 IU is complex and should be discussed individually. Non-responders should be tested for past or current HBV infection. Most adults with acute hepatitis B clear the virus (i.e. become HBsAg negative) within 6 months of infection and can practice normally thereafter. When a healthcare worker is found to be HBsAg positive the sample should be tested urgently for HBeAg and the HBV viral load quantified. HBeAg positive and HBeAg negative staff with a viral load greater than 1000 genome equivalents per ml are *not* allowed to continue doing EPP. Likewise, carriers of hepatitis C and HIV should not perform EPPs. Prior to 2005, the identification of a surgeon BBV carrier was often followed by an extensive look-back exercise, attempting to identify and test any patients who may have been exposed. These were generally costly and distressing for both patients and staff, and in many cases were of limited benefit. The decision to undertake a look-back is now taken on a case by case basis by the Director of Public Health and the Primary Care Trust involved. Effective vaccines against HCV and HIV are many years away, as both of these are RNA viruses, with a high rate of mutation.

Risk-reduction strategies

Most surgical injuries are caused by suture needles, usually to the non-dominant index finger. Many are caused to the assistant by the operator. The rate varies between procedures, e.g. the rate of percutaneous injury has been quoted as 10% for abdominal and 21% for vaginal hysterectomy. Double gloving reduces the rate of inner glove puncture, and is believed to reduce the risk of viral transmission by wiping the external surface of the needle. Blunt-tipped needles are the safest option where they can be used.

Management of inoculation injuries

All UK Health Authorities and NHS Trusts are required to have a designated doctor and local policy for the management of blood exposure incidents. The detail of where to seek advice, availability of testing and post-exposure prophylaxis will vary between centres, and surgeons should familiarize themselves with their local arrangements, as uncertainty about immediate action after an incident is stressful, and delay may increase the risk of transmission. Immediately following an exposure, the wound should be washed with soap and water but without scrubbing. Exposed mucous membranes should be irrigated copiously. Puncture wounds should be gently encouraged to bleed, but not sucked. Our local practice is for the injured member of staff to go to the Accident and Emergency Department where a blood sample is collected for long-term storage. Another doctor or nurse will seek consent from the source patient for urgent hepatitis B surface antigen, HIV and hepatitis C antibody testing in all cases. It is exceptionally rare for this request to be refused. It is not usually considered necessary for UK surgeons to cease operating pending serological follow up after an exposure to bloodborne viruses, though they should not donate blood or carry an organ donor card. Advice should be taken from local experts about considering safe sex practices until a final negative result is obtained.

Potential HIV exposure

If the patient is in an at-risk group for HIV infection, post-exposure prophylaxis should be made available as soon as possible, ideally within 1 hour. It is not usually possible to HIV test the source patient within this time frame, so the exposed healthcare worker will need to decide whether to start antiretroviral therapy on the basis of incomplete data. Guidelines on the management of this dilemma have been drawn up by the Expert Advisory Group on AIDS. These suggest the use of a starter pack of antiretroviral treatment, together with antiemetics and antidiarrhoeals. This treatment can cause significant gastrointestinal upset, and a high proportion of recipients discontinue the drugs early. The standard combination may not be optimal if the exposure is from a patient who has been on antiretroviral therapy as they may be carrying a resistant virus. Contacting the GU physician managing the index patient may be very helpful.

Inoculation injuries may occur while treating unconscious patients, or those who may not have capacity to consent to BBV testing. In many countries outside the UK testing the source patient without consent is considered ethically acceptable, but the UK General Medical Council and Expert Advisory Group on AIDS (EAGA) have unequivocally stated this is not permissible unless done in the direct medical interests of the patient. Some additional guidance is available on the GMC website, but this is limited, and rarely helpful in practice. In such cases it may be necessary to start taking PEP before exploring the issues around testing, as expert occupational health and legal advice will not be available within the relevant timeframe.

HBV exposure

In contrast to HIV, management of hepatitis B exposure is straightforward. All surgeons should know their HBV immune status; known responders to the vaccine are often given a booster dose as a precaution, though there is no evidence that this is necessary. Known non-responders to HBV vaccine will need intramuscular hepatitis B immunoglobulin as soon as possible after the injury, and careful follow-up.

HCV exposure

At present there is no post-exposure prophylaxis for hepatitis C. Our policy is to test any anti-HCV-positive source patients by PCR. If this is negative, the risk of transmission is virtually non-existent. If the source patient is PCR-positive, the healthcare worker is tested by PCR 6 weeks after the injury and for anti-HCV at 6 months. The aim is to detect transmission as early as possible, as interferon and ribavirin treatment early in the course of infection is highly effective at permanently eradicating the virus.

Specific infections

Postoperative pneumonia

Pneumonia is the leading cause of infectious mortality in hospitalized patients. Surgery and prolonged intubation are the main predisposing factors; others include age, reduced level of consciousness, use of proton pump inhibitors and underlying medical illnesses. Aspiration is the main method of entry of organisms into the lower respiratory tract. Many reports, particularly from US studies, suggest that aerobic Gram-negative bacilli and *Staphylococcus aureus* are the predominant cause. Defining the aetiology of postoperative pneumonia is difficult, as most patients are unable to produce an adequate sputum sample. The preponderance of Gram-negatives may partly reflect colonization of the oropharynx, and the after-effects of perioperative antibiotics. Antibiotics should be started after blood cultures and ideally sputum have been collected in patients who are pyrexial with no other focus, with new infiltrates on chest X-ray, or clinical signs of consolidation. The choice of agent depends on previous antibiotics and local resistance data; our local recommendation is piperacillin-tazobactam, adding a glycopeptide to cover MRSA unless the patient has had a recent negative screen. Cephalosporins and fluoroquinolones have been widely used in the past, but carry a significant risk of *C. difficile* colitis. Legionnaire's disease has caused major nosocomial outbreaks in the past; this is no longer a significant risk with adequate maintenance of hospital water supplies and cooling towers.

Aspiration pneumonitis is an inflammatory response to gastric acid aspiration. It may be subsequently complicated by infection, but there is no evidence to support the use of antibiotics in the acute stage. Selective decontamination of the digestive tract (SDD) is a strategy which aims to prevent ventilator-associated pneumonia (VAP). It involves prophylactic use of a cephalosporin for 3 days after ICU admission, with application of a mixture of non-absorbed antibiotics to eliminate aerobic gut organisms. The anaerobic bowel flora is unaffected by this regimen, and may provide a natural barrier to colonization with multi-resistant hospital-acquired organisms. Numerous studies have shown a reduction in culture-positive VAP with this strategy, but its effect on mortality is controversial, and its use has not extended beyond centres with a specialist interest in the strategy.

A more widely accepted prevention strategy is the use of the Ventilator Care Bundle, pioneered in the US as part of the Saving 100,000 lives campaign. Deceptively simple in concept, this strategy involves ensuring compliance with five steps:

- elevating the bed head to between 30 and 45 degrees
- actively lightening sedation on a daily basis
- actively assessing the potential to wean or extubate on a daily basis
- avoiding antacids and H2 blockers unless clearly indicated
- DVT prophylaxis.

While diagnosis of VAP is to some degree subjective, there is a general consensus that rates have fallen in units which implement these steps, and it is likely that they will become mandatory in the UK.

Surgical site infection (SSI)

Many of the specific infections described below can complicate the surgical wound, though most infections are minor and may not require antibiotic treatment. Microbial contamination of the wound is inevitable in a small proportion of cases, even with modern aseptic techniques and filtered air. Overall, up to 5% of patients undergoing surgery will develop an SSI. A number of factors influence whether infection will become established – the patient, the nature of the surgery, prophylactic antibiotics, and the virulence of the contaminating organism. The usual local signs of inflammation are present, and the presence of a purulent discharge is the best single indicator of infection. The incubation period of *S. aureus* wound infection is 5–7 days; consequently many patients will have been discharged from hospital before these are clinically apparent. SSI is conventionally classified into superficial incisional, deep incisional and organ space infections. The UK Health Protection Agency has been running a surveillance scheme for these infections for many years; summary data can be accessed at their website. Surgeon-specific infection rates are fed back to Directors of Infection Prevention and Control and, in the event of an abnormally high rate in a particular setting, these can be shared with Clinical Governance Directors if appropriate. Confidential data on local wound infection rates are available to participating centres, together with anonymous overall results. Results are stratified by known risk factors.

Management of most surgical wound infections is straightforward. In many cases, drainage of the collection is all that is required. A swab or ideally aspirated pus should *always* be sent for culture even if antibiotics are not being used immediately. This will enable early detection of resistant organisms or cross-infection. *S. aureus* is the commonest cause; aerobic Gram-negatives and anaerobes may be involved after bowel surgery. NICE has issued guidance on the prevention and treatment of surgical site infection; the full document is available on their website, and key priorities for implementation are reproduced in Table 3.4.

Cellulitis

This is an acute, progressive infection of the skin and subcutaneous tissues. The usual local signs of inflammation are present, though the advancing margin of erythema often has an indistinct, impalpable edge. Patients are systemically unwell, and bacteraemia may occur. It is a complication of peripheral oedema, trauma and leg ulcers. The microbiology of cellulitis is straightforward in most cases, though as

Table 3.4 NICE Clinical Guideline CG74 Prevention and treatment of surgical site infection

Key priorities for implementation

Information for patients and carers
- Offer patients and carers clear, consistent information and advice throughout all stages of their care. This should include the risks of surgical site infections, what is being done to reduce them and how they are managed.

Preoperative phase
- Do not use hair removal routinely to reduce the risk of surgical site infection.
- If hair has to be removed, use electric clippers with a single-use head on the day of surgery. Do not use razors for hair removal, because they increase the risk of surgical site infection.
- Give antibiotic prophylaxis to patients before:
  - clean surgery involving the placement of a prosthesis or implant
  - clean-contaminated surgery
  - contaminated surgery.
- Do not use antibiotic prophylaxis routinely for clean non-prosthetic uncomplicated surgery.
- Use the local antibiotic formulary and always consider potential adverse effects when choosing specific antibiotics for prophylaxis.
- Consider giving a single dose of antibiotic prophylaxis intravenously on starting anaesthesia. However, give prophylaxis earlier for operations in which a tourniquet is used.

Intraoperative phase
- Prepare the skin at the surgical site immediately before incision using an antiseptic (aqueous or alcohol-based) preparation: povidone-iodine or chlorhexidine are most suitable.
- Cover surgical incisions with an appropriate interactive dressing at the end of the operation.

Postoperative phase
- Refer to a tissue viability nurse (or another healthcare professional with tissue viability expertise) for advice on appropriate dressings for the management of surgical wounds that are healing by secondary intention.

immunocompromised patients may be infected with a wider range of organisms the advice of a medical microbiologist should be sought prior to starting treatment.

Common causes of cellulitis

- *Staphylococcus aureus*
- Group A streptococcus
- Groups C and G streptococci (rarely)
- anaerobes and *Pasteurella multocida* (after bite injuries).

The most useful investigation is blood culture, though this is only helpful if collected before starting antibiotics. Swabs of any wounds may reveal the infecting organism; it is also worth swabbing between the toes in cellulitis of the lower limb, as even very mild athlete's foot can lead to Group A streptococcal infection. Attempts to isolate the causal organism by aspiration from the advancing edge are painful and rarely helpful, though this may be worth attempting if an unusual organism is suspected. Group A streptococcal infection in culture-negative cases may be confirmed by testing paired sera for anti-streptolysin O and anti-DNAase B. This is useful in recurrent cases, as continuous prophylaxis with oral penicillin can be helpful. Anti-staphylococcal antibody testing is insensitive and not widely used.

Treatment of cellulitis

Under-dosing in severe cellulitis is common; adults with normal renal function should be given 2 g of flucloxacillin 6-hourly. This is because antibiotic levels in the infected tissue will only be a fraction of blood levels. Elevation of the affected limb and adequate analgesia are essential. Treatment of penicillin-allergic patients is complex, and a vague history of penicillin allergy should always be verified with the patient's general practitioner before committing the patient to suboptimal therapy. Erythromycin is poorly absorbed orally, and causes phlebitis when given intravenously. Oral clindamycin is well absorbed and very effective, but associated with pseudomembranous colitis, particularly in the elderly. First-generation cephalosporins such as cephradine have good activity against common causes of cellulitis, but may also cause colitis and have a small risk of cross-allergy with penicillin. In severe cases, an intravenous glycopeptide such as vancomycin or newer agents such as linezolid or daptomycin may be required.

Response to antibiotics in severe cellulitis is slow, and incomplete response 3–4 days into treatment is not an indication to change treatment. Marking the margin of erythema early on provides an objective assessment of response.

Necrotizing fasciitis

This is a rapidly progressive, necrotizing infection of subcutaneous tissue and fascia. It encompasses a wide spectrum of infections, including Fournier's and Meleney's gangrene, though these subdivisions are of little practical importance. It is divided into two types by the causal organisms.

Type I is a mixed infection, with anaerobes, enterobacteriaceae and other organisms. It occurs in patients immunocompromised by age, diabetes or renal failure, and may rarely complicate abdominal and pelvic surgery in otherwise healthy patients. The affected area is extremely tender; the margin of erythema is diffuse. It progresses rapidly and subcutaneous necrosis extends beneath normal skin. This may lead to thrombosis of small blood vessels with ischaemic necrosis and anaesthesia of skin outside the area of erythema. Patients are markedly systemically toxic, and in the early stages this will appear out of proportion to the severity of the skin lesions. Thrombocytopenia or leucopenia may be a clue to the diagnosis. The mortality is high, up to 43% if diagnosis is delayed. Immediate surgical debridement to healthy tissue is essential. It often has to be repeated after 24 hours. Urgent microscopy and culture of debrided tissue should be performed, though the mixed infection means that full culture results may not be available for some days. Broad-spectrum antibiotics are used; a widely used combination is meropenem and clindamycin intravenously until culture results are available. Hyperbaric oxygen therapy and intravenous immunoglobulin have been used as adjunctive therapy; there is no compelling evidence for benefit from these treatments.

Type II fasciitis involves Group A beta-haemolytic streptococci, usually alone, occasionally in combination with other organisms. It may affect patients with underlying medical conditions, but can also cause a devastatingly rapid infection in young, previously fit people. Clusters of infection have been described, but these have been found to involve different strains of streptococci, and there is no evidence that hypervirulent strains cause outbreaks of this infection. The clinical features are similar to type I fasciitis, though it often affects the limbs, head or neck. Bullae are common but not diagnostic. Once again the mainstay of therapy is complete surgical debridement. Group A streptococci are invariably highly susceptible to benzyl penicillin, which should be given in combination with clindamycin. Clindamycin is believed to reduce the production of exotoxins by Group A streptococci and is more active than penicillin where organisms are multiplying most rapidly, i.e. at the advancing edge of the lesion.

Gangrene

More accurately described as clostridial myonecrosis, this condition occurs when clostridial spores germinate in ischaemic or traumatized muscle. *C. perfringens* is the commonest cause, particularly after limb trauma. *C. novyi* can cause a similar problem after intramuscular injection of heroin, and *C. septicum* can cause local infection arising from colonic cancers or diverticulitis.

The cardinal symptom is severe pain and tenderness, associated with marked systemic toxicity. Gas in the soft tissues can be seen on plain X-rays, and may be palpable. The infection is rapidly progressive and fatal unless the infected tissue is urgently debrided. Antibiotics are used as for necrotizing fasciitis, but are of secondary importance to aggressive surgery. The appearance and odour of infected tissue is diagnostic, but as mixed infection may occur samples should always be sent urgently for microscopy and culture.

Intra-abdominal sepsis

The only intra-abdominal infection which can always be managed with antibiotics alone is primary peritonitis. This occurs in patients with ascites, and is diagnosed by finding a polymorph count greater than 500/microlitre in ascitic fluid, and positive culture from ascites or blood. Co-amoxiclav is a suitable treatment unless the patient has received previous antibiotics which may have altered the gut flora.

Other infections, such as diverticulitis or postoperative abscesses, may respond to antibiotics alone, but only if they are diagnosed early, are unusually small, and if there are significant risks associated with drainage. They are usually mixed, and penetration of antibiotics is slow and incomplete. Some antibiotics such as gentamicin are inactivated at the pH found in pus, others such as glycopeptides are large molecules and diffusion across tissue planes is poor. The bowel flora found in community-acquired abscesses is likely to be susceptible to simple antibiotics such as co-amoxiclav; however, microbiological advice should be taken in patients who have had multiple operations and antibiotics, where multi-resistant Gram-negatives and candida infection are common.

Tetanus

Vaccine coverage for tetanus in the UK is universal, and consequently this infection is extremely rare, with fewer than 10 confirmed cases each year. Most occur in the elderly or in unvaccinated immigrants. It occurs when spores of *Clostridium tetani* become implanted deep into a wound where conditions are anaerobic. A powerful exotoxin is produced which causes muscle spasm, initially apparent at the site of the injury and in the facial muscles, but also involving the back, neck, abdomen and extremities. Autonomic dysfunction also occurs and is the leading cause of death. Most cases occur within 2 weeks of the injury, but some have occurred after several months. The diagnosis is clinical, and can occasionally be confirmed by inoculation of immune and non-immune mice with serum collected from the patient early in their illness, but this is insensitive and a negative result does not exclude the diagnosis.

Treatment of tetanus

- Debridement of the wound
- Intramuscular tetanus immunoglobulin
- Intravenous metronidazole
- Benzodiazepines
- Ventilatory support.

Adequate surgical debridement of the wound site is essential to prevent further systemic diffusion of the toxin. There may be no local signs at the site of the injury so an accurate collateral history is essential. Remarkably, the amount of toxin required to produce life-threatening symptoms is insufficient to produce immunity, and vaccination after recovery is necessary. Immunization in the UK was introduced in 1961 (1938 for members of the armed forces) and consists of three doses of adsorbed tetanus vaccine 1 month apart, starting at 2 months of age. Booster doses are given at school entry and before leaving school. Further booster doses are unnecessary and may cause local reactions. Tetanus-prone wounds include puncture wounds, wounds or burns left unattended for over 6 hours, and wounds with dead tissue, evidence of sepsis or soil contamination. A dose of human tetanus immunoglobulin is recommended if the risk of infection is particularly high or if the patient may be unimmunized.

Further reading

Mandell GL, Bennett JE, Dolin R. *Principles and Practice of Infectious Diseases.* 7th edn. Churchill Livingstone, 2010.

Török E, Moran E, Cooke F. *Oxford Handbook of Infectious Diseases and Microbiology.* 1st edn. Oxford University Press, 2009.

Chapter

4

Fundamentals of radiology

Arvind Pallan

Key learning objectives

Describe basic principles of plain X-ray, fluoroscopy, computed tomography (CT), magnetic resonance imaging (MRI), nuclear medicine including PET and ultrasound (USS) as used in diagnostic imaging.

Describe the basic principles of image guided biopsy and interventional radiology techniques.

Highlight the potential risks and hazards related to diagnostic imaging techniques.

Plain film radiography

Wilhelm Conrad Röntgen first discovered X-rays in November 1895, with his work earning the 1901 Nobel Prize in Physics. Initial photographic images, using the newly discovered rays, quickly demonstrated potential for medical application, especially in the localization of foreign bodies and diagnosis of fractures. Plain radiographs are still regularly used in initial assessment of patients, especially after trauma and for the acute abdomen.

In order to obtain a plain radiograph, the area of interest is positioned between a beam of electromagnetic radiation and a radiosensitive detector. The radiation is produced by the interaction between high-energy electrons produced by a heated tungsten cathode with a tungsten anode. The energy of the photons in this radiation beam lies within the X-ray spectrum of energy. The patient's tissue interacts with the photons, either absorbing or scattering (deflecting) them. The degree and type of interaction depends on the thickness, density and atomic density of the matter as well as the energy of photons in the beam with the net effect of attenuating the beam, i.e. reducing beam intensity.

The attenuation of the radiation beam is a sum of the attenuation by the various anatomical structures the radiation must traverse between source and detector. Passage through dense or high average atomic number tissues, e.g. bone will diminish the amount of radiation reaching the detector. Structures which cause less beam attenuation will allow greater detector exposure (Figure 4.1). The greatest distinction between tissues is obtained when there is significant difference in their attenuation characteristics, e.g. between soft tissue and pneumatized lung (attenuation similar to air) or between soft tissue and calcified bone. Tissues of similar attenuation characteristic, e.g. soft tissue structures will cause only minimal variation in detector exposure by transmitted radiation. Any observed differences in the image would be subtle. The ability of plain film radiographs to resolve between similar tissues is therefore limited (poor contrast resolution). The ability of plain films to resolve small objects of a given density is good (good spatial resolution).

The traditional detector used in radiography has been a cassette containing a phosphor screen to absorb X-ray radiation and then emit visible light photons. These in turn are trapped by photosensitive film which is then chemically developed to generate an image for review. Film-screen combinations are now being replaced by computed radiography (CR) and digital radiography (DR) technologies allowing a digital output, more rapid image generation and a reduction in the use of processing chemicals and other consumables.

Portable X-ray machines allow images to be acquired outside the imaging department, enabling the imaging of the unstable patient. Mammography equipment is designed to optimize contrast and spatial resolution to allow the differentiation between soft tissue densities and visualize microcalcification.

Fundamentals of Surgical Practice, Third Edition, ed. Andrew N. Kingsnorth and Douglas M. Bowley.
Published by Cambridge University Press. © Cambridge University Press 2011.

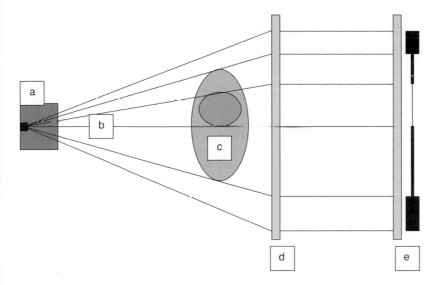

Figure 4.1 Process of plain radiography. A radiation source (a) emits a diverging X-ray beam. This beam is orientated towards the imaging subject (b). The beam is attenuated within the subject dependent upon the atomic number and density of tissue through which it passes (c). The beam exposes a radiosensitive detector (d). Variation in the radiation intensity reaching the detector are revealed when the detector is read or processed (e).

Fluoroscopy

Fluoroscopy is the practice of using dynamic and moving radiographic images to perform a diagnostic investigation or guide an interventional procedure. Fluoroscopy requires the ability to view a real-time image, precluding the use of film-screen combinations. The equipment generating the radiation beam must be reliable and capable of continuous function without overheating. Until the 1960s the image was formed on a fluorescent phosphor-coated screen by the transmitted radiation beam. The images obtained were limited by very low brightness, requiring the radiologist's eyes to become fully acclimatized prior to the study by spending 10–20 minutes in complete darkness.

Electronic amplification by image intensifiers subsequently allowed brighter, more useful images to be generated. By using an image intensifier and video camera system or more recently a digital flat plate detector, real-time images can be electronically displayed and captured. Portable image intensifiers are commonly used to guide orthopaedic surgeries especially involving bone fixation or joint replacement.

Contrast agents in fluoroscopy

Contrast agents are high density materials which can easily be differentiated from soft disuse densities on radiography. They are further described later. Contrast agents are utilised in many fluoroscopic examinations to demonstrate the surface contours of a hollow lumen which would not otherwise be differentiated from the soft tissue density of surrounding structures. Single contrast techniques use a contrast agent to opacify an anatomical structure and therefore demonstrate its contours. Double contrast techniques first require a dense contrast agent to coat mucosal surfaces with a second radiolucent agent then used to fill and distend the lumen. Double contrast techniques allow much improved demonstration of surfaces to enable the identification of mural lesions.

The majority of gastrointestinal tract fluoroscopy examinations utilise barium sulphate suspensions with either single or double contrast techniques. Water-soluble contrast agents are used if there is risk of underlying mural perforation as barium leakage can cause peritonitis or mediastinitis. If there is a possibility of pulmonary contrast aspiration, ionic water-soluble contrast agents, e.g. sodium amidotrizoate and meglumine amidotrizoate (gastrografin, Bayer), must not be used due to risk of pneumonitis. A non-ionic water-soluble contrast agent, e.g. iopamidol (gastromiro, Bracco), must be used in this situation.

Gastrointestinal tract fluoroscopy

The accuracy of barium swallow and meal examinations is less than oesophago-gastroscopy but they retain a role in the assessment of patients who decline endoscopy. High-frame-rate imaging of the oropharynx (videofluoroscopy) allows assessment of the swallowing mechanism. Dynamic information regarding oesophageal motility can provide an alternative or complement to oesophageal manometry. Contrast

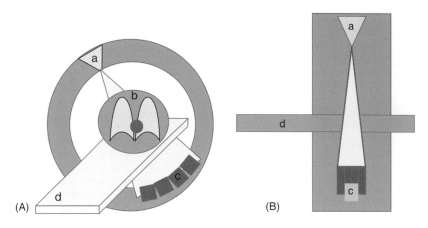

Figure 4.2 Process of CT scanning (A) Frontal diagram of CT scanner: The radiation source (a) generates a fan shaped beam of radiation which is attenuated by the image subject (b) prior to reaching the array of detectors (c). The image subject is resting upon the mobile table (d). (B) Lateral diagram of CT scanner. The beam of radiation originating at the radiation source (a) is detected by four rows of detectors, allowing the generation of four image slices with each rotation of the gantry about the table (d).

swallow studies may demonstrate subtle strictures or pouches not seen at endoscopy.

The small bowel may be imaged when filled with contrast. If the contrast enters the small bowel following oral administration, the study is termed an enterography, small bowel meal or follow-through. Direct injection into the jejunum via a nasojejunal catheter is termed small bowel enteroclysis or small bowel enema. This allows optimal distension of the small bowel with greater accuracy in the detection of stricture, mucosal lesion or obstruction. Double contrast enteroclysis uses high density barium to coat the bowel wall followed by low density material, e.g. methylcellulose solution or even carbon dioxide gas to distend the bowel and optimize mucosal demonstration.

Double contrast barium enema allows good evaluation of the colonic mucosa though its accuracy, especially for subcentimetre lesions, is lower. These studies require formal bowel cleansing to remove faecal material. Unprepared barium enemas may be used to document the extent of active colitis but are now infrequently performed, with cross-sectional imaging or colonoscopy preferred. In single contrast studies the ability to identify small mural lesions is limited but obstructing bowel lesions can be confirmed and localized. Water-soluble contrast studies are used to confirm surgical anastomotic integrity. Water-soluble enema can be useful to allow the planning of colonic stent placement.

Urinary tract fluoroscopy

Retrograde opacification of the urinary tract with water soluble contrast via a urethral catheter allows the identification of mucosal disruption following surgery or trauma. Vesicoureteric reflux and urethral stricture may be demonstrated with some adaptation of technique. Antegrade opacification of the renal tract via a nephrostomy catheter may be undertaken to define the level of renal tract obstruction.

Other fluoroscopy

Further commonly performed fluoroscopy investigations include hysterosalpingography, used primarily to assess tubal patency in the investigation of infertility; herniography, used in the assessment of clinically occult or uncertain hernia and arthrography, used to identify deficiencies in specific joint capsule components.

Computed tomography

Computed tomography [CT] was developed in the 1970s, with the first clinical CT scanner installations in 1974. The 1979 Nobel Prize was shared between Allan Cormack of Tufts University, Massachusetts, USA, and Geoffrey Hounsfield of EMI laboratories, London, UK, for their pioneering work in the field. Whilst the first generation of scanners was limited to producing grainy images of the brain, modern scanners can produce detailed, three-dimensional images of the whole body in only a few seconds.

The major components of a CT scanner are the table, gantry and the image-processing computer. The scanner table is built within the open bore of a circular gantry. This contains a source of ionizing radiation fixed opposite to a curvilinear sector array of detectors (Figure 4.2A). The patient lies upon the table, which can be moved to allow the region of interest to be placed between source and detectors. Ionizing radiation in the form of a tightly focused, fan-shaped, high-energy X-ray beam is generated, which passes through the patient and table to the detectors. In the same manner as plain film radiographs, the degree of beam attenuation depends upon the density and atomic number of tissues between the source and detector. The radiation source and detectors rotate about the patient generating data from multiple projections. These data are analysed (reconstructed) by the image processing computer to calculate the degree of attenuation caused by individual structures between source and detector.

The number of images, known as slices, that can be acquired with a single rotation of the gantry is dependent upon the arrangement of the detector array (Figure 4.2B). If detectors are arranged four rows deep in the long axis of the table a single rotation of the gantry components will allow the generation of four slices. Detector banks capable of acquiring up to 320 slices at each rotation are currently commercially available. The thickness or width of each slice can be altered by summating information from adjacent detector rows. For example, if an array consisted of four 1 mm thick rows of detectors it could produce either four 1 mm thick slices, two 2 mm thick slices or one 4 mm thick slice with each rotation.

If the table remains static only, the volume of the patient between source and detector array will be imaged. If the table is moved between rotations, a series of slices would be built up, which would allow the coverage of a larger anatomical region. In modern scanners the table is moved smoothly through a continuously spinning gantry. The radiation beam therefore passes in a helix through the patient, accumulating a volume of data. This process is termed a helical or spiral scan.

The values calculated by the image processing computer are transformed onto a linear scale of radiodensity. This is known as the Hounsfield Scale and has two fixed points: pure water, which has a density value of 0, and room air, which has density value of −1000. This linear scale facilitates image display via a grey scale. Each image is a mosaic of two-dimensional picture elements (pixels) within a matrix. As the image slice has a depth corresponding to the slice width, each pixel represents an average radiodensity of all the tissue contained in the corresponding three-dimensional volume element (voxel). The human eye can differentiate a finite number of shades on a grey scale so these shades must be distributed to facilitate useful assessment of the image. Pixels with greater densities are conventionally displayed as lighter shades of grey. In order to allow assessment of a specific tissue type, the grey scale is spread between the range of radiodensities most relevant in the assessment. This spread is defined by its centre point (window level) and the range between maximum and minimum grey scale Hounsfield unit values (window width). The distributions (windows) used can be altered at any stage during the image viewing process to allow assessment of each tissue type. (Figure 4.3).

Following a helical scan, a volume of contiguous data is obtained and it is possible to manipulate this data to create an image in any orthogonal or non-orthogonal plane that is required (multiplanar reconstruction). Selective display of the highest or lowest densities within a volume or density interfaces allows the generation of maximum or minimum intensity projections and surface rendering which are used in advanced imaging display techniques, e.g. angiography and colonography.

CT techniques

Non-enhanced CT

CT without the use of contrast agents is often termed non-enhanced CT (NECT). In many circumstances there are sufficient inherent radiodensity differences to allow a clinically useful assessment of the image to be made, e.g. brain imaging for infarction or haemorrhage, assessment of the pulmonary parenchyma and renal tract assessment for calculi. NECT may also have a role as part of a multiphase study to document appearances before the use of contrast agents and quantify subsequent change, e.g. in adrenal lesion characterization. NECT enables the identification of hyperdensity as can be seen in hepatic cirrhotic nodules or following haemorrhage. NECT can be used as an alternative to contrast enhanced study when factors such as patient choice, allergy to contrast media or renal dysfunction, prevent contrast administration (see later section on contrast media specific risks). In this situation it may still be possible to make limited assessment of structures which are associated with inherent radiodensity differences, e.g. surrounded by fat such as retroperitoneal lymph nodes. The assessment of otherwise relatively homogenous structures such as the upper abdominal solid viscera will become significantly impaired.

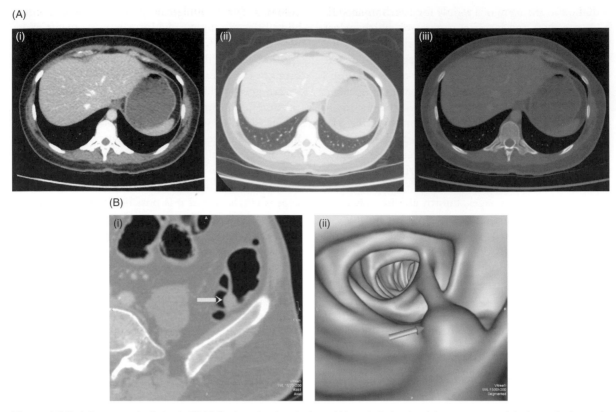

Figure 4.3 Basic image manipulation in CT. (A) By changing the window width and window level the appearance of the image is changed. The image below is optimised to demonstrate (i) the soft tissues, (ii) the lung parenchyma and (iii) the bony skeleton. This process is termed 'windowing'. (B) A colonic polyp (arrowed) as demonstrated on (i) original axial and (ii) virtual colonoscopy surface rendered images.

Contrast-enhanced CT

Many CT studies utilize contrast agents to increase the amount of useful information obtained in the study. Contrast agents are commonly administered intravenously or orally. Contast-enhanced CT (CECT) usually relates to the use of an intravenous contrast agent.

The timing of a CT scan after an intravenous contrast agent injection is optimized to maximize the useful changes which will be seen in the image. If the scan is performed soon after injection and the majority of contrast remains in the arterial lumen, the scan can be described as an arterial phase study. If the scan is timed later, the images will reflect the redistribution and eventually the excretion of the contrast agent. Most routine CT scans of the abdomen and pelvis are timed for optimal enhancement of the hepatic parenchyma, known as the portal venous phase. To answer some clinical questions, a region may require scanning more than once following contrast agent injection, e.g. in the characterization of liver lesions. As each additional scan acquisition within an examination will entail an additional radiation dose, their added value must be carefully considered before scanning. The types, uses and hazards of contrast agents are further described later in this chapter.

CT angiography

To assess vascular patency and anatomy, an acquisition in the arterial phase (5–40 seconds post-injection dependent upon the clinical question) is common. Arterial phase scans can also provide valuable information regarding organs which maximally enhance more rapidly than the liver, e.g. the pancreas or small bowel. They may also be valuable in the assessment of focal lesions (e.g. hypervascular liver metastasis, hepatocellular carcinoma and neuroendocrine tumours).

CT colonography and enterography

By distending the lumen of hollow viscera, their walls can be assessed well.

CT colonography is a widely used technique with high sensitivity and specificity for colonic polyps. Most patient preparation regimes require formal bowel preparation with its accompanying risks and inconveniences to the patient. Faecal tagging can be used as an adjunct or alternative to formal bowel preparation. High density oral contrast agents are administered prior to the study, often over a few days. The density of residual faecal material at the time of the scan is therefore increased which allows easy identification and potentially electronic subtraction by imaging software. Good bowel distension achieved with either room air or carbon dioxide insufflation via a rectal catheter is vital. The administration of a smooth muscle relaxant, either glucagon or hyoscine butylbromide (Buscopan, Boehringer Ingelheim), is useful. The patient is imaged in the prone and supine positions to facilitate the redistribution of gas and retained faecal matter. Images are viewed both as multiplanar reconstructions and surface-rendered volumes of the colonic lumen to optimally demonstrate any mural abnormality.

In a similar manner, distending the small bowel lumen allows assessment of the small bowel wall. The distending agent is commonly a high osmolality solution, e.g. mannitol, polyethylene glycol or locust bean gum, to prevent absorption. Distension can be promoted by high-volume oral intake (CT enterography) or by direct injection into the small bowel following passage of a nasojejunal tube (CT enteroclysis).

CT urography

A scan acquisition can be timed to image contrast excreted into and filling the pelvicalyceal systems, ureters and bladder. This will allow the demonstration of filling defects, e.g. calculi, urothelial lesions and tumours. A CT urogram examination will usually also contain a non-contrasted scan to allow the identification of renal tract calcification and a scan at maximal renal cortical enhancement (nephrographic phase).

Magnetic resonance imaging

Building upon the development of nuclear magnetic resonance in the 1940s, for which Edward Mills Purcell of Harvard University, Massachusetts, USA, and Felix Bloch of Stanford University, California, USA, were awarded the Nobel Prize in Physics in 1952, Paul C. Lauterbur of New York, USA, and Sir Peter Mansfield of Nottingham, UK, developed and refined the technology so that it could be used for imaging the human body. They in turn were awarded the Nobel Prize in Medicine in 2003.

The major components of an MRI scanner are a magnet, electromagnetic (gradient and shim) coils, radiofrequency coils and the image reconstruction hardware.

The spinning, charged, unpaired proton of each hydrogen nucleus produces its own magnetic field called a moment. This magnetic pole spins or precesses around an axis, much like the rotation of a child's spinning top about a vertical axis. The speed of precession depends upon the strength of the background magnetic field. Usually moment has a random orientation but when placed in a strong, homogeneous external magnetic field they are aligned along the axis of the external field. The number aligned parallel to the external field is slightly in excess of the number aligned opposite, or antiparallel, to the external field, creating a small net magnetization force or vector. The size of this vector is determined by the external field strength.

A precise radiofrequency pulse applied by the scanner radiofrequency coils can transiently realign the net magnetic vector. This vector will then decay back to its resting state (relaxation), influenced by the macromolecular environment of the proton and releasing electromagnetic radiation which can be detected by radiofrequency coils. Two types of relaxation occur, T1 and T2, each of which will vary by tissue type.

Minor precise local fluctuations in the magnetic field are managed by the gradient coils. Controlling these fluctuations allows the spatial origin of the emitted radiofrequency signal to be established. The information received can therefore be reconstructed into an image. It is the rapid switching of electrical coils in the high-strength magnetic field which causes vibrations, manifesting as the loud noises associated with MRI scanning with most MRI scanners.

The signal intensity received varies with the relative density of protons in the tissue as well as the local macromolecular environment. By varying the intensity, sequencing and timing of radiofrequency pulses applied by the scanner the signal can be further altered to maximize the difference between tissue types. Each of these permutations of user-defined imaging parameters is termed a sequence. Many sequences are known by an acronym, often specific to an MRI scanner manufacturer. A T1 weighted sequence maximises the effect of tissue T1 relaxation characteristics on the image. Tissues such as fat and melanin appear bright or hyperintense on these images with water appearing dark or hypointense. Similarly a T2 weighted sequence maximizes the effect of T2 relaxation upon the image, with fluid appearing bright.

The majority of MRI examinations, including most musculoskeletal and neuroaxis imaging studies, do not require any addition of contrast media. This is due to the high inherent difference in relaxation characteristics between tissues, i.e. their high inherent contrast.

MRI techniques

Contrast-enhanced MRI

Intravenous contrast agents are used to increase the difference in relaxation characteristics between tissue types, most commonly to enable lesion localization. Regions of blood–brain barrier breakdown will allow the local retention of contrast agents to highlight intracranial lesions. Contrast agent use allows the differentiation between recurrent intervertebral disc herniation and postoperative fibrosis. The dynamic use of contrast agents allows lesion assessment in a manner similar to contrast-enhanced CT studies. MRI contrast agents are discussed in more detail later in the chapter.

Magnetic resonance cholangiopancreatography (MRCP)

By using highly T2 weighted, fluid-sensitive imaging sequences, images of the biliary tree can be generated to give an endoscopic retrograde cholangiopancreatography (ERCP)-like image. Hepatobiliary ductal anatomy can therefore be assessed without the risks associated with ERCP examinations. The presence of calculi can be identified as filling defect within the otherwise homogenous intraductal bile.

MRI urography

Similar fluid-sensitive sequences of the renal tracts generate intravenous urogram equivalent images without the need for contrast administration.

MR angiography

Advances in manufacturer-specific imaging technology allow high-resolution MR angiography over significant lengths of the body or even angiography without contrast agent injection.

MR arthography

The injection of contrast agent into a joint allows imaging its related soft tissue structures, e.g. joint capsule and labrum.

Dynamic MRI

By repeatedly acquiring identically orientated sequences the effect of movement upon a lesion or anatomic site can be assessed. If useful, a 'stop motion' effect movie can be generated. There are many potential applications including the characterization of dynamic musculoskeletal impingement in joints or the spine, characterizing small bowel stricture or visualising the pelvic floor. MR defaecography is an accurate and holistic tool for identifying pelvic floor pathology. The rectum can be filled during the study to facilitate imaging of a defaecatory effort.

Nuclear medicine

The decay of unstable radioisotopes generates radiation and ionizing particles. Whilst radioisotopes have been used in therapy since the 1930s, the technology to enable imaging of radioisotope distribution developed in the 1950s with the first scintillation camera invented in 1958 by Hal Anger of the University of California. Radioisotopes can be combined with ligands to form radiopharmaceuticals for administration to patients. Dependent upon the in vivo redistribution of the radiopharmaceutical specific physiological processes can be imaged.

The most commonly used radioisotope in nuclear medicine imaging is technetium 99m, which decays with a half-life of 6 hours with the release of gamma radiation. Dependent upon the ligand used, the distribution of radioisotope will vary. In this way myocardial perfusion, renal function or regions of increased skeletal osteoblastic activity may be assessed. The gamma radiation produced by radioactive decay travels in random directions from its point of origin. It is consequently difficult to generate images of high spatial resolution despite the use of collimators and images generated in more than one projection.

By using technologies to systematically move the detector system around the patient, a higher-resolution single photon computed tomography (SPECT) study can be obtained. Positron emission tomography (PET) studies detect the formation of high-energy gamma photons following positron emission decay of certain radioisotopes, most commonly fluorine-18. This isotope is usually administered as a glucose analogue, fluodeoxyglucose (FDG), which is actively imported into metabolically active cells but not metabolized, leading to further accumulation in these tissues. Images are generated with high spatial resolution and often fused to CT or MRI images obtained during the same examination to allow anatomical localization of the FDG uptake and image optimization.

Ultrasound

Ultrasound is defined as sound waves beyond the audible range, taken to be above 20 000 hertz. Inspired by military sonar technologies, diagnostic ultrasound was developed in the 1940s and 1950s with practical applications in a clinical setting described by Professor Ian Donald of Glasgow in 1958.

In the ultrasound transducer, vibrating piezoelectric crystals generate sound waves. The speed of sound wave transmission in vivo varies will vary according to the type of tissue it is passing through. The speed of sound, in combination with the tissue density allows the calculation of the tissue acoustic impedance. When sound waves reach an interface with tissue of different acoustic impedance they can be reflected or refracted in a similar way to light waves. The reflected waves returning to the transducer are detected by the piezoelectric crystal. The time taken for sound to return from deep interfaces is greater than from superficial interfaces, allowing the calculation of the interface depth from the transducer. Due to ultrasound absorption, signal returning from deeper structures is also generally reduced in amplitude. An image is built up by allocating pixel intensity values dependent upon the calculated position and intensity of the reflection.

A coupling agent is needed to exclude air between the transducer and skin surface which would otherwise cause reflection of the sound waves and prevent useful image generation. Similarly there is essentially complete reflection of ultrasound from interfaces with high acoustic impedance materials, e.g. gas or dense calcification in bony cortex or calculi. These interfaces are brighter or hyperechogenic on the ultrasound image. Little ultrasound penetrates beyond the interface, with a reduction in echoes from deeper interfaces resulting in the phenomenon of distal acoustic shadowing. There are no acoustic interfaces in fluid-filled structures such as simple cysts, which will therefore appear anechoic. Increased ultrasound wave transmission through anechoic structures will increase the amplitude of signal returning from distal structures, resulting in the phenomenon of distal acoustic enhancement.

Ultrasound is a highly operator-dependent modality with sound technique and persistence required

to maximize the information obtained. It is common practice to archive representative images from the examination to demonstrate findings rather than recording the entire examination. It must be recognized that the absence of abnormality on these images may potentially only reflect a lack of recognized or visualized abnormality rather than guarantee the absence of significant pathology. It can be impossible to accurately orientate the plane and position of images acquired if recognizable anatomical landmarks are absent.

In abdominal imaging, the majority of imaging is performed with curvilinear arrays of crystals which together generate a sector-shaped image. The ultrasound frequency used is often between 2 and 5 MHz, with lower frequencies enabling greater penetration through tissues and imaging at greater depths from the skin surface. These advantages must be balanced with a reduction in the spatial resolution of the image. High-frequency linear arrays are capable of high resolution imaging but are limited to the imaging of superficial soft tissue structures.

Ultrasound is commonly used in the assessment of soft tissues, particularly within the neck, abdomen and pelvis. Small bowel ultrasound enables the diagnosis and follow up of Crohn's disease without radiation exposure. Musculoskeletal ultrasound utilizes high frequency probes to demonstrate soft tissue abnormality. Intraoperative ultrasound allows high-frequency probes to be used in identifying focal lesions and organ vasculature, most commonly in hepatic surgery.

In order to generate clinically useful information, the ultrasound waves must be able to penetrate the relevant anatomical structure. If sound transmission is prevented by intervening highly reflective interfaces such as gas within the lungs or bowel, the deeper structures will not be visualized. Ultrasound studies can therefore be limited unless a viable route, or acoustic window, for the ultrasound waves is found. The volume of adipose tissue that must be traversed will also tend to impact negatively upon image quality.

As images are generated in real time, ultrasound is a valuable tool in guiding percutaneous intervention, as will be discussed later in this chapter.

Doppler ultrasound

When sound waves are reflected from a moving structure there is a consequent change in the wavelength and frequency of the sound waves returning to the transducer. The difference between the transmitted and received frequencies, termed the Doppler shift, can be used to calculate the velocity of the moving interface. If ultrasound is reflected by intravascular erythrocytes the Doppler shift is essentially dependent upon blood flow velocity. This can be depicted graphically as a spectral analysis or as coloured pixels in a colour Doppler image. Whilst colour Doppler allows rapid assessment of vascular flow it does not allow the accurate quantification of velocity that is obtained with spectral analysis.

In a normal vessel flow is laminar. If the vessel lumen becomes progressively stenotic, the laminar flow pattern is lost with turbulence becoming increasingly apparent. The volume of blood flowing through a stenosis is constant until the stenosis is severe (90%). In order to compensate for a reduction in cross-sectional area the flow velocity increases. Techniques for estimating the degree of stenosis in the carotid artery most commonly use the measured peak systolic velocity in the internal carotid artery to categorize the stenosis, though end diastolic velocities and the peak systolic internal carotid artery : common carotid artery velocity ratio may also be utilized.

Doppler vascular assessment is integral to the investigation of arterial stenosis, notably in the carotid arteries and peripheral arteries. Ultrasound assessment of varicose vein anatomy, venous occlusions and suspected deep venous thrombus is common.

Endoscopic and endovascular ultrasound

Advances in probe technology and image processing serve to improve image quality. Endoscopic ultrasound (EUS) has developed since the 1980s, allowing high-frequency, high-resolution probes to be placed close to structures of interest. Diagnostic probes generally have a circular array producing a 360° radial image. Therapeutic echoendoscopes have a therapeutic channel and most commonly a linear array to allow fine needle aspiration or core biopsy.

Endobronchial probes allow access to the bronchi and much of the mediastinum. Gastro-oesophageal EUS allows assessment of the mediastinum, oesophagus, stomach, retroperitoneum and hepatopancreatobiliary system, and is now part of the standard staging pathway of oesophageal malignancy. Endoanal EUS allows high resolution assessment of the rectal wall with the ability to accurately assess the depth of tumour invasion in malignancy. Intravascular probes

can be used to generate high-resolution images of vascular plaque and to assess stent stenosis.

Contrast-enhanced ultrasound

Contrast-enhanced ultrasound allows high temporal resolution continual imaging of the solid viscera, especially the liver, in a manner similar to dynamic contrast enhanced CT or MRI studies. Other described indications include the differentiation of high-grade carotid stenosis from occlusion and the investigation of vesicoureteric reflux. The utility of contrast-enhanced studies is affected by the same factors of body habitus and anatomy as conventional ultrasound. If baseline ultrasound is limited in its quality due to patient factors, it is likely that any attempt at contrast-enhanced studies will be similarly degraded.

Interventional radiology

Interventional techniques have developed rapidly since percutaneous vascular catheterization was first described by Sven-Ivar Seldinger of the Karolinska Institute, Stockholm, in 1953. Prior to this, angiography had predominantly relied on vascular access following cut-down procedures and the use of rigid needles. The Seldinger technique involves vascular puncture with a hollow needle. Through this needle a flexible guidewire is passed to secure vascular access, and the needle is removed. A flexible catheter can then be passed over the guidewire into the vessel and the guidewire removed. The catheter can then be used and will allow injection or aspiration. The Seldinger technique remains the cornerstone of interventional access, having been translated throughout vascular and nonvascular procedures. The development of fluoroscopy greatly facilitated catheter manipulation and placement.

Analgesia with adequate local anaesthetic is mandatory. Sedation may be required to facilitate cooperation, especially for lengthy or painful procedures.

Angiography

Intravenous contrast agents are is used to allow visualization of the vessel lumen. The majority of interventions utilize iodinated contrast media as will be described later in this chapter. Carbon dioxide is an alternative intravascular contrast agent which is less commonly used but avoids the risks associated with iodinated contrast media.

The added density of intravascular contrast agents may be difficult to define accurately when included in an image with the bony skeleton and soft tissue densities. Subtraction techniques were therefore developed. Here at least two images are obtained; the first a mask image prior to the injection of contrast and a subsequent image following intravascular injection to demonstrate the opacified vessel. Prior to digital imaging technologies the mask would be photographically subtracted from the post-injection images to leave only the image of the intravascular contrast. Modern digital subtraction angiography (DSA) allows high-resolution, real-time demonstration of the subtracted angiographic study.

Catheters and guidewires

The catheters used in vascular intervention are varied in their material and shape. Non-selective catheters, e.g. straight or pigtail shaped catheters, are used to inject contrast into large blood vessels. Selective catheters facilitate cannulation of branch vessels by holding complex three-dimensional forms that more easily engage with specific branches of the aorta. For example sidewinder and headhunter catheters are used for the cannulation of visceral and aortic arch vessels respectively.

There is similar variation in the guidewires available. Non-steerable guidewires are used for intravascular manipulation but not crossing luminal strictures. The guidewire tips are varied in the shape that they adopt. Steerable guidewires are often covered in hydrophilic material to reduce intravascular resistance in stenoses. Guidewires are available in several lengths to enable catheter exchanges. Different guidewire stiffnesses will allow the negotiation of tortuous vessels or provide support for the introduction of other larger catheters.

Vascular access techniques

The most common vascular access is retrograde common femoral artery puncture, which allows easy access to the iliac arteries and abdominal aorta. The ideal puncture is below the inguinal ligament at the site of maximal femoral pulsation, as the vessel passes over the medial femoral head. This reflects the optimal site to secure post-procedure haemostasis by direct pressure. A puncture of the superficial femoral artery is at higher risk of causing arteriovenous fistula or false aneurysm complication.

Antegrade femoral puncture will allow access to the ipsilateral superficial femoral and more distal arteries. Access via the upper limb (axillary, brachial or radial arteries) generally allows easier post-procedure puncture site monitoring and quicker patient mobilization but the size of catheters which can be used is limited. The intraluminal distance from percutaneous access point to the site of any intervention may be a factor in selecting the most suitable access site, with longer distances limited by the available equipment and also by the limited ability to manipulate catheters accurately the longer they become.

Angioplasty

Angioplasty is used to increase the luminal diameter of a stenosis. An ovoid balloon-tipped catheter is passed through the stenosis over a guidewire. Angioplasty balloons are available in several lengths, profiles and calibres to cater for the different locations, lengths and severity of stenoses. To minimize local complications the fully inflated balloon diameter should not exceed the diameter of the adjacent normal vessel lumen. Typical balloon diameters used are 10–15 mm, 7 mm and 4 mm in the aorta, external iliac artery and popliteal artery, respectively.

Inflating the balloon within a stenotic diseased segment causes a series of splits in concentric plaque which may extend into the intima and media with stretching of the adventitia. The plaque itself is not flattened or reduced in volume; the increase in the cross-sectional diameter of the lumen is caused by the adventitial stretch. Angioplasty of eccentric plaques causes stretch of the normal vessel wall. In either case, the damaged intima subsequently remodels to re-form a smooth surface. Less than 30% residual stenosis is desirable on post-angioplasty images.

Endovascular stents

Vascular stents are either placed following unsuccessful angioplasty (secondary stenting) or as a primary therapeutic manoeuvre if there is high risk of distal embolization or failure due to vessel wall recoil or re-stenosis. Each stent is a metal framework delivered to the stenosis in a tightly collapsed state over a catheter. The desired calibre of an expanded stent is generally 1–2 mm greater than the post-angioplasty vessel diameter to ensure friction between wall and the stent and prevent stent migration. The stent may either require expansion by a balloon catheter or be self-expanding, in which case it is actively held in the collapsed state by a sheath or membrane on the delivery catheter. When this mechanism is withdrawn the stent will spontaneously expand.

Covered stent grafts exclude the vessel wall and allow the treatment of aneurysm, most commonly of the aorta, and may have a role in the management of acute arterial perforation or dissection.

Venous Intervention

Venous intervention follows similar principles to arterial intervention. Venous angioplasty is widely used in the treatment of renal dialysis fistula or graft stenosis. The superficial position of these vessels enables ultrasound-guided angioplasty as an alternative to fluoroscopically guided procedures, particularly in patients with contraindication to intravenous contrast media injection. Venous angioplasty and stenting is also used in central venous stenosis.

Inferior vena cava filters are mesh-like devices, which are placed in the infrarenal inferior vena cava and are an option in the management of thromboembolic disease. Absolute indications for filter placement include the presence of pulmonary embolus or deep venous thrombus with inability to maintain adequate anticoagulation, recurrent thromboembolic disease despite anticoagulation, complications of anticoagulation or contraindication of anticoagulation.

Embolotherapy

Embolotherapy is used to reduce blood flow and tissue perfusion. This may be in order to stop bleeding, especially from the gastrointestinal tract or following trauma; as a therapeutic intervention, e.g. treatment of intracranial aneurysm or varicocele; or as an adjunct to surgery or radiofrequency ablation. To prevent unintended, non-target embolization the vascular anatomy must be well examined and a catheter placed within the vessels supplying the target. The embolic agents selected for use will depend upon the access obtained, size of vessels involved and degree of permanence required from the intervention. Metal coils are used to occlude large–medium vessels. Smaller target vessels can be occluded permanently by injection with polyvinyl alcohol particles or temporarily by the injection of gelatine sponge pledgets (Gelfoam, Pfizer). Where the target for embolization has dual vascular supply, e.g. the gastroduodenal artery, each must be embolized.

Complications of vascular intervention

The complications of vascular intervention can be divided into immediate and delayed. These may be related to the puncture site or the site of the intervention.

At the puncture site, haemorrhage, haematoma, vessel thrombosis or formation of false aneurysm or arteriovenous fistula may occur. At the intervention site, dissection, vessel occlusion or rupture can occur. The rates of complication will vary with the severity of disease treated, the site of intervention, type of intervention and experience of the operator. Delayed complications include the sequelae of distal embolization of atherosclerotic plaque fragments and complications involved with the use of intravenous contrast. The latter will be further described later in this chapter.

Image guided biopsy and drainage

Percutaneous procedures require the ability to accurately visualize and therefore manipulate biopsy or drainage equipment. The most widely used techniques are using ultrasound or CT guidance although fluoroscopy and MRI can also be used.

In ultrasound guided techniques a safe access route is identified to minimize trauma and complications. The transducer is then placed to allow the simultaneous visualization of the target, access path and the access needle itself. Whilst keeping these findings on the image the access needle is advanced to the target. The use of needle guides can make the process easier but the majority of procedures are performed without this aid, using a freehand technique.

If CT is used the process of finding a safe access route is replicated, but limited to the plane of slice acquisition. Unless the gantry is tilted, this is therefore the transaxial plane. To avoid unnecessary irradiation the access needle is moved in a stepwise manner with a repeat localised scan after each adjustment. CT fluoroscopy allows rapid scan acquisition to speed this process. Real time imaging is also possible but is likely to increase the radiation dose to the operator.

There is no such restriction to the scan plane with MRI guided intervention and cine type dynamic imaging can potentially once again be used. An 'open' magnet MRI scanner is needed to allow access to the patient whilst scanning. The equipment used will clearly need to be compatible and safe for use in the high field MRI environment.

The use of fluoroscopy has declined with the increased utilization of other guidance techniques. Unless the radiation beam, target, access needle and skin puncture site are aligned it can be difficult to orientate needle manipulation in terms of tip depth.

Percutaneous biopsy

Percutaneous imaging-guided biopsy (core biopsy or fine needle aspiration) is indicated when histological, cytological or occasionally microbiological assessment of tissue will further patient management. Due to the risk of tumour seeding (the incidence of which is estimated at approximately 3% in hepatocellular carcinoma) confirmatory liver biopsies should be avoided in resectable focal hepatic lesions, e.g. colorectal carcinoma metastasis or hepatocellular carcinomas. If there is any doubt, a discussion with local hepatobiliary surgical teams will prevent the potentially adverse consequences of biopsy. Similarly the biopsy of focal bone lesions, which may require subsequent limb-sparing surgery, should be performed by appropriately trained individuals, as unnecessary contamination of additional compartments could preclude effective surgery in the future.

Percutaneous drainage

Image-guided percutaneous placement of drainage catheters is undertaken for many indications. Infected fluid collections and abscesses may be drained as a definitive therapeutic measure or to temporize until definitive surgical management. The anatomical location of the collection will determine the approach taken and modality of image guidance. Drainage catheters are available in a range of sizes and designs.

Whilst clear fluid will usually drain through a 6F catheter, thick pus may require a 12F catheter with larger catheter lumens needed if the collection contains debris. The majority of drainage catheters have an integrated mechanism of coiling the distal end into a pigtail shape to prevent accidental removal. The technique for forming and releasing the pigtail is dependent upon the catheter used. The catheter must be able to uncoil in order to be removed safely. A Seldinger technique is most commonly used to introduce the drainage catheter over a guidewire following serial soft tissue dilatation. A single-stage 'single-stab' technique utilizing a sharp central stylet may be used as an alternative, especially in large superficial collections.

An initial aspirate should be sent for microscopy and culture. Post-insertion catheter care must be meticulous, with regular flushing of the catheter with sterile saline (especially if the fluid drain is thick or contains debris to prevent blockage). Catheter removal must be considered when drain volumes reduce (e.g. to not more than 10 ml/24 h). The collection may need reimaging to ensure complete resolution prior to catheter removal. If drainage ceases prematurely a kink in the external drainage tubing should be excluded first. Gentle flushing of the drain may clear debris. If neither manoeuvre restarts drainage the catheter position must be checked, with repositioning or replacement if necessary. If the drain catheter is in a satisfactory position but does not flush, a blockage could be cleared by the gentle use of a guidewire, but if this is not successful the drain may need to be removed or replaced. In this circumstance discussion with the relevant radiologist is strongly recommended.

In percutaneous nephrostomy and percutaneous transhepatic biliary drainage, catheters are introduced into obstructed renal pelvicalyceal or hepatic biliary systems to improve renal or hepatic function. Catheter injection with contrast media generates nephrostogram or cholangiogram images, potentially identifying the site and cause of obstruction. After passing a guidewire through the obstruction, internal ureteric or biliary drainage catheters provide a more physiological drainage channel for the previously obstructed system. Long-term internal drainage of inoperable malignant biliary obstruction may require metal stent placement in a similar manner to obstructing vascular disease. Removal of the external drainage catheter can only be considered when there is satisfactory internal drainage and no further percutaneous intervention is planned. Re-access of pelvicalyceal or biliary systems is significantly more difficult when they are not distended.

Percutaneous ablation

Localised cytotoxic therapies rely upon the precise local delivery of heat, cold or microwave energy to initiate cell death. The most commonly used of these is considered to be radiofrequency ablation (RFA). This involves intense, cytotoxic heating generated by alternating electrical current passing between the electrodes of specifically designed probes. Having had its origins in cardiology electrophysiology intervention, radiofrequency ablation is now utilized in bone, lung, liver and renal tumours either as an adjunct to surgical management or as definitive treatment. The indications for radiofrequency ablation continue to grow. Non-tumour indications include the treatment of varicose veins and Barrett's oesophagus.

Stent placement

Oesophageal and colonic stenting can be performed under colonoscopy, fluoroscopy or combined guidance to manage obstructing lesions.

Complications of non vascular intervention

Complications of non-vascular intervention can be divided into the immediate and delayed, local and distant in the same manner as vascular intervention. Immediate complications include haemorrhage, haematoma, arteriovenous fistula formation and target organ damage. Hepatic intervention has specific risks of haemobilia and bile leak, renal intervention has risks of haematuria and clot retention.

The post-procedure care required will depend upon the intervention performed. A period of observation and bed rest is needed following any vascular or organ puncture.

Contrast agents

Contrast agents are compounds administered to improve visualization of structures in an image or study, i.e. increase the difference, or contrast, between regions of the image. A positive contrast agent increases the 'brightness' within a study. Similarly a negative contrast agent causes a reduction in brightness.

In investigations which utilize ionizing radiation, contrast agents contain materials of different atomic number or density from the region being examined. Positive contrast agents contain barium or iodine, which are more effective in attenuating the radiation beam than soft tissue. Negative contrast agents are of low density, e.g. water or gas, which are less attenuating to the radiation beam than soft tissue.

In MR studies the behaviour of contrast agents is more complicated, dependent upon the particular agent and imaging sequence used. Positive MRI contrast agents contain gadolinium (which speeds up T1 relaxation following the imaging radiofrequency pulse), which can be visualized as an increase in signal on T1 weighted images. The MRI characteristics of water allow its use as a positive contrast agent in T2 weighted imaging sequences. When water is used, to distend the bowel certain additives, e.g. polyethylene glycol, mannitol or locust bean gum, can be added to increase its osmotic pressure and prevent rapid absorption. Negative MR contrast agents, e.g. iron or barium, cause inhomogeneity of the local magnetic field which manifests as a reduction in signal on T2 weighted sequences.

Intraluminal contrast agents

Intraluminal contrast agents used in fluoroscopy contain barium or iodine, both of which are effective in attenuating medical ionizing radiation. Cross sectional modalities may similarly utilize luminal contrast agents to allow the clear identification of anatomical structures such as the large or small bowel.

Intravenous contrast agents in CT and MRI

The iodinated contrast agents used in CT and the gadolinium-based agents used in MRI are most commonly intravascular, extracellular agents which rapidly enter the extravascular, extracellular space and then are passively excreted via glomerular filtration. This process generates the phenomenon of vascular and visceral enhancement, organ enhancement characteristics being dependent upon the vascular anatomy of the organ.

Phases of enhancement

Due to the hepatic dual vascular supply both arterial and portal venous blood contribute to enhancement as seen in Figure 4.4. Other organs, e.g. the kidneys, small bowel and spleen, have a uniphasic enhancement pattern with each requiring a different time post contrast injection for optimal appearances. Due to the relative importance of hepatic appearances a typical contrast enhanced abdominal study is acquired in the hepatic portal phase, approximately 70 seconds following the start of injection. To enable more reproducible enhancement between patients bolus tracking software will allow image acquisition to be triggered a pre determined interval following the intravascular arrival of contrast.

Hepatocyte-specific contrast agents

Gadobenate (Gd-BOPTA, Multihance, Bracco) and gadoxetic acid (Gd-EOB DTPA, Primovist, Schering) and gadolinium-based agents have significant

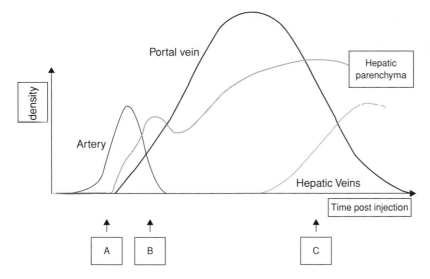

Figure 4.4 Graph representing changes in hepatic radiodensity following intravenous injection of contrast agent. Intravenous contrast agent reaches the liver initially reaches the liver via the aorta and hepatic artery. A larger volume of contrast then reaches the liver via the portal vein. At time A imaging would demonstrate hepatic artery enhancement with very little parenchymal enhancement (early arterial phase). At time B arterial and early parenchymal enhancement would be demonstrated (late arterial phase). At time C contrast via the portal vein has perfused the hepatocytes with subsequent filling of the hepatic veins (hepatic portal phase) with optimal enhancement of the normal hepatic parenchyma.

hepatocyte uptake and biliary excretion. Mangafodipir trisodium (Mn-DPDP, Teslascan, GE-Amersham) is taken up by tissue with an active aerobic metabolism. In the liver the manganese is bound to intracellular molecules before biliary excretion. These agents demonstrate further differences between normal and abnormal hepatic parenchyma, facilitating lesion uptake and characterization.

Reticulo-endothelial system contrast agents

Super paramagnetic iron oxide (SPIO) agents are cleared from plasma by Kupfer cells. This causes a focal disruption of the magnetic field with loss of MR tissue signal only in regions of the liver containing Kupfer cells. The only SPIO currently commercially available in the UK is ferumoxide (Endorem, Guebert), with ferucarbotran (Resovist, Bayer) recently withdrawn by the manufacturer.

Ultrasmall super paramagnetic iron oxide (USPIO)

These agents are cleared by peripheral phagocytes and progressively accumulate in peripheral lymph nodes where they cause local magnetic field disruption. Whilst showing promise in differentiating benign from pathological lymph nodes in trials no SPIO agent is currently commercially available.

Ultrasound contrast agents

Contrast agents for use in ultrasound initially consisted of agitated saline used in echocardiography. Modern agents are formed of microbubbles with a gaseous core and hydrophobic shell. These are small enough to pass through the microcirculation (1–10 mm diameter). Due to resonant properties when exposed to diagnostic ultrasound waves they significantly increase the signal returned to the probe. By imaging a lesion continuously following intravenous injection real-time dynamic changes in echogenicity are demonstrated dependent upon lesion vascularity, similar to the effects of intravenous contrast during multiphase CT or MRI examinations but without the need to preselect specific times for image acquisition.

The agents are safe in renal dysfunction, permitting lesion detection and characterization when contrast enhanced CT and MRI are contraindicated.

Managing imaging related risks

An examination is useful only if the result influences patient care. Unfortunately a significant number of investigations performed are not of use, leading to unnecessary use of resources and potentially unnecessary ionizing radiation exposure. Before requesting an investigation it is important to consider whether it is going to influence patient management (Table 4.1). Resources including local departmental IRMER proceedures and the Making the best use of clinical radiology services (MBUR) referral guideline document published by the Royal College of Radiologists provide information on optimal referral practice and the radiation associated with imaging studies to facilitate the appropriate us of imaging services.

Table 4.1 Important considerations when requesting imaging studies

1. Is there previous imaging which will provide the necessary information?

This is especially important when caring for patients who are acutely admitted to the hospital. There may be relevant imaging performed in the emergency department, during a previous health care episode or by a different healthcare provider. If the report of previous imaging does not answer the current clinical question it is often beneficial to review those images before requesting a similar study.

2. Is this investigation going to change clinical management of the patient?

Whilst it may be valid to image in order to reinforce a clinical impression it is not valid to image 'because it would be nice or interesting to know'.

If it is clinically unlikely that imaging will demonstrate a relevant abnormality or if the presence of abnormality is clinically irrelevant imaging is not required.

If sufficient information is available from other investigations will further studies add anything to the patient's care?

3. Is this the best investigation to answer the clinical question?

In addition to the permutations of modality and technique the timing of the investigation in the natural history of disease should be appropriate.

4. Is the request providing enough relevant information?

By providing pertinent clinical information and posing specific questions the relevance of the report generated can be maximized. Risks to the patient can be minimized if information regarding previous adverse events and contraindications to modality or contrast are provided.

Table 4.2 Relative radiation dose involved in common imaging investigations

Procedure	Typical effective dose (mSv)	Equivalent number of chest X-rays	Approximate equivalent period of natural background radiation
Chest radiograph	0.02	1	3 days
Abdomen radiograph	0.7	35	4 months
Barium swallow	1.5	75	8 months
Barium enema	7.2	360	3.2 years
CT head	2	100	10 months
CT chest	8	400	3.6 years
CT abdomen or pelvis	10	500	4.5 years
Tc-99m bone scan	4	200	1.8

The risks involved in imaging studies can be grouped into radiation-specific, modality-specific, contrast-agent-related and logistical risks.

Radiation protection

It is the net benefit of the information gained over the associated risks that justifies the exposure to ionizing radiation. Ionizing radiation is used in plain film, fluoroscopy, nuclear medicine and CT examinations.

The Ionizing Radiation (Medical Exposure) Regulations (IR(ME)R) 2000 (GB Parliament 2000) control medical radiation exposure in the UK. These regulations require any individual requesting imaging involving ionizing radiation to have undergone suitable training including the risks of radiation exposure. To minimize radiation exposure each request for imaging must be assessed and justified by an IRMER practitioner to ensure that the benefit of the investigation far exceeds the risk of the radiation involved. Sufficient information to assess and justify the request must be provided to the IRMER practitioner by the requestor. If justified the exposure must be optimized to ensure

that the radiation dose is as low as reasonably achievable (the ALARA principle) when the operator undertakes the investigation. Every imaging investigation must be interpreted and a written opinion documented in the patient's notes. The imaging protocols and techniques used must be optimized and kept under review. Unnecessary repeat imaging must be prevented.

Radiation from medical imaging sources is estimated to have increased its contribution to average annual radiation dose by 10% between 1999 and 2005. Typical radiation doses for a variety of investigations are shown in Table 4.2. A 10 mSv radiation dose (e.g. CT scan abdomen) carries an estimated excess cancer mortality of 1:2000. Children are more susceptible to the effects of radiation, with estimated lifetime cancer mortality risks attributable to the radiation exposure from a CT scan in a 1-year-old being 0.18% (abdominal) and 0.07% (head). Public awareness of radiation risks is growing, particularly in the USA. Ultrasound and MRI provide options to image even acutely unwell patients without ionizing radiation.

Females in whom pregnancy cannot be excluded are specifically identified in the IR(ME)R 2000, which identifies specific responsibilities related to them. Related advice on the protection of pregnant females was published in 2009 by the Health Protection Agency, UK. In the majority of diagnostic procedures, fetal radiation exposure will not be significant enough to cause intrauterine death, growth retardation, malformation or impairment of mental development. The additional risk of childhood cancer following such exposure is below 1 in 10 000 (which is low compared to the natural incidence of approximately 1 in 500). In higher-dose examinations the added risk is usually below 1 in 1000 and certainly below 1 in 200. High-dose examinations, e.g. CT of the pelvis, are considered to double the risk of childhood cancer when the fetus is exposed in the first 3 or 4 weeks of pregnancy.

In order to minimise the potential irradiation of pregnant females all imaging centres must have protocols and procedures in place. In any female undergoing a nuclear medicine investigation or an investigation involving direct irradiation of the pelvis with the radiation beam (i.e. irradiation between diaphragm and knees) pregnancy status should be indicated on the imaging request and rechecked at the time of imaging. If pregnancy cannot be excluded, the patient must be asked whether her menstrual period is overdue. Further management then falls into one of four groups.

(a) If there is no possibility of pregnancy the imaging can carry on as planned subject to the usual justifications.
(b) If the patient is definitely pregnant the investigation can still be undertaken provided that the benefit to the mother and/or fetus exceeds the risks involved.
(c) If pregnancy cannot be excluded but the patient's menstrual period is not overdue the imaging may proceed.
(d) If pregnancy cannot be excluded, the patient's menstrual period is overdue and the planned investigation would generate a low fetal dose the patient must be regarded as probably pregnant as above. In the case of high-dose examinations, due to the potential doubling of childhood cancer risk, consideration of deferring the examination until the first 10 days of the next menstrual cycle is needed. Alternatively arrangements could be made to ensure all high-dose imaging of the female is booked within the first 10 days of the menstrual cycle, but clearly this may have logistical implications. Investigations should only be deferred if it is safe to do so. Discussion between the referring clinician and radiologist is likely to be needed in these cases.

MR-specific risks

MR scanning is contraindicated if there is an intraocular metallic foreign body, a ferromagnetic haemostasis clip in the central nervous system or an implanted device which could be compromised by exposure to either the high-strength magnetic field or radiofrequency pulses required during scanning. Databases of device-MR compatibility are available. Missile effects of ferromagnetic objects brought into the scanner's magnetic field have been well documented as a cause of adverse events.

MRI examinations should only be undertaken in pregnancy if the benefit exceeds the risks, and avoided in the first trimester. Discussion with the radiology department is needed on these occasions.

Contrast-specific risks

Contrast reaction

Following the administration of intravenous nonionic iodinated contrast the incidence of severe contrast reactions is 0.04%, with very severe reactions in 0.004%. Individuals at increased risk of reaction should be identified at the time of imaging request, e.g. those with a history of previous contrast reaction, unstable asthma, allergy requiring medical treatment, untreated hyperthyroidism and interleukin-2 treatment.

Contrast-induced nephropathy

Contrast-induced nephropathy (CIN) is defined by the European Society of Urogenital Radiology (ESUR) as a condition in which an impairment in renal function (an increase in serum creatinine by more than 25% or 44 mol/l (0.5 mg/dl)) occurs within 3 days of the intravascular administration of iodinated contrast medium in the absence of an alternative aetiology.

Contrast-induced nephropathy is associated with an excess in morbidity and mortality. The management of CIN is largely preventative. High-risk groups can be identified by identifying a combination of risk factors (Table 4.3). For these high-risk groups the volume of contrast media administered must be reduced – optimally by utilizing an alternative imaging modality or un-contrasted examination to answer the clinical question. Effective pre- and post-contrast hydration is the most important method of limiting contrast-induced nephropathy. The patient's drug history must be examined with nephrotoxic medications identified

Table 4.3 Risk factors for contrast-induced nephropathy

- Pre-existing renal failure
- Old age
- Diabetes mellitus
- Congestive heart failure
- Concurrent administration of nephrotoxic medication, e.g. non-steroidal anti-inflammatory drugs
- Volume of contrast material administered

and reviewed. Many institutions have local guidelines/protocols which should be consulted.

Metformin

Impairment to renal function can lead to reduced clearance of metformin and consequent accumulation with theoretical risk of lactic acidosis. Guidelines published by the Royal College of Radiologists in 2009 state that if the patient's renal function is normal and the volume of intravenous contrast administered is small (not more than 100 ml) metformin does not need to be discontinued. If the volume of intravenous contrast is more than 100 ml or intra-arterial contrast is used, metformin should be withheld for 48 h from the time of the injection and then can be restarted. If there is renal dysfunction the requirement to use iodinated contrast media should be reviewed and if needed metformin should be withheld for 48 h and restarted after renal function is rechecked and confirmed as unchanged.

Nephrogenic systemic fibrosis

An association between nephrogenic systemic fibrosis and gadolinium-containing MRI intravascular contrast media was first made in 2006. Risk of this rare, potentially fatal condition appears limited to individuals with severe renal impairment and those who have had or are awaiting a liver transplant who have been exposed to an intravascular gadolinium containing contrast agent, gagodiamide (Omniscan, GE healthcare). Children up to 1 year of age could theoretically also be at risk as they have immature renal systems.

Logistical risks

The acutely ill must continue to be resuscitated during cross-sectional imaging with interruptions to active resuscitation potentially reducing the relative benefit of the examination. In MRI scanning, compatible equipment including gas cylinders, ventilators and clamps must be used.

Summary

The permutation of imaging modality, contrast media usage and scanning parameters should be optimized in every case to maximize the benefit of the imaging study whilst ensuring the given radiation dose is as low as reasonably possible and the patient is not exposed to any other unnecessary risk.

The imaging request must therefore include the relevant information to allow the best test to be undertaken and optimal interpretation of the images. Both the requesting clinician and the radiology department must be prepared to enter discussions to determine the most appropriate imaging option.

Risk factors for contrast media reaction should be disclosed at the time of the imaging request rather than at the time of scanning to allow elective management. Similarly, risk factors for contrast-induced nephropathy or nephrogenic systemic fibrosis need to be managed prior to the patient reaching the department.

Further reading

Athanasoulis CA. Vascular radiology: looking into the past to learn about the future. *Radiology* 2001;**218**(2): 317–322.

European Society of Urogenital Radiology. ESUR guidelines on contrast media. Available from http://www.esur.org/Contrast-media.51.0.html

Garden OJ, Rees M, Poston GJ *et al.* Guidelines for resection of colorectal cancer liver metastases. *Gut.* 2006; **55**(Suppl 3): iii1–iii8.

Gillams A. Tumour ablation: current role in the kidney, lung and bone. *Cancer Imaging.* 2009;**9** Spec No A:S68–70.

HPA, RCR and CoR (2009). *Protection of Pregnant Patients during Diagnostic Medical Exposures to Ionising Radiation.* Chilton. HPA

Kessel D, Robertson I. *Interventional Radiology: A Survival Guide.* London, Churchill Livingstone 2010.

Liu PT, Valadez SD, Chivers FS *et al.* Anatomically based guidelines for core needle biopsy of bone tumors: implications for limb-sparing surgery. *RadioGraphics* 2007;**27**;189–205.

Rosch J, Keller FS, Kaufman JA. The birth, early years, and future of interventional radiology. *J Vasc Interv Radiol* 2003;**14**:841–853.

Royal College of Radiologists (2007). *Making the Best Use of Clinical Radiology Services* (MBUR), 6th edition: London.

Zealley IA, Chakraverty S. The role of interventional radiology in trauma. *BMJ.* 2010;**340**:c497.

Surgical techniques and technology

Michael A. Scott and Mark G. Coleman

Skin preparation

Traditional skin preparation involved fastidious cleansing with preoperative bathing, shaving of the surgical area and, particularly for orthopaedic operations, cleaning of the skin with antiseptic solutions and covering with sterile bandages. Some of these practices have been abandoned, largely due to the fact that patients are now often admitted on the morning of their planned day for surgery; however, those for which good supportive evidence exists form the basis for best practice today.

Preoperative bathing in antimicrobial solutions lowers skin colonization and reduces wound infection rates particularly when combined with not shaving the surgical site. Evidence suggests that routine surgical shaving may actually increase the incidence of wound infections by producing microscopic skin abrasions at the surgical site. Hair removal should therefore be limited to the immediate surgical site and be performed either with depilatory agents or by clipping, as close to the time of surgery as possible.

Immediately prior to any procedure the skin is cleaned with an antiseptic solution, commonly either povidone iodine or chlorhexidine. A small number of patients are allergic to these solutions and therefore careful attention to known hypersensitivities is essential. Testing on a remote area of skin 24 h beforehand will exclude any resulting hyperaemia; however, this is often difficult to achieve in practice and therefore in any patient in whom there is clinical suspicion of hypersensitivity 10% alcohol on its own can be used. There have been a number of reports of explosions and burns to patients caused by the use of diathermy in the presence of alcohol, therefore it is mandatory to ensure that the alcohol has evaporated from all areas of the skin prior to the use of electrical devices.

The skin is cleansed using a sterile swab soaked in antiseptic solution. It is important to clean the centre of the surgical field and extend outwards in ever-widening circles to prevent recontamination of the field by a swab that has touched the skin at the periphery. Self-adhesive sterile skin towels are then applied to isolate the surgical field. These are water-resistant and are increasingly disposable. A sterile plastic adhesive dressing is often applied to cover the whole area, reducing the amount of exposed skin, thus lowering the risk of potential contamination.

Local anaesthesia

(For more details refer to Chapter 1 for dosage and toxicity.)

The required equipment and knowledge to carry out resuscitation must be available. Adrenaline solution 1 in 1000 should also be to hand. Except for the most trivial procedure, an adequately trained assistant should be present. The volume of local anaesthetic agent used, and any reactions to it, must be recorded. Local anaesthesia may be combined with premedication drugs such as midazolam or temazepam. However, they may mask the side-effects of local anaesthetics and should be used sparingly, especially in day case surgery, so that the patient can achieve early full recovery.

Topical

Lignocaine 4% and prilocaine 4% are effective when applied to mucous membranes within the mouth, urethra, conjunctival sac and also in wounds.

Local infiltration

Lignocaine 0.5–2% is often used but it is also effective in more dilute solution. The effect is prolonged if

Fundamentals of Surgical Practice, Third Edition, ed. Andrew N. Kingsnorth and Douglas M. Bowley.
Published by CAMBRIDGE UNIVERSITY PRESS. © Cambridge University Press 2011.

it is given in adrenaline solution, up to 1 in 200 000, which causes vasoconstriction and also reduces bleeding. No more than 3 mg/kg body weight should be used, except when given with adrenaline, in which case up to 7 mg/kg body weight may be given. However, adrenaline must be avoided if the local blood supply is prejudiced. Lignocaine anaesthesia lasts up to 90 min. This may be extended by adding 0.25% bupivacaine to 0.5% lignocaine. If the operation site is painful or tender, a bleb is first raised in normal skin a short distance away, such as 1 cm. The needle is inserted and anaesthetic gently injected as the tender area is approached. The local anaesthetic spreads ahead of the needle. Initially the solution is infiltrated superficially to produce a wheal along the line of the proposed incision. If the exposure is deepened, infiltration is taken progressively deeper to create a field block. The injection is given slowly to avoid pain caused by hydrostatic pressure. Each time the needle is in a new area, aspiration is performed to guard against intravenous injection. It is often wise to inject deeper progressively as the operation proceeds, rather than attempt a complete field block at the beginning. Local infiltration of anaesthetic agent is commonly used to enable the manipulation of fractures. Perhaps the commonest such use is for setting a recently acquired Colles' fracture of the wrist. The level of the fractured radius is identified and infiltration of the fracture haematoma with 10–15 ml of plain 1% lignocaine can begin. After 10 min, the fracture may be reduced. The amount of anaesthetic agent used should be checked constantly to ensure the maximum amount has not been exceeded. The patient should be asked to report pain or untoward symptoms and signs of cerebral toxicity such as drowsiness and slurred speech, and myocardial depression, such as slowing or irregularity of the pulse, should be closely monitored.

Sufficient time (5–10 min for lignocaine and up to 20 min for bupivacaine) should be allowed for the anaesthetic to act before starting the operation. It should be explained to the patient that touch sensation remains after pain sensation has been abolished, but discomfort or pain should be reported as soon as it is felt. Additional anaesthetic should be retained to use if there is discomfort.

Nerve blocks

These reduce the amount of local anaesthetic that needs to be used and they can sometimes be injected at

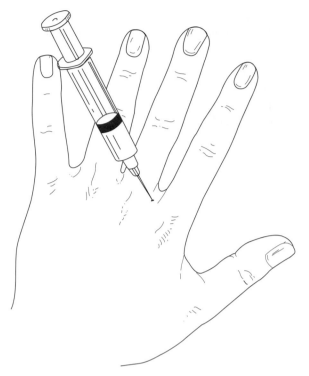

Figure 5.1 Blocking digital nerves in the web space to avoid raising tissue tension.

a distance from the operation site. Digital nerve block can be injected from the dorsal surface of the fingers and toes. There is a risk of ischaemia if the circumferential tension is raised by injecting a large volume or from digital artery spasm if adrenaline is added and as such, adrenaline must never be used. The nerves in the web space are blocked so the tension does not rise (Figure 5.1). As an extra precaution an ampoule of hyalase, the spreading enzyme, may be added to the local anaesthetic; this reduces the volume of fluid needed to achieve anaesthesia and encourages the fluid to spread and be reabsorbed quickly. The two dorsal nerves are injected first, on either side of the first phalanx; the injection is then deepened from the dorsum to catch the palmar branch on either side.

The pain of a fractured rib can be alleviated for several hours by injecting 1–2 ml 0.25% bupivacaine posteriorly beneath the affected rib to block the intercostal nerve. Aspiration is carried out before injecting it to avoid intravascular injection.

When carrying out certain operations, nerve block can be combined with field block. A common example is in repair of inguinal hernia under local anaesthesia. Field block is augmented by infiltrating around the ilioinguinal and iliohypogastric nerves as they lie between internal and external oblique muscles about 2 cm medial to the anterior superior iliac spine.

Intravenous regional anaesthesia

This is also known as Bier's block and is valuable for producing anaesthesia in a limb. The limb is exsanguinated using an Esmarch bandage or rubber roller sleeve, or simply elevated. A proximal tourniquet is then inflated to higher than systolic pressure to isolate the blood vessels of the distal limb. Dilute local anaesthetic is injected through a previously placed intravenous cannula and perfuses the venous system, producing anaesthesia. This should not be attempted without special training and appropriate equipment and assistance.

Regional nerve block

This entails injecting local anaesthetics proximally into the nerves supplying a region or a limb. It requires specialized knowledge of anatomy, the technique and the dangers involved.

Incisions and their closure

Incisions

These may be made for procedures on the skin or through the skin to reach deeper structures. They require careful planning and placement. Whenever possible, incisions should be made along tension lines, not across them. The tension lines on the face can be identified by getting the patient to smile or grimace. Critical incisions may be marked with ink before incision.

For most incisions a scalpel with a large blade is used and the belly of the knife is drawn along in a smooth line, cutting at right angles to the skin surface. For very small and crucial incisions, it may be better to use a small-bladed scalpel held like a pen. Skin is elastic and the drag of the knife distorts it. To avoid this, the skin is fixed with the non-dominant hand and the edges slightly separated as the knife cuts through (Figure 5.2).

The depth of cut is as important as the line. A fold of skin can be picked up to estimate its thickness. When making the incision, the correct depth should be reached as soon as possible and cutting then continued at that depth. One of the crucial surgical skills

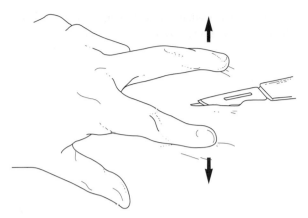

Figure 5.2 Steadying the tissue when making an incision and separating the edges with the fingers of one hand.

is the knowledge of tissues and tissue planes. The plane that has been reached must be carefully identified.

Bleeding is encountered as the incision is made and can be reduced or abolished in several ways:

- for very fine surgery of the extremities, the blood may be drained and a tourniquet applied
- the skin and subcutaneous tissues can be infiltrated with a weak (e.g. 1 in 250 000) solution of adrenaline, which produces vascular constriction
- simple pressure on the cut edges for a few minutes usually controls small vessel bleeding.

Neurosurgeons traditionally apply the tips of fine haemostatic forceps to the dermis and evert the edges to slightly compress them and control bleeding. Haemostatic forceps can be applied to individual vessels which may be sealed by compression, by twisting or by ligature. Cutting diathermy is becoming increasingly popular for making skin incisions. Avoid using coagulation diathermy near the skin surface for fear of causing burns that heal slowly and leave ugly scars. Bleeding from small vessels can also be avoided by using a laser beam to cut through the skin; the depth of cut determines the choice of laser.

Deep exposures

To approach deep regions, intermediate structures must be divided or displaced. There are standardized approaches to various parts of the thorax, abdomen and pelvis, joints, bones, nerves, blood vessels, the central nervous system and special sense organs. There are well-documented anatomical anomalies that should be remembered as well as the pathological processes that can distort the normal anatomy.

Closure

Healing will take place and produce the best scar if the wound edges, retaining a good blood supply, are apposed accurately, without tension or trauma, in the absence of infection, and with the minimum foreign material present.

Healing cannot take place if the blood supply is deficient. Ischaemic edges must be cut back until bleeding is seen at the cut edges and the colour appears normal. As in many circumstances in surgery, good and absent blood supply make decisions easy. It is in the 'grey areas' between these extremes that difficulty arises. In case of doubt it is usually best to leave the wound open until the viability of the edges is clear; if they then appear healthy, delayed primary suture is appropriate. If the blood supply is poor, the skin edges can be cut back until they appear healthy and the defect closed with a flap or skin graft.

Traumatized or crushed skin may show little evidence of non-viability at the time of repair but will subsequently die and scar. Rough handling and grasping the skin with dissecting forceps will add to the trauma; rather the closed blades of the forceps should be used to move the skin and exert counterpressure, or use skin hooks. Suture material mounted in eyeless needles should be used.

Tension not only pulls the wound edges apart but also aggravates any deficiency of the blood supply. In wounds that are oedematous, closure should be deferred until the oedema has resolved. If the blood supply is good, the tension can be spread by undermining the edges in the subcutaneous tissue, or by forming a flap that can be swung in. Very occasionally after undermining, a relieving incision can be made so that the defect is transferred to a more convenient area – in some instances the relieving incision may further prejudice the blood supply of the skin which has already been undermined. Sometimes skin tension can be reduced by drawing together the deeper layers of the wound.

Infection or heavy contamination is inimical to good wound healing. It is much safer to leave the wound open and wait until the tissues are clean and healthy before closing it. Local antiseptics and antibiotics are usually of less benefit than exposure. In some circumstances, appropriate systemic antibiotics may

be indicated. Foreign material causes tissue reaction that retards healing and the material may harbour, or form a suitable nidus for, infecting organisms. In this context dead tissue is foreign material. For this reason, when dealing with wounds, every particle of dead or foreign material must be removed, by gentle exploration. Foreign material in the form of sutures should be kept to a minimum.

When closing a simple, straight incision made along tension lines, apposition is easy but for more complex closures, the progression should be planned carefully. If the edges are not of similar length, the extra length of one edge should be evenly distributed along the whole length of the wound. This can usually be achieved by inserting stitches across the middle of the wound, then halving this and continuing until the wound is closed (Figure 5.3).

Perfect apposition implies the edges are united across the gap so that the living layers are brought together. Overlapping brings together dissimilar layers. Inversion of skin apposes dead, keratinized layers. The method of uniting the edges influences the perfection with which they are apposed.

Stitches

Stitches vary in type and size, and in the distance from the edges and from each other, depending upon the circumstances. For closing the skin of large abdominal wounds, they may be 2/0 nylon or polypropylene, placed 5 mm apart, up to 5 mm from the wound edges. In cosmetically important areas they may be 4–6/0 nylon or polypropylene, placed 2–3 mm from the edge and 2–3 mm apart. The thread is usually mounted in a half circle cutting edge, eyeless needle, held in a needle holder. Each stitch must cross the wound exactly at right angles and emerge at the same distance from the edge as it entered on the opposite side. It should be tied with a reef knot, and an extra half hitch added to form a reef knot with the second hitch. The first hitch should be tightened just sufficiently to appose the edges, the second just to secure it, and the third tightly, otherwise the first hitch will be overtightened, with consequent ischaemia. The ends should be cut short so they do not interfere with subsequent stitches. Stitches may be interrupted or continuous. Each type has advantages and disadvantages; the use of one or the other is a matter of personal choice.

If the skin edges tend to invert, they can be everted using mattress sutures. These are double stitches that may cross the wound parallel to each other (horizontal

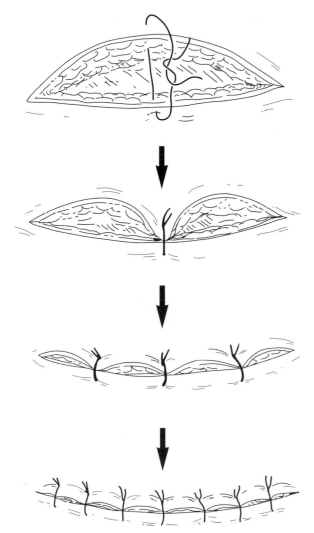

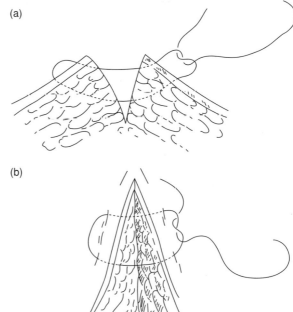

Figure 5.4 Everting mattress sutures. (a) Vertical section through a longitudinal mattress suture. (b) View of a longitudinal mattress suture.

Figure 5.3 Accommodating disparity in the length of the wound edges by successively halving the wound with sutures.

mattress), or in the same line (vertical mattress) (Figure 5.4). These stitches must be removed at varying times. On the face they can often be removed after 48 h to avoid producing ladder-type marks across the scar. On the other hand, abdominal wound skin stitches are sometimes left in for 8–10 days.

Subcuticular stitches avoid the cross marks that may mar a scar sutured conventionally (Figure 5.5). Non-absorbable monofilament nylon or polypropylene is inserted through the skin about 5 mm from one end of the wound to emerge through the deeper part of the skin in the angle of the wound. It then takes horizontal bites of the deep epidermis on alternate sides until the far end is reached. The needle is then passed through the far angle to emerge on the surface about 5 mm from the end of the wound. The two ends of the suture are then drawn apart to tighten the stitch and draw the skin edges together. The suture ends can be taped to the skin at each end. When the suture is to be withdrawn, it is gently tautened and freed by gently drawing on the ends alternately, then pulling through intact from one end.

Absorbable subcuticular sutures, for example, metric 1 or 1.5 (5/0 or 4/0) multifilament polyglactin 910 or polyglycolic acid, do not need to be removed. A subcuticular stitch at one end, uniting both sides, begins the process, then a knot should be tied, which will be buried. The subcuticular suture is then inserted until the other end is reached, a loop being retained before the last encircling stitch is inserted, catching both sides. This loop is then tied to the thread end, forming a knot that will be buried.

Staples

Staples are useful in some circumstances but are not as versatile as sutures. Staples are usually dispensed from a cartridge which thrusts the ends of a U-shaped metal staple into the apposed edges on each side of the wound, then deforms the shape into a nearly closed

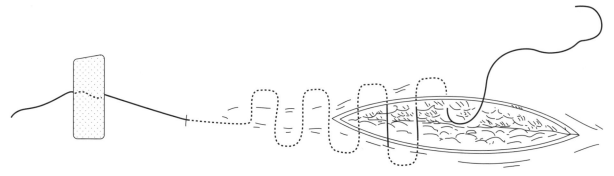

Figure 5.5 Subcuticular stitches inserted in the deep dermis. A non-absorbable suture is inserted a short distance from the end of the wound to emerge within the wound and then the edges are picked up alternately. When drawn taut, as shown on the left, the edges are opposed. The ends of the non-absorbable suture are fixed using adhesive tape as shown on the left. The ends can be freed and drawn out.

'O'. These disposable staplers are more expensive than sutures but allow very rapid closure of long surgical incisions. They are easily removed.

Adhesive strips

Adhesive strips can often be used to avoid stitching when the edges lie accurately together. Make sure the skin surface is absolutely dry. Adhesion is improved if a plastic spray is first applied and allowed to dry. Alternatively, paint the edges with Whitehead's varnish. Place the strips across the wound at right angles, pressing them into place. These strips may be spaced or placed contiguously, forming a dressing for the wound. Care must be taken to avoid excessive skin traction as this may result in blistering or superficial abrasions or blistering.

Abdominal wound closure

Most abdominal wounds incorporate peritoneum, muscles, aponeuroses, subcutaneous tissues and skin. In the past these have been closed as individual layers – and this is still appropriate for many incisions. Catgut was the traditional suture material but has now been abandoned due to the potential transmission of prions. Peritoneum can be sutured with size 3 or 3.5 metric absorbable synthetic suture and the muscles and aponeurotic sheaths with metric size 4 non-absorbable monofilament polyamide or size 4 or 5 monofilament or multifilament braided absorbable synthetic suture. A continuous suture at least four times the length of the abdominal incision is loosely inserted through peritoneum, aponeuroses and muscles but not the subcutaneous tissues and skin. Wound dehiscence is virtually abolished. The skin is usually closed with 3/0 monocryl, vicryl rapide, or metal clips.

Table 5.1 Metric suture material sizes

| Metric gauge (mm) | Previous gauges | |
	Catgut	Non-absorbables Synthetic absorbables
0.1		
0.2		10/0
0.3		9/0
0.3		8/0 virgin silk
0.4		8/0
0.5	8/0	7/0
0.7	7/0	6/0
1.0	6/0	5/0
1.5	5/0	4/0
2.0	4/0	3/0
3.0	3/0	2/0
3.5	2/0	0
4.0	0	1
5.0	1	2
6.0	2	3&4
7.0	3	5
8.0	4	5

For suture and ligature materials see Table 5.1.

All known threads have been used in surgery, including silk, cotton and linen, and are all only partially destroyed by the tissues. They can be twisted or braided. These materials are easy to handle and knot reliably. For many years monofilament or multifilament stainless steel was used because of its strength and because it causes little tissue reaction but it is difficult to handle and later tends to fragment.

The classic absorbable material is catgut, which is composed of twisted strips of the submucous coat of sheep's or cow's intestine. It soon loses strength within days. Plain catgut is rapidly, but irregularly, absorbed. If the protein is denatured by tanning, usually with chromic acid, absorption is delayed. Natural threads cause inflammatory reaction, may harbour infection and lose their strength capriciously and have almost completely been replaced by synthetic materials. Among the non-absorbable threads are polyamides, polypropylene and polyesters produced as monofilaments or braids. The monofilamentous threads often have 'memory' – they tend to return to their original shape after being deformed, as in a knot. They cause very little tissue reaction and retain their strength reliably. However, they are very susceptible to weakening by surface damage. Never grasp any part except the ends with a metal instrument and never snatch or snag them.

Absorbable polymer threads have been synthesized which cause relatively little tissue reaction, retain their strength and are absorbed slowly and reliably by hydrolysis rather than by inflammatory reaction. They are also produced in monofilament and multifilament, braided forms. Polyglyconate (Maxon) and polydioxanone (PDS) are monofilaments; polyglactin 910 (Vicryl) and polyglycolic acid (Dexon) are multifilaments.

Ligatures

The reliability of synthetic absorbables has made these ligatures increasingly popular and many vessels are routinely secured with vicryl. The vessel to be ligated is preferably isolated and doubly ligated in continuity before being divided between the ligatures. Alternatively the isolated vessel is doubly clamped with haemostatic forceps, divided and then ligated. When a vessel is already divided, it should be carefully picked up with haemostatic forceps and then ligated.

Sutures

Suture threads are also made from silk, linen, cotton or catgut. Those that are to be removed, such as skin sutures, are made from non-absorbable silk or synthetic polyamide, polyethylene or polyester. These sutures are usually dyed so that they are easily seen against the skin.

Buried sutures of catgut are still popular and extensively used in economically poor countries but increasingly the synthetic materials are employed because of their reliability. The braided synthetic absorbable materials do not retain their strength as long as monofilament PDS, which retains its strength for about 50 days and takes about 6 months to be reabsorbed.

Where permanent retention of sutures is important, then synthetic non-absorbable sutures are usually chosen because they evoke little tissue reaction. Polyamide, polypropylene and polyester are frequently used. Monofilaments are less likely to retain microorganisms because they have a smooth exterior surface. Strong threads are ideal for abdominal wound closure and for uniting fascia and tendons. Fine synthetic materials are used for vascular sutures.

Needles

Nearly all needles are now 'eyeless', the thread having been attached to the needle during manufacture. This is done either by swaging or crimping the needle onto the thread, or drilling a hole into the shank of the needle and inserting the thread end after first dipping it into an adhesive substance.

In the past, many surgeons used hand-held straight or curved needles with incomparable facility. Unfortunately, the risks of needlestick injury and consequent viral transmission make hand-held needles dangerous. In addition, many such needles were of large cross-section and produced large stitch holes. All needles should now be held in a needle holder and for this reason the majority are curved needles.

Round-bodied needles penetrate soft tissues that can be dilated by the passage of the needle and then close around the thread to form a leak-free stitch. For this reason they are used for intestinal and cardiovascular sutures. Cutting needles penetrate tough tissues such as aponeuroses, tendons and skin. These needles are triangular in the cutting section, with edges laterally and on the inside of the curvature. If such needles carry through threads that need to be tied under tension, the suture may tear towards the edge. Reverse cutting needles have the third cutting edge on the outside of the curvature to avoid this (Figure 5.6). Other shapes include trocar-, spear- and spatula-pointed needles. In the hope of reducing the number of needlestick injuries, modified blunt-pointed needles have been introduced and these penetrate the tissues remarkably well but do not easily penetrate surgical gloves.

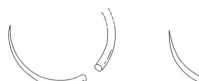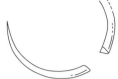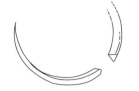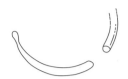

Figure 5.6 From left to right: round bodied, cutting, reverse cutting and blunt pointed needles.

Dressings

Wound dressings serve many functions but not necessarily all of them on every occasion. A dressing should be chosen to suit the need.

Seal

A clean, dry, perfectly apposed wound seals itself rapidly and often requires no dressing if it is on an area where it is not exposed to damage, such as the face. For extra protection such wounds can be sprayed with a plastic sealant or painted with Whitehead's varnish. Proprietary adhesive strips of thin porous material can be applied over the wound; they allow moisture to evaporate through them.

Protection

It may be necessary to protect the wound from inspection or picking by the patient or from inadvertent damage during movement or activity. The amount of protection varies. A neonate or infant cannot easily be restrained; an active boy who is not in pain soon forgets that he has a wound; an elderly, confused person may attempt to remove the dressing. A cotton gauze pad can be laid over the wound and held with adhesive plaster. Additionally, a pad of cotton wool can be applied and held with elastic, adhesive plaster or an encircling crepe bandage. In a few cases, a part can be temporarily immobilized by binding it; for example, an arm can be bound to the body with an encircling bandage to protect a wound over the shoulder that might be stretched and torn. Hand wounds can be protected by placing a large pad or roll of wool in the palm and binding the fingers over it in the shape of a fist, with crepe bandages.

Pressure

Some wounds require compression if oozing of blood, collection of tissue or joint fluid, or oedema are likely. Compression must be applied evenly without producing constriction. Seal the wound and protect it with a cotton dressing. Apply evenly laid cotton wool or compression wool. Depending on the circumstances, compression may be applied using crepe bandage, stretch adhesive plaster, elastic corset or other methods.

Absorbance

Throughout the operation every effort should be made to prevent bleeding, collection of pus or tissue fluid. If, in spite of this, considerable oozing or discharge is expected, drainage or the application of a stoma-type bag should be considered. Controlled and closed collection is better than incurring the risk and inconvenience of soaked dressings that need to be changed frequently.

When the discharge is likely to be minimal and temporary, the wound is covered with material that will protect the skin and allow the discharge to pass through into an absorbent dressing. Traditionally, this was achieved by placing tulle gras (literally, greasy net) onto the wound. The original tulle gras tends to make the tissues soggy; proprietary non-adherent preparations are available that allow the skin to remain healthy. Now apply absorbent cotton gauze followed by cotton wool, held in place with adhesive plaster, crepe bandage or a corset. Ensure that the thickness of absorbent cotton is sufficient to last until the next projected dressing or the cotton wool will become soaked and produce an uncomfortable caked, wet pack.

Cavities and raw areas

Whenever there is a raw area, some exudation takes place, whether or not there is infection. The raw area can be covered with a layer of non-adherent porous dressing to allow the discharge to pass through and be absorbed in layers of cotton gauze. In the presence of infection, unhealthy granulation tissue or necrotic tissue that has been excised, gauzes soaked in flavine emulsion, or Edinburgh University solution of lime (Eusol) alternating daily with hypertonic saline dressings, are often used. Eusol is considered to be harmful to the tissues but many surgeons still prefer it.

New wound dressings such as alginate hydrophilics, hydrogels and hydrocolloids absorb or transmit fluids and exudate and maintain a moist environment. Some proprietary preparations are impregnated with antibiotics.

It is sometimes important to keep a cavity open while it granulates up from the base, rather than allowing the skin to bridge across. It can be packed with a dressing. Alternatively, it can be packed with a plastic material that sets into polymerized foam which can be washed and reapplied.

Haemostasis

Having anticipated the possibility of abnormal bleeding preoperatively, great care must be taken to prevent bleeding at operation by using good technique. Hoping for the best is not enough. Stagnant blood separates tissues that are intended to unite. It attracts infection and creates tissue tension, resulting in anoxia.

Prevention

- A tourniquet safely prevents bleeding in the distal limbs provided there is no ischaemia or venous thrombosis. This offers a bloodless field for very fine surgery. A tourniquet is applied proximally. The limb is elevated and can then be further exsanguinated by winding an Esmarch or Martin bandage from the extremity, proximally. The tourniquet is inflated above systolic pressure by 50–70 mmHg in the arm and 90–100 mmHg in the leg. The constricting bandage is then unwound. The tourniquet is released after a maximum of 1 hour in the arm and 1.5 h in the leg. The tourniquet should not be re-inflated for at least 30 min. At the end of the procedure, the tourniquet should be released before closing the wound, so that missed open vessels can be identified and sealed.
- Fluid infiltration of the tissues with sterile physiological saline increases the local tissue pressure and bulk so that blood vessels are easily visible. If adrenaline diluted even as much as 1:400 000 is added, it produces vascular constriction.
- Diathermy current seals vessels by coagulation.
- Laser, which is a high-energy coherent light beam, vaporizes tissues while simultaneously coagulating small vessels.
- Ligature: intact blood vessels can be isolated, doubly ligated and then divided between the ligatures. Alternatively, apply two haemostatic

forceps across the vessel, divide it between the haemostats and ligate it. Secure very major vessels using a double ligature or suture–ligature which impales the vessel and is then tied as a ligature which is thus prevented from slipping off.

Control

- Pressure between finger and thumb, against a firm base with a finger or swab, or gentle compression using a non-crushing clamp stops bleeding. Sometimes a confined region can be packed with one or more swabs to compress one or several bleeding vessels. If bleeding is severe, pressure should not be relaxed for 5 min, timed by the clock. Arterial bleeding that is difficult to reach can often be controlled by compressing the proximal supplying vessel.
- Ligature control of a divided vessel must be preceded by capture with a haemostatic forceps.
- Sutures can be used to constrict a vessel that is difficult to isolate. They are also useful to appose oozing surfaces after completing all other appropriate measures.
- Diathermy current can also be applied once a small vessel is captured with a forceps.
- Coagulating agents may be applied over areas of capillary oozing. Gelatine foam, absorbable gauze and powdered collagen are usually effective, or a small piece of excised, crushed muscle can be sewn over the area.

Excision of cysts of the skin and subcutaneous tissues

The commonest subcutaneous cysts encountered are epidermoid, often called sebaceous cysts. They are most frequently seen on the scalp, face and scrotum and are sometimes infected. The only indication for operation on an infected epidermoid cyst is if it forms an abscess that needs draining; otherwise the infection should be treated first. True dermoid cysts are seen at the outer end of the eyebrows or in the midline. Implantation dermoids occur where skin has been driven deeply as occurs in the fingers of seamstresses.

Before excising a simple, uninfected epidermoid cyst, written, informed consent must be obtained and all the required materials and instruments and good light secured. If hair interferes with the procedure, it should be shaved or trimmed. The skin is cleaned. A

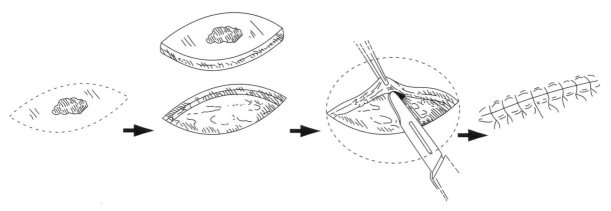

Figure 5.7 Elliptical biopsy. On the left, an ellipse is marked out with its long axis parallel to the skin tension lines. A boat-shaped full-thickness specimen is excised. If necessary, the edges are undermined to allow linear closure without tension.

short distance from the normal skin near the cyst, 1% lignocaine is injected through a fine needle, raising a wheal extending to and over the cyst. The crown of the cyst where the punctum lies should be avoided in order not to penetrate the cyst and burst it. The injection is then extended around and under the cyst. The hydrostatic pressure should separate the cyst from all its attachments except at the punctum.

Five minutes is allowed for the local anaesthetic action of lignocaine to take effect. An incision is then made over the cyst, to one side of the crown, and extended a few millimetres at each end beyond the cyst, taking care to avoid opening the cyst. Control of bleeding is achieved by simple pressure. The two sides of the incision are separated with the tips of haemostatic forceps and the white cyst is now visible, free of attachments. Using the forceps blades as levers, the cyst is gently mobilized and freed until it is attached only at the punctum. Once free, the intact cyst is removed by cutting its attachment to the skin. If the cyst is ruptured, sebaceous material should be carefully removed, the cyst wall identified and dissected free.

Simple pressure is applied or persistent bleeding vessels picked up and tied. The wound is carefully sutured using fine metric 1.5 or 1 (4/0 or 5/0) black monofilament polyamide or similar material. The wound usually requires only a plastic spray seal. The sutures can be removed after 4–5 days.

Biopsy and cytological sampling

Always fully explain the procedure and its implications to the patient and obtain consent.

Biopsy

This implies a viewing of living tissue but dead tissue is also included. Specimens are taken for examination, usually histologically. Those for routine histology should be placed in 10% formalin but not those for electron microscopy. Some specimens are later divided so that part can be sent for microbiological or chemical investigation. Advice should be taken from the laboratory staff and the correct specimen bottles and media used and the correct forms filled in.

Elliptical biopsy

This entails removing a full thickness boat-shaped specimen of skin. If it is an excision biopsy, ensure the ellipse is completely clear of the margins of the lesion. The ellipse is aligned with the skin tension lines. With the scalpel cutting vertically into the skin, crossing the cuts at the ends is avoided (Figure 5.7). Some normal skin is included, together with the junctional tissue at the edge of the lesion. For potentially malignant lesions, ensure that you have adequate clearance in depth.

To close the ellipse, the skin edges may be gently undermined. The wound is sutured to bring the edges together, forming a linear scar. It is often valuable to place the first stitch across the centre of the ellipse where the gap is greatest and insert the other stitches subsequently. If the first stitch is now lax, it can be removed and a replacement inserted. If the ellipse is short and wide, closure will be difficult. Long, narrow ellipses are easy to close and produce the best scars.

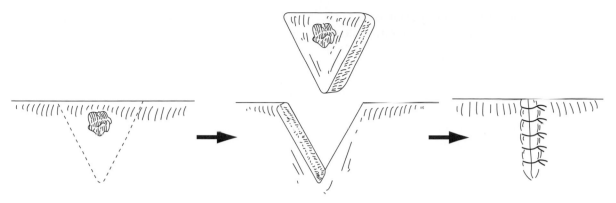

Figure 5.8 A wedge biopsy removed near an edge, followed by linear closure.

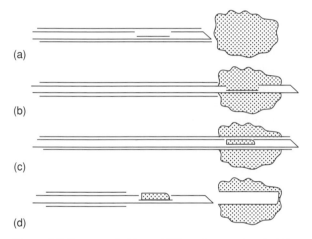

Figure 5.9 Trucut needle biopsy. (a) The stylette, enclosed within a hollow needle, has a thinned segment. (b) When the needle reaches the lesion, it is held still while the stylette is advanced into the lesion. (c) The stylette is then held still while the needle is advanced, cutting off the tissue that has bulged into the thinned segment. (d) The closed needle and stylette are withdrawn, the needle is drawn back, freeing the biopsy specimen.

Wedge biopsy

This is indicated where the lesion is near an edge such as a lip or an ear. It can be used to remove part of a lesion or as an excision biopsy. It can be closed as a linear scar (Figure 5.8).

Needle biopsy

This allows for a core of tissue to be removed at a depth. The most usual needle is the Trucut (Travenol) instrument (Figure 5.9). The lesion and its depth must be confirmed. Adjacent important structures must not be at risk. The skin is cleaned and a bleb raised with local anaesthetic. A nick is then made with a sharp-pointed scalpel at the insertion point of the needle. With the fingers of one hand, the lump is fixed, if necessary, while inserting the closed needle into it. The cannula is held still while the stylette (which has a flattened area behind the sharp tip into which some tissue bulges) is advanced. The stylette is held still and the needle advanced over it, cutting off a thin core of tissue that bulges into the flat part of the stylette. The needle is kept closed and withdrawn to reveal the excised core of tissue, which is gently placed in the fixative. As a rule the entry point in the skin requires a simple dressing only.

Cytological sampling

In a number of areas, diagnosis can be made from specimens of cells. An example is the simple aspiration of ascitic fluid in the abdomen that may on cytology reveal metastatic carcinoma, sparing the patient extensive, distressing investigations of no further benefit. After the skin is cleaned, a size 12 needle is gently inserted through the full thickness of the abdominal wall in one quadrant. Fluid is aspirated and the syringe emptied into a container that will be sent immediately, with a completed form, to the cytology laboratory. If necessary, aspiration is performed in each of the four quadrants. This technique can be used wherever there is fluid that may contain diagnostically important cells. Sometimes elusive fluid can be identified and aspirated using imaging by ultrasound or CT.

Cells may be removed from solid lumps for cytological examination. A well-developed technique is used for breast lumps. The fixative pot and microscope slides should first be made ready. After the skin is cleaned and the patient made aware of the procedure, the lump is fixed with the fingers of the non-dominant hand. A fine, for example, 23-gauge needle attached to a 10 ml syringe is advanced into the lump. The syringe plunger is strongly withdrawn while the needle tip is jerkily moved within the lump. The technique is facilitated by fitting the syringe into an apparatus that allows it to be controlled with one hand. The syringe and needle is withdrawn, the contents ejected onto several prelabelled microscope slides and fixative immediately applied. Finally, some fixative is drawn up into the syringe through the needle and the contents emptied into a specimen bottle for centrifugation. The specimen and completed form are sent immediately to the cytology laboratory.

Drainage of superficial abscesses

An abscess is a collection of pus confined within a cavity. Sometimes the abscess resolves spontaneously; a 'blind boil' is an example. Abscesses may also become chronic and remain static. If the abscess is superficial it causes local swelling and inflammation. The fact that it contains fluid can be detected by fluctuation. Others track towards internal or external surfaces. The tracking of an abscess to the external surface is described as 'pointing'. There is often a swelling with central tenderness. The centre of the swelling softens and often turns white, later becoming necrotic and turning black, and may break down so that the contained pus can discharge. If the overlying skin is macerated by applying moist dressings, this facilitates the breakdown and discharge of pus. Abscesses in some places increase the dangers; an example is the 'danger triangle' between the root of the nose and the corners of the mouth where infection may spread via the veins to the cavernous sinus.

Abscess cavity walls are relatively impervious to systemically administered antibiotics. If an abscess is localized and superficial but does not show signs of pointing, it is usually best to drain it. It is important to know the anatomy and be aware of important structures in the region. The necessary instruments and materials, including receptacles for collecting the pus for culture, should be available before the procedure is started.

Aspiration

The contents of a very soft abscess may be fluid, in which case a large-bore needle can be introduced under local anaesthesia and the pus aspirated. This method is often successful provided there is no continuing cause. It is a frequently used technique in the treatment of breast abscess. More than one procedure may be required to allow the abscess to fully resolve and the efficacy of this treatment is enhanced by the use of ultrasound guidance.

Incision

Superficial abscesses can be incised under local anaesthesia. Infiltration is started a short distance from the central, tender spot. A bleb in the skin is raised and the needle is gradually advanced. The anaesthetic is injected into the skin over the crest of the swelling. Five minutes is allowed for the local anaesthetic to take effect.

A small elliptical incision is made over the crest of the swelling and a specimen of the pus collected for culture and determination of antibiotic sensitivities. The inside of the cavity is then explored. If it is small, closed dissecting forceps or sinus forceps should be used. If it is large, a gloved finger may be inserted to examine the inside.

The contents of the abscess cavity are emptied using gentle suction, flushing with physiological saline or by swabbing. In some cases, such as a perianal abscess, a portion of the abscess wall is removed for histology, to aid in determining the cause of the abscess.

The hand offers particular difficulties in diagnosis and treatment. The pus may lie beneath thick, tense tissues through which it is difficult to detect the relatively small abscess. The tension causes severe pain, especially in the distal pulp space. It may be necessary to rely on finding the tenderest spot. However, paronychia is obvious, as are web space infections. Subungual infections can often be drained by cutting or drilling a panel or hole out of the nail. Palmar space abscesses often produce oedema of the dorsum of the hand or tendon sheaths; these demand expert treatment.

Basic principles of anastomosis

In surgery, anastomosis is usually union between tubes, especially the digestive tract, blood vessels or other ducts. These may be united end-to-end, end-to-side or side-to-side (Figure 5.10).

Digestive tract

Anastomoses are used to reconnect bowel after resection of a segment or to bypass a diseased portion. It is critical for a successful anastomosis for the tissues to have both an adequate blood supply and to be tension-free. It was shown by Lembert that if the serous

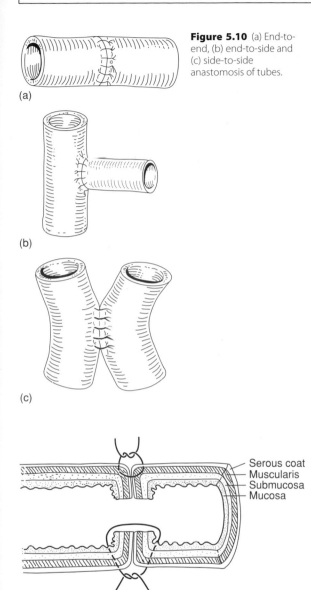

Figure 5.10 (a) End-to-end, (b) end-to-side and (c) side-to-side anastomosis of tubes.

(a)

(b)

(c)

Figure 5.11 Lembert's inverting seromuscular stitch (above) and all-coats intestinal stitch (below).

- Serous coat
- Muscularis
- Submucosa
- Mucosa

a second time, either as a continuous or interrupted stitch. This is then continued onto the front wall to complete the union. Finally, the seromuscular stitch on the back wall is continued onto the front wall as an inverting suture to complete the encircling and inverting anastomosis. It has been shown that single-layer can be as safe as two-layer anastomoses. Edge-to-edge union is also safe; in theory, bringing together the layers that will unite seems sensible. Finally, many surgeons exclude the mucosa from the traditional all-coats stitch. The technique that can best be applied to all gastrointestinal anastomoses is a single layer of extramucosal interrupted sutures of synthetic absorbable thread, with edge-to-edge union.

Mechanical sutures have been used in surgery since the early 1900s. Hutl, a Hungarian surgeon, developed a mechanical stapling device which he used for stapled closure of the upper gastrointestinal tract with success. Further development largely by Russian scientists and subsequently the American surgeon Ravitch led to the creation of reloadable stapling devices. Evolutions of these instruments are commonly used in clinical practice today for anastomoses throughout the gastrointestinal tract.

Circular staplers

After the diseased segment of the gastrointestinal tract has been resected a circular anvil is inserted into the proximal lumen and it is secured using a purse-string suture. For a colorectal anastomosis the stapling gun is inserted through the anus into the rectum. The instrument is then 'unwound', delivering a sharp spike through the centre of the distal rectal staple line. The spike is then removed and the anvil can then be securely located into the handpiece and the proximal and distal ends of the bowel approximated. The instrument allows the operator to carefully control the degree of approximation and therefore tissue compression at the level of the anastomosis. The instrument is activated by squeezing the handles firmly as far as they will go. This inserts a double staggered row of titanium staples inverting the serosal edges of the bowel. Immediately after staple formation, the knife blade resects the excess tissue, creating a circular anastomosis. The resected tissue, in the form of circular doughnuts, is then inspected to ensure a complete ring of tissue has been obtained and the integrity of the anastomosis can be checked with an air test. Saline is introduced to the pelvis and air is insufflated into the rectum via the anus. Any leak of air bubbles is readily detected. This

(visceral peritoneal) coats of bowel are apposed, they fuse and seal the junction. From this developed the convention of inverting bowel ends when they are united with a seromuscular stitch. The important stitch holding the bowel is a stitch which picks up the strong, collagenous seromuscular layer (Figure 5.11).

Historically, the anastomosis was performed in four successive layers. The bowel ends were apposed and their back layers united with a continuous seromuscular suture of metric 3 or 2 (2/0 or 3/0) size synthetic absorbable thread. The back layers are united type of anastomosis is also commonly used for distal oesophageal anastomoses after total gastrectomy. The circular stapling guns have also been used in the treatment of prolapsing haemorrhoids. A circular cuff of mucosa above the haemorrhoidal tissue is created with a pursestring suture. Introduction of the stapling gun allows this tissue to be resected whilst a circular ring of staples is inserted to restore mucosal continuity.

Linear staplers

Linear staplers can be used both for sealing the ends of bowel during a resection and for the creation of anastomoses. They typically insert four rows of staggered titanium staples and a blade integral to the stapling device is then triggered which divides between the second and third rows of staples. The enterotomy through which the two blades of the stapling device are introduced can then be closed with either sutures or a second stapling device. It has been common practice to reload and reuse the first stapler but there are reports which suggest the use of an instrument with an integral blade can cause structural disruption to any staple line that it crosses. It is therefore safer to either suture this enterotomy or use a bladeless linear staple gun. This technique can provide an anatomical side-side but functional end-end anastomosis. There is some evidence to suggest that creation of a stapled side-side or functional end-end anastomosis is particularly beneficial in the treatment of Crohn's disease as it may afford a longer disease-free interval at the anastomosis.

It is important to pause for 15 seconds prior to firing any stapler to ensure time has been given to allow proper tissue approximation. If considering using a stapling device to fashion an anastomosis it is essential that care is taken in assessing the bowel at the planned site. In the emergency setting the altered calibre of thickened oedematous bowel can reduce the ability of the staples to secure an adequate amount of tissue and as the oedema resolves the potential for anastomotic leaks is heightened.

Vascular anastomosis

The union of blood vessels must be carried out not by inversion but by eversion, in order to bring into apposition the inner endothelial layers. If this is not done, clots form at the anastomosis and block the lumen. Classically, the ends of vessels are first united by three stay sutures that divide the circumference into thirds (Figure 5.12). A running stitch of fine (metric 0.7–

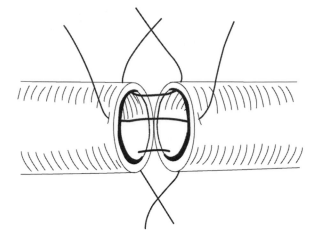

Figure 5.12 Triangulation method of performing vascular anastomosis.

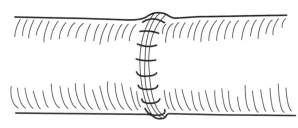

Figure 5.13 Everted edges in vascular anastomosis to bring the inner, endothelial surfaces into contact.

0.4) monofilament polyamide or polypropylene suture is then carried round the circumference of the stoma (Figure 5.13).

Very small vessels can be united but this requires an entirely different technique. The anastomosis is carried out using very fine instruments and the procedure is performed using an operating microscope. If it is not possible to evert the vessels, instead, the anastomosis is formed using a series of interrupted sutures bringing the ends together, edge-to-edge.

Laparoscopic surgery

Since the first laparoscopic cholecsytectomy 20 years ago the role of laparoscopic surgery as both a diagnostic and therapeutic tool has increased substantially and it now forms an integral part of a general surgical practice. The benefits of laparoscopic surgery in terms of faster recovery time, less postoperative pain and fewer wound complications have been demonstrated in large randomized controlled trials. More recent studies have suggested that laparoscopic surgery may be associated with less adhesion formation, which is particularly important in reducing the incidence of postoperative adhesion obstruction. Initial concerns regarding poorer oncological outcomes associated with laparoscopic colorectal cancer surgery have not been proven to be true. Hand-assisted laparoscopic surgery (HALS) is advocated as a way of providing the tactile feedback that is absent with totally laparoscopic surgery. HALS potentially reduces operating time and improves the operator's ability to deal with unexpected adverse events. Proponents believe that utilization of the incision which will ultimately be made to remove the resected specimen is not detrimental to the patient; however, there is increasing evidence that the physiological insult to the patient is greater with HALS than with totally laparoscopic surgery. HALS may remain a useful adjunct in selected cases and may have a role as a training tool in the transition to totally laparoscopic surgery. The current focus of laparoscopic surgical development is the move towards less invasive surgery with fewer and smaller incisions with less physiological insult to the patient.

Pneumoperitoneum

Integral to laparoscopic surgery is safely establishing a pneumoperitoneum. Insufflation of carbon dioxide into the peritoneal cavity provides a working space within which a wide range of surgical procedures can be performed. Safe use of laparoscopic surgery requires an understanding of the cardiovascular and respiratory effects of pneumoperitoneum as well as the often steep position changes during surgery. Carbon dioxide is utilized as it is an inert, readily excreted gas but CO_2 pneumoperitoneum causes hypercapnia and respiratory alkalosis. Continuous end-tidal CO_2 monitoring is essential and minute volumes will need to be adjusted to maintain normocapnia. Steep position changes, particularly common in laparoscopic colorectal procedures, have both respiratory and cardiovascular effects. Head-down positioning reduces pulmonary compliance and increases potential ventilation-perfusion mismatches. Head-up positioning combined with raised intra-abdominal pressure reduces venous return from the lower limbs and therefore compression stockings or boots are recommended for all laparoscopic procedures.

Pneumoperitoneum can be established either by an open technique or by utilization of a veres needle. Both approaches can be performed at any site on the anterior abdominal wall but are most commonly performed at the umbilicus. Randomized controlled trials have not demonstrated any significant difference in major complication rates between closed and open access techniques; however, both techniques offer advantages in selected patients and the skilled surgeon will be familiar with both approaches. The intra-abdominal pressure required to produce a safe working space varies between individuals and will be affected by the degree of relaxation of the anterior abdominal wall and patient body habitus. It is important to ensure that the lowest possible pressure is used to maintain an adequate pneumoperitoneum so that the associated deleterious effects on cardiovascular and respiratory function are minimized. Traditionally routine urinary catheterization and naso-gastric tube insertion were advocated to reduce inadvertent visceral injury. Surgeons utilizing the open technique often omit these steps due to direct visualization of entry but it is important to be aware of any comorbid pathologies which may place the bladder or stomach at increased risk of injury. Safest practice would suggest that those employing the veres needle technique should routinely empty the bladder and stomach.

Veres needle

The veres needle consists of a spring-loaded, blunt-tipped insufflation cannula encircled by a needle. The instrument is designed so that on insertion the blunt-tipped cannula retracts, as resistance from the tissue is encountered, allowing the needle to penetrate the tissues. Upon entering the peritoneal cavity the cannula springs forward thereby reducing the risk of visceral injury. It is essential that the mechanism is checked prior to use to ensure the cannula functions satisfactorily and is patent. It was previously suggested that confirmation of entry into the peritoneal cavity could be achieved by one of the following:

(i) Double click test – as the veres needle passes through the abdominal wall the blunt-tipped cannula will spring forward as the needle passes through the linea alba and the peritoneum. These two characteristic clicks can be detected by the operator.

(ii) Droplet test – this test is performed by placing 1 ml of saline on the blunt end of the veres needle after it has been inserted into the peritoneal cavity. The anterior abdominal wall is physically lifted by the operating surgeon. The

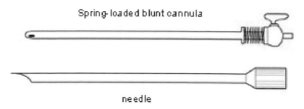

Figure 5.14 Veres needle.

resulting negative intra-abdominal pressure will draw the saline down through the veres needle if the veres needle is correctly positioned.

(iii) Aspiration test – 10 ml of saline is injected through the veres needle. If the tip is free within the peritoneal cavity the fluid will be delivered with ease but it will not be possible to aspirate the saline.

(iv) Insufflation pressures – insufflation should be monitored closely to ensure that the pressure generated with CO_2 insufflation falls within expected norms. Abnormally high pressures suggest extra-peritoneal or intra-visceral insufflation.

There is increasing evidence to suggest that none of the tests used to confirm veres needle placement is specific enough to guarantee accurate needle placement although monitoring insufflation pressures seems to be the most reliable. 'Waggling' the veres needle to check that it moves freely within the peritoneal cavity should be strongly avoided as this manoeuvre may increase a 1.6 mm puncture injury to up to 1 cm in diameter in viscera or blood vessels if inaccurately placed (Figure 5.14).

Open technique

A mini-incision is made in the skin, linea alba and the peritoneum using a No 15 or No 11 blade. Stay sutures are inserted into the rectus sheath and the blunt-tipped Hasson cannula is then inserted into the peritoneal cavity under direct vision. The port is then secured using the stay sutures. A modified-Hasson or 'umbilical stalk' technique is frequently used whereby a non-bladed trocar is inserted through a small incision at the base of the umbilical stalk. A small curvilinear incision is made in the skin just below the umbilicus. The subcutaneous fat is cleared to expose the umbilical stalk and its junction with the rectus sheath. A tissue-holding forceps, e.g. littlewoods, elevating the

umbilical stalk can help to display this junction. A small incision is made in the fibres of the linea alba as they encircle the stalk extending onto the base of the umbilical cicatrix which is large enough to enable port placement under direct vision without the need for securing sutures to prevent port displacement or carbon dioxide leak. Proponents of this technique suggest it affords rapid establishment of pneumoperitoneum without the potential need for what some consider to be cumbersome stay sutures or the potentially life-threatening complications from a blind veres needle insertion.

Optical access trocars

An alternative method to the above two commoner approaches is to employ an optical access trocar. In this technique a 5 mm laparoscope is inserted and secured within a hollow trocar. It is then possible to directly visualize the layers of the abdominal wall as the trocar is introduced and the individual layers are traversed and the peritoneal cavity is entered. As with any technique experience is essential to avoid potential visceral injury, which is a recognized complication particularly in the presence of intra-abdominal adhesions. A large US series evaluating this technique has shown it to be safe (<1% complication rate) in experienced hands and it is a common choice for establishing pneumoperitoneum.

It is essential that whatever method employed the operator is familiar with that technique and is aware of the potential pitfalls of establishing a safe pneumoperitoneum.

Natural orifice transluminal surgery (NOTES)

Kalloo first published his work on the feasibility of transgastric peritoneoscopy in 2004. Further animal model studies showed that a flexible endoscope could be safely introduced into the peritoneal cavity through a number of natural body orifices, i.e. stomach, vagina and anus. In 2007 the first transvaginal cholecsytectomy was reported with excellent results. This area of surgery remains very much in its evolutionary phase; however, scarless surgery offers obvious benefits in terms of cosmesis and absence of postoperative pain; however, any potential advantages remain to be proven and critics challenge the safety and advantages of NOTES over existing laparoscopic techniques.

Robotic surgery

Robotic surgery was developed to improve on conventional laparoscopic surgery by providing superior visualization, enhanced ergonomics and greater precision. Although termed robotic surgery at no time is the machinery autonomous, always requiring surgical input from a trained clinician. The most commonly used robotic system, the Da Vinci surgical system, comprises a surgeon's console, the interactive robotic arms which are located in a stack at the patient's side and a high-performance 3D high-definition imaging system. The system allows the surgical inputs on a remote console to be scaled and filtered, thus eliminating tremor, and transmitted to the interactive robotic arms where the precise micro-movements of the instruments are carried out. The system affords the surgeon high-definition three-dimensional magnification due to the binocular nature of the eyepiece on the surgeon's console, unlike the conventional two-dimensional image obtained with a laparoscopic monitor. The robotically controlled instruments also have greater dexterity, with 'wrist' joints which mimic the range of movement possible with the human hand. This is a significant advancement over the restricted range of movement available with existing laparoscopic instruments. A wide range of procedures have now been carried out using robotic surgery with excellent results; however, the financial outlay involved in setting up and maintaining robotic surgery is largely prohibitive in the NHS and to date only a few UK centres offer this surgical approach.

Telesurgery

Telesurgery is where a surgical procedure is performed by an operator at a site distant from the patient. This offers huge potential for patients in remote or inaccessible locations as well as military application in areas of conflict. Subsequent to the development of robotic surgery the possibility of telesurgery became apparent and research into its possible applications proceeded rapidly through the 1990s. One of the earliest reported human telesurgical procedures was performed by Marescaux in September 2001. He carried out a laparoscopic cholecsytectomy on a female patient in Strasbourg, France, whilst controlling a Zeus robotic system from an office in New York. This was the first reported trans-Atlantic surgery and was named Operation Lindbergh. Telesurgery remains limited by the reliability and speed of current communication systems. However, as this technology improves the usage and scope of telesurgery will inevitably increase.

Laparoscopic equipment

Insufflators

A number of automatic insufflators are currently in use and it is vital that the user is familiar with their own particular model. In general insufflators will display intra-abdominal pressure (mmHg), CO_2 insufflation rates (l/min) and total volume of gas insufflated (l). It is usual to set the limit for abdominal pressure to between 10 and 12 mmHg. This enables a satisfactory working space to be created without the deleterious cardiovascular and respiratory effects of an elevated intra-abdominal pressure for the majority of patients. Lower pressures may be acceptable in thinner patients and the aim is to proceed with the lowest pressure at which good views can be obtained. A pressure of 10–12 mmHg does not produce clinically relevant effects in patients of ASA grade I–II.

Insufflation rates can be controlled manually or by selection of a number of pre-set flow rates. These typically include 'veres' (0.5 l/min), 'low-flow' (1 l/min), which is used on initial establishment of pneumoperitoneum during which time pressures will be closely monitored to ensure safe trocar placement, and 'high-flow' (up to 35 l/min), which is selected for the remainder of the procedure. Total volume insufflated when combined with insufflation pressures is an important tool for monitoring the establishment of a pneumoperitoneum. Abnormally high intra-abdominal pressures generated with only a small insufflated volume should warn the surgeon that the first trocar is inaccurately placed and commonly CO_2 is being insufflated into the extra-peritoneal space. Every insufflator has in-built alarms which alert the surgeon if any of the predefined limits are breached.

Port types

Laparoscopic ports are inserted through the patient's abdominal wall to provide access for instruments to the peritoneal cavity. These ports may be either single-use or sterilizable and reusable. Ports range from 5 to 15 mm to allow insertion of a variety of different instruments. Ports have either a blunt- or sharp-tipped trocar and the choice of port depends on the method of pneumoperitoneum, the site of insertion and the planned surgery (Figure 5.15).

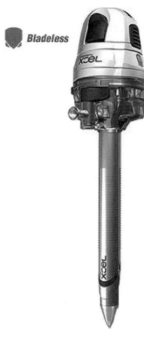

Figure 5.15 Bladeless optical trocar.

Disposable ports have been manufactured with either a bladeless trocar, which splits the muscle fibres, or bladed trocars which have a knife which retracts on entry in a similar way to the veres needle for ports inserted under direct vision. Bladeless trocars are believed to make smaller wounds and may obviate the need for fascial closing off the midline. Optical trocars allow an endoscope to be placed within the shaft of the port to enable direct visualization of the layers of the abdominal wall as the port is introduced. Standard reusable ports have smooth cylindrical exterior surfaces to facilitate cleaning and sterilization; however, this frictionless surface can lead to port slippage during lengthy procedures. Newer single-use ports utilize 'corkscrew' or 'ridged' exterior surfaces to provide friction against the surrounding tissues and provide greater port stabilization. Some ports have inflatable balloon sections which when inflated can be drawn back against the abdominal wall to provide a secure port position whilst affording the optimum viewing angle. Hand-assisted laparoscopic surgery requires the use of specific ports which, whilst allowing entry of a hand into the peritoneal cavity, create a tight seal to maintain the pneumoperitoneum. This can be achieved by the use of either an inflatable cuff which fits snugly around the user's forearm or 'Gelpad' ports which produce a seal via a rubbery jelly-like pad through which a hand can be introduced. It is recommended that the fascial layer of all port sites >10 mm is closed primarily to avoid the potential complication of a port site hernia.

Single insertion or single port laparoscopic surgery

Single insertion (SILS) or single port laparoscopic surgery (SPLS) is an evolution of existing surgical technology and has become possible due to improvements in laparoscopic instrument design. Traditional laparoscopic instruments allowed rotation in a 360° axis but there was no facility to angulate the tip. Development of a range of shears, graspers and stapling devices with a 'roticulating' tip has allowed greater dexterity within the peritoneal cavity and the possibility of single port surgery has become a reality. These instruments will allow up to 80° of angulation at the 'wrist' joint, which enables the surgeon to achieve the required triangulation from within a single port to safely perform laparoscopic procedures. Two techniques are currently being developed.

> Single incision laparoscopic surgery – through a single incision at the umbilicus three 5 mm ports are introduced.
> Single port laparoscopic surgery – a specifically designed shaft-less port is inserted at the umbilicus. This sheath allows the introduction of either three (triport) or four (quadport) instruments through a single port on the abdominal wall.

A number of procedures have now been performed using these techniques including cholecsytectomy, splenectomy, hysterectomy, nephrectomy, nissen fundoplication and colonic resection. This innovative evolution of laparoscopic surgery is a very exciting prospect for the future.

Laparoscopes

Most laparoscopes are constructed of a rod and lens system. The scope is simply a conduit through which the light is transmitted via a series of lenses to a video camera which displays the image on a viewing monitor. These scopes were particularly vulnerable to 'misting' or 'fogging' due to cooling of the air within the scope. Condensed water on the end of the scope would regularly impair the image obtained. Developments in video chip design and particularly chip size have enabled scopes in which the video chip is mounted on the end to be produced (Figure 5.16).

This has led to two significant advantages. Firstly the heat generated by the chip reduces condensation

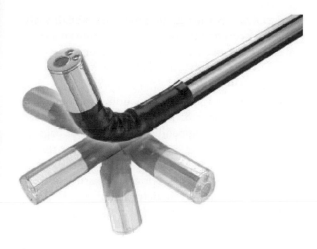

Figure 5.16 Flexible-tip laparoscope.

on the lens thereby reducing image impairment but more importantly since the image can now be transmitted through the scope via flexible fibre-optic cables the tip of the scope can now be flexible. This offers considerable advantages for laparoscopic surgery. The viewpoints offered by the flexible tip scope were traditionally provided by angled lenses at the tip of the scope, i.e. 30°, 45°; however, the flexible tip now affords a greater freedom of movement and larger viewable field. Improvements in image resolution and display capabilities have enabled high-definition laparoscopes and monitors to be created. Recent studies have shown that these HD systems offer superior resolution, increased image brightness, increased depth of field and reduced distortion. Depth perception is critical in laparoscopic surgery and this appears to be a key limiting factor particularly for intricate tasks. The use of HD systems in clinical trials has shown a reduction in the time taken to perform intricate tasks such as laparoscopic knot tying and it has been suggested that it is the increased depth of field which has enabled this. Despite the improvements in laparoscope and image display technology surgeons continue to operate using two-dimensional images for the majority of laparoscopic procedures. Further development in imaging technology may well afford 3D displays for all future laparoscopic surgery.

Laparoscope control devices

The most commonly used laparoscope control device is the surgical trainee and it is essential that experience is gained to enable the young trainee to attain the most basic of laparoscopic skills; however, a number

of laparoscope control devices have been developed which give the surgeon direct control of the laparoscope whilst leaving both hands free for manipulating surgical instruments. These devices can be either fixed or mobile.

Fixed

A 'goose-neck' scope holder has numerous ball-joints which once positioned can be locked in place. For procedures where scope movement is limited, i.e. laparoscopic cholecsytectomy, this instrument can afford a rock-steady camera image and obviate the need for a surgical assistant. It is possible to reposition the scope if required but this necessitates further physical input from the surgeon.

Mobile

More recently electronically controlled devices have been developed which can be controlled without direct manual input by the surgeon or assistant. They can be controlled by a pedal at the surgeon's feet or by a head-mounted device, enabling the laparoscope to be moved in response to either pedal inputs or movement of the surgeon's head. In practice some of these devices remain slightly cumbersome to use and the bulky control system renders them impractical when a large number of ports are employed. As technology progresses and the control system enables the laparoscope to move more intuitively this will free both the surgeon and assistant to be actively involved in the surgical procedure.

Accessories
Clip/stapler appliers

Reusable re-loadable single clip applicators were developed at the inception of laparoscopic surgery and have been used frequently in cholecystectomy. It is necessary to remove these instruments from the peritoneal cavity for reloading and it is not uncommon for clips to become displaced from the jaws during usage. Newer disposable multi-fire clip or staple application devices have been manufactured delivering a number of clips which are contained within the shaft of a single instrument. This negates the need to remove and reload the instrument between firings. They have been produced to fit down either a 5 mm or 10 mm port and have been used reliably and safely to secure large blood vessels, e.g. inferior mesenteric artery.

Evolution in staple design and the delivery system has enabled self-securing cork-screw or helical-shaped clips to be developed which can be used to secure prosthetic mesh against the flat surface of the abdominal wall during laparoscopic hernia repair. Originally these were of titanium construction due to its strength and inert nature but more recent staples are made from an absorbable synthetic polyester copolymer derived from lactic and glycolic acid.

Laparoscopic versions of the open linear staplers fire long rows of titanium staples and are used to either divide the bowel or if a specific vascular cartridge is selected to seal and divide major arteries. Some versions of these staplers have ends which can 'flex' or roticulate, which can be particularly useful when stapling in areas more difficult to access, e.g. when trying to cross staple the rectum in the pelvis.

Prefabricated ligatures

Laparoscopic suturing is one of the more advanced laparoscopic skills. To facilitate control of divided vessels, the appendicular stump or, on occasion during cholecystectomy, prefabricated ligatures have been developed which enable structures to be controlled and sealed with ease. They consist of an 18 inch ligature, of either vicryl or PDS, enclosed within a plastic tube. The ligature has a prefabricated knot at one end which protrudes from the plastic tube. Once the ligature has been introduced into the peritoneal cavity and positioned around the target structure it can be tightened and secured extra-corporeally by pushing on the plastic tube. The suture can be divided with laparoscopic shears and both the excess suture and the plastic tube are removed.

Wound protectors

Shortly after the introduction of laparoscopic colorectal surgery concerns arose regarding the possibility of port site and incision site metastases. These initial concerns seem unfounded; however, the majority of surgeons use a wound protection device to cover the exposed skin at the site of tumour extraction to prevent seeding of tumour cells. A number of different models are commercially available. The simplest consists of a plastic ring, which is introduced through the surgical incision to secure it against the peritoneal surface, with a large plastic sheet attached. This can be unfolded to cover the skin of the anterior abdominal wall. More complex designs have twin rings joined by a cylindrical sheet. These can be twisted to fit snugly and maximize the size of the incision in the abdominal wall. It is also possible by rotating the outer ring to create an airtight seal and re-establish a pneumoperitoneum.

Tissue-extraction bags

Bags may be used for the extraction of tissue following a large number of procedures, e.g. cholecsytectomy, splenectomy, appendicectomy. Simple bags are introduced via a 10 or 12 mm port and once the tissue to be removed has been placed within the bag are drawn back into the port. For occasions where tissue or fluid spillage would be detrimental more complicated extraction bags exist. These bags have a dedicated delivery system which enables the bag to be opened using an extra-corporeal control system. They are then held open by a metal ring until the required tissue has been placed within the bag. The bag can then be closed and sealed and extracted via either a 10 or 15 mm port.

There are a large number of different adjuncts available for laparoscopic surgery and they are rapidly increasing and evolving. It is important to consider, however, the huge cost implications for the National Health Service of the rapidly expanding surgical equipment budget. All surgeons must be confident they can provide a safe high-quality service but also consider the costs of technology and equipment utilized.

Energy devices

Electrosurgery (diathermy)

Electrosurgery was developed in the early 1900s and was first used in a surgical procedure in the 1920s. It is important to distinguish between electrocautery, which uses direct current and tissue damage only at the site of contact, and electrosurgery, which uses high-frequency alternating current and can be used to cut, coagulate, fulgurate or desiccate tissues. In electrosurgical practice two electrode configurations are commonly used, monopolar and bipolar.

Monopolar

Monopolar diathermy machines have one large electrode attached, with good contact to the skin, usually of the thigh. This is the return electrode. The active electrode is small and is applied directly or indirectly to a blood vessel to coagulate and seal it, usually as a pair of forceps or needle-point.

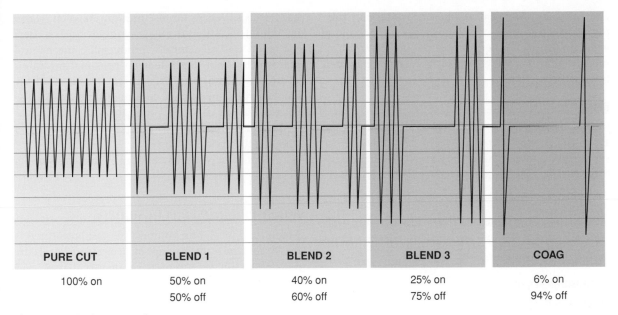

PURE CUT	BLEND 1	BLEND 2	BLEND 3	COAG
100% on	50% on 50% off	40% on 60% off	25% on 75% off	6% on 94% off

Figure 5.17 Diathermy waveforms.

Standard electrical current alternates at 60 Hz. At this frequency there is excessive neuromuscular stimulation. This stimulation ceases at frequencies in excess of 100 kHz. Electrosurgical generators convert current alternating at 60 Hz to a current which can be used safely alternating at over 200 000 cycles per second (200 kHz). At this frequency there is negligible neuromuscular stimulation.

This high-frequency alternating current produces heat, not by the effect of electrical resistance but by oscillation of the ions in the tissues. Variation of the waveform alters the amount of heat generated and the modality of the monopolar instrument.

A pulsed high-frequency alternating current coagulates the tissues with minimal disruption. Continuous output disrupts the tissues because an arc is struck between the electrode and the tissues. It produces only minimal coagulation. A blended current of cutting and coagulation frequencies improves haemostasis, but beware of using coagulation current close to the skin surface for fear of causing burns (Figure 5.17).

It is important to be aware that the use of diathermy coagulation of blood vessels entails risks and particular care must be taken when using diathermy in laparoscopic surgery.

Direct coupling

This is where current applied to the active electrode arcs to an adjacent metal instrument. The adjacent instrument becomes energized and the current will then seek an alternative route back to the return electrode. The risk of inadvertent visceral injury is high.

Capacitive coupling

The conductive active electrode is surrounded by non-conductive insulation. This, in turn, is surrounded by a conductive metal cannula. A capacitor creates an electrostatic field between the two conductors and, as a result, a current in one conductor can, through the electrostatic field, induce a current in the second conductor. This current can then pass through tissue at a distance from the surgical site, potentially resulting in burns or visceral injury.

Insulation

All laparoscopic instruments are insulated throughout the shaft length. This is designed to prevent accidental injury to viscera in contact with the instrument when current is applied. The routine cleaning and sterilization process which all reusable instruments undergo can potentially damage this insulation and it is the surgeon's responsibility to check the integrity of this insulation before any instrument is used.

Explosions

Explosions have occurred when alcoholic substances have been used to prepare the skin followed soon afterwards by the use of diathermy, which may produce an electric arc. Similarly, bowel gases may explode when polyps are diathermized at colonoscopy. Anaesthetic vapours such as ether can also explode if ignited by a diathermy spark.

Bipolar

In bipolar surgery the two tines of a pair of forceps act as the active and return electrodes. Only the tissue grasped between the forceps is included in the electrical circuit. This has the advantage of delivering current and therefore heat to a very localized area and can therefore be readily used under local anaesthetic. It is important to note, however, that if the two electrodes are allowed to touch the circuit is completed and no current will pass through the tissue.

Electrosurgical generators

Original generators used a grounded current from a mains outlet. It was assumed that the current would return to earth via the return electrode plate. Unfortunately the current would always seek the path of least resistance. Any metal object touching the patient may serve as a preferential route to earth and if the surface area of contact is small, current concentration results in heat and burns. Isolated generators were introduced in the late 1960s. In these generators the electrosurgical current will not recognize grounded objects as pathways to complete the circuit, reducing the risk of alternate site burns. The generators are also fitted with alarms which alert the user if there is inadequate contact between the return plate and the patient's skin or the circuit is for some other reason disrupted. However, as with any technology utilized it is essential that all precautions are taken to minimize inadvertent injury.

Further generator development has produced machines which are computer-controlled and continuously measure the tissue impedance and resistance at the electrode contact site. This allows them to provide instant response to any changes measured and ensure, by modifying power output, that they deliver a constant tissue effect. They also control maximum output voltage, which limits the development of capacitive coupling and minimizes video interference.

Pressure/electrosurgery

Ligasure^{TM} (Valleylab) uses a combination of pressure and energy to reform the collagen and the elastin in vessel walls to achieve an autologous seal and reliable haemostasis. Vessels up to 7 mm can be safely sealed with this device. The advantage of this device is it alters the vessel wall structurally, producing a mechanical seal which is not dependent on proximal thrombus to achieve haemostasis. This device uses a low-voltage bipolar-type generator. It continuously monitors tissue response to choose appropriate energy settings as well as sensing that the tissue response is complete and stopping the cycle.

This process is effective but can be time-consuming in lengthy procedures.

Argon-enhanced electrosurgery

Argon is an inert, non-combustible gas; however, it is readily ionized by the passage of an electrosurgical current. When ionized it is more conductive than air and therefore makes an ideal gas for use in electrosurgery. Argon gas is delivered through the tip of an electrosurgical instrument. An electrosurgical current is passed through the tip of the instrument and by ionizing the argon gas around the tip is delivered to the tissue. This form of non-contact electrosurgery causes less tissue damage, produces less smoke and odour than conventional electrosurgery, and is suggested to cause less blood loss and reduce the risk of re-bleeding by producing a more flexible eschar.

Radiofrequency coagulators

Radiofrequency devices rely on the same principle of molecular excitation by an alternating current resulting in heat around the tip of the active electrode. This heat rapidly denatures and coagulates proteins. The radiofrequency generators measure tissue impedance in the same way as monopolar diathermy generators, delivering the optimum amount of radiofrequency energy. Circulation of water around the active electrode cools the tissue, lowering tissue impedance. Lowered impedance enables maximum energy delivery for a larger ablation volume.

Ultrasonic dissection

One of the more commonly used ultrasonic dissectors is the harmonic scalpel. This is an ultrasonic cutting and coagulating surgical device. Piezo-electric crystals in the hand-piece become excited by electricity and transfer electrical energy into mechanical energy. This motion is amplified in the hand-piece shaft. The mechanical energy generates heat which tamponades small vessels and the active blade, vibrating at 55 000 Hz, cuts through the tissue and seals it by denaturization of the proteins forming a protein coagulum. Secondary heat formation with prolonged usage can seal larger vessels. This device functions at lower heat levels (50–100°C) than conventional electrocautery (150–400°C) with minimal lateral thermal damage. The next challenge will be to produce a device which utilizes ultrasonic technology but is deliverable via a flexible instrument.

CUSA (Cavitron ultrasonic aspirator) is frequently used in liver resection. Acoustic vibrations selectively disrupt the liver parenchyma by producing a cavitating force. The relevant blood vessels and bile ducts can be identified and ligated separately. This technique, combined with a better understanding of the liver anatomy, has enabled blood loss during major hepatic resections to be significantly reduced.

Laser

The name is an acronym for Light Amplification by Stimulated Emission of Radiation. The atoms of a medium, often a gas, are excited so that the electrons reach a higher-energy state. As they revert to their lower-energy state, they emit photons. The photons are reflected back and forth between two opposed mirrors, which amplifies the light until some of it escapes as a coherent beam. The coherent beam of high-intensity light vaporizes tissues and simultaneously coagulates small blood vessels. There are several mediums, such as argon, CO_2 or neodymium yttrium aluminium garnet (NdYAG), resulting in beams of differing wavelengths and therefore different tissue absorptions. Argon and NdYAG laser light can be transmitted through optic fibres. NdYAG light is used to destroy lesions in the gastrointestinal tract and urinary bladder through endoscopes and in ophthalmology to destroy a thickened lens capsule and to treat lesions of the retina. CO_2 laser light has very low penetration and can be used to act at a surface, such as the destruction of cervical and vulval lesions in gynaecology. It may be passed into diseased, blocked blood vessels to perform laser angioplasty. Ruby laser light is valuable for the destruction of

certain skin lesions. Excimer laser light is used in ophthalmology to reshape the cornea to correct myopia. The name excimer derives from a contraction of the words 'excited dimer'. Dimers are molecules that can unite and dissociate. When they dissociate they emit high-energy photons which break surface molecules – photoablation; because this is non-thermal, no deep damage is caused.

Dangers

When using lasers there is danger of damaging tissues that lie in the path of the beam. This is a particular risk during minimal access surgery since the field of view may be limited. Another risk with penetrating laser light is that deep tissues may be damaged or perforation of vessels or hollow viscera may ensue. The operator must take precautions not to accidentally expose skin or eyes to damage by laser light. Lasers are classified by their manufacturers by the degree of risk they engender. Wherever these instruments are used there must be proper supervision by a trained laser protection officer and only nominated, properly trained people may use them.

Each energy device has its own unique properties and it is therefore important to choose a device for which the user is trained and which best suits the task at hand.

Further reading

Amid PK, Shulman AG, Lichtenstein IL. Local anaesthesia for inguinal hernia repair; step by step procedure. *Ann Surg* 1994;**220**:735–737.

Jenkins TPN. The burst abdominal wound: a mechanical approach. *Br Med J* 1976;**131**:130–140.

Kirk RM. *Basic Surgical Techniques*. 4th edn. Churchill Livingstone, 1994.

Kirk RM, Mansfield AO, Cochrane J (eds). *Clinical Surgery in General*. 2nd edn. Churchill Livingstone, 1996.

MacGregor IA, MacGregor AD. *Fundamental Techniques in Plastic Surgery*. 9th edn. Churchill Livingstone, 1995.

Memon AA. Surgical diathermy. *Br J Hosp Med* 1994;**52**:403–408.

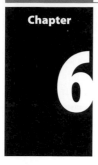

Professionalism – including academic activities: clinical research, audit, consent and ethics

Evangelos Mazaris, Paris Tekkis and Vassilios Papalois

Introduction

Surgical practice of the highest standards has always been based on sound knowledge of applied anatomy, sharp clinical judgment and excellent operative skills. In modern times, surgical practice is also integrated with basic and translational research in which the surgeon has to be actively and creatively involved.

Tight monitoring of the outcomes of surgical practice and the development of evidence-based surgery is a central theme in modern surgery. Clinical audit is an important process for the continuous evaluation of care provided to patients, leading to the acknowledgement of drawbacks, and has become a driving force for future improvement. Thus, it is necessary for surgeons to familiarize themselves, as early as possible during their careers, with the basic principles.

Acquiring informed consent is a crucial part of the daily practice of a surgeon. In modern healthcare, the patients rightly have a very strong say regarding their care and medical-legal problems arise more frequently. Therefore, surgeons have to be trained properly regarding the width and depth of the information they need to provide to the patients and their families prior to surgery regarding the type of operation, the potential problems and alternative treatments and allow them sufficient time and space to 'digest the information', ask questions and finally consent without coercion.

Last, but most certainly not least, in the modern world, the provision of healthcare is a complicated partnership between the healthcare professionals, the patients and their families and the healthcare organizations and all this in the context of multicultural open societies (with a variety of values, ideas, religious beliefs, etc.) which makes the role of clinical ethics absolutely paramount for surgical as well as any other clinical practice.

Principles of clinical research

In the past, research experience and practice were considered to be nothing more than a bonus for a good surgeon while in modern surgery they are absolutely mandatory for practising surgery at the highest level. Typically, at least 1 or 2 years of research are undertaken after completing basic surgical training and membership exams, in order to increase the chances of entering into higher specialist training.

Research is designed and conducted to create new knowledge, while audit is designed to assess whether a certain practice reaches a predetermined standard. Another difference is that clinical research requires approval after review by an NHS Research Ethics Committee (REC). There are two ways to conduct research: creating a new research project or applying for a research post with an ongoing research project. Setting up a new project has the advantages of choosing a specific area of personal interest, choosing a supervisor, unit, university, gaining experience of writing grant proposals and obtaining funds as well as demonstrating the confidence, motivation and skills necessary for a surgeon. The participation in an ongoing project has the advantages of usually a respectable salary, the lack of the stress of applying for funding, using tested methods and techniques and thus being an easier start in a research effort.

All research projects require a protocol. This should include sufficient detail not only to inform about the design and methodology of the study but also to provide the opportunity for someone to replicate or continue the study. All research conducted

Fundamentals of Surgical Practice, Third Edition, ed. Andrew N. Kingsnorth and Douglas M. Bowley.
Published by Cambridge University Press. © Cambridge University Press 2011.

within the NHS requires a sponsor. This is the organization which assumes responsibility for the quality and conduct of the research. Sponsors are also responsible for the scientific review of the study. They should be identified at the early stages of a research project since they may have special requirements regarding the study protocol in order to assess the quality of the study. The next step is applying for funding. There are organizations which offer prestigious research fellowship grants such as the Medical Research Council, the Wellcome Trust, the Royal College of Surgeons, etc. The final step before starting a project is gaining ethical approval by the NHS REC and research and development (R&D) department approval by the trust where the research is going to be conducted. This process may take up to 3 months and most of the time involves revisions of the research project according to the requirements of the REC. The RECs have lay and expert members whose role is to ensure that the project will cause no harm to the research subjects but will also not create any problems for the investigators. One of the most important parts of an application going through a REC is the Patient Information Leaflet (PIL). It is important because it is the main channel of communication between the investigators and the potential research participants. Therefore it has to be written clearly and in lay terms. The guidelines of the National Research Ethics Service (NRES) in the UK highlight that the PIL has to be written in such a way that an intelligent 12-year-old child can understand it. The PIL must also be truthful, explain the potential advantages of participating in the study as well as (very importantly) any potential risks and problems, allow the participants to have free access of communication to the investigators and explain to the participants their rights and options should something go wrong with the study. Proper independent scientific peer review of the study, the protection of the anonymity of the research participants and of the confidentiality of the data collected, the legitimacy of the funding of the study and ensuring that research subjects participate in the study freely and without coercion are some of the other main concerns of a REC.

Essentially there are two types of research methods: quantitative and qualitative research, although both methods may be used in the same research project. In quantitative research information is collected in the form of measurements or numbers that can be analysed statistically in order to determine whether there is a difference between them. Data may be collected

Table 6.1. Levels of evidence and grade of guideline recommendations

Level	Type of evidence:
1a	Evidence obtained from meta-analysis of randomized trials
1b	Evidence obtained from at least one randomized trial
2a	Evidence obtained from one well-designed controlled study without randomization
2b	Evidence obtained from at least one other type of well-designed quasi-experimental study
3	Evidence obtained from well-designed non-experimental studies, such as comparative studies, correlation studies and case reports
4	Evidence obtained from expert committee reports or opinions or clinical experience of respected authorities

Grade	Nature of recommendations:
A	Based on clinical studies of good quality and consistency addressing the specific recommendations and including at least one randomized trial
B	Based on well-conducted clinical studies but without randomized clinical trials
C	Made despite the absence of directly applicable clinical studies of good quality

in a retrospective manner, which offers speed since the results are already present but with lower scientific value compared with prospective studies, which are designed to accumulate results in the future and have a higher scientific validity. Qualitative research consists of the investigation of processes between patterns of behaviour, people's emotions or their responses to certain situations. It uses different ways than quantitative analysis for data collection such as words or phrases expressed by people in interviews or focus groups and employs specialized non-mathematical analysis.

There are several types of quantitative research related to different levels of evidence and leading to different grades of guidelines/recommendations (Table 6.1).

• A case study is a report of a single case, i.e. how one patient responded to treatment.
• A cross-sectional study involves the observation of a specific population at one point in time, e.g. how a group of patients responded to treatment.
• Cohort studies involve the following up of the same group of subjects over a period of time in order to observe how their condition is progressing or to investigate whether exposure to a particular risk results in a health problem later.

- Clinical trials compare the way different groups of patients respond to a new treatment.
- A controlled clinical trial compares patients receiving a course of new treatment with others receiving conventional, no treatment or placebo (controls), in order to assess the effects of the new treatment. The scientific validity of such a trial is increased by assigning participants to each group in random order in a process called randomization. Another step of ensuring that a study is objective is the process of blinding (or masking). Blinding is used to eliminate bias from either the patient or the researcher. In a single-blind study, patients are not aware whether they are assigned to the treatment or the control group but researchers have this information. In a double-blind study neither patients nor researchers have such information, which is known to a third party not directly involved in the trial. Double-blind, randomized controlled trials have very high scientific validity.
- A meta-analysis has the highest level of evidence in scientific research (Table 6.1). It is a statistical technique for amalgamating, summarizing and reviewing previous quantitative research. The reported results of primary studies are entered into a database and they are meta-analysed in order to test certain hypotheses. It provides a systematic overview of quantitative research which has examined a particular question with maximum objectivity. The main advantage is that it combines all the available research in one topic into one large study; however, the disadvantage of combining a large set of different studies may be imprecise results and difficulty in their interpretation. A meta-analysis is a study of studies and it can be as good or as bad as the studies which are meta-analysed.

Clinical trials for testing innovative treatments or new medicinal products are conducted in three phases. In Phase I trials, researchers test a new treatment or product in a small group of research subjects in order to evaluate its safety. In Phase II trials a larger number of subjects are involved and the trial aims mainly to test the effectiveness and secondarily the safety of the treatment or product. In Phase III trials much larger groups of research subjects are involved, aiming to confirm the treatment's or drug's effectiveness and monitor its side effects. Pharmaceutical companies also conduct post-marketing or Phase IV studies to examine longer-term and more widespread use of a new drug.

Principles of clinical audit

Clinical audit is a quality improvement process, which systematically compares current practice with available scientific evidence. Its aim is to improve patient care and treatment outcomes. Aspects of structure, processes and outcomes of care may be systematically evaluated. Changes are implemented and further monitoring is necessary to confirm improvement in healthcare delivery.

A classic historical example is the efforts of Florence Nightingale in the Crimean War, who managed to reduce mortality from 40% to 2% in a military hospital in Scutari, by using clinical audit. In a hospital setting someone may encounter a list of audits of particular importance such as the National Institute for Health and Clinical Excellence's (NICE) guideline audits, re-audits of previous projects or national audits, without excluding a young doctor's own fresh ideas. A basic audit project consists of five components:

- selecting standards
- collecting data
- comparing the data collected with standards
- identifying changes
- implementing changes.

A clinical audit project may have positive implications not only for patients' care but for a surgeon-in-training's curriculum vitae as well. The first crucial step that a surgeon should take to conduct a robust audit is the generation of a specific and clinically interesting idea. Such ideas are usually the result of debate or concern among clinicians following review of complicated clinical cases (especially those with unfortunate outcome), reviewing of complaints, attending risk management or clinical governance meetings. The next step is to find the appropriate supervisor who will not only be willing to guide a young surgeon to undertake such a project but also have the necessary expertise to assist in all stages. Another step is to find a team interested in the same project. Colleagues may get involved by either sharing the same enthusiasm about a specific idea or by being potentially affected by the outcomes of the clinical audit project. Furthermore, standards of care have to be set according to the existing evidence. These usually are described in the NICE guidelines, the

Royal Colleges' guidelines, trust or departmental local policies and guidelines produced by special bodies and associations for every specialty. Most audit projects do not require ethical approval as long as they do not alter patients' care in any way and protect their confidentiality. The next step is data collection and data analysis. Data may be recorded either prospectively, which produces better quality, or retrospectively, which may have adequate power if a bigger sample is generated in less time. Results should be either presented in meetings or turned into publications. Implementing the results of an audit programme is the most difficult part. Opinion leaders and people with influence as well as the whole team of healthcare professionals involved in the audit process should support such results in order for them to be put into practice effectively. Re-evaluation is the final step, aiming to re-assess the changes that have taken place as a result of the audit in order to consolidate the implementation of such practice.

Informed consent

The process of obtaining informed consent requires surgeons to provide a patient with all relevant information about a proposed treatment/procedure/operation, allow him/her to freely ask questions and offer him/her adequate time and space to understand the information and sign the consent form without pressure/coercion. Obtaining consent is one of the most important aspects of daily surgical practice, which puts the trust and relationship between doctor and patient to the test and affects the communication between the surgeon and patient, including the latter's family or friends. The essential information that should be provided is:

- the nature of the procedure
- the benefits
- the risks
- the availability of alternative treatment (including no treatment) and its risks and benefits.

The surgeon should explain clearly and in detail the steps of a certain procedure (including information about the type of anaesthetic that is going to be used), as well as any alternative therapeutic means available. The patient needs to be informed clearly regarding the potential benefits of the proposed surgical intervention. Although it is totally inappropriate and unethical to raise expectations and 'paint a rosy picture' regarding the potential benefits, it is very important

to present to the patient a clear and positive idea as to what he/she should expect from the proposed surgical procedure. In general, the patient should be informed of common risks even if they are not serious, as well as of very serious risks such as death, even if they are not common. For the process to be more clinically sound and ethically acceptable, data should be presented to the patient not only from the literature but also from the actual results of the specific surgical team. Patients should be respected as competent and equal partners with different areas of expertise. Patients' perception of their experience of their illness should be respected. At the end of the fact and evidence presentation, the patient should be asked whether he/she requires any more general or specific information on the topic discussed, often not obvious to the surgeon. When discussing risk with patients, one has to understand that the mere citation of statistical figures may be meaningless to them, while the relation to more meaningful facts may be more helpful, e.g. the approximately 1 in 100 000 risk of death during general anaesthesia in a healthy patient can be compared to the risk of death in a car accident (of about 1 in 20 000 per year in the UK).

The influence exerted by the surgeon on a patient during the informed consent process may appear in three forms:

- coercion
- manipulation
- persuasion.

Coercion is the presentation of credible threat to the patient and is always clearly unethical. Manipulation involves the presentation of incomplete or untruthful information such as lying, deliberately omitting vital facts or deceiving the patient. This is equally unethical and inappropriate. Persuasion is the presentation of a rational argument regarding a choice and is permissible and, one might argue, even desirable during the consent process. Patients recognize that surgeons have expertise and their advice is most of the time welcomed and respected. Sometimes surgeons may have to respect a patient's choice of 'not wanting to know anything about a procedure' by exhibiting confidence in their surgeon's skills. Patients have the right to refuse to obtain information and their autonomy must be respected. Furthermore, patients may ask their surgeon about his/her choice if he/she had to face the same treatment/procedure/operation. In that case the response should be truthful since usually such a suggestion is the one the patient will choose. The idea that information may harm patients and cause distress is often cited as a reason for making the discussion regarding the risks of anaesthesia and surgery superficial and without detail. Patients should be asked whether it is their personal will to receive information in such a way, although it has never been proved that patients who receive detailed information experience increased stress levels.

In emergency situations, patients have the right to make choices regarding their treatment just as in elective cases. When patients are incapacitated it is important to seek the advice of surrogate decision-makers such as family members, or others who know the patient and his or her personal preferences. If it is impossible to obtain consent from such individuals, the surgeon should act in the best interests of the patient until such a surrogate is found. Apart from the incapacitated or sedated patient, other situations in which a patient's ability to make treatment decisions is questioned are:

- patients with known mental illness
- patients with organic brain disease
- minors or patients with learning difficulties.

In such cases a surrogate or a carer of the patient should be given the necessary information in order to decide on the course of treatment. Patient immaturity can be relevant when the patient is of a very young age and presumed not to have the mental and cognitive capacity to make meaningful decisions or has serious learning difficulties which impair cognitive development. Neither condition in itself precludes the participation of the patient in decision-making. However, expert consultation may be needed in order to determine whether the patient is capable of understanding his/her health status and options and any information should be presented to such patients in an appropriate, tactful and meaningful way. Legislation determines when a minor can give legal consent; however, it does not address the issue of when it is ethically acceptable for a minor patient to be invited to participate in the informed consent process.

In summary, informed consent protects the patient by providing him/her with adequate and appropriate information based on which he/she can agree that an operation should go ahead. It also protects the surgeon from financial liability provided that the procedure is properly executed according to the prevailing standard of care and without negligence.

Principles of clinical ethics

Medical ethics are 'those obligations of a moral nature which govern the practice of medicine'. Ethical codes and guidelines date back to the origins of medicine in virtually all civilizations. Medical practitioners of each era and culture have developed oaths and codes that bind new physicians to the profession through agreement with the principles of conduct towards their patients and colleagues as well as society. The Hippocratic Oath, which medical students in many countries take upon graduation, is probably the most enduring medical code of practice in Western civilization. Surgeons are increasingly encountering clinical issues in the constantly changing clinical, technical, legal and economic landscape of modern surgical practice. In the last decade, interest in the field of medical ethics has expanded rapidly and this is reflected in the marked increase in the relevant textbooks, journals and public seminars.

Many of the ethical issues mentioned in the Hippocratic Oath, such as beneficence, non-maleficence, confidentiality, prohibition of abortion, euthanasia and relationships with patients, influence the basis for contemporary codes of practice. The first universal code on human research, the Nuremberg Code, was developed after World War II, as a consequence of the human experiments performed by the Nazis. This Code emphasizes the patient's right to know, to choose and the right not to be harmed. In modern practice there are mainly four principles governing the healthcare professional–patient relationship:

- autonomy
- non-maleficence
- beneficence
- justice.

Autonomy is the first principle, which is the capacity to think and act independently without any obstacle, in other words self-governance without constraint from another individual. Non-maleficence is the intentional avoidance of causing harm to a patient and beneficence is not only the protection of a patient from harm but also the provision of benefit after some form of treatment. Justice is the fair and equitable provision of available medical resources. There are three types of moral conduct:

1. Deontological or duty-based moral conduct is based on the principle that 'I am doing something because I believe it is the right thing to do'. As an

extreme example, a doctor committed to such moral principles would try to preserve human life at all costs (human life is sacred and has to be prolonged by using all means available to us) even if the patient has most probably nothing to gain and can even suffer because of such a decision; he/she will try even invasive treatments in an elderly and terminally ill patient with generalized carcinomatosis who will probably benefit more from just palliative care.

2. Utilitarian or goal-based moral principles accept as ethical any action that aims to achieve the best possible outcome with the minimum possible cost. Based on these principles, and again as an extreme example, healthcare resources should be allocated to a treatment that allows longer survival of more patients even if this means seriously depriving and disadvantaging other patients.

3. The dominant contemporary approach, which is also the cornerstone of medical law and clinical practice, is rights-based morality. Such an approach condemns any violation of the patient's rights, gives paramount emphasis to the respect of the patient's autonomy and accepts as ethical any clinical action that aims to serve the patient's best interests. In modern times emphasis is also given to the importance and the effectiveness of the partnership between all parties involved: patients and their families, healthcare professionals and the institutions (national or private) involved in healthcare provision.

As a characteristic example of the application of clinical ethics in modern surgical practice we will examine one of the 'hottest' ethical debates regarding the issue of commercialization of live donor kidney transplantation, which is clearly considered as the treatment of choice of end stage renal failure.

In the United Kingdom, an Act of Parliament in 1990 made the sale of organs illegal. This Act was produced after a General Medical Council enquiry into the case of a British physician's involvement in transplants involving Turkish peasants. In the United States, the transplant team is responsible for determining and assessing the motives of the donor and the sale of organs is illegal, as is the case in most countries around the world. Yet, the shortage of cadaveric organs has led to a worldwide black market in living donor organs, with patients who possess the necessary means travelling to distant locations in order

to purchase a kidney for transplantation. For example in Bombay, India, the price for a woman's kidney is alleged to be $1000; in Manila, the Philippines, a man's kidney is said to be $2000; and in urban Latin America a kidney can be sold for more than $10 000, with additional payments to the brokers in all these cases. While Americans are purchasing kidneys from strangers in China, Peru and the Philippines, the current federal law does not prevent these patients from returning back to the United States for post-transplantation care. Furthermore, there are also allegations that affluent patients from other countries have paid at least $200 000 to undergo transplantation at US centres, as part of a package prearranged outside the United States by international brokers, including compensation of unrelated donors.

On one hand we consider the purchase of organs a hideous act (deontological ethical approach), yet on the other hand we are obliged to consider ways to increase the live donor pool (utilitarian ethical approach). Some of the arguments and counter-arguments related to the commercialization of organ donation are as follows:

(a) It is unethical to sell your body or your organs since life is sacred and every human being is special. Organs cannot be regarded as commodities for sale. For the same reasons that we cannot accept prostitution and child trading, we cannot endorse commerce in human organs. Some might counter-argue that in a free society, one is entitled to do anything one wants, including selling one's organs, as long as one is not restricting the liberty of one's fellow citizens.

(b) A poor donor is compelled by his financial status to donate, thus making his action not voluntary. Yet, he may be choosing the best from a list of bad options, since it carries significantly less risk than working, for example, under harsh and dangerous conditions, as well as offering him the satisfaction of contributing to the well-being of the recipient. Although the recipient may be taking advantage of the donor's difficult economic situation, this will not improve by refusing donation.

(c) Paid donors are, in the majority, poor and less educated, thus possibly unable to understand the risks involved. But someone could easily argue that it is the surgeon's duty to explain the whole procedure as simply and clearly as possible, as well as to clarify every question raised by the potential donor.

(d) Another argument against the commercialization of donation is that the rich will eventually have access to organs while the poor will not. However, it is also a fact of life that since private healthcare exists, the rich are able to buy better conditions of care than the poor.

(e) The sale of organs may also cause exploitation of donors and recipients by unscrupulous middlemen and surgeons. Yet, such practice may increase even more in an illegal uncontrolled environment, resulting in the provision of inferior medical care. The financial exploitation of donors could be avoided if donation was supervised and controlled by a national agency which would allocate organs nationally according to best tissue type match and clinical need criteria as well as maintaining the anonymity of the donor–recipient relationship. In such a setting, safety for the donor and the recipient would be guaranteed with better pre-, intra- and postoperative care for them. However, if such a policy is applied on a larger scale it may lead to differences in financial compensation between transplant centres and even countries, resulting in 'donation tourism' from poor to wealthy areas of the world. Other researchers have also proposed a closely regulated and supervised market of organs, claiming that we do not regard it as any the less caring a profession because doctors are paid. Since the long-term cost of kidney transplantation is less than that of dialysis, the government or medical insurance organizations would save money. It has also been proposed that wealthier patients could make financial contributions to a general and independent fund that would pay the potential donors, thus reducing the cost for the government even more. The initial selection and screening of the potential donor could be performed by an independent physician/surgeon and then the transplant centre could have the right to reject him/her, after consulting a specialist on medical ethics. The paid donor would not be able to select a specific recipient.

(f) Another argument against commercial donation is that the poor will be unable to handle money, comparing this with some experience gained from lottery winners, thus making in the long term no difference to their poverty. The possibility of misuse of the money paid for donation, although difficult to predict, could not justify overriding the donor's decision.

(g) Transplantation has always relied on the altruism of donors and paid donation may lead to the disappearance of altruistic donation since it is possible that eventually all donors will request to be paid.

(h) Even if we manage to regulate the sale of organs, there is always the fear that some people will take it to the extreme and add to the existing stories of street children from the developing world who have been kidnapped and killed for their organs.

(i) It is argued that living donation involves a 'highly artificial enforced altruism' according to which everyone is paid, including the transplant team, the transplant coordinator and the recipient, who gains an important benefit, and only the donor is required to be altruistic. However, we have to acknowledge that those involved professionally with the transplant procedure do not receive extra payment for every transplant they perform and ultimately it is their job to perform it.

(j) We could consider the scenario of an impoverished father who has a daughter ill with leukaemia, to whom if she had renal failure he would have donated his kidney. It could be morally acceptable for some clinical ethicists to sell his kidney in order to earn money to pay for her treatment. However, the counter-argument is that in such cases a well organized national health service should be able to provide the necessary resources and financial assistance for them.

(k) Others consider as an act of paternalism the fact that the rich are free to engage in dangerous sports for pleasure and the poor are denied the smaller risk of selling a kidney which may even save another life and help them with their financial situation. It is true that if kidney sales are allowed rich people will have opportunities for medical care unavailable to the poor, but this is a reality in many areas of medical care around the world and by outlawing such sales the social inequities will not be corrected.

The debate is tough and interesting and, as is always the case in clinical ethics, there is no straightforward right or wrong answer. What is of paramount importance is the active, genuine and ever evolving participation of all parties involved.

Another characteristic example of intense ethical debate is the use of stem cells in modern research and clinical practice. There is not much debate regarding the use of adult stem cells since they are retrieved from blood/bone marrow of adults who can give a properly informed consent. The debate can get particularly heated regarding the use of stem cells derived from embryos. Embryonic stem cells are primitive cells which possess distinct properties. These cells are unspecialized and so can either renew themselves through cell division or have the ability to become cells with a specific function by differentiation, if induced under appropriate conditions. Theoretically, they have much more potential compared to adult stem cells; they can potentially differentiate into any type of cell and cure any type of disease. The biggest ethical clash is regarding the very principle of the use of embryonic stem cells. There is the camp with the strong deontological views: an embryo is life in whatever stage of development, life is sacred and therefore embryos cannot be used for stem cell research even if this aims to help suffering humans. The other camp with equally strong feelings is the utilitarian camp: using embryos which are going to be discarded anyway (i.e. unused IVF embryos or spontaneously aborted fetuses) is totally ethically acceptable since it is going to advance research that has the potential to offer better treatment for a wide range of diseases. The deontological camp present stories of unused IVF embryos being adopted by couples and finally beautiful babies came to life giving enormous and unexpected joy to their parents. The utilitarian camp present the shocking stories of young people on wheelchairs after an accident or suffering from Parkinson's disease who can potentially have their lives changed completely should something positive come out of embryonic stem cell research. There is obviously no easy solution or compromise. What is of utmost importance for any healthcare professional and especially surgeons is to actively join the debate. We would consider this not to be optional, but rather a duty toward our patients.

Another aspect of modern surgery with a significant ethical dimension is the introduction of new innovative surgical technologies. By definition surgical innovation is 'the execution of a previously untried and untested procedure in the hopeful expectation that it will help the patients concerned while also being aware that it may endanger them'. But is the application of new surgical technologies aimed always for the benefit of the patients? Examples are not hard to find since the introduction of laparoscopic surgery; robotic surgery was considered by many to be corporate-driven in the beginning. Results of randomized trials comparing old and new techniques become known sometimes many years after their application. Thus, although innovation should not be discouraged, scientific principles and ethical guidelines should be followed. Patients should be informed whether a procedure is innovative or research and provided with data regarding the actual experience of a specific surgeon or centre. Sometimes companies advertise new techniques and instruments so vigorously that patients ask for them without being aware of the results, believing that modern is better. Surgeons must be honest regarding the outcomes for their patients as their experience increases with new techniques and modalities.

Conclusion

Modern surgery is not just about 'cutting and stitching'. Surgical trainees need to develop a broad and robust persona, being able to advance their clinical practice through their own research, monitor and evaluate their work and practice evidence-based surgery, develop proper interpersonal skills so that they can develop healthy channels of communication with their patients and get involved actively and positively in the important ethical debates regarding modern surgical practice. Only then will they come much closer to becoming, as Albert Schweitzer said, 'one of those that the world truly needs'.

Further reading

Choudhry S et al. Unrelated living organ donation: ULTRA needs to go. J Med Ethics 2003;**29**(3):169–170.

Delmonico FL et al. Ethical incentives–not payment–for organ donation. N Engl J Med 2002;**346**(25):2002–2005.

de Wert G, Mummery C. Human embryonic stem cells: research, ethics and policy. Hum Reprod 2003;**18**(4):672–682.

Dickstein E, Erlen J. Ethical principles contained in currently professed medical oaths. Acad Med 1991;**66**: 622–624.

Harris J. In praise of unprincipled ethics. J Med Ethics 2003;**29**(5):303–306.

Hou S. Expanding the kidney donor pool: ethical and medical considerations. *Kidney Int* 2000;**58**(4):1820–1836.

Levine DZ. Kidney vending: 'Yes!' or 'No!' *Am J Kidney Dis* 2000;**35**(5):1002–1018.

Lo B, Zettler P, Cedars MI, Gates E, Kriegstein AR, Oberman M *et al.* A new era in the ethics of human embryonic stem cell research. *Stem Cells* 2005;**23**(10): 1454–1459.

Mansell MA. The ethics of rewarded kidney donation. *BJU Int* 2004;**93**(9):1171–1172.

Radcliffe-Richards J, Daar AS, Guttmann RD, Hoffenberg R, Kennedy I, Lock M *et al.* The case for allowing kidney sales. International Forum for Transplant Ethics. *Lancet* 1998;**351**(9120):1950–1952.

Scheper-Hughes N. The global traffic in human organs 1. *Curr Anthropol* 2000;**41**(2):191–224.

Schlitt HJ. Paid non-related living organ donation: Horn of Plenty or Pandora's box? *Lancet* 2002;**359**(9310):906–907.

Towns CR, Jones DG. Stem cells, embryos, and the environment: a context for both science and ethics. *J Med Ethics* 2004;**30**(4):410–413.

Tung T, Organ CH. Ethics in surgery. Historical perspective. *Arch Surg* 2000;**135**:10–13.

Chapter

7

Fundamentals of palliative and end of life care

Chantal Meystre and Riffatt Hussein

Introduction

The palliative care patient is not defined by disease process, body system, age, or care setting, but by entry to the final common pathway of dying, expected to do so within the next 12 to 18 months. Palliative care professionals therefore require wide-ranging clinical skills and experience, with access to a range of expertise within an extended team.

Palliative care grew out of the modern hospice movement established by Dame Cecily Saunders (1918–2005) with the opening of St Christopher's at Sydenham, London, in 1964. Seeing the need, when practising as an almoner and nurse at St Thomas's Hospital, London, she decided change in care of the dying would only come from within the medical profession and retrained as a doctor. She gained postgraduate experience at St Joseph's in Hackney, observing the efficacy of opioids for end of life pain relief. Stepping outside the norms of medical care, Dame Cecily established an organization with a flatter hierarchical structure and multi-professional teams. St Christopher's took the most complex cases and developed an expertise in caring for the dying that has now been replicated in hospices throughout the world. In 1967, she coined the term 'Total Pain' having observed the physical, psychological, social, emotional and spiritual dimensions of pain, each of which may need addressing to effect resolution and control. This formed the ethos of holistic palliative care now enshrined in the World Health Organization's (2008) definition.

WHO definition of palliative care

Palliative care is an approach that improves the quality of life of patients and their families facing the prob-lems associated with life-threatening illness, through the prevention and relief of suffering by means of early identification and impeccable assessment and treatment of pain and other problems, physical, psychosocial and spiritual. Palliative care:

- provides relief from pain and other distressing symptoms
- affirms life and regards dying as a normal process
- intends neither to hasten nor postpone death
- integrates the psychological and spiritual aspects of patient care
- offers a support system to help patients live as actively as possible until death
- offers a support system to help the family cope during the patient' illness and in their own bereavement
- uses a team approach to address the needs of patients and their families, including bereavement counselling, if indicated
- will enhance quality of life, and may also positively influence the course of illness
- is applicable early in the course of illness, in conjunction with other therapies that are intended to prolong life, such as chemotherapy or radiation therapy, and includes those investigations needed to better understand and manage distressing clinical complications.

The success of palliative care and the paucity of hospice provision has led to the outreach of skilled palliative care personnel into acute and community settings over the last three decades. Palliative Medicine was accepted as a subspecialty by the Royal College of Physicians in 1987 and now has a defined curriculum and career pathway of training.

Fundamentals of Surgical Practice, Third Edition, ed. Andrew N. Kingsnorth and Douglas M. Bowley.
Published by Cambridge University Press. © Cambridge University Press 2011.

The palliative care team (PC team)

Palliative care is included in the Cancer Network organization as laid out in the Cancer Plan in 2000 and the NICE Guidance for Supportive and Palliative Care in 2004. This means service specification and team components were defined but the constituents of teams vary considerably between settings and geographical areas. This is largely due to the piecemeal development of services and the mix of statutory and voluntary providers that is peculiar to palliative care.

Core team members are usually:

palliative medicine consultant
clinical nurse specialist
administrative support.

Extended team members may include:

pharmacist
social worker
occupational therapist
physiotherapist
chaplain
psychologist/counsellor
dietician
complementary therapist
volunteers.

It would be usual to have access to:

pain services
oncology
neurosurgery for metastatic spinal cord
    compression
orthopaedics for bone metastases
speech and language therapy.

The function of the PC team is to support and improve the palliative care skills of all groups of hospital staff through outreach and education and to provide expert specialist advice for patients and families with complex physical, psychological emotional, social and spiritual concerns. The aim of palliative care is to work holistically with the patient in the context of his/her social relationships, improving what is amenable to change in all spheres and promoting acceptance and endurance of what cannot be altered. Scrupulous attention to detail in clinical care can lead to an overall improvement for the patient with surprising results. One of the highest skills of palliative care is to continue to see the patient as a person to the end and assisting them to maintain their social roles. Practised effectively, this transferable skill is enabling and contagious. Most hospital PC teams act as an advisory service and do not take over the care of the patient but become an extended part of the surgical team.

Teamwork

Fundamental to palliative care is effective teamwork. Multidisciplinary teams work by each individual discipline contributing its expertise, with hierarchical leadership weaving all the interdependent inputs into the plan of care. Success requires cooperation, shared values and defined goals. When teams work well a wide range of problems can be addressed, engendering confidence and containing distress. Interdisciplinary teams work by team identity being more important than the professional role of team members. Leadership is shared and passes between team members, depending on the problem in hand. Team members share learning and are able to participate in each other's roles. These teams are the most effective although professional maturity is required to ensure that the most able professional deals with the most challenging problems.

Self-care

Avoiding distancing as a defence and being open to the vicissitudes of dying patients exposes clinicians to death, to a degree that is unusual within our modern schema, where death is more usually seen as part of entertainment, often with attendant violence, and unlikely to affect the reality of life. Working closely with death in a death-denying culture can cause distress and isolation, reactivate old grief, and cause confusion if an unconscious transferential attachment to a patient becomes painful. Unaddressed emotional pain encountered in the course of duty can cause loss of efficacy and function. Clinical supervision, beyond the technical learning for our chosen specialty, is unusual in medicine; although mandatory within the talking therapies and social work. Supervision aims to promote the professional development of the supervisee and their patient relationships. Whilst it may benefit the supervisee therapeutically this is not the main aim. Many doctors regard psychological supervision as suspect and those requiring it flawed. The high rates of stress, burnout, alcohol and drug abuse, divorce and suicide amongst surgeons suggest attention to self-care in supervision may not be a wasted effort.

Demographics and strategy

The NHS has been in existence for more than 60 years. This cradle to grave service is having to adapt to the changing demographics brought about by advances in medical care. In 1948, the product was largely cure and if cure were possible, there was little argument to withhold treatment. Now, increasingly, the product is care and just because a treatment is possible it may not be the appropriate course of action. Demographic changes are leading to an increase in sections of the population classed as old (>65) and very old (>80) and a decrease in the 40–60-year-old population who bear the burden of care for the elderly as volunteers and lay carers. Falling rates of cardiovascular deaths in those over 65 years of age are leading to an increase in the very old and the emergence of higher rates of death from diseases that have increased prevalence in very old age, e.g. dementia. The baby boomer effect will increase the very old population after 2028. It is estimated that by 2050 the percentage of population over 80 will have doubled to 10% and of those over 65 almost 40% will be over 80.

In July 2008, the Department of Health (DoH) launched its first End of Life Care Strategy. The strategy addresses the need for forward planning in commissioning and developing quality services with secure funding. The strategy also addresses the disappointment of many over the delivery of end of life care, as reflected in complaints, and the mismatch between patients' preferred place of death (70% would choose to die at home) and the place they actually die (58% die in hospital). It notes that care of the dying is a societal litmus test; death with dignity and respect and support for carers should be universal. The Strategy includes engagement of the population in discussion about death and dying in its aims. Choice, care planning, education and training with measurement and research and development of joined-up community services are given profile.

What is the relevance of this to the trainee surgeon? Surgeons diagnose and care for many patients who are incurable from the outset, or later become so. In the course of this care patients come to trust their surgeon and to look to them for advice about treatment, perhaps particularly when further treatment has

a reversed benefit/burden ratio and the focus is changing to palliation of symptoms.

Advance care planning

Despite increasingly open requests for euthanasia it remains unlawful in the UK and the new advice regarding prosecution for assisting suicide is as yet untested. There is, however, clear guidance on advance care planning and advance decisions to refuse treatment that is helpful in forward planning with patients and relatives who have clear views about their future care. As public engagement increases these tools will be useful to surgeons planning with patients and carers, but will be invaluable to the surgeon faced with an ill patient without mental capacity. The Mental Capacity Act (MCA) (2005) for England and Wales gives legal force to patient autonomy and, if conditions are fulfilled, gives a patient who may lose capacity in the future a mechanism to refuse treatment in foreseen circumstances that has equal legality to a current refusal of consent. The MCA does not give the right to opt into treatments.

Advance care planning (ACP) is a function applicable to all patients and is used to increase the chance of patient choice being fulfilled. It is known to be acceptable to patients whose condition is stable; it increases patient satisfaction with care but can be distressing if tackled at points of transition. Sixty to ninety per cent of the general public agree with ACP but only 8% have addressed it in writing. Some terminal and hospitalized patients find the discussion difficult. ACP is not mandatory and patients should not be traumatized by a staff imperative to have pathway objectives fulfilled for outcomes measurement. Experience of such targets may be why doctors are the group that have the most reservations about ACP being helpful.

Advance care planning is best approached within managed realization of incurability. It should be a partnership between patient, care provider and informal carers so that realistic options are planned for as specifically as possible. It may take many discussions, with time for thought between, to achieve a robust plan. Outpatient visits may be an ideal opportunity to plan with stable patients. Surgical advice is key for many patients, especially to understand nuances such as the impossibility of resection of a bowel cancer but the relevance of palliative defunctioning surgery in the case of bowel obstruction. Such a patient should rightly present to acute services for further intervention. It is often plain to surgeons that for many patients even if bowel obstruction occurs there will be no benefit from surgical intervention. The latter patient, forewarned, can be prepared to receive conservative management and may prefer to plan not to be moved away from home. In this way ACP helps to allow patients the choice of a home death and has benefits in effective service utilization.

Different forms of advance statements are acceptable and do not need to be in writing. They should always be taken into consideration, but patient preferred goal/outcome statements, rather than specific preferences in specific circumstances, may be hard to interpret in the surgical context.

The MCA provides a mechanism for advance decisions to refuse treatment (ADRT) that are specific to foreseen circumstances and, if valid and applicable, are binding upon clinicians. They come into force if capacity is lost. Despite clinician fears, as yet there are no data showing increased death rates or worse care where ADRTs have been used.

ADRTs are valid if the patient is over 18 and not detained under the Mental Health Act (1983). If the ADRT is a refusal of life-saving treatments this needs to be explicitly stated, including recognition that death may be the outcome, and in this circumstance they need to be written, signed, dated and witnessed. ADRTs are applicable only to the circumstance for which they are written, so conferring with a clinical advisor to ensure clarity and applicability is wise.

When considering a valid ADRT the surgeon needs to test its applicability to current circumstance and investigate whether recent behaviour demonstrates consistency of expression of the view. Friends and family may be a valuable source of information if time permits seeking them out. One-third of ADRTs change over time so note needs to be taken of the date it was signed and whether the person would have been aware of advances in treatment outcomes in the interval.

ADRTs can refuse artificial nutrition and hydration but cannot refuse other basic care. Specific treatments cannot be demanded; neither can a place of care be specified, nor can an ADRT be used to justify an illegal procedure such as euthanasia.

Next of kin decisions have no formal authority in English law, but an alternative to an ADRT is available within the MCA by lodging a Lasting Power of Attorney (LPA) for a specific person with the Office of the Public Guardian. This has considerable cost implica-

tions, and as at January 2010 only 100 000 have been registered.

The rights invested in the LPA can be specified to cover serious medical decisions as well as social and welfare. A registered LPA covering health decisions invalidates a pre-existing ADRT. A person invested with a LPA has the legal right to make decisions on behalf of the patient. Careful choice and regular discussion is therefore important.

Where capacity is lost, and no ADRT or LPA is available, the surgeon can apply directly to the Court of Protection (available 24/7) for a court-appointed deputy (CAD) to make decisions on the patient's behalf. In less urgent circumstances, or where no family or friends are available, or care is disputed, an independent mental capacity advocate (IMCA) can be contacted through Trust governance departments to advise on best-interest discussions within NHS and local authority care about residence or treatment. IMCAs do not make proxy decisions, and independent hospices and independent hospitals are not obliged to access their services.

The MCA introduced criminal offences of wilful neglect and ill treatment that can carry prison sentences. Faced with this knowledge how does a surgeon respond to an incapacitated patient with an urgent surgical problem?

The MCA is drafted to support doctors preserving life. Where capacity is in doubt there is helpful guidance on procedure (see Figure 7.1). Each individual decision requires a separate capacity assessment. Individuals who lack the capacity to choose between complex treatment options may well be capable of less complex decisions such as choosing between types of anaesthetic and their place of care. Efforts to enable capacity are to be used and supported by communication aids in accessible, understandable form. Eccentric or unwise decisions do not, per se, imply lack of capacity; neither do age, religion, class, behaviour or beliefs different from the norm.

The healthcare professional is protected from prosecution if practical and appropriate steps have been taken, an ADRT has not been found, or its validity and/or applicability is suspect, and the patient has been treated. Equally where it was reasonable to believe an ADRT to be valid and applicable and a patient was not treated, the surgeon has a defence. Where any doubt exists, an existing advance statement should be considered and a best-interest decision made with

Making best interest decisions in serious medical conditions in patients over 18 years.

Adapted from Regnard, © Regnard, Dean and Hockley, *A Guide to Symptom Relief in Palliative Care* 6e. Oxford: Radcliffe Publishing; 2009. Reproduced with the permission of the copyright holder.

Start by assuming that the patient has capacity. If there is doubt, proceed to the two stage test of capacity:

Stage 1: Does this person have an impairment of, or a disturbance in the functioning of, their mind or brain?

Stage 2: Does the impairment or disturbance mean that the person is unable to make a specific decision when they need to? This is tested as follows:

1 Can they understand the information?
NB this must be imparted in a way the patient can understand

2 Can they retain the information?
NB this only needs to be for long enough to use and weigh the information

3 Can they use or weigh up that information?
NB they must be able to show that they are able to consider the benefits and burdens of the alternatives to the proposed treatment

4 Can they communicate their decision?
NB the carers must try every method possible to enable this

The result of each step of this assessment should be documented, ideally by quoting the patient.

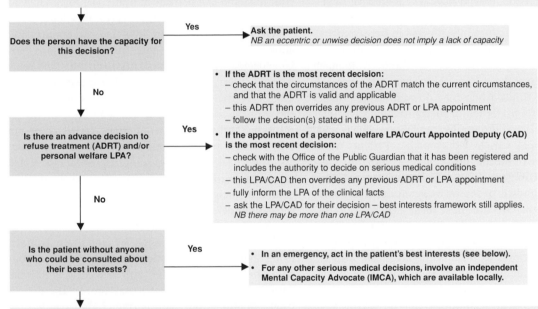

Does the person have the capacity for this decision? — Yes → **Ask the patient.**
NB an eccentric or unwise decision does not imply a lack of capacity

No ↓

Is there an advance decision to refuse treatment (ADRT) and/or personal welfare LPA? — Yes →

- **If the ADRT is the most recent decision:**
  – check that the circumstances of the ADRT match the current circumstances, and that the ADRT is valid and applicable
  – this ADRT then overrides any previous ADRT or LPA appointment
  – follow the decision(s) stated in the ADRT.

- **If the appointment of a personal welfare LPA/Court Appointed Deputy (CAD) is the most recent decision:**
  – check with the Office of the Public Guardian that it has been registered and includes the authority to decide on serious medical conditions
  – this LPA/CAD then overrides any previous ADRT or LPA appointment
  – fully inform the LPA of the clinical facts
  – ask the LPA/CAD for their decision – best interests framework still applies.
  NB there may be more than one LPA/CAD

No ↓

Is the patient without anyone who could be consulted about their best interests? — Yes →

- **In an emergency, act in the patient's best interests (see below).**
- **For any other serious medical decisions, involve an independent Mental Capacity Advocate (IMCA), which are available locally.**

↓

- **Appoint a decision maker** (usually after an interdisciplinary team discussion) who should:
  – encourage the participation of the patient
  – identify all the relevant circumstances
  – find out the person's views (ie wishes, preferences, beliefs and values): these may have been expressed verbally previously, or exist in an ADRT or advance care plan made when the patient had capacity
  – avoid discrimination and avoid making assumptions about the person's quality of life
  – assess whether the person might regain capacity
  – if the decision concerns life-sustaining treatment, not be motivated in any way by a desire to bring about the person's death
  – consult others (within the limits of confidentiality): this may include friends, family, carers, an LPA, IMCA or CAD
  – avoid restricting the persons rights
  – take all of this into account, ie weigh up all of these factors in order to work out the person's best interests.
- **Record the decisions.**

↓

If there are unresolved conflicts, consider involving:

– the local ethics committee
– the Court of Protection, possibly through a CAD.

Figure 7.1 Making best- interest decisions in serious medical conditions in patients over 18 years. Adapted from Regnard, © Regnard, Dean and Hockley, A Guide to Symptom Relief in Palliative Care (6th edn). Oxford: Radcliffe Publishing, 2009. Reproduced with the permission of the copyright holder. CAD = court-appointed deputy; LPA = lasting power of attorney. From Advance Care Planning: National Guidelines Number 12, February 2009. Copyright Royal College of Physicans. All rights reserved.

reference to the family or application for a CAD made to the court at the earliest possible moment.

Communication

To be able to talk openly with patients and their carers requires communication skills so the surgeon can not only help a patient plan for their death, preserving their right to choice, but also influence effective service utilization with cost reduction by avoiding needless hospitalization and reducing life-sustaining intervention where it is not wanted. End of life discussions help patients accept terminal conditions and opt for less intervention. Patients who have less aggressive intervention maintain better quality of life and their relatives are less psychologically affected in bereavement. Whilst patients do not want to talk about the meaning of their illness all the time and may employ avoidance, normalization and comfort-seeking within their social structures at times, when they do want to talk or be given news they prefer senior specialists who have time for them, sit down, use understandable language and are professional, caring and empathic. Patients want full disclosure of the diagnosis and help with information and choosing treatments. The majority of patients are given diagnostic bad news by a consultant surgeon. Junior surgeons are the most likely non-consultant-grade doctors to be involved. Even if not breaking bad news, the junior doctor is likely to be the person the patient chooses to discuss the diagnosis with as they are accessible and informed by contact with the consultant.

Just as surgical techniques can be learnt and improve with practice, delivering satisfying success with patients, so investment in communications skill training pays dividends in promoting the relationship with patients and protecting the clinician from litigation and burn-out. There is evidence that poor communication in cancer care causes psychological distress and morbidity, reduced quality of life and poor adherence to treatment by patients.

Clinicians can fear communicating with patients in case the patient becomes upset and emotional, causing themselves distress and unleashing emotions the clinician will not be able to contain, and questions that are difficult to answer. Clinicians also fear saying the wrong thing and that the consultation will take too long. Being faced with psychological, social and spiritual issues in a busy clinic where there may be no other supportive professional to call on is also a cause for

concern. Lack of emotional support for staff, uncertainty about whose role it is to disclose information and team conflict may all compound the issue.

Patients avoid disclosure of concerns to doctors because they fear losing control and crying. They do not want to burden or upset the doctor who they deem to have an important and exacting job, and would not wish to appear inadequate or ungrateful. When they do try to communicate they fear not having the right words, not knowing the questions to ask, and are often met by distancing from the professional. For example: 'Doctor I am wondering why I am taking so long to get better.' 'Don't worry we will keep you here till your husband can manage at home.' Unfortunately as a result only 20% of patient concerns are elicited.

Gathering information involves open enquiry and allowing the patient enough time to finish answers. Unexpectedly, allowing patients to finish their reply without interruption with a further question usually takes less than one minute and does not prolong the surgical consultation. It will help the patient feel respected and give them confidence in disclosing not only answers to the questions of physical health, but also the social, psychological and spiritual issues that give meaning to their illness and may influence the course of their disease and recovery. Understanding the patient perspective is a crucial part of the two-way communication required in clinical consultations.

Disclosure is encouraged by good eye contact, using open directive questions such as 'How does your pain affect your daily life?' and reflecting emotional answers as encouragement to say more, 'The pain is tragic, doctor.' 'Your pain is tragic? Can you tell me more about that?'

Moments of silence allow patients to take in information and to assess its meaning within their context. Silences feel much longer to the doctor than they do to the patient, who is thinking about what has been said. Silence often precedes a disclosure. A prolonged silence may need to be addressed directly 'I notice you are very quiet, I am wondering if you need time to think or would like to ask a difficult question?'

Patients may frequently give a cue by using emotive language or by tears, body language or anger. Often a simple enquiry reflecting what is observed is enough to help them express their affect. 'I notice you are crying, would you be able to tell me why?' or 'Just at the moment you look very angry. Is that how you are feeling?' When perplexed, honesty can be helpful. 'I can see you are upset and I would like to help but I don't understand what is going on for you just at the moment. Would it help to explain it to me?'

In our experience, patients are rarely rude or undisciplined when faced with distressing circumstances and a professional motivated to help. Teaching communication skills has become a *sine qua non* of undergraduate medical training but it is more likely to be effective once the doctor is practising, when theoretical knowledge can be applied in daily practice.

General principles of breaking bad news:

What constitutes bad news varies between people. It is usual to consider a diagnosis of cancer, progression of disease, death in utero and sudden death of a relative as bad news but for some a diagnosis of cancer that is treatable may be less bad than they had expected, and being told there is no abnormality to be found will stress dysmorphophobic patients. So any discourse may require skilled communication.

Prior to the interview prepare by:

- reading the clinical notes and collating results
- making the appointment and inviting a companion if the patient wishes; it is also helpful to both the patient and the doctor to have a nurse present
- ensuring as much privacy as possible and provide chairs and tissues; this is a challenge on wards but if a separate room is truly out of the question, draw the curtains and sit close to the patient to demonstrate some acknowledgement of confidentiality; where perfection of environment is not attainable patients appreciate most the demonstration of a caring attitude and a listening, competent professional
- avoiding interruptions by having a colleague take the bleep or phone.

At the consultation:

- introduce yourself and any nurse companion
- ascertain relationships of those present and whether the patient would prefer them to stay or have a private consultation
- maintain an attitude of listening and observation for verbal and non-verbal cues
- check the patient understands why you are meeting and find out what they already know; this defines the knowledge gap: 'I wanted to see you both today to talk about your illness. What have you understood about it so far?'

- explain that there is new information, give the patient a cue it may not be what they wish to hear, and ask whether they wish you to continue: 'We have your test results back now and it may not be as good as you were expecting. Would you like me to tell you what they are?'
- use plain language, avoiding jargon such as lesion, shadow, tumour. 'The X-ray looked abnormal and the piece of tissue we took when you had the bronchoscopy unfortunately shows that you have cancer in your lung'
- STOP. At this point it is tempting to soften the blow and rush on to tell the patient all the things that can be done to help, but at this moment the patient is still assimilating the word 'cancer'. If he has had a relative die of lung cancer in the last year he will be distracted by devastating thoughts. If he has friends with successful prostate cancer treatment he may not realize the import of the diagnosis of lung cancer. Check out concerns and questions. 'I have just told you that you have a cancer in your right lung and before we continue I am wondering what your thoughts and reactions are at present.' Then give an opportunity for the patient to ask questions. Summarize what you think are the concerns and questions and ask for clarification if you are correct. 'I understand that your wife has dementia and her care is your main concern, especially as both your sons are studying away from home, so you would like to be in hospital as little as possible. Have I understood you correctly?'
- elicit any unexpressed feelings: 'You looked quite upset when talking about your wife, is that how you are feeling?'
- having heard and responded to the patient's concerns use a transitional statement to go back to the purpose of the interview: 'Caring for your wife is clearly your top priority and we will arrange some help and advice for you both, but now I would like to discuss the best treatment for your cancer. Is that OK with you?'
- give treatment advice and reassurance
- give written information about the disease and self-help contacts
- check understanding and whether the person is ready to end the interview
- it is helpful to allow the patient and carer a few minutes of privacy after the consultation to

recover before having to cope in public; the offer of a nurse to stay with them may be helpful

- once the patient has left, document the discussion and make referrals, including informing the general practitioner within 24 hours if the diagnosis of cancer is a new one; if the news broken is of incurable recurrence the GP needs to know to enter the patient on the primary care end of life register (Gold Standards Framework: see below)
- check out how you are yourself and whether you are ready to go on to the next patient.

It is tempting to soften the bad news with a positive message at the end of the consultation, but not always helpful to the overall objective. 'The good thing is your blood tests are normal' is often interpreted as a cue that the patient has less of a problem than they believed at first, and denial may be encouraged.

It can be difficult to acknowledge the fear a patient expresses but it does not need to be brutal honesty for a therapeutic effect. Here are some examples of helpful replies when tempted to use a distancing platitude:

Patient: 'I do not seem to be getting over this illness.' Tempted to say: 'It's early days yet.' Instead try: 'That must be quite a worry for you, would you like to talk more about it?'

Patient: 'I do not feel life is worth living any more.' Tempted to say: 'Oh but look the sun's out and it's a lovely day.' Instead try: 'That must be very hard for you. Can you tell me what is the worst thing?'

Patient: 'The consultant said I am dying.' Tempted to say: 'Well, we are all dying.' Instead try: 'Does that frighten you? May I sit with you for a while?'

Symptom control

Most patients entering the end of life phase of their illnesses will have physical symptoms the management of which optimizes quality of life and maintenance of activities of daily living. In dying people, symptom control poses a particular challenge due to declining organ systems. Best practice in medicine is based on evidenced intervention. In palliative care populations, research and evidence-gathering is particularly difficult due to the attrition rate of research subjects and the ethical and social implications of studying patients with only a short time to live. There is, however, a body of published evidence and consensus best practice on

which this chapter is based. Much of this relates to patients dying of cancer but is increasingly being found to be applicable to the suffering in non-malignant terminal conditions.

Pain

Pain is defined by The International Association for the Study of Pain as

'an unpleasant sensory and emotional experience associated with actual or potential tissue damage, or described in terms of such damage'.

Nociceptors occur in skin, bone, connective tissue, muscle and viscera, producing an electrical charge in response to noxious stimuli that is carried centrally by fast, myelinated A-delta fibres, and slower, unmyelinated C nerve fibres. After synapsing in the dorsal horn the impulse is transmitted centrally to the thalamus and cortex. The ascending impulse may be modulated at both spinal cord and higher levels by excitation and inhibition.

Pain is both a physical and affective experience which is integrated and given meaning by the patient. So pain and the attendant degree of suffering is an individual experience and may be influenced therapeutically not only by drugs and physical intervention, but also by psychological, social and emotional treatments.

Classification

Pain may be nociceptive when produced by somatic or visceral nociceptors. Somatic nociceptors respond to mechanical, thermal and chemical stimuli producing a well-localized aching-type pain. Visceral nociceptors respond to stretch, distension, distortion and tumour invasion producing a deep pressure-like pain that may be gnawing or cramping and referred to a surface area.

Neuropathic pain is produced by peripheral or central nerve dysfunction and damage. It produces an often severe pain of unpleasant nature associated with altered sensation and intermittent lancinating, shooting exacerbations or continuous burning sensations (see Figure 7.2).

Whether pain is nociceptive or neuropathic is important as it dictates likely successful therapeutic options.

Pain may be classified temporally as acute or chronic when present for more than 3 months, but more helpfully acute pain may be thought of as pain

NOCICEPTIVE PAIN

•Somatic Pain
  - Arises from bone, muscle, cutaneous and connective tissue
  - Localized
  - Typically clinically described as throbbing, aching or stabbing

•Visceral Pain
  - Arises from internal organs
  - Generalized / diffuse
  - Associated with autonomic response e.g. nausea and vomiting
  - Clinically, typically described as cramping or gnawing

NEUROPATHIC PAIN

•Arises from neural tissue

•Clinical descriptions are variable
  - Continuous: 'burning'
  - Spontaneous: 'lancinating' or 'electric'

•Associations
  - Allodynia [pain from stimuli that are not normally painful]
  - Hyperalgesia [increased sensitivity to pain]
  - Hyperpathia [nociceptive stimuli provoke exaggerated pain]

Figure 7.2 Pain classification.

Table 7.1 Causes of pain in cancer patients

Cancer	Iatrogenic
Soft tissue infiltration	Post-op neuralgia
Visceral involvement	Post-XRT fibrosis
Bone metastases	myelopathy
Nerve compression	Post-chemo neuropathy
Raised intra-cranial pressure	Phantom limb pain
Ulceration	Drug side effects
Infection	

Cancer debility	Second diagnosis
Constipation	?
Bedsore	
Lymphoedema	
Candidiasis	
DVT	
Embolus	
Herpetic neuralgia	
Psychological sequelae	

that has an ongoing nociceptive input and chronic pain where the nociceptive input has stopped but there is a persistent pain reaction without biological cause; this is a chronic pain state.

Acute pain evokes a sympathetic autonomic response with pallor, sweating and hypertension. Once pain is present for a prolonged period the patient adapts and no longer has observable signs of pain. Instead the patient may be withdrawn, depressed, isolated and display vegetative symptoms of anorexia, asthenia (weakness) and poor sleep. This should be remembered when assessing pain.

Incidence

Cancer pain occurs in 30–50% of patients at diagnosis and increases in incidence as the disease progresses such that 90% of patients have pain at some point in their illness. Half of these patients report pain as moderate or severe and 30% as very severe or excruciating. It is a salutary message that one-third of cancer survivors report ongoing pain.

Pain may be caused by the cancer, its treatment, associated debility or another unrelated cause; some patients have pre-existing chronic pain (see Table 7.1). Patients may have more than one pain; one-third of cancer patients have three or more pains and treatment of one pain may unmask others.

Assessment

Pain should be characterized fully by taking a comprehensive pain history and where possible using a validated assessment tool for severity and recording over time such as a visual analogue scale. The simplest tool is to ask the patient to rate their pain out of 10, zero being no pain and 10 the worst pain imaginable. To gauge temporal fluctuations, asking for the worst pain rating and the best in the last 24 hours, and how long the pain lasted at the worst intensity is useful (see Table 7.2).

Pain can only be assessed by patient self-reporting. Pain is what the patient says it is. That a patient who says they are in pain is watching the TV or talking to friends does not make the patient a liar. Clinicians are poor assessors of patient pain and there are no investigations that quantify pain. Where the patient is unable to speak for himself observational scales are available. Assessment should be repeated at least daily in patients with uncontrolled pain in hospital.

Patients should be fully examined with attention to tenderness, deformity, organomegaly, abnormal sensations, muscle spasm, incoordination and the effect of mobility on the pain. Whilst for many patients investigations may not determine the cause of the pain and its management, some will benefit from X-ray diagnosis of a pathological fracture or a bone scan showing metastases. Where possible the cause of the pain should be determined to maximize the benefit of treatment.

Table 7.2 Based on Suggested Core Elements of a Pain Assessment Tool: Edinburgh Cancer Centre 2003

Location	Identify and record painful areas with a body outline chart
Severity	Measure with a visual analogue scale or a score out of 10, recording best and least
Duration, diurnal variation	When did it start? When does the pain come and how long does it stay?
Description of type of pain	What words describe your pain? Ache, dull, sharp, burning, sore, hot, numb, electric shocks, tingling, pins and needles.
Aggravating and relieving factors including medication and side effects	Is there any position or movement that makes a difference; better or worse? What drugs have helped? Have the drugs suited you?
Effect on sleep	Does the pain wake patient from sleep, interfere with dreams?
Effect on activities of daily living	How is mobility, shopping, caring for others, caring for self affected?
Associated psychological or social distress	Does it distress or worry you? Does it affect your job, income, relationships? Any financial impact?
What does it mean existentially to the patient?	What does having the pain mean to you? (Some patients see pain as a punishment for wrong doings.)

Management of pain

Management strategies for pain require attention to psychological, social and spiritual factors as well as physical aspects and a multi-modal approach is often necessary to achieve acceptable pain relief. Non-specific pain-modifying interventions are aimed at raising the pain threshold and include:

- explanation to reduce anxiety and increase patient compliance
- environment modification for safety and to enhance function
- information about stage of disease to help modify goals
- psychological support
- financial assistance
- complementary therapies
- diversional therapy.

These inputs need not delay more specific treatments but pain control may be delayed if they are not addressed. They are aimed at the subjective perception of pain that is affected by mood and morale.

Tumour-modifying treatments such as chemotherapy, radiotherapy, hormones and surgery may be of benefit for pain relief.

Analgesic drugs

In the UK, pain relief has been a subject of study for decades but many patients remain undertreated. This is more likely in the young, those with early stage disease or better functional status and those from ethnic minorities. Other poor prognostic features for pain relief are neuropathic pain, incident or episodic pain, psychological distress, cognitive impairment, severe pain at presentation and substance misuse disorder.

Globally access to services and drugs led to consensus statements from the World Health Organization that form the basis of pain management. These are expressed in terms of a three-step ladder (see Figure 7.3 and Table 7.3):

The first step of the ladder is for patients presenting with mild pain. Paracetamol and/or a non-steroidal anti-inflammatory drug (NSAID) with or without an adjuvant may suffice. Many of the drugs used following the WHO ladder require careful titration and management of side effects but NSAIDs can be the most dangerous in terms of catastrophic gastrointestinal side effects and renal impairment in this vulnerable group of patients. All palliative care patients require gastroprotection with acid-suppressing agents when taking NSAIDs, particularly when they are also taking steroids.

The second step of the ladder is for patients with mild to moderate pain or who have not responded to step 1. Non-opioids and adjuvant drugs are continued and a weak opioid is started in regular divided doses. Even weak opioids require management of opioid side effects. If pain persists do not add a second weak opioid but go to step 3 of the ladder and replace the weak opioid with a strong opioid and consider an adjuvant drug if the patient is not taking one already. The WHO approach to analgesia has been summarized by Robert Twycross as:

- by the clock – analgesics should be given regularly to abolish pain not taken once the pain returns
- by the ladder – using the stepwise escalation of analgesia
- by mouth – the oral route is preferred as pharmacokinetics demonstrate no benefit of opioids given parenterally, and to maintain patient confidence

Analgesic Ladder WHO 1996

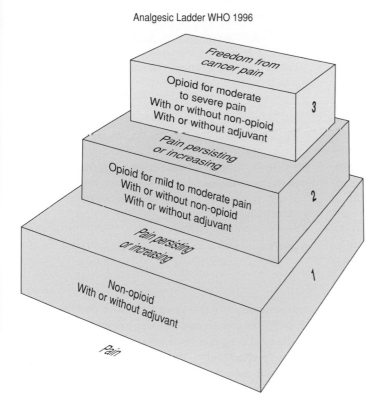

Figure 7.3 WHO three-step pain relief ladder. From: Cormie PJ, *et al.* BMJ 2008;337:a2154. Copyright ©2008 BMJ Publishing Group Ltd.

Table 7.3 Drugs used at each step

Step 3. Strong opioids Morphine, diamorphine, oxycodone, fentanyl, hydromorphone
Step 2. Weak opioids Codeine, dihydrocodeine, tramadol
Step 1. Non-opioids Paracetamol NSAIDs
Adjuvant drugs Anti-depressants Anti-convulsants Anti-arrhythmics Anti-spasmodics Steroids Bisphosphonates

- for the individual – there is great inter-individual variation in required dosing to achieve pain control
- with attention to detail – side effects require careful management and monitoring.

It is wise (and reflected in hospital formularies) to be familiar with one or two drugs in each class. Despite the increasing availability of alternative strong opioids and the lack of randomized double-blind controlled trial evidence the number-needed-to-treat (NNT) evidence remains favourable to morphine as the first-line strong opioid orally and diamorphine subcutaneously.

There is up to 1000-fold inter-individual variation in dose requirements of morphine, thought to result from genetic polymorphism of opioid receptors. Most analgesic effect of strong opioids is mediated at the mu receptor, which has a linear dose–response curve. This means as the dose of strong opioid increases so does the analgesic effect, and there is therefore theoretically no ceiling dose. Prescribing starts with a low dose depending on the prior use of opioids and is increased until the patient is pain-free or the dosage is limited by intolerable opioid side effects. This regimen ensures patients are not put off using strong opioids by being opioid-toxic when starting the drug but also requires vigilance on the part of the prescriber to ensure the doses are increased until the patient is pain-free. Many patients believe their pain is untreatable with strong opioids because they remain underdosed. This is often due to the professional becoming uncomfortable with the doses the patient requires. Audit experience suggests a median total daily dose of morphine between 200 mg and 300 mg and 100 μg of transdermal fentanyl but some individuals will require far more. Whatever the dose the principle remains the same: if the patient is in pain, not opioid-toxic, and without unacceptable side effects, the dose can be increased. Even specialists, at times, have to remember to look at and listen to the patient, not at the dose of opioid drugs.

Breakthrough and incident pain

Breakthrough pain is the emergence of pain during the day in a patient whose pain is otherwise controlled. Incident pain is caused by a volitional or non-volitional action that causes precipitated pain in an otherwise pain-controlled patient.

It is custom and practice when prescribing strong opioids to always prescribe an equivalent 4-hourly dose of an instant-release form of the maintenance drug to be taken for breakthrough pain. Some patients adjust this dose according to effect. Experience with newer preparations of strong opioids for breakthrough and incident pain suggests that the same scrupulous titration for the individual should be applied to breakthrough dosing.

Incident pain is harder to prescribe for as it requires a fast-onset, short-acting strong opioid so the patient is not obtunded by higher than required doses of the drug once the incident causing the pain has passed. The newly licensed sublingual and buccal fentanyl preparations are marketed for this purpose but caution is advisable with their use until the hedonic and possibly addictive side effects of such fast-acting strong opioids are known.

Starting a strong opioid

It is usual to start a patient with uncontrolled pain on a regular instant-release strong opioid 4 hourly to facilitate titration of dosing. If they have been on a full dose of a weak opioid they will have had the equivalent of approximately 20 mg of morphine in 24 hours so their dose will need to be at least 5 mg morphine 4 hourly. Pragmatically in hospital where drug rounds are not timed to suit 4-hourly dosing the patient is often started on a low dose of sustained-release morphine 10 mg or 20 mg twice daily so that they have some continuous background pain relief. Titration is done by adding up the total dose of morphine in 24 hours, including the breakthrough doses, and assessing how the patient's pain was during that time. If the pain was well controlled the 12-hour sustained-release dose of morphine is calculated by dividing by

> *Example:*
>
> Mrs B has breast cancer with painful bone metastases. She is on 30 mg sustained release morphine but in the last 24 hours she has had moderately severe pain that interfered with sleep and required five breakthrough doses of 10 mg oral morphine solution.
>
> Total dose last 24 hours:
>
> 60 mg sustained-release + 50 mg instant release = 110 mg
>
> New dose:–
>
> 110 mg + 33 mg (30%) = 143 mg. This approximates to 70 mg sustained-release morphine b.d. and 20 mg instant release morphine as required for breakthrough pain

Figure 7.4 Worked example of morphine adjustment.

two yesterday's total dose of morphine, and the breakthrough dose is adjusted to approximately one-sixth of the total dose (i.e. the 4-hourly dose) as an instant-release preparation.

If the pain was not controlled and moderately severe, the total dose is increased by between 20% and 30%, with one-sixth of the total daily dose prescribed for breakthrough medication (see Figure 7.4). If the pain in the previous day was severe the total dose is increased by 50% and breakthrough dosage altered accordingly. Opioid dosing should not be increased by more than 50% in one single change. Patients undergoing dose titration in hospital should be seen daily for pain assessment and monitoring for toxicity and side effects.

Changing doses of opioids requires diligent arithmetic and note-making. Many hospital errors are due to wrongly prescribed or administered opioids. Handover to the next team of carers needs to be given. In the example in Figure 7.4 the dose of sustained-release morphine has gone from 30 mg b.d. to 70 mg b.d. and at first glance it would be easy to presume an error.

Opioid side effects

Starting a strong opioid can be time-consuming as most patients fear the meaning of needing one, believing that opioids should be reserved for when the pain becomes really bad and that death is near once opioids are started. Patients also require information and support about side effects to avoid them believing they are allergic to morphine because they vomit, or

Table 7.4 Differential diagnosis of constipation

Iatrogenic
- Opioid analgesia
- Antacids
- Calcium channel blockers
- Anti-cholinergics
- Ferrous sulphate
- Ondansetron

Metabolic disturbances
- Hypercalcaemia
- Hypokalaemia

Immobility

Reduced oral intake (fluids and food)

Hypothyroidism

Intestinal obstruction
- Intra-luminal tumour
- Extra-luminal tumour

Post-radiation fibrosis

Strangulated hernia

Malignant pseudo-obstruction

untreatable because the pain is not abolished by the first few doses.

Constipation is almost universal and requires treatment with the first dose of opioid, titration of laxatives, and close monitoring of bowel function throughout the illness. Opioids specifically inhibit gut motility and increase fluid absorption. Patients frequently require two or three laxatives, at least one of which should be a stimulant. Despite this rectal measures are needed in one-third of patients. Other important contributing factors to constipation in palliative care (see Table 7.4) should be excluded, or treated as appropriate.

Usually, combination treatment with a stool softener and a stimulant laxative is successful. Bulk-forming laxatives and bran should be avoided, as patients may be unable to consume sufficient volumes of fluid to facilitate their action and they may increase the risk of intestinal obstruction.

There are now specific opioid antagonists available to counter opioid-induced constipation. Subcutaneous methylnaltrexone is an opioid antagonist that does not cross the blood–brain barrier and is intended to be used with best laxative therapy. It produces a bowel motion in 50% of patients within 4 hours. Oral naloxone is marketed in a combined product with low-dose oxycodone. Taken by mouth it is poorly absorbed, acting as an opioid antagonist locally in the gut. Both products are new and the complexity of

receptor response to opioid antagonism, with a possible bi-polar action, means use is restricted, and prescribing in discussion with the specialist palliative care team is advisable.

Nausea and vomiting occurs in >60% but tolerance develops over 5–7 days in many. Antiemetics should be prescribed with the first opioid dose. Haloperidol may be prescribed either as a single night-time dose of 3–5 mg or 0.5–1.5 mg orally tds. Cyclizine 50 mg orally tds is an alternative. For severe or prolonged vomiting other causes should be sought. It is important to note that if the opioid is withdrawn for a period and then restarted, nausea and vomiting will recur for the first few days as tolerance will have been lost.

Dry mouth is an autonomic side effect of opioids and other drugs frequently prescribed in palliative care, e.g. anticholinergics. This may be compounded by oral candidiasis and vitamin deficiencies. The mouth has a disproportionately large representation at the somato-sensory homunculus, which explains the misery associated with oral symptoms. Good hygiene, hydration, saliva replacement, sugar-free gum and antifungals produce relief.

Drowsiness and other central nervous side effects such as decreased cognitive function, dreams and shaded vision are more frequent in the first week, after which tolerance develops. Hallucinations and delirium may represent too rapid an escalation of dose. Opioids titrated carefully in a well-hydrated patient are less likely to cause a problem. These are much-feared side effects of morphine and it can be helpful to warn the patient of drowsiness and explain that they may well have been short of sleep in the last few days and weeks, so catching up will do no harm; but if they remain drowsy there are alternative opioids that can be tried. Medication review and stopping other sedating drugs is helpful. For prolonged opioid sedation there is some evidence of benefit from methylphenidate.

Myoclonus is particularly a feature of doses above 500 mg oral morphine or at lower doses when prescribed in conjunction with other drugs or in renal impairment.

Pruritis and urinary retention are rare side effects.

Respiratory depression is rarely a problem in palliative care patients as pain is a stimulant and opioids are individually titrated. Expert advice should be sought before reversing opioids with naloxone in patients on long-term treatment as it will very suddenly reverse not only respiratory depression but also all pain relief, with a traumatic effect on both patient and doctor. Protocols for naloxone infusion for palliative care patients are available at www.//palliativedrugs.com.

Opioid switching

Morphine is the pragmatic choice for a first-line opioid but some undoubtedly have residual pain whilst experiencing difficult side effects. In this circumstance, opioid switching involves swapping from one strong opioid to another, in the hope of exploiting cross-tolerance and achieving improved pain relief with reduced side effects. About a quarter of patients require a switch, far fewer require a second. Uncontrolled pain without problematic side effects is not a good reason to switch strong opioids; it is a reason to increase the opioid dose. Following clear guidelines can deliver more than 90% of patients good pain control in expert hands.

Relative potency of opioids

Empirical estimates of relative potency (the amount of drug required to achieve a given effect) have been developed. These are summarized in equi-analgesic tables, i.e. doses of different opioids which can be expected to have an equivalent analgesic effect. Conversion ratios vary between publications and significantly simplify what is actually complex pharmacology. Note that dose equivalents are estimations only, and dose conversion is not an exact science. There may be significant differences between published conversion tables, and any one individual table may give a wide range. It is best to err on the side of caution in the arithmetic conversion, and make sure that breakthrough pain relief is available as necessary and the patient re-titrated. It is custom and practice to convert doses to oral morphine equivalents even if converting between two other strong opioids. Careful handover to ward staff is essential during opioid switches. If in doubt specialist advice is available. Excellent conversion charts are available at www.//palliativedrugs.com and in the British National Formulary.

Opioids in renal failure

Patients on dialysis and those living with impaired renal function require caution with codeine and morphine as active metabolites accumulate with prolonged half-lives and toxicity. The doses can be titrated down and effects monitored regularly but many units prefer to prescribe drugs that are not renally excreted.

Drugs safe in renal failure include:

non-opioid: paracetamol

weak opioid: tramadol

strong opioids: fentanyl, alfentanil, buprenorphine, hydromorphone

adjuvants: use individual drugs as indicated, taking into account knowledge of potential renal effects and balancing risk against the patient's prognosis

NSAIDs are contraindicated in renal failure but they are used for symptom relief when the renal failure is irretrievable and symptoms severe and responsive to NSAIDs. They may also be indicated on the same basis in the last few days of life.

Opioids and driving

Whilst pain relief is being titrated the patient should not drive but once established on a stable dose, if they are not sedated, feel well, lucid and able, there is no bar to driving. Regular review of driving capability is sensible in anyone with end-stage disease.

Opioid addiction and pain relief

Physical dependence is seen universally when opioids are used; a sudden cessation will precipitate a withdrawal syndrome. Opioid addiction is a psychological state and very rare in palliative care. More frequent is the patient with a history of opioid misuse who presents with a painful condition. The principles of pain relief remain the same, with what the patient says being the gold standard of pain assessment. When staff are aware of the previous misuse, there is an understandable concern about prescribing strong opioids that leads to patients not receiving adequate doses of pain relief.

Confusion can occur if the patient is on maintenance methadone in the community and requires additional pain relief. Whilst methadone is a good painkiller it is simpler to keep the methadone maintenance dose stable, and use a second strong opioid for pain. Difficulties can arise in keeping track of the drugs if the patient is discharged home to live with other addicts. Constant communication with primary care and giving small, regular prescriptions with surveillance from the community specialist nurses are advised. In hospital drug rationalization is easier. If needed, methadone can be given by subcutaneous infusion for care at the end of life. In these circumstances referral for shared care with specialist palliative care is advisable.

Neuropathic pain

Neuropathic pain management is required in up to 20% of pain cases and starts with opioids, but with adjuvant drugs as an early co-prescription as the higher opioid doses required often have limiting side effects. Adjuvant analgesics are drugs that are not primarily painkillers but that relieve pain in certain circumstances. The choice of adjuvant drug is based on likely tolerance of side effects as all have a similar NNT of 3.

Anti-depressants block the central monoamine reuptake, which causes more descending inhibition to dorsal horn synapses. Tricyclics such as low-dose amitriptyline (NNT 3.6) 25 mg nocte (10 mg in the elderly) rising to 50 mg nocte are often used first-line. Venlafaxine (NNT 3.1), a dual serotonin and noradrenaline reuptake inhibitor, and the newer duloxetine in the same class, are superior to selective serotonin reuptake inhibitors and have the added benefit of being used at doses effective in depression.

Gabapentin and pregabalin are anti-convulsants licensed for neuropathic pain; their mode of action is neuronal calcium channel blockade. Anti-arrhythmics influence pain transmission by blocking neuronal sodium channels. Evidence (at the level of case series) exists for mexiletine and flecainide, although the latter is contraindicated in ischaemic heart disease. High-dose steroids are often used to ease painful nerve compression.

Ketamine, an NMDA receptor antagonist, inhibits dorsal horn neuron depolarization and reduces central sensitization; it can cause an unpleasant dysphoria. Specialist advice should be sought to use this anaesthetic drug off licence and careful monitoring is required as it returns the patient to opioid sensitivity with the risk of toxicity.

Topical lidocaine plasters have been licensed for post-herpetic neuralgia and are indicated when there is an alteration in skin sensitivity. They produce skin analgesia, not anaesthesia, and, when successful, limit the drug side effect burden as only 3% of the dose is absorbed parenterally.

As treatment of neuropathic pain is challenging, requiring polypharmacy, close liaison with the interventional pain team to access nerve blockade and the physiotherapy department for transcutaneous nerve stimulation early in the course of the pain management is beneficial.

Bone pain

NSAIDs and opioids are both useful in bone pain. Bisphosphonates reduce cytokine production, so inhibiting metastatic bone pain. Given intravenously they have a NNT of 6 for pain relief at 12 weeks but radiotherapy remains the treatment of choice, with a NNT of 4.2 for complete remission of pain and opioid dose sparing. Both bisphosphonates and radiotherapy can cause an increase in pain in the first few days post-treatment which will need careful management. Resolution of the pain over the next 2–4 weeks may lead to opioid toxicity if doses are not reviewed.

Where bone metastases are widespread such that conventional radiotherapy is not possible, radionucleides have demonstrable benefit and radiofrequency ablation has also been used to treat pain from bone metastases.

Bisphosphonates are also used prophylactically to reduce skeletal related events in breast, prostate and myeloma patients with bone metastases. They have been shown to reduce pathological fracture, hypercalcaemia and the requirement for radiotherapy. Bisphosphonates do not reduce the incidence of metastatic spinal cord compression and, as yet, there is no firm evidence of survival benefit.

Hepatic capsule pain

Pain from a stretched hepatic capsule presents in the upper abdomen, is worse on deep breathing and exquisite as the liver is palpated during inspiration. It responds only partially to opioids and NSAIDs but usually responds well to dexamethasone 6 mg o.d.

Nausea and vomiting of cancer

Nausea and vomiting (N+V) are considered together as the neural control pathways are similar, although those controlling vomiting are more neuroanatomically defined. Nausea is an unpleasant, invisible, subjective sensation and autonomic response which many patients find hard to describe. Nausea is more debilitating than retching and vomiting. Retching is rhythmic, laboured and spasmodic muscle movements often leading on to vomiting, which involves sustained abdominal muscle action with opening of the gastric cardia resulting in the forceful expulsion of gastric

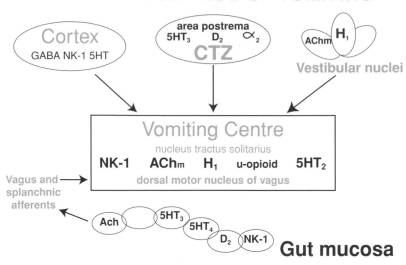

NEURAL CONTROL OF VOMITING

Figure 7.5 Based on the Palliative Care Formulary (3rd edn) (PCF3).

contents via the mouth. Patients describe nausea and vomiting as demeaning, demoralizing and as distressing as pain; it reduces quality of life and induces carer stress.

Nausea occurs in 30% of patients with advanced malignancy, rising to 70% in the last week of life. Vomiting occurs in 30% and is more common in females, those under 65 years of age, and in gynaecological and gastric malignancy. N+V is the cause of one-third of palliative care admissions.

Pathophysiology of nausea and vomiting

The brainstem vomiting centre (VC), composed of the medullary reticular formation's nucleus tractus solitarius and the dorsal motor nucleus of the vagus, is a neuronal network that functions as a physiological control centre integrating input from:

- higher cortical pathways
- the chemoreceptor trigger zone (CTZ)
- vestibular labyrinthine pathways via the eighth cranial nerve
- the gut via vagal and splanchnic afferents.

Neural messaging is expressed via neurotransmitters, although this is complex and a rapidly expanding field of research. Knowledge of the neurotransmitter activation in N+V is helpful to direct effective treatment. Within the vomiting centre neurotrans-mitter receptor expression includes anticholinergic muscarinic (Ach_m), histamine (H_1), mu opioid, serotonin $5HT_2$ ($5HT_2$) and neurokinin-1 (NK-1) (see Figure 7.5).

Higher centres

The cortex, diencephalon and limbic system input to N+V is via serotonin $5HT_3$ ($5HT_3$) and gamma-aminobutyric acid (GABA) receptors. NK-1 receptors are a more recent discovery within the cortex. Cortical receptors are stimulated by fear, anxiety, memory and olfactory and visual stimuli as well as meningeal irritation and raised intracranial pressure.

Chemoreceptor trigger zone

The CTZ is situated at the dorsal surface of the medulla oblongata and the caudal end of the fourth ventricle. There is no blood–brain barrier so it detects chemical stimuli directly from blood and cerebrospinal fluid. Its receptors are $5HT_3$, $5HT_2$, dopamine (D_2), ACh_m, mu opioid and NK-1. Receptor activation occurs in metabolic upsets, e.g. hypercalcaemia, hyponatraemia, uraemia; by drugs, e.g. opioids, antidepressants, chemotherapeutic agents, antibiotics, antiepileptics, and digoxin; by toxins – either chemical or bacterial; and inflammatory products such as tumour necrosis factor-alpha.

Table 7.5 Causes of nausea and vomiting in cancer patients

Cancer	Iatrogenic
Infiltration/obstruction	Post-op
Visceral involvement	Post-XRT
Hypercalcaemia	Post-chemo
Raised intra-cranial pressure	Drug side effects
Hepatic metastases	NSAIDs, antibiotics
Squashed stomach syndrome	Opioids, antidepressants
Pain	Iron, steroid withdrawal
Infection	
Cancer debility	**Second diagnosis**
Constipation	?
Bedsore, fungating wound, odour	
Gastric stasis, autonomic	
Peptic ulcer	
Candidiasis	
DVT and embolus	
Pain	
Fear and psychological upset	

Table 7.6 Antiemetic drug receptor site of action

Antihistamine H1	Cyclizine
	Promethazine
	Levomepromazine
Dopamine D2 antagonists	Haloperidol
	Metoclopramide
	Domperidone
	Does not cross BBB
	Levomepromazine
Anticholinergic muscarinic	Cyclizine
	Levomepromazine
Serotonin ($5HT_3$) antagonists	Ondansetron
	Granisetron
	Levomepromazine
	Metoclopramide in high dose 100–200 mg in 24 hours
Neurokinin-1	Aprepitant

Vestibular pathways

Motion induces nausea via the labyrinthine responses of the inner ear; this is sensitized by opioids. Nausea and vomiting has a higher incidence in ambulant palliative care patients than those who are sedentary. Local infections are also emetogenic. Receptors in the vestibular nuclei are ACh_m and H_1.

Gut afferents

N+V may also be mediated by afferent signals from the gut and intra-abdominal organs via the vagus and splanchnic nerves. Stimulation anywhere in the gut, including the pharynx, may generate nausea and vomiting. Causes of gut-induced N+V include mechanical and chemical stimuli such as constipation, obstruction, distortion, compression, drugs, bacterial endotoxins and radiotherapy, which releases $5HT_3$ from enterochromaffin cells.

Management of nausea and vomiting

High-quality trial evidence is lacking but the management of N+V in palliative care is based upon expert opinion and experience. The efficacy of treatment improves with careful assessment based on the timing, persistence, content of vomit and exacerbating and relieving factors. Disease status and antiemetic drug history is the starting point and will help choice of treatment by giving a guide to side effects best avoided. Knowing the meaning of the N+V to the patient can be useful due to the contribution of cortical mechanisms. Associated constitutional upset as in syncope or early satiety may point to autonomic dysfunction.

General measures

Environmental control of smells and body odours from wounds, in addition to mouth hygiene, explanation and psychological support develops confidence in expert care and improves nausea and vomiting. Complementary therapies can be a useful adjuvant treatment.

Drug treatment

A clear history may establish a cause (see Table 7.5) and suggest the likely neuroreceptor involved at which to direct drug treatment (see Table 7.6). This mechanistic approach is popular and effective but only 25% of nausea and vomiting has a single known cause, 50% is multifactorial and in 25% the cause is unknown. As the cause may not be clear and neural networks lead to complex neurotransmitter interaction, empirical approaches to treatment have also been defined and found successful (see Figure 7.6). Sixty per cent of nausea and vomiting resolves with one drug and a further 30% with a second.

Levomepromazine is a good broad-spectrum antiemetic but its sedative effects can be a problem for patients already on other sedating drugs who wish to live the time they have to the full. In the last few days of life sedation may be an advantage.

Use of the syringe driver

Drug delivery by subcutaneous infusion via the syringe driver has advantages which may override the inconvenience to the patient. The drugs are delivered in constant dose so control is better throughout the

- Evaluate and document
- Treat reversible causes
- First-line antiemetic chosen for most likely cause of N+V
- Use parenteral route if unlikely to absorb drug orally due to vomiting
  - Prokinetic: metoclopramide 10 mg tds
  - CTZ effect: haloperidol 1.5–3 mg as single or divided doses
  - Vomiting centre: cyclizine 50 mg tds

Review 24 to 48 hours later. If little or no improvement:

- Are dose and route optimized?
- Review cause
- Add or substitute second-line antiemetic and consider steroids as adjuvant

Second-line antiemetics

- Large-volume vomits: hyoscine butylbromide 20 mg qds
- Broad-spectrum: levomepromazine 6.25–25 mg od

Figure 7.6 Empirical treatment guideline for nausea and vomiting.

24 hours. Fewer injections are required and the oral drug burden is reduced. Syringe drivers are indicated where nausea and vomiting is uncontrolled despite compliance, the patient has dysphagia or intestinal obstruction, or the patient is comatose. Rarely syringe drivers are used to overcome poor absorption of drugs. There is a requirement for staff training and at least once-daily intervention. Patients with cachexia or reduced immunity may suffer increased site reactions. Information about compatibility of drug combinations in the syringe driver is available at http://www.palliativedrugs.com.

Malignant bowel obstruction

Malignant bowel obstruction (MBO) is a well-recognized complication of advanced abdominal or pelvic malignancies occurring in up to 20% of colorectal cancer and 50% of ovarian malignancies. It is usually due to diffuse intraperitoneal carcinomatosis but may be the presenting complaint of a solid tumour or treatment complications (see Table 7.7).

MBO occurs more rarely due to isolated gastrointestinal metastases (e.g. from breast cancers or

Table 7.7 Causes of malignant bowel obstruction

Mechanical obstruction	
Extrinsic compression	Increasing tumour size
	Masses
	Adhesions
	Post-irradiation fibrosis
Intrinsic compression	Tumour growth through bowel wall, impairing intestinal transit
Intraluminal obstruction	Primary or secondary tumour deposits causing obstruction or foci for intussusception
Functional obstruction	
Motility disorders	Electrolyte abnormalities
Inflammation	Secondary to tumour burden
Dehydration	Reduced oral intake
Paraneoplastic	Autoimmune pathophysiology
Drugs	E.g. opioid analgesics delaying peristalsis Anticholinergics: reduced parasympathetic nerve transmission

melanoma). There may be multiple partial occlusions which may be intermittent, but perforation is rare.

Obstruction is thought to lead to four distinct pathophysiological processes:

- accumulation of secretions (these stimulate further secretion proximal to the obstruction)
- decreased absorption of sodium and water from the gut
- increased secretion of sodium and water, with increasing distension
- inflammatory responses in the bowel wall, leading to oedema and further obstruction.

The last two factors cause the vicious cycle of distension and secretion.

Presentation

As with any bowel obstruction, symptoms vary depending on the extent and level of the obstruction. Alternating constipation and diarrhoea from subacute obstruction may herald the development of complete obstruction, when the patient will present with cramping abdominal pain, nausea, vomiting and abdominal distension. Overflow diarrhoea secondary to bacterial liquefaction of bowel contents may complicate the picture.

Management

Initial assessment and imaging to exclude emergencies amenable to surgical intervention by stenting, defunctioning or bowel resection are required. Surgery is most likely to be of benefit in patients with a life expectancy greater than 2 months.

Indicators of poor surgical outcome include multiple obstruction, diffuse carcinomatosis, diffuse intra-abdominal masses, distant metastases, pleural effusions, ascites, age > 63 years, low serum albumin, poor nutritional status, prior radiotherapy, prolonged intestinal transit times, comorbidities and short time from diagnosis to obstruction. Explanation of risks and benefits is key, as patients in the late stages of cancer and their relatives may decline operative treatment even where there is a chance of benefit.

The definitive treatment options for MBO used to be either palliative surgery or conventional 'drip and suck' management with intravenous fluids and nasogastric tube (NGT) insertion. Both of these approaches may be unsuitable for palliative patients, due to their invasive nature and need for hospitalization. Prolonged NGT placement, as well as being a traumatic procedure, may be uncomfortable, it may block or require frequent suctioning, and NGTs can reduce quality of life. Furthermore, NGTs may cause oesophagitis, erosion or oesophageal bleeding, sinusitis, otitis media and aspiration pneumonia. Research on the management of malignant bowel obstruction using non-interventional care and limited post mortem studies at St Christopher's Hospice has demonstrated the efficacy of medical management.

Medical management

Medical management, started in hospital, facilitates discharge and ongoing management of obstruction at home or in a hospice setting. The aims of medical treatment are to:

- relieve obstruction if possible
- relieve pain
- relieve nausea
- reduce frequency of vomiting
- support the patient and family as they cope with the final illness.

Corticosteroids, e.g. dexamethasone

Corticosteroids reduce inflammation and oedema around tumour deposits, and increase salt and water reabsorption. They also act as antiemetics and adjuvant analgesics. Corticosteroids are given in high dose for 5–7 days, and discontinued if there is no appreciable improvement, to limit their side effects.

The role of corticosteroids in the management of MBO is complex, and not well understood, but they deliver a trend for improvement in symptoms of MBO with a NNT of 6. There is no increase in mortality at 1 month after corticosteroid use.

Custom and practice in palliative care is to use dexamethasone 8–12 mg as a single morning dose or as a subcutaneous infusion. Started early it can delay complete obstruction and maintain enough oral absorption of fluids to allow management at home without a drip.

Pain relief

Pain is managed with opioids via a subcutaneous syringe driver following the principles outlined above. Management of constipating side effects is a challenging problem. Specific opioid antagonists have not been tried in MBO and remain contraindicated. If the obstruction is not total a lubricant laxative, liquid paraffin or faecal softener sodium docusate are least likely to produce colic.

Nausea and vomiting

Either cyclizine or haloperidol is added to the syringe driver to control nausea although it is likely that anti-secretory drugs will be required to reduce the vomiting. Metoclopramide and domperidone are prokinetic and therefore should be avoided.

Anti-secretory drugs

Hyoscine butylbromide (scopolamine butylbromide) is used for relief of colicky pain and reduction of nausea and vomiting by decreasing intestinal secretions and inhibiting peristalsis in intestinal smooth muscle. It can be given as 20 mg bolus doses subcutaneously, or continuously via a syringe driver (80–160 mg in 24 hours). It is safe to mix diamorphine, haloperidol and hyoscine butylbromide in the same syringe. The butylbromide salt of hyoscine does not cross the blood–brain barrier, therefore avoiding centrally mediated side effects such as drowsiness, blurred vision, dry mouth or mydriasis (cf. the hydrobromide salt).

Octreotide, a synthetic analogue of somatostatin, reduces gastric acid secretion, intestinal motility, bile flow and splanchnic blood flow. Fluid secretion in bowel obstruction is mediated by vasoactive intestinal peptide (VIP), which octreotide inhibits. Sodium and water secretion from the intestinal epithelium is decreased and electrolyte absorption from the intestinal lumen is improved. The reduction of the hypertensive state in the intestinal lumen breaks into the distension–secretion cycle. The resultant reduction of gastrointestinal volume and distension leads to improvement in pain and vomiting. The duration of action of octreotide is 12 hours; it can be given twice daily subcutaneously, or via a continuous subcutaneous infusion (CSI). Doses of 0.3–1.6 mg daily (SC or by CSI) have been used, with good relief of pain and vomiting. Usually the patient is started on 0.5 mg daily and the dose increased to 1 mg if large-volume vomiting persists. Octreotide is generally well tolerated; common side effects include dry mouth, and mild hyperglycaemia when used long-term.

Venting procedures

If decompression is required for symptom relief, this may be better achieved by insertion of a PEG tube as a venting gastrostomy. These improve nausea and vomiting in up to 90% of patients. However, PEG tubes should be avoided in patients with complications of end-stage liver failure, such as portal hypertension, large-volume ascites or increased bleeding risk. A PEG tube may later be used for feeding if a patient's symptoms improve, but they do not improve survival.

Prognosis

Death can supervene very quickly and good preparation should be part of the management of MBO as it is an incurable terminal event. Some patients live as long as 4 months. Supervision by the specialist palliative care team across organizational boundaries is beneficial.

Feeding

For many patients eating is part of social and family life as well as a daily pleasure. In palliative care we rarely forbid eating in MBO as many people would wish to have one last bacon sandwich, or similar request. Explanation of the common sense that 'what goes down will have to come back up, if it does not pass through the gut because of the "blockage"' helps the patient make their own decision about eating. Families also need support, and permission to eat, when their relative is seen to be starving to death. Parenteral feeding is unlikely to be of any benefit and fraught with risk. It should only be considered for patients with

Table 7.8 Malignancies associated with hypercalcaemia

Common	Uncommon
Lung – squamous cell	Lung – small cell
Breast	Large bowel
Myeloma	Stomach
Head and neck	Prostate
Kidney	
Cervix	
Lymphoma	

complete gut obstruction who have a prognosis in the region of 3–6 months, a very good performance status and no distant metastases.

Hypercalcaemia of malignancy

Calcium ions are involved in neuromuscular transmission and cell function. Serum calcium is tightly controlled between 2.02 and 2.6 mmol/l. The majority is protein-bound, with the active ionized portion available for metabolic function. In cancer patients blood proteins are frequently low and hypercalcaemia will be missed without the serum level being corrected for concomitant protein. Most labs quote the corrected calcium; where this is not available the following formula may be used:

Mesured serum calcium (mmol/l)
$$+ 0.02 + (40 - [\text{albumin g/l}])$$
$$= \text{corrected calcium}$$

Hypercalcaemia of malignancy (HM) causes a rapidly rising serum calcium. The rapid rise results in a highly symptomatic condition which is fatal if left untreated.

HM has a prevalence of up to 30% in cancer patients, with squamous cell lung cancer, breast cancer, and myeloma being the most common (see Table 7.8). It may occur as the presentation of malignancy in renal cancers or feature late in the progression of the disease.

HM can complicate any cancer type but is less common with adenocarcinomas and small cell lung cancer. Other causes of hypercalcaemia should be considered as primary hyperparathyroidism (PPT) and cancer coexist in 15%; particularly in colon and breast cancer, associated with MEN type 1, and lymphoma. Rarely ionizing radiation may cause hyperparathyroidism. In the presence of raised calcium, a normal or increased serum parathyroid hormone (PTH) is pathological. The prognosis of hypercalcaemia in a cancer patient with coexistent hyperparathyroidism is years, but a true HM has a median survival of 2 months. Careful assessment and care planning will avoid the trauma of patients being told their cancer has recurred when it has not, and allow others to prepare appropriately for death.

A quick guide whilst awaiting PTH assays is:

$$\times \frac{[\text{serum chloride (mmol/l)} - 84]}{\dfrac{[\text{albumin (g/l)} - 15]}{\text{Serum phosphate (mmol/l)}}}$$

This formula is a reliable guide for 95% of cases; those with values under 400 suggest malignancy, those greater than 500 suggest hyperparathyroidism.

Raised serum calcium may be found in renal disease, sarcoidosis, vitamin D toxicity and thyrotoxicosis, amongst other causes, but PPT and HM account for 90% of cases.

There is more than one mechanism of HM. One-fifth of cases are caused by osteoclastic activation by cytokines leading to bone lysis in the presence of bone metastases, as in breast cancer; but the majority are due to paraneoplastic endocrine humoral secretion of parathyroid hormone-related peptide (PTHrP), common in cancers of squamous origin. Calcitriol (1,25-dihydroxy vitamin D3) is thought to be a cause of hypercalcaemia in certain lymphomas, which may explain the unusually good response of HM in these cases to treatment with high-dose steroids.

Presentation

The classic presentation of 'stones, bones, abdominal groans and psychic moans' describes the patient with a slowly rising calcium. The presentation of a patient with a rapid rise in serum calcium due to HM is more acute as homeostatic mechanisms attempt to excrete calcium, causing polyuria and loss of sodium, potassium and magnesium in the proximal renal tubule. Loss of concentrating ability by the nephron leads to worsening dehydration. Further direct damage to the renal tubule itself is possible when the serum calcium exceeds 3 mmol/l. The rate of and degree of the rising calcium correlates with severity of symptoms. Patients complain of anorexia, nausea, vomiting, constipation, thirst and mental changes early in the course of the HM, leading on to a presentation with dehydration, renal insufficiency, obtundation, twitching, fit-

ting, coma and cardiac arrest as the calcium rises above 4 mmol/l.

Despite the acute presentation and poor prognosis, treatment is often rapidly effective and worthwhile. All palliative care teams can cite instances of moribund patients transformed by treatment with good subsequent quality of life, and will be aware that HM is a rare instance where one can misdiagnose dying in a patient with an advanced malignancy.

It is important, however, to assess the stage of disease and discuss with the patient, and if not competent the relatives or advocate, the context of the current exacerbation and whether treatment would be acceptable and appropriate.

Treatment

The patient will have lost fluid and electrolytes and the immediate treatment is rehydration with saline and potassium. Intravenous fluids reverse the dehydration cycle and increase renal excretion of calcium such that the serum calcium falls by up to 0.5 mmol/l. The patient improves at this point and a common error is to declare them better and take the drip down. The process that caused the hypercalcaemia is, however, unresolved and the condition rapidly recurs.

Bisphosphonates are the drugs of choice to treat HM. They are analogues of inorganic pyrophosphate that bind to hydroxyapatite crystals in bone and are released by bone resorption. Once taken up by the osteoclast they are cytotoxic and inhibit signalling pathways. When given for HM bisphosphonates stop the release of calcium from the bones, allowing the rehydrated patient to normalize their serum calcium by excretion of excess calcium in the urine. Turning off the tap of an overflowing bath and allowing it to empty via the plughole is a useful analogy. The manufacturer gives a schedule of dosing for Pamidronate dependent upon the serum calcium but systematic review evidence suggests 90 mg should be given whatever the serum calcium level to effectively combat the ongoing HM process.

The dose of any bisphosphonate should be adjusted in renal insufficiency and attention paid to rehydration and ongoing monitoring of renal function because the drug itself can cause renal tubular damage and acute renal failure.

Bisphosphonates are well tolerated such that even a seriously ill patient has the option of a trial of therapy. The main side effects are mild pyrexia and flu-like symptoms for 24–48 hours; fatigue, headache, myalgia, bone pain and hypocalcaemia which occasionally requires calcium replacement if the patient has excreted large amounts of calcium whilst serum levels were high. A very rare but challenging side effect is osteonecrosis of the jaw but this usually develops only in patients on long-term bisphosphonate treatment.

Patients who have been treated for hypercalcaemia require careful handover for ongoing monitoring in other care settings as the condition will recur and can be treated early to prevent a recrudescence of symptoms.

Cachexia

Cachexia is a composite word from 'kakos' meaning bad and 'hexis' meaning condition. It is a hypercatabolic state causing skeletal muscle wasting, lipolysis and altered carbohydrate metabolism. It is associated with nausea, anorexia, decreased mobility and poor quality of life. It occurs in up to 80% of cancer patients, shortens survival and predicts poor treatment outcomes to oncological intervention. Cachexia occurs independently of tumour mass, metastases or nutritional intake. It is common in cancers of the pancreas, stomach, colon and lung. Cachexia is also seen in non-malignant conditions such as acquired immunodeficiency disorder, congestive cardiac failure, prolonged sepsis and other chronic disease states.

Mechanism

The catabolic state with lipolysis and proteolysis develops due to the production of cytokines produced in lymphocytes, monocytes, macrophages and other tissues, including skeletal muscle. These stimulate nuclear transcription factors and alter the regulation of skeletal muscle proteozomes, leading to breakdown of muscle proteins, which causes each individual muscle cell to become smaller. The cause of the anorexia cachexia syndrome is multi-factorial but cytokines implicated in the inflammatory state include:

- tumour necrosis factor alpha (TNF, cachectin)
- interleukin 1
- interleukin 6
- interferon gamma
- proteolysis induction factor
- oxidants
- renin-angiotensin system.

TNF acts centrally at the hypothalamus and also acutely on skeletal muscle contractability. Proteolysis occurs over hours and days, the timelag allowing for gene expression and protein transcription. Both TNF-induced effects are reversible in vitro and in animal studies with antioxidants.

Management

- General measures of comfort, and eating away from smells in a peaceful environment
- Dietary advice to patient and family about small portions of calorie-rich food
- Orexigenic agents, e.g. aperitifs, appetizing food
- Patient and family counselling to relieve the stress of family members trying to feed the patient to prevent death, and to address the patient's altered body image
- Graded exercise and rest periods to combat fatigue and maintain muscle strength; exercise has been shown to protect muscle against proteolysis induced by oxidation
- Consider ibuprofen for the pro-inflammatory state
- Drug treatment with some evidence of efficacy as in Table 7.9.

Fatigue

Fatigue is a commonly experienced symptom in patients with cancer; some studies suggest the majority of patients will experience fatigue at some stage during their illness or treatment. Cancer-related fatigue is defined by the National Comprehensive Cancer Network as 'a persistent, subjective sense of tiredness related to cancer and/or its treatment', which interferes with normal activities of daily living, and impairs quality of life. Fatigue is more common in patients undergoing active treatment and those with advanced disease. Fatigue is also common in non-cancer terminal illnesses such as COPD, HIV/ADS, multiple sclerosis and heart failure. Patients' experience of fatigue may be subjective with emotional changes or physical tiredness; or objective with changes in mental and physical performance. Many patients find fatigue distressing.

Despite its prevalence in palliative care, the mechanisms underpinning the syndrome are poorly understood. Primary fatigue is thought to be caused by tumours, and resultant high levels of pro-inflammatory cytokines. Secondary fatigue may

Table 7.9 Drugs with evidence of benefit in the treatment of cachexia

Progestogens	Megestrol acetate: systematic review demonstrated improved appetite and increased body weight. Some doubt that muscle is increased. Start at 160 mg a day as a single dose and regulate by response up to 1600 mg a day. Optimal dose 480 to 800 mg. Medroxy progesterone 1 g daily. Evidence less clear. Side effects: thromboembolism 5%, oedema, vaginal bleeding, impotence in men at high dose, raised blood pressure. Mild catabolic effect on skeletal muscle may be from glucocorticoid effect or anti-androgen.
Immunomodulator	Thalidomide inhibits TNF-alpha and is licensed for HIV and cancer-related cachexia. Antiemetic and anti-angiogenesis agent. Not for use in pregnant females as teratogenic.
Corticosteroids	Dexamethasone improves appetite, food intake, well-being and performance status, but not muscle mass or weight gain. Effects last 2–4 weeks only. Dexamethasone promotes catabolism and proteolysis. If the patient has a prognosis of months, prednisolone may be substituted for a better side effect profile. Progestogens have fewer side effects, so steroids are best avoided in cachectic patients, or preserved for the last 2–4 weeks of life.
NSAIDs	Ibuprofen is anti-inflammatory and may have an anti-tumour effect. There is some evidence of weight gain and possible survival advantage.
Omega 3 fatty acids	Block inflammatory pathways and shown to produce weight gain in patients with pancreatic cancer. Available as food supplement Prosure.

be caused by comorbid conditions, such as cachexia, anaemia, infection or drug side effects.

Fatigue should be carefully assessed before considering treatment, as current therapeutic options have a burden of side effects and fatigue may be protective for patients in end-stage disease. At present, there is no licensed treatment for primary fatigue.

Non-pharmacological treatment

Physical activity: this helps reduce fatigue and improve mood. Patients are advised to plan activities that are important to them, and pace themselves to avoid over-exertion and resultant fatigue. Day centres have graded exercise programmes within fatigue and breathlessness clinics.

Pharmacological treatment

Stimulant drugs –– Methylphenidate and modafinil are under investigation in palliative care patients.

Erythropoietin –– This improves fatigue in patients with chemotherapy-related anaemia. It is unclear whether the reduction in fatigue is due to increased haemoglobin or other mechanisms. Patients with squamous cell tumours respond best. However, the cost of treatment must be considered, in addition to the delay in onset of effect (approximately 4–6 weeks). Overall benefit is unproven and the possible promotion of tumour growth may limit its use.

Dexamethasone –– It is always tempting to use a steroid for fatigue as the early euphoric effect that lasts

2–4 weeks is encouraging. Steroids are counterproductive in the longer term due to myopathy, skin thinning and other, often severe, side effects and are not recommended.

Pathways for end of life and terminal care

Crucial to dying patients and their lay carers is coordination of care across boundaries. The Gold Standards Framework (GSF) is a systematic, evidenced-based framework that establishes a register of patients entering the last year of life and supports multidisciplinary review in general practice meetings. The tool is designed for generalists with underpinning education. The GSF is linked to specialist palliative care by outreach staff. It has graded, increasing, assessment and support for patients and carers as death approaches. Information sharing from secondary care is very important. The GSF is being extended currently with pilots into secondary care.

The Liverpool Care Pathway (LCP) is a tool that guides generalist staff in the intensive palliative care for patients, and lay carers, in the last few days of life. It has goals for physical comfort, with guidance on anticipatory prescribing, together with psychological, spiritual, and social care goals. Assessment and communication of the bereavement risk for carers is included. Communication of outcomes to primary care is part of the pathway.

Versions of the LCP are available for hospital, hospice, nursing home and community. It is constantly improving with annual national audits and is agreed good practice.

Conclusion

Palliative and end of life care is a broad field. In this text we have chosen some commonly encountered problems on the surgical wards in the hope of enthusing surgeons to extend the precision and science of their specialty to include the delivery of excellent palliative and end of life care. Similar to obstetrics, when as term approaches the doctor has two patients to consider when planning intervention, care of the dying is almost always delivered in the presence of distressed carers or relatives. Their experience of this death may influence not only the coming bereavement, but also the way they approach and plan for their own death in the future. Expert care of both parties is not only humane, but good healthcare prevention.

Further reading

Berger AM, Shuster JL Jr, **Von** Roenn JH (eds). *Principles and Practice of Palliative Care and Supportive Oncology.* 3rd edn. Lippincott Williams and Wilkins, 2007.

Speck P (ed). *Teamwork in Palliative Care: Fulfilling or Frustrating?* Oxford University Press, 2006.

Twycross R, Wilcock A (eds). *Palliative Care Formulary.* 3rd edn. Palliativedrugs.com Ltd., Nottingham.

Chapter

8

Preoperative assessment

Jeffrey L. Tong

The preoperative assessment (POA) of a patient presenting for surgery is a crucial component of management and embraces medical, surgical and anaesthetic care. The preoperative assessment should contribute to the patient's management and in particular to the decision-making process. For high-risk patients a multidisciplinary decision regarding the risk–benefit of the proposed surgery should be encouraged. An accurate preoperative assessment should allow the team to:

- determine the need for surgery based on the patient's general status (should we operate; what should be performed; when should it be done?)
- identify and optimize co-existing disease
- select the best anaesthetic technique and perioperative management.

Assessment should be directed towards the individual patient and may be divided into: history, physical examination and investigations.

History

The best source of information relevant to any subsequent anaesthesia is obtained from a thorough history. A questionnaire can be given to the patient prior to clerking as a starting point, followed by more direct interrogation on receiving positive responses.

History of previous anaesthesia

The presence of co-existing disease and certain conditions are particularly relevant to anaesthesia. Warning notices following adverse reactions or complications during anaesthesia may be visible on patient records. Previous anaesthetic records should be examined for more detailed explanations.

Malignant hyperthermia/hyperpyrexia

Malignant hyperthermia/hyperpyrexia (MH) is a rarely encountered inherited disease (autosomal dominant) which can be triggered by all inhalational anaesthetic agents and suxamethonium. It is a potentially fatal disorder of muscle with uncontrolled muscle contraction and increased metabolism. Its occurrence is more likely in the presence of muscular disorders, e.g. strabismus, scoliosis and muscular dystrophies. It presents with muscle rigidity, hypercapnia and increased temperature during anaesthesia. Cardiovascular instability, increased oxygen consumption and metabolic acidosis also occur. Reactions have been reported up to 11 hours postoperatively. Treatment involves discontinuing the triggering agent (and if feasible the abandonment of surgery), cardiovascular support and the administration of intravenous (IV) sodium dantrolene. Survivors and screened relatives usually carry 'medical alert' bracelets.

Suxamethonium apnoea

Suxamethonium is a depolarizing muscle relaxant of short duration, which is usually rapidly metabolized by the plasma cholinesterase enzyme. Muscular fasciculation may be seen following administration. In the presence of a recessive abnormality or insufficient enzyme, it is metabolized slower than normal, prolonging the period of apnoea and paralysis. There is a delay in restoring respiratory effort after surgery, requiring ventilation and prolongation of anaesthesia or sedation to avoid awareness.

Anaphylaxis

This is a severe life-threatening, systemic hypersensitivity reaction. Investigation will determine whether the reaction was allergic (immunoglobulin E

Fundamentals of Surgical Practice, Third Edition, ed. Andrew N. Kingsnorth and Douglas M. Bowley.
Published by Cambridge University Press. © Cambridge University Press 2011.

(IgE)-mediated or non-IgE-mediated) or non-allergic anaphylaxis. Immunological reactions to anaesthetic drugs are usually commoner within families and may be more serious in atopic patients or in those with pre-existing sensitivities to other classes of drugs. A history of post-induction cardiovascular collapse, severe bronchospasm requiring admission to intensive care or cardiac arrest is highly suggestive. The term anaphylactoid reaction is no longer used.

Porphyria

This is a group of inherited disorders in haem synthesis, characterized by overproduction and excretion of porphyrins and their precursors. Acute attacks may present with abdominal pain, cardiovascular instability or neuropsychiatric manifestations. Known precipitants include: barbiturates (thiopental), phenytoin, sulphonamides and alcohol.

Sickle cell disorders

This is a group of autosomally inherited abnormalities in haemoglobin structure and function (haemoglobinopathy) caused by a single amino acid substitution. Sickle is characterized by polymerization of haemoglobin (Hb) in the presence of hypoxaemia, which causes a distortion (sickle-shaped) and increased rigidity of the erythrocyte, which can lead to microvascular occlusion, organ infarction and haemolysis. Manifestations include ischaemic pain, haemolytic anaemia, susceptibility to infection and organ dysfunction. It is prevalent in sub-Saharan Africa, the Caribbean, Asia, the south-eastern Mediterranean and Arabian peninsula. Heterozygotes (sickle cell trait) possess both normal (HbA) and abnormal haemoglobin (HbS), whilst homozygotes (sickle cell disease) possess only abnormal haemoglobin (HbSS). Diagnosis involves Hb electrophoresis which distinguishes between different Hb abnormalities (AS, SS, SC and SD). It can be screened by an agglutination test, e.g. sickledex, which induces sickling in susceptible cells but it cannot distinguish between the different variants (Table 8.1). If in doubt about the diagnosis it is safer to treat the patient as though they had sickle cell disease (SS). In the absence of haemorrhage or chronic disease, sickle cell disease (SS) patients are likely to be anaemic.

For elective surgery, a preoperative diagnosis is important, but Hb electrophoresis should never delay life-saving surgery. Perioperative and anaesthetic

Table 8.1 The relationship between haemoglobin polymerization and PO_2

Haemoglobin genotype	Critical PO_2 (kPa)
Hb AS	2.5–4
Hb SC	4
Hb SS[a]	5–6

[a] May see continuous sickling at venous PO_2.

management is based on efforts to minimize those factors known to precipitate sickling: hypoxaemia, dehydration, hypothermia, blood stasis and acidaemia. If a bloodless surgical field is essential, tourniquets have been used without complication, but as a general rule they should be avoided. Postoperative analgesia should be appropriate to the pain score, and may be achieved using a patient-controlled analgesia system (PCA). Opioid addiction can occur. Precautions against venous thrombosis are important as blood stasis and thrombosis may occur postoperatively.

Difficult tracheal intubation

This is an important cause of morbidity and mortality in emergency anaesthesia, as the difficulty encountered during intubation may not have been anticipated. Difficult intubation has an incidence of about 1–3% in the general population. Although many of these patients have common features, difficulty may also occur in otherwise unremarkable patients.

Past medical history

The presence of coexisting disease may adversely affect organ systems, resulting in functional limitations, which may affect the administration and recovery following anaesthesia:

Respiratory disease

Chronic obstructive airway disease (COAD), restrictive disorders and bronchial asthma can potentially have great limitations on the conduct of anaesthesia. Dyspnoea, cough, haemoptysis, wheeze and excessive smoking are important aspects of the history and disease severity may be estimated by the restriction of daily activities and immobility. Home oxygen and the use of non-invasive methods of optimizing gas exchange should be identified. It is essential that any deterioration in disease control and the presence of active respiratory tract infection be promptly identified and evaluated. The use of steroids for management of exacerbations should be recorded.

Cardiovascular disease

Questioning should focus on the presence of angina pectoris, palpitations or rhythm disorders, dyspnoea and syncope. Effort tolerance may provide a useful guide to disease severity. Further questioning should be aimed at identifying the symptoms of congestive heart failure and peripheral vascular disease. Previous acute coronary syndrome (ACS) events or myocardial infarction and their subsequent management are extremely important. The presence of valvular disorders or pacemakers should be confirmed. In patients with cardiac pacemakers, the indication for insertion, setting and most recent service date are required.

Gastrointestinal disease

Gastro-oesophageal reflux disease and hiatus hernia increase the risk of regurgitation of gastric contents and pulmonary aspiration. In the presence of these diseases a modification to the anaesthetic technique is required, which influences the choice of induction drugs and airway device selected. A thorough history will help determine whether these precautions are necessary.

Endocrine disease

Diabetes mellitus is a common coexisting disease which can affect multiple organ systems. The efficiency of glycaemic control should be established by questioning and by biochemical investigation. In the presence of obesity, the likely cause should be explored and the body weight measured. Hyperthyroid patients may require further investigation and optimization prior to surgery.

Hepatic and renal disease

Previous episodes of jaundice, bleeding disorders, encephalopathy and symptoms of uraemia and bone disease should be confirmed. Questions directed at urine volume may help determine renal function. The method and frequency of dialysis together with the location of functioning and older arteriovenous fistulae are relevant. Renal and hepatic disease may influence the choice of anaesthetic drugs due to their significant effect on pharmacokinetics.

Table 8.2 Drug interactions and anaesthesia

Drug	Effect	Comment
Beta-blockers	Hypotensive effect enhanced Bradycardia may be refractory	Caution if treatment recently started
Angiotensin-converting enzyme inhibitors (ACEI)	Hypotensive effect enhanced Hyperkalaemia	Risk of renal impairment
Calcium channel antagonists	Additive effect with inhalational anaesthetic agents (which also reduce calcium entry into cells)	Continue perioperatively as severe interactions are rarely a problem
Clopidogrel Aspirin	Platelet aggregation inhibited	Consider stopping 1 week preoperatively (discuss with surgeon)
Monoamine oxidase inhibitors (MAOI)	Hypertensive response to pethidine and sympathomimetics drugs exaggerated	Do **not** stop drug before surgery. Alternative antidepressants may not be effective

Musculo-skeletal disease

A careful assessment is required in patients with connective tissue diseases, e.g. rheumatoid arthritis and systemic lupus erythematosus (SLE), as they may have systemic manifestations which can have widespread effects during the perioperative period.

Drug history

A thorough list is required of prescribed, over-the-counter and recreational drugs, with dosages, frequency and route of administration. Knowledge of known allergy to specific substances or groups of substances is essential. Medication that should be discontinued or omitted preoperatively should be identified. Many different classes of drugs can have pharmacokinetic and pharmacodynamic interactions with anaesthetic agents (Table 8.2), which may be a cause of morbidity and mortality.

Social history

Alcohol and tobacco use should be quantified and the symptoms of diseases associated with their use sought.

Table 8.3 An AMPLE history

A	Allergies
M	Medication
P	Past medical history
L	Last meal or drink (time of)
E	Events and environment leading to the injury

Table 8.4 Tests to predict difficult airways

Test	Method	Scoring
Modified Mallampati classification	Assesses the view of pharyngeal structures on maximal mouth opening and tongue protrusion	Class I–IV
Upper lip bite test	Assesses forward movement (subluxation) of the mandible	Class I–III
Thyromental distance (Patel distance)	Distance from tip of mandible to top of thyroid cartilage. Ideally >6.5 cm	Critical distance 6 cm
Sterno-mental distance (Savva distance)	Distance from tip of mandible to sternal notch. Ideally >12.5 cm	Critical distance 12.5 cm
Delilkan warning signs	Assesses movement of the occiput on the atlas	Normal or abnormal

AMPLE

In emergency and trauma surgery there may be insufficient time to obtain a detailed history from the patient. The mnemonic AMPLE provides a helpful reminder in extracting the essential components from the patient's history (Table 8.3). When patient confusion or reduced consciousness restricts history-taking, information should be requested from the ambulance crew, relatives and general practice or hospital records.

Physical examination

A systematic and full clinical examination should be performed on every patient before anaesthesia.

Airway

There are many syndromes and diseases which are associated with difficult tracheal intubation but these may be anticipated preoperatively, e.g. Pierre-Robin syndrome. Identifying physical features and performing specific bedside tests may allow potential airway problems to be predicted preoperatively (Table 8.4). A single airway test or measurement is insufficient to accurately predict a difficult airway (Figure 8.1), so to improve the predictive power all of the tests should be performed. The Wilson difficult intubation scoring system incorporates five individually scored predictive risk factors: weight, head and neck movement, jaw movement, receding mandible and buck teeth. High scores are associated with an increased incidence of difficult intubation.

Dental irregularity may make tracheal intubation difficult, e.g. buck teeth and maxillary overbite, but teeth may also be damaged or displaced. Loose teeth and crowns should be carefully documented and loose-fitting dentures removed prior to anaesthesia.

Respiratory system

Infection of the respiratory tract in association with pyrexia, purulent nasal discharge or productive cough is a clear indication to postpone elective surgery. Many children frequently present with pyrexia of viral origin, tonsillitis or ear infections. These cases require thorough assessment with parental discussion of the risk–benefits, before the child is fed or sent home. In chronic conditions evidence of recent deterioration should be identified.

Cardiovascular system

Untreated or poorly controlled hypertension increases the risk of cardiac, renal and cerebrovascular

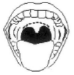 Class 1
 Class 2
 Class 3
 Class 4

Figure 8.1 The modified Mallampati classification of pharyngeal appearance. Class 1, full view of structures; Class 2, base of uvula obscured by tongue, faucial pillars seen; Class 3, soft palate still visible; Class 4, only hard palate visible.

Table 8.5 Revised cardiac risk index

Active cardiac conditions
Unstable coronary syndromes
   unstable angina
   acute myocardial infarction (within 7 days)
   recent myocardial infarction (within one month)
Decompensated heart failure
Significant arrhythmias
Severe valvular disease

Clinical risk factors
History of ischaemic heart disease
History of compensated or prior heart failure
History of cerebrovascular disease
Diabetes mellitus
Renal insufficiency

complications. Any cardiac rhythm other than sinus rhythm is associated with increased cardiac morbidity. Valvular lesions carry the risk of arrhythmias, embolism and endocarditis and warrant careful assessment. Angina may be classified according to the New York Heart Association (NYHA) classification. Recent myocardial infarction increases the risk of perioperative re-infarction or cardiac morbidity. If present, arteriovenous fistulae should be afforded appropriate perioperative protection.

Cardiac risk

A revised cardiac risk index has been developed for assessing the risk of perioperative death or severe cardiovascular complications following non-cardiac surgery. The presence of one or more active cardiac conditions mandates intensive management unless the surgery is emergent (Table 8.5).

In patients who have not had a previous myocardial infarction (MI) the perioperative infarction rate is 0.1–0.2%. However, following previous MI the perioperative reinfarction rate is 6%, but it has a mortality up to 70%, and is commonest on the third postoperative day. This risk is related to how recently the infarct occurred, being greater during the first 3–6 months, but it is also influenced by the degree of residual damage, which may be limited by thrombolytic therapy and angioplasty. Traditionally the advice has been to delay surgery for up to 6 months, but the risk of cardiac complication must be balanced against the benefit of surgery.

Obesity

All patients should have their weight (kg) and height (m) measured, which allows body mass index (BMI)

to be calculated. Morbid obesity is defined as a BMI $>35 \text{ kg/m}^2$. Obesity is associated with many complications and technical challenges, which combine to produce a patient with an increased risk of perioperative morbidity and mortality. Associated endocrine disorders may require perioperative optimization.

Investigations

Preoperative clinical investigations provide a tool for assessing a patient's fitness for surgery, but the history and examination are generally considered more useful when screening for disease. Investigations may be used to demonstrate that further preoperative optimization is required and they provide an important baseline for subsequent testing. Inappropriate investigations are time consuming and are a waste of resources. Consequently guidelines for ordering investigations are related to the:

- specificity and sensitivity of the test
- incidence of abnormality in the population
- clinical significance if result is abnormal
- cost-effectiveness.

ECG

A relationship exists between abnormalities detected on the preoperative 12-lead ECG and adverse postoperative cardiac outcome. ECG evidence of dysrhythmia, myocardial ischaemia and previous infarction is a clear indication for further investigation. In an exercise ECG test, the patient performs a graded increase in exercise to achieve a maximum heart rate or until ischaemic changes occur. A combination of inability to achieve 75–85% of maximal heart rate response with ischaemic ECG changes is associated with a higher incidence of postoperative cardiac events.

Cardiac function

Measurements of the ventricular ejection fraction have been used as a preoperative predictor of compromised cardiac function. Radionucleotide ventriculography studies established that an ejection fraction (EF) $<35\%$ had a 75% risk of postoperative complications. An EF of 35–56% had an intermediate risk.

Transthoracic echocardiography is frequently performed to assess ventricular filling and ejection, ventricular wall thickness and contractility. Stress echocardiography improves the assessment by identifying wall motion abnormalities in ischaemic areas.

This may be achieved by infusing dobutamine to produce a graded increase in heart rate to a predetermined level.

Dipyridamole-thallium scintigraphy (DTS) is able to identify areas of infarction or reversible myocardial ischaemia, which have been used to predict postoperative cardiac problems, but it is insufficiently specific to be applied to all patients.

Chest X-ray

Chest X-rays should **not** be routinely requested as part of hospital admission, preoperative, pre-anaesthesia or postoperative assessment. In a previous review, only 1.3% of routine preoperative chest X-rays showed an unexpected abnormality. A chest X-ray is indicated when there is a clinical suspicion of active chest disease based on the history and physical examination. Indications recommended by the radiologists include:

- cardiorespiratory disease (unless recent (6–12 months) films available)
- new respiratory symptoms
- possible pulmonary metastases
- severe trauma
- immigration from tuberculosis (TB) region.

Pulmonary function tests

In patients with known pulmonary disease, simple lung function tests significantly contribute to the preoperative assessment. The forced vital capacity (FVC) and forced expiratory volume in one second (FEV 1) can be measured using a spirometer. In obstructive lung disease both the FEV 1 and the FEV 1 / FVC ratio are reduced. In restrictive disease the FEV 1 may be normal but the FVC is reduced.

In asthmatic patients the peak expiratory flow rate (PEFR) should be measured using a peak flowmeter before and after the administration of bronchodilators. Any improvement following the administration of bronchodilators indicates that preoperative optimization is required.

Haematology

If indicators are identified from the history and examination, a full blood count should be performed preoperatively. Anaemia and thrombocytopaenia may require further investigation and treatment. For major surgery intraoperative transfusion is often preferred. In certain types of surgery a preoperative leukocy-tosis may necessitate treatment with antibiotics and the rescheduling of the procedure. Coagulation studies should be performed selectively in patients scheduled to receive spinal or epidural analgesia.

Biochemistry

Metabolic diseases, drug therapy and dehydration are known to alter biochemistry. Electrolyte abnormalities should be corrected and optimized preoperatively. Daily maintenance can be provided by intravenous electrolyte solutions when nil by mouth. Further fluid and electrolyte replacement may be necessary with large gastric aspirates or other intestinal losses.

Arterial blood gas analysis may provide information on the adequacy of oxygenation, gas exchange and acid base balance. Modern measuring devices also provide information on haemoglobin, electrolytes, glucose and lactate. Providing the blood sample has been heparinized, venous and capillary blood can also be loaded into the device.

Autonomic dysfunction

An autonomic neuropathy may occur in up to 40% of patients with long-standing diabetes mellitus, resulting in an increase in cardiorespiratory morbidity, which may lead to intraoperative haemodynamic instability and sudden death. In addition to identifying factors from the history, clinical tests can be performed to measure the integrity of the autonomic nervous system, e.g. heart rate response to a Valsalva manoeuvre.

Scoring systems

ASA classification

The definitions of the American Society of Anesthesiologists (ASA) physical status classification provides a grading system to assess the patient's physical state prior to anaesthesia and surgery. The modern classification system consists of six categories (Table 8.6). The grading system is not intended for use as a measure to predict operative risk, but ASA class IV and V patients invariably require postoperative admission to an intensive care unit (ICU). It is crucial that prompt resuscitation is commenced once critically ill patients are identified, as early organ system support and preoperative optimization may reduce the risk of subsequent organ system failure.

Numerous scoring systems exist which may be used for classifying patients according to preoperative

Table 8.6 ASA classification system

Category	Status	Comments
ASA I	Normal healthy patients	Excludes extremes of age
ASA II	Patients with mild systemic disease	Well-controlled disease of one body system
ASA III	Patients with severe systemic disease	Controlled disease with some functional limitation
ASA IV	Patients with severe systemic disease that is a constant threat to life	Poorly controlled or end stage disease
ASA V	Moribund patients who are not expected to survive without the operation	Not expected to survive more than 24 hours
ASA VI	A declared brain-dead patient whose organs are being removed for donor purposes	Ongoing organ harvest

The addition of an 'E' indicates emergency surgery.

status: New York Heart Association (NYHA) classification, Glasgow coma scale (GCS), Ranson score, MELD score, Acute Physiology and Chronic Health Evaluation (APACHE) etc.

Further reading

Aitkenhead AR, Smith G, Rowbotham DJ. *Textbook of Anaesthesia.* 5th edn. Churchill Livingstone Elsevier, 2007.

Archer C, Levy AR, McGregor M. Value of routine preoperative chest X-rays: a meta-analysis. *Can J Anesth* 1993;**40**:1022–1027.

Hines RL, Marschall KE. *Stoelting's Anesthesia and Co-Existing Disease.* 5th edn. Churchill Livingstone, 2008.

Khan ZH, Kafshi A, Ebrahimkhani E. A comparison of the upper lip bite test (a simple new technique) with modified Mallampati classification in predicting difficulty in endotracheal intubation: A prospective blinded study. *Anesthesia and Analgesia* 2003;**96**:595–599.

Lee TH, Marcantonio ER, Mangione CM *et al.* Derivation and prospective validation of a simple index for prediction of cardiac risk of major noncardiac surgery. *Circulation* 1999;**100**:1043–1049.

Roa TLK, Jacobs KH, El-Etr AA. Reinfarction following anaesthesia in patients with myocardial infarction. *Anesthesiology* 1983;**59**:499–505.

Smith T, Pinnock C, Lin T *et al. Fundamentals of Anaesthesia.* 3rd edn. Cambridge University Press, 2009.

Vaughan RS. Predicting difficult airways. *Br J Anaesth CPD Rev* 2001;**1**:44–47.

Chapter

9

Fundamentals of anaesthesia

Jeffrey L. Tong

Anaesthesia may be defined as a pharmacologically induced state of reversible unconsciousness, during which the patient neither perceives nor recalls noxious stimuli. Anaesthetic drugs depress all excitable tissues and the central neurons are amongst the most sensitive. At sufficient anaesthetic depth conscious awareness and recall are lost, and normal sensory, somatic and autonomic responses to surgical stimulation are absent.

Anaesthesia is a non-therapeutic intervention, performed within a dedicated environment. The complications of anaesthesia may be poorly tolerated, so all patients must be individually assessed to evaluate the benefits versus potential risks. The maintenance of maximum perioperative safety is of significant importance during the administration of anaesthesia.

Stages of clinical anaesthesia

In 1937, four stages of progressively deeper anaesthesia were described by Guedel in unpremedicated patients during inhalational induction with diethyl ether. Modern advances have resulted in considerable changes to techniques and available drugs, so that the early stages of anaesthesia often occur too rapidly to be easily distinguished. The stages may be seen in reverse on emergence from anaesthesia.

Analgesia

In stage 1, inhalational sedation occurs prior to the loss of the eyelash reflex and unconsciousness.

Excitement

During stage 2, the breathing gradually becomes more irregular and airway irritability increases. The pupils become more dilated and uncontrolled limb movements may occur. The eyelid reflex is lost.

Surgical anaesthesia

Stage 3 classically consists of four 'planes' (I–IV):

1. Breathing is regular with large tidal volumes (automatic breathing). The pupils are small and the conjunctival reflex is lost. Swallowing and vomiting reflexes are depressed.
2. Regular deep breathing remains, but intercostal muscle paralysis begins. The corneal reflex is lost and the pupils become larger.
3. Shallow diaphragmatic breathing occurs due to intercostal paralysis. Pupils are large with depressed light reflex. Lacrimation and the laryngeal reflexes are depressed.
4. Breathing becomes irregular and shallow until diaphragmatic paralysis occurs. The pupils are dilated and the carinal reflexes are depressed.

Surgery is normally conducted in plane III of stage 3, which is also called surgical anaesthesia.

Overdose

In stage 4 brainstem activity is reduced, with profound cardiorespiratory depression and apnoea. The pupils are fixed and dilated.

Awareness

The primary duty of the anaesthetist is to maintain patient safety during anaesthesia – 'in somno securitas'. Failure to maintain adequate intraoperative anaesthetic depth and appropriate analgesia may lead to conscious awareness with recollection. It is rare for a patient to remember intraoperative events, but 0.1–0.2% of all patients undergoing general anaesthesia may report being 'awake during an operation'. This may cause considerable patient stress with both psychological and medico-legal consequences,

Fundamentals of Surgical Practice, Third Edition, ed. Andrew N. Kingsnorth and Douglas M. Bowley.
Published by Cambridge University Press. © Cambridge University Press 2011.

Table 9.1 The aims of premedication prior to anaesthesia

Reduce anxiety
Alleviate pain
Facilitate intravenous cannulation
Reduce salivation and secretions
Reduce nausea and vomiting
Reduce autonomic reflexes
Increase gastric emptying and pH

especially if the provision of intraoperative analgesia was inadequate.

Awareness has been reported following general anaesthesia in patients with minimal cardiac reserve and hypovolaemic shock, e.g. cardiac, trauma and obstetric surgery. It has a higher incidence when muscle relaxants are used, as the patient is unable to move or respond to pain when anaesthetic depth decreases. However, 'moving' under general anaesthesia does not necessarily correlate with awareness, just as 'not moving' under general anaesthesia does not necessarily correlate with amnesia!

Awareness may be due to poor anaesthetic technique or equipment malfunction, but clinical assessment of the patient for signs of light anaesthesia (tachycardia, hypertension, sweating, lacrimation and reactive pupils) and appropriate monitoring, e.g. endtidal anaesthetic agent and bispectral index (BIS) monitoring, can help avoid inadequate anaesthesia.

Premedication

The aim of premedication is to prepare the patient for surgery and reduce the risk from coexisting diseases and anaesthesia-specific complications (Table 9.1). It is important that certain regular medication is continued prior to surgery, e.g. anticonvulsants, bronchodilators and cardiac drugs. In adult practice routine oral premedication is rarely administered, as many anaesthetists prefer to give drugs intravenously in the anaesthetic room.

Topical anaesthesia

Local anaesthetic creams can provide good anaesthesia at venepuncture and cannulation sites, and are used primarily in infants and children. They should be applied to intact skin and be covered with an occlusive dressing. Amethocaine 4% (Ametop) should be removed after 45 min. Hypersensitivity has been reported. EMLA (eutectic mixture of local anaesthetic) is a mixture of lidocaine 2.5% and prilocaine 2.5% and should be applied at least an hour before anaesthesia. Methaemoglobinaemia may occur.

Sedation

Anxiolysis, light sedation and amnesia (anterograde) may be achieved using oral benzodiazepines, e.g. temazepam 1–2 h before surgery. Some benzodiazepines have a long elimination half-life and active metabolites, which can delay recovery. Midazolam and chloral hydrate have been used in children. Intramuscular ketamine has been used for sedation when efforts to facilitate intravenous access are challenged. Procedural consent should be obtained before administration of sedative premedication.

Analgesia

In the presence of acute pain, appropriate analgesia should be administered. Opioid premedication is unnecessary in the absence of pain, due to the risk of predictable side effects: respiratory depression, dysphoria, sedation, nausea and vomiting. Histamine release may also cause bronchospasm and cardiovascular instability. A loading dose of oral paracetamol is occasionally given to children.

Aspiration

Pharmacologically increasing gastric pH, gastric emptying and oesophageal sphincter pressure are important when the risk of regurgitation of gastric contents is high. Metoclopramide can achieve some of these effects and has the added benefit of antiemetic properties. Histamine H_2-receptor antagonists and antacids (sodium citrate) have a supplementary role. A specialized anaesthetic technique which involves the application of cricoid pressure helps minimize the risk of pulmonary aspiration.

Anticholinergics

Bradycardia may be associated with surgery, airway instrumentation and certain drugs, e.g. suxamethonium. To improve cardiovascular stability anticholinergic drugs are used for their vagolytic action, which protects against bradycardia. Anticholinergics also have an antisialogue effect that decreases airway secretions and salivation, resulting in a dry mouth. Atropine and hyoscine both cross the blood–brain

Table 9.2 Preoperative fasting prior to anaesthesia

Food type	Rules
Water Clear fluids Black tea or coffee	Can be given up to 2 hours pre-induction
All solids Formula baby milk[a] Hot drinks with milk All sweets Chewing-gum[a]	Can be given up to 6 hours pre-induction

[a] The rules for breast milk and chewing-gum are variable.

barrier, which has a sedative effect, but this may cause confusion in the elderly.

Preoperative fasting

Anaesthesia abolishes the airway protective reflexes, so if gastric contents regurgitate into the pharynx, pulmonary aspiration may occur. Therefore for all non-emergency surgery, anaesthesia is contraindicated in patients with a full stomach. In an emergency, the balance of risk between delaying surgery and aspiration needs to be determined. Patients should be kept nil by mouth (NBM) prior to anaesthesia or sedation, and protocols have been developed at departmental level to deal with preoperative fasting. A typical protocol is shown in Table 9.2.

To reduce the risk of dehydration and other metabolic consequences, prolonged periods of fasting should be avoided and IV fluids provided as appropriate. Despite being NBM, important medication, including analgesia, should not be omitted and may be given up to 1 hour pre-induction. Diabetics should be placed at the start of an operating list and glycaemic control is improved using an insulin sliding scale. Normal gastric emptying may be delayed by pain, anxiety and following the administration of opioids, and these patients require special anaesthetic precautions.

Preanaesthesia checks

Checking the availability and correct functioning of anaesthetic equipment is a mandatory procedure before administering any anaesthetic and represents an important aspect of patient safety. Following completion of the checklist, a record is made in a logbook kept with each anaesthetic machine. Some of the important checks and requirements prior to anaesthesia include:

- a trained assistant
- IV cannulae
- emergency and routine drugs
- minimum monitoring standards (AAGBI working party 2007) in the anaesthetic room and theatre:
  - continuous ECG
  - non-invasive blood pressure (NIBP)
  - capnography
  - pulse oximetry
  - suction apparatus
- a range of airway equipment
- a checked anaesthetic machine and ventilator
- oxygen and medical gases
- breathing system and filters
- vaporizers
- a tipping trolley and operating table
  - the patient:
  - identity confirmed
  - appropriately consented
  - site of surgery marked
  - NBM status confirmed.

The WHO Safe Surgery Initiative has introduced a preoperative checklist that has been shown to improve compliance with standards and decrease complications from surgery.

Preoxygenation

Once the patient has been checked in, IV access and monitoring are established (ECG, NIBP and pulse oximetry). The patient is then given 100% oxygen via an anaesthetic breathing system and facemask. The purpose of preoxygenation is to denitrogenate the functional residual capacity (FRC), which increases the amount of oxygen in the lungs, blood and tissues. This allows more time for post-induction airway management and may prevent arterial desaturation and hypoxaemia. Preoxygenation is an essential procedure prior to rapid sequence induction of anaesthesia and when difficult airway management is anticipated. Anaesthetic facemasks may exacerbate anxiety and fear in some patients, but, in general, preoxygenation should always be attempted prior to anaesthesia.

Induction

Following a period of preoxygenation, induction of anaesthesia should normally be performed in a dedicated environment. Induction describes the transition from the awake to the anaesthetized state and represents a period of great physiological change during which the following may occur:

- airway obstruction and laryngospasm
- hypoventilation and apnoea
- hypotension and arrhythmias
- regurgitation and aspiration
- adverse drug reactions.

The most commonly used induction techniques are intravenous and inhalational, although other routes of drug administration (rectal or intramuscular) are possible.

Intravenous induction

An estimated dose of IV anaesthetic agent should be given slowly and the effect observed before injecting more (titration to effect). Unconsciousness is usually achieved in one arm–brain circulation time, due to the drug rapidly crossing the blood–brain barrier to interact with the receptors in the central nervous system (CNS). Unconsciousness may be delayed when the arm–brain circulation time is prolonged, e.g. in those with cardiovascular disease and the elderly. The duration of effect of an induction agent is not limited by its rate of metabolism, but by its redistribution within the body. The characteristics of IV induction depend largely on the physicochemical and pharmacological properties of the agent used. Extravasation and intra-arterial injection may occur.

Inhalational induction

Spontaneous ventilation is maintained and the inhalational anaesthetic agent is gradually introduced in increasing concentrations. The different stages of anaesthesia may be seen, which may be prolonged. Inhalational induction occurs at a slower rate than with IV agents, and the factors that influence this are the inspired anaesthetic concentration, alveolar ventilation and cardiac output. Unconsciousness may occur more rapidly in infants because of their greater alveolar ventilation and smaller FRC per unit body weight. The technique may be associated with breath-holding, laryngospasm and coughing. It is an important method of induction in uncooperative children, and when presented with difficult IV access or airway.

Rapid sequence induction

When the risks of regurgitation of gastric contents and aspiration are high a rapid sequence induction (RSI) is indicated. The technique involves administering a predetermined dose of an intravenous induction agent, followed by suxamethonium to achieve rapid muscle relaxation. Alternatives are available if suxamethonium is contraindicated. Pressure applied to the cricoid cartilage by an assistant compresses the oesophagus against the body of the sixth cervical vertebra, which minimizes the risk of aspiration. Cricoid pressure is maintained until tracheal intubation has been completed and the cuff inflated. The procedure is performed promptly and, with adequate preoxygenation, significant arterial desaturation and hypoxaemia are uncommon. An action plan in the event of a difficult or failed intubation is essential.

Airway management

Once anaesthesia has been induced, oxygenation and ventilation of the lungs is performed using the anaesthetic facemask. Loss of muscle tone may result in an obstructed airway which may be improved using airway-opening manoeuvres and adjuncts. A head-tilt and chin-lift (extending the head and lifting the chin) or a jaw-thrust manoeuvre, in combination with an oropharyngeal (Guedel) airway, can restore airway patency by clearing the tongue off the pharyngeal wall. When cervical trauma is suspected, a jaw-thrust is the only acceptable airway opening manoeuvre. Whilst airway patency using an oropharyngeal airway and facemask can be continued intraoperatively, it is rarely practised.

Supra-glottic airway devices

The laryngeal mask airway (LMA) and other supra-glottic devices are frequently used to maintain airway patency when tracheal intubation is unnecessary or difficult. They do not prevent aspiration and so should only be used when the stomach is empty. It consists of an inflatable oval mask attached to a connecting tube. The mask is inserted blindly into the pharynx where it rests against the glottis and cuff inflation creates a seal. They can be safely used during intermittent positive pressure ventilation (IPPV) and techniques using muscle relaxation. A modification to the classic LMA design has incorporated a drain tube to protect against gastric insufflation and minimize the risk of aspiration, by providing an escape route for air and unexpected regurgitation. Devices are available with reinforced connecting tubes to prevent kinking.

Tracheal intubation

Inserting a cuffed tube into the trachea provides a secure airway, protection to the endobronchial tree from aspiration, a means of performing endobronchial suctioning and a conduit for IPPV. Following induction, ideal intubating conditions are achieved using muscle relaxants, but non-relaxant techniques using potent opioids are also effective. Traditionally a laryngoscope with a curved blade (Macintosh) is inserted between the teeth and advanced until the tip is in the vallecula, anterior to the epiglottis. Traction applied to the thyro-epiglottic ligament displaces the tongue into the sub-mandibular space, which provides a direct line of sight from the incisors to the vocal cords. The view of the glottis may be improved by optimal positioning of the head and neck and external pressure to the thyroid cartilage.

The aetiology of difficult intubation is multifactorial, and although unanticipated difficulty has a low incidence in the general population, protocols are an essential component of failed intubation plans. Fibreoptic endoscopy remains the gold-standard method of managing a difficult airway and intubation may be performed in a conscious patient following local anaesthesia to the airway.

The pressor response associated with laryngoscopy and tracheal intubation (hypertension and tachycardia) may be diminished by providing adequate analgesia and depth of anaesthesia. Conversely, parasympathetically mediated bradycardia and asystole may occur following laryngo-pharyngeal stimulation in children. In paediatric patients a non-cuffed tube is preferred as sub-glottic mucosal oedema can occur following extubation, which significantly increases the work of breathing, which may result in the development of pulmonary oedema.

Ventilation

Intraoperative ventilation may be controlled or spontaneous.

Spontaneous

Following induction, apnoea is common but spontaneous ventilation may be re-established providing paralysis and controlled ventilation are not required. Normally an LMA or facemask technique is used, but patients can also breathe spontaneously through a tracheal tube. As muscle relaxants are not required during spontaneous ventilation, reflex movements may follow surgical stimulation. This can be minimized with a balanced technique of higher anaesthetic concentrations and potent analgesia, whilst avoiding decreased alveolar ventilation and prolonged emergence from anaesthesia. Spontaneous ventilation is often used for minor surgical procedures of short duration.

Controlled

Positive pressure ventilators are widely used to deliver IPPV via a tracheal tube, but this usually requires the intermittent administration of muscle relaxants. Controlled ventilation may be achieved without formal paralysis, as anaesthetic and analgesic drugs promote relaxation of skeletal muscle and depress respiratory drive. In suitable patients undergoing certain procedures, IPPV may be performed via supra-glottic airway devices.

IPPV involves the delivery of positive pressure to the airway during an inspiratory phase and passive exhalation during the expiratory phase, when the lungs recoil elastically to atmospheric pressure. Ventilators may be employed as:

1. Flow generators: these produce high generating pressures and flow is unaffected by patient characteristics. They can produce high inflation pressures required to ventilate non-compliant lungs, but barotrauma may occur.
2. Pressure generators: these produce low generating pressures and flow is affected by patient characteristics. The peak airway pressure is preset so the risk of barotrauma is reduced.

The delivered tidal volume is dependent on the airway resistance and compliance. This type of ventilator is used in paediatric anaesthesia.

High-frequency ventilation (HFV) may be necessary during specialized procedures, e.g. rigid bronchoscopy. This includes high-frequency jet ventilation (HFJV), which delivers high-frequency tidal volumes (up to 150 ml), producing positive airway pressures of approximately 5 cmH_2O. Exhalation is through the open system. Gas exchange is maintained without barotrauma and other adverse effects of IPPV.

Positive end-expiratory pressure

At the end of exhalation there is no pressure gradient between the lungs and the atmosphere. Positive end-expiratory pressure (PEEP) is an adjunct to IPPV, and is produced by maintaining a positive airway pressure during expiration. This increases the FRC, which minimizes alveolar collapse and terminal airway closure and increases compliance. Thus alveolar gas exchange is improved and pulmonary shunt is reduced, which may allow a reduction in inspired oxygen concentration. Adverse effects are related to the increase in intrathoracic pressure and include decreased venous return, reduced cardiac output, increased air trapping and barotrauma. When ventilation is spontaneous, maintaining a positive airway pressure during expiration is called continuous positive airway pressure (CPAP). The following terms describe PEEP adjustment:

- best PEEP: produces the least shunting without significant deterioration in cardiac output
- optimum PEEP: produces maximal O_2 delivery with the lowest dead space/tidal volume ratio.

Maintenance of anaesthesia

Following induction, the depth of anaesthesia-induced CNS suppression must be constantly monitored and maintained until surgery has been completed. Close vigilance of muscle paralysis and analgesic requirements are also necessary. Although no absolute monitor of depth of anaesthesia exists, electroencephalogram (EEG) and BIS monitoring may be helpful. Anaesthesia can be maintained using either inhalational agents or IV anaesthetic drugs.

Inhalational maintenance

The concentration of inhalational anaesthetic agent delivered into the breathing system is controlled by vaporizers attached to the anaesthetic machine. During ventilation, anaesthetic vapour enters the alveoli and the capillary blood down a partial pressure gradient. When the blood reaches the CNS, the high concentration of anaesthetic agent diffuses out of the blood to reach its site of action. With continuous administration of inhalational agent a steady state is reached after 20 min, but this is dependent on numerous factors and is agent-specific.

Inhalational maintenance is popular because it is simple to administer and alveolar levels (and blood levels) can easily be controlled by adjusting the inspired concentration. Clinical observations to exclude signs of inadequate anaesthetic depth are required, but it is customary to administer inhalational agents at concentrations known to provide CNS suppression. The concentration may then be titrated according to the individual patient response.

Intravenous maintenance

Total intravenous anaesthesia (TIVA) describes the technique of using intravenous anaesthetic agents to induce and maintain general anaesthesia. Propofol was introduced in 1986 and is the only available IV agent that has the pharmacological profile to be used in this way.

Technological advances in drug infusion systems and pharmacokinetics have enabled calculated blood concentrations to be achieved and controlled during intravenous anaesthesia. Specialized software within the infusion pump automatically alters the infusion rate according to validated pharmacokinetic models. Target controlled infusion (TCI) systems enable the anaesthetist to set and adjust the target blood concentration, so that the depth of anaesthesia can be adjusted intraoperatively according to the level of surgical stimulus and clinical responses.

Simultaneous opioid infusions are often administered, e.g. remifentanil, providing a balanced technique. Onset and offset of anaesthetic effects are rapid and reliable, and the technique has a low incidence of postoperative nausea and vomiting (PONV).

Analgesia

Intravenous analgesia is administered at induction and intraoperatively. Potent opioids are administered at induction to depress the pressor response associated with airway instrumentation and intubation. The duration of analgesia provided by these agents is short and additional intraoperative analgesia is often required according to the degree of surgical stimulation and response. Selecting agents with a longer duration of action provides analgesia during recovery and the immediate postoperative period. The choice of agent is often influenced by:

- pharmacological properties of the drug
- contraindications and adverse drug effects
- coexisting organ system dysfunction, e.g. hepatic and renal.

A multimodal approach often provides superior analgesia and this may involve the administration of non-opioid agents, e.g. local anaesthetic agents, non-steroidal anti-inflammatory drugs (NSAIDs), paracetamol and tramadol.

Muscle relaxation

Neuromuscular blocking drugs are used to impair neuromuscular transmission and provide skeletal muscle relaxation during anaesthesia or critical care. Following induction of anaesthesia, they are used to facilitate tracheal intubation, IPPV and provide optimal conditions for surgery. Neuromuscular function should be monitored with a peripheral nerve stimulator, which assesses the muscle response following stimulation of a peripheral nerve, via skin electrodes.

At the conclusion of surgery, residual neuromuscular function is assessed and antagonized by administering a reversal agent, e.g. neostigmine. This can precipitate unwanted muscarinic effects, e.g. bradycardia, excessive salivation and bronchospasm, so glycopyrronium or atropine is given with neostigmine.

Pharmacology

Inhalational agents

Modern inhalational agents are fluorinated hydrocarbons. They are liquid at room temperature and have a high saturated vapour pressure (SVP), so are often called volatile anaesthetic agents.

The potency of volatile agents depends on their lipid solubility (solubility in the CNS), which is estimated by the oil/gas solubility coefficient. Potency is gauged by the MAC or minimal alveolar concentration, and is defined as the alveolar concentration of inhalational anaesthetic agent that prevents movement in response to skin incision in 50% of patients. It is inversely related to anaesthetic potency and may be used to guide dose adjustment when monitoring the end-tidal concentration of agent. MAC values can be monitored, which provides useful information on anaesthetic depth. At 1.5 MAC, response is abolished in 95% of the population. The MAC may be influenced by many factors, and its value is lower in the elderly and higher in infants.

The speed of uptake of an anaesthetic depends on its solubility in blood, which is estimated by the blood/gas solubility coefficient. When agents with low solubility diffuse from the lungs into arterial blood, relatively small amounts are required to saturate the blood, so the arterial tension (and brain tension) rises quickly. More soluble agents require the solution of much more anaesthetic agent before the arterial tension approaches that of the inspired gas, so induction is slower. Emergence from anaesthesia is also slower with increasing anaesthetic solubility. Metabolism of inhalational agents occurs to a variable extent, but they are mostly eliminated unchanged during exhalation.

Modern inhalational agents have many similar characteristics, but each agent affects the systems to different degrees. They commonly decrease myocardial contractility, heart rate and arterial blood pressure, dilate vascular smooth muscle and alter the conducting system. Their effects on the respiratory system include bronchodilatation and respiratory depression. Airway irritability varies from coughing to bronchospasm.

Older agents

Halothane is a potent, non-irritant agent which provides a smooth inhalational induction. It can cause arrhythmias by sensitizing the myocardium to circulating catecholamines. Up to 20% is metabolized via hepatic oxidative pathways and a major toxic effect of halothane is hepatic necrosis (1 in 35 000). Minor hepatic dysfunction is common, especially after repeated use, so its use has declined. Enflurane causes the greatest depression of cardiac output and arterial blood pressure. Two per cent is metabolized, releasing fluoride ions which may be associated with renal impairment after prolonged use. Epileptiform activity may occur at high doses. Isoflurane is a pungent agent that is associated with the least increase in cerebral blood flow (CBF) and intracranial pressure (ICP), so has been used for neuroanaesthesia. It is a potent vasodilator and may cause coronary steal of blood from diseased arteries to healthy ones. Less than 0.2% is metabolized.

Newer agents

Sevoflurane is non-irritant and has a low blood/gas solubility coefficient, so induction and recovery are rapid. It causes less hypotension and tachycardia. It is currently the agent of choice to induce inhalational anaesthesia in children. Desflurane is less pungent than isoflurane but it has an extremely low blood/gas solubility coefficient. Thus uptake and recovery are very rapid. Delivery is via a specialized vapourizer.

Table 9.3 The adverse effects of nitrous oxide

Increases CBF and ICP
Diffusion hypoxia
Nausea and vomiting
Expansion of air-filled spaces
Bone marrow depression
Megaloblastic anaemia
Peripheral neuropathy

Nitrous oxide

This sweet-smelling gas is not potent enough to be used as a sole anaesthetic agent. Nitrous oxide (N_2O) is commonly used as an anaesthetic carrier gas with oxygen, allowing lower concentrations of volatile agent to be used. It is relatively insoluble and diffuses out of the alveolus faster than nitrogen diffuses in, which increases the alveolar concentration of the remaining substances (second gas effect). During recovery the reverse happens, causing a reduction in alveolar oxygen concentration (diffusion hypoxia). Supplementary oxygen may prevent the development of hypoxaemia. N_2O is a good analgesic and may be used with a 50% mixture in oxygen (Entonox). It has many side effects and many anaesthetists prefer using air (Table 9.3). Xenon is an inert gas that has anaesthetic properties, being 50% more potent than N_2O.

Intravenous agents

A variety of single IV agents or a combination of agents, e.g. benzodiazepines or opioids, may be used to induce anaesthesia. Intravenous induction agents are contraindicated in all patients with upper airway obstruction. Multiple factors influence the choice of an IV anaesthetic drug.

Propofol

This is an emulsion of phenol formulated in intralipid (soyabean oil and egg phosphatide), which is highly lipophilic and extensively protein-bound. Pain on injection has an incidence of 50% when administered into small veins on the dorsum of the hand. It causes a marked reduction in peripheral vascular resistance (PVR), a variable fall in cardiac output and is associated with bradycardia. Apnoea may occur with varying doses, so when used to provide sedation, appropriate airway management equipment must be readily available. Excitatory myoclonic activity may occur, which

has been mistaken for epileptiform activity. Pharyngeal and laryngeal reflexes are rapidly depressed after administration, allowing airway adjuncts or supraglottic devices to be inserted early. Its elimination is fairly constant, so there is less accumulation after large doses or prolonged use and rapid recovery occurs after cessation of an infusion. Its use is associated with a low incidence of PONV.

Thiopental

Previously known as thiopentone, this sulphur (thio) containing barbiturate is highly lipophilic and protein-bound, and is commonly used worldwide. Pain on injection is uncommon; therefore pain should provide warning of the possibility of extravasation or intra-arterial injection, which can cause tissue necrosis and distal ischaemia. Vasodilatation and decreased myocardial contractility commonly cause a reduction in mean arterial pressure (MAP), which in hypovolaemic patients may lead to cardiac arrest. Laryngeal spasm may occur if airway manipulation is performed before the protective reflexes are lost. Thiopental is metabolized in the liver and has a long elimination half-life, so a hang-over effect is often experienced during recovery.

Etomidate

This compound is more cardiovascularly stable and releases less histamine than other agents. However, it is associated with pain on injection, thrombophlebitis, myoclonia and suppression of adrenal steroidogenesis. The incidence of PONV is high.

Ketamine

This phencyclidine derivative is a racemic mixture, and is unique in that it produces both anaesthesia and analgesia. It has a hyperdynamic effect on the circulation, increasing heart rate, blood pressure and cardiac output. This effect is centrally mediated via the blocking of noradrenaline uptake mechanisms and noradrenaline release from sympathetic ganglia. Administration may be accompanied by increased salivation and psychological side effects, e.g. hallucinations and nightmares. It has an important role in high-risk patients, following pre-hospital trauma and in field anaesthesia.

Opioids

These provide the analgesic component in a balanced anaesthetic technique, and are routinely used as supplements during general anaesthesia to obtund the sympathetic response to tracheal intubation and the metabolic response to surgery. Opioids have a general anaesthetic agent-sparing or MAC-lowering effect, but they are unable to reliably produce anaesthesia alone. Opioid receptors are located in the CNS and gastrointestinal tract. All subtypes are antagonized by naloxone. Common side effects include: respiratory depression, cough suppression, euphoria, pruritus, constipation, urinary retention, miosis, nausea and vomiting. Histamine release and muscle rigidity may also occur.

Naturally occurring agents

Morphine is an alkaloid derived from poppy seeds and is the standard against which other opioids are compared. It undergoes significant first-pass metabolism following oral administration. The IV dose is 0.1–0.2 mg/kg, but in practice it should be titrated to response in 1 or 2 mg boluses. Peak effect occurs 15 min after IV and 60 min after IM injection. It has active metabolites (analgesic properties) that are excreted in the urine, and may prolong the effect in renal impairment or following chronic use.

Codeine has a similar effect to morphine, but with less potency and efficacy. Classically used following head injury and neurosurgery as the side effects are less than with other opioids. Some metabolism to morphine may occur.

Synthetic agents

Alfentanil and fentanyl are both more potent than morphine and have a rapid onset of action (1–2 min). Further boluses or infusions are required as they have short durations of action. The pharmacokinetics of alfentanil makes it suitable for use as an infusion, but fentanyl may accumulate, prolonging the duration of effect. Residual respiratory depression may persist postoperatively, necessitating respiratory support. Bradycardia and hypotension are more common following alfentanil.

Remifentanil is a potent ultra-short-acting opioid that causes a dose-dependent reduction in heart rate and blood pressure. It is metabolized by tissue and non-specific esterases so it does not accumulate following an infusion. The context-sensitive half-time of remifentanil (the time for the plasma concentration to decrease by 50% after an intravenous infusion has stopped) is less than 5 min. Its pharmacokinetics is perfectly suited to a continuous intraoperative infusion and TCI, but once the infusion is stopped, analgesic levels will rapidly decline unless supplementary analgesia is given. Chest wall rigidity has been reported and may necessitate muscle relaxation and IPPV.

Neuromuscular blocking drugs

At the neuromuscular junction (NMJ), muscle relaxants compete with acetylcholine (ACh) for receptor sites and block neuromuscular transmission. They may be classified into two main types.

Depolarizing

Suxamethonium has the most rapid onset of any muscle relaxant and has a brief duration of action. It causes depolarization by mimicking the action of ACh at the post-synaptic membrane, which may be seen as fasciculations. A brief transmembrane ion flux occurs but this rapidly stops and the action potential fails to propagate. Suxamethonium is hydrolysed slower than ACh, which prolongs the period of depolarization, blocking neuromuscular transmission. A tachycardia often occurs following single use, but repeated doses can cause bradycardia.

Suxamethonium cannot be reversed; administering an anticholinesterase would only potentiate the block. Recovery occurs spontaneously when sufficient plasma cholinesterase is available. Giving fresh frozen plasma would also increase the rate of hydrolysis. If large or repeated doses of suxamethonium are administered a non-depolarizing block may follow the initial depolarizing block (dual block), resulting in prolonged paralysis. The use of suxamethonium is limited to emergency airway management, but with the release of sugammadex its use may decline further. It has a significant side effect profile that includes:

- hyperkalaemia (may be severe in renal failure, burns and neuropathies)
- anaphylaxis
- postoperative muscle pains
- raised intraocular pressure
- MH trigger
- sustained muscular contraction (myotonia).

Non-depolarizing

These are competitive antagonists that prevent ACh from activating the postsynaptic ACh receptors. They have a slower onset of action than suxamethonium. Agent selection is influenced by speed of onset, duration of action and side-effect profile.

Rocuronium is an aminosteroid compound that has the fastest onset of the non depolarizing agents. It is cardiovascularly stable but high doses have a vagolytic effect. In common with atracurium and vecuronium, it has an intermediate duration of action. Pancuronium is another aminosteroid compound which has a long duration of action. It has sympathomimetic and vagolytic effects that can cause hypertension and tachycardia.

Reversal agents

Anticholinesterases are used to reverse the effects of non-depolarizing agents by increasing the ACh concentration at the NMJ. Neostigmine acts quickly and its effects last for up to 30 min. Its muscarinic side effects include bradycardia, salivation, increased GIT motility and bladder contractility, which can be minimized using an anticholinergic.

Sugammadex is a selective relaxant binding agent (SRBA) that can be used to rapidly reverse the effects of non-depolarizing agents such as rocuronium. It is a modified γ-cyclodextrin, which encapsulates and binds muscle relaxant molecules, destroying their ability to antagonize the ACh receptor. This newly introduced compound provides the ability to quickly restore neuromuscular transmission, which should contribute to improving patient safety and reduce adverse airway events.

Perioperative fluid management

Fluid balance is normally regulated to maintain the extracellular fluid volume and osmolality, compensatory mechanisms being initiated when the baroreceptors and osmoreceptors detect change. Balance may be disrupted in patients presenting for surgery, and estimations of pre-existing deficits, normal maintenance requirements and ongoing losses are used to guide perioperative fluid management:

Deficit –– Modern preoperative starvation policies allow water to be taken up to 2 h before surgery, but a water deficit of almost one litre may exist. Patients

Table 9.4 The electrolyte composition (mmol 1^{-1}) of common intravenous fluids

	Na$^+$	Cl$^-$	K$^+$	Ca$^+$	HCO$_3^-$
Sodium chloride 0.9%	154	154	–	–	–
Sodium chloride 0.45%	75	75	–	–	–
Hartmann's solution	131	111	5	2	29
Gelofusine	154	120	–	–	–
Haemaccel	145	145	5.1	6.25	–
Volplex	154	125	–	–	–

with dysphagia, nausea and increased GIT losses often require volume and electrolyte resuscitation.

Maintenance –– In adults normal maintenance requirements may be achieved with 40 ml/kg per day (1.6 ml/kg per h). Paediatric patients have greater requirements. Electrolyte maintenance should be guided by body weight and organ dysfunction.

Losses –– Blood-conservation methods, e.g. cell salvage and lowering the haemoglobin trigger value for transfusion, help reduce the need for homologous blood transfusions. Third-space losses vary and may be 10–15 ml/kg per h following major abdominal surgery. Nasogastric aspirate volume may also be considerable.

Careful attention to fluid balance, electrolyte abnormalities and cardiovascular parameters may prevent complications. An understanding of the electrolyte composition of commonly prescribed crystalloids and colloids is essential (Table 9.4). Body weight is an important supplement to fluid balance calculations and may be used to guide volume replacement therapy.

Monitoring

The most important monitor during the course of an anaesthetic episode is the continuous presence of a trained anaesthetist. In addition to patient assessment and good clinical judgement, an array of modern monitoring devices is available. When monitoring parameters stray outside predetermined limits an audible alarm is activated. The range of these preset factory limits is different for adult and paediatric patients. Manual adjustment is also possible.

The monitoring software records data at regular intervals and trends can be displayed over adjustable time periods. This patient-specific data may be printed and used as a component of the anaesthesia record.

Recommendations for monitoring standards during anaesthesia have been described and routinely used devices are discussed below.

Pulse oximetry

This non-invasive device allows arterial oxygen saturation of haemoglobin to be determined by measuring the absorbance of light by the blood. Oxygenated and deoxygenated haemoglobin have different absorbance spectra and the positions at which the lines cross are called isobestic points. The relative concentrations of oxy- and deoxyhaemoglobin may be estimated by comparing absorbance at different wavelengths, light absorbance by the tissues being separated from that of blood. In the presence of carboxyhaemoglobin, methaemoglobin and severe hypoxaemia pulse oximetry readings may be inaccurate. The device may fail to give a reading if digital perfusion is limited.

Capnography

A sample of gas from the breathing system is collected and the concentration of carbon dioxide (CO_2) is measured by infrared absorption. The value may be displayed in graphical form against time. End-tidal CO_2 monitoring is able to detect many life-threatening conditions and thus is a crucially important anaesthetic monitor.

1. Oesophageal intubation: failure to detect CO_2 following tracheal intubation after five breaths is an immediate indication to remove the tube and to recommence mask ventilation and oxygenation. Single-use devices that change colour when exposed to CO_2 are available for use outside theatres.
2. Disconnection: a sudden loss of end-tidal CO_2 will trigger the apnoea alarm.
3. Efficiency of ventilation: the CO_2 curve has a characteristic shape in obstructive airway disease. During rebreathing the CO_2 value fails to return to the base-line during inspiration.
4. MH: a sustained rise in end-tidal CO_2 despite an increase in minute volume may be an important early warning sign.
5. Cardiac arrest: a decrease in expired CO_2 occurs when pulmonary perfusion falls (ventilation continues normally diluting the alveolar gas) and this may occur following cardiac arrest, low

cardiac output, pulmonary embolism and venous air embolism.

Arterial blood pressure

Non-invasive methods involve attaching an appropriately sized cuff to the upper arm or limb. Specialized software is used to compare consecutive pulsations. The systolic and mean arterial blood pressures are measured and the diastolic is calculated. They tend to over-read when the pressure is high (or cuff too small) and under-read when pressures are low. Sudden changes to the blood pressure, arrhythmias and external pressure to the cuff will affect their accuracy.

Invasive blood pressure measurement involves cannulating a peripheral artery and provides a direct beat-by-beat value. At the wrist, Allen's test should be performed before radial artery puncture, to ensure adequate collateral circulation via the ulnar artery. The pressure transducer should be calibrated and located level with the heart. Damping may be caused by air bubbles, thrombus and kinking of the catheter. Systolic pressure variation (SPV) may be calculated to provide an estimation of intravascular volume. Arterial blood may also be sampled from the measuring catheters.

Electrocardiography

The cardiac rhythm and rate may be continuously monitored in real-time through three surface electrodes. Correctly positioned (over bone rather than muscle and on hair-free skin) they will enable monitoring using modified limb leads I, II or III. Modified lead II is routinely selected as it usually displays good-amplitude P waves and QRS complexes. Intraoperative myocardial (left ventricular) ischaemia is more likely to be detected (up to 80%) using the CM5 configuration: the right arm electrode (red) is placed on the manubrium and left arm electrode (yellow) placed at the V5 position. The left leg lead (green or black) acts as a neutral and is often placed on the clavicle, but may be placed anywhere.

Temperature

Hypothermia is defined as a core temperature below 35°C. Excessive heat loss should be avoided during anaesthesia and efforts to maintain the core temperature should be routinely practised. Modern devices are very efficient and overheating may occur. When cerebral protection is required, deliberate hypothermia may be induced intraoperatively. A decrease in cardiac output and arrhythmias are more common as the temperature falls. The difference between the core and peripheral temperature (temperature gradient) may be used to provide an indication of cardiac output.

Airway gas and pressure monitoring

Oxygen concentration in the breathing system may be measured using a variety of analysers. These are designed to alarm before hypoxic concentrations are delivered. A separate device on the anaesthetic machine has been designed to alert the anaesthetist to failure of the oxygen supply.

Inhalational agent concentrations and MAC are measured, which helps minimize the risk of delivering insufficient or excess inhalational anaesthetic agent. In addition to the apnoea alarm, the disconnection alarm is an important safety feature. Following ventilator failure or disconnection within the breathing system, the cyclical pressure fluctuations will no longer be detected, causing the alarm to trigger.

Recovery

Originally described by Florence Nightingale, the recovery room or post-anaesthetic care unit (PACU) ideally should be located close to the operating theatre and intensive care unit. It must be equipped with appropriate monitoring (similar to that used in theatre), oxygen and suction apparatus. A continuous patient to staff ratio of 'one-to-one' is essential until the patient can maintain their own airway. Resuscitation equipment and anaesthetic drugs should be available, with an emergency call system to request assistance.

All patients who have received general, regional or local anaesthesia /sedation should receive appropriate post-anaesthesia care. On arrival in recovery, monitoring will be established and the patient re-evaluated. A verbal report must be given to the recovery staff, providing information concerning the intraoperative course and the preoperative condition of the patient.

The modified Aldrete score (Table 9.5), which is based on the Apgar score, provides a tool to assess recovery following anaesthesia. The score ranges from zero in a comatose patient to ten for complete recovery. The score should be calculated and documented on admission and at 10–15 min intervals. When the score is >9 the patient may be discharged to ward.

Table 9.5 Criteria for discharge from recovery – the modified Aldrete score

Activity
2 = Moves all extremities spontaneously or on command
1 = Moves two extremities
0 = Unable to move extremities

Respiration
2 = Breathes deeply and coughs freely
1 = Dyspnoeic
0 = Apnoeic

Circulation
2 = BP +/− 20 mm of preanaesthetic level
1 = BP +/− 20–50 mm of preanaesthetic level
0 = BP +/− 50 mm of preanaesthetic level

Consciousness
2 = Fully awake
1 = Arousable on calling
0 = Not responding

Oxygen saturation
2 = SpO_2 > 92% on room air
1 = Supplemental oxygen required to maintain SpO_2 >90%
0 = SpO_2 < 90% with oxygen supplementation

Postanaesthetic complications

Pain

A plan for managing postoperative pain should be agreed with the patient during the anaesthetic assessment. The use of patient-controlled analgesia (PCA) systems, epidural infusions and continuous peripheral nerve blocks (CPNB) has contributed to improving pain control. A multimodal pharmacological approach should be adopted, as the quality of analgesia achieved is likely to be superior to single agents. Rescue analgesia appropriate to the severity of the pain should be available during the recovery period.

Up to 50% of patients may experience a mild sore throat following airway instrumentation and tracheal intubation. Myalgia is common following the administration of suxamethonium but it is generally transient and may be controlled using simple analgesics.

Postoperative nausea and vomiting

This occurs in about 20% of all surgical patients, but is more common in females and following specific procedures, e.g. gynaecological surgery. Causative factors include: opioids, nitrous oxide, previous PONV, motion sickness, dehydration and sudden movement or postural change. Some individuals are more susceptible and may be difficult to treat, requiring a polypharmacy approach.

In high-risk patients the anaesthetic technique should include avoidance of causative factors and the prophylactic administration of an IV antiemetic. If prophylaxis is ineffective, an additional class of antiemetic should be given with a different mechanism of action to that used for prophylaxis. The 5-HT antagonists (e.g. ondansetron and granisetron), dexamethasone and cyclizine have fewer side effects than the dopamine antagonists, e.g. procholorperazine and metoclopramide.

Airway obstruction

Following anaesthesia airway muscle tone is reduced, and the tongue may approximate to the pharyngeal wall. As this residual airway obstruction may persist, maintaining airway patency is essential until consciousness and airway protective reflexes have been restored. Oropharyngeal airways or LMAs should be removed as the patient emerges from anaesthesia, but some patients may bite on airway devices, restricting airflow and delaying their removal. Suction will clear vomit or blood clot. Meticulous technique and in-theatre documentation should minimize the need to remove broken teeth and retained pharyngeal packs. The risk of laryngospasm may be reduced by clearing secretions and avoiding stimulation to the laryngopharynx.

Hypoxaemia

Atelectasis causes alveolar hypoventilation and is the most common postoperative complication. The collapse of alveoli and terminal airways often accompanies anaesthesia due to a reduction in the FRC. Following thoracic or upper abdominal surgery the aetiology of atelectasis is due to smaller tidal volumes and the inability to take a deep breath (or sigh). Pain due to inadequate analgesia or residual sedation from opioids will affect the efficiency of normal tidal ventilation, and exposes the patient to the risk of hypoxaemia and respiratory infection.

When the ability to cough is impaired, sputum retention may follow, which can lead to collapse and consolidation. Management includes supplementary oxygen, adequate analgesia, physiotherapy and the appropriate use of antibiotics. A well-managed epidural can provide superior postoperative analgesia, which may minimize pain associated with coughing and sighing.

Low cardiac output states increase alveolar dead space, which compromises alveolar gas exchange due to poor perfusion through well-ventilated areas of the lungs. Diffusion hypoxia can be prevented by administering supplementary oxygen using a variable-performance facemask.

Following upper abdominal and thoracic surgery, vital capacity falls, creating a restrictive deficit on pulmonary function testing that may last for a week. The changes are less following lower abdominal surgery. In smokers and patients with COAD, bronchodilator therapy, antibiotics and the cessation of smoking may help reduce the risk of postoperative atelectasis.

Hypertension

During emergence from anaesthesia, hypertension and tachycardia commonly occur prior to removal of the LMA or oropharyngeal airway. This may persist for several minutes, but rarely requires treatment.

Confusion, anxiety and agitation may accompany hypertension, and these may provide information as to the likely cause. Inadequate analgesia will lead to an elevation in the blood pressure, but it responds to appropriate pain relief. Urinary catheterization may relieve the pain from bladder distension. Residual neuromuscular paralysis due to incomplete reversal, hypercapnia and hypoxaemia all cause sympathetic stimulation. Vasodilators may be required when postoperative blood pressure values need to be controlled, e.g. following carotidendarterectomy. Omitting regular antihypertensive medication, due to rigid enforcement of preoperative starvation rules, may lead to poor postoperative control of the blood pressure.

Hypotension

Common postoperative causes include residual cardiodepressant effects of opioids or anaesthetic drugs, recent epidural boluses of local anaesthetic or opioid, hypovolaemia and reduced cardiac output. Management may require the administration of intravenous fluids, vasopressors, inotropes or anticholinergics. If haemorrhage is suspected, surgical re-exploration and volume resuscitation may be necessary.

Prolonged unconsciousness

The use of sedative premedication may prolong the effect of anaesthesia and a synergistic effect between anaesthetic agents and opioids may also extend the period of hypnosis. Oxygenation and ventilation must be maintained at all times when unconsciousness is prolonged, but it is important to differentiate between postoperative coma and neuromuscular paralysis. Residual muscular paralysis may be assessed using a peripheral nerve stimulator prior to reversal. Modern inhalational anaesthetic agents are relatively insoluble and rapid awakening occurs when they are discontinued, but a marked reduction in alveolar ventilation may delay emergence. Bradypnoea and miosis may provide an indication of excessive opioid administration, which may be antagonized with small IV boluses of naloxone. Once normoglycaemia has been confirmed, patients may be allowed to recover spontaneously from anaesthesia. Doxapram may result in rapid restoration of breathing and consciousness, but it causes global CNS stimulation and has many side effects.

Hypothermia

Hypothermia may delay awakening and efforts to minimize heat loss should commence prior to induction of anaesthesia and be continued intraoperatively. Preventing hypothermia is more practical than treatment. Keeping the patient covered and avoiding unnecessary exposure are simple measures. The use of warm skin-prep solutions, IV fluids and forced air warming blankets may minimize intraoperative temperature loss.

In recovery a warm ambient temperature is important and intraoperative warming devices may be continued. Warm and humidified oxygen should be administered as shivering significantly increases oxygen consumption. Recurarization has been described during rewarming.

Local anaesthetic agents

The maximum safe doses of the local anaesthetic (LA) agents are often quoted. Whilst body weight is an important factor, the presence of coexisting disease, the site of injection and use of vasoconstrictors also influence the maximum safe dose. Cocaine is an ester LA which is used to induce nasal vasoconstriction and analgesia; it has numerous cardiovascular side effects, and alternative drugs are widely available, e.g. lidocaine with phenylephrine. The commonly used amide LA agents are discussed below (maximum safe doses are shown in parentheses):

Lidocaine (3 mg/kg) has the most rapid onset and shortest duration of action. It can be given in higher dosage (doubled) when used with a vasoconstrictor. Bupivacaine (2 mg/kg) has a slower onset but longer duration of action than lidocaine. Cardiac toxicity may lead to malignant dysrhythmias and cardiac arrest. L-Bupivacaine (2 mg/kg) has a similar speed of onset and duration to bupivacaine but is associated with less severe toxic side effects than bupivacaine. Prilocaine (5 mg/kg) is equipotent with lidocaine and is the agent of choice for IVRA. Higher doses may be used with a vasoconstrictor. Methaemoglobinaemia may occur.

Regional anaesthesia

Regional anaesthesia involves the administration of LA solutions, which block nervous conduction in a specific anatomical region. It may be performed as the sole technique or in combination with sedation or general anaesthesia. The advantages of regional anaesthesia include:

- reduced surgical haemorrhage
- lower incidence of thromboembolic events
- preservation of organ function
- prolonged postoperative analgesia
- preservation of consciousness.

Thorough preoperative checks and patient assessment are required prior to regional anaesthesia. Factors that influence the choice of technique include: coexisting disease, concurrent medication, patient consent, type and duration of surgery, and speed of onset.

Complications

Sympathetic block –– This may lead to significant hypotension and bradycardia, depending on the height of the block. Preloading with IV fluids and the use of vasoconstrictors help achieve cardiovascular control.

Motor block –– This commonly encountered complication may be avoided by using lower doses (less concentrated solutions) of LA, but this may compromise the quality of analgesia. It can delay postoperative mobilization.

Failure –– Any regional technique may fail or be partially effective, requiring supplementary analgesia or conversion to general anaesthesia.

Local anaesthetic toxicity –– High plasma concentrations of LA may follow accidental IV administration or excess administration. Circumoral paraesthesia and tinnitus are early signs which may progress to convulsions and cardiac arrest. Intralipid 20% has an important therapeutic role in LA induced cardiac arrest.

High block –– Cephalad spread of local anaesthetic may result in intercostal and phrenic nerve paralysis. Higher spread may cause brainstem paralysis causing profound cardiovascular collapse and apnoea. Airway management and cardiovascular support must be immediately available.

Spinal and epidural blocks

A spinal or subarachnoid block involves injecting a LA bolus into the cerebrospinal fluid (CSF). In the UK hyperbaric bupivacaine is preferred as the spread within the CSF is more predictable. An epidural block involves injecting LA through a percutaneous epidural catheter. The epidural space is located by a loss of resistance (LOR) technique, which requires a low-resistance syringe and specialized tuohy needle. The epidural space may be approached via the caudal route, but this does not utilize the LOR technique. Complications include:

Postdural puncture headache –– A postural head-ache occurs due to CSF leakage through a perforation or tear in the arachnoid matter. The incidence is less when narrow-gauge needles are used. Management involves simple analgesia, but refractory headache may require an autologous epidural blood patch.

Total spinal –– This complication may occur when LA intended for injection into the epidural space is accidentally injected into the subarachnoid or subdural space. Rapid spread to the brainstem will require airway intervention and cardiovascular support.

Intravenous regional anaesthesia

Intravenous regional anaesthesia (IVRA) was first described by Bier in 1908 (Bier's block), to provide distal analgesia to a limb. Following IV cannulation, the limb is exsanguinated and a proximal pneumatic tourniquet inflated above systolic blood pressure. Prilocaine is injected into the vein, which then diffuses down its concentration gradient through the tissues to reach the nerves. It provides analgesia suitable for minor surgery, e.g. fracture reduction.

Patients should be fasted and have IV access in the opposite limb. The standard preoperative checks should be applied. Pain may be experienced at the level of the tourniquet, which may be reduced by using double-cuffed devices. To avoid potentially toxic plasma levels of LA, the tourniquet should be deflated at least 20 min after injecting the prilocaine. Premature deflation of the tourniquet should be avoided.

Continuous peripheral nerve block

Continuous peripheral nerve blockade (CPNB) may be used to provide opioid-sparing postoperative analgesia. LA solutions are infused through a peripherally inserted catheter, which blocks single nerves or a plexus. Side effects may be minimized using lower concentrations of LA.

Contraindications

The following conditions are not absolute contraindications to regional anaesthesia, but they are associated with significant risk:

Local or systemic infections –– Infection over the injection site, pyrexia and an elevated white cell count may cause bacterial translocation through the injection tract or to the site. LA solutions are bacteriocidal, and abscess formation, meningitis, arachnoiditis and myelitis are rare complications.

Anticoagulation and bleeding diathesis –– Haemostasis may be difficult when coagulation is impaired, leading to haematoma formation or hypovolaemia. Urgent neurosurgical decompression may be necessary.

Low molecular weight heparin –– Following administration for prophylaxis against DVT, regional anaesthesia should be delayed for 6 hours. The same safety period should be allowed prior to removal of epidural catheters.

Fixed cardiac output states –– Sudden changes in arterial blood pressure and heart rate must be avoided. When the cardiac output is fixed, e.g. aortic stenosis, hypotension and tachycardia can significantly reduce myocardial perfusion, leading to ischaemia, dysrhythmia and cardiac arrest.

Sedation

This describes a state of reduced consciousness in which verbal contact is maintained. It is used to decrease anxiety and recall and enhance cooperation during uncomfortable procedures, e.g. GI endoscopy. Drugs with a short duration of action should be administered as IV boluses, infusions or by patient-controlled systems. The level of sedation required depends on the procedure and varies between patients. Analgesia may also be required for painful procedures. Commonly used drugs include midazolam, propofol, remifentanil and ketamine.

As for general anaesthesia, full monitoring and preoperative checks should be employed during sedation procedures. Supplementary oxygen is administered to reduce the risk of hypoxaemia. Scoring systems are used on intensive care to assist titration of sedation.

Anaesthetic emergencies

Failed tracheal intubation

Following no more than four failed attempts at direct laryngoscopy (Plan A), further efforts to intubate the trachea should be postponed and the priority must return to maintenance of adequate oxygenation, ventilation and anaesthesia. Prior to arterial desaturation and the development of hypoxaemia, intubation may be attempted using an intubating laryngeal mask airway (ILMA) or via a classic LMA (Plan B). If oxygenation fails and arterial saturation is <90%, anaesthesia must be discontinued, the patient woken up and surgery postponed (Plan C).

If ventilation is difficult in association with worsening hypoxaemia, rescue techniques for a 'can't intubate, can't ventilate' situation must be employed immediately (Plan D). The first step is to perform a cannula cricothyroidotomy to reestablish oxygenation and ventilation. If this intervention fails then a surgical cricothyroidotomy must be performed and a cuffed tube inserted into the trachea. Following successful cricothyroidotomy, a definitive airway must be established as soon as possible.

An urgent call for additional anaesthetic assistance is crucial once the initial attempts to intubate the trachea have failed (Plan A).

Cardiac arrest

Primary cardiac arrest is uncommon in healthy patients, but unexpected complications may occur that can compromise myocardial perfusion and oxygenation. Hypotension and cardiac arrhythmias often provide advance warning and if treated promptly and appropriately, the peri-arrest patient may be stabilized and cardiac arrest averted.

Following confirmation of cardiac arrest (apnoea and absent carotid pulse) obtaining additional assistance is crucial and involves initiating a cardiac arrest alert. In adults, external cardiac compressions and ventilation should be commenced at a ratio of 30:2 respectively. Oxygen (100%) should be delivered ideally via a tracheal tube. Subsequent management is determined by the cardiac arrest rhythm, which may be classified as shockable (ventricular fibrillation and pulseless ventricular tachycardia) or non-shockable (pulseless electrical activity and asystole). When appropriate, defibrillation must be delivered safely and promptly. The energy selected for the asynchronous shock varies according to the type (biphasic or monophasic) and manufacture of the defibrillator.

Pulseless electrical activity (PEA) has many causes, which may be memorized using the 4Hs and 4Ts mnemonic: Hypoxia, Hypovolaemia, Hypothermia and Hyperkalaemia, Tension pneumothorax, cardiac Tamponade, Thromboembolic phenomena and Toxicity. Management of PEA involves maintenance of cardiopulmonary resuscitation (CPR) and the rapid identification and treatment of the most likely cause. Adrenaline (1 mg) boluses are administered IV every 3 min during cardiac arrest. Atropine (3 mg IV) is indicated during asystole, which completely antagonizes vagal innervation to the sino-atrial node.

Tourniquets

Tourniquets are used to create an operative field with minimal haemorrhage. Following exsanguination, pneumatic cuffs are inflated above the systolic blood pressure, which prevents limb perfusion.

Limb ischaemia is associated with nerve and muscle injury, but excessive tourniquet pressure is more likely to cause injury than long ischaemic times. Ideally the tourniquet pressure should be 50 and 100 mmHg above the systolic for upper and lower limbs respectively. Tourniquet times may vary, but 3 hours should be regarded as the upper limit of safety, although most deflate the cuff after 2 hours.

Following reperfusion of the limb, microemboli, anaerobic metabolites and potassium are released into the circulation. Arrhythmias and vasodilatation may occur, which may compromise organ perfusion and function. Reactive hyperaemia may increase blood loss at the surgical site.

Further reading

AAGBI working party. Checking anaesthetic equipment. 3rd edn. 2004. http://www.aagbi.org/publications/guidelines.htm.

AAGBI working party. Guidelines for the management of severe local anaesthetic toxicity, 2007. http://www.aagbi.org/publications/guidelines/docs/latoxicity07.pdf.

AAGBI working party. Recommendations for standards of monitoring during anaesthesia and recovery. 4th edn. 2007. http://www.aagbi.org/publications/guidelines.htm.

Haynes AB, Weiser TG, Berry WR, Lipsitz SR, Breizat AH, Dellinger EP, Herbosa T, Joseph S, Kibatala PL, Lapitan MC, Merry AF, Moorthy K, Reznick RK, Taylor B, Gawande AA. Safe Surgery Saves Lives Study Group. A surgical safety checklist to reduce morbidity and mortality in a global population. *N Engl J Med* 2009 29;**360**(5):491–499.

Henderson JJ, Popat MT, Latto IP *et al.* Difficult Airway Society guidelines for the management of the unanticipated difficult intubation. *Anaesthesia* 2004;**59**: 675–694.

Joint Commission on Accreditation of Healthcare Organizations (JCAHO). Sentinel Event Alert 6 October 2004;32.

Peck T, Hill S. *Pharmacology for Anaesthesia and Intensive Care.* 3rd edn. Cambridge University Press, 2008.

Sebel PS *et al.* The incidence of awareness during anesthesia: a multicenter United States study. *Anesth Analg* 2004;**99**:833–839.

Smith T, Pinnock C, Lin T *et al. Fundamentals of Anaesthesia.* 3rd edn. Cambridge University Press, 2009.

Resuscitation Council (UK). *Advanced Life Support Manual.* 5th edn. 2006.

Chapter 10

Fundamentals of cancer management

Mark Duxbury

The objective of this chapter is to summarize the biological processes that drive cancer development and progression together with the key principles of clinical cancer management.

Cancer biology

Defining cancer

Neoplasia (Greek 'new growth') is the formation of abnormal tissue, the growth of which is not coordinated with that of normal tissues, and that persists after the cessation of the stimulus which induced the change. These features are accompanied by genetic abnormalities that alter cell growth. Although neoplasia commonly manifests as a tumour (Latin 'abnormal mass'), neoplasia and tumour are not synonymous. Some neoplastic processes do not result in tumour formation, e.g. leukaemia. Conversely, not all clinically tumorous lesions are neoplastic, e.g. abscesses. Neoplasia may be benign or malignant, cancer being a malignant neoplasm. Malignant neoplasms are distinguished from benign neoplasms by the presence of cellular invasion and metastasis.

Cancers are named according to the embryological origin of the tissue from which they arise. Carcinoma is a malignant neoplasm arising from endodermal or ectodermal epithelial tissue. This group includes most common human cancers. Adenocarcinoma refers to a carcinoma originating from glandular epithelium. Sarcomas are malignant neoplasms of mesodermal origin. While mesoderm is capable of producing epithelium, mesothelium which lines pleural, peritoneal and pericardial cavities, a tumour of mesothelial origin is usually referred to as a mesothelioma.

Premalignant disease

A range of lesions are now recognized to be precursors of human cancer. The adenoma–carcinoma sequence in colorectal cancer is well-described. Intraepithelial neoplasia (carcinoma *in situ*) is an immediate precursor of cervical (CIN) and anal (AIN) carcinoma. Pancreatic adenocarcinoma has also been shown to have an intraepithelial precursor lesion (PanIN). Many of the microscopic cellular abnormalities that cancer cells display do not necessarily define cancer. These morphological changes are accompanied by characteristic genetic changes. Dysplasia (Greek 'abnormal formation') refers to cellular abnormalities of the type seen in cancer, e.g. nuclear atypia, abnormal nuclear:cytoplasmic ratio, disordered cellular distribution, but without evidence of invasion or metastasis.

Although not inevitable, carcinoma *in situ* may progress to invasive carcinoma over a period of months to years. Dysplasia is distinct from metaplasia (Greek 'change in form') which is the reversible replacement of one differentiated cell type with another mature differentiated cell type. Dysplasia may occur on a background of metaplasia and lead to invasive carcinoma. A metaplasia–dysplasia–carcinoma sequence is believed to be responsible for distal oesophageal adenocarcinoma arising on a background of Barrett's oesophagus. Detection of pre-cancerous lesions is one of the rationales behind screening programmes.

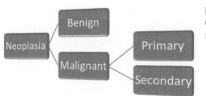

Figure 10.1
Classification of neoplasia.

Fundamentals of Surgical Practice, Third Edition, ed. Andrew N. Kingsnorth and Douglas M. Bowley.
Published by Cambridge University Press. © Cambridge University Press 2011.

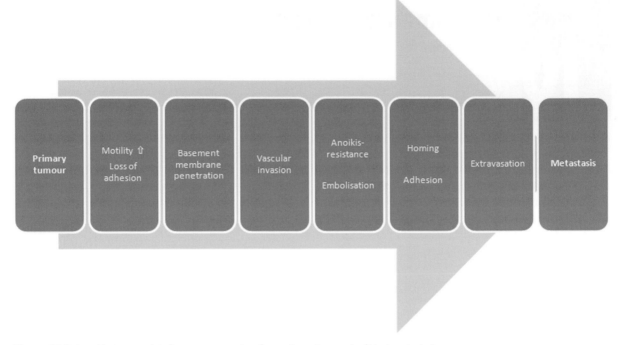

Figure 10.2 A multi-stage model of cancer progression, from primary tumour to distant metastasis.

Cancer biology and the molecular genetics of cancer cells

Invasion and metastasis

Metastases do not develop passively, but as a result of a cascade of tumour–host interactions caused by a series of genetic and epigenetic events which cause the cancer cells to detach from their neighbours, migrate through the interstitial tissues, intravasate through a blood or lymphatic vessel wall, survive the mechanical stress of circulating in the blood stream, target a new capillary and invade new host tissues where they proliferate and grow. Normal cells can also invade, e.g. trophoblast and vascular endothelium, but this is a regulated process during which 'arrival' cues are sensed. Only a very small fraction of cells in a tumour are able to survive in the circulation and even fewer are capable of forming metastases. These cells can be regarded as having accumulated the essential phenotypic changes required for invasion and metastasis.

Cells normally adhere to each other by a macromolecular 'glue' which binds to specific adhesion receptors. Inadequate or inappropriate adhesion between cell and substrate induces anoikis, a specific form of apoptosis. Under normal circumstances, anoikis prevents ectopic cellular proliferation, maintains tissue architecture and guards against metastasis. Transformed cells are characteristically resistant to anoikis. Several families of cell adhesion molecule have been described which mediate cell-to-cell and cell-to-matrix binding. These include integrins, cadherins, the immunoglobin superfamily, hyaluronate receptors and mucins. Best characterized are the integrins, which are transmembrane glycoproteins, and provide a functional and structural chain between extracellular matrix molecules, e.g. collagen, fibronectin and laminin, and cytoskeletal components within the cell. Before the cells can separate, the ligand–integrin interactions must be disrupted enzymatically or by inhibitors. This event is critical to both invasion and metastasis.

To gain access to the interstitial tissues, the cells must penetrate the basement membrane and become mobile. The basement membrane is a specialized layer of extracellular matrix containing proteoglycans (chondroitin and heparin), matrix proteins (laminin and fibronectin) and type IV collagen. The cell first attaches to the basement membrane through surface laminin receptors. Release of proteolytic enzymes, such as calcium- and zinc-dependent

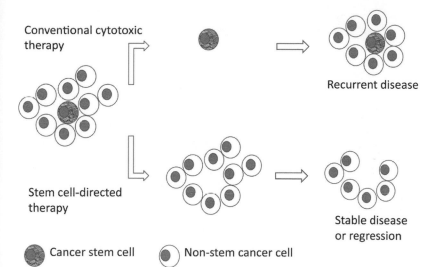

Conventional cytotoxic therapy

Recurrent disease

Stem cell-directed therapy

Stable disease or regression

Cancer stem cell   Non-stem cancer cell

Figure 10.3 The cancer stem cell concept. Conventional cytotoxics may not target the cancer stem cell, resulting in residual disease and tumour recurrence due to repopulation by cancer stem cells. It is argued that stem cell-directed therapy may limit the ability of the tumour to repopulate, leading to stable disease or even regression.

metalloproteinases, type IV collagenase, cathepsin and stromolysin from cancer and neighbouring fibroblasts degrade the matrix. This allows the cell to migrate by active contractions of its cytoskeleton. By pushing out pseudopodia, studded with matrix receptors which act as a 'sense organ', the cell advances by attaching and subsequently releasing itself from the matrix proteins of the interstitium. Motility-stimulating cytokines (autocrine motility factors – AMF) have been identified.

Once in the blood or lymphatic systems, tumour cells are free to circulate. As the lungs receive 100% and the liver 73% of the cardiac output, these organs are first encountered by the tumour cell. In order to survive, tumour cells must resist anoikis, surviving to become attached to the capillary endothelium, but only a few cells adhere and grow. Most freely circulating cells are arrested at points of vascular branching and are destroyed by host defence mechanisms (see Ch. 11), but some continue their onward passage to other sites.

Having targeted a capillary in a new site, the malignant cells attach to its endothelial wall. Cells within a clump are relatively protected by the outer layer and may be more likely than single cells to proliferate within the capillary, bursting out into the interstitial tissues and degrading the capillary subendothelium. Having migrated through the tissues of the new host site, the cells initially receive nourishment by diffusion, but their growth is limited to a spheroid of 1–3 mm in size. For further proliferation they must acquire new vessels (neovascularization), which are

formed through release of angiogenic factors from stromal cells, e.g. vascular endothelial growth factors (VEGFs), platelet-derived growth factor (PDGF) and fibroblast growth factors (FGF). The tumour cell proliferation is modulated by factors acting in autocrine, paracrine and endocrine fashions.

Considering the complexity of this metastatic cascade, and the hazards that the tumour cells encounter at every step, it is not surprising that only a few of the millions of cells that are shed from a tumour survive to form metastases. Many aspects of this process are poorly understood, including the varying distribution of metastases in different types of cancer, the long periods of time that may pass before they become clinically evident and the mechanism by which they cause death in the absence of obvious organ failure. A number of 'check-points' in the metastatic process, e.g. inhibitions of cell surface and secreted proteins, offer sites for regulatory restoration by novel therapies. These various processes are under the genetic control of 'metastasis-promoting' genes which may have dominant positive effects. Metastases-suppressor genes have also been identified, e.g. nm23 on chromosome 17q.

The cancer stem cell

Specialized cells occupy a unique differentiation compartment within the organism and, once 'committed' to that lineage, generally cannot change to another cell type. A limited number of progenitor 'stem cells' occupy each compartment and are genetically controlled to proliferate and repopulate it. As

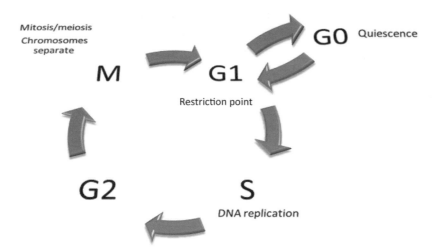

Figure 10.4 The cell cycle.

differentiating genes take over control, proliferative activity usually decreases. Once fully differentiated, cells enter a third sequence of genetic events, that of apoptosis or programmed cell death. Interest has focused on the 'cancer stem cell' and a potential mediator of disease recurrence, chemoresistance and as a target for novel therapies.

Cell cycle

A characteristic of neoplastic cells is their unregulated progression through the cell cycle. It is now known that this cycle is driven by a family of proteins, cyclins, which form complexes with cyclin-dependent protein kinases. The most important trigger for mitosis occurs during the G1 phase of the cycle, which is effected by cyclins A, D and E in combination with a range of regulatory protein kinases, of which CDK2 is particularly important. Once the cells pass through the synthetic phase and reach G2 they are committed to mitosis, which is initiated by the action of cyclin B complexed to CDK1. Regulatory steps, termed checkpoints, occur between G1–S and G2–M which, should there be damage to DNA, allows time for repair so that errors in replication are avoided. Repair of DNA is brought about by topoisomerase I and II, enzymes which unwind the helix, and re-align the strands. Inhibition of these enzymes causes cell death.

Chemotherapeutic drugs may be classified according to their cell-cycle specificity. Type 1 drugs, which include alkylating agents and platinum derivatives, act by complexing DNA to cause irreparable damage by intercalation. Type 2 drugs specifically inhibit

Table 10.1 Examples of cytotoxic chemotherapeutic agents

Class of agent	Examples
Alkylating agents	Cyclophosphamide, cisplatin, dacarbazine, cholambucil, gemcitabine
Antimetabolites	Methotrexate, 5-fluorouracil
Antibiotics	Doxorubicin, bleomycin
Plant-derived agents	Taxanes, vinca alkaloids

the 'engine' driving the cycle and are termed antimetabolites.

Telomeres

Repeat sequences of TTAGGG (telomeres) form on ends of chromosomes and protect them from enzyme digestion, stopping end replication and loss of DNA. As a cell ages, the length of these telomeres shortens. Telomeres are constructed by reverse transcription from RNA by the enzyme telomerase, which is expressed in highly proliferative cells, such as those of the basal epithelium of the small intestine, sperm and marrow stem cells. Although not expressed by mature normal cells, telomerase is expressed by 80% of cancers, when it may be detected as a marker of early malignant change or used as a target for novel therapies.

Apoptosis

Like cell growth, apoptosis (Greek apo 'from', ptosis 'falling'), that is cell death other than that resulting from necrosis or degeneration, is an active phenomenon which programmes cells towards their self-execution.

Unlike necrosis or degeneration, which affects groups of adjoining cells, apoptosis characteristically affects single cells scattered throughout a tissue. The earliest recognizable changes are compaction of the nuclear chromatin into finely granular masses which become distributed peripherally close to the nuclear membrane. The cytoplasm also becomes condensed, so that cell density is markedly increased. The nuclear membrane convolutes and breaks up into segments, which enclose small fragments of nucleus. These structures are extended from the cell as buds or form clusters (apoptotic bodies) which include cytoplasmic organelles. They are rapidly ingested by nearby cells and degraded. Unlike necrosis, apoptosis does not evoke an inflammatory response.

Expression of a number of genes and their protein products have been linked with both stimulation and inhibition of apoptosis. These include the proto-oncogenes c-*MYC*, c-*FOS* and *BCL*-2 and the *P*53 tumour suppressor gene, suggesting that mitosis and apoptosis may share signalling pathways.

The importance of apoptosis in the control of normal tissue growth during development is well established in both slow and fast proliferating tissues. In the latter, such as intestinal epithelium and spermatogonia, shedding of cells from the surface accounts for the greater part of cell loss, but in those which proliferate slowly, mitosis and apoptosis balance each other. Apoptosis counts for a number of involutional processes, e.g. that of the lactating breast, and can be recognized in virtually all untreated malignant tumours. Apoptosis is enhanced by ionizing radiation and chemotherapy, particularly in stem cells, possibly to prevent transfer of mutant DNA. Abnormalities of apoptosis may have a role in drug resistance, the effects of hyperthermia, withdrawal of trophic hormonal stimulation and immune-mediated killing of cancer cells.

Metabolic abnormalities in cancer

Cancer cells exhibit many abnormalities of cellular metabolism. Cancer cells are often more metabolically active than surrounding normal cells. This characteristic may contribute to the catabolic state that is associated with cancer cachexia. Expression of glucose transporters and hexokinase may also be altered. Functional imaging in the form of positron emission tomography (PET) exploits these metabolic abnormalities to demonstrate metabolically active tumour deposits.

Carcinogenesis

Cancer develops as a result of a complex interaction between reversible and non-reversible (genetic and non-genetic) patient-specific factors and environmental factors. The discovery that viruses containing specific genes could induce tumours led to the concept of oncogenes, which has radically altered our understanding of the role of genetic factors in cancer.

Oncogenes and tumour suppressor genes

Oncogenes function by altering transcriptional events either directly or through control of the cell-signalling pathways. Proto-oncogenes are normal cellular genes that function as regulators of cell growth and can be converted into oncogenes by mutation, deletion or overexpression. Oncogenes can be classified as nuclear or cytoplasmic.

Nuclear oncogenes –– These oncogenes regulate transcription and other interactions within the growth control network. As proto-oncogenes they are the original developmental genes for proliferation and differentiation in normal cells, but when mutated or inappropriately expressed, they cause uncontrolled cell division and transformation. Examples include MYC, JUN, FOS and ERB-A.

Cytoplasmic oncogenes –– A number of classes of cytoplasmic oncogenes have been described. Some are homologous to growth factors, e.g. *SIS* and platelet-derived growth factor, *HIS* and *INT-2* and fibroblast growth factor; others activate growth factors, e.g. *RAS* and TGF-A, a member of the epidermal growth factor family. Some have receptor tyrosine kinase activity, the most prominent of which is *ERB-B2*, which codes for the epidermal growth factor (EGF) protein; others may code for non-receptor protein kinases. Examples that have been implicated in human cancer include *RAS* (colonic and pancreatic adenocarcinoma), *ERB-B2* (breast carcinoma) and *ABL* (leukaemia).

Oncogenes act on the cell in a dominant fashion. Mutation of one copy of the gene can drive a cell towards malignancy, even when the other copy is normal. Despite the complex genetic and epigenetic abnormalities found in cancer cells, their growth and survival can often be impaired by the inactivation of a single oncogene. This phenomenon, called 'oncogene

Table 10.2 Tumour suppressor genes associated with hereditary tumours

Condition	Gene	Location
Retinoblastoma	RB	Chromosome 13
Li–Fraumeni syndrome	P53	Chromosome 17
Wilms' tumour	WT1	Chromosome 11
Neurofibromatosis	NF1	Chromosome 17
Hereditary polyposis coli	APC	Chromosome 22

addiction', provides a rationale for molecular targeted therapy.

Tumour suppressor genes

In addition to oncogenes, the recognition that loss of genetic material through chromosomal deletions might also be associated with carcinogenesis implicated a second set of cancer genes: tumour suppressor genes, whose normal function is to suppress growth. The first suggestion that human cancer might be associated with loss of suppressor genes came from studies of the genetic epidemiology of retinoblastoma, a highly malignant tumour of the retina. Retinoblastoma occurs in hereditary and sporadic forms. Hereditary tumours occur at an earlier age and are multifocal: sporadic cases occur later as a single focus in one eye. Studies of affected families suggested that two 'hits' were required, each affecting one allele of the suppressor gene. In the inherited form of the disease, the first 'hit' mutation or loss of a single allele occurs in the retinal germ cells, predisposing daughter cells to neoplastic growth. Tumour formation occurs only with a second 'hit' causing mutation or loss of the remaining normal allele which takes place during the time of maximum proliferation of retinal cells. In the sporadic form of the disease, both inherited alleles are intact, so that their disruption requires two somatic events. This explains occurrence in older individuals and single-site distribution. Discovery of the Rb gene confirmed this 'two-hit' action of tumour suppressor genes (Figure 10.5). Although inherited in dominant fashion, their biological action is recessive, one normal copy of the gene being sufficient to maintain normal function.

Mutations or loss of tumour suppressor genes have now been identified for a number of hereditary tumours (Table 10.2). Loss of P53, a tumour suppressor gene, is one of the most common genetic defects observed in human tumours. It is evident that the con-

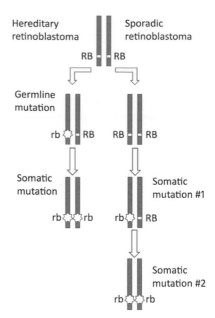

Figure 10.5 Two-hit hypothesis. Knudson proposed that multiple 'hits' to DNA were necessary to cause cancer. In the children with hereditary retinoblastoma, the first 'hit'/mutation was inherited. A second 'hit' would rapidly lead to cancer. In sporadic retinoblastoma, two 'hits' are necessary for tumour development, hence sporadic retinoblastoma occurs in older patients. In 1987, the retinoblastoma gene was identified, confirming the hypothesis. See Knudson (1991) for general overview.

version of a normal to a cancer cell does not occur in a single step, but requires a number of sequential genetic and possibly 'epigenetic' events, which do not involve changes to the genetic sequence, e.g. DNA hypermethylation.

Age

Cancer is primarily a disease of old age, although cancer can develop at any age. Certain cancers, e.g. nephroblastoma (Wilm's tumour), typically occur in the paediatric population. However, the fact that cancer becomes more common with advancing age probably reflects cumulative exposure to carcinogens over the individual's lifetime. As the population ages, the incidence of cancer will continue to increase.

Race

Racial groups exhibit differing levels of malignant disease. Hepatocellular carcinoma is markedly more common in Asian and African populations than in Western populations, where carcinoma of the bronchus is the most common fatal malignancy. Migrant populations tend to assume the risk profile of their new geographical location over time, although genetically determined differences may persist in migrant groups.

Reproductive factors

Gender is an important factor in determining risk from individual types of cancer. Differing male and female hormone levels determine some of this differential risk. Other factors relate to gender-dependent environmental factors. Sexual behaviour may affect cancer risk through the acquisition of sexually transmitted infections. Transmission of human papilloma virus and the human immunodeficiency virus predispose to cancer of the uterine cervix, Kaposi's sarcoma and some other tumours. Cancer of the uterus is more common in women cohabiting with men who have multiple sexual partners. Penile cancer is more common in the uncircumcized and in those with poor hygiene.

Exposure to exogenous hormones, e.g. anabolic steroids and oestrogens, is associated with the development of hepatocellular adenomata in which hepatocellular carcinoma can develop. Historically, in utero exposure to diethylstilbestrol increases the risk of normally rare clear cell carcinoma of the female genital tract.

Environmental factors

Carcinogens may be classified as *non-biological*, comprising chemical and physical carcinogens, and *biological*, i.e. caused by organisms.

A multi-stage model of chemical carcinogenesis

The natural history of experimental tumours caused by chemical carcinogens consists of three phases:

1. Initiation – an irreversible interaction between the chemical carcinogen and the normal target stem cells. An initiated cell acquires the phenotypic features of a transformed cell.
2. Promotion – unlike initiation, promotion is, in general, reversible and ceases when the promoting agent is no longer applied. This effect is analogous to the hormone dependence of experimental mammary tumours. Promotion is modulated by the frequency with which the agent is applied and by environmental alterations such as diet and age.
3. Progression – includes such changes as increase in growth rate, invasiveness and metastatic potential, which imply increasing genetic instability.

Endogenous and exogenous chemical agents are the cause of the majority of human cancers. Lifestyle, diet and reproductive history exert their carcinogenic effects through chemical processes. Chemical carcinogens may be direct or indirect and complete or incomplete. Direct carcinogens interact with DNA in their original state. Indirect carcinogens require modification by the body before they exert their carcinogenic effect. A complete carcinogen affects stage 1 and 2 in the multistage model. An incomplete carcinogen requires a promoter.

Tobacco smoke is one of the principal sources of chemical carcinogens, causing in the UK each year approximately 100 000 male and 50 000 female cancers. While cancer of the lung receives greatest prominence, tobacco use is also associated with buccal, pharyngeal, oesophageal, pancreatic and urinary cancers. In Asia, chewing betel nut is popular and has similar hazards to tobacco chewing, resulting in an increased risk of oropharyngeal carcinoma.

Alcohol consumption is associated with cancer. Habitual consumers of strong alcoholic drinks have an increased risk of cancer of the mouth and oesophagus. While this may be due to a promoting effect of ethanol through cytochrome P450 enzyme systems, initiation from aromatics in alcoholic drinks cannot be ruled out.

Metals may be carcinogenic. In haemochromatosis iron overload leads to cirrhosis and increases the risk of hepatocellular carcinoma. Industrial nickel exposure is associated with nasopharyngeal and bronchial carcinoma. Other industrial carcinogens include benzene, chromium compounds, coal tar, mineral oils and solvents used in the rubber industry. Their effects are site-related. Coal tar and mineral oils cause cancer of the skin, lung and bladder. Arsenic exposure is associated with skin, lung and liver tumours. Improvements in industrial hygiene since the Second World War with constant surveillance for potential 'clusters' of cases of cancer around factories have greatly reduced these hazards. As the latent period between exposure and cancer is generally long, the hazard may have disappeared before its association with cancer can be identified.

Diet

Obesity is recognized as an increasingly important risk factor for developing cancer. Low-calorie diets inhibit tumour formation in experimental animal models and this is possibly one reason for the lower incidence of breast and colorectal cancer in those of poorer socioeconomic status. There is increasing evidence that nutrition in early life may be an important factor for human breast cancer risk. A strong positive correlation between height and breast cancer risk has been observed (the risk of breast cancer increasing by 7% for each 5 cm increase in height for postmenopausal women. Fetal development within the uterus may also influence breast cancer risk. Variations in the normal constituents of the diet may explain the international differences in the incidence of such common cancers as breast and colon, which are positively correlated with the intake of dietary fat. Migration from a country of low cancer risk to one of high risk alters the incidence of certain cancers in migrants.

Aflatoxin is a direct carcinogen with relevance to human cancer that is produced by the fungus *Aspergillus flavus,* which affects grain and groundnuts stored in the damp, a common situation in the developing world. Aflatoxin is a possible cofactor to hepatitis B virus for hepatocellular carcinoma. *N*-Nitroso compounds, proven to be carcinogenic in experimental animals, can occur in the primary form in cured meats and are potential causes of nasopharyngeal and gastric cancer. Nitrosamines may also be formed in the mouth or stomach by bacterial action, which combines secondary and tertiary amines in the diet with dietary or endogenous nitrites. These reactions are enhanced in the achlorhydric stomach, providing an explanation for an increased risk of gastric cancer in pernicious anaemia. Ascorbic acid lowers the intragastric formation of *N*-nitroso compounds.

Micronutrients

Green-yellow vegetables, e.g. pumpkin, carrot, spinach, contain over 600 mg of β-carotene/100 g. This may protect against cancers of the lung, stomach and breast by directly restraining proliferation and promoting differentiation through antioxidant activity. Similar properties have been reported for the retinoids, synthetic analogues of vitamin A, which are under trial for the chemoprevention of breast cancer. There is some evidence that lack of 1–2,5-dihydroxyvitamin D may promote carcinoma of the prostate and that vitamin E may enhance epithelial cell adhesion. Trace elements such as selenium may be protective against cancer.

Iatrogenic cancer and immunosuppression

An intact immune system is important for prevention of cancer development as well as influencing the outcome of established cancer. Patients undergoing solid organ transplantation usually receive potent immunosuppressive drugs, e.g. calcineurin inhibitors such as tacrolimus and antimetabolites such as azathioprine and steroids. Transplant patients are at increased risk of a range of malignancies, most notably skin and cervical cancer, Kaposi's sarcoma and haematological malignancy. Cytotoxic chemotherapy and radiotherapy may increase the risk of developing additional malignancy, e.g. breast cancer following mantle radiotherapy for Hodgkin's disease. The potential cancer risk of diagnostic radiological investigations must be put in context with the potential benefit of the diagnostic test. A single full-body CT examination in a 45-year-old adult has been estimated to result in an estimated lifetime attributable cancer mortality risk of around 0.08%.

Physical carcinogens

Ionizing radiation

Many pioneers of radiation research, including Madame Curie, died from cancer. Historically, a variety of cancers followed radiotherapy for benign conditions (e.g. ankylosing spondylitis), most notably cancer of the breast, thyroid and liver. In Hiroshima and Nagasaki there has been an excess mortality from cancer as a result of the nuclear weapons detonated over these cities. Leukaemia accounts for half of these cancer deaths, but a small but significant increase in the incidence of tumours affecting lung, gastrointestinal tract, bladder, breast and ovary has also been recorded. Radiation exposure during early life is particularly hazardous for breast cancer and leukaemia.

Ionizing radiation includes electromagnetic irradiation, X-rays and γ-rays and subatomic particles (α particles, neutrons and electrons). As X-rays and γ-rays liberate electrons, their final effects are the same through direct damage to DNA or indirect damage as a result of the formation of free radicals, e.g. OH^-. Neutrons interact with atoms within tissues to liberate ionizing protons and other nuclear particles. The ionizing properties of these various types of radiation and their damaging effects vary according to penetration and absorption in tissues and the capacity for tissue repair.

The biological effects of radiation on tissues include loss of proliferative capacity, gene mutations, chromosomal abnormalities and neoplastic transformation. These have been extensively studied in experimental systems, but the variation in sensitivity of different tissues prevents a uniform approach. The potential dangers of chronic exposure to low-dose radiation, such as that around nuclear establishments, from diagnostic investigations, from cosmic radiation and from low-frequency electromagnetic radiations emitted from power cables and electrical appliances, are of current concern. Ultraviolet radiation as a cause of melanoma in white-skinned individuals is well recognized.

Other physical forms of tissue damage may lead to the development of cancer. Chronic ulcers such as those resulting from burns or venous insufficiency predispose to skin cancer: the Marjolin ulcer.

Biological carcinogens

Oncogenic viruses

Both DNA and RNA viruses can harbour oncogenes, which transform cells in a dominant fashion. It is estimated that 20% of human cancers are associated with viruses. Established associations include:

- genital cancer with human papilloma viruses (HPV)
- T-cell leukaemia with human T-cell leukaemia virus type 1 (HTLV-1)
- Burkitt's lymphoma and nasopharyngeal cancer with Epstein-Barr virus (EBV)
- liver carcinoma with hepatitis type B and C viruses (HBV and HCV).

A number of specific tumour types are also associated with human immunodeficiency virus (HIV). Although in experimental systems infection by virus can directly transform a cell, it is unlikely that in humans this is the sole event. It is more likely that viral infections initiate a cascade of events which include activation of cellular oncogenes and loss of tumour suppressor genes. Viruses can also act in an indirect fashion, increasing susceptibility to malignant disease, as in those rendered immunodeficient.

Retroviruses

The family of retroviruses consists of three groups: spumaviruses, lentiviruses (of which HIV types 1 and 2 are members) and oncogenic viruses. Oncogenic viruses are further divided into acutely transforming and slow-transforming viruses. The genome of acutely transforming retroviruses contains an oncogene, originally hijacked from a host cell, which, on reinsertion in mutated form or under novel transcriptional control, disrupts normal growth control mechanisms. While the discovery of oncogenes has been central to the understanding of the mechanism of transformation, there is no record of a human cancer being caused in this way. Slow-transforming viruses do not contain a classic oncogene, but exert their effect through the insertion of viral material (pro-virus) into the host genome near to the coding region of a cellular proto-oncogene, which leads to over-expression of normal gene products. T-cell leukaemia is caused by the HTLV-1 retrovirus.

DNA viruses

These contain double-stranded DNA. A number of groups, the hepadana viruses (hepatitis B), papillomaviruses (human papilloma virus) and herpes viruses (Epstein-Barr virus), are associated with hepatocellular carcinoma, uterine cervical cancer, Burkitt's lymphoma and nasopharyngeal carcinoma, respectively.

Hepatocellular carcinoma

This cancer is particularly prevalent in sub-Saharan Africa, China, Japan and East Asia. More prevalent in males, 80% of cases develop in livers affected by multinodular cirrhosis. Carriers of HbSAg have higher rates of both multinodular cirrhosis and hepatocellular carcinoma than non-carriers. Viral antigens have been identified in the liver cells of affected patients and the viral genome in cancer cells, suggesting that viral DNA may play a central role in the transforming process. The exact mechanism underlying this process is unknown, but promotion by later exposure to mycotoxins (e.g. aflatoxin) or alcohol excess has been implicated. Unlike in the Western world, in which infection with HBV occurs through contact with blood and blood products or sexual activity (horizontal transmission), in the East it is transmitted vertically from mother to child during the first year of life. As 250 million humans worldwide are chronic carriers of the virus (10% of the population in some endemic areas), the scale of the problem is immense. Eradicating HBV infection is key and large-scale programmes of vaccinating newborn infants, using a recombinant vaccinia virus carrying the HBV gene, are being evaluated. Public health programmes to minimize exposure to aflatoxin have also been established.

Carcinoma of the cervix

Human papilloma viruses (HPV) have small double-stranded circular genomes of DNA which cause benign infective skin warts. They infect basal cells during their proliferative phase which on full differentiation complete the life cycle of the virus. Genital warts, the third commonest form of sexually transmitted disease, are also due to infection by HPV, and are associated with carcinoma of the cervix. Approximately 30% of all women are infected with HPV. HPV DNA sequences have been identified in the majority of cervical carcinomas. Over 70 types of HPV are known to infect genital sites, but only a few (predominantly types 16 and 18) are associated with neoplasia. Cofactors are smoking, infection by herpes simplex virus and, possibly, oral contraceptives. A new programme of HPV vaccination has commenced in the UK.

Burkitt's lymphoma and nasopharyngeal cancer

Epstein-Barr virus (EBV) is a member of the herpes virus group. Its primary human target is the B-cell lymphocyte, in which it establishes a latent infection. It may also infect cells of the nasopharynx, the parotid gland and the uterine cervix, and is present in saliva and cervical secretions. The discovery of EBV in cells cultured from Burkitt's lymphoma suggested that this virus was the causative agent, but the disease can occur in its absence. Furthermore, EBV infection affects >95% of the world population. The restricted geographical distribution of Burkitt's lymphoma implicates a cofactor and this is believed to be constant antigen stimulation from malarial infection stimulating the continuous recruitment of new B cells which, under the influence of virus, avoid programmed cell death.

Nasopharyngeal cancer is common in South-East Asia. EBV DNA can be detected in most tumour samples. Its restricted geographical distribution again indicates the importance of cofactors which are believed to be related to smoking and a diet of salt-cured fish and preserved meats rich in nitrosamines.

Human immunodeficiency virus (HIV)

In AIDS patients, Kaposi's sarcoma occurs 20 000 times more frequently than in the general (HIV seronegative) population. The initial stimulus for transformation is a specific viral protein (tat) to which is added cell proliferative factors (cytokines) released from activated T-cells, and possibly from the Kaposi cells themselves. As the risk of Kaposi's sarcoma is greater in those infected by AIDS as a result of sexual rather than other forms of contact, an additional sexually transmitted agent may be a cofactor.

Non-viral biological carcinogens

The Gram-negative bacterium *Helicobacter pylori* is associated with chronic gastritis and mucosal intestinal metaplasia. Dysplasia and ultimately gastric carcinoma may develop. *H. pylori* is also associated with mucosa-associated lymphoid tissue (MALT) lymphoma. Interestingly, MALT lymphoma has been shown to regress in some cases following *H. pylori* eradication. In this context, *H. pylori* may be a growth-promoting factor rather than a conventional carcinogen.

Chlonorchis sinensis, the Chinese liver fluke, is a risk factor for cholangiocarcinoma. Infestation with the trematode *Schistosoma haematobium* leads to an increased risk of bladder cancer, usually of the squamous type rather than the transitional cell carcinoma more commonly occurring in the bladder.

Managing patients with cancer

Clinical presentation

Symptomatic cancer patients present due to the local or systemic effects of the tumour, or as a result of paraneoplastic syndromes.

Local tumour effects

Patients may seek medical advice following the development of symptoms due to local tumour effects such as the presence of a mass, haemorrhage, hollow viscus obstruction, compression of adjacent structures or pain.

Systemic effects and paraneoplastic syndromes

Initial presentation may be with systemic features. Systemic effects such as fatigue may result from a large or rapidly proliferating primary tumour. Metastatic disease may lead to cachexia, characterized by anorexia, weight loss, lethargy or anaemia. Less commonly, patients present with paraneoplastic syndromes, which are features that arise due to presence of neoplasia in the body, but are not directly attributable to the local presence of cancer cells.

Paraneoplastic syndromes may be divided into endocrine, neurological, mucocutaneous and haematological disorders. Syndromes may result from hormonal mediators secreted appropriately for the affected organ, e.g. hypoglycaemia due to an insulin-secreting islet cell tumour, or 'ectopically', e.g. parathyroid-related hormone secreted in lung cancer. Non-hormonal mediators are also recognized.

Patients may be identified by an established screening programme. Others may present because of anxiety, perhaps related to an affected family member or friend.

Cancer prevention and screening

There are three levels of general disease prevention.

Primary prevention is aimed at avoiding the development of cancer. Primary prevention includes most population-based health promotion activities, e.g. smoking prevention and cessation and immunization against human papilloma virus in childhood.

Secondary prevention is aimed at early cancer detection or the detection of premalignant disease, thereby maximizing the potential for interventions to cure disease or prevent progression, e.g. national breast and bowel screening programmes.

Tertiary prevention reduces the impact of an established disease by restoring function and reducing disease-related morbidity, e.g. follow-up after colorectal cancer surgery.

Screening is a population-based strategy employed to detect disease in asymptomatic individuals. Screening may be unstratified (the whole population) or stratified (targeted to the population at risk). The objective of screening is to identify disease early, thus allowing earlier intervention on the basis that this may reduce mortality and morbidity from the disease. Screening is a potentially expensive process and cost-effectiveness must be demonstrated before widespread implementation. In order to achieve cost-effectiveness, most screening programmes target a stratified section of the total population at risk. Any screening programme should fulfil criteria set out by Wilson and Jungner (Table 10.3; see also http://www.screening.nhs.uk/criteria). The criteria apply to the disease, the screening test, the treatment and the programme as a whole.

When evaluating the benefits of screening programmes, potential inherent sources of bias must be taken into account.

Table 10.3 The Wilson and Jungner criteria for a screening programme

1. The condition being screened for should be an important health problem
2. The natural history of the condition should be well understood
3. There should be a detectable early stage
4. Treatment at an early stage should be of more benefit than at a later stage
5. A suitable test should be devised for the early stage
6. The test should be acceptable
7. Intervals for repeating the test should be determined
8. Adequate health service provision should be made for the extra clinical workload resulting from screening
9. The risks, both physical and psychological, should be less than the benefits
10. The costs should be balanced against the benefits

Selection bias -- Those engaging in screening programmes may be more health-conscious and the programme may be more accessible to younger healthy people. This may result in an artificial 'benefit' to the screened population. Conversely, those with a family history of cancer may be more likely to participate in the programme.

Lead time bias -- Although the disease may be detected earlier through screening, this may not affect the time of death.

Length bias -- Screening is more likely to detect slower-growing cancers with a longer pre-clinical period and a potentially more favourable prognosis.

Overdiagnosis bias -- Detection of cancer that may never become clinically relevant, e.g. indolent prostate cancer, may artificially improve the apparent value of a screening programme.

There is considerable evidence that screening programmes are effective. In the UK, established cancer screening programmes include the NHS Breast Screening Programme (3-yearly two-view mammography from 50 to 70 years), cervical cancer screening (3-yearly cervical smear cytology until 60 years) and colorectal cancer screening programmes. Other malignancies that may be suitable for population-based screening include prostate and ovarian cancer.

Genetic testing

As a result of the identification of a number of mutated genes in hereditary non-polyposis colon cancer (MSH2, MSH1, PMS1 and PMS2) and in breast and ovarian cancer (BRCA1 and 2), the genetic testing of individuals for common cancers has become a

161

reality. As over 20% of all cases of breast cancer have a family history (usually only a mother or aunt with the disease), breast cancer has become the spearhead for genetic testing. In the study of a family with a suspected inherited genetic disorder, it is best to define the mutation of the disease gene, which, as it may only affect one base-pair, requires sequencing of the whole gene from an index case. For a large gene such as BRCA1 this is impractical, but likely sites of mutation have been identified on which limited sequencing can be performed. Having identified the specific mutation, it can be sought in other members of the family. For the genetic testing of 'familial' rather than dominantly inherited cancer, e.g. those with one or two first-degree relatives affected, a less specific test seeking alterations in the expressed product, e.g. a 'protein truncation test', can be used.

The indiscriminate use of genetic testing is to be avoided. Young women who know that they have a family history of breast cancer must be made aware of the benefits and risks before having a test, and care should be taken to minimize psychological distress, stigmatization and discrimination. This has led to the development of the genetic clinic, where a geneticist, with the support of a nurse counsellor, will compile a detailed family pedigree, recognizing that most people have knowledge of at most two generations. At this clinic the woman should be fully informed about the concept of inheritance, the extent to which this contributes to general population risk, and the benefits and risks of genetic testing. This should include the nature of the gene to be tested, its mode of inheritance and associated cancer risk, and the advantages and limitations of the test to be used. The implications of a positive test must be fully described, in particular the effect it might have on employment and insurance. Potential monitoring or preventative measures should be explained. Emotional and psychological support may be necessary at this first session. Once the result of the test is known, further counselling is necessary. Consultation with a surgeon may be required if prophylactic surgery is being considered.

Screening for inherited cancer

Approximately 5% of patients with colorectal cancer develop the disease due to an autosomally inherited defect in mismatch repair genes, e.g. MSH2 and MLH1 (hereditary non-polyposis colorectal cancer, HNPCC) or, less frequently, the APC (polyposis coli) gene on

Table 10.4 Members of the cancer multidisciplinary team (MDT)

Medical
Surgeon
Physician
Radiologist
Oncologist (clinical/medical)
Radiotherapist
Palliative care physician
General practitioner

Nursing
Clinical nurse specialist (surgical/medical/oncological)
Ward staff
Outpatient staff
Hospice

Paramedical
MDT coordinator
Secretary
Dietician
Physiotherapist
Occupational therapist
Social worker
Spiritual

chromosome 5. A similar proportion of breast cancer arises due to mutations in the BRCA1 and BRCA2 genes. These genetic abnormalities predispose to a range of cancers. Criteria exist for the diagnosis of these diseases, e.g. Amsterdam criteria for HNPCC, and for the selection of patients for genetic screening, e.g. the Bethesda criteria.

The patient's 'cancer journey' and the multidisciplinary team

Patients may enter the cancer pathway at different points, e.g. symptomatic, asymptomatic via screening programme, or following an incidental finding (Figure 10.6).

Patients may be referred from primary (general practitioner), secondary (general hospital), tertiary or quaternary (specialist or ultra-specialist centres) care. Even in cancer where the treatment is principally non-surgical, surgeons may still be required, e.g. to perform diagnostic biopsy. Current organization of cancer services relies on the multidisciplinary team (MDT) approach (Table 10.4).

The MDT approach relies on team-working but with individual healthcare professionals undertaking specific aspects of the patient's care. Staging and treatment plans are discussed at a regular MDT meeting. Following initial assessment and MDT discussion, further staging and other investigations may be coordinated. Where discrepancies occur between assessment

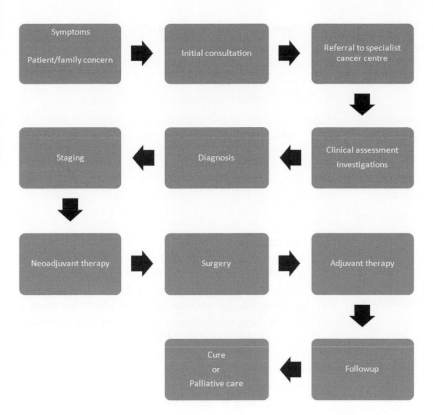

Figure 10.6 The patient's 'cancer journey'.

modalities, e.g. a clinically malignant lesion from which benign cytology is obtained, appropriate steps must be taken to ensure the correct diagnosis is established. Ideally the MDT should synthesize and apply available information in a way that optimizes patient outcome. Clinicians involved in cancer management have a responsibility to ensure that audit of process and outcome identifies and rectifies deficiencies in the service. Throughout the often complex cancer journey, communication with the patient and their family remains key.

Investigating the patient with cancer

The objectives of investigation are the diagnosis and clinicopathological staging of cancer, as well as the assessment of comorbidities which may alter the therapeutic options open to the individual patient.

Diagnostic investigations

Where the diagnosis remains to be established, investigation should proceed logically using simple non-invasive investigations, e.g. blood investigation and plain radiography, progressing through more complex imaging investigations, e.g. computerized tomog-

raphy. Further more complex imaging, e.g. nuclear medicine, and invasive investigations, e.g. endoscopic or image-guided biopsy, may be required to obtain tissue in some cases. In cases where biopsy may adversely affect outcome through tumour seeding, e.g. liver lesions, biopsy should only be undertaken following discussion within the relevant MDT. Once a cytological or histological diagnosis is established, staging can proceed. In some cases, e.g. suspected pancreatic cancer, preoperative tissue diagnosis may be impossible or undesirable. In this setting imaging-based diagnosis may be sufficient for the patient to be offered surgery.

Clinicopathological staging and grading cancer: the TNM system

Cancer staging relies on the synthesis of clinical (examination, radiology) and pathological (cytology, histology) information. The nature of staging is site-specific, e.g. magnetic resonance imaging for rectal cancer staging and endoscopic ultrasound for oesophageal cancer staging. The Union Internationale Contre le Cancer (UICC) TNM system for the

Table 10.5 The TNM system

Four degrees of primary tumour (T1–4) depending on size and local extent, in addition to which Tis indicates carcinoma *in situ*

Four degrees of node status (N0–3) representing increasing involvement

Two degrees of distant metastatic disease (M0–1) indicating absence or presence

The suffix 'x' is used where a variable cannot be assessed, e.g. T1N0Mx

Table 10.6 Cytology grades

C1. Inadequate/not useful
C2. Benign
C3. Probably benign
C4. Probably malignant
C5. Malignant

Table 10.7 Tumour histological grading

GX. Grade of differentiation cannot be assessed
G1. Well differentiated
G2. Moderately differentiated
G3. Poorly differentiated
G4. Undifferentiated

classification of malignant tumours was developed during the 1950s with the following objectives:

1. aid the clinician in the planning of treatment
2. give some indication of prognosis
3. assist in the evaluation of the results of treatment
4. facilitate exchange of information between treatment centres
5. contribute to the continuing investigation of human cancer.

The TNM system facilitates unambiguous communication by concentrating on the anatomical extent of the disease at the time of initial presentation. For prognostic purposes, many other variables need to be taken into account. The division of the disease into stages was an attempt, by merging of TNM factors, to define groups which are more or less homogeneous in terms of the extent of the disease.

The same basic principles are applied to all sites and coded as T to classify the extent of the primary tumour, N to determine the condition of the regional nodes and M to indicate the presence or absence of distant metastases. With some exceptions, the broad subdivisions in each category are as shown in Table 10.5.

Several revisions have taken place since the original TNM system. With the realization that the relationships between clinical findings and outcome may not reflect those found on pathological examination, the TNM system of classification became more complex. In 1987 a revision was accepted by all national TNM committees, by the American Joint Committee on Cancer and by the European Organization for Research on Treatment of Cancer as a standard classification.

Current TNM systems

The basis of the TNM system remains the assessment of three components: the extent of the primary tumour (T), the presence or absence of metastases in regional lymph nodes (N) and the presence or absence of distant metastasis (M), these being separately classified for pre- (clinical, cTNM), postoperative (pathological, pTNM) and following alternative treatment (yTNM). Following determination of each category, they are grouped into stages, the limits of which are stage 0 representing *in situ* cancer and stage 4, distant metastases. As the extent to which detailed clinical, surgical and pathological findings contribute to the stage varies, there is a regrettable lack of uniformity for staging cancers at different sites. For some cancers (e.g. thyroid), simple clinical findings are still used, whereas for others (e.g. uterine, cervix or prostate) detailed pathological findings predominate.

A certainty or 'C factor' has been introduced which attempts to determine the certainty with which the findings have been recorded at different sites. C1 reflects a diagnosis made using standard diagnostic tests, while C5 reflects a diagnosis made at autopsy. The 'C factor' should not be confused with the more commonly used C1–5 grading of fine-needle aspiration cytology, shown in Table 10.6.

Tumour grade is a microscopic assessment of differentiation. In general, cancer is graded according to the scheme shown in Table 10.7.

All staging systems have limitations in that microscopic disease may not be identified, especially in cancer where micrometastasis is a common early event. However, the current system is a pragmatic attempt to provide a meaningful framework on which to base each patient's therapy.

General physiological assessment and investigation

History will often give a good indication of a patient's functional capacity. The concept of metabolic equivalents (METs) allows a patient's capacity to perform common activities to be quantified. One MET is equivalent to an oxygen uptake of 3.5 ml/kg per min in a 70 kg 40-year-old at rest. One MET equivalents include dressing oneself, walking at 2–3 mph and doing light housework. More strenuous activities are allocated higher MET scores. Functional capacity is regarded as excellent in those able to perform > 7 METS, moderate 4–7 METS and poor < 4 METS. Perioperative and long-term risk is increased in those unable to achieve 4 METs during normal daily activities, particularly in those less than 65 years of age.

Specific investigations aimed at assessing the patient's fitness for intervention will often be required. Assessment of cardiorespiratory function is important in patient selection for major surgery. More recently, dynamic techniques such as cardiopulmonary exercise (CPX) testing, which determines the patient's anaerobic threshold during a standardized exercise protocol, have gained popularity as a more meaningful assessment of patient functional capacity. Patient investigation must be based on individual requirements and risk factors.

Tumour markers

A tumour marker is a tumour-associated deviation from normal of a substance or process that can be detected by assay of tissue or body fluid. Tumour markers can be produced directly by the tumour, or by non-tumour cells as a response to the presence of a tumour. Tumour markers are classified into cancer-specific and tissue-specific markers.

Cancer-specific markers

These markers are produced by certain types of cancer. Their principal use is the monitoring of disease, as overlap between tumour types limits their diagnostic utility. Carcinoembryonic antigen (CEA) is one such example, which is produced by colorectal adenocarcinoma as well as other tumours, e.g. breast adenocarcinoma. Circulating tumour cells and DNA may also have application as cancer-specific tumour markers. Polymerase chain reaction (PCR) techniques are particularly useful for detecting single tumour cells or tiny amounts (of the order of pg) of abnormal genetic material against a background of normal cells or DNA.

Tumour-specific markers

These markers are released by tissues that contain tumour, but not necessarily by the tumour cells.

Prostate specific antigen (PSA) is a serine protease that is produced by normal prostate cells. Abnormalities of the prostate, e.g. benign prostatic enlargement, prostatitis or tumour, may all result in elevated serum PSA levels. Elevated levels of tissue-specific markers also require careful interpretation.

Tumour markers can also be classified as prognostic or predictive.

(1) Prognostic markers predict the future behaviour of the disease independent of the effect of treatment. Prognostic markers can be grouped as markers of:

Proliferation, e.g. Ki-67 immunoreactivity useful for predicting gastrointestinal stromal tumour behaviour;

Receptor and growth factor activity, e.g. oestrogen-receptor protein status in breast cancer, oestrogen-receptor negative tumours having a poorer prognosis;

Invasiveness, e.g. pro-cathepsin D, heat shock proteins and laminin receptors.

(2) Predictive markers determine the outcome of treatment. They can be defined in terms of survival, quality of life following treatment and even of the cost of healthcare. HER-2 status predicts response to Herceptin and is also an index of prognosis in breast cancer.

Treating cancer: defining cancer cure

The logical objective of cancer treatment is the destruction of all cancer cells, i.e. a 'clinical cure'. This definition of cure is impractical as it requires the complete search for asymptomatic deposits of tumour on death. Freedom from cancer recurrence during the remainder of a patient's lifetime constitutes an arguably more relevant 'personal cure'. This definition of cure also has limitations, as the patient killed in a road accident on the way home from hospital following the palliative resection of an incurable cancer could be classified as 'cured'. 'Statistical cure' refers to a group of disease-free survivors whose annual death rate from all causes is the same as that of a group of the normal population of similar sex and age distribution. Five-year survival is widely used as an arbitrary indicator of 'cure'. However, five-year survival is only relevant to cancer that exhibits initial rapid progression. In some more indolent cancers, excess mortality from metastatic disease may persist for over 30 years, hence five-year survival does not equate to cure.

Table 10.8 Classification of surgical resection

RX. Presence of residual tumour cannot be assessed
R0. No residual tumour
R1. Microscopic residual tumour
R2. Macroscopic residual tumour

Local therapy

Surgical management

Radical cancer surgery implies the excision of all cancer tissue together with a margin of surrounding normal tissue. In cancers where lymph node metastasis occurs, this approach includes excision of a variable number of the locoregional draining nodes. The sequential spread of primary tumour cells to locoregional lymph nodes is an over-simplistic model of cancer progression, but offers the best opportunity for cure in those who have isolated nodal metastases. In some cases, e.g. breast cancer and melanoma, where routine en bloc removal of locoregional nodes may result in unacceptable morbidity, a node sampling approach may be adopted. The sentinel node is the hypothetical node which is the first node or group of nodes reached by metastasizing tumour cells. Dye and radioisotope techniques have gained popularity for identifying sentinel nodes, allowing a targeted nodal sample to be obtained. This approach theoretically maximizes diagnostic yield while minimizing morbidity, e.g. limb lymphoedema and nerve injury.

Surgery for cancer may be curative or palliative. Successful outcomes from surgery require accurate staging to allow selection of patients most likely to benefit. Under the TNM system, surgical resection is classified according to an 'R factor' which defines the likelihood of residual disease following surgical resection. Based on macroscopic and microscopic features, the resection is assigned an R value (Table 10.8).

The aim of radical surgery performed with curative intent must be an R0 resection. Surgery resulting in non-R0 resection may be acceptable in some situations in which palliation is intended. In cases where a tumour appears adherent to an adjacent structure, the usual principle is to perform an en bloc resection of the tumour together with all or part of the adherent structure. The temptation to develop a plane of dissection between tumour and adherent adjacent structure should be resisted if R0 resection is to be achieved, although histological studies show that such adhesions are often inflammatory in nature, rather than malignant infiltration.

Radiotherapy

Radiation therapy may be classified as adjuvant (given following surgery) or neoadjuvant (administered before local treatment, reducing the bulk of the primary tumour before surgery). Postoperative adjuvant radiotherapy is used discriminately when there is a high likelihood of residual disease or when the potential problems associated with recurrence exceed the morbidity caused by irradiating normal tissues. The radiosensitivity of a tumour is also relevant and some primary tumours, e.g. upper oesophageal squamous carcinoma, may be managed better by radiotherapy than by surgery. Radiation tends to fail at the centre of a tumour where the cells are hypoxic. Tumours contain areas of anoxic cells which require greater doses of radiation for 'kill' than do well-oxygenated cells. In the belief that these anoxic cells are likely to cause relapse, treatment during exposure to hyperbaric oxygenation was introduced, but was found to have a beneficial effect only when the radiation was given as a small number of fractions. Other radiosensitizers such as halogenated pyrimidines and nitroimidazoles are also used. Conversely, surgery is more likely to fail at its perimeter, due to the need to preserve anatomical boundaries.

Ionizing radiation consists of subatomic particles or photons which cause ejection of an orbital electron. In clinical practice they are generated by machine or from a decaying radioactive source. The amount of energy absorbed by tissue is known as the 'absorbed dose', which is measured in gray, each Gy equalling 100 rads. The intensity of radiation varies inversely to the square of the distance from the source (inverse square law). Beams of ionizing radiation are described as superficial if their energy lies between 10 and 125 kV, orthovoltage if between 125 and 400 kV and megavoltage if over 400 kV. As the energy increases, so does the penetrating power. For orthovoltage therapy the skin is the limiting factor, while megavoltage radiation is skin-sparing, the maximum dose being delivered to tissues below the surface.

Radiotherapy can be delivered by applying the source within or near to the tumour (brachytherapy) or from a distance (teletherapy). Radium needles were first used for interstitial and intracavitary radiotherapy, but have been superseded by iridium-192, caesium-137 and cobalt-60, which emit γ-rays, and by yttrium-90, which emits β-rays. For teletherapy of other than superficial sites, beams of 4–8 MeV from cobalt-60 sources are normally used. Higher-energy beams can be generated from a linear accelerator.

In planning treatment, the radiotherapist must ensure accurate localization of the beam to the tumour site, modifying its intensity and shape by the use of filters, and develop a treatment plan to give the best distribution and homogeneity of the radiation. This is tested on a simulator which utilizes superficial radiation to reproduce the effect of treatment on radiographs, or through an image intensifier. The fields are marked in indelible ink on the patient and the treatment is usually given in a series of fractions spread over several weeks.

The important target molecule for radiation is DNA, but reaction between electrons and water produces free radicals which also may cause cell damage. As the effect of radiation varies during the cell cycle, not all cells are killed; others evoke repair mechanisms. There is also recruitment of new cells. Fractionation of the total dose of radiation achieves higher cell kill while sparing normal tissues from excessive radiation.

The effect of radiation on normal tissues is variable. Tissues which do not require renewal, such as muscle, nerve, bone and liver, are relatively resistant compared to the skin, gastrointestinal tract, reproductive organs and exocrine glands, which are constantly repopulated and most sensitive to damage. Tissues such as the lung fall in between. Adverse effects include inhibition of the immune response, mutagenesis and, through damage to cell membranes, oedema. The ataxia-telangectasia (AT) gene is autosomal recessive, and one defective gene is carried by 1.4% of the population. In those who are homozygous for the gene there is a high incidence of new cancers in childhood and adolescence and an exquisite sensitivity to radiation which causes lethal necrosis of normal tissues.

Photodynamic therapy

Photodynamic therapy (PDT) utilizes a combination of light and photosensitizing drugs to treat accessible deposits of cancer. The photosensitizing drug is concentrated in all cells but, unlike normal cells, tumour cells retain it for several days. Drug activation by the light source leads to cell death. The main advantage of PDT over other forms of treatment is its relative mildness, making it suitable for some patients unfit for surgery. Its main side effect is to render the skin hypersensitive to the sun. A new generation of photosensitizers is being developed which are cleared from normal cells within minutes, and this prevents this side effect and offers the possibility of repeated treatments. A disadvantage of current photosensitizers is that they absorb light best in the red area close to that of haemoglobin and melanin, which limits the penetration of light. New agents with different spectra for light absorption allow greater depths of light penetration.

Systemic therapy

Adequate local treatment of the primary tumour and its lymph nodes is an essential part of the total treatment of cancer. Exceptions are those in which systemic therapy leads to complete remission of the local disease, as with lymphomas. However, once a cancer has disseminated, effective systemic therapy is required. As with radiotherapy, systemic therapy may be classified as adjuvant or neoadjuvant. Subtypes of systemic therapy include general cytotoxic chemotherapy, target-specific biological agents, hormonal therapy and immunotherapy. In sites where the size of a tumour may be measured, response to systemic treatment may be assessed and, if ineffective, changed.

Cytotoxic chemotherapy

Although in Western countries the administration of chemotherapy lies within the province of the non-surgical oncologist, all surgeons must be aware of its advantages and shortcomings. Initially used for the palliation of advanced cancers, the first critical evaluation of the role of chemotherapy in early cancer arose from the observation that the course of acute lymphoblastic leukaemia in children, a uniformly fatal disease, could be dramatically altered by the administration of the folic acid antagonist aminopterin. Although early hopes of 'cure' were not realized, the development of new agents that could be given in combination, recognition of the principles of their action and the ability to monitor objectively responses by marrow aspiration led to successful and often curative treatment. Although this success has been extended only to a small number of solid tumours, e.g. lymphomas and testicular and ovarian cancers, the principles are equally applicable to other forms of cancer and should be understood.

Dosage

Experimental studies in mouse leukaemia indicated that chemotherapy acted in a logarithmic fashion on cancer cells according to 'first-order kinetics'. A given dose of drug kills the same fraction, not the same number, of cells. The fractional reduction of tumour cells following chemotherapy is constant, irrespective of the size of the tumour burden. The amount of treatment required to effect a 99% reduction of a tumour of 1 mg (from 10^6 to 10^4 cells) is the same as that for one of 1 kg (from 10^{12} to 10^{10} cells). This finding suggests that the induction of an apparent complete remission is only the first step in treatment. To eradicate all leukaemia cells and maintain remission, more intensive, prolonged and potentially lethal therapy is required. This in turn requires measures to counteract its effects.

Marrow transplantation

The potentially lethal problems associated with intensive chemotherapy are infection and haemorrhage due to destruction of marrow cells. Initially these were countered by intensive antibiotic treatment, laminar-flow isolation and granulocyte and platelet transfusions, but with the development of marrow transplantation a more lasting solution evolved. Supralethal cytoreductive therapy followed by salvage allogeneic marrow transplantation, when practised during the initial remission of acute leukaemia, results in a high proportion of disease-free and treatment-free survivors.

During developmental studies in experimental animals it was noted that stem cells from the buffy coat of the peripheral blood, when injected into recipients, could repopulate marrow spaces. Following the discovery of the colony-stimulating factors, CSF and GCSF, which control the proliferation of granulocytes, monocytes, macrophages and related haemopoietic cells in human marrow, it became practical to 'shift' stem cells from the marrow into the peripheral blood, from where they could be harvested and stored for re-infusion at a later date. Peripheral stem-cell rescue has now largely replaced marrow transplantation in the initial management of leukaemias and lymphomas and increasingly in other cancers in which high-intensity dose regimens of chemotherapy are being used. However, as chronic graft-versus-host reaction may attack the host's leukaemic as well as normal cells of skin, liver and/or intestinal tract, allogeneic marrow transplantation still has a place in the long-term management of this disease.

Chemoresistance

Combinations of chemotherapeutic drugs are more effective than single agents, and their scheduling is of primary importance to the duration of their effect. Resistance to cytotoxic chemotherapy is well established in the laboratory, and it is believed that similar mechanisms may operate in some human tumours.

In the clinical situation, resistance may be temporary due to physiological barriers such as the blood–brain and blood–testicular barriers already referred to. Temporary resistance may also follow sojourning of the cells in the G0 (resting) phase of the cell cycle when they are no longer sensitive to cell-cycle-specific drugs. Permanent resistance implies alteration of the phenotype of the cancer cell. Drug-resistant phenotypes may be inherent in the initial cell population so that only sensitive cells are eliminated, but these more commonly develop due to mutations in the genetically unstable cells. As the mutated pool of cells increases, so does the resistance of the tumour. Such mutations may be spontaneous or, as in laboratory situations, result from continuous exposure to the relevant drug.

Although developed in vitro by exposure to a single agent such as doxorubicin, resistance to anthracyclones is characteristically shared with other seemingly unrelated agents, e.g. vinca alkaloids and colchicine. This 'pleomorphic' drug resistance is due to overexpression of a 170 kDa protein, P-glycoprotein, which forms a molecular marker for resistant cells. The gene encoding this protein, *MDR 1,* has been sequenced. It belongs to a superfamily of genes which are highly conserved in plants, bacteria, insects and mammals, and express ATP-dependent transport proteins. P-glycoprotein spans the cell membrane. An internal ATP-binding domain couples the energy to pump a number of diverse hydrophobic compounds through transmembrane ion channels to the exterior of the cell. It is normally expressed in the adrenal, gravid uterus, colon and capillary endothelium of the brain where, as in the testicle, it may be concerned with blood–brain barrier function. Overexpression in tumour cells may be due to amplification of the *MDR* gene or to abnormal transcriptional or translational events.

Targeted biological agents

While conventional antineoplastic approaches such as surgery, radiotherapy and cytotoxic chemotherapy remain the mainstay of cancer treatment, the essential need is to reassert normal controlling mechanisms that regulate growth, invasion and metastasis. Dissecting the molecular pathways responsible for the dysregulation of cell function shows promise for identifying new targeted agents.

Examples of targeted therapies that have been investigated include:

- The development of inhibitors of enzymes such as topoisomerase and telomerase which are concerned with repair and integrity of the genome. Drugs which over-ride the checkpoints in the cell cycle apparently sensitize the cells to DNA damaging agents.
- The infusion of genetically modified immunocompetent cells which over-express cytokines (e.g. interleukin-2) and mount an exaggerated immune response against the tumour.
- The enhancement of protection against the toxic effects of chemotherapeutic agents by the insertion, into normal cells, of a drug-resistance gene. This applies particularly to bone-marrow stem cells into which the *mdr*1 gene can be inserted. Through stimulation of the P-glycoprotein efflux pump, daughter cells expressing this gene are protected against the cytotoxic effects of the drug, which can then be given in higher dose.
- The development of strategies to enable tumour cells to activate selectively a 'pro-drug', normally inert, into a highly toxic metabolite. An example is the insertion of the thymidine kinase gene, the product of which can convert ganciclovir into its cytotoxic triphosphates. This gene can be inserted into neurological tumours using a herpes simplex virus vector.
- The synthesis of 'antisense' DNA oligonucleotides which have complementary coding to mRNA but which, being inert, block the normal process of translation.
- Small interfering RNA which potently inhibits gene expression at a post-transcriptional level with an apparently high degree of potency and specificity.

The objective of gene therapy is the replacement or correction of a defective oncogene or tumour-suppressor gene which is causally associated with the cancer in question. Delivery of the replacement gene has proven to be problematic. To date most attention has focused on viral vectors, particularly retroviruses, but alternative non-viral vectors are also being studied. These include liposomes and synthetic molecular complexes as well as 'naked' and modified oligonucleotides. Attachment of tumour-specific ligands may improve selectivity.

Other forms of non-genetic biological therapy have entered clinical use. These include monoclonal antibodies directed against kinases e.g. EGFR. Antibodies specific for tumour antigens, carrying a radioactive isotope (e.g. yttrium-90) or a cell toxin (e.g. saporin) which can penetrate the cell membrane, have also been investigated. Inhibitors of 'downstream events' that affect the metabolism, proliferation of the cancer cell and its invasive properties are also being developed. Targeted agents such as small molecule kinase inhibitors have revolutionized the treatment of some malignancies e.g. Imatinib, a c-KIT/ABL inhibitor used in GIST and leukaemia. This exciting area of cancer research holds promise for future drug development.

Patient follow-up

Patients undergoing surgical treatment for cancer usually undergo follow-up to identify complications of surgery and disease recurrence. There are few standardized protocols for this follow-up, and the benefit of intensive follow-up over more rudimentary arrangements remains controversial. The potential benefit to systematic intensive follow-up is that those patients with disease recurrence that is amenable to potentially curative surgery will be more reliably identified at an early stage. Despite aggressive investigation and follow-up it remains difficult to identify disease recurrence in many patients and such an approach may adversely affect quality of life in those who will not derive any benefit. Intensive follow-up also has significant cost implications. Currently, trials are assessing the contribution of follow-up to cancer patient outcome.

Prognostication and counselling

Key determinants of patient outcome following the surgical management of cancer include physiological and performance status, tumour histological type, disease stage and grade, achieving an R0 resection and avoidance of postoperative complications. Other disease-specific prognostic markers have been developed that give useful prognostic information, e.g.

HER2 in breast cancer, Ki67 proliferation index in gastrointestinal stromal tumours. Despite significant advances, our ability to prognosticate has significant deficiencies. Effective communication with patients regarding prognostic information as well as sharing uncertainty where it exists remain a critical and challenging component of the doctor–patient relationship.

Quality of life

The success of cancer treatment cannot be measured only in terms of freedom from disease and survival. Of equal importance to the patient is the quality of well-being during remaining life. This is of particular importance to those with advanced cancer, in whom the unpleasant side-effects of treatment must never exceed potential benefit. A number of patient-completed questionnaires have been developed to assess the functional quality of the day-to-day life of the cancer patient. These include the Functional Living Index for Cancer (FLIC), the Cancer Rehabilitation Evaluation System (CARES), as well as the more traditional Karnovsky Performance Status and General Health Questionnaire. Profiles of mood states and scales for global adjustment to illness are also available.

Pain control and palliative care

The surgeon may be involved in aspects of palliation, e.g. relieving bowel obstruction. Surgeons should also have a rational approach to the management of cancer-related pain.

Cancer-related pain

Pain at diagnosis is experienced by 20–50% of cancer patients. By the time the disease is advanced, this proportion has risen to 75%. Pain may be acute or chronic. Acute pain may be catastrophic and accompanied by autonomic and psychological responses, drawing attention to an acute pathological process which needs to be remedied. Chronic pain is continuous, recurring at intervals of months or years, and is associated with vegetative disturbances such as lack of sleep, anorexia, decreased libido and personality change. Unlike acute pain it does not serve any useful purpose. Pain associated with cancer may be caused by the cancer itself, when it may be somatic or visceral in origin, or due to associated factors such as muscle spasm, bedsores, constipation or complications of treatment. It may also arise from an unrelated disorder. Cancer pain can be differentiated from other forms of pain by its chronicity and by overwhelming associated features of insomnia, reduced appetite, irritability, depression, rage and spiritual or social disturbance.

The mainstay of the successful treatment of cancer pain is the use of non-opioid, opioid and a number of adjuvant drugs. The WHO 'ladder' ascends from the prescription of non-opioid drugs, through 'weak opioids' to 'strong opioids' as control is lost. Opioid is a generic term which refers to codeine, morphine and other natural and synthetic drugs which act on specific receptors in the central and peripheral nervous systems. With correct administration of appropriate drugs, pain can be controlled in 90% of cases. Unwarranted fear of opioid addiction and lack of knowledge of alternative remedies may present management problems. Following assessment, a specific pain management plan should be identified for each patient, which must be fully discussed with him or her, and his or her family. The aim of treatment and the risk of adverse effects should be explained. Optimum requirements for non-opioids and opioids, laxatives and psychotropic drugs are planned. As these will require adjustment, continuing assessment is necessary.

The commonest complications of morphine administration are nausea, vomiting, constipation, drowsiness and confusion. Difficulty with micturition, ureteric spasm and a variety of other autonomic effects may also occur. Large doses of morphine can cause respiratory depression and hypotension, leading to circulatory failure and deepening coma. Unless there is a definite reason for not doing so, a laxative should be prescribed for all patients receiving morphine. Best is a combination of a contact laxative (e.g. senna) and a faecal softener (e.g. docusate). Vomiting must be controlled. Haloperidol or fluphenazine are preferable to prochlorperazine, which is more likely to cause drowsiness. Vomiting secondary to delayed gastric emptying or to a 'functional' opioid-induced intestinal ileus usually responds to metoclopromide.

Opioid-resistant pain

A number of measures are available to treat opioid-resistant pain. Local anaesthetics administered either orally or by intravenous injection may have a general analgesic effect. The alpha-receptor antagonist clonidine administered transdermally, orally or by

Table 10.9 Key aspects of the surgical management of cancer

Early detection
MDT assessment
Accurate staging
Radical (en bloc) surgery
(Neo)adjuvant therapy
Communication with patient/carers
Audit
Effective follow-up/surveillance

injection, either alone or combined with morphine, may provide relief. Subcutaneous infusions of the dissociative anaesthetic ketamine may be used.

A variety of non-drug treatments is also available for the management of intractable pain. These may consist of simple counter-irritation with cold compresses, hot water bottles or ointments. Transcutaneous electrical nerve stimulation (TENS) is of benefit in a wide range of conditions which cause localized pain, particularly of muscle origin. This is believed to be due to stimulation of large nerve fibres which release the inhibitory neurotransmitter γ-aminobutyric acid (GABA) in the dorsal horn. A similar effect may account for the success of acupuncture whether by deep needling alone or combined with electrostimulation. A number of psychological methods of pain relief, e.g. relaxation therapy, are also employed.

A particular pathological process, e.g. bone metastases, may respond to direct treatment by prophylactic internal fixation, radiotherapy or bisphosphonates. Mobility must be preserved. A local anaesthetic block may give temporary relief of localized pain arising from a myofascial 'trigger point', rib metastases, sacroiliac joint or other local site. More permanent destruction of nervous tissue can be achieved by phenol, alcohol, thermocoagulation or cryodestruction. Abdominal visceral pain can be relieved by coeliac plexus block or somatic pain by intrathecal lysis of nerve roots, but at the risk of producing bladder and anal dysfunction.

Members of the palliative care team will often play a key role in the management of cancer patients both in the perioperative period and following discharge. It is important to involve the palliative care team early to allow plans to be made and a constructive relationship to develop. Most patients with incurable disease will wish to die either at home with support of the community palliative care team, or in a hospice. Palliative care physicians will often be able to address cancer-related

pain and other symptoms with good effect. A holistic approach addressing not only biological problems but also psychological, social and spiritual issues is one most likely to be of benefit to the patient.

Acknowledgements

This chapter has been developed from the first and second edition versions, authored and co-authored by A. Patrick Forrest.

I am very grateful to SJ Duxbury for assistance in preparing the text and to RW Parks for reviewing this chapter.

Further reading

Blanks RG, Moss SM, McGahan CE, Quinn MJ, Babb PJ. Effect of NHS breast screening programme on mortality from breast cancer in England and Wales, 1990–8: comparison of observed with predicted mortality. *BMJ* 2000;**321**(7262):665–669.

Castells A, Bessa X, Daniels M, Ascaso C, Lacy AM, Garcia-Valdecasas JC *et al.* Value of postoperative surveillance after radical surgery for colorectal cancer: results of a cohort study. *Dis Colon Rectum* 1998;**41**(6):714–723.

Fidler IJ, Poste G. The 'seed and soil' hypothesis revisited. *Lancet Oncol* 2008;**9**(8):808.

Knudson AG Jr. Overview: genes that predispose to cancer. *Mutat Res* 1991;**247**(2):185–190.

Mandel JS, Church TR, Ederer F, Bond JH. Colorectal cancer mortality: effectiveness of biennial screening for fecal occult blood. *J Natl Cancer Inst* 1999;**91**(5):434–437.

Van Den Brandt PA, Spiegelman D, Yaun SS, Adami HO, Beeson L, Folsom AR *et al.* Pooled analysis of prospective cohort studies on height, weight, and breast cancer risk. *Am J Epidemiol* 2000;**152**(6):514–527.

Visvader JE, Lindeman GJ. Cancer stem cells in solid tumours: accumulating evidence and unresolved questions. *Nat Rev Cancer* 2008;**8**(10):755–768.

Selected internet resource links

http://www.sign.ac.uk/pdf/SIGN106.pdf SIGN Guidelines: Control of pain in adults with cancer

http://www.nice.org.uk/nicemedia/pdf/csgspmanual.pdf NICE Guidance on Cancer Services Improving Supportive and Palliative Care for Adults with Cancer

171

http://www.ukgtn.nhs.uk/gtn/digitalAssets/0/277_UKGTN_
Framework_March_06.pdf Genetic testing guidance

http://www.library.nhs.uk/HealthManagement/
ViewResource.aspx?resID=301251 Tackling cancer:
improving the patient journey

http://www.uicc.org/index.php?option=com_content&
task=view&id=14296&Itemid=428 An introduction to
the UICC TNM classification

http://www.egtm.eu/general_information_on_tumor_
markers.htm European Group on Tumour markers

Chapter

11

Fundamentals of intestinal failure and nutrition

Tim Campbell Smith and Alistair Windsor

Introduction

Intestinal failure (IF) exists when a patient cannot maintain their fluid balance and nutritional needs independently through the enteral route (i.e. orally). This is due to a loss of functioning gut. In most patients this loss of function is temporary, for example, immediately following abdominal surgery when intravenous fluids and or PN are required until gastrointestinal function returns. This resolves without any long-term sequelae. However, some patients develop a long-term reduction in functioning intestine. The management of these cases is complicated and care under a specialist multidisciplinary team maximizes the likelihood of an optimum outcome. Some of these patients may require long-term intravenous nutrition or bowel transplantation. Shaffer recently set out a classification of IF identifying the differences in duration and severity.

Type 1 – self-limiting IF as occurs following abdominal surgery
Type 2 – IF in severely ill patients with major resections of the bowel, with septic, metabolic and nutritional complications requiring multidisciplinary intervention with metabolic and nutritional support to permit recovery
Type 3 – chronic IF requiring long-term nutritional support.

Such a devastating condition has a huge impact on their lives and ability to live independently as well as considerable cost and resource implications for the healthcare provider. In the UK there are several supra-regional centres caring for these patients.

Epidemiology

The number of patients suffering with intestinal failure in the UK is very difficult to quantify. In 1998 the British Artificial Nutrition Survey (BANS) estimated that there were 12 000 patients on home enteral tube feeding (HETF) and more than 360 on home parenteral nutrition (HPN). The annual growth of these is up to 20% for HETF and approximately 5% for HPN. The prevalence of HPN is 6–8 per million with an incidence of 2–3 per million. The variability in prevalence between health authorities is large (0–30 per million), and probably reflects the referral of these patients to supra-regional centres. This growth in provision of nutritional support and the complex care of this group and their prolonged hospital stay has significant implications for the resourcing of these services.

The incidence of intestinal failure in hospitals is likely to be much higher, as many of the patients requiring PN are successfully weaned off it. As small bowel transplantation improves with improvement in survival and morbidity, more patients on lifelong PN may be offered this. At present approximately half of those on long-term PN may be suitable.

Causes

The causes of intestinal failure vary between adults and children. Children, however, often have an impressive capacity to adapt, especially neonates and toddlers.

Adults
- Massive enterectomy due to:
  - Mesenteric infarction
  - Small bowel volvulus
  - Trauma

- Crohn's disease
  - Fistulating disease
  - Recurrent resection resulting in short gut

- Mesenteric desmoid disease

Fundamentals of Surgical Practice, Third Edition, ed. Andrew N. Kingsnorth and Douglas M. Bowley.
Published by Cambridge University Press. © Cambridge University Press 2011.

- Pseudo-obstruction
- Radiation enteritis

  Children
- Small bowel volvulus
- Gastroschisis
- Necrotizing enterocolitis
- Congenital atresia
- Hirschprung's disease
- Pseudo-obstruction

Anatomically short bowel

Surgery may result in significant loss of small bowel length. This may be over the course of years with recurrent resections for Crohn's disease or from a massive enterectomy following mesenteric thrombosis or embolus, volvulus or trauma. The reduction of absorptive capacity leads to loss of fluid and electrolyte balance and malnutrition. It is the amount of remaining bowel, rather than how much is removed, which is important. At operation it is important to accurately document what remains, in terms of both length and its anatomical position. The amount of small bowel resulting in SBS varies between individuals. The presence of the colon in continuity influences this. The length of small bowel varies from 300 to 800 cm. With less than 200 cm of small bowel some patients will have a degree of intestinal failure; however, less than 100 cm without the colon or 50 cm with colonic continuity will result in IF and dependence on PN.

Functional short bowel

The amount of bowel in continuity may be reduced despite being anatomically present. Fistulae, bypassing large segments of bowel, result in reduced absorption and increase intestinal losses of fluids and electrolytes. These may be overt as in enterocutaneous fistulae or be internal between bowel loops. Most (75–85%) of these occur in postoperative patients. The commonest cause is an anastomotic leak, but other postoperative causes include unrecognized bowel injury at the time of primary surgery (certainly a concern with laparoscopic surgery with instruments out of the field of view), breakdown of an enterotomy repair or breakdown of exposed bowel in a laparostomy wound. Disease processes leading to fistulation include Crohn's disease, diverticular disease, radiation enteritis, cancer and pancreatitis. There is often a surgical procedure preceding the fistula, and it is particularly

dangerous reopening an abdominal wound after about 10 days when adhesions and oedema increase the risk of further bowel injury. Enterovaginal fistulae, seen occasionally after surgery and radiotherapy for cervical cancer, are particularly distressing and are associated with discharge of caustic bowel content *per vaginam*. This may necessitate early re-entry in to the abdomen to defunction the fistula to prevent serious skin damage to the perineum. Small bowel loops embedded in a frozen pelvis may necessitate the formation of a proximal stoma to relieve their symptoms, but a manageable high-output stoma is preferable to uncontrolled PV discharge.

Absorptive capacity can also be reduced by inflammatory conditions including coeliac disease, sprue, amyloidosis, scleroderma and giardiasis.

As well as having an adequate surface area for optimum small bowel function, gut motility is essential for adequate absorption to occur. Loss of function is seen in pseudo-obstruction, postoperative ileus, visceral myopathies and autonomic neuropathy. The principles of nutritional support for these patients are the same as for other causes.

Pathology

A patient with intestinal failure passes through three stages during its progression.

Stage 1: hypersecretion
Stage 2: adaptation
Stage 3: stabilization.

Hypersecretory stage

The hypersecretory phase is usually fairly short-lived, lasting 1–2 months. It is dominated by high-output diarrhoea or high stoma/fistula effluent, causing fluid depletion and a loss of electrolytes. Gastric hypersecretion accompanies this, exacerbating the losses and contributing to dehydration and malnutrition. Management is directed at correcting the fluid and electrolyte imbalances, and intravenous feeding is usually needed as enteral feed worsens the output.

Adaptation stage

Adaptation varies with the age of the patient and the pathology underlying the cause of IF. It lasts from 3 to 12 months and enteral feeding can usually be reintroduced. Some patients can be maintained entirely with

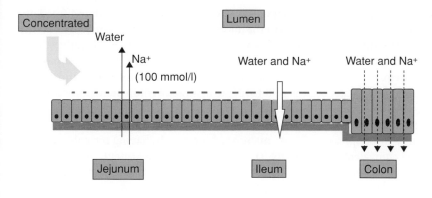

Figure 11.1 On ingesting food under normal anatomical circumstances a concentrated fluid enters the jejunum. The jejunum, being freely permeable, allows sodium into the lumen, which equilibrates at a concentration of 100 mmol per litre. A substantial volume of water moves along with the sodium into the lumen of the gut. Active sodium reabsorbed in the ileum and proximal colon allows most of this water to be recovered.

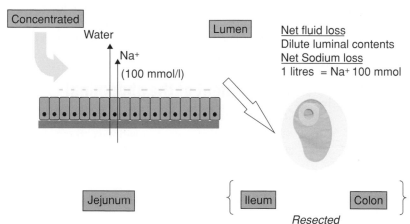

Figure 11.2 Loss of ileum and colon prevents the normal recovery of sodium and water, thus net water and sodium loss lead to rapid dehydration and sodium depletion.

enteral feed and supplements, whereas others need fluid and/or TPN supplementation.

Stabilization stage

Once the patient has adapted to their full extent, the aim of treatment is to maintain as normal and independent a life as possible, ideally at home. Depending on their adaptation, extra support may be required, in some cases involving a home parenteral nutrition team.

Gut physiology

Fluid and electrolyte balance

The bowel handles about 7 litres of fluid each day. This is secreted by the stomach, liver, pancreas and small bowel, most of which is reabsorbed in the ileum, leaving approximately 800 ml presenting to the colon, of which only 200 ml is lost in the stool. Thus with disturbances in gut function, and in particular with proximal stomas or fistulae, there is the potential to lose huge amounts of fluid and electrolytes, which, left untreated, would be fatal.

Sodium is key in the reabsorption of water. It is actively absorbed in the ileum together with glucose and some amino acids. Monosaccharide absorption in the ileum is via sodium-dependent glucose and galactose co-transporters (SGLT 1 and 2). Driven by the concentration gradient of sodium and glucose, water follows passively. The jejunum is freely permeable to water and therefore its contents are isotonic. If luminal sodium is low then sodium moves into the lumen together with water, exacerbating gut losses and further depleting the patient. For sodium to be absorbed from the jejunum its concentration needs to be greater than 100 mmol/l; as it is absorbed, water follows. It can be seen, therefore, that a proximal small bowel stoma or fistula will result in substantial losses, of the order of 3–4 litres of fluid and 300–400 mmol Na^+ per day. If oral sodium intake is low then more Na^+ will diffuse from the extracellular space in to the lumen, resulting in further losses. Patients are restricted in their free fluid intake and encouraged to drink fluid with high

175

sodium and glucose content (double-strength diora-lyte or St Mark's solution) to reverse this flux and increase Na^+ and water reabsorption. The difficulty for the patient is the palatability of these solutions; the addition of squash to flavour them can help.

The colon usually reabsorbs 800–1500 ml of water a day, but can reabsorb up to 6 litres and 700 mmol Na and 40 mmol K^+; leaving about 150 ml of water in the stool. Having the colon in continuity in the presence of short small bowel is roughly the equivalent of an additional 50 cm of small bowel and may make the difference between a patient being independent of oral supplement and having lifelong TPN.

K^+ losses become marked with less than 60 cm of small bowel, when IV replacement of 60–100 mmol per day is required. Similarly, loss of the distal jejunum and ileum will result in significant Mg^{2+} loss with knock-on effects with cardiac dysrhythmias and Ca^{2+} deficiency, as PTH release is impaired by hypomagnesaemia.

Nutrition

Nutrition of the patient with intestinal failure is fundamental to their survival and recovery. A nutrition team caring for them as a part of the multidisciplinary team is vital.

Most protein, carbohydrate and water-soluble vitamins are absorbed in the upper 2 metres of the jejunum. Protein absorption is least affected by short gut and 98% of small gut intestinal protein is absorbed. Half of this is derived from shed epithelial cells and digestive juices. Faecal protein is minimal and is mainly derived from bacterial cell walls and colonic epithelial cells.

Fats in food are a challenge to digestion. Even in health, due to their lipophobic nature, only 95% of it is absorbed. In malabsorption states, steatorrhoea is prominent. Fats, together with fat-soluble vitamins, are absorbed over the entire length of the small bowel, hence, loss of significant length affects not only fat absorption, but fat-soluble vitamin levels as well (A, D, E and K). Disruption to the enterohepatic circulation of bile salts, reabsorbed in the ileum, will worsen fat absorption as bile-salt-activated lipases act to hydrolyse cholesterol and phospholipid esters. The use of cholestyramine to alleviate steatorrhoea may in fact worsen it by binding dietary fats as well as worsening vitamin deficiencies. Most patients with IF have lost their terminal ileum and vitamin B12 and K

injections will be needed. Luminal acid and free fatty acids in the duodenum stimulate the entero-endocrine glands to secrete CCK and secretin. Secretin stimulates the release of pancreatic juice and CCK stimulates the release of enzymes from acinar cells and causes the gallbladder to contract. Proton pump inhibitors are therefore of use in elevating luminal pH and limit these secretions as well as reducing gastric acid secretion.

As mentioned previously, having the colon in continuity (i.e. after surgical treatment of an entero-cutaneous fistula) not only slows intestinal transit, thus improving time for absorption, but also contributes to energy intake by reabsorbing fatty acids, adding up to 500 kcal per day. Diarrhoea from both high carbohydrate load and from unabsorbed bile salts delivered to the colon can be difficult to manage.

Management of the abdominal catastrophe

All gastrointestinal surgeons will have to manage this difficult and stressful situation during their career. Sometimes IF is secondary to mesenteric infarction and massive enterectomy or due to Crohn's disease, but more commonly it follows a surgical disaster: an anastomotic leak, unrecognized small bowel injury or broken-down enterotomy closure. This only adds to the emotional toll on both patient and surgeon.

Early re-entry into the abdomen within the first week may be required to form a defunctioning stoma and to treat peritonitis, but surgery after this and before about 3 months is perilous and risks further injury. It is important, however, not to delay local surgical procedures to drain uncontrolled sepsis which cannot be percutaneously managed.

A clear management strategy is required for an optimal outcome for these patients. It consists of the four Rs:

Resuscitation, **R**estitution, **R**econstruction, **R**ehabilitation.

Resuscitation

Fluid resuscitation, correction of electrolyte imbalances and drainage of sepsis are fundamental in gaining control of the severe metabolic disturbance these patients present with. Uncontrolled sepsis is the single most important factor contributing to their mortality. This phase is often performed at the hospital at which the patient initially presents prior to transfer to a tertiary centre if needed. Control of sepsis may require laparotomy, but often radiologically guided percutaneous drainage is successful.

Restitution

Two acronyms are commonly used to summarize the key steps in managing this phase: SNAPP – standing for sepsis, nutrition, anatomy (of the fistula and bowel), protection of the skin, planned surgery, and SOWATS – sepsis, optimization of nutrition, wound care, anatomy, timing of surgery and surgical strategy. The principles are exactly the same.

Sepsis

There is no apology for repeating how important control of sepsis is. Reber *et al.* showed that with ongoing sepsis at one month from onset, the mortality was as high as 85%, compared to 8% in those with septic foci drained successfully. Secondary sepsis is common and vigilance is needed with aggressive investigation with ultrasound, CT or MRI to identify and drain subsequent collections together with early use of appropriate antibiotics. If percutaneous drainage is not possible then local open drainage, laparotomy or even laparostomy may be required.

Nutritional support

Fluid and electrolyte replacement is guided by careful measurement of losses, which can be considerable during the hypersecretory phase.

Guide to replacement:

Water: losses + 1 litre
Na+: 100 mmol/l of effluent + 80 mmol
K+: 80 mmol per day
Mg^{2+}: 10 mmol per day.

Nutritionally these patients are often already malnourished at presentation, exacerbated by sepsis, malignancy, inflammatory bowel disease and the trauma of surgery. Initially parenteral nutrition is used until fluid losses are stabilized and sepsis is controlled. Ideally a nutrition team manages the requirements for IV nutrition, which vary with height, weight and the activity of the patient and their metabolic status. IV nutrition will provide calories from carbohydrate and fat, protein in the form of amino acids, vitamins and trace elements. Additional IV fluid may be required depending on losses and is given as normal saline.

Fluid losses may be high and steps to reduce these include restriction of 'free fluids' to 500–1000 ml per day; instead they may have electrolyte solutions (dioralyte or St Mark's solution). Loperamide (up to 16 mg four times daily) and codeine phosphate (up to 60 mg four times daily) can slow transit and PPIs reduce gastric secretions. Octreotide may also reduce secretions, but is expensive and is often found to be of little benefit. If there is no effect on output within 3 days, it should be discontinued. Regular medications should be reviewed with respect to site of absorption and enteric coated tablets replaced with alternatives.

Enteral feeding can usually be reintroduced whilst carefully monitoring outputs. Fluid restriction remains. Antidiarrhoeals continue and are given 30–60 minutes before meals and oral fluids avoided at meal times. Eating little and often increases the time for absorption and overnight nasogastric feeding utilizes this 'dead time'.

Requirements for IV nutrition vary widely, but those with outputs of less than 1500 ml/day can usually be managed with oral replacement. Losses of 1500–2000 ml often require sodium and water replacement intravenously or subcutaneously, and losses greater than 2000 ml will require IV nutrition. As adaptation occurs these needs will change.

As well as measuring fluid and effluent losses, serum electrolytes, renal and liver function and trace elements must be regularly measured to guide replacement. Urinary sodium is a useful guide as to whether adequate sodium is being replaced; it should be >20 mmol/l.

Even if a patient cannot be maintained without IV nutrition, some enteral feeding is beneficial. It helps maintain normal gut flora and has a trophic effect on the mucosa. With appropriate support and planning patients can be managed at home with TPN.

With sepsis resolved and balance in electrolyte and nutritional intake established, time is now required to allow resolution of the intra-abdominal inflammation and softening of adhesions before surgery is undertaken.

Anatomy

Understanding the anatomy of the patient's GI tract is useful in planning surgery. This is particularly true of fistulating disease, be it following a surgical disaster, radiotherapy-induced or as a complication of Crohn's or diverticular disease. It may not alter what happens at operation, but is beneficial in discussing the planned surgery with the patient. CT, MRI and contrast studies via the mouth or anus, any stomas or fistulas define a 'road map' of the GI tract and additionally may identify unexpected problems:

- internal fistulas
- strictures
- distal obstruction
- residual disease
- associated abscess cavities
- can the distal small bowel be used for feeding?

Close liaison between the team and a radiologist with an interest in GI pathology is essential.

Protection of the skin

Small bowel contents are caustic and will rapidly damage the skin, causing excoriation and ulceration. Stoma and wound management bags not only protect the skin, they make nursing easier, prevent spillage of enteric content, which is very distressing and embarrassing, and allow accurate measurement of fistula output. Occasionally early surgical intervention is required to defunction upstream of the site of a fistula to gain control. This is especially true of entero-vaginal fistulas, which very quickly damage the vulva and perineum and are incredibly distressing. Recovery of the skin requires protection, good nutrition and time. The stoma care team are invaluable in this regard.

Planned surgery

A proportion of fistulas (16–25%) will close spontaneously, without surgery. Factors which influence the chances of spontaneous closure should be considered, as a number of patients will not require any further surgical procedures. They are:

- low output (<200 ml/day)
- simple fistulas
- lack of comorbidities.

The vast majority of those which do heal spontaneously do so within the first month. After 3 months there is almost no chance of closure without surgery. For the majority of patients, however, surgery will be needed to rid them of their fistula. Surgery is planned once sepsis is eradicated, nutrition optimized, and time has elapsed to allow for resolution of the inflammatory process in the peritoneal cavity. It is essential to be patient and not to be tempted to 'dive in' too early.

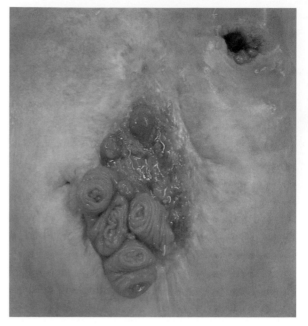

Figure 11.3 Delay in surgery allows for a clean, granulating, non-infected and prolapsing wound. These are all signs of a mature entero-cutaneous fistula ready for surgical reconstruction.

Early surgery before these problems have resolved not only commonly results in failure, but is associated with a high mortality. Timing is essential, and counselling and careful explanation is needed for patients to come to terms with the prolonged nature of their illness. Most surgeons wait at least 3 months, but preferably 6 or more until the abdomen becomes soft and 'wobbly'. A prolapsing stoma or fistula is a good sign that the internal adhesions have softened.

Early surgery maybe unavoidable for the following reasons:

- drainage of sepsis
- removal of infarcted bowel
- laying open of superficial abscess cavities
- formation of a proximal defunctioning stoma
- following an anastomotic dehiscence to exteriorize both ends of the bowel.

Reconstruction

Surgical reconstruction is undertaken in the stable, well-nourished patient, once time has elapsed to allow adhesions to soften.

The exact detail of the operation undertaken is individual to each case, and will vary with the nature of the causative pathology and what bowel remains.

It may be a matter of anastomosing small to large bowel, excising a fistulated segment en bloc and re-anastomosing the ends or it may require specialist surgery in a tertiary referral centre for surgery to alter bowel length, transit times or for small bowel transplant. A stoma may be required if there is residual sepsis at the site of anastomoses.

As well as addressing the fistula itself, the patients often have large abdominal wall defects which can be equally challenging to treat. A combination of component separation of the layers of the abdominal wall and modern meshes are used to achieve the optimum abdominal closure.

Rehabilitation

Patients who have developed intestinal failure require constant psychological support. Many are terrified by what has happened to them and may feel that there is no hope of recovery. Those with catastrophic anastomotic failure and enterocutaneous fistulation were expecting to be in hospital for 1–2 weeks and are then faced with prolonged hospitalization, loss of self-esteem, poor body image, depression, isolation and, for some, institutionalization. This has serious knock-on effects on employment, finances and relationships. It is easy for staff looking after them to become engrossed with the myriad of problems which need managing and to forget about the huge psychological stress they are under. On a hard-pressed, busy surgical ward it can be difficult to meet these needs and some patients will benefit from referral to a tertiary centre with expertise in the management of IF and ECF.

The aim of treatment is to enable the patient to resume as normal a life as possible. As their condition stabilizes, attention changes from that of resuscitation and the acute management of sepsis and fluid and electrolyte imbalance, to that of coping and coming to terms with their situation. Patients may have high-output stomas or fistulas or diarrhoea due to short bowel and some will require long-term PN. The services of specialist stoma nurses, dietitians, physiotherapists, occupational therapists and social workers are all invaluable.

The professional body supporting this work is the British Association of Parenteral and Enteral Nutrition (BAPEN: www.bapen.org.uk). The organization keeps a census of all patients requiring long-term nutritional support; the British Artificial Nutritional Survey (BANS). The annual report is published and can be found on the BAPEN website.

Organizations providing support and advice to patients are PINNT (Patients on Intravenous and Nasogastric Nutrition Therapy: www.pinnt.com) and the children's support arm of it Half-PINNT (www.pinnt.com/halfpinnt-new).

When to refer to a tertiary centre?

1. Intestinal failure continuing for more than 6 weeks
2. Multiple intestinal fistulas with laparostomy
3. A fistula beyond the expertise of the referring unit; particularly second or third recurrences
4. Massive small bowel enterectomy resulting in <30 cm of remaining small bowel
5. Recurrent severe venous access problems, including thrombosis or sepsis
6. Persistent intra-abdominal sepsis and metabolic derangement not responding to radiological or surgical drainage
7. Metabolic complications from high-output stomas or fistulas and intravenous feeding not responding to regimen alterations and medication
8. Hepatic and/or renal dysfunction due to intravenous feeding
9. Chronic intestinal failure in a hospital without experience or expertise to manage it

Summary

The management of intestinal failure continues to develop, with significant improvements in the mortality and quality of life of these patients being achieved over the past 20–30 years. There are two supra-regional centres (St Mark's Hospital at Northwick Park in London, and Hope Hospital in Salford, Manchester) as well as other tertiary referral centres such as UCLH in London which have expertise in caring for these patients.

There are three stages to intestinal failure: the hypersecretory phase with diarrhoea or high stoma output and fluid and electrolyte depletion; an adaptation phase; and a stabilization phase during which the aim is to enable as normal a life as possible. An understanding of gastrointestinal physiology is essential in understanding the pathophysiology and management of intestinal failure. Management is summarized as the four Rs: resuscitation, restitution, reconstruction and rehabilitation. Restitution is divided into Sepsis control, Nutritional support, Anatomy, Protection of the skin and Planned surgery (SNAPP). Control of sepsis is the single most important step in the management of these patients.

A multidisciplinary approach to these complicated patients is essential to achieve the optimum outcome for them, and referral to a specialist unit may be required.

Further reading

Annual BANS report, 2008; Artificial Nutrition Support in the UK 2000–2007. Available at http://www.bapen.org. uk ISBN 978-1-899467-26-6.

Berry SM, Fischer JE. Classification and pathophysiology of enterocutaneous fistulas. *Surg Clin North Am* 1996;**76**:1009–1018.

Draus JM Jr, Huss SA, Harty NJ, Cheadle WG, Larson GM. Enterocutaneous fistula: Are treatments improving? *Surgery* 2006;**140**:(4).

Dudrick SJ, Maharaj AR, McKelvey AA. Artificial nutritional support in patients with gastrointestinal fistulas. *World J Surg* 1999;**23**:570–576.

Haffejee AA. Surgical management of high output enterocutaneous fistulae: a 24-year experience. *Curr Opin Clin Nutr Metab Care* 2004;**7**:309–316.

Hollington P, Mawdsley J, Lim W, Gabe SM, Forbes A, Windsor AJ. An 11-year experience of enterocutaneous fistula. *Br J Surg* 2004;**91**:1646–1651.

Levy E, Frileux P, Sandrucci S. Continuous enteral nutrition during the early adaptive stage of short bowel syndrome. *Br J Surg* 1988;**75**:549–553.

Lloyd DA, Gabe SM, Windsor AC. Nutrition and management of enterocutaneous fistula. *Br J Surg* 2006;**93**(9):1045–1055.

Lynch AC, Delaney CP, Senagore AJ, Connor JT, Remzi FH, Fazio VW. Clinical outcome and factors predictive of recurrence after enterocutaneous fistula surgery. *Ann Surg* 2004;**240** (5).

Mawdsley JE, Hollington P, Bassett P, Windsor AJ, Forbes AS, Gabe M. An analysis of predictive factors for healing and mortality in patients with enterocutaneous fistulas. *Aliment Pharmacol Ther* 2008;**28**(9):1111–1121.

Nightingale JM, Lennard-Jones JE, Gertner DJ, Wood SR, Bartram CI. Colonic preservation reduces the need for parenteral therapy, increases incidence of renal stones, but does not change the high prevalence of gallstones in patients with a short bowel. *Gut* 1992;**33**:1493–1497.

Robinson MK, Ziegler TR, Wilmore DW. Overview of intestinal adaptation and its stimulation. *Eur J Pediatr Surg* 1999;**9**(4):200–206.

Staun M, Pironi L, Bozzetti F, Baxter J, Forbes A, Joly F, Jeppesen P, Moreno J, Hébuterne X, Pertkiewicz M, Mühlebach S, Shenkin A, Van Gossum A. ESPEN guidelines on parenteral nutrition: Home parenteral nutrition (HPN) in adults. *Clin Nutr* 2009 May 22 [Epub ahead of print].

Visschers RGN, Olde Damink SWM, Winkens B, Soeters PB, Van Gemert WG. Treatment strategies in 135 consecutive patients with enterocutaneous fistulas. *World J Surg* 2008;**32**(3):445–453.

Wallis K, Walters JR, Gabe S. Short bowel syndrome: the role of GLP-2 on improving outcome. *Curr Opin Clin Nutr Metab Care* 2009 May 26 [Epub ahead of print].

Enhanced recovery after surgery

John Evans and Robin H. Kennedy

Introduction

History of gastrointestinal surgery

Gastrointestinal surgery in one form or another has been described since the writings of Hippocrates in the fourth century BC. By the twelfth century AD, the seminal work *Regimen Sanitatis Salerni* was published by the School of Salerno and became one of the most influential medical texts ever produced. In it, Roger Frugardi (also known as Roger of Salerno) described suturing wounds of the intestine and laid out rules of hygiene. In the early 1890s, Maunsell described the preoperative preparation of patients by washing out the stomach and rectum, and this principle of mechanical bowel cleansing has been widely followed to this day. However, the art and science of surgery are constantly evolving and many doctrines that were rigorously adhered to in the past have not stood the tests of time and scientific evaluation. Even Hippocrates' teachings have not been immune to subsequent correction; in his 'Apology and Treatise', the sixteenth-century French surgeon Ambroise Paré argues against Hippocratic treatment of volvulus.

'Moreover, I should be sorry to follow the saying of the sayd Hippocrates, in the third booke, De Morbis, who commands in the disease called Volvulus to cause the belly to bee blowne with a pair of Bellowes, putting the nosell of them into the intestinum rectum, and then blow there till the belly be much stretcht, afterwards to give an emollient glister, and to stop the fundament with a sponge. Such practise as this is not made now a dayes therefore wonder not if I have not spoken of it.'

The ability to change practice in the light of new evidence is fundamental to the development of medicine and surgery. Many of the ideas central to an enhanced recovery protocol challenge teaching that has been dogmatically adhered to in the past.

'Starve, stress and drown'

Fearon has stated that the perceived wisdom in perioperative management was to ensure the patient was sufficiently fasted (starved) prior to administering powerful laxatives and then performing major surgery (stressed). Postoperatively, the patients were starved until the passage of flatus per rectum occurred, whilst copious quantities of intravenous fluids were administered in order to maintain a urine output greater than 0.5 ml/kg per h (drowned). This results in average hospital stays of between 10 and 14 days prior to a long convalescence at home. There has been a great deal of interest in reducing both the length of hospital stay and the time to resumption of normal activities through a variety of 'fast-track', 'multimodal' or 'accelerated' recovery programmes.

In 2000, Kehlet published 'A Clinical Pathway to Accelerated Recovery after Colonic Resection' and a year later the European Society of Clinical Nutrition and Metabolism (ESPEN) set up a working party, leading to the publication of a consensus view of enhanced recovery after surgery (ERAS).

An enhanced recovery programme (ERP) seeks not only to reduce the time until discharge, but also to minimize the physiological insult caused by surgery and the perioperative process. We define this process as follows:

An ERP involves improvements in preoperative, operative and postoperative care that reduce the side effects of surgery and the pathophysiological response to stress – consequently both the magnitude of the physical insult and the duration of recovery decrease. ERPs have evolved as a result of evidence-based advances and important aspects include patient education, physiological optimization, improved anaesthesia and analgesia, modifications in surgical technique and an improved understanding of early feeding and mobilization. The intervention may also be referred to as fast-track surgery,

Fundamentals of Surgical Practice, Third Edition, ed. Andrew N. Kingsnorth and Douglas M. Bowley.
Published by Cambridge University Press. © Cambridge University Press 2011.

but we prefer the term 'enhanced recovery' as merely emphasizing reduction in hospital stay does not reflect the full patient benefits.

Central tenets of enhanced recovery

Preadmission counselling

The foundations of an ERP are laid well before the patient is admitted to hospital. When the decision to operate is made in the outpatient department, the concept of enhanced recovery can be briefly discussed. More importantly, at the preadmission clinic the whole process should be explained in detail, preferably by a dedicated enhanced recovery facilitator, to the patient and a relative or friend. It is vital that the patient understands what is expected of them as well as what to expect from the healthcare team. A full ERP depends upon well-motivated and well-informed patients. Setting recovery targets at this point gives the patient something to aim for, enables them to be proactive in their rehabilitation and increases compliance with the ERP. Such targets include oral intake after surgery and aspects of postoperative mobilization, such as time out of bed and walking distances.

The idea that talking to people might improve their recovery is not new. In 1964 Egbert demonstrated that by counselling patients, their experience of pain was greatly reduced. Kiecolt-Glaser went further, investigating the link between patient anxiety and recovery. In addition to behavioural differences, laboratory work in psychoneuroimmunology has shown that stress delays wound healing, and that pain has pronounced effects on endocrine and neurological function. Taking the time in the preadmission meeting to explain the process can reduce the level of stress and pain experienced later on, consequently aiding recovery.

Avoidance of mechanical bowel preparation

The logic behind mechanical bowel preparation for colorectal surgery has been to attenuate the consequences of an anastomotic leak and to reduce the risk of infection due to faecal spillage. Many oral and rectal purgatives have been used for this purpose, but the majority cause significant fluid loss per rectum and subsequent fluid shifts throughout the body compartments. Electrolyte disturbance and dehydration are common, particularly in elderly or infirm patients. Even in the young and fit, the whole process of bowel

preparation is deeply unpleasant, causing one to experience a loss of control and increasing stress.

The evidence suggests that the theory behind the use of bowel preparation is flawed. Bucher performed a meta-analysis of seven randomized, controlled trials analysing this process in nearly 1300 patients. The results surprised many: anastomotic leakage was significantly more frequent in patients who had received preparation and the incidence of wound infection, intra-abdominal infection and reoperation all tended to be higher in this group.

The Association of Coloproctologists of Great Britain and Ireland now recommend that bowel preparation is not routinely used prior to colorectal cancer resection. However, perhaps the one situation in which it is still appropriate is the planned defunctioning stoma above a low anastomosis. Matthiessen demonstrated that after total mesorectal excision (TME) a proximal stoma reduces leak rates. If bowel prep is not used for these patients then a column of faeces will remain between the stoma and the anastomosis. This might be presumed to have the same potential for leakage as if the stoma had not been formed in the first place.

Preoperative carbohydrate loading

The traditional approach of fasting for 8 hours or more prior to a general anaesthetic is aimed at avoiding aspiration of gastric contents. It has now been accepted that clear fluids can be continued up to 2 hours prior to the induction of anaesthesia, without increasing the risk of aspiration (providing the patient is not having emergency surgery and they have normal gastric emptying, without previous gastric surgery or severe reflux). Excessive starvation preoperatively places the patient in a catabolic state before they enter the operating theatre, thereby increasing their postoperative insulin resistance. Insulin resistance, or the lack of insulin sensitivity, has been extensively studied by Ljungqvist and colleagues in Stockholm. It, along with the type of surgery and blood loss, is an independent factor predicting length of hospital stay. Postoperatively, as glucose production rises, insulin resistance causes impairment of peripheral glucose uptake. In addition, when glucose is transported to muscles, glycogen is not formed in the normal way – the patient behaves like an untreated type II diabetic.

Insulin resistance is seen in many catabolic situations including burns, major trauma and elective surgery, and has been shown to be associated with a worse outcome. In order to prevent insulin resistance, a randomized, controlled trial of oral carbohydrate loading was undertaken in Sweden. In this trial, patients undergoing elective total hip replacement were randomized to receive either 800 ml of a complex carbohydrate drink (12.5 g/100 ml) or a placebo the night before surgery. The drink has a low osmolality (260 mOsmol/kg water) and clearance from the stomach has previously been shown to be similar to water. On the morning of surgery, a further 400 ml drink was given, to be finished 2 hours prior to the induction of anaesthesia. Insulin sensitivity was measured by the hyperinsulinemic/euglycemic clamp technique both 1 week prior to surgery for a baseline reading, and at 40–60 minutes postoperatively. Insulin, glucose and lactate levels were measured at several points throughout the perioperative period. Glucagon, cortisol, glycerol and nonesterified fatty acids were also measured. Intraoperative insulin levels were found to be similar in both groups. Despite this, the placebo group had significantly higher glucose levels. The difference in relative glucose resistance between the two groups was of the order of 20–25%. Preoperative CHO loading works on two key factors to prevent hyperglycaemia: significantly reducing endogenous production of glucose and almost halving the postoperative decline in glucose uptake.

In addition to attenuating insulin resistance, the administration of carbohydrate-rich drinks prior to surgery does much to alleviate hunger, thirst and anxiety in the preoperative patient. Hausel *et al.* randomized patients to receive carbohydrate-rich beverage or a placebo of flavoured water or to remain nil by mouth on the night prior to surgery. The trial was double-blinded and randomized, and the treatment group showed decreased levels of hunger and anxiety compared to both of the other groups, whilst gastric fluid volumes and acidity levels were unaffected.

Optimal anaesthesia and analgesia

Premedication

Sedatives and anxiolytics have been used as an adjunct to anaesthesia and to alleviate anxiety in the preoperative period. They are usually given on the ward prior to transfer to the operating theatre, but the use of long-acting drugs potentiates many anaesthetic agents and may cause a 'hangover' effect postoperatively. Seda-

tion in the postoperative period may interfere with an enhanced recovery protocol and with modern anaesthetic agents we expect patients to be able to eat, drink and mobilize on the day of surgery, thus reducing their period of recovery. As discussed earlier, administration of oral carbohydrate-rich drinks preoperatively can help to alleviate stress without the need for anxiolytics.

Intraoperative agents

Long-acting anaesthetic agents are best avoided if the patient is to wake promptly. Analgesics such as morphine not only have a long duration of action, but they are opiates that contribute to postoperative nausea and vomiting, and will also delay the return of bowel function. However, a single dose of intravenous morphine at the end of the surgical procedure can be used to provide analgesia in the immediate postoperative period. By using short-acting volatile or intravenous anaesthetic agents, the patient should be awake enough on the day of surgery to sit out of bed and begin oral intake. In addition, the routine use of antiemetics during anaesthesia helps to reduce postoperative nausea and vomiting, allowing the patient to recommence oral intake earlier than they would otherwise do.

Avoidance of postoperative opiates

Opiate analgesia is not only sedating, but is strongly emetogenic and constipating. It should therefore be avoided where possible. We would routinely use a multimodal approach to analgesia, with a combination of paracetamol and an epidural following open surgery, commencing non-steroidal anti-inflammatory drugs (NSAIDs) immediately the epidural is discontinued. One has to bear in mind that NSAIDs should be avoided when renal function is compromised and that creatinine should be monitored daily. Some of the newer, synthetic opiates are an alternative, having fewer side effects than morphine and avoiding renal dysfunction.

Epidural analgesia

There is evidence from a large meta-analysis showing that epidural use reduces the incidence of deep-vein thrombosis, pulmonary embolism, respiratory depression, transfusion requirements and chest infection. However, this large meta-analysis contained a heterogeneous collection of 141 trials, and the authors accept that it is not apparent whether the benefits were entirely due to the use of epidurals or to the avoidance of general anaesthesia. In two more recent meta-analyses concerning colorectal surgery, clear benefits from epidural use were only demonstrated for reduction of pain and ileus. Provided epidurals are placed high enough in the thoracic region, their postoperative use allows early mobilization, which in turn has beneficial effects on gut function, the incidence of respiratory complications, deep-vein thrombosis and pulmonary embolism. Thoracic epidurals also allow patients to cough, clearing secretions from the lungs and further improving respiratory function. This concept of epidurals which facilitate mobility has been referred to as 'dynamic pain relief', and requires avoidance of lower limb motor block.

The benefits of epidurals are not totally attributable to superior postoperative analgesia. There is evidence to suggest that the use of epidural anaesthesia attenuates the inflammatory and physiological responses to surgical stress. Surgical trauma renders the body catabolic in the postoperative period, leading to hyperglycaemia, lipolysis and a loss of body protein. This is probably mediated through a central release of catecholamines, adrenocorticotrophic hormone, cortisol and cytokines. Use of an epidural during and immediately after surgery leads to a decrease in protein breakdown, nitrogen excretion, and lipolysis. Postoperative hyperglycaemia has been shown to be reduced by the use of epidural analgesia in several studies, although the effects described above are at their most pronounced in the first 48 hours.

Neurological reflexes are a major contributor to postoperative ileus, and the use of a mid-thoracic epidural can inhibit these reflexes. There are three levels of reflexes that mediate this effect: ultrashort gut wall reflexes, prevertebral reflexes, and longer, spinal reflexes. The latter reflexes are probably the most significant, and are most affected by spinal and epidural anaesthesia. In a review of eight randomized, controlled trials of epidural anaesthesia, a reduction in the duration of postoperative paralytic ileus was seen in six. It is possible that in the two trials that did not show a reduction, the epidural catheters were either placed too low or were not left *in situ* for a sufficient duration. Postoperative ileus is a major contributor to prolonged hospital stay and anything that can be done to reduce it is to be encouraged.

Drugs used in the epidural infusion are usually a combination of an opioid and a local anaesthetic.

The local anaesthetic alone can provide analgesia and block the sympathetic outflow, helping to prevent postoperative ileus when the catheter is placed in the mid-thoracic region. If an opioid is used in the epidural space it should be in a low concentration in order to avoid the systemic effects of nausea and constipation.

Epidurals, however, are not without risk. Combined complication and failure rates of up to 40% have been quoted, although the risk of catastrophic complications is extremely small. Epidural abscesses or haematomas can cause permanent, disabling neurological damage and are the most feared complication of epidural placement; fortunately, their occurrence is exceptional. Epidural abscess affects approximately 1:1000 patients, although it may be more common after emergency surgery. It can present at any time postoperatively with lower back pain and pyrexia, and if left untreated can lead to irreversible neurological damage within 24 hours. Not all abscesses present in a classic way, and some can be delayed by up to a month. Other presentations include headache, photophobia and meningism. A high index of suspicion is important, and urgent investigations should be commenced if a patient develops any of these signs or symptoms. Epidural haematomas occur in around 1:2700 cases and predictably the risk is greater in patients with a coagulopathy, or those receiving anticoagulant therapy. A more common problem is a dural tap, which leads to cerebrospinal fluid leakage into the epidural space. This causes severe postural headaches, and in extreme cases can lead to coning. Most dural taps can be treated by bed rest, intravenous fluids, analgesia and, if necessary, a 'blood patch' – injecting a few millilitres of the patient's blood into the subdural space in order to seal off the puncture site.

The published literature suggests that the benefits of epidurals far outweigh the risks in the setting of an enhanced recovery programme, and it is therefore recommended that mid-thoracic epidurals are routinely sited for major abdominal surgery.

With the advent of laparoscopic surgery the place of epidurals has become less clear, since some authors feel patients can be well managed using a multimodal analgesic approach with a combination of patient-controlled opiate analgesia (PCA), paracetamol and either a NSAID or a synthetic oral opiate once the PCA has been discontinued. Some of the available analyses attempting to define the postoperative benefit of an epidural in this situation do show trends in favour of it, but the few studies published are probably all underpowered and we await further research to clarify this. Most authors agree that a multimodal approach to pain is important, incorporating pain scoring and regular medication rather than the use of an 'on demand' (PRN) approach, which tends to undertreat patients.

Goal-directed fluid therapy

Exact assessment of intra-operative fluid requirements can be a difficult skill even for the most experienced anaesthetist. Factors taken into consideration include total fluid in the suction device, the weight of used swabs to estimate blood loss, fluid evaporation from the open abdomen, urine output and other losses. Central venous pressure monitoring is a guide to right heart filling pressure, but its use is confounded by issues such as a pneumoperitoneum or head-down positioning. Trans-oesophageal Doppler can be used intraoperatively to measure the cardiac output and is a more accurate method of assessing fluid requirements and monitoring the effect of replacement. A 2007 review looked at nine studies comparing goal-directed fluid therapy to standard perioperative fluid regimes. In seven of the nine studies, hospital stay was reduced, although interestingly only three of the studies showed a reduction in paralytic ileus or postoperative nausea and vomiting. The improvement in postoperative recovery may result from the administration of fluid earlier during an anaesthetic than would otherwise occur, as some research has not demonstrated a significant difference in the amount of fluid given, but merely its timing. Further work is necessary to understand fully this effect.

Excess fluid administration can be just as harmful as dehydration. It was shown as far back as the 1930s that fluid administration caused gut wall oedema and slowed gastric emptying times. More recently, Lobo demonstrated that delivering 3 or more litres of fluid per day, combined with a moderate amount of sodium (154 mmol), was detrimental to the recovery of gut function. When compared to a similar group of postoperative patients in whom replacement was restricted to 2 litres of water and 77 mmol of sodium per day, the unrestricted group had significantly slower gastric emptying times, a longer time until passage of flatus and first stool, and hospital stays on average 3 days longer.

The daily requirement for sodium is 0.9–1.2 mmol/kg and the explanation for Lobo's findings would seem to be excess sodium and fluid administration, which causes water retention and subsequent deleterious effects. The delivery of 'normal saline' (containing 154 mmol of sodium and chloride/litre) may also induce a hyperchloraemic acidosis, but whether this contributed to the outcomes in the above study is unclear.

In Lobo's work, the unrestricted group had a greater incidence of peripheral oedema, hyponatraemia, confusion, wound infection, respiratory tract infection and readmission. Although the numbers in this study were small, similar differences in complication rates were observed in four of the studies reviewed by Bundgaard-Nielsen et al. Today we should be aiming to replace the correct amounts of sodium and potassium at surgery and ensure that there is euvolaemic fluid management rather than restricting fluid or overloading. Brandstrup et al. randomized patients to receive either standard fluid therapy, or a replacement regime aimed at maintaining preoperative weight. In this randomized and observer-blinded trial, both cardiopulmonary and tissue-healing complications were reduced in the goal-directed group.

Peripheral nerve blockade

In order to further reduce the amount of postoperative analgesia (and in particular opiate analgesics) required by the patient, the use of local anaesthetic for peripheral nerve blockade is encouraged. This can be either by direct infiltration of the largest wound or by an appropriate regional block. The technique of transversus abdominis plane (TAP) block has recently been described and involves injecting local anaesthetic into the neurofascial plane between the transversus abdominis and internal oblique muscles. In a randomized, controlled trial, TAP block was found to reduce visual analogue pain scores at 2, 4, 6 and 24 hours postoperatively, reducing opiate requirements by more than 70%. The anatomical location for placement of this block can be found in the lumbar triangle of Petit – a triangle on the lateral abdominal wall bounded by the iliac crest inferiorly, the external oblique anteriorly and the latissimus dorsi posteriorly. Injecting anaesthetic into the correct plane at this point blocks the first lumbar and lower six thoracic nerves, which supply the skin and musculature of the abdominal wall.

Other methods of nerve blockade include a continuous infusion of local anaesthetic using an indwelling catheter.

Optimal surgery

Whilst individual elements of enhanced recovery care have been in use for years, it was Henrik Kehlet's work in the late 1990s that created the concept of a multimodal rehabilitation package. His observation in 2000 that one would not see the maximal benefits that laparoscopic techniques can potentially offer patients stimulated the use of ERP in combination with minimal access surgery. This type of surgery often has greater theatre costs and can be more time-consuming than open surgery, but has many potential benefits. These include a reduction in the trauma of access to the abdominal cavity, leading to less postoperative pain, earlier mobilization and decreased complications. Meta-analysis of the largest randomized trials has shown that laparoscopic surgery is safe and comparable to open surgery in terms of oncological outcome. Early concerns about the safety of laparoscopic surgery in the resection of rectal cancer have not translated into increased local recurrence, and the benefits outweigh the risks.

Laparoscopic surgery is not always possible, but the principle that wounds should be the smallest necessary to undertake the procedure safely is one to which all surgeons should adhere. Transverse rather than longitudinal incisions cross fewer dermatomes and probably reduce postoperative pain and improve recovery. Accurate dissection in the correct tissue plane is essential to performing laparoscopic surgery, and equal precision in open surgery is desirable. Modern combined coagulation and dissection devices utilize either ultrasonic or bipolar energy to minimize blood loss in both open and laparoscopic surgery. This in turn reduces transfusion requirements, preventing loss of clotting factors, and helps to maintain thermoregulation. Maintenance of body temperature is another important principle of enhanced recovery, as it has been shown to reduce cardiovascular complications and wound infections. The failure to maintain normothermia can lead to a downward spiral of bleeding, impairment of clotting, blood transfusion with further impairment, and more bleeding. All intravenous fluids given intraoperatively should be through a warming device, and the patient also actively warmed.

It is arguable whether open surgery per se leads to a longer ileus than the laparoscopic equivalent. It is reasonable to assume, and experimental work supports the concept, that excess handling of the bowel leads to the release of inflammatory mediators that prolong gut paralysis. Handling of the bowel should therefore be reduced to a minimum, and in laparoscopic surgery it is possible to perform virtually all manipulation by handling only the mesentery or fatty appendages. Drying of bowel by its exposure to the atmosphere leads to heat and fluid loss in traditional open surgery that does not seem to occur to the same degree in minimal access surgery.

Early mobilization and stimulation of gut function

Early mobilization is encouraged following surgery to counteract the increased risk of thromboembolic disease associated with bed rest and immobility. In addition, prolonged bed rest increases insulin resistance, decreases muscle mass and strength, impairs pulmonary function and lowers tissue oxygenation. It is questionable whether early mobilization alone leads to earlier restoration of gut function but we encourage it for that reason too. With adequate analgesia, patients can be mobilized on day one after surgery; we aim for 6 to 8 hours out of bed and four 60 metre walks per day thereafter. It is essential that this part of the programme is explained to the patient at the preoperative visit so they understand what is expected. Serving meals in a separate dining room can encourage mobility as well as restoring a feeling of independence. A further measure to aid mobility is early removal of the urinary catheter, and this is usually performed on the first postoperative day, provided the patient is mobile. The exception to this is in low rectal surgery, where damage to autonomic nerves may increase the likelihood of urinary retention. In this case it is prudent to leave the catheter *in situ* for 24–48 hours longer.

Nasogastric drainage is uncomfortable and makes eating difficult. A meta-analysis has also shown that there is an increased incidence of basal atelectasis, fever and chest infection when nasogastric tubes are used postoperatively. If there is a requirement for a nasogastric tube to be passed intraoperatively to decompress the stomach, then it should be removed at the end of the procedure. The nasogastric tube is also another impediment to early mobilization as it, along with all other tubes, restricts independent movement.

Stimulation of gut function is encouraged by early oral intake and avoidance of opiate analgesia. Many other techniques have been tried in order to supplement these measures. Chewing gum has been suggested as a gut stimulant, with variable results. A recent meta-analysis has concluded that chewing gum reduces the time taken to first flatus and the passage of faeces, although any effect on hospital stay was not statistically significant. Cisapride was used in the past as a prokinetic with some success. It enhances acetylcholine release from the myenteric plexus and also acts as a serotonin agonist. However, it has been withdrawn in the UK as it could cause prolongation of the QT interval and cardiac arrhythmias and is probably only of historical interest. One of the simplest measures to encourage the return of gut function is the use of oral laxatives, and these are routinely prescribed postoperatively to patients undergoing surgery within an ERP.

Antiemetics are a valuable adjunct and are particularly important in patients who are known to suffer postoperative nausea and vomiting. Metoclopramide is both an antiemetic and prokinetic, acting mainly on dopamine receptors, but also on cholinergic and serotonin receptors throughout the gastrointestinal tract. Despite this, six controlled trials have been performed to examine the effect of metoclopramide on the resolution of paralytic ileus, and none showed any significant effect.

Audit of results and discharge data

When an enhanced recovery programme is introduced results should be audited, as they would be with other changes in care. Once a unit has chosen the elements of an ERP that it wishes to introduce it should then audit the compliance with each of the elements. This assessment allows one to address compliance when it is low, and, by increasing it, improve ER care and clinical outcomes.

We routinely organize outpatient review 2 weeks after surgery and also provide contact telephone numbers for patients to use should a problem arise within 2 weeks of operation. As part of the preoperative information we advise that, should there be symptoms suggesting anastomotic leakage following early discharge, people re-attend the ward, rather than visit their general practitioner.

Challenges of enhanced recovery

An enhanced recovery programme is a radical change from traditional perioperative management, and it is important that this is a multidisciplinary approach. The introduction of the service is undermined if staff are not conversant with, and supportive of, the changes. This can best be achieved by involving key team members in a specific multidisciplinary training day and then regular review of outcomes. In addition, the introduction of such a change is much more likely to succeed if a specific ER facilitator (usually a relatively senior ward nurse) is available on the ward each morning, at least during the first year or two of the programme.

A challenging aspect of this new approach can be the recognition of a patient who is deviating from the pathway. Relatively subtle signs, such as a persistent or slight tachycardia, may be the only indication that someone is developing acute gastric dilatation and needs the passage of a nasogastric tube to exclude this potentially serious complication. Renal function needs to be closely monitored, as decreased fluid intake and the use of a non-steroidal anti-inflammatory could lead to acute tubular necrosis. By addressing such problems early it is hoped that they will be pre-empted and their impact lessened.

The future

Enhanced recovery care is the adoption of a package of measures that are essentially best practice and there will always be unanswered questions regarding individual components. Laparoscopic colorectal surgery has had an impact on recovery and reducing postoperative stay; some have suggested that open surgery, optimized with an ERP, will produce comparable results. In order to answer this King et al. randomized 62 patients to receive either open or laparoscopic surgery, all within the setting of an ERP. Outcomes improved after laparoscopy such that length of hospital stay was reduced by 32%, and, if convalescent or readmission stay were included, by 37%.

The EnROL (Enhanced Recovery Open versus Laparoscopic) trial will analyse this issue further within a multicentre setting, randomizing patients between laparoscopic and open surgery and blinding both patients and carers to the treatment allocation. Similarly the LAFA Trial (Laparoscopy and/or FAst track multimodal management versus standard care), is a 2×2 factorial trial, with patients randomized both to the type of surgery (laparoscopic versus open) and to the type of perioperative care. Unfortunately, as the trial designers point out, it is impossible to blind patients or assessors to whether the postoperative care is traditional or 'fast-track', and therefore patients will be managed on different wards according to their randomization group.

The benefits of enhanced recovery care are such that this approach is likely to be instituted for many other surgical specialities. Past research has usually involved unimodal changes in perioperative care, but the emphasis on multimodal care packages has produced quite startling improvements in recovery. Further components are likely to be added as new developments occur and it will be important to develop measures that accurately reflect the true recovery experienced by a patient, so that modifications can be accurately analysed.

Further reading

Abraham NS, Young JM, Solomon MJ. Meta-analysis of short-term outcomes after laparoscopic resection for colorectal cancer. *Br J Surg* 2004;**91**(9):1111–1124.

Bardram L *et al.* Recovery after laparoscopic colonic surgery with epidural analgesia, and early oral nutrition and mobilisation. *Lancet* 1995;**345**(8952): 763–764.

Basse L *et al.* A clinical pathway to accelerate recovery after colonic resection. *Ann Surg* 2000;**232**(1):51–57.

Brandstrup B *et al.* Effects of intravenous fluid restriction on postoperative complications: comparison of two perioperative fluid regimens: a randomized assessor-blinded multicenter trial. *Ann Surg* 2003;**238**(5):641–648.

Bucher P, Mermillod B, Gervaz P, Morel P. Mechanical bowel preparation for elective colorectal surgery: a meta-analysis. *Arch Surg* 2004;**139**(12):1359–1364; discussion 1365.

Bundgaard-Nielsen M, Holte K, Secher NH, Kehlet H. Monitoring of peri-operative fluid administration by individualized goal-directed therapy. *Acta Anaesthesiol Scand* 2007;**51**(3):331–340.

Cheatham ML, Chapman WC, Key SP, Sawyers JL. A meta-analysis of selective versus routine nasogastric decompression after elective laparotomy. *Ann Surg* 1995;**221**(5):469–476; discussion 476–478.

Christie IW, McCabe S. Major complications of epidural analgesia after surgery: results of a six-year survey. *Anaesthesia* 2007;**62**(4):335–341.

Egbert LD, Battit GE, Welch CE, Bartlett MK. Reduction of postoperative pain by encouragement and instruction of patients. A study of doctor-patient rapport. *N Engl J Med* 1964;**270**:825–827.

Fearon KC *et al.* Enhanced recovery after surgery: a consensus review of clinical care for patients undergoing colonic resection. *Clin Nutr* 2005;**24**(3):466–477.

Gendall KA, Kennedy RR, Watson AJ, Frizelle FA. The effect of epidural analgesia on postoperative outcome after colorectal surgery. *Colorectal Dis* 2007;**9**(7): 584–598; discussion 598–600.

Graney MJ, Graney CM. Colorectal surgery from antiquity to the modern era. *Dis Colon Rectum* 1980;**23**(6): 432–441.

Hausel J *et al.* A carbohydrate-rich drink reduces preoperative discomfort in elective surgery patients. *Anesth Analg* 2001;**93**(5):1344–1350.

Holte K, Kehlet H. Postoperative ileus: a preventable event. *Br J Surg* 2000;**87**(11):1480–1493.

Kehlet H, Holte K. Effect of postoperative analgesia on surgical outcome. *Br J Anaesth* 2001;**87**(1):62–72.

Kiecolt-Glaser JK *et al.* Psychological influences on surgical recovery. Perspectives from psychoneuroimmunology. *Am Psychol* 1998;**53**(11):1209–1218.

Lobo DN *et al.* Effect of salt and water balance on recovery of gastrointestinal function after elective colonic resection: a randomised controlled trial. *Lancet* 2002;**359**(9320):1812–1818.

King PM *et al.* Randomized clinical trial comparing laparoscopic and open surgery for colorectal cancer within an enhanced recovery programme. *Br J Surg* 2006;**93**(3):300–308.

Matthiessen P *et al.* Defunctioning stoma reduces symptomatic anastomotic leakage after low anterior resection of the rectum for cancer: a randomized multicenter trial. *Ann Surg* 2007;**246**(2):207–214.

McDonnell JG *et al.* The analgesic efficacy of transversus abdominis plane block after abdominal surgery: a prospective randomized controlled trial. *Anesth Analg* 2007;**104**(1):193–197.

Noblett SE, Snowden CP, Shenton BK, Horgan AF. Randomized clinical trial assessing the effect of Doppler-optimized fluid management on outcome after elective colorectal resection. *Br J Surg* 2006;**93**(9): 1069–1076.

Rodgers A *et al.* Reduction of postoperative mortality and morbidity with epidural or spinal anaesthesia: results from overview of randomised trials. *BMJ* 2000; **321**(7275):1493.

Soop M *et al*. Preoperative oral carbohydrate treatment attenuates immediate postoperative insulin resistance. *Am J Physiol Endocrinol Metab* 2001;**280**(4):E576–583.

Thorell A, Nygren J, Ljungqvist O. Insulin resistance: a marker of surgical stress. *Curr Opin Clin Nutr Metab Care* 1999;**2**(1):69–78.

Vasquez W, Hernandez AV, Garcia-Sabrido JL. Is gum chewing useful for ileus after elective colorectal surgery? A systematic review and meta-analysis of randomized clinical trials. *J Gastrointest Surg* 2008;**13**(4):649–656.

Fundamentals of intensive care

Angela L. Neville

Introduction

Intensive care generally refers to the care of patients who are critically ill or injured, thereby requiring constant monitoring, frequent assessment and thoughtful intervention to facilitate a successful recovery. A thorough understanding of human physiology and how to support or correct alterations from the norm is essential in the treatment of such patients. Critical illness often affects the entire body and a multisystem approach must be considered. This chapter will address fundamentals of physiology, pathology and treatment of patients you will encounter in an intensive care setting.

Cardiovascular system

Simply, the cardiovascular system is composed of the heart and an extensive network of blood vessels. Its function is to deliver oxygen (perfusion) and nutrients to the entire body and take away the by-products of the body's utilization. While seemingly elementary, returning to this basic concept helps make the complexities of this intricate process understandable.

Physiology

The heart

The heart has four chambers, four valves, and is composed of specialized conduction tissue; its purpose is to pump blood throughout the body. The heart itself is perfused by right and left coronary arteries arising directly from the aorta. The left coronary artery leaves the aorta and is referred to as the 'left main stem' before it bifurcates into the circumflex artery and the left anterior descending (LAD) artery. The branches of the circumflex artery are referred to as obtuse marginal

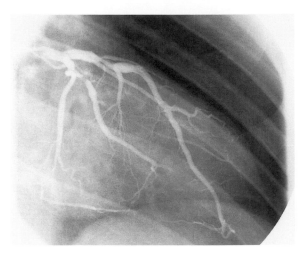

Figure 13.1 Right anterior oblique angiographic view of left coronary artery and major branches. Note the stenotic lesion in the LAD and the obstructed obtuse marginal artery arising from the circumflex. The posterior descending artery, which in this case arises from the right coronary artery, is filled in a retrograde fashion by dye from the LAD.

(OM) branches and individual branches as OM1, OM2, etc. (Figure 13.1).

Classically, the right coronary artery gives rise to the marginal branches of the right ventricle, before terminating as the posterior descending artery (PDA). However, in 10–15% of cases, the right coronary artery is small and the PDA may arise as a terminal branch of the left circumflex artery; this is referred to as 'left dominant' circulation. If the right coronary artery gives rise to the PDA, the right coronary is said to be dominant. It should be noted that regardless of the origin of the PDA, the bulk of the blood supply to the heart is borne by the left coronary artery.

Knowledge of coronary anatomy is important, as occlusion of any of these arteries can result in

Fundamentals of Surgical Practice, Third Edition, ed. Andrew N. Kingsnorth and Douglas M. Bowley.
Published by Cambridge University Press. © Cambridge University Press 2011.

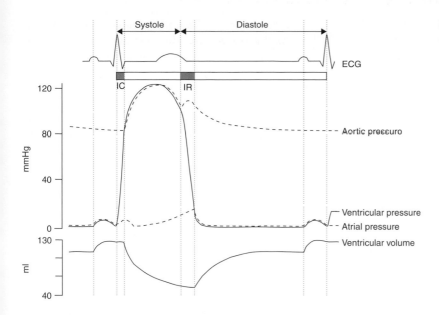

Figure 13.2 The cardiac cycle.

cardiac ischaemia and ultimately infarction. Critical illness often increases the demand of the heart and partially occluded vessels may not be able to meet this demand. Coronary blood flow occurs mainly during diastole, because during systolic contraction intramyocardial coronary arteries are compressed and blood flow is reduced. Conditions which result in a low diastolic blood pressure or which increase the intramyocardial tension during diastole (e.g. an increase in cardiac filling) can compromise coronary blood flow. In these situations, subendocardial muscle is particularly vulnerable.

Cardiac muscle consists of specialized striated muscle cells with an intrinsic, involuntary ability to contract known as automaticity. Pacemaker cells within the sinoatrial node establish the heart rate and are influenced by innervation from the autonomic nervous system. Cardiac cells are dense in myofibrils consisting of sarcomeres and their actin and myosin components. The cells are branched, intertwined and in tight communication via gap junctions and desmosomes. This arrangement allows depolarization to occur rapidly throughout the heart such that it acts as a single unit or syncytium.

Cardiac troponins (cTn) have received significant attention for their use in evaluating acute coronary syndromes. The cardiac troponin 'complex' regulates cardiac muscle contraction and consists of three protein subunits – Ca^{2+} binding (cTnC), inhibitory (cTnI) and tropomyosin binding (cTnT). In the absence of

calcium, the troponin–tropomyosin complex inhibits cross-bridge formation between actin and myosin filaments. When calcium is present, it binds to the troponin complex, changing its conformation and allowing for the formation of actin/myosin cross-bridges and cardiac contraction.

While the majority of cardiac troponin is within the myofibril, a small fraction of cTnI and cTnT is found within the cardiac cytoplasm. When cardiac cells are injured, cytoplasmic troponin is released. Because cardiac troponin is specific to cardiac cells, serum assays of cTnI or cTnT can provide early, sensitive information about cardiac injury.

Cardiac cycle

The cardiac cycle refers primarily to the function of the ventricles and is divided into two phases: systole and diastole (Figure 13.2). Systole begins with a period of isovolumetric contraction during which the intraventricular pressures rise until the aortic and pulmonary valves are pushed open by the force of ejected blood. Blood is ejected, and systole ends as the aortic and pulmonary valves close. Diastole commences with a period of isovolumetric relaxation. The atrioventricular valves then open and there is a period of rapid inflow of blood into the ventricle. Atrial contraction follows and contributes up to 25% of ventricular filling. For optimal cardiac function, the mitral valve must remain shut, avoiding regurgitation, during

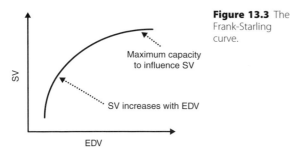

Figure 13.3 The Frank-Starling curve.

systole, whereas the aortic valve must remain shut during diastole.

Cardiac output

The purpose of the heart is to effectively pump blood to the body to meet its metabolic demands. We describe such cardiac work as 'cardiac output.' Cardiac output (CO) is the volume of blood pumped from the heart each minute. It is a function of stroke volume (SV) and heart rate (HR).

$$CO \propto SV \times HR$$

It follows that increasing either the stroke volume or the heart rate will increase cardiac output. Stroke volume is the amount of blood ejected from the heart during each systole. It is defined by end diastolic volume (EDV) (full heart) minus the end systolic volume (ESV) (empty heart).

$$SV = EDV - ESV$$

Unfortunately, it is clinically 'impossible' to measure heart volumes so stroke volume is usually a derived number based on measuring the patient's cardiac output and heart rate.

$$SV \propto CO/HR$$

Clearly cardiac output and stroke volume are intricately related. Yet it is much more important to comprehend that the amount of cardiac filling has a profound effect on the heart's overall performance, rather than try to know any particular numeric value of stroke volume.

The body modulates cardiac output both intrinsically and extrinsically. Intrinsically, cardiac output is affected by the Frank-Starling mechanism (Figure 13.3). Starling found that 'the energy of contraction is a function of the initial length of the muscle fibre'. The more the heart fills (EDV), the more the fibres lengthen, resulting in a greater force of contraction and stroke volume. The ascending limb of the Starling curve was initially attributed solely to a length–tension relationship of the sarcomeres – the greater the overlap of the thick and thin filaments, the greater the force of contraction. It is now realized that myofilaments become more easily activated when they are stretched and that this also increases the contractile force.

Extrinsic regulation of the heart is performed by the autonomic nervous system. Input to baroreceptors and chemoreceptors leads to discharges of the sympathetic and parasympathetic nervous system. The sympathetic response is to increase heart rate and contractility whereas the vagal (or parasympathetic) response is the reverse.

Using these concepts, clinicians have found ways to modulate cardiac output –by affecting either heart rate or stroke volume. The body's ability to accommodate an increase in heart rate decreases with age. Maximum heart rate (MHR) is approximated by a simple formula: MHR = 220 − age. Thus, for an 80-year-old, the maximum heart rate is only 140. (This is useful to remember in that heart rates greater than a patient's MHR generally reflect pathological arrhythmias (such as atrial fibrillation, etc.).) Furthermore, such high heart rates put a huge demand on the cardiac muscle and may not be tolerated for extended periods of time – particularly in elderly patients. Another point to consider is that with increased heart rate, diastolic filling time decreases. Above a heart rate of 160, the diastolic filling time decreases to a point that stroke volume diminishes and cardiac output begins to drop. Thus, heart rate manipulation is limited and not a mainstay of influencing cardiac output.

Stroke volume is impacted by three factors: preload, afterload, and contractility. Preload is the 'load' or quantity of blood that is entering the heart from the venous circulation. Its value is reflected by the central venous pressure (see invasive monitoring section). To increase cardiac output, one of the first interventions done is to optimize preload by giving fluid challenges. As intravascular volume increases, preload increases, EDV increases, and cardiac output improves. Alternatively, situations such as heart failure may be improved by 'off-loading' the heart. Here, preload can be decreased by using a venodilator such as nitroglycerine. By decreasing venous tone, blood is redistributed peripherally, and the amount of blood returning to the overloaded heart is diminished.

Afterload is the 'load' or impedance that the heart must pump against during systole to deliver its stroke volume. Afterload is estimated by the patient's systemic vascular resistance (SVR). SVR is a calculated value that depends heavily on the patient's mean arterial blood pressure (MAP) and is inversely related to the cardiac output. The calculations for these are as follows:

$$SVR = (MAP - CVP)/CO$$
$$MAP = P_{diastolic} + 1/3(P_{systolic} - P_{diastolic})$$

To make this easier to understand, notice that MAP relies heavily on the diastolic blood pressure. The higher the resting diastolic blood pressure, the more difficult it is for the heart to generate a pressure to open the semi-lunar valves and deliver its volume. The result is a decreased stroke volume. By decreasing afterload, the heart is able to pump a larger volume without needing to generate such a large pressure. Afterload reduction is a significant way in which clinicians augment cardiac output. Agents that decrease arterial pressure, for example arterial dilators such as hydralazine or minoxidil, are useful in this regard. Angiotensin-converting enzyme (ACE) inhibitors, the mainstay of heart failure treatment, work through afterload reduction. ACE inhibitors disrupt the renin-angiotensin pathway and thus decrease the amount of angiotensin II (a potent vasoconstrictor) produced and diminish the salt (and fluid) retentive effects of aldosterone.

Enhancing the heart's contractility is the final way in which we can manipulate cardiac output. Optimizing preload and taking advantage of the cardiac muscle's intrinsic contractile properties (Starling's law) should be the first mechanism employed to improve cardiac output. Once the heart has been optimally filled, inotropes can be utilized to further augment cardiac output. Inotropes are agents that increase cardiac contractility by increasing intracellular calcium. They are discussed further in the section on cardiovascular support.

The vasculature

An equally important component of the cardiovascular system is its vasculature. The systemic vasculature is an exquisite network extending from the aorta, to the arteries, capillaries, veins, and back through the venae cavae. Arteries and veins contain a varying amount of smooth muscle in their middle layer (tunica media) which the body (and the clinician) manipulates to maintain its goal of perfusion. Vascular smooth muscle contracts as a result of increased intracellular calcium which is released from the cytoplasmic reticulum.

Contraction of vascular smooth muscle – vasoconstriction – is mediated by a variety of factors. Sympathetic nerve endings directly release noradrenaline (norepinephrine) to affect α-1 adrenergic receptors on the vessel wall. Even at rest, this phenomenon results in partial contraction of the smooth muscle and 'vascular tone'. The sympathetic nervous system also modulates the release of adrenaline (epinephrine) from the adrenal medulla. This circulating catecholamine causes vasoconstriction via β-adrenergic receptors. Hormones such as vasopressin (released from the hypothalamus in response to hypovolemia) and angiotensin II (a consequence of renin production by the kidney) also lead to vasoconstriction. Finally, paracrine factors such as endothelin or thromboxane cause local vasoconstriction.

Alternatively, vasodilatation, vascular smooth muscle relaxation, occurs when the sympathetic discharges cease. Locally, factors such as nitric oxide and prostaglandins cause vasodilatation.

Blood pressure

Blood pressure is the pressure that circulating blood exerts against the walls of the arterial blood vessels. Blood pressure is a critical vital sign because we often think of blood pressure as a marker of perfusion. While this is not always a correct assumption, it is very important to understand the components of blood pressure so we can modulate it.

Blood pressure is directly related to cardiac output and total peripheral resistance (TPR).

$$BP \propto CO \times TPR$$

Exemplifying a key concept of physics, pressure is directly related to flow (cardiac output) and resistance. In the body, total peripheral resistance is the sum of resistances from the vessels from the left side to the right side of the heart. The factors that influence resistance include the viscosity of the blood (η), the length of the blood vessels (L), and predominantly the radius of the blood vessel (r). The relationship is as follows:

$$R \propto \frac{\eta \times L}{r^4}$$

The radius of the blood vessel impacts resistance to the fourth power. Furthermore, the viscosity of the blood and the length of the blood vessels are fairly constant. Thus, vessel diameter is the major contributor to resistance. Anything that decreases the radius of the blood vessel (vasoconstriction) is going to have a profound effect of increasing peripheral resistance.

Putting these concepts together, blood pressure can be increased either by increasing cardiac output or by vasoconstriction. We have already discussed the methods the body uses to increase cardiac output and increase vascular tone. We will address pharmacological ways to provide cardiovascular support later in this chapter.

Mean arterial blood pressure

The concept of mean arterial blood pressure (MAP) was introduced in the section above on afterload. It is the average blood pressure that occurs during an entire cardiac cycle (systole and diastole). MAP is often considered a 'better' blood pressure by intensivists for several reasons. MAP is the true driving force of peripheral blood flow or perfusion pressure. It is also less influenced by the site of the reading than are systolic and diastolic pressures.

The MAP can be measured continuously when arterial cannulation is performed. Arterial cannulation provides an arterial waveform, and area under the curve analysis with specialized software derives a continuous MAP.

The MAP can also be estimated from the equation:

$$MAP = P_{diastolic} + 1/3(P_{systolic} - P_{diastolic})$$

as it is usually presented, or in another form:

$$MAP = 1/3P_{systolic} + 2/3P_{diastolic}$$

The second equation clearly reveals that MAP is more heavily dependent upon the diastolic pressure. In looking at the cardiac cycle (refer back to Figure 13.2), you will notice that about a third of the cardiac cycle is systole and two-thirds of the cardiac cycle is diastole, hence the equation is our best estimate of the MAP.

Maintaining a MAP above 60 mmHg is important for organ perfusion. Below this, risk of systemic ischaemia and shock becomes real and life-threatening. Targeting a perfusing MAP will be a goal in our treatment of shock. As was previously mentioned, a continuous MAP and other important values would not be obtainable without the assistance of invasive haemodynamic monitoring. We will focus on this in the following section.

Haemodynamic monitoring

Arterial catheterization

Continuous blood pressure monitoring allows the clinician to closely track responses to interventions in critically ill patients. Indications for arterial lines include:

- the need for continuous blood pressure monitoring (e.g. shock or hypertensive crisis), or
- frequent arterial blood gases (e.g. DKA or respiratory failure).

While the usual site of insertion of arterial catheterization is the radial artery, the dorsalis pedis, femoral, axillary and rarely brachial artery can be used. The most significant complications of arterial lines are thrombosis and infection. When a radial line is planned, an Allen's test should first be performed to test for collateral flow to the hand via the ulnar artery and palmar arch. Multiple punctures, catheters greater than 20G and prolonged line duration should be avoided to minimize the risk of thrombosis. Cannulation of the brachial artery has a significant risk of distal emboli (5–41%) and should be avoided if at all possible.

Central venous catheterization

Central venous catheters are placed in one of the major veins leading to the heart: subclavian, internal jugular or femoral. Indications for a central venous line include high volume resuscitation, continuous monitoring of the central venous pressure (CVP), infusion of multiple medications or vasoactive drugs, need for parenteral nutrition or inability to secure peripheral venous access. Complications of central venous catheters include infection, venous thrombosis, arterial puncture, bleeding and air embolism. Pneumothorax is a complication of subclavian and, less commonly, internal jugular line insertion.

Central venous pressure (CVP)

The CVP is a pressure reading obtained from a central venous catheter whose tip is ideally situated in the vena cava at the level of the right atrium. Subclavian and

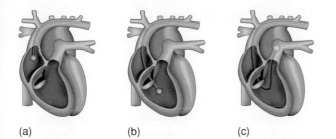

(a)　　　　　　　(b)　　　　　　　(c)　　　　　　　(d)

Figure 13.4 Floating a pulmonary artery catheter. The catheter is introduced through a central vein and the balloon inflated. The flow of blood pulls the balloon and thus catheter via the right atrium and RV to its final resting position in the PA. As the catheter is floated, its position can be followed by evaluating pressure tracings on the monitor. Once the balloon has 'wedged' itself in the PA, the balloon should be deflated to avoid complications such as a ruptured PA or pulmonary infarct.

internal jugular lines are usually employed. Correct placement should be confirmed with a post-procedure chest X-ray. A pressure transducer is then attached to the line and a CVP recording may be performed.

The CVP reflects the adjacent right atrial pressure (RAP). Because blood is in continuity between the heart and the cavae, the CVP reading is useful in helping gauge intravascular volume and cardiac filling. Intuitively, CVP is directly proportional to venous return and inversely proportional to cardiac contractility. It follows that CVP can be used to guide fluid replacement.

In order for the CVP to be an accurate guide for fluid management, the patient's heart should be normal with right ventricular (RV) function paralleling left ventricular (LV) function. Starling's law reminds us that cardiac output is optimized as left ventricular filling is optimized. Because we cannot measure ventricular end diastolic volume, we rely on the ventricular end diastolic pressure (VEDP) as a surrogate. When the heart is normal, right ventricular filling parallels that of the left. Furthermore, in a normal heart, RVEDP equals RAP (as the tricuspid valve is open in diastole). Thus, RVEDP = RAP = CVP. To summarize, in the normal heart, CVP can be used as a guide to resuscitation because it ultimately reflects LVEDP. If we optimize the CVP, we are optimizing cardiac filling and then cardiac output by engaging the intrinsic contractility properties of the heart.

The problem is that the vast majority of critically ill patients do not have normal hearts. Thus, as an absolute value, CVP can be unreliable for a variety of reasons. CVP will be numerically elevated in any situation where intrathoracic pressures are increased (mechanical ventilation), but in actuality venous return is impaired. Pulmonary vascular disease, RV disease, LV failure or valvular heart disease will also affect the CVP reading. Keeping such limitations in mind, looking at the dynamic changes of the CVP in response to fluid therapy can still be extremely useful. If the CVP remains low in a hypotensive septic patient after receiving a fluid challenge, they are likely to need more fluid. If the CVP rises rapidly in response to a fluid challenge, it implies the patient may already be appropriately filled and alternative measures to maintain blood pressure should be sought.

Pulmonary artery catheterization

Pulmonary artery (PA) catheters are long catheters which are introduced through large-bore central venous lines usually in the subclavian or internal jugular veins. The catheters have a balloon at their tip which allows them to be carried via the flow of blood or 'floated' to their resting position within the pulmonary artery (Figure 13.4). The catheter has a distal lumen that measures pulmonary artery pressures and obtains mixed venous (SvO_2) blood samples. A proximal lumen permits fluid infusions and manometric measurement in the right atrium (CVP).

PA catheters allow for measurement of a number of haemodynamic parameters which can be useful in characterizing a patient's illness and guiding therapy. The most important of these are cardiac output, pulmonary artery occlusion pressure (PAOP) and SvO_2.

PA catheters measure cardiac output via a technique known as thermodilution. A small bolus of cold 5% dextrose is quickly injected into the right atrium via the proximal lumen of the PA catheter. The injectate mixes with the blood and causes a fall in temperature which is recorded by a temperature probe at the catheter tip. The change in temperature over time is

195

recorded as a curve. Cardiac output is inversely proportional to the area under the curve and is calculated using the Hamilton–Stewart equation (performed by computer software).

Complications of PA catheters include arrhythmias, pulmonary infarction, pulmonary embolism, pulmonary artery rupture, infection and knotting of the catheter within the heart. Furthermore, with regard to patient outcome, multiple studies have failed to show a benefit with PA catheter use; hence today, PA catheterization is rarely used.

Doppler ultrasound

Doppler ultrasound is increasingly utilized to provide a less invasive way of monitoring cardiac output. A Doppler probe positioned in the suprasternal notch or oesophagus detects changes in the frequency of reflected ultrasound waves when blood moves through the ascending aorta (suprasternal notch) or descending aorta (oesophagus). From an analysis of the velocity waveform and aortic diameter, an estimate of the stroke volume and hence cardiac output can be made.

Echocardiography

Echocardiography (ECHO) has become an increasingly utilized modality in ICUs. An ultrasound beam is transmitted to the heart and the reflections are analysed and integrated to create an image or echocardiogram. Two methods of imaging are available, transthoracic ECHO (TTE) and transoesphageal ECHO (TOE). In TTE, the ultrasound probe is placed on the chest wall and ultrasound waves are emitted through the intercostal spaces. TOE obtains images with a transducer on the end of a flexible endoscope in the oesophagus; it is useful for visualizing the thoracic aorta as well as the heart.

In the ICU, ECHO can be utilized to assess cardiac filling and correlate this observation to pressure readings. ECHO is useful in characterizing right and left heart interactions. For example, in a patient with right heart failure, ECHO can help determine whether this is secondary to a failing left heart or otherwise. Measurements of ventricular size and function (ejection fraction) can be made. ECHO can identify myocardial ischaemia, pericardial effusion and valvular abnormalities. When ECHO is used in conjunction with Doppler technology, intracardiac blood flow can be studied and cardiac output estimated.

Pulse contour analysis

Pulse contour analysis (often known as PiCCO) is a novel method of haemodynamic monitoring that employs a specialized femoral or axillary arterial line and a central venous catheter. With PiCCO, an arterial pulse contour (obtained via arterial catheter) in conjunction with a thermodilution technique is used to estimate variables such as cardiac output, stroke volume and systemic vascular resistance. Unlike the thermodilution technique utilized with the PA catheter, PiCCO depends on transpulmonary thermodilution. The injectate is administered via the central venous line, travels through the heart (and lungs) and is analysed at the specialized arterial line site. Once the initial thermodilution technique is performed, the system is able to determine a continuous cardiac output reading from the arterial waveform. Haemodynamic values obtained from PiCCO technology correlate well to conventional PA catheterization and avoid the complications associated with catheterizing the right heart.

Cardiac arrest and resuscitation

Cardiac arrest is sudden cessation of the pumping action of the heart (loss of heartbeat) resulting in the loss of effective circulation. Causes include:

- cardiac arrhythmias, conduction disturbances, myocardial infarction
- respiratory failure
- shock
- metabolic and electrolyte disturbances – hyperkalemia, metabolic acidosis
- hypothermia – especially <32°C.

Clinical presentation

When patients arrest, they almost immediately lose consciousness. If the arrest occurs whilst the patient is being monitored in the ICU or operating theatre, an arrhythmia or asystole may be seen on the monitoring screen. Four situations are possible:

- pulseless ventricular tachycardia (VT)
- ventricular fibrillation (VF)
- pulseless electrical activity (PEA)
- asystole.

Recognition of VT/VF is important (Figure 13.5), because these arrhythmias respond to defibrillation, whereas PEA and asystole do not.

(a)

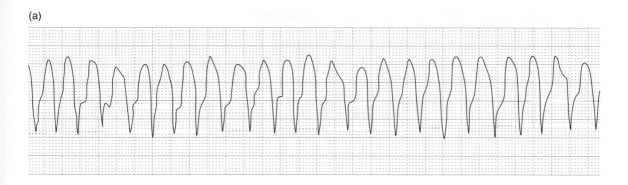

(b)

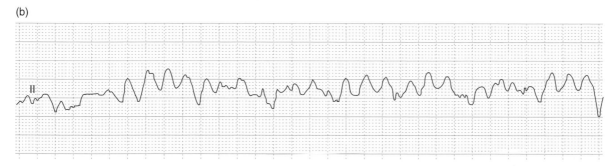

Figure 13.5 Shockable arrhythmias associated with cardiac arrest. A, ventricular tachycardia; B, ventricular fibrillation.

Resuscitation

The European Resuscitation Council has established well-developed guidelines for patients with sudden cardiac arrest. In hospitalized patients, advanced life support (ALS) with early, effective cardiopulmonary resuscitation (CPR) and defibrillation (when indicated) are of critical importance.

Adult advanced life support

When cardiac arrest occurs, ALS is initiated immediately; after ensuring a lack of responsiveness, the healthcare provider should begin the ABCs. Attach a monitor-defibrillator as soon as possible.

A – AIRWAY: tilt the head backwards, lift the chin and clear the airway. If need be, consider an oro-pharyngeal airway. Begin preparations for a definitive airway via tracheal intubation; however do not delay the initiation of CPR. Laryngeal mask airway (LMA) is an acceptable, temporary alternative to tracheal intubation if the healthcare provider is more familiar with this type of airway.

B – BREATHING: bag-valve-mask ventilation should be performed until tracheal intubation is possible. Tidal volume recommendations are 500–600 ml per breath with high flow oxygen. The desired rate is 10 breaths per minute. Hyperventilation is detrimental as it can increase intrathoracic pressure and ultimately decrease venous return and cardiac output.

C – CIRCULATION: once the absence of a carotid pulse is confirmed, initiate chest compressions immediately! Vascular access (either peripheral or central venous) needs to be secured as soon as possible. Intraosseous access can be used alternatively.

Cardiopulmonary resuscitation (CPR) combines external cardiac massage (cardio) with intermittently administered breaths (pulmonary). Effective cardiac massage involves compression of the chest in the centre of the sternum while the patient is lying on a firm surface. Current recommendations for both one and two person CPR are 30 chest compressions for 2 breaths. Once the patient's airway is secured, continuous chest compressions should be done at a rate of 100 times per minute. Continuous, effective chest compressions improve the effectiveness of drug administration and defibrillation.

External cardiac massage usually results in a cardiac output sufficient to achieve systolic pressures between 60 and 80 mmHg. Though higher pressures may be achieved by greater compression, the risk of myocardial contusion is increased. Diastolic pressures during CPR are low (0 to 20 mmHg). This means that perfusion to all organs will occur largely during systole. Coronary blood flow, which usually occurs in diastole, now must also occur in systole. As ventricular fibrillation raises intramyocardial tension and increases resistance to blood flow, the heart is particularly vulnerable to ischaemia.

Throughout resuscitation, evaluation of potentially reversible causes of arrest should be sought and corrected. These include the four 'Hs' (Hypoxia, Hypovolaemia, Hypothermia, and metabolic causes – Hypo/hyperkalemia, hypocalcaemia, and acidaemia) and the four 'Ts' (Tension pneumothorax, Tamponade, Thromboembolic event, and Toxic/therapeutic substance overdose). (In actuality, it may be helpful to think of it as seven 'Hs' with the potassium counting as two, the hypocalcaemia as one, and the acidaemia (H+) as one.) In any case, administration of IV fluids, high-flow oxygen, checking for clinical signs of pneumothorax and tamponade, an ABG evaluating for hypoxia, acidosis or electrolyte disturbance, and review of the drug chart are essential components of any arrest situation.

VF/VT

The defibrillator should be connected to any cardiac arrest patient as soon as it is available. If the monitor shows VF or VT, the heart should be defibrillated immediately. CPR needs to be continued just before and immediately after defibrillation. Do not pause to check the rhythm after defibrillation, but continue CPR for 2 more minutes. Hold CPR after 2 minutes and check for return of an organized rhythm and pulse. If VF/VT persists, then re-shock. Adrenaline (1 mg) should be administered after the second shock and every 3–5 minutes thereafter to increase blood pressure and perfusion to the heart. If the patient remains in VF/VT, then amiodarone may be administered after the third and fourth shock. Continue the cycle of CPR, defibrillation, and medication administration, until defibrillation is achieved – in the form of either a survivable rhythm or asystole.

ALS guidelines suggest that patients with a witnessed arrest be given a single precordial thump before moving quickly to the algorithms of resuscitation if a defibrillator is not available. The precordial thump is occasionally effective in converting pulseless VT to sinus rhythm.

Asystole/PEA

The ABCs should be initiated immediately, while the cause of the arrest is sought (Hs and Ts). Survival of a non-shockable arrest is unlikely unless the underlying cause is identified and corrected. Adrenaline (1 mg) should be administered and this dose repeated every 3 minutes while the resuscitation is in progress. A single 3 mg dose of atropine is given for patients with asystole/PEA. Sodium bicarbonate can be given if the arrest is thought to be a result of hyperkalemia or to correct a severe acidosis (pH < 7.1). Hold CPR every 2 minutes to check for a rhythm and pulse.

Arrhythmias

Sinus rhythm is initiated by the sinoatrial node and is recognized by the presence of a P wave, a QRS complex and a T wave. In sinus rhythm, the heart rate is between approximately 60 and 100 beats per minute (bpm). Occasionally, other 'ectopic' foci within the heart will discharge spontaneously, causing a premature heartbeat. Atrial ectopy is frequent, occasionally symptomatic and usually benign. It is characterized by an abnormal P wave followed by a normal QRS complex. Treatment is reassurance, avoiding caffeine and occasionally beta or calcium blockade. Junctional ectopy has a normal-looking QRS complex but is not necessarily preceded by a P wave; the P wave may immediately precede, follow or be located within the QRS complex. Ventricular ectopy lacks a P wave and often has a bizarre, wide QRS complex. Such premature ventricular contractions usually also occur in the absence of any cardiac pathology, are self-limited, but may be treated with beta-blockade if patients are severely symptomatic.

Tachycardia

Sinus tachycardia is a fast heart rate (greater than 100 bpm) that is generated by the sinoatrial node in response to autonomic or catecholamine stimulation. By definition, a normal P-wave should precede each QRS. It is a 'benign arrhythmia' in that there is no intrinsic abnormality of the heart. However, sinus tachycardia is a response to physiological stress, be it exercise and anxiety or hypotension, anaemia, sepsis, pulmonary embolism, etc. Thus, in any patient with sinus tachycardia, a pathological source of stress should be sought and treated.

Narrow complex tachycardias are arrhythmias initiating above the A-V node which result in a narrow QRS complex on the ECG. They include atrial fibrillation, atrial flutter and varying conduction or re-entry abnormalities often grouped together broadly as 'SVTs'. Atrial fibrillation is characterized by rapid, random depolarizations of the atria (up to 600/min) which are irregularly transmitted to the ventricles. This accounts for the lack of a P-wave as well as the irregular rate and rhythm. Treatment of atrial fibrillation depends on patient stability, underlying disease and duration of the arrhythmia; expert consultation is recommended. In any unstable patient (HR >150 bpm, chest pain, poor perfusion) synchronized cardioversion should be performed. The management of stable atrial fibrillation is either by rate control (beta- or Ca^{2+}-channel blockade or digoxin) or rhythm control (amiodarone). Anticoagulation (to prevent the potential complication of dislodging an atrial clot) is usually required in patients who are rate-controlled but still irregular or in patients with atrial fibrillation of greater than 48 hours duration who are candidates for rhythm control.

Patients with other narrow-complex tachyarrhythmias are often categorized together for treatment purposes. Pulseless narrow complex tachycardias require immediate synchronized cardioversion. In patients with a pulse, initial treatment involves vagal manoeuvres and adenosine administration. If the patient fails to convert to sinus rhythm, expert advice should be sought; less stable patients may need cardioversion, whereas stable patients may benefit from amiodarone, beta- or Ca^{2+} channel blockade, or digoxin.

Broad-complex tachycardia is usually ventricular in origin but can be supraventricular with an aberrant conduction (such as a bundle branch). Pulseless VT is treated with defibrillation as was discussed in the previous section. VT in the unstable patient (chest pain, heart failure, hypotension) is treated with cardioversion and amiodarone. VT in the stable patient is treated with amiodarone (and potentially cardioversion). Expert evaluation is critical as certain patients may benefit from automatic implantable cardiac defibrillators (AICDs). Electrolyte levels should be checked in all cases, keeping in mind that potassium and magnesium supplementation may be indicated. If the broad-complex tachycardia is supraventricular in origin, then treatment is as discussed above.

Bradycardia

Bradycardia is defined as a heart rate of less than 60. While this may be normal in a well-trained athlete, it may be pathological in others, not allowing for a sufficient cardiac output. Bradycardia usually results from either sinus node dysfunction or from atrioventricular (heart) block. First-degree heart block is characterized by a prolonged PR interval (>0.21 s). In second-degree heart block, there is failure to conduct all atrial impulses to the ventricle. In Mobitz I, the PR interval increases until there is a dropped beat. In Mobitz II, there is a normal PR interval but not all atrial impulses are conducted to the ventricle such that the ratio of atrial to ventricular beats may be 2:1 or 3:1. Third-degree heart block is also known as complete heart block; P waves and QRS complexes occur independently as no atrial impulses are transmitted to the ventricle. Patients showing adverse signs of bradycardia should be given 500 μg of atropine IV, repeated as needed every 3–5 minutes to a maximum dose of 3 mg. If this fails to relieve symptoms, then external pacing or a low-dose adrenaline drip should be considered. Expert advice is recommended to determine whether the patient is a candidate for more permanent pacing options.

Cardiac tamponade

Cardiac tamponade is compression of the heart due to fluid accumulation within the pericardial space. The lower-pressure, thin-walled atria are most vulnerable to compression. Atrial compression leads to impaired venous return and overall decreased cardiac filling. Compression of the heart as a whole impairs diastolic filling. If not corrected urgently, the result is low cardiac output failure and shock.

Surgical causes of tamponade include penetrating cardiac wounds, blunt trauma to the chest, or postoperative accumulation after open-heart surgery. Tamponade can also occur as a complication of central line placement. Medical causes include malignancy, pericarditis, post-MI ventricular rupture and uraemia.

Clinical presentation and diagnosis

Presentation may be acute when fluid or blood accumulates in the heart very rapidly or it may be late when the rate of fluid accumulation has been slow. Beck's triad of muffled heart sounds, hypotension and elevated jugular venous distension may be evident

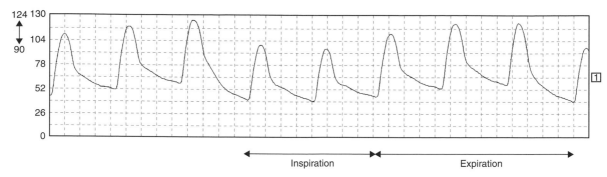

Figure 13.6 Pulsus paradoxus. Arterial waveform of a patient with pulsus paradoxus. Note the exaggerated fall in systolic pressure (>10 mmHg) seen on inspiration.

particularly in the acute setting. Haemodynamically compromised patients are tachycardic and hypotensive. They may be sitting up and extremely anxious. Evidence of right heart failure with jugular venous distension and hepatomegaly may be apparent. Decreased heart sounds or a pericardial friction rub may be noted in up to a third of patients.

Pulsus parodoxus is a classic finding in patients with tamponade. It is defined as an exaggerated fall in arterial systolic pressure (>10 mmHg) during inspiration (Figure 13.6). Kussmaul described this 'paradox' by noting a disappearance of the pulse during inspiration, although the heartbeat was still audible. Here is how it works. During inspiration, intrathoracic pressure falls and allows for increased venous return and increased RV filling. However, in tamponade, because the heart is compressed and there is no room to accommodate the increased RV filling, the intraventricular septum becomes displaced to the left. The bulge of the septum inhibits LV filling and, as a result, stroke volume actually decreases with a subsequent decrease in cardiac output and arterial pressure.

In the acute setting, diagnosis should be suspected clinically. In a postoperative cardiac patient, hypotension, tachycardia and low urine output should put the surgeon on instant alert. Diagnosis is now made quickly and easily with ultrasound. Bedside ultrasound is becoming increasingly available, even in A & E departments. In the absence of ultrasound, pericardiocentesis may be performed as a diagnostic and potentially therapeutic measure. Nevertheless, pericardiocentesis has associated risks (arrhythmias, cardiac laceration, coronary artery laceration, tamponade and pneumothorax) and is ideally performed only once pericardial fluid is confirmed or very highly suspected.

Management

Management involves draining the cause of tamponade. In a patient who has undergone cardiac surgery, emergency sternal reopening and evacuation of blood may be life-saving. Patients with penetrating chest wounds and tamponade should be taken for immediate sternotomy. Incidentally, these patients are rarely stable and may require resuscitative thoracotomy (and opening of the pericardial sac) in A & E. Pericardiocentesis has a role in providing urgent symptomatic relief in tamponade due to more chronic conditions such as uraemia or malignancy. Successful pericardiocentesis is done with the patient sitting up and the needle introduced at a 15° angle just to the left of the xiphoid. The needle is directed slowly toward the left shoulder while drawing back the syringe. Ultrasound guidance is now the norm. Surgical creation of a 'window' or small hole in the pericardium to communicate with the pleural space is a useful option for draining chronic pericardial effusions causing tamponade.

Cardiovascular support

Cardiovascular support can be pharmacological and/or invasive. The goal is to restore perfusion to physiological levels. Adding cardiovascular support usually occurs in a step-wise fashion, such that least-invasive modalities are employed first.

Inotropes

Inotropes are drugs that work directly on the heart to increase its output by increasing the heart rate and contractility. Inotropes fall into two broad categories:

Table 13.1 Catecholamines, adrenergic activity, and clinical effects

Catecholamine	Property	Beta-1	Beta-2	Alpha-1	Clinical effect
Noradrenaline	Endogenous catecholamine	++	–	++	Predominantly increases MAP. Increase in SVR limits inotropic effects
Adrenaline	Endogenous catecholamine	++	++	++	Predominant effect is inotropy at low doses and vasoconstriction at high doses. May cause tachyarrhythmias
Dopamine	Endogenous catecholamine	++	–	++	Dose-dependent. 2–5 (mcg/kg/min): dopaminergic receptor activation increases splanchnic blood flow. 5–10: predominant beta/inotropic effect. >10: predominant alpha/vasoconstrictor effect.
Dobutamine	Synthetic catecholamine	++	++	–	Potent inotrope. May cause significant hypotension, particularly in hypovolaemic patients.

++, potent agonist; –, minimal agonist.

- cyclic adenosine monophosphate (cAMP)-dependent (β-adrenergic agonists and phosphodiesterase inhibitors)
- cAMP-independent (α-adrenergic agonists and digoxin).

The vast majority of inotropes are cAMP-dependent; their primary action is to increase second messenger cAMP. In the heart, cAMP activates a protein kinase which opens a sarcolemma calcium gate allowing calcium to influx into the cytoplasm. Calcium then binds troponin C and cardiac muscle contraction is facilitated (see physiology section).

Importantly, cAMP activation causes the opposite effect in vascular smooth muscle. In smooth muscle, cAMP leads to calcium uptake by the sarcoplasmic reticulum and resultant smooth muscle relaxation. These contrasting effects of cAMP account for the inotropy and systemic and pulmonary vasodilatation (inodilation) seen with a majority of inotropes.

Adrenergic receptor agonists (catecholamines)

Naturally occurring catecholamines and synthetic amines act via β-adrenergic and α-adrenergic receptors. The different amines have varying affinities for the receptors, leading to their variable effects.

β-1 receptors in cardiac muscle account for 80% of inotrope activity. Catecholamines bind β-1 receptors on the cardiac muscle sarcolemma. The β-1 receptor acts via a G protein to activate adenylate cyclase and convert ATP to cAMP. As described above, increased cAMP causes enhanced cardiac muscle contraction. β-1 receptor activation also causes an increase in sino-atrial node firing (chronotropy), an increase in atrio-ventricular conduction and a decrease in the muscle cell excitation threshold.

β-2 and α-1 adrenergic receptors also exist in the heart and probably contribute to inotropy. β-2 receptors also work via cAMP-dependent pathways. They have an important role in patients with chronic heart failure who have persistently elevated levels of catecholamines and thus down-regulation of their β-1 receptors. α-1 receptors are cAMP-independent. The alpha-receptor is linked to the phospholipase C, GTP, inositol phosphate pathway. Ultimately, calcium is released to aid in cardiac muscle contraction, but cAMP is not required.

Catecholamines used for inotropic support include dobutamine, dopamine, adrenaline and noradrenaline. These catecholamines, their receptor affinities and primary clinical effects are listed in Table 13.1.

Phosphodiesterase inhibitors

Phosphodiesterase (PDE) is responsible for the breakdown of cAMP. PDE inhibition limits the breakdown of cAMP and thus increases cardiac contractility (and vascular smooth muscle relaxation). PDE inhibition evokes the same physiological response as the β-1 pathway, but is independent of β-1 receptor occupation. Thus, PDE inhibitors can be particularly useful in patients who are likely to have down-regulation of their β-1 receptors (chronic failure). It is useful to note that there are a variety of PDE inhibitors available; phosphodiesterase III is the active PDE in the heart, thus agents specific to PDE III are used for inotropy.

Amrinone, milrinone and enoximone are examples of PDE III inhibitors. Amrinone was the first PDE used for inotropic support, but it has fallen out of favour as the result of causing GI side effects and thrombocytopenia. Milrinone is currently the most widely used PDE inhibitor.

Digoxin

Digoxin increases intracellular calcium and thus cardiac contractility via inhibition of a sodium/potassium membrane pump. Digoxin is of limited use in the critically ill patient because of its narrow therapeutic index and increased potential for toxicity (electrolyte disturbances, hypoxia and acidosis).

Vasopressors

Vasopressors are agents that cause vasoconstriction of the peripheral vasculature. Their main purpose is to increase mean arterial pressure. This is done predominantly via α-adrenergic mechanisms.

Catecholamines

As previously discussed, catecholamines vary in their receptor activity. Those which strongly influence alpha receptors (noradrenaline, high adrenaline and dopamine) can be used to support a failing blood pressure.

Phenylephrine

Phenylephrine is a strong vasopressor with almost exclusive α-1 receptor activity. It has minimal beta activity and only at very high doses. Its primary use is treating refractory hypotension in patients with neurogenic shock (loss of pure alpha-mediated vasomotor tone).

Vasoregulatory agents

Vasoregulatory agents are endogenous mediators that have a role in maintaining vascular tone. In sepsis and multiple organ dysfunction syndrome, there can be loss of the body's responsiveness to these agents.

Vasopressin

Vasopressin is a peptide hormone normally secreted by the posterior pituitary. It helps regulate intravascular fluid volume by facilitating water reabsorption by the renal collecting tubules (hence its other name – anti-diuretic hormone), but it also has direct vasoconstrictor effects. Decreased vasopressin levels have been noted in patients in septic shock. Vasopressin infusions have been shown to decrease catecholamine requirements in patients with septic shock. Vasopressin's effect on mortality has not yet been established.

Steroids

Stress-dose steroids (300 mg hydrocortisone per day) may improve vascular responsiveness to catecholamine infusion in patients with septic shock. This has been a controversial topic, but current recommendations are that IV steroid administration be considered in patients with septic shock who are poorly responsive to both fluid resuscitation and vasopressors.

Intra-aortic balloon pump

The intra-aortic balloon pump (IABP) is an invasive device utilized to increase cardiac output and myocardial perfusion. The IABP consists of a balloon which is connected to a long catheter. The catheter is inserted via the femoral artery and positioned such that the balloon sits in the descending thoracic aorta (Figure 13.7). The balloon is also connected to a pump that allows it to be inflated and deflated at designated intervals.

The pump is synchronized with the ECG so that the balloon is deflated in systole and inflated in diastole. When the heart ejects in systole, rapid deflation of the balloon creates an 'empty space' in the aorta, thus decreasing afterload and hence myocardial work. This improves cardiac contractility and output. During diastole, inflation of the balloon displaces a volume of blood equal to the volume of the balloon. Some of the blood will be pushed 'forward' and by this means the output of the heart is further augmented. As coronary blood flow occurs largely during diastole, inflation of the balloon during diastole also displaces blood 'backward' and thus enhances coronary blood flow.

Use of the IABP is indicated in selected cases of cardiogenic shock. It is particularly used for support of cardiac failure after CABG and as a bridge to intervention for patients with acute coronary syndromes, mitral regurgitation or septal defects. The device is not useful at very rapid heart rates (>150 beats/min), since there is insufficient time for inflation and deflation of the balloon. It is contraindicated in aortic regurgitation as it exacerbates valvular insufficiency and heart failure. The IABP is also not useful in

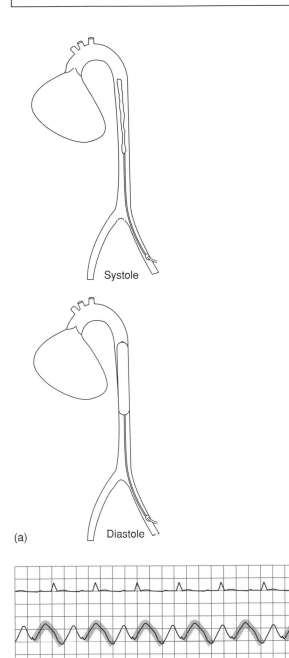

(a)

Systole

Diastole

(b)

Figure 13.7 Intra-aortic balloon pump. (a) The intra-aortic balloon pump *in situ*. (b) The arterial waveform showing augmented diastolic blood pressure (highlighted section of the trace).

children because of their relatively rapid heart rates and because the major vessels in children are more distensible than in adults; inflation of the balloon in diastole simply distends the aorta without augmenting flow.

Extracorporeal membrane oxygenation

Extracorporeal membrane oxygenation (ECMO) is a technique of providing a temporary external circulation to a patient with severe, reversible cardiopulmonary failure. In ECMO, blood is removed from the body via a special cannula, pumped through the ECMO circuit where it is oxygenated in an oxygenator, and then returned back to the body.

ECMO use in the adult ICU is exceedingly rare, but it is being studied internationally. ECMO does have a confirmed role in critically ill children. Improved outcomes are seen in neonates with disorders such as meconium aspiration, respiratory distress syndrome, congenital diaphragmatic hernia, pneumonia and persistent pulmonary artery hypertension. It also has use in paediatric patients with congenital heart defects. In the UK, there are four centres within the NHS that provide ECMO; acceptance for transfer for therapy is approved on an individual case basis.

Shock

Definition

Shock is defined as circulatory failure resulting in inadequate tissue perfusion with consequent end organ/cellular hypoxia. Shock occurs when the cardiovascular system is unable to deliver a necessary amount of oxygen to meet the metabolic demands of the body. Understanding how oxygen is delivered and consumed is critical to comprehending shock and our approach to its treatment.

Oxygen delivery

Oxygen delivery (DO_2) is defined as the amount of gaseous oxygen delivered to the body per minute. It is determined by the cardiac output and oxygen content of the blood (CaO_2).

Oxygen delivery (ml O_2/min)
$$= \text{cardiac output(ml blood/min)}$$
$$\times \text{oxygen content (ml } O_2\text{/dl blood)}$$
$$DO_2 = CO \times CaO_2$$

The oxygen content of the blood is the amount of oxygen that is carried by the blood. It includes both the oxygen that is bound to haemoglobin and that which is dissolved in the blood.

Oxygen content (CaO_2)

    = Oxygen bound to haemoglobin

      + Oxygen dissolved in the blood

The amount of oxygen bound to haemoglobin will depend on the patient's haemoglobin (Hb), the oxygen saturation (SaO_2), and a constant which reflects the amount of oxygen in millilitres carried by a gram of fully bound haemoglobin.

Oxygen bound to Hb (ml O_2/dl)

    = $SaO_2 \times Hb(g/dl)$

      $\times 1.34$ ml O_2/g saturated Hb

The amount of oxygen dissolved in the blood is relatively insignificant, as oxygen is not very soluble in blood. Nevertheless, it is determined by the product of the partial pressure of oxygen in the blood (PaO_2) and the solubility coefficient of oxygen.

Oxygen dissolved in blood (ml O_2/dl) = $PaO_2 \times 0.0031$

To summarize:

$CaO_2 = (SaO_2 \times Hb \times 1.34) + (PaO_2)(0.0031)$

    Oxygen delivery then can be augmented either by increasing cardiac output or by improving oxygen content. Increasing cardiac output was explained in the above section. As is evidenced by the formulas, oxygen content is improved primarily by increasing the haemoglobin (transfusion) or by providing additional oxygen.

Oxygen consumption

Oxygen consumption (VO_2) is the volume of gaseous oxygen consumed by the body per minute. It is a calculated value that is obtained by knowing how much oxygen is delivered to the tissue (DO_2) and how much oxygen is returned to the heart by the venous blood. The volume of oxygen returned to the heart in venous blood is referred to as the venous oxygen content (CvO_2). Its equation is identical to that of the arterial oxygen content, except that a venous haemoglobin saturation and partial pressure of oxygen is required.

$CvO_2 = (SvO_2 \times Hb \times 1.34) + (PvO_2)(0.0031)$

    Obviously, different organs extract oxygen in different quantities. For example, the heart extracts much more oxygen from the same quantity of blood than does the resting bicep muscle. Drawing venous blood

from the arm then might not give a true representation of the body's consumption. The most sensitive sample of venous blood to detect the amount of oxygen being utilized by the entire body is a sample coming from the right heart itself. This technique is indeed used in critically ill patients. Venous samples can be drawn from catheters that sit in the pulmonary artery (see invasive monitoring section). These 'mixed venous' oxygen (SvO_2) saturations are utilized to most accurately determine the body's CvO_2. Normal SvO_2 is 75%, because about 25% of oxygen delivered to the body is utilized.

    Putting these factors together, we conclude:

Oxygen consumption

    = Oxygen delivered − Oxygen returned to the

      heart in venous blood

$VO_2 = DO_2 −$ Oxygen returned to heart

$VO_2 = [CO \times CaO_2] − [CO \times CvO_2]$

$VO_2 = (CO)(CaO_2 − CvO_2) \times 10$ dl/l

Oxygen extraction ratio

Knowing how much oxygen the body is utilizing and how much oxygen the cardiovascular system is delivering allows us to calculate a ratio. The oxygen extraction ratio (O_2ER) is determined by comparing oxygen consumption to oxygen delivery.

$O_2ER = VO_2/DO_2$

    Normally, the body consumes approximately 25% of the oxygen that is delivered. Thus, the normal oxygen extraction ratio is 0.25. When oxygen delivery decreases, in order to maintain a constant level of tissue oxygenation, cells extract more oxygen from the available blood than usual (increased oxygen consumption). The result is a decreased mixed venous oxygen saturation and increased extraction ratio (e.g. SvO_2 65% and O_2ER 0.35). Improving oxygen delivery to normalize the mixed venous saturation (and oxygen extraction ratio) is an important goal of resuscitation.

    A summary of the above oxygenation values and their reference ranges is provided in Table 13.2.

    While there seems a multitude of equations, awareness of the concepts of oxygen consumption and delivery is fundamental to the understanding of critical care. If the patient consumes more oxygen than the circulatory system can deliver, the patient is in oxygen

Table 13.2 Haemodynamic variables, formulas, and reference ranges

	Abbreviation	Formula	Reference range	Units
Measured variables				
Cardiac output	CO		4–8	l/min
Central venous pressure	CVP		0–8	mmHg
Pulmonary artery occlusion pressure	PAOP		<18	mmHg
Mixed venous saturation	SvO_2		75%	
Calculated variables				
Arterial oxygen content	CaO_2	$(Hb \times SaO_2 \times 1.34) + (PaO_2 \times 0.003)$	18–20	ml/dl
Mean arterial pressure	MAP	$DBP + 1/3\ (SBP - DBP)$	70–110	mmHg
Oxygen consumption	VO_2	$(CaO_2 - CvO_2) \times CO \times 10$	100–280	ml/min
Oxygen delivery	DO_2	$CaO_2 \times CO \times 10$	640–1200	ml/min
Oxygen extraction ratio	O_2ER	VO_2 / DO_2	0.22–0.30	
Stroke volume	SV	CO / HR	60–130	ml
Systemic vascular resistance	SVR	$[(MAP - CVP) \times 80] / CO$	800–1400	dynes s/cm^5
Venous oxygen content	CvO_2	$(Hb \times SvO_2 \times 1.34) + (PvO_2 \times 0.003)$	13–16	ml/dl
Indexed variables				
Cardiac index	CI	CO / BSA	2.8–4.2	l/min per m^2
Oxygen delivery index	DO_2I	DO_2 / BSA	500–600	ml/min per m^2
Oxygen consumption index	VO_2I	VO_2 / BSA	120–160	ml/min per m^2
Stroke volume index	SVI	$(CO / HR) / BSA$	40–60	ml/m^2
System vascular resistance index	SVRI	$[(MAP - CVP) \times 80] / CO / BSA$	1700–2400	dynes s/cm^5 per m^2

debt. If this persists, the end result will be cellular hypoxia and by definition, shock. Understanding that optimizing cardiac output and oxygen content are the two ways in which we can improve oxygen delivery allows for a systematic way of treating the shocked state.

Diagnosis

Patients in shock will demonstrate evidence of end organ hypoperfusion. Thinking of this systemically will allow one not to be fooled by less obvious signs. Confusion or altered mental status may be one of the most subtle and least appreciated signs of cerebral hypoxia; in the late stage, shocked patients are often obtunded. Patients are tachypnoeic and show increased work of breathing as they attempt to meet the body's oxygen demands. Their extremities may be cool and they may appear 'clamped down' with delayed capillary refill as the periphery vasoconstricts to divert blood flow to the more important splanchnic organs. Urine output diminishes as the kidneys are hypoperfused. Ultimately, cells receiving inadequate oxygen resort to anaerobic metabolism and systemic lactic acidosis results.

Patients in shock may have a low blood pressure and compensatory tachycardia. These can be very mis-leading signs for a variety of reasons and thus should not be used to define shock. For example, in a usually hypertensive elderly patient, a 'normal' blood pressure may not provide adequate tissue perfusion. Likewise, a patient on a beta-blocker may not be capable of mounting an expected tachycardia. It is important not to count on these classic signs when approaching a patient with suspected shock.

Types of shock

Thinking of shock as either pump (cardiac output) failure or peripheral circulatory failure can be a useful starting point in approaching the shocked patient. With this in mind, four main types of shock are described (Table 13.3):

1. Cardiogenic – the heart intrinsically is not providing the output required to meet the demands of the body.
2. Hypovolaemic – the heart is under-filled because of an inadequate circulating blood volume and is thus not able to deliver adequate output to the body.
3. Obstructive – the heart itself is healthy and there is adequate blood volume, but the heart is still not able to deliver adequate output because of impedance. This is due to either inflow

Table 13.3 Classification of shock

Cardiogenic shock	Hypovolaemic shock	Obstructive shock	Distributive shock
Heart failure	Haemorrhage	Pericardial tamponade	Sepsis/SIRS
Myocardial infarction	Fluid depletion	Constrictive pericarditis	Neurogenic
Arrhythmia	(vomiting, diuretics, diarrhoea)	Tension pneumothorax	Anaphylaxis
Valvular failure	Fistula/stoma losses	Pulmonary embolism	
Cardiac contusion		Air embolism	

obstruction (e.g. pericardial tamponade, constrictive pericarditis) or outflow obstruction (e.g. pulmonary or air embolism).

4. Distributive – loss of systemic vascular tone resulting in difficulty perfusing critical organs. Patients often develop a compensatory increase in cardiac output to try and maintain perfusion.

Thus, the first three types of shock listed are considered low cardiac output shock (pump failure), whereas distributive shock is truly a peripheral vascular failure.

It should be noted that patients may have more than one type of shock at any given time. While the initial management of the shocked patient is the same regardless of its cause, early recognition of the type of shock affecting the patient is paramount to providing further appropriate treatment. In the following sections, we will first discuss early resuscitation of the shocked patient followed by a look at strategies for managing the particular types of shock.

Resuscitation

Treatment of shock begins with the Airway, Breathing, and Circulation model of treating any critically ill or injured patient. Airway and breathing may be intact, but this is not always the case. Obtunded patients or haemorrhaging, severely injured patients may need airway protection and control. Intubation is often necessary in ventilatory failure and also decreases work of breathing thus decreasing the body's oxygen demands.

Improving circulation and perfusion is the cornerstone of shock treatment. It begins with early goal-directed fluid resuscitation, which has been shown to improve survival. Fluids should be administered immediately with the goal of improving deranged physiological parameters. In its initial stages the clinician should aim for mental status improvement, urine output increase, lactic acidosis correction, normalization of capillary refill and blood pressure rise.

Fluid administration can be in the form of crystalloid (normal saline or Hartmann's solution) or colloid (albumin, Gelofusine). While there was some concern that colloid solutions might lead to a slightly increased mortality, a larger and more recent meta-analysis disputed this claim. Furthermore, a well-designed multi-centre randomized controlled study of critically ill patients failed to find a difference in outcome in patients resuscitated with normal saline versus albumin. Thus, it is the appropriate administration of fluid rather than the fluid itself that is important. Blood and blood products may also be judiciously used as resuscitative fluids in patients in shock. Certainly, blood replacement should accompany fluid replacement in an actively haemorrhaging patient. Red blood cell transfusion can also be useful to increase oxygen delivery.

After fluid resuscitation begins, the clinician should quickly assess the patient's response. In addition to improvement, patients should also be monitored for any signs of volume overload (such as pulmonary oedema or increased jugular venous distension). If physiological markers are not improving, then more objective parameters and invasive monitoring will probably be needed to guide further therapy. Central venous pressure monitoring or echocardiogram can be very useful in determining fluid status. Echocardiogram has the additional benefit of looking at cardiac function. Cardiac output monitoring may be necessary for shock that is unresponsive to treatment and may aid in determining the type of shock encountered. (Please refer to invasive monitoring section.)

Vasoactive drugs should not routinely be part of initial resuscitation efforts. Vasoconstrictors increase blood pressure and thus may cause clinicians to prematurely limit needed fluid resuscitation. Such drugs should be utilized when patients remain shocked despite adequate filling and often should be used with invasive monitoring.

In the following section, we will address the major categories of shock. A summary table of the

Table 13.4 Summary of haemodynamic variables in different types of shock

	Cardiogenic shock	Hypovolaemic shock	Obstructive shock (tamponade)	Obstructive shock (PE)	Distributive shock (neurogenic)	Distributive shock (sepsis/SIRS)
HR	↑ → ↓	↑	↑	↑	↑ → ↓	↑
BP	↓	↓	↓	↓	↓	↓
CVP	↑ →	↓	↑	↑ →	↓	↓
CO	↓	↓	↓	↓	↑	↑
PAOP	↑	↓	Equalization of diastolic pressure with CVP	↑ → ↓	↓	↓
SVR	↑	↑	↑	↑	↓	↓

↑, increased; ↓, decreased; →, neutral; ↑→↓, variable.

haemodynamic disturbances associated with each type of shock is provided for a reference in Table 13.4. Recognizing trends is important in helping to distinguish a patient's type of shock and administering appropriate treatment. Nevertheless, it should also be recognized that patients may have several aetiologies for their haemodynamic compromise (e.g. cardiogenic and hypovolaemic shock). Keeping an open mind and frequently re-assessing responses to therapy will ensure the best outcome in this critically ill group.

Cardiogenic shock

Cardiogenic shock refers to intrinsic pump failure, or failure of the heart to generate a sufficient cardiac output despite adequate filling (preload). Cardiogenic shock may be due to a variety of causes including myocardial infarction, cardiac contusion (trauma), arrhythmia, or valvular abnormality. In cardiogenic shock, patients' extremities are cold and have delayed capillary refill. Patients often demonstrate clinical signs related to the aetiology of their cardiac failure. They may have an elevated jugular venous pressure (RV failure), pulmonary crackles (LV failure), an irregular heartbeat (arrhythmia) or murmur. Invasive parameters reveal a decreased cardiac output and increased SVR (a reflection of their compensatory increase in vasomotor tone). CVP varies, but is generally elevated as the heart fails and cannot adequately distribute the venous return.

The classic cause of cardiogenic shock is systolic dysfunction or left ventricular heart failure. With LV failure, left heart stroke volume is diminished and there is subsequent increase in left atrial pressure and pulmonary artery pressure. This manifests clinically as

pulmonary oedema, but will be demonstrated as an increase in the PAOP in patients with PA catheters. Acute coronary syndromes (ischaemia) are the most common cause of such dysfunction with cardiogenic shock occurring in up to 10% of patients sustaining an acute MI. If possible, early revascularization either by interventional cardiology or surgery has demonstrated survival benefits.

Treatment:

- Ensure adequate preload. Central venous catheter may be needed for guidance of fluid resuscitation
- Inotropes
- Reduction of afterload
- Intra-aortic balloon counterpulsation
- Correction of the cardiac abnormality. Modalities may include early revascularization (ischaemia), correction of the valvular abnormality (valvuloplasty, valve replacement), anti-arrhythmic, etc.

Hypovolaemic shock

Hypovolaemic shock occurs as a result of haemorrhage or severe dehydration. Patients at highest risk of dehydration are children and the elderly. Causes of dehydration may include diarrhoea, vomiting, heat (including burns), diuretic use, prolonged operation and fistula losses. A patient in hypovolaemic shock will have cold extremities with delayed capillary refill. They are often initially anxious and later somnolent. Invasive monitoring demonstrates a low CVP, a low CO and a high SVR.

Haemorrhagic shock has been divided into four classes based on the amount of blood lost and the

Table 13.5 Classification of haemorrhagic shock.

	Class 1	Class 2	Class 3	Class 4
Estimated blood loss (ml)	<750	750–1500	1500–2000	>2000
Estimated blood loss (% total blood volume)	<15%	15–30%	30–40%	>40%
Respiratory rate	14–20	20–30	30–40	>35
Heart rate	<100	>100	>120	>140
Blood pressure	Normal	Normal	Decreased	Decreased
Urine output (ml/hour)	>30	20–30	5–15	Negligible
Mental status	Slightly anxious	Mildly anxious	Anxious, confused	Confused, lethargic
Fluid replacement	Crystalloid	Crystalloid	Crystalloid + blood	Crystalloid + blood

Modified from Committee on Trauma of the American College of Surgeons, *Advanced Trauma Life Support*. 2004.

body's compensatory response [Table 13.5]. The body has significant ability to compensate for blood loss; hypotension is a late sign of haemorrhage, not occurring until 30–40% of the circulating blood volume is lost. Compensatory mechanisms include baroreceptor reflexes leading to an autonomic increase in myocardial contractility, tachycardia and peripheral vasoconstriction. Humoral mediators (vasopressin, aldosterone and renin) are released in an attempt to stabilize intravascular volume.

Ongoing bleeding should be treated with surgical control of the source and blood replacement. If there is difficulty or delay in controlling haemorrhage, initial compensatory mechanisms begin to fail. Myocardial depression occurs and vasomotor reflexes are lost. Hypoxic cells develop an altered membrane potential, allowing sodium and water influx into the cell and with subsequent cellular oedema. Organ failure may follow. A vicious triad of metabolic acidosis, hypothermia and coagulopathy begins to perpetuate itself, ultimately leading to arrhythmia and death.

Treatment:

- Fluid replacement
- Blood replacement in haemorrhagic shock. Of note, if massive transfusion (greater than 10 units of blood in a 24 hour period) is anticipated, patients should begin early transfusion of fresh frozen plasma and platelets to help avoid coagulopathy
- Surgical control of the bleeding source.

Obstructive shock

In obstructive shock, the heart is not able to deliver adequate output because of impedance of either blood inflow or outflow. Because the end result is a low cardiac output, the patient will be cold and clamped down. SVR will be increased with a compensatory tachycardia.

Inflow obstruction (tamponade and tension pneumothorax)

Inflow obstruction is primarily due to cardiac tamponade or tension pneumothorax. In tamponade, CVP will be dramatically increased as there is impedance to inflow and back up of venous return. Because the heart is being compressed externally, all of the pressures within the heart at rest (diastole) will be the same. Such 'equalization of pressures' is reflected by the PAOP (a reflection of left atrial pressure), pulmonary artery pressure, RV pressure and RA (or CVP) being the same in diastole. This finding is highly suggestive of cardiac tamponade. Please refer to the previous section for the causes, diagnosis and treatment of tamponade.

Tension pneumothorax is another source of inflow obstruction. In tension pneumothorax, the positive intrathoracic pressure pushes the heart toward the opposite side of the chest (away from the pneumothorax), distorting anatomy and impairing venous return. Treatment involves emergency needle decompression followed by thoracostomy drain placement.

Outflow obstruction (thromboembolism and air embolism)

Outflow obstruction is usually secondary to a pulmonary embolic event. In outflow obstruction, the right heart outflow tract (pulmonary arteries) is obstructed with emboli. This leads to impaired emptying of the right heart and right heart strain. Invasive monitoring will demonstrate an increased CVP. The PAOP is highly variable in this situation and is in no way diagnostic. Venous thromboembolism is the most common cause of outflow obstructive shock; it is discussed in detail later in this chapter.

Of note, air embolism is another embolic phenomenon seen in surgical patients. Air embolism occurs when a bolus of air travels through the venous system and becomes lodged in the right ventricular outflow tract. This bolus can occur if pressurized gas is forced into a body cavity, or it can occur when there is disruption of the venous system above the level of the heart. In this last situation, the pressure differential causes air to be 'sucked' into the vasculature. Air embolism most commonly occurs in the setting of neurosurgery or head and neck surgery when patients are in a seated operative position. Nevertheless, it can also be seen as a complication of central venous access, in penetrating vascular trauma or with an injury to the pulmonary hilum involving both vessel and bronchus. Approximately 50 ml of air is needed to cause haemodynamic compromise; the lethal dose is probably around 100–300 ml of air. Treatment of air embolism is to first suspect it. Next, the patient should be positioned in the head down and left lateral decubitus position (Durant's manoeuvre) such that the bolus of air drifts to the apex of the right ventricle away from the outflow tract. After this, the aims are to prevent further air entry (clamp the pulmonary hilum, if due to an injury), if possible aspirate the air versus give it time to reabsorb, and provide haemodynamic support. Some authors recommend a trial of aspirating the air from a central venous catheter positioned at the level of the right atrium.

Distributive shock

There are three types of distributive shock; they are neurogenic, anaphylaxis and sepsis/SIRS. The clinical picture of distributive shock differs from other forms of shock as the mechanism is loss of peripheral vascular tone. Patients tend to be peripherally warm and may even have an increased capillary refill. The diastolic blood pressure is low. The heart compensates by increasing its rate and contractility, thus resulting in a high cardiac output state. Invasive monitoring demonstrates a low CVP, low SVR and a high CO. Of note, there is a small subset of septic patients who demonstrate myocardial depression; the reason behind this is still uncertain.

Neurogenic shock

Neurogenic shock occurs because of disruption of sympathetic innervation to peripheral vessels leading to venodilatation and venous pooling. It is seen in high spinal anaesthesia and more commonly in injury to the cervical or high thoracic spinal cord. Most patients will demonstrate reflexive tachycardia; however, injuries of the cervical cord tend to be associated with sinus bradycardia. Neurogenic shock occurs immediately after a spinal cord injury and is self-limiting, generally resolving several days after the insult.

Treatment:

- Volume expansion to fill the expanded intravascular space
- Vasopressors. This is the one shock state where a pure alpha-agonist (phenylephrine) may be judiciously used to counteract the loss of vascular tone. Adequate filling should be ensured prior to initiation of such agents.

Anaphylactic shock

Anaphylactic shock is the severest form of an allergic reaction in which a sensitized individual releases histamine in response to antigen exposure. This response leads to peripheral vasodilatation and potentially haemodynamic instability (shock). Other symptoms include wheezing and respiratory distress, swelling of the throat and mucous membranes, itching, and urticaria.

Treatment:

- ABCs (patients may have airway and breathing compromise as well)
- Volume expansion to fill the expanded intravascular space
- Intravenous epinephrine
- Anti-histamines
- Steroids.

Septic shock

Septic shock is the extreme end of the spectrum in the entities of systemic inflammation. It is defined as hypotension – unresponsive to fluid resuscitation or requiring the use of vasopressors – in a patient with a severe inflammatory response to a source of infection. Please refer to the section on SIRS, sepsis and MODS for a detailed discussion of the definition and treatment of these complicated disorders.

Respiratory system

Physiology

Work of breathing

During quiet respiration, inspiration occurs through diaphragmatic contraction decreasing the intrathoracic pressure and drawing air into the respiratory tree. This pressure must be great enough to overcome airway resistance and the compliance of the lungs and chest wall. Elastic recoil is responsible for expiration and the whole process of breathing utilizes very little energy – only 1–2% of the total body oxygen consumption. During active respiration, the accessory muscles are used for inspiration and the abdominal muscles and internal intercostals are used for expiration. Much more energy is required and the work of breathing may consume as much as 25% of the body's total oxygen consumption. It is little wonder that compromised patients quickly fatigue with such an increased work of breathing.

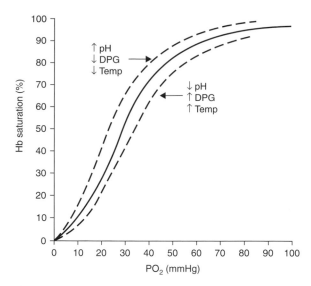

Figure 13.8 The haemoglobin dissociation curve. Note the effects on pH, DPG, and temperature allowing for alterations in oxygen unloading at a given partial pressure of oxygen. A shift of the curve to the right indicates that haemoglobin will remain less saturated for a given pO₂.

Regulation of respiration

The respiratory system supplies O_2 and removes CO_2 over a wide range of metabolic demands. Control is exercised by the respiratory centre located in the medulla oblongata and pons. There is a dorsal and a ventral group of neurons in the medulla. The dorsal group within the medulla functions during quiet respiration and acts as the pacemaker by initiating inspiration. The ventral group is more important during active respiration. The pons contains the apnoeuistic and pneumotaxic centres. The apnoeuistic centre responds to stimuli by enhancing inspiration and helps control the depth of respiration. The pneumotaxic centre inhibits inspiration so that it does not continue too long.

The respiratory centre receives input from higher brain centres and from chemo- and mechanoreceptors. There are two major stimuli to breathe – acidosis and hypoxia. Central chemoreceptors are located in the medulla and are sensitive to acidosis in the form of CO_2 (as hydrogen ions cannot cross the blood–brain or blood–CSF barriers directly). The CO_2 binds with water and produces hydrogen ions, which act on the pacemaker (dorsal group of neurons) and stimulate respiration. Peripheral chemoreceptors are located in the carotid and aortic bodies and respond to falls in arterial pO_2 below 8 kPa (60 mmHg).

They provide input to the higher brain centres and brainstem to increase respiration. Mechanoreceptors include stretch receptors, irritant receptors and juxtacapillary receptors. Stretch receptors inhibit the level of inspiration and juxtacapillary (or J) receptors are thought to be important in the sensation of dyspnoea.

Haemoglobin dissociation curve

There are four iron atoms in a haemoglobin molecule and each can bind one molecule of oxygen in a reversible interaction. As haemoglobin binds oxygen it changes its conformation and takes up oxygen more readily. This accounts for the sigmoid-shaped haemoglobin dissociation curve (Figure 13.8). As demonstrated by the curve, haemoglobin binds oxygen rapidly to a PaO_2 of 8 kPa (60 mmHg) and then levels off, requiring higher partial pressures of oxygen to remain fully saturated. Another way of looking at it is that a PaO_2 of 60 mmHg is required to maintain saturations above 90%. This is important physiologically, because it allows for the easy off-loading of oxygen in the peripheral capillary beds where oxygen is needed (i.e. if the PaO_2 is low in the periphery, haemoglobin gives up its oxygen molecule easily). Factors such as acidosis, increased temperature and increased 2,3-DPG shift the haemoglobin dissociation

Table 13.6 Causes of metabolic acidosis

High anion gap metabolic acidosis		Non-anion gap metabolic acidosis	
Methanol/metformin	Lactic acidosis	Gastrointestinal	Renal
Uraemia	Ethylene glycol	Diarrhoea	Renal tubular acidosis
Paraldehyde	Rhabdomyolysis	Hyperalimentation	Mineralocorticoid deficiency
Isonizaid	Salicylates	Ureteral diversion (ureteroileostomy)	Acetazolamide

curve to the right, resulting in easier unloading of oxygen for a given PaO_2.

Interpretation of special investigations

Arterial blood gas (ABG)

An arterial blood gas (ABG) is one of the most important and heavily utilized tests in the ICU. It provides rapid information about the patient's respiratory status (oxygenation and ventilation) and acid-base status. An ABG can be withdrawn from any artery and should be analysed immediately (or immersed in iced water) to provide accurate information.

Normal values for an ABG from a healthy adult are:

pH	7.35–7.45
PO_2	10–13 kPa (75–100 mmHg)
PCO_2	4.8–6.1 kPa (36–46 mmHg)
Actual HCO_3	22–26
Base deficit	0–2.5

Oxygenation is assessed by the patient's PaO_2 and O_2 saturation (SaO_2). Arterial hypoxaemia occurs when the PaO_2 is <8 kPa (60 mmHg). Because of the haemoglobin dissociation curve (see above), patients with a PaO_2 <8 kPa are at significant risk of hypoxic respiratory failure. Ventilation is assessed by the $PaCO_2$. If the patient is hyperventilating, the $PaCO_2$ will be low. If the patient is hypoventilating, the $PaCO_2$ will be elevated. Patients with a $PaCO_2$ >6.7 kPa may be demonstrating ventilatory failure.

ABG interpretation is critical in assessing a patient's acid-base status and should be performed systematically. First, the arterial pH indicates whether the patient is acidaemic or alkalaemic. Next the $PaCO_2$ and the bicarbonate are inspected. In respiratory acidosis, the $PaCO_2$ will be elevated. A primary respiratory acidosis occurs when patients are hypoventilating such as in the event of a narcotic overdose. In respiratory alkalosis, the $PaCO_2$ will be low as the patient is hyperventilating and blowing off CO_2 rapidly. An acute event such as a PE or early sepsis will often induce tachypnoea, with respiratory alkalosis being a first early sign on the ABG.

The bicarbonate tells you of the metabolic component of the patient's acid-base status. Metabolic acidosis occurs as a result of increased hydrogen ions or loss of bicarbonate. Either way, on the ABG, the bicarbonate is low. Metabolic acidosis needs to be evaluated further with a determination of the anion gap (AG). The AG is a measure of the unmeasured anions in the plasma that result in an accumulation of hydrogen ions. Reference range is 8–16 mmol/l.

$$AG = Na^+ - (Cl^- + HCO_3^-)$$

Causes of elevated anion gap acidosis and non-anion gap acidosis are listed in Table 13.6. You will note that anion gap acidosis arises from exogenous acids being introduced into the body, whereas non-anion gap acidosis is due to bicarbonate loss from either the gastrointestinal or renal system.

Metabolic alkalosis is reflected by an elevated serum bicarbonate. Causes of metabolic alkalosis include vomiting or nasogastric tube suction, hyperaldosteronism, iatrogenic administration of alkali (hyperalimentation or citrate from banked blood transfusion) and contraction alkalosis (often associated with diuretic use).

Importantly, the primary acid-base disturbance will generally be accompanied by a compensatory response. For example, if a primary metabolic acidosis occurs, the body responds by increasing ventilation (respiratory alkalosis). However, not uncommonly in severely ill patients, mixed disorders may be present. For example, a patient who has sustained cardiac arrest may have both a metabolic and respiratory acidosis, the metabolic acidosis occurring as a result of the absence of perfusion and the respiratory acidosis from the absence of respiration.

Oxygenation assessment

Pulse oximetry

Pulse oximetry measures arterial oxygen saturation. It utilizes a spectrometric method in which light of two known wavelengths is transmitted through a pulsating vascular bed. The amount of light transmitted through the vascular bed depends on the proportions of oxygenated and deoxygenated haemoglobin. By evaluating the amount of light absorption, it is possible to obtain an estimate of the relative proportion of oxygenated haemoglobin (i.e. saturation). Fingers, toes and earlobes have good vascular beds that can be used for oximetry. Pulse oximetry is an extremely useful tool, but does have limitations. Readings can be difficult to obtain in patients with poor perfusion (hypotensive) or may be inaccurate in patients with very dark skin/nail polish (falsely low) or haemoglobinopathies (falsely high in metHb and COHb). An ABG should be checked in such patients to ensure adequate oxygenation.

Transcutaneous oxygen monitoring

Electrodes applied to the skin can estimate PaO_2 (and $PaCO_2$) in a non-invasive manner. The electrodes are heated, inducing a local hyperperfusion, PO_2 readings are obtained, and calibration and correlation to formal blood gases are established. Good correlation between transcutaneous PO_2 and PaO_2 is found in neonates, who have very thin epidermal layers; thus, this technology has been utilized for years in neonatal ICUs. Thicker epidermal layers in adults lead to increased variability in readings and blood gas correlations, making it a less utilized but still actively studied tool in adult ICUs.

Alveolar gas equation and alveolar-arterial gradient

One way to evaluate the cause of hypoxia is to look at the difference in the partial pressure of oxygen within the alveolus (PAO_2) compared to the partial pressure of oxygen within the arteries (PaO_2). Normally, the difference between alveolar and arterial oxygen pressures is relatively small. However, when there is significant lung pathology, there is a disconnect between ventilation and perfusion. When V/Q mismatch occurs, as the FiO_2 (and therefore PAO_2) is increased, PaO_2 does not increase accordingly.

PAO_2 is calculated by the alveolar gas equation. The partial pressure of oxygen within the alveoli equals the amount of oxygen inspired minus the amounts of water and CO_2 within the alveoli. The equation is as follows:

$$PAO_2 = [FiO_2(P_{atm} - P_{H20})] - PaCO_2/0.8$$

From here, the alveolar to arterial (A-a) gradient can be determined.

$$A\text{-a gradient} = PAO_2 - PaO_2.$$

Often, the A-a gradient will be reported on the ABG. The normal A-a gradient is age-dependent and is estimated by the equation (Age + 10) / 4. Nevertheless, for ease of recollection, a normal A-a gradient is <25 mmHg. An A-a gradient > 25 mmHg indicates significant V/Q mismatch and the cause of lung pathology should be sought and treated. Hypoxaemia with a normal A-a gradient is usually secondary to hypoventilation, but may be a function of altitude as well.

Capnography

Capnography is the continuous monitoring of CO_2 in the respiratory gases of intubated patients. A CO_2 sensor is attached to the endotracheal tube and the CO_2 in the expired gas is measured by an infrared absorption spectrometer. When CO_2 is recorded over time, a 'capnogram' is produced. A value known as the end tidal CO_2 ($ETCO_2$) can be determined from capnography. $ETCO_2$ is the measurement of CO_2 at the end of expiration, just before inspiration is initiated.

In normal subjects, the $ETCO_2$ closely reflects the $PaCO_2$, though there should be a difference of 2–5 mmHg (1 kPa). The $ETCO_2$ will always be slightly lower than the $PaCO_2$ because there is mixing of the alveolar air with air in the physiological dead space. An ABG is done at the time that capnography is set up to see how the two correlate. The difference between the arterial CO_2 and the $ETCO_2$ reflects V/Q mismatch.

Lung pathology exacerbates V/Q mismatch and will be manifested in a change in $ETCO_2$. For example, if a patient suddenly develops a mucus plug and stops ventilating several segments of lung, the $ETCO_2$ will decrease and the difference between arterial CO_2 and $ETCO_2$ increases as a result of the V/Q mismatch. $ETCO_2$ also changes with alterations in cardiac output and pulmonary blood flow; decrease in cardiac output/pulmonary blood flow will cause a decrease in

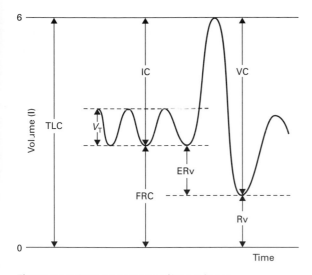

Figure 13.9 Spirometric tracing of lung volumes.

$ETCO_2$. Evaluation of the capnographic waveform can give clues to alterations of the ventilator circuit or airway obstruction. Overall, $ETCO_2$ monitoring can contribute significantly to evaluating minute-to-minute cardiopulmonary changes in a ventilated patient and is frequently used by anaesthetists. It is also being increasingly used as a tool to confirm correct intubation in emergency situations.

Pulmonary function tests (PFT)

Lung volumes are measured by spirometry and once quantified can be compared against predicted values for the size, age and gender of the patient. An example of a spirometry tracing is provided in Figure 13.9 and an explanation of these volumes is provided below.

Tidal volume (V_T) is the volume of air inspired or expired per breath.
  Normal tidal volume = 500 ml.
Minute ventilation is the volume of air inspired or expired over 1 min.
  Minute ventilation = V_T × Respiratory rate.
  Normal minute ventilation = 5–7 l/min.
Total lung capacity (TLC) is the volume of air in the lungs after maximal inspiration (6 l). TLC equals the sum of the vital capacity and the residual volume.
Vital capacity (VC) is the maximal volume of air that can be exhaled after a maximal inspiration. It depends on the strength of the respiratory muscles and the resistance of the lungs and chest wall.
  Normal vital capacity is approximately 4.8 l.

Forced expiratory volume in 1 s (FEV_1) is the volume of air that can be forcibly exhaled in one second.
Functional residual capacity (FRC) is the volume of air left in the lungs after exhalation (2.2 l). It is a critical volume because it allows for gas exchange throughout the entire respiratory cycle. FRC decreases with anaesthesia, obesity, surgery (particularly thoracic and abdominal) and increasing age. When the FRC is too low, atelectasis occurs resulting in hypoxaemia. Recruitment manoeuvres to open alveoli (e.g. PEEP) are aimed at increasing FRC.
Residual volume (RV) is the amount of air remaining in the lungs after a maximal expiration (1.2 l).

Diffusion capacity of carbon monoxide (DL_{CO}) is the ability of CO to diffuse across intact alveoli. This study is often performed in conjunction with spirometry. The patient inhales a small known quantity of CO, holds his breath for 10 seconds, and then exhales. The expired gas is analysed for CO. A low DL_{CO} implies that there is a ventilation perfusion mismatch and is often seen in disorders that disrupt normal alveolar architecture (emphysema or pulmonary fibrosis). It can also be present in severe anaemia. Alternatively, DL_{CO} may be increased in patients with polycythaemia.

Measurements of VC and FEV_1 are useful in determining whether obstructive, restrictive or mixed airway disease is present. FEV_1 is also one of the best predictors of outcome for patients about to undergo pulmonary resection (for example in lung cancer). In general, a patient with a FEV_1 greater than 2 l or 60% predicted and DL_{CO} >60% is at low risk of complications even for pneumonectomy.

Respiratory failure

The respiratory system has two major functions: provide oxygen to meet the metabolic demands of the body (oxygenation) and remove carbon dioxide, the byproduct of metabolism, from the body (ventilation). As such, respiratory failure is the failure of oxygenation, ventilation, or both.

Hypoxaemic respiratory failure is failure of oxygenation. It is characterized by a PaO_2 <8 kPa (<60 mmHg). There are four causes of hypoxaemic respiratory failure (Table 13.7). The most common

Table 13.7 Causes, pathophysiology, and examples of respiratory failure

V/Q mismatch	Shunt	Hypoventilation	Diffusion abnormalities
Ventilation to areas of lung which are not adequately perfused	In essence, blood bypasses alveoli such that gas exchange does not occur	Decreased ventilation due to a variety of causes	Thickened alveolar membrane impairs diffusion
Pulmonary embolism	Pulmonary consolidation (pneumonia, oedema, ARDS)	Neurological event	Pulmonary fibrosis
Obstructive airway disease	Atelectasis Cardiac R→L shunt	Drugs/narcotic overdose Muscular weakness	ARDS

cause of hypoxaemia is ventilation/perfusion (V/Q) mismatch. V/Q mismatch occurs when ventilated portions of the lung are not being perfused or when perfused portions of the lung are not being ventilated. Either way, the alveolar PO_2 will be greater than arterial PaO_2 with a resultant increase in the alveolar-arterial gradient. V/Q mismatch affects oxygenation more than ventilation. Because CO_2 diffuses much more easily (and quickly) than oxygen, when hypoxia causes respiratory stimulation CO_2 is rapidly cleared. Thus, PCO_2 may be normal or decreased.

In discussing hypoxaemic failure, the term 'V/Q mismatch' is usually reserved for a situation in which ventilation occurs, but not in areas that are being perfused. Classic examples are pulmonary thromboembolism or air embolism. Alternatively, 'shunting' refers to a situation in which the alveoli are perfused, but not ventilated. This can occur because the alveoli are collapsed (atelectasis) or full of fluid (pneumonia or pulmonary oedema). Intracardiac defects that result in blood flow from the right to left heart bypassing the lungs are also a form of shunt. Hypoxaemia due to V/Q mismatch improves with the administration of supplemental oxygen. On the other hand, in shunting, deoxygenated blood essentially bypasses alveoli. Thus, supplemental oxygen is much less useful in correcting hypoxaemia secondary to shunt pathology.

Hypoventilation is a less common cause of respiratory failure, but is always associated with hypercapnia. In hypoventilation, the patient has insufficient minute ventilation, but the alveolar and arterial relationship is maintained. Thus, there is a normal alveolar-arterial gradient in hypoventilation. Hypoxia due to hypoventilation responds to supplemental oxygen as it increases the alveolar PO_2.

Hypercapnic respiratory failure is failure of ventilation. It is characterized by a $PaCO_2$ >6.7 kPa (>50 mmHg). As was just discussed, hypoventila-

tion tends to cause both hypercapnia and hypoxaemia. Hypoventilation may be caused by CNS depression (drugs, opiates) or by pathology of the brainstem (infarction, compression). Peripheral nervous system involvement (spinal cord injury, myasthenia) and respiratory muscle or chest wall abnormalities may also cause ventilatory failure.

It should be noted that in late stages of any cause of respiratory failure combined failure of oxygenation and ventilation is the norm. Thus, even causes of primarily hypoxaemic respiratory failure (ARDS, COAD) will lead to hypercapnia as the disease progresses. Patients who develop acute respiratory failure are often anxious and complain of feeling short of breath. Alternatively, they may be confused or even somnolent. On examination, signs of respiratory failure include cyanosis, use of accessory muscles and stridor. Patients may be tachypnoeic or hypoventilating. Tachycardia is also a common sign. Work-up of a patient with acute respiratory failure involves a thorough history and physical examination, chest radiograph, ECG and ABG. Supplemental studies such as CT scan, bronchoscopy and V/Q scan can be done at the evaluator's discretion.

Mechanical ventilation

Indications for mechanical ventilation (MV) include:

- Inadequate oxygenation
  - PaO_2 <8 kPa (<60 mmHg) despite maximal supplemental oxygen

- Inadequate ventilation
  - Apnea or hypoventilation resulting in $PaCO_2$ >8 kPa (>60 mmHg)
  - Rapid shallow breathing (respiratory rate >35 breaths per minute with a tidal volume <5 ml/kg) – indicating inadequate ventilation and fatigue.

- Elective ventilation perioperatively in high-risk surgical cases
- Airway protection
- Airway obstruction (trauma/oedema/burn)
- Loss of ability to protect airway due to neurological event (CVA/head injury)

The clinical objectives of MV are to support a patient who is unable to meet the demands of the respiratory system until the cause of respiratory failure is identified and corrected. MV should relieve respiratory distress and decrease work of breathing. Correction of oxygenation and ventilation to physiological levels is ideal.

Establishing mechanical ventilation

In setting up MV, it is important to consider the amount of support that a patient requires, pulmonary mechanics, patient sedation/cooperation and underlying pathology. Ventilator settings are chosen with optimization of oxygenation and ventilation in mind.

Oxygenation is improved by providing more oxygen (increasing the fraction of inspired oxygen – FiO_2) or by recruiting more alveoli to be involved in gas exchange. Alveolar recruitment involves adding pressure through the ventilator circuit so that the alveoli do not collapse during expiration – positive end expiratory pressure (PEEP). PEEP keeps alveoli open so that gas exchange occurs through the duration of the respiratory cycle. FiO_2 should be reduced to the lowest possible level to maintain a PaO_2 >8 kPa (or SaO_2 ≥92%) to reduce complications of oxygen toxicity.

Adequate CO_2 exchange is based on appropriate minute ventilation. Minute ventilation depends on tidal volume and respiratory rate, both of which can be manipulated in MV. A normal tidal volume in a spontaneously breathing individual is about 5–7 ml/kg. While this volume is generally too small in mechanical ventilation (due to increased dead space), large tidal volumes have been associated with alveolar injury. Setting initial tidal volumes in the 7–8 ml/kg range is appropriate (unless acute lung injury is present – see below). Respiratory rates can be adjusted to obtain appropriate PCO_2 levels but are usually started at 10–14 breaths per minute.

Intermittent positive pressure ventilation (IPPV)

Patients with insufficient breaths (sedation, sepsis, trauma, etc.) or who cannot generate their own breaths (anaesthesia, paralysis) require the ventilator to do it for them. This is referred to as intermittent positive pressure ventilation (IPPV). 'Intermittent' refers to the cyclic nature of the machine-generated breaths and allows for gas exchange. 'Positive pressure' is the way in which the machine gives the breath. In normal breathing, inspiration occurs when the diaphragm contracts downward and a negative pressure is created, drawing air in. Ventilators 'force' air into the lungs during inspiration utilizing positive pressure.

IPPV employs either volume-cycled or pressure-cycled modes. In volume-cycled modes, a set tidal volume is administered during each inspiration. In pressure-cycled modes, air is administered until a preset pressure level is reached. With these fundamentals in mind, there are four main modes of IPPV.

Controlled mechanical ventilation (CMV)

CMV is a volume-cycled mode in which tidal volume and rate are fixed. All breaths are delivered by the ventilator and the patient does not contribute. CMV is used for the completely apnoeic (anaesthetized or paralysed) patient. It is poorly tolerated by a conscious or even moderately sedated patient; thus CMV is essentially an obsolete mode in the ICU setting.

Pressure control ventilation (PCV)

PCV is a pressure-cycled mode. Rate and airway pressure are set and the ventilator delivers a volume of air to achieve the preset pressure. PCV is useful when there is a need to restrict the upper airway pressure, but can lead to variability in tidal volume. In PCV, tidal volume changes based on pulmonary compliance; as the lungs become more compliant, a larger tidal volume will be administered per the same preset pressure. PCV is preferred by some for the ventilation of small children in order to reduce the risk of barotrauma. It seems to be a less comfortable mode for most adults.

Assist control (AC) ventilation

In AC, a breath is delivered when triggered by the patient's inspiratory effort or after a preset time if the patient does not breathe. Thus, each time the patient attempts to take a breath, the slight negative pressure is sensed by the ventilator and fully supported breath is given by the machine (Figure 13.10). AC is available in volume-cycled 'volume control' or pressure-targeted 'pressure control' modes. In 'volume control AC', volume and rate are set and a fixed tidal volume is

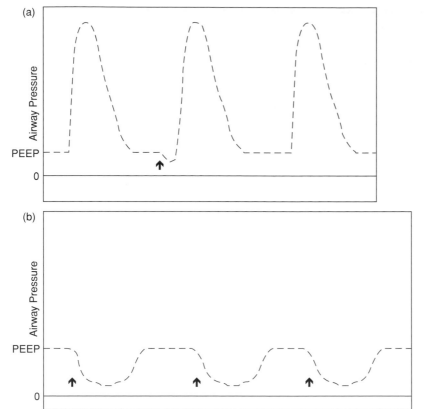

Figure 13.10 Airway pressure curves in IPPV (A) and CPAP (B). (↑) indicates a patient-initiated breath. (A) Positive pressure inspiration in IPPV. The represented mode is 'Volume control AC + PEEP'. The patient receives supported breaths at the pre-set rate, but additionally gets a fully supported breath with each effort (↑). (B) CPAP delivers supportive continuous positive pressure with airway pressures maintained above zero. Note how patient-initiated breaths are always associated with a negative deflection.

delivered with each breath, triggered or set. This is a highly supportive mode of ventilation that is better tolerated by conscious or semiconscious patients.

Intermittent mandatory ventilation (IMV) and synchronized intermittent mandatory ventilation (SIMV)

IMV and SIMV are volume-cycled modes, thus a tidal volume and rate are set. IMV delivers a preset tidal volume according to the rate that is set, and it allows for additional spontaneous breaths in between the mandatory breaths. In SIMV, mandatory breaths are delivered at regular time intervals synchronized with the patient's respiration. Thus, if the patient makes an inspiratory effort, the ventilator delivers its mandatory breath for that time interval. Additional patient breaths may be taken in between mandatory breaths but, unlike A/C, these breaths are on the patient's own and not fully supported. IMV and SIMV were originally designed to function as weaning modes in that the number of mandatory breaths could be slowly reduced, allowing the patient to assume more and more responsibility for the work of breathing.

Aside from the standard modes of IPPV, additional amounts of pressure support can be given to mechanically ventilated patients. These are discussed below.

Pressure support ventilation (PSV)

PSV is supplemental positive pressure administered to assist the spontaneously ventilating patient. When the patient makes an inspiratory effort, the fall in airway pressure triggers the ventilator to assist inspiration. The ventilator supplements the patient's effort by supplying gas to a preselected pressure. As its name suggests, it supports ventilation. PSV can be administered independently or be incorporated into an IPPV mode. For example, isolated PSV may be used for ventilator weaning; support is gradually decreased as the patient assumes more of the work of breathing. Alternatively, in SIMV with pressure support, a patient's spontaneous, unsynchronized breaths are augmented with this extra positive pressure.

Positive end expiratory pressure (PEEP)

As discussed above, with PEEP, airway pressures are maintained above atmospheric pressure at the end of expiration. This is done by attaching a valve to the expiratory end of the ventilator circuit to create resistance and prevent the airway pressure from ever reaching zero. PEEP means that a positive pressure is applied even during expiration. PEEP recruits alveoli, increases the functional residual capacity and thus improves oxygenation. PEEP can supplement the previously discussed modes of mechanical ventilation. Addition of PEEP often allows for decreased levels of FiO_2.

Continuous positive airway pressure (CPAP)

CPAP is a continuous positive pressure administered through the ventilator circuit (Figure 13.10). It is, essentially, pressure support (inspiratory positive pressure) plus PEEP (expiratory positive pressure). CPAP provides supplemental pressure to patients who are breathing spontaneously. Patients can be weaned from the ventilator using steadily decreasing levels of CPAP.

Complications of mechanical ventilation

While MV is critical to the supportive care of patients with respiratory failure, it is not without its own complications.

Animal and human studies have found that MV can actually cause lung injury. Ventilator-induced lung injury (VILI) is probably secondary to over-distension of alveoli caused by the tidal volume delivered by the ventilator – volutrauma. The previous notion that VILI is related to ventilatory pressures – barotrauma – is being challenged. Low tidal volume strategies are being studied with increased interest and have become standard of care in the treatment of ARDS (see below). Shear injury – caused when completely collapsed alveoli are popped open by positive pressure volumes of air – may also be a contributing factor to VILI. Repeated popping open and collapse ultimately causes injury to the delicate alveoli, leading to their disruption. Adding PEEP helps keep alveoli from collapsing completely and has been shown to reduce shear-related injury.

Intubated patients are also at risk for ventilator-associated pneumonia (VAP), with the chance of developing pneumonia increasing the longer the patient is ventilated. Risk of VAP is 3% per day for the first 5 days of ventilation, 2% per day for days 5–10, and 1% per day for days 10–15. The diagnosis of VAP is based on clinical and radiological findings. Two of the following suggest VAP: fever $>38°C$, leukocytosis, purulent tracheal secretions, or worsening oxy-

genation. Additionally, a new or progressive infiltrate should be apparent on chest radiograph. Once VAP is suspected, cultures need to be obtained and broad-spectrum antibiotics initiated immediately. VAP can be difficult to treat since the organisms may be drug-resistant and patients immunocompromised.

MV can cause haemodynamic instability because positive pressure increases intrathoracic pressure and can impede venous return to the heart. The decreased preload can lead to hypotension, especially with PEEP >15. Respiratory muscle dysfunction and wasting can occur with prolonged periods of MV and technical complications (tube dislodgement, kinking, disconnections) are possible.

Discontinuing mechanical ventilation

The daily evaluation of any intubated patient should include the thought: is the patient ready for extubation and if not, why not? Seeking and reversing any contributing factors to ongoing respiratory failure is an important part of the ventilatory discontinuation process. Witholding sedation daily to assess level of cognition and potential for extubation has also been shown to decrease time of ventilation.

Discontinuation of MV should be considered when the patient displays:

- evidence of reversal for the underlying cause of respiratory failure
- adequate oxygenation (PaO_2/FiO_2 ratio >27, PEEP $<5–8$ cmH_2O, $FiO_2 \leq 40–50\%$)
- adequate ventilation and correction of acid-base status (pH ≥ 7.25)
- haemodynamic stability
- capability to initiate an inspiratory effort
- capability to clear secretions.

Accurately determining whether or not a patient requires MV is important. There is currently no reliable predictor of weaning success. Several of the most promising predictors of successful extubation include a respiratory rate <38 breaths per minute and a rapid shallow breathing index (RSBI) of <105 breaths per minute per litre. RSBI is calculated as the ratio between the patient's spontaneous breathing rate and his spontaneous tidal volume (RSBI $=$ rate/V_T). Intubated patients who breathe spontaneously at a lower rate and a larger tidal volume have greater extubation success than those who exhibit rapid, shallow breathing.

Tracheostomy

A tracheostomy is a surgically created opening within the trachea which can be cannulated to allow for long-term MV. Indications for tracheostomy include:

- prolonged ventilatory insufficiency (>2 weeks)
  - may be secondary to prolonged pulmonary insufficiency (multiple chest injuries or ARDS), long-term unconsciousness (coma), or paralysis (spinal cord injury)

- airway obstruction (e.g. maxillofacial trauma, pharyngeal oedema)
- post-laryngectomy or pharyngo-laryngectomy
- paralysis of the swallowing apparatus to prevent aspiration (e.g. bulbar palsy)
- to facilitate weaning from mechanical ventilation.

Tracheostomies have certain advantages over orotracheal intubation. They improve patient comfort, decrease sedation requirements, allow for easier pulmonary toilet and facilitate ventilator weaning. Tracheostomies can be done via a standard open or percutaneous technique. In either situation, the tracheostomy is ideally positioned between the second and third tracheal cartilage. Complications of tracheostomy placement include bleeding, injury to local structures, misplacement of the tube and loss of airway. Long-term complications are tracheitis, tracheal stenosis, tube dislodgement and tracheo-innominate artery or tracheo-oesophageal fistula.

Pulmonary embolism

Pulmonary emboli primarily originate from lower extremity deep venous thrombosis, but embolization from other veins (axillary, subclavian, iliac, and pelvic) does occur. Risk factors for pulmonary embolism (PE) are listed in Table 13.8. Critically ill surgical patients are at particularly high risk and daily prophylaxis with either subcutaneous heparin or low molecular weight heparin (LMWH) is in order.

Clinical presentation and diagnosis

Patients with PE most commonly present with acute shortness of breath and hypoxia, with or without associated pleuritic type chest pain. They may have a new-onset tachycardia and low-level pyrexia is not uncommon. Clinically, patients tend to have unremarkable examinations unless they have new findings of right

Table 13.8 Risk factors for pulmonary embolism

Immobilization	Pregnancy	Surgery
Bed rest	Increasing age	(particularly orthopaedic, pelvic,
Trauma	Obesity	and major abdominal)
Spinal cord injury	Central venous access	
Malignancy	Hypercoagulable states	

heart failure. Occasionally, unilateral leg swelling will be supportive of the diagnosis.

ECG most commonly shows sinus tachycardia or non-specific ST changes. Right heart strain with the classic S1Q3T3 pattern may be seen with a large PE (Figure 13.11). CXR findings vary widely. A peripheral wedge-shaped infiltrate may suggest pulmonary infarction, yet non-specific cardiomegaly, infiltrates, effusions or atelectasis may also be seen. Incidentally, a normal CXR in the presence of new hypoxaemia may be one of the most suggestive signs of a pulmonary embolism. Thus, the major role of the ECG and CXR in the evaluation of PE is to exclude other primary cardiopulmonary pathology.

D-dimer assays have become an important tool in the evaluation of PE. The test is highly sensitive in the outpatient setting, with approximately 95% of patients with PE testing positive. Unfortunately, D-dimer assays are of limited use in postoperative patients or surgical trauma patients who already have an increased level of fibrinolysis present due to their primary insult. A positive result is essentially meaningless in this patient group. However, a negative D-dimer does virtually exclude PE as a cause of sudden-onset hypoxia in this setting.

Diagnostic modalities include computerized tomography pulmonary angiography (CTPA), ventilation perfusion (V/Q) scanning, duplex ultrasound, ECHO or pulmonary angiogram. CTPA has replaced V/Q scanning as the diagnostic modality of choice in evaluating a patient with PE. If the CTPA is negative, no further work-up is required. V/Q scan is still a useful diagnostic modality in some centres. V/Q scan results are reported as high, intermediate or low probability of PE. High-probability scans offer a reliable result in patients with a good clinical history. Unfortunately, only a minority of patients will have a high-probability scan. Conversely, patients with a low-probability scan and low clinical suspicion have

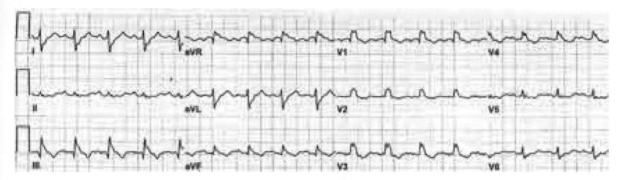

Figure 13.11 ECG findings in acute pulmonary embolism. The S1Q3T3 findings represent the volume and pressure overload experienced by the obstructed right ventricle ('right heart strain'). The S wave in lead I represents a complete or incomplete bundle branch block. The strain on the right ventricle leads to conduction abnormalities which account for the Q wave, mild ST segment elevation and T wave inversion seen in lead III.

a low probability of PE. The vast majority of patients however, fall into a 'non-diagnostic' category with intermediate-probability scans or low-probability scans and higher clinical suspicion. These patients will require further imaging.

Lower extremity Doppler can be a confirmatory study in a patient with clinical signs of DVT, because treatments for DVT and PE are the same. ECHO can detect massive pulmonary emboli. Pulmonary angiogram, while originally the gold standard, is less utilized with the improved accuracy of CT scanning and invasive nature of the angiogram.

Treatment

Anticoagulation is the treatment for PE and should be initiated once the thromboembolic event is suspected. A heparin infusion (goal PTT 1.5–2.0 above control) or subcutaneous LMWH is started immediately. LMWH is preferable to unfractionated heparin because of ease of use. Once the diagnosis is established, long-term anticoagulation with warfarin (target INR 2.0–3.0) should be organized. Thrombolysis is the treatment of choice in patients with massive PE manifested by haemodynamic instability or severe hypoxia. Alteplase 50 mg IV bolus is recommended. Surgical embolectomy may be considered in the unstable patient who has contraindications to or fails thrombolytic therapy.

Acute lung injury (ALI) and acute respiratory distress syndrome (ARDS)

ALI and ARDS are sudden-onset inflammatory-mediated conditions of the lungs resulting in pulmonary oedema and subsequent hypoxia. In 1994 the American–European Consensus Conference Committee established clinical criteria to define these conditions.

ARDS is defined by the following:

1. Acute onset
2. Bilateral pulmonary infiltrates on chest radiograph (Figure 13.12)
3. Pulmonary artery occlusion pressure <18 mmHg or absence of clinical evidence of left atrial hypertension
4. PaO_2/FiO_2 ratio $\leq$27 kPa (200 mmHg).

Evaluating these criteria closely, bilateral pulmonary infiltrates on chest X-ray are the clinical manifestation of pulmonary oedema. The critical aspect of the definition is the requirement that the PAOP is less than 18 or that there is lack of clinical evidence of left atrial hypertension. These criteria eliminate the heart as a cause of the observed oedema, and point to an inflammatory a etiology.

Pulmonary oedema leads to tissue hypoxia. Normally, an individual has a PaO_2 of 13 kPa on 21% FiO_2 (room air). The PaO_2/FiO_2 ratio then is 13/0.21 or 62. In ARDS, pulmonary oedema and disruption of the pulmonary architecture severely impair gas exchange (shunt pathology). Consequently, oxygenation remains poor despite increasing levels of oxygen. Mathematically, the PaO_2 is very low despite high levels of FiO_2, driving down the ratio to less than 27. For example, a patient with ARDS may require a FiO_2 of 70% to get a PaO_2 of 10 kPa. The PaO_2/FiO_2 ratio is 10/0.70 = 14. ALI implies a less severe form of lung injury and shares the definition of ARDS with

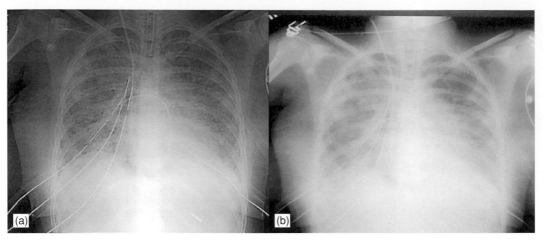

Figure 13.12 Chest radiographic findings in ARDS. (a) Note the bilateral patchy infiltrates necessary to make diagnosis of ARDS. (b) This CXR is of the same patient 12 hours later. It emphasizes how rapidly such patients can deteriorate and helps illustrate why oxygenation can be extremely difficult.

the exception that the PaO_2/FiO_2 ratio is ≤ 40 kPa (300 mmHg).

Aetiology

ARDS is seen in both medical and surgical patients and has an extensive list of causes. The most common cause of ARDS is sepsis. Sepsis may be pulmonary-related (pneumonia), but any septic focus can trigger the inflammatory cascade leading to ARDS. Other causes of ARDS in surgical patients include aspiration, inhalation injury, transfusion, pancreatitis and trauma.

Pathogenesis

Regardless of the inciting factor for ARDS, the lungs respond characteristically. Normally, alveoli are composed of an epithelial cell layer lying adjacent to a capillary endothelial cell layer. These thin layers permit necessary diffusion of oxygen and carbon dioxide. A prominent feature of early ARDS is epithelial and endothelial cell injury. Endothelial injury leads to a markedly increased vascular permeability and the influx of a protein-rich fluid into the alveolar space. Injured epithelial cells are unable to remove the fluid and do not make needed surfactant. As these cells are sloughed, denuded alveolar surfaces are lined by a thick hyaline membrane. Fluid-filled alveolar spaces and disruption of the alveolar architecture explain the problem with gas exchange seen in these patients. This

phase of ARDS is known as the acute or exudative phase and generally lasts 1–3 days.

A complex interplay of cytokines and inflammatory cells probably both causes this alveolar disruption as well as helping to resolve it. Neutrophils are prominent in early ARDS. Cytokines (such as IL-1, IL-6, IL-8, IL-10 and TNF-alpha) are secreted by macrophages and activate neutrophils. Inflammatory mediators also stimulate fibroblast activity and can lead to increased collagen deposition in the interstitial spaces.

While some patients quickly resolve their lung injury after the acute phase, others may go on to develop fibrotic lung changes and move into what is know as the proliferative phase of ARDS. In these patients at approximately 5–7 days, mesenchymal cells proliferate and there is increased collagen deposition in the alveolar spaces. This histological finding is known as fibrosing alveolitis and is associated with an increased mortality.

Ultimately, the injured alveoli enter a complicated process of repair. Type II alveolar epithelial cells differentiate into Type I cells to repopulate the alveolar lining. Fluid and protein are cleared from the alveolar space. Inflammatory cells are removed most likely by a combination of apoptosis and phagocytosis. Finally, remodelling of the fibrosis reestablishes normal alveolar architecture. While this process is successful in some patients, others are left with areas of tissue destruction, emphysema and fibrosis. At the current time, we cannot predict who will progress to long-term lung injury or how to prevent it.

Table 13.9 Classification of sepsis and systemic inflammatory response syndromes

Systemic inflammatory response syndrome (SIRS):
Two or more of the following:
Temperature >38°C or <36°C
Tachycardia – HR >90
Tachypnoea – RR >20 breaths/min or $PaCO_2$ <4.3 kPa (32 mmHg)
White cell count >12 000 or <4000 or >10% immature (band) cells
Sepsis
SIRS + established focus of infection
Severe sepsis
Sepsis + associated organ dysfunction and hypoperfusion as evidenced by one of the following:
Acute mental status change
Systolic blood pressure <90 mmHg or decreased normal systolic pressure by >40 mmHg
Lactic acidosis
Hypoxaemia
Oliguria
Hyperbilirubinaemia
Coagulopathy
Septic shock
Severe sepsis and
Hypotension not responsive to intravenous fluid resuscitation *or*
Need for inotropes or vasopressors to maintain blood pressure.

Table 13.10 Non-infectious causes of systemic inflammation

Pancreatitis	Burns
Ischaemia	Haemorrhagic shock and transfusion
Trauma	

Management

Management of ARDS involves treating the underlying cause and supportive care while the lungs recover. Mechanical ventilation is necessary in the vast majority of patients because of the profound hypoxia. To date, the biggest breakthrough in the management of ARDS came in 2000 in a landmark multi-centre, randomized controlled trial put forth by the US National Institutes of Health-funded ARDS Network. A total of 861 patients were randomized to either a conventional ventilator strategy using a 12 ml/kg body weight tidal volume or a low tidal volume strategy of 6 ml/kg. Mortality was 39.8% in the conventional group and 31% in the low tidal volume group, a reduction of 22% ($P = 0.007$). The trial was stopped early because of the significant findings. Low tidal volume ventilation has become standard of care in the ventilatory management of ARDS. Studies evaluating optimal PEEP, prone positioning, recruitment manoeuvres and alternative ventilation styles are ongoing.

Fluid management can be complicated in ARDS patients. Because the central pathology is pulmonary oedema, some people have advocated fluid restriction. The caveat to this is that the majority of these patients are systemically unwell and fluid restriction may come at the cost of reducing preload, cardiac output and thus organ perfusion. The randomized, multi-centre FACTT (Fluid and Catheter Therapy Trial) Study published in 2006 by the ARDS Network addressed these issues. The study concluded that conservative fluid management did reduce the number of ventilator days, but did not change overall survival. It also concluded that use of a pulmonary artery catheter to guide fluid resuscitation did not change outcome relative to using a standard central venous line. Current recommendations are to try and utilize a conservative volume strategy – resuscitating patients with the lowest possible volume to still maintain adequate tissue perfusion.

SIRS, sepsis and multiple organ dysfunction syndrome (MODS)

Definitions

In 1992, a consensus conference of the American College of Chest Physicians and the American Society of Critical Care Medicine published definitions of the systemic inflammatory response syndrome (SIRS) and sepsis syndromes (Table 13.9). In SIRS and sepsis, the body initiates an inflammatory response to an insult (Table 13.10) or infection. As the inflammatory process progresses, there is loss of vasomotor tone resulting in sepsis-induced hypotension and hypoperfusion. Hypoperfusion induces organ dysfunction and is termed 'severe sepsis'. If hypotension is unresponsive to fluids, the patient is in 'septic shock'. These definitions have been adopted worldwide and provide a universal language through which clinicians can discuss, research and improve outcomes in one of the most challenging entities we encounter. Sepsis remains the leading cause of mortality in critically ill patients.

MODS is the culmination of inflammatory events associated with SIRS and/or sepsis which leads to organ failure. It is characterized by the sequential failure of organs, usually starting with the lungs and progressively involving other organ systems. The mortality rate is high and increases with the number of organs involved: 30% when one organ fails and 100% when four organs fail.

Treatment

Significant international research is slowly leading to improved outcomes in septic patients. In 2004, the 'Surviving Sepsis Campaign' was established to assess available literature and expert opinion and produce evidence-based recommendations for the management of severe sepsis and septic shock. This campaign was a worldwide initiative of the European Society of Intensive Care Medicine, the International Sepsis Forum and the Society of Critical Care Medicine. The campaign concluded its funding at the end of 2008 and final recommendations were recently published. The recommendations are summarized below. The major components of treating sepsis are: resuscitation, source (infection) control, antibiotics and supportive care.

Resuscitation:

- Resuscitation should begin immediately with the goal of optimizing tissue perfusion. Early goal-directed resuscitation starts with administering fluids to target a CVP of 8–12 mmHg and improve perfusion parameters (MAP $\geq$65 mmHg, UOP $\geq$0.5 ml/kg per h, and mixed venous O_2 saturation $\geq$70%).
- Fluid challenges with either crystalloid (1000 ml) or colloid (300–500 ml) should be given as long as they result in haemodynamic improvement.
- Fluid administration should be reduced when filling pressures increase without haemodynamic improvement.

Antibiotics:

- Intravenous antibiotics should begin within the first hour of recognizing severe sepsis. Initial coverage should be broad and then narrowed as culture results become available.
- Prior to starting antibiotics, culture the blood (peripheral and from any existing line) and any other potential source of infection (e.g. sputum, urine, wound).

Source control:

- Controlling the source of infection is a critical part of sepsis treatment. This includes catheter removal, tissue debridement, abscess drainage, etc.

- Imaging studies to evaluate for the source of sepsis may be necessary.

Supportive care:

- Sepsis is a systemic disease and when severe often requires ICU admission so that all systems are monitored and supported as needed.

Neurological:

- Sedation and analgesia should be utilized for patient comfort, particularly if intubated. Use daily interruption to ensure that the patient is not over-sedated and assist with ventilator weaning.

Cardiovascular:

- Vasopressor therapy (noradrenaline or dopamine) should be introduced when fluid challenges fail to restore blood pressure and perfusion.
- Dobutamine may be added in patients with elevated cardiac filling pressures and low cardiac output.
- Patients with refractory hypotension (despite fluid and vasopressor therapy) should be considered for intravenous hydrocortisone 200–300 mg/day.

Respiratory:

- Many patients with severe sepsis develop ALI/ARDS and require mechanical ventilation. They should be managed with the low tidal volume ventilation strategies discussed above.
- Daily spontaneous breathing trials are appropriate to help expedite extubation.

Gastrointestinal:

- Provide stress ulcer prophylaxis with an H2 blocker or proton pump inhibitor.

Renal:

- If renal failure develops, use haemodialysis or continue renal replacement therapy as needed (see below).

Haematological:

- Recombinant human activated protein C (rhAPC) – Xigirs – is recommended in patients at high risk for death (sepsis-induced MODS or APACHE II $\geq$25) with no contraindication for bleeding. rhAPC is the first licensed therapy for the treatment of severe sepsis and associated multi-organ failure. Studies found an absolute

Table 13.11 Causes of ischaemic acute renal failure

Hypovolaemia	Decreased 'effective' intravascular volume	Hypotension	Renal vascular disease	Medications
Bleeding	Cirrhosis	Shock	Renal artery cross clamp	IV contrast
Renal losses	Heart failure	Medication-related	Malignant hypertension	NSAIDS
GI losses	Third spacing (pancreatitis)		Renal artery thrombosis	Cyclosporine

mortality reduction of 6.1% (from 31 to 25%) in patients receiving rhAPC.

- Red blood cell transfusions should be administered to target a haemoglobin between 7 and 9 g/dl. A higher haemoglobin concentration may be needed in patients with myocardial ischaemia, hypoxia, ongoing bleeding, etc.

Endocrine:

- Maintain blood glucose 4.5–8.0 mmol/l using continuous intravenous insulin and glucose infusions as needed. This simple intervention has significantly reduced in-hospital mortality. It also resulted in significant decreases in length of ICU stay, duration of ventilatory support, need for renal replacement therapy, incidence of septicaemia and incidence of polyneuropathy.

These guidelines elucidate the intensive care that is involved in caring for a patient with sepsis/MODS. More detailed discussions of shock and ARDS (manifestations of sepsis/MODS) were discussed in previous sections. Further manifestations of MODS are expanded upon in the sections below.

Acute renal failure (ARF)

ARF is the sudden development of renal insufficiency resulting in the body's inability to excrete nitrogenous waste and maintain fluid and electrolyte balance. While a straightforward concept, defining renal failure in the clinical setting remains more challenging. Commonly used definitions include: an increase in serum creatinine by 20–50% over baseline, a creatinine clearance of <50% or the need for renal replacement therapy (RRT).

The incidence of ARF thus varies depending on the definition used. Based on the definition of a raised serum creatinine, up to 15–35% of critically ill patients will develop ARF. However, only approximately 1% will need RRT. Development of ARF in critically ill patients is a poor prognostic indicator, associated with up to a 50% mortality rate. Despite major advances in

critical care, this mortality rate has not changed in the past 50 years.

Aetiology

The causes of ARF are classified as pre-renal, renal (intrinsic) or post-renal (obstructive). Seventy-five per cent of ARF is related to renal hypoperfusion resulting in the reversible 'pre-renal' state or acute tubular necrosis. Renal hypoperfusion can come from a variety of sources in the surgical patient (Table 13.11) and many patients in the ICU will demonstrate a combination of these.

Pre-renal ARF

Although the kidney has an auto-regulatory mechanism to maintain the glomerular filtration rate (GFR), when renal perfusion decreases below a critical level the GFR decreases and urine output falls.

Intrinsic ARF

Acute tubular necrosis (ATN) may occur after prolonged hypoperfusion or as a result of the toxic effects of certain drugs or pigments. Histological examination reveals multiple areas of focal necrosis along the nephron with rupture of the basement membranes and occlusion of the lumen by casts.

Post-renal ARF

Obstruction anywhere along the urinary tract may cause postrenal ARF. Common causes include calculi and prostatic hypertrophy.

Diagnosis

The diagnosis of ARF is usually made because of either oliguria or derangement of laboratory values. Oliguric ARF (>400 ml urine/day) is often seen in ARF secondary to radiological contrast or aminoglycoside toxicity. Alternatively, anuric ARF (<100 ml urine/day) occurs in complete obstruction, severe ATN, glomerulonephritis or vascular injury. An obstructive aetiology can usually be ruled out quickly with placement of a

Table 13.12 Diagnosis of acute renal failure. The most sensitive and specific determination of ARF is the fractional excretion of sodium (FENa)

	Pre-renal	ATN
Urea/Cr ratio	>15–20:1	<15:1
Urine Na (mmol/l)	<20	>30
Urine osmolality (mosmol/l)	>350	<350
FENa (%)	<1	>1

FENa = ratio of the amount of sodium excreted to the amount of sodium filtered = (urine Na/serum Na) / (urine Cr/serum Cr).

urinary catheter and ultrasound looking for any signs of either bladder distension (urethral obstruction) or hydronephrosis (ureteral obstruction).

Because the vast majority of ARF (particularly in surgical patients) is secondary to renal hypoperfusion, the next important step is determining whether the patient has pre-renal failure or ATN. Pre-renal failure is reversible if perfusion to the kidney is restored promptly. In the pre-renal state, the still functioning kidney actively absorbs sodium and urea in an attempt to retain as much water (and thus intravascular volume) as possible. This results in an increased urea:creatinine ratio, decreased urinary sodium, high urine osmolality, and decreased fractional excretion of sodium (FENa). Conversely, when the kidney has been subjected to prolonged ischaemia and ATN ensues, the kidney loses its concentrating ability. The urinary sodium increases, urine osmolality decreases and the FENa raises. A summary of these parameters is available in Table 13.12.

Of note, while the FENa is the most sensitive and specific tool for evaluating AFR, the urinary sodium is a quick and reliable test to begin assessing a patient with suspected ATN. Evaluating urinary sediment may also be an easy adjunctive test in patients with AFR. Patients with pre-renal failure will often have bland hyaline casts. On the other hand, 80% of patients with ATN will have brown casts and tubular epithelial cells.

Treatment

Despite the medical advances of the past 50 years, mortality of patients developing AFR in the ICU has remained unchanged. Probably this is because there are still no real treatments for ARF. The two mainstays of therapy in ARF are appropriate volume expansion and avoidance of any further nephrotoxic insults. What is appropriate volume expansion in a patient

whose kidneys are failing and is oliguric? Excellent question. Optimizing tissue perfusion (see shock section) without pushing the patient into fluid overload is the main objective. If the patient's renal failure progresses to acidosis, hyperkalaemia, fluid overload and/or severe uraemia, then renal replacement therapy will be required.

Two potential therapies, dopamine and loop diuretics, which have received intensive study in past years are worth mentioning. Dopamine has potential advantages in ARF because it increases renal blood flow, increases the glomerular filtration rate and increases sodium and water excretion (diuretic property). Nevertheless, a multitude of studies have consistently found that dopamine does not prevent ARF in at-risk patients, nor does dopamine change the outcome (particularly mortality or need for RRT) in patients with ARF. Thus, at this time, there is a growing consensus that dopamine should not be utilized for either the prevention or treatment of ARF.

Loop diuretics have potential advantages of decreasing oxygen consumption in tubular cells (by inhibiting sodium transport) to limit cellular injury, causing vasodilatation of arterial vessels to improve oxygenation, and augmenting tubular flow via their diuretic action. Nevertheless, studies have also failed to find diuretics beneficial in either the prevention or treatment of ARF. In fact, one well-designed, prospective, cohort study found that diuretics were actually associated with an increased risk of death and non-recovery of renal function. Thus, at this time, the use of diuretics in ARF cannot be advocated.

Many novel therapies for ARF continue to be studied. We are learning that ARF in humans is more complicated than originally thought and that sub-lethal cell damage and apoptosis play a predominant role. The fact that most previous animal models were those of widespread necrosis may explain why promising interventions in animal models have not awarded the same success in human studies.

Renal replacement therapy (RRT)

When the kidneys ultimately fail, RRT is needed. There are generally two forms of RRT in the intensive care setting: haemodialysis and haemofiltration. In haemodialysis, blood is pumped through a semipermeable filter which is bathed in a dialysate fluid. Electrolytes and fluid move down a concentration gradient into the dialysate fluid and it is removed, carrying

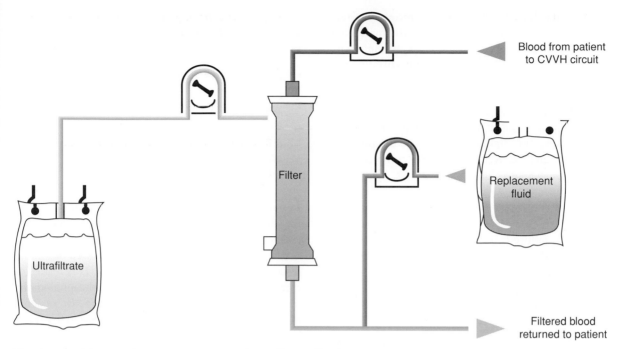

Figure 13.13 Schematic of continuous veno-venous haemofiltration. Blood is pumped from the patient through a filter while ultrafiltrate is removed and discarded. Replacement fluids are added to the concentrated blood before it is returned to the patient.

off potassium, phosphate, urea, water, etc. Haemodialysis utilizes rapid blood flow rates over a 2–4 hour duration and is performed on a daily or every other day basis. As such, it is felt to be associated with haemodynamic instability and large fluid shifts, which may not be tolerated in an unstable patient. Peritoneal dialysis is generally not utilized in the ICU.

In haemofiltration, blood is pumped through highly permeable fibres with hydrostatic pressure driving water, urea and electrolytes out to be collected as an 'ultrafiltrate'. There is no concentration gradient, so it is based on pressure. Generally, 1–6 litres of ultrafiltrate are generated each hour. At the same time that ultrafiltrate is being drawn off, fluid and electrolytes (in the amount the clinician determines) are added back to the now highly concentrated blood before its return to the body (Figure 13.13). The blood flow for haemofiltration is approximately 200 ml/hour (slower than haemodialysis) and thus has the potential advantage of providing more haemodynamic stability. Proponents have advocated that it provides better control over volume status and that it may help clear inflammatory mediators, hastening the recovery from SIRS/sepsis. The disadvantages of haemofiltration are that it is a continuous 24-hour process with specialized

machinery. This makes it labour-intensive and cumbersome when a critically ill patient needs to be mobilized for surgery or studies.

Haemofiltration was initially done by withdrawing blood from the arterial side and returning it to the venous side (continuous arterial venous haemofiltration – CAVH). This was fraught with complications such that continuous veno-venous haemofiltration (CVVH) is now the standard mechanism of filtration. CVVH can be done utilizing a standard haemodialysis catheter. A counter-current of dialysate fluid can also be run through the CVVH circuit to enhance electrolyte clearance. This is known as continuous veno-venous haemofiltration dialysis (CVVHD).

Prognosis

ARF is associated with a mortality rate of 50% in critically ill patients. In general non-oliguric ARF has a much better outcome than oliguric ARF. The cause of ARF also influences outcome. ARF related to trauma, abdominal sepsis or burns has an associated mortality of 70–90%. Conversely, patients with aminoglycoside or contrast-induced ARF do much better, with a mortality rate in the 25–30% range.

If the pateint with ARF survives, recovery of renal function is common (75–95%). Approximately half of these patients will have long-term, asymptomatic, minor reductions in GFR or renal concentrating abilities. The typical clinical course of ARF is a 10–14 day period of oliguria. This may be followed by a 'diuretic phase', lasting 3–7 days, in which concentrating ability is impaired. During this phase, patients may require fluid support, but dialysis can often be discontinued. Complete renal recovery is generally complete by 30 days, but may take as long as 60–90 days.

Acute liver failure

Acute liver failure is the sudden development of liver parenchymal injury resulting in coagulopathy (INR >1.5) in a patient who lacks underlying chronic liver disease. Progression to encephalopathy in such a patient is known as fulminant hepatic failure (FHF).

The aetiologies of acute liver failure include:

- viruses: hepatitis viruses A, B, C, D and E, rarely herpes simplex, varicella-zoster and CMV
- drugs/toxins: paracetamol, isoniazid, phenytoin, halothane, carbon tetrachloride, mushrooms (*Amanita* spp)
- ischaemia: blood flow to the liver may be reduced in shock, resulting in hepatocellular damage
- MODS: ischaemia and endotoxaemia stimulate Kupffer cells to produce cytokines which then act on the hepatocytes, resulting in injury.

The leading causes of fulminant hepatic failure, in order of frequency, are paracetamol toxicity, cryptogenic (unknown), other drug toxicity, hepatitis B and hepatitis A.

Clinical features

Patients with acute liver failure are jaundiced as the liver fails to conjugate and excrete bilirubin. Their laboratory values demonstrate marked transaminase elevation (AST and ALT in the range 1000–5000), as liver cells are injured. Synthetic function is compromised and coagulopathy occurs as a consequence of clotting factor depletion. DIC can also contribute to clotting abnormality.

Life-threatening hypoglycaemia may develop secondary to impaired gluconeogenesis and depletion of glycogen stores.

Hepatic encephalopathy is a key feature of fulminant hepatic failure. Four clinical grades are recognized:

- grade 1: awake, mild confusion, altered personality
- grade 2: awake, agitated, disoriented, hallucinations
- grade 3: stuporous, but may be aroused
- grade 4: comatose, but with intact pupillary reflexes and usually ability to withdraw to pain.

Importantly, hepatic encephalopathy in the acute setting differs from that of encephalopathy related to cirrhosis and chronic liver failure. In chronic hepatic failure, encephalopathy is related to increased ammonia levels. Conversely, encephalopathy in FHF is related to cerebral oedema. Thus, worsening of encephalopathy in patients with FHF is a sign of progressive oedema and a poor prognostic indicator. Progression to central herniation is possible in these patients.

Management

The cornerstone of management of acute hepatic failure is treating the source of failure (if possible) and systemic support. Liver transplantation is indicated in patients with FHF and grade 3 or 4 encephalopathy. Only 10–20% of these patients will survive without transplant; transplant improves survival to 60–80%.

Supportive care for less severe acute hepatic failure or as a bridge to transplant for those awaiting transplant can be quite intensive. These patients may be haemodynamically compromised, thus close monitoring of CVP, arterial pressure, oxygen saturation and urine output may be needed to ensure optimal tissue perfusion. Vitamin K administration is used to correct coagulopathy; transfusions should be restricted to patients with active bleeding. Glucose infusions are often needed to correct hypoglycaemia. Early, aggressive treatment of sepsis with antibiotic therapy is recommended. Oral lactulose and reduction of dietary protein may reduce the load of nitrogen metabolism and assist in management of encephalopathy. Even though encephalopathy in FHF is related to cerebral oedema, ammonia may play a role in the development of this oedema. Management of cerebral oedema is critical in encephalopathic patients; mechanical ventilation may be needed for airway protection and an ICP monitor placed to guide therapy. Liver support devices such as the extracorporeal liver assist device (ELAD) are still being developed and evaluated.

Prognosis

Prognosis in acute liver failure is related to the cause of the failure and the severity of the failure. Patients with acute liver failure due to paracetamol toxicity demonstrate an overall 50% survival rate. Liver failure caused by hepatitis A or B has survival rates in the 30–50% range. Finally, in FHF secondary to non-A, non-B, non-C hepatitis or Wilson's disease the survival rate may be less than 10%. Progressive encephalopathy is associated with a worse prognosis. Metabolic acidosis, renal failure, severe jaundice, or marked coagulopathy also suggest a worse prognosis.

Chronic liver disease

Superimposed acute hepatic failure also occurs in patients with chronic liver disease. Often an event such as a new infection (spontaneous bacterial peritonitis) or GI bleed will tip a previously stable cirrhotic into fulminant liver failure. Treatment is supportive as described above. Generally such patients may have already been candidates for liver transplant, and this acute event may increase their priority on the organ recipient waiting list. Each healthcare system must prioritize organ allocation to those individuals who most urgently need it.

Principles of intensive care

Organization

In 2000, an expert panel supported by the UK's Department of Health put forth an executive summary on adult critical care services. In this manuscript, recommendations for the organization and delivery of critical care were made. They recommended classifying critically ill patients according to their clinical need (examples are provided for readers' understanding and are not part of the recommendations):

- Level 0: patient needs can be met on normal ward care in an acute hospital.
  (e.g. post-op 4–6 hourly observations, PCA, IV fluids and medications)
- Level 1: patient is at risk of a deteriorating condition or has recently relocated from a higher level of care. Patient needs can be met on an acute

ward with support from the critical care team. (e.g. abnormal vital signs, observations more than 4 hourly, tracheostomy or epidural care)
- Level 2: patient requires more detailed observation or intervention. Patient may need support for a single failing organ system, postoperative care, or 'step down' from a higher level of care.
  (e.g. non-invasive ventilation, invasive monitoring or infusion of vasoactive drug)
- Level 3: patient requires advanced respiratory support or basic respiratory support plus support of at least two other organ systems. This includes all complex patients requiring support for multi-organ failure.
  (e.g. mechanical ventilation with vasoactive drug infusion and renal replacement therapy)

These recommendations provide a framework that may replace the traditional division of high-dependency and intensive care units, emphasizing level of care required rather than patient location. Ideally, critically ill patients should be located in a unit in close proximity to diagnostic facilities and operating theatres. Consultants with specialized training in intensive care medicine should be responsible for directing patient care.

Indications for admission and discharge

Since intensive care is limited and expensive, it is useful to have guidelines for admission and discharge to such units. The most recent guidelines put forth by the Department of Health are from 1996. Formulation of guidelines is difficult and the aforementioned executive summary recommended that these be reviewed and revised. At the present time, the following algorithm (adapted from the Department of Health guidelines) should be used to consider admission to high-dependency or intensive care units:

Is the illness reversible?	no → Continue ward care
yes ↓	
Does the patient have significant comorbidity?	yes → Continue ward care
no ↓	

(cont.)

Has patient made a stated or written statement against intensive care? no ↓	yes → Continue ward care
Does the patent need advanced respiratory support? no ↓	yes → **Intensive care**
Does the patient need acute organ support? yes ↓	no → Can patient be safely observed on ward? yes → **Ward care** no ↓
Does patient need more than one organ supported? yes ↓ Intensive care	no → **High-dependency unit**

Table 13.13 APACHE II

Acute physiology score (APS)
Normal values score 0, abnormally low or high values score from 1 to 4 (except creatinine and GCS)

	Scores
1. Score temperature	0–4
2. Mean blood pressure	0–4
3. Heart rate	0–4
4. Respiratory rate	0–4
5. Oxygenation	0–4
6. Arterial pH	0–4
7. Serum Na^+	0–4
8. Serum K^+	0–4
9. Serum creatinine	0–8
10. Haematocrit	0–4
11. White cell count	0–4
12. Neurological score obtained by subtracting the GCS score from 15	

'Age' (eliminate the '44–75 score range from') CHS Surgical cases	0–6

	Score
• Elective admission to ICU postoperatively	2
• Admission to ICU after emergency surgery	5

Medical cases
• Admission to ICU with any of the following:
   1. cirrhosis
   2. chronic heart failure
   3. chronic hypertension
   4. dialysis-dependent renal disease
   5. immunosuppression

APACHE II score	Approximate hospital death rate (%)
0	2
10	10
20	30
30	70
40	95
>50	100

CHS, chronic health score.

In general, patients are candidates for intensive care when they are unstable or require multi-organ monitoring and support. These patients should have a reversible illness, an anticipated meaningful quality of life, and limited comorbidities. Patients with anticipated poor outcomes or significant comorbidities may not be intensive care candidates. These can be difficult decisions and often require dialogue between primary and ICU consultants as well as discussions with patients or their family members.

Discharge from intensive care occurs when the patient's condition improves or irreversibly deteriorates. Ideally, patients will stabilize, no longer require respiratory support, and have their underlying illness corrected. If the patient is not improving and organ support is only deferring death, if the patient enters a persistent vegetative state or if the patient or the family wish to pursue palliative care, then discharge from intensive care should be considered. Sometimes discharge from intensive care will mean a step down in the level of care and transfer to a high-dependency unit. Other patients are well enough to be transferred directly to ward care.

Scoring systems

A number of scoring systems have been developed for use in the ICU. Scoring systems use statistical modelling techniques to assess patient variables and prognosticate on patient outcome.

Scoring systems can be broadly grouped as follows:

Assess severity of physiological derangement

The acute physiology and chronic health evaluation (APACHE) score is a physiologically based score used to measure illness severity. The APACHE II score, a modification of the original, is based on 12 acute physiological variables (acute physiology score), a chronic health score and the patient's age (Table 13.13). Scores are totalled, providing a value between 0 and 71; the higher the APACHE II score, the more severe the illness. APACHE II remains the most widely studied and utilized scoring system. APACHE III, a 'refinement' of APACHE II, includes more variables, but may underestimate mortality. APACHE IV, released in 2005, is showing promise and continues to have studies validate its accuracy. Another example, the SAPS II (simplified acute physiology score), is also commonly used to assess severity of illness.

Assess severity of injury

The injury severity score (ISS) quantifies a patient's anatomical injury. The revised trauma score (RTS) looks at physiological parameters (GCS, systolic blood pressure and respiratory rate) to assess injury severity.

Predict outcome

The mortality prediction model (MPM) has undergone a number of modifications but essentially uses variables available at the time of ICU admission to predict the probability of hospital mortality. APACHE II has been shown to be a good predictor of mortality outcome in large patient groups, but a poor one in individual patients and some subgroups that were not represented in the original database (e.g. AIDS or trauma patients). SAPS II is an accurate predictor of mortality and is the most widely used score for mortality prediction in Europe. SAPS III is in the process of being validated.

Assess utilization of resources

The therapeutic intervention scoring system (TISS) was originally devised to quantify the intensity of care and use this to predict illness severity. For TISS, points are assigned based on the complexity of interventions performed on a patient (e.g. 1 for dressing change, 5 for mechanical ventilation). While no longer used to predict illness severity, TISS has proven a very useful index of utilization of ICU resources such as staffing and costs.

Assess outcome of ICU care

An example is the perceived quality of life (PQ$_O$L) score. This is a questionnaire that gauges patients' satisfaction with life after they have left the ICU.

While scoring systems can be used to evaluate patients individually, no scoring system is accurate enough to predict the outcome of a given patient and should not be used as such. Scoring systems have greater merit in evaluating patient populations. They can serve as an important research tool by helping stratify patients for randomized clinical trials.

Scoring systems also help standardize illness severity in patients with highly complicated and varying disorders; this allows for comparisons between predicted and actual outcomes.

Further reading

2009 Focused update: ACCF/AHA Guidelines for the Diagnosis and Management of Heart Failure in Adults. A report of the American College of Cardiology Foundation/American Heart Association Task Force on Practice Guidelines: Developed in Collaboration With the International Society for Heart and Lung Transplantation. *Circulation* 2009;**119**:1977–2016. Public access to these guidelines is available on the American Heart Association *Circulation* web site hhttp://circ.ahajournals.org.

A Collective Task Force Facilitated by the American College of Chest Physicians; the American Association for Respiratory Care; and the American College of Critical Care Medicine. Evidence-based guidelines for weaning and discontinuation of ventilatory support. *Chest* 2001; **120**:375S–396S.

British Thoracic Society Guidelines for the management of suspected acute pulmonary embolism. *Thorax* 2003;**58**: 47–84.

Dellinger RP, Levy MM, Carlet JM *et al*. Surviving Sepsis Campaign: International guidelines for management of severe sepsis and septic shock: 2008. *Intensive Care Med* 2008;**30**:536–555. Public access to this extensively referenced international consensus statement is available via website hhttp://www.suvivingsepsis.org.

Department of Health. Comprehensive Critical Care: a Review of Adult Critical Care Services. Department of Health: London. May 2000.

Department of Health. Guidelines on Admission to and Discharge from Intensive Care and High Dependency Units. London. March 1996.

Hilton R. Acute renal failure. *BMJ* 2006;**333**:786–790.

Nolan J, Deakin C, Soar J *et al*. European Resuscitation Council Guidelines for Resuscitation 2005. Section 4. Adult advanced life support. *Resuscitation* 2005;**67S1**;S39–S86. Public access to guidelines and algorithms for cardiac arrest and arrhythmias is available on the European Resuscitation Council web site hhttp://erc.edu.

NHLBI ARDS Clinical Network. Public access to previous studies and ongoing projects available via web site hhttp://www.ardsnet.org.

Wheeler AP, Bernard GR. Acute lung injury and the acute respiratory distress syndrome: a clinical review. *Lancet* 2007;**369**:1553–1564.

Chapter

14

Caring for surgical patients: complications and communication

Douglas M. Bowley

'Every surgeon carries about him a little cemetery, in which from time to time he goes to pray. A cemetery of bitterness and regret, of which he seeks the reason for certain of his failures.'
La Philosophie de la Chirurgie.
René Leriche, 1879–1955

Introduction

Surgery creates a unique relationship between patient and practitioner. The impact of serious illness, particularly cancer, and the surgery required to treat it may impose lifelong physical and psychological burdens. These consequences are unlikely to be confined to the individual, as the patient's family and even wider society may be affected.

Establishment and maintenance of trust and the relationship of care between a surgeon and his or her patients facilitates the necessary physical and psychological transitions after major surgery. Optimal outcomes depend on this relationship as well as good preoperative preparation, optimum surgery and meticulous postoperative management.

Outcomes after surgery are influenced by:

- preoperative physiological status
- operative severity and
- the provision of appropriate care.

Surgeons can minimize the deleterious effects of the surgical insult by careful preoperative planning, meticulous intraoperative technique and by accurate postoperative care.

Preoperative physiological status

Preoperative co-existing medical problems translate into increased operative risk. The simplest tool to assess patient risk factors is the American Association of Anesthetists (ASA) scale. This is a subjective assessment of the patient's operative risk based on the presence and severity of co-existing medical problems, which are detected by routine history and physical examination. Increasing ASA grade correlates with increased risk of postoperative complications.

One simple method of assessing a patient's functional reserves is to ask about stair climbing. In a prospective study of patients undergoing thoracotomy, sternotomy or upper abdominal laparotomy, the subjects were asked preoperatively to climb stairs until limited by their symptoms. Complications after surgery occurred in 25% overall; however, of those unable to climb one flight of stairs, 89% developed a postoperative cardiorespiratory complication and no patient able to climb the maximum of seven flights of stairs had a complication. The inability to climb two flights of stairs was associated with a positive predictive value of 82% for the development of a postoperative complication.

The **P**hysiological and **O**perative **S**everity **S**core for the en**U**meration of **M**ortality and morbidity (POSSUM) was developed in 1991. POSSUM variables include physiological markers and other factors related to operative severity. These variables have been tested extensively and have resulted in a central database of over 200 000 patients. POSSUM scoring has been used to predict the outcome of patients undergoing a broad range of operations and has been recognized as being the most appropriate available score for assessing risk in surgical patients. However, POSSUM over-predicts mortality for those patients at the low-risk end of the spectrum. The Portsmouth group revised the scoring and the so-called P-POSSUM is now widely used.

A useful online resource that allows doctors to use P-POSSUM scoring is Risk Prediction in Surgery

Fundamentals of Surgical Practice, Third Edition, ed. Andrew N. Kingsnorth and Douglas M. Bowley.
Published by Cambridge University Press. © Cambridge University Press 2011.

(www.riskprediction.org.uk). The site has been developed by the association of Coloproctology of Great Britain and Ireland (with their partners) to allow surgeons to estimate risk online for their patients undergoing surgery. P-POSSUM scoring, and other risk prediction models, are provided to help surgeons more fully consent their patients by giving mortality and other surgical risk predictions based on relevant prognostic factors including age, disease severity and comorbidity. Risk-adjusted operative mortality can also be used as an objective measure of outcome for monitoring performance within a centre or between centres.

Operative severity

Surgery (or trauma from injury) has been shown to result in immune suppression and organ failure is the leading cause of death in surgical patients. A causal relationship exists between the extent of the surgical or traumatic injury, the postoperative metabolic and immunological changes and the predisposition of patients to develop infectious complications and multiple organ dysfunction.

Provision of appropriate care

In a study in 2003, postoperative mortality was compared between centres in the UK and the USA with patients matched according to POSSUM criteria. The risk-adjusted mortality rates following major surgery were four times higher in the UK cohort. The reasons behind this difference are complex, but the authors speculate that the difference may be due to differences in the quality of patient care.

Higher-risk surgery performed independently by doctors in training correlates with poor postoperative outcomes. In the UK's National Confidential Enquiry into Perioperative Deaths (NCEPOD) published in 2000, of 1518 operations that resulted in postoperative death, 4.2% were conducted by a doctor with as little as 1 year of specialist training and 41% of the anaesthetics were administered by trainees.

The nature of postoperative nursing care is also important; in a study involving over 200 000 surgical patients in the state of Pennsylvania, higher patient to nursing staff ratios were associated with a higher risk-adjusted postoperative mortality rate.

If we believe that high-dependency care is the optimum environment for an at-risk surgical patient then it is sobering to realize that over 50% of patients who die after surgery in the UK are never admitted to an ICU.

Recognition of the ill surgical patient

The ability to recognize an ill surgical patient is a fundamental skill of a good surgeon and, unfortunately, can be harder than it might seem. History and examination remain the cornerstone, but understanding the definition of the systemic inflammatory response syndrome (SIRS) is helpful. A postoperative surgical patient is said to be exhibiting SIRS if two or more of the following are present and action should be taken immediately:

> temperature $<36°C$ or $>38°C$
> respiratory rate >20 breaths per minute
> pulse rate >90 beats per minute
> white blood count >12 or $<4 \times 10^9/l$.

Postoperative monitoring

The patient's response to a surgical procedure is assessed by measurement of vital signs. Observations that must be monitored by medical and nursing staff include:

- conscious state
- temperature, pulse, blood pressure and respiratory rate
- urinary output
- drainage from the nasogastric tubes, T-tubes, or wound drains, stomas or fistulae.

More intensive monitoring may be needed for high-risk surgical patients and after major surgery; these include one-to-one nursing by highly trained nurses, continuous electrocardiographic monitoring and invasive haemodynamic monitoring (arterial line, central venous pressure (CVP) monitoring and a method of monitoring cardiac output) in a high-dependency or intensive care unit.

Vital signs

Heart rate

Tachycardia is defined as a heart rate > 90 beats/min. When premature ventricular contractions or other irregularities are present, the heart rate may be determined by auscultation at the apex; the difference between apical and radial rates represents the number of dropped beats. Tachycardia occurs with hypovolaemia, infection, anxiety, fear, fever and pain. Bradycardia (a heart rate <60 beats/min) may occur with heart block associated with myocardial ischaemia.

Blood pressure

Blood pressure falls after hypovolaemia due to blood or fluid loss, during cardiac failure from primary myocardial dysfunction or tamponade, or as a result of severe sepsis or anaphylaxis. Hypotension is often a late manifestation of shock, especially in children.

The pulse pressure is the difference between the systolic and diastolic pressures. A reduced pulse pressure may precede a fall in systolic pressure in a patient developing hypovolaemic shock and is a clinical sign of hypovolaemia. Mean arterial pressure (MAP) may be calculated from the formula: MAP = [(2 × diastolic) + systolic]/3.

Body temperature

Body temperature is measured orally, rectally or more commonly by use of a device that analyses the tympanic membrane. Temperature elevations are associated with infection, tissue necrosis, late-stage carcinomatosis and malignant hyperthermia. Low-grade fever is also present after accidental or surgical trauma and particularly when haematoma, a foreign body, urinary extravasation or stasis or bronchial secretions are present. Hypothermia (temperature <34°C) may occur in some patients with septic shock, reduced metabolism associated with hypothyroid state, severe anaemia and exposure to cold. Hypothermia is of particular relevance to patients undergoing major operations. Muscle relaxants abolish the shivering response and the opening of a body cavity causes loss of large amounts of heat. Hypothermia causes platelet dysfunction and abnormalities of the enzymatic clotting cascade and can lead to a clinically relevant coagulopathy. Hypothermia also prolongs the action of neuromuscular blocking drugs.

Ventilatory monitoring

Clinical monitoring of ventilation consists of observation of the patient's colour, respiratory rate and adequacy of chest movements. Auscultation of both lungs should be performed to detect equality of air entry and the presence of secretions or consolidation. Pulse oximetry estimates the percentage of saturation of circulating haemoglobin. An arterial oxygen saturation of 95% represents a PaO_2 value of approximately 85 mmHg. In the recovery period oxygen supplementation should be given to patients whose saturation falls below 13 kPa (95 mmHg).

Urinary output

Urinary output is easily measured after bladder catheterization. The hourly rate of urine output is a rough marker of end-organ perfusion, and is typically used as a marker of the (in)adequacy of resuscitation.

Central venous pressure (CVP)

A central venous catheter with the tip in the lower superior vena cava or right atrium provides valuable information concerning the volume status of the circulation. CVP monitoring can be used to guide fluid therapy after major surgery. A healthy person in the supine position typically has mean CVP values that range from 0 to 3 mmHg.

Arterial blood gases

Measurement of arterial blood gases is extremely useful to evaluate surgical patients: the first laboratory signs of early lung problems are arterial blood gas abnormalities, such as arterial partial pressure of oxygen (PaO_2) values lower than 9.4 kPa (70 mmHg), arterial partial pressure of CO_2 ($PaCO_2$) values higher than 6 kPa (45 mmHg) and pH values <7.3 or >7.5. Respiratory failure is suggested by PaO_2 values lower than 6–7 kPa (50 mmHg) in a patient breathing room air.

Acute respiratory acidosis in the postoperative period is most commonly a complication caused by the respiratory depressant effect of anaesthesia and narcotics. Other causes are pneumothorax, airway obstruction (foreign body, laryngospasm, severe bronchospasm) and ventilator malfunction. Treatment of acute respiratory acidosis comprises adequate ventilation. In the case of respiratory depression, this may mean administering a narcotic antagonist (naloxone). Maintaining an adequate airway is critical and intubation and mechanical ventilation may be required. Respiratory alkalosis is due to hyperventilation and there is a decrease in $PaCO_2$. Hyperventilation can occur due to diverse causes (respiratory disease such as pneumonia, pulmonary embolism or oedema, shock, pain, anxiety and disturbed ventilatory control). The treatment entails tackling the underlying cause.

Metabolic acidosis may be due to impaired perfusion of the tissues, as in hypovolaemic shock, or due to diabetic ketoacidosis or renal failure. It is critically important to recognize metabolic acidosis in a surgical patient.

Critical care

Organ failure is the leading cause of death in surgical patients. Critical care is best provided by a multidisciplinary team focused on resuscitation, monitoring, and life support (see Chapter 13 for full discussion). The fundamental goals of critical care are early restoration and maintenance of tissue oxygenation and prevention and treatment of infection and multiple organ failure.

Multi-organ dysfunction syndrome (MODS) is a clinical syndrome characterized by progressive failure of multiple and interdependent organs. It occurs along a continuum of progressive organ failure, rather than absolute failure. The lungs, liver and kidneys are the principal target organs; however, failure of the cardiovascular and central nervous system may occur. Specific therapy for MODS is currently limited, apart from providing adequate and full resuscitation, treatment of infection and general ICU supportive care.

Goal-directed therapy

After major trauma or surgical illness, hypoperfusion of tissues leads to cellular hypoxia and the initiation of the factors that lead to organ dysfunction. The fundamental defect is a failure of adequate delivery of oxygen to the respiring tissues. Traditional attempts at resuscitation have been guided by normalization of vital signs, such as pulse, blood pressure and urine output, and only when haemodynamic instability has been recognized has the patient been considered for invasive monitoring in a critical care environment. However, these vital signs fail to identify the important group of patients with occult hypoperfusion, whose outcomes are likely to be poor unless adequate oxygen delivery is restored.

Shoemaker and his co-workers from the University of Southern California discovered that survivors after major trauma had significantly higher cardiac output, oxygen delivery and oxygen consumption compared to those patients who died. This led them to introduce the concept of 'goal-directed therapy' in which they attempted to manipulate the circulation of patients and achieve target values for cardiac output, oxygen delivery and consumption. In a group of high-risk patients who had required major surgery for trauma, they were able to achieve significant reductions in mortality. However, other studies were unable to reproduce these results.

In 2001, a randomized controlled trial of early goal-directed therapy compared to standard therapy was published in a group of patients arriving at hospital with severe sepsis or septic shock, but in whom organ dysfunction was not yet established. This study demonstrated significant survival advantage for the 'goal-directed group'. The conclusion that haemodynamic optimization as soon as possible in the perioperative period is helpful has been further strengthened by the publication of a meta-analysis, which has confirmed that optimization before organ failure has occurred leads to a substantial reduction in deaths in high-risk surgical patients. Invasive monitoring is required in order to record the necessary haemodynamic variables; a pulmonary artery catheter is the traditional method of gathering these data, although less invasive techniques such as oesophageal Doppler probes are now being used.

Intensive blood sugar control

Hyperglycaemia and insulin resistance are common in critically ill patients, even if they have not previously had diabetes. A prospective, randomized, controlled study randomly assigned adults admitted to a surgical intensive care unit to receive intensive insulin therapy (maintenance of blood glucose at a level between 4.4 and 6.1 mmol/l) or conventional treatment (infusion of insulin only if the blood glucose level exceeded 11.9 mmol/l and maintenance of glucose at a level between 10.0 and 11.1 mmol/l). This, so-called, 'tight glycaemic control' significantly reduced mortality during intensive care; the greatest reductions in mortality were in patients with a proven septic focus. However, subsequent work has shown that such tight control may not offer as much benefit as thought and exposes the patient to the risks of hypoglycaemia. Current best practice guidelines suggest paying close attention to control of blood sugar, avoiding both hypo- and hyperglycaemia (goal of therapy BM of 8 mmol/l).

Steroids in severe sepsis

It is now well established that severe sepsis may be associated with reversible failure of the hypothalamic-pituitary-adrenal axis. In a randomized, double-blinded, placebo-controlled multicentre trial a 7-day treatment with low doses of hydrocortisone and fludrocortisone significantly reduced the risk of death in patients with septic shock and relative adrenal insufficiency without increasing adverse events. Stress doses of hydrocortisone (hydrocortisone 50 mg 6 hourly and fludrocortisone 50 μg tablet per day) are indicated in all inotrope-dependent patients with septic shock who have a stress (random) cortisol level of <25 μg/dl.

Activated protein C

Activated protein C, an endogenous protein that promotes fibrinolysis and inhibits thrombosis and inflammation, is an important modulator of the coagulation and inflammation associated with severe sepsis. Activated protein C is converted from its inactive precursor, protein C, by thrombin coupled to thrombomodulin. The conversion of protein C to activated protein C may be impaired during sepsis as a result of the down-regulation of thrombomodulin by inflammatory cytokines. Reduced levels of protein C are found in the majority of patients with sepsis and are associated with an increased risk of death. In a randomized, double-blind, placebo-controlled, multi-centre trial, treatment with activated protein C significantly reduced mortality in patients with severe sepsis. Consistent with the antithrombotic activity of activated protein C, bleeding was the most common adverse event associated with the administration of the drug; serious bleeding tended to occur in patients with predisposing conditions, such as gastrointestinal ulceration. According to the trial results, one additional serious bleeding event would occur for every 66 patients with severe sepsis treated with activated protein C. However, one life would be saved for every 16 patients treated.

Further understanding of the optimal treatment for patients with sepsis has been elaborated and published by the Survive Sepsis collaboration (see Chapter 5).

Blood transfusion

Allogeneic (bank) blood

Allogeneic blood is used after grouping and cross matching and is available for use in the postoperative period as:

- whole blood
- packed red cells (plasma reduced cells).

Red cells for transfusion are usually depleted of leukocytes as this is thought to reduce the possible immunological consequences of transfusion.

Blood stored at 4°C in a citrate-dextrose preservative solution has a shelf life of about 5 weeks; however, storage of blood causes abnormalities in red cell structure and function and results in a shortening of the red cell lifespan. These 'storage lesions' are caused by:

- a fall in 2,3-DPG (which increases the red cells' affinity for oxygen)
- red cell membrane changes leading to spherocyte formation and leakage of potassium.

Upon transfusion, a proportion of the red cells in the transfused blood do not survive and this proportion rises the longer the blood has been stored (30% or even more are lost as the blood approaches the end of its shelf life).

The volume and rate of transfusion will depend on the clinical state. In general for a stable, euvolaemic adult patient, the transfusion of 1 unit of packed cells raises the haemoglobin concentration by 1 g/dl and each unit of blood is transfused over 4 hours. More rapid transfusion may be needed especially with cases of acute haemorrhage requiring blood transfusion in the postoperative period. If it is anticipated that more than 2 units of blood will need to be transfused, a blood warmer should be used to prevent hypothermia. Massive blood transfusion can be defined as the transfusion of ten or more units within 24 hours.

Complications of blood transfusion

To analyse the risks of transfusion, a confidential voluntary reporting system was instituted in the UK in 1996 entitled the Serious Hazards of Transfusion (SHOT) initiative. Major morbidity and deaths were analysed and categorized into three major sections:

- incorrect blood or component transfused
- immunological interaction between donor and patient
- transfusion-transmitted infection.

Incorrect blood or component transfused

Major ABO incompatability reactions and rhesus D sensitization in young female patients still occur due to errors leading to failure to detect the correct identity of blood or patient. Collection of the wrong blood from the blood fridge is the most common primary error.

Immunological interaction between donor and patient

Immunological reactions were reported in five categories: acute and delayed transfusion reactions, post-transfusion purpura, transfusion-associated graft versus host disease and transfusion-associated acute lung injury. In addition, even in the absence of acute reactions, allogeneic blood transfusion leads to immunomodulation, which has been implicated in increasing the risk of postoperative infection, organ failure and worsened long-term survival after surgery for malignant disease.

Transfusion-transmitted infection

Transfusions may lead to infectious disease in the recipient if the component is contaminated during collection and storage, or if the transfusion unwittingly transfers a biological agent from the donor pool to the recipient.

Red cells are kept refrigerated, so bacterial contamination is usually by agents that survive at low temperature, such as *Serratia liquifaciens*. Platelets have to be kept at room temperature and so may be contaminated with skin organisms (*Staphylococci*) or coliforms. However, contamination by *Salmonella* species due to asymptomatic donor bacteraemia has been recorded; in one case the source of the salmonella infection was the donor's pet boa constrictor.

The risk of transfusion-transmitted viral infections is primarily due to the failure of serological screening tests to detect recently infected donors in the 'window' phase of infection. Hepatitis B and C and HIV have all been transmitted by blood transfusion. A fatal case of cerebral malaria was also recorded by the SHOT initiative after blood transfusion. There is currently great concern about the possibility of transfer of prion proteins by blood transfusion.

Autologous blood

Autologous blood may be collected preoperatively or intraoperatively and used for transfusion in the postoperative period. Some of the hazards of homologous transfusion are eliminated although these techniques also create problems of their own.

Preoperative autologous donation

In this technique, an otherwise fit patient who is to undergo an elective operation which is anticipated to need several units of blood may donate up to four units of blood in the preoperative period. Recombinant erythropoietin may be used to restore a normal haematocrit in the interval between donation and surgery.

Intraoperative haemodilution

Up to two units of blood may be withdrawn from the patient after induction of anaesthesia and prior to commencement of the surgical procedure; intravascular volume is replaced with crystalloids or colloids.

Intraoperative blood salvage

Where it is anticipated that considerable bleeding is likely to occur intraoperatively (such as elective aortic aneurysm surgery), salvage of red cells with an apparatus such as the cell saver helps to reduce wastage of blood. In this system, blood shed into the intraoperative field is aspirated and washed to remove debris. The cells are then suspended in saline and retransfused. Platelets and plasma proteins including clotting factors are lost during the washing process.

Other blood products

Platelet concentrates

The platelets recovered from a unit of freshly donated blood can be transfused into patients who are bleeding and who have a low platelet count. The risk of bleeding increases as the platelet count falls below 50 000/mm^3.

Fresh frozen plasma

This contains all the coagulation factors. It is used to reverse the effects of anticoagulation with warfarin and in patients who are bleeding and require transfusion. It provides the Factors V and VIII, which are not present in banked blood. Each unit is 150–250 ml.

Cryoprecipitate

Cryoprecipitate contains Factors XIII, VIII, fibrinogen and von Willebrand's factor and is used in cases of massive haemorrhage, disseminated intravascular coagulopathy (DIC) and fibrinogen deficiency. Each unit is 10–20 ml.

Transfusion requirements in critical care (TRICC study)

An important trial was recently undertaken by the Canadian Critical Care Trials Group. Critically ill patients with euvolaemia after initial treatment were randomly assigned to either a restrictive strategy of transfusion, in which red cells were transfused if the haemoglobin concentration dropped below 7 g/dl and haemoglobin concentrations were maintained at 7 to 9 g/dl, or a liberal strategy, in which transfusions were given when the haemoglobin concentration fell below 10.0 g/dl and haemoglobin concentrations were maintained at 10.0 to 12.0 g/dl. The mortality rate during hospitalization was significantly lower in the restrictive-strategy group. This reduction in mortality was not seen among patients with clinically significant ischaemic heart disease.

Massive transfusion protocols for patients with exsanguination

Bleeding remains the leading cause of preventable death after major injury. Early resuscitation of these maximally injured patients has changed significantly, guided by recent military experience. The overwhelming conclusion of the data available supports the administration of a high ratio of plasma and platelets to packed red blood cells for patients with massive blood loss. Several large retrospective studies have shown that ratios close to 1:1:1 (FFP:PRBCs:platelets) will result in higher survival. These complex transfusion regimens need to be delivered within the context of massive transfusion protocols.

Postoperative pain

Pain as defined by the International Association for the Study of Pain is 'an unpleasant sensory and emotional experience associated with actual or potential tissue damage, or described in terms of such damage'. Nociception (perception of a painful stimulus) elicits physiological responses even in anaesthetized individuals and minimization of pain can improve clinical outcomes. An individual's response for months after injury may be determined by processes that occur within the first day. Even brief intervals of acute pain can induce long-term neuronal remodelling and sensitization ('plasticity'), chronic pain, and lasting psychological distress.

Factors which influence postoperative pain include the:

- site and size of the incision
- anaesthetic management
- psychological makeup of the patient
- mental preparation (this includes a full explanation from surgeon and anaesthetist).

Pain pathways and mechanism

Injury causes the local release of bradykinin, arachidonic acid and prostaglandin, which stimulate peripheral receptors that in turn transmit impulses via peripheral afferent fibres (A and C) to the spinal cord where they terminate in the dorsal horn and synapse with second-order neurons. Modulation occurs in the spinal cord through action of beta-endorphins and opiates and inhibitory interneurons (the Gate mechanism), which act to inhibit transmission of painful impulses. Fibres of the second-order neurons cross over to the contralateral spinothalamic tract and ascend to the midbrain (thalamus and other nuclei) where they synapse with the third-order neurons and are relayed to the sensory cortex where the location of pain is perceived.

Postoperative pain management

Preemptive treatment

There is evidence to suggest that a powerful stimulus such as an incision sensitizes the CNS to further stimuli and thus pre-incision analgesia should be beneficial. However, the majority of trials have shown that timing of analgesia does not affect postoperative pain control. A recent study has shown, however, that multimodal treatment with opiates, anti-inflammatories, local anaesthetics and a *N*-methyl-D-aspartic acid (NMDA) antagonist (ketamine) diminishes pain and analgesic requirement after hernia surgery. NMDA receptors are thought to mediate central sensitization pathways for pain.

Postoperative analgesia

Intramuscular opiates

Intermittent intramuscular opiates used to be the mainstay of postoperative pain therapy, but the quality of analgesia provided by this regime is often unsatisfactory and it has generally been replaced by patient-controlled techniques.

Intermittent infusion of opiates – patient-controlled analgesia

In this technique, an infusion pump is used to inject a preset bolus dose of analgesic (morphine or pethidine) intravenously whenever the patient activates it. A 'lockout interval' is incorporated in the system to ensure against accidental activation and opiate overdosage. A loading dose is needed, as is a maintenance dose. This technique provides very satisfactory control of pain in the postoperative period. Patient-controlled analgesia is widely used and improves patient satisfaction; however, meta-analysis has shown that PCA does not reduce postoperative morbidity compared to intermittent opioid therapy. Morphine is metabolized by the kidney and caution must be exercised in patients with renal impairment.

Non-opiate drugs

Non-steroidal anti-inflammatory drugs (NSAIDs) have an opioid-sparing effect of 20–30%, which may be important in reducing opioid-related side effects. NSAIDs act by inhibiting prostaglandin synthesis. Paracetamol acts centrally and has analgesic and antipyretic effects, but no anti-inflammatory activity. These preparations may be used alone for intermediate analgesic needs or combined with opiates and may be given orally or rectally.

Local, regional and epidural anaesthetic techniques

Local anaesthetic agents inhibit the sodium channels along nerve fibres. Commonly used local anaesthetic agents are lignocaine, which is short-acting (up to 2 hours), and bupivacaine, which is longer-acting (up to 8 hours). Bupivacaine (0.25% or 0.5%) is the drug of choice for peripheral nerve blockade and epidural block. The toxic systemic side effects of the local anaesthetic agents, particularly on the CNS (convulsions), and cardiac dysrhythmias limit the volume of agent that can be used.

Local anaesthetic infiltration is effective in reducing postoperative pain and subfascial infiltration is more effective than simple subcutaneous infiltration in operations where muscle has been divided (such as hernia repair).

Continuous epidural blockade reduces surgical stress responses and autonomic reflexes; in addition it has been shown to be the most effective method of providing dynamic pain relief (analgesia during patient movement, such a coughing) after major procedures. Epidural analgesia significantly reduces the incidence of postoperative ileus, with consequent reduction in respiratory morbidity, and allows earlier introduction of enteral feeding, which may be beneficial. In major abdominal and vascular procedures, epidurals lead to a significant reduction in pulmonary complications. Postoperative epidural analgesia, especially thoracic epidural analgesia, continued for more than 24 hours reduces postoperative myocardial infarction. In contrast to the beneficial effects of epidural in lower limb procedures on the incidence of thromboembolic complications, in an analysis of six randomized controlled trials there was no significant difference in the incidence of thromboembolic complications in major abdominal and thoracic surgery with epidural or without.

A recent multicentre trial randomized 915 high-risk patients undergoing major abdominal surgery to intraoperative epidural anaesthesia and postoperative IV opioid analgesia for 72 hours or control. Mortality at 30 days was no different between the groups and only respiratory failure occurred less frequently in patients managed with epidural techniques. Postoperative epidural analgesia was, however, associated with lower pain scores during the first 3 postoperative days and there were no major adverse consequences of epidural-catheter insertion.

The risks in placement of an epidural catheter are low; nerve damage, epidural haematoma, and infection of the central nervous system all have an incidence of less than one per 10 000. Permanent neurological injury is very rare (0.02 to 0.07%); however, transient injuries do occur and are more common (0.01 to 0.8%). Disturbances of micturition are a common accompaniment of epidurals, especially in elderly males. Hypotension is the most common cardiovascular disturbance associated with epidural blockade.

Postoperative fluid and electrolyte balance

Intraoperative fluid requirement is usually based on an assumption of maintaining a euvolaemic state. This requires assessment of:

- preoperative circulatory status (euvolaemic/dehydrated/overloaded)

Table 14.1 Electrolyte content of intravenous fluids

Intravenous fluid	Na$^+$ (mmol/l)	K$^+$ (mmol/l)	Cl$^-$ (mmol/l)	HCO$_3^-$ (mmol/l)	Ca^{2+} (mmol/l)
0.9% saline	150	–	150	–	–
0.18% saline + 4% dextrose	30	–	30	–	–
Hartmann's	131	5	111	29	2
Normal plasma	140	4.5	103	26	2.5

Table 14.2 Daily volume and electrolyte composition of gastrointestinal fluids

Fluid	Volume (ml)	Na$^+$ (mmol/l)	K$^+$ (mmol/l)	Cl$^-$ (mmol/l)	H$^+$ (mmol/l)	HCO$_3^-$ (mmol/l)
Gastric	2500	30–80	5–20	100–150	40–60	
Bile	500	130	10	100		30–50
Pancreatic	1000	130	10	75		70–110
Small bowel	5000	130	10	90–130		20–40

- intraoperative losses of blood and insensible fluid loss during the operation.

Intraoperative monitoring of the circulation is used to determine fluid requirement. Postoperative fluid therapy can be difficult to judge and is often delegated to the most junior member of the surgical team. It is helpful to keep the following factors in mind:

- pre-existing circulatory deficit
- ongoing losses (if any)
- daily maintenance fluid requirements.

Assessment of the pre-existing circulatory deficit

Each surgical patient should be assessed with the state of the circulation in mind. The patient should be asked whether he or she is thirsty and physically examined, looking at the peripheries and the state of hydration of mucous membranes. A review of vital signs and urine output and an examination of jugular venous pressure, chest and abdomen should enable the doctor to establish whether the patient is euvolaemic, over-loaded or dehydrated.

An estimate of current status and likely ongoing losses (if any)

The fluid chart must be examined to assess fluid input and output, including urine, nasogastric, stoma or drain losses. Blood count and serum electrolytes should be ascertained. Tables 14.1 and 14.2 provide details of the approximate composition of some gastrointestinal secretions and typical intravenous fluids.

An estimate of maintenance fluid requirements

Maintenance fluid requirements are estimated for replacement of:

- insensible losses from the skin and respiratory system (about 750 ml)
- obligatory losses in urine (about 1 litre).

A rough guide for maintenance fluid requirement for an adult is 30 to 40 ml/kg body weight per day. The following are approximate daily requirements of some electrolytes in an adult:

- 1 mmol/kg per day for sodium
- 1 mmol/kg per day for potassium
- 5–7.5 mmol/kg per day for calcium
- 4–10 mmol/kg per day for magnesium.

Choosing replacement and maintenance fluids

For daily maintenance requirements 500 ml of Hartmann's solution and 1500 ml of dextrose 5% is sufficient to supply electrolytes and fluid but it should be noted that it only provides 600 kcals.

If the operation was a relatively straightforward procedure not involving the gastrointestinal tract, and associated with little blood loss and a short general anaesthetic, in an otherwise fit patient, e.g. hernia repair, cystoscopy or pinning of a fracture, intravenous fluids may not be required at all. The patient may be allowed to drink when fully conscious after the operation and be able to have a normal diet as soon convenient.

Dangers of potassium infusion

It should be noted that Hartmann's solution and Haemaccel contain potassium and these should be used sparingly, if at all, in a patient whose urine output is reduced. It is not necessary to replace potassium if the anticipated need for intravenous fluids is likely to last for 1–2 days as the body's store of potassium (3000 mmol) is more than sufficient.

Postoperative complications

Haemorrhage

Haemorrhage is usually the result of a failure of technique but coagulation disorders may also play a role. Occult blood loss, e.g. postoperative haemoperitoneum, should be suspected when unexplained tachycardia, decreased blood pressure, decreased urine output and peripheral vasoconstriction occur. A fall in the haematocrit is useful in making the diagnosis but this may not occur until quite late and consequently is of limited diagnostic help. The differential diagnosis of immediate postoperative hypotension includes myocardial infarction, cardiac arrhythmia, pulmonary embolism, pneumothorax, pericardial tamponade and severe allergic reaction. Infusions to expand the circulatory volume should be started as soon as other diseases have been ruled out. If hypotension persists, reoperation should be performed.

Respiratory complications

Postoperative respiratory complications (atelectasis and pneumonia) occur significantly more often than cardiac complications and are associated with significantly longer hospital stays. An accurate history and examination is central to the identification of patients at risk for respiratory complications. Approximately one-third of patients with respiratory complications will also have cardiac complications.

Risk factors can be patient- or procedure-related.

Patient-related risk factors

- chronic lung disease

- current cigarette smokers even in the absence of chronic lung disease
- morbid obesity.

Procedure-related risk factors:

- surgical procedures lasting longer than 3 to 4 hours
- general anaesthesia compared to regional anaesthesia
- the rate of complications is inversely related to the distance of the incision from the diaphragm.

Routine preoperative spirometry does not accurately predict the risk of postoperative pulmonary complications in individual patients; however, remember to assess the patient's functional reserves by asking about stair climbing or tolerance for other effort.

Treatment

Cessation of smoking, weight reduction and prophylactic treatment of at-risk patients is helpful; oral and inhaled bronchodilators, systemic steroids and antibiotics can decrease respiratory complications. Good postoperative analgesia, physiotherapy and provision of humidification to loosen secretions are vital; incentive spirometry can be helpful and chest physiotherapy is more effective if started preoperatively.

Cardiac complications

The normal physiological response to surgery is an increase in circulating catecholamines, which leads to an increase in heart rate, myocardial contractility and peripheral vascular resistance, all of which increase myocardial oxygen demand. Also, myocardial oxygen supply may be decreased by hypotension, tachycardia, anaemia and hypoxia. A patient with significant coronary artery disease may not be able to cope with this and may develop myocardial ischaemia. Diagnosis of a perioperative MI can be difficult as the majority of postoperative myocardial ischaemic events are not associated with anginal pain. When present, features of perioperative MI include dysrhythmias, heart failure, hypotension and impaired mental status especially in the elderly.

In patients with significant ischaemic heart disease, coronary artery bypass grafting (CABG) prior to noncardiac surgery is significantly protective against adverse cardiac events. The protection afforded by CABG appears to last for many years; however, the operative mortality of CABG is approximately 1%.

Percutaneous transluminal angioplasty has also been advocated to alleviate myocardial ischaemia prior to noncardiac surgery and also as an emergency intervention in perioperative patients with evolving acute MI in whom thrombolysis is clearly contraindicated.

Various interventions have been shown to reduce cardiac morbidity; a meta-analysis, reported in 2001, showed that postoperative epidural analgesia, especially thoracic epidural analgesia, continued for more than 24 hours reduces postoperative MI and maintenance of perioperative normothermia has also been shown to reduce cardiac morbidity in patients with known coronary artery disease undergoing major noncardiac surgery.

In a randomized, double-blind, placebo-controlled trial comparing atenolol with placebo on overall survival and cardiovascular morbidity in patients with or at risk for coronary artery disease who were undergoing noncardiac surgery, overall mortality after discharge from the hospital was significantly lower among the atenolol-treated patients than among those who were given placebo.

Heart failure

Heart failure is a syndrome where the cardiac output is insufficient for the body's need. The best predictor for the development of postoperative heart failure is symptoms and signs of its existence preoperatively. However, heart failure can be precipitated by an increase in demand for cardiac output, such as anaemia, hypoxia and sepsis or through deterioration in pump function through MI, perioperative volume overload, pulmonary embolus, or cardiac dysrhythmia. Treatment is directed at the primary cause and provision of medical therapy directed at normalizing intravascular volume and cardiac output.

Cardiac dysrhythmias

Cardiac dysrhythmias are common in the perioperative period; transient dysrhythmias are said to occur in approximately 80% of patients if continuous ECG monitoring is employed, but only 5% are significant. Atrial fibrillation is the commonest rhythm disturbance seen in patients undergoing noncardiac surgery, occurring in 10% of patients admitted to a surgical ICU.

The guiding principle in the treatment of perioperative cardiac dysrhythmias and conduction disturbances is that the cause of the dysrhythmia should be identified and reversed if possible. Common causes

Table 14.3 Analysis of infection rates related to wound types

Wound type	Total number	Number infected	%
Clean	47,054	732	1.5
Clean contaminated	9370	720	7.7
Contaminated	442	676	15.2
Dirty	2093	832	40
Overall	62,939	2960	4.7

Cruse PJ, Foord R. The epidemiology of wound infection. A 10-year prospective study of 62,939 wounds. *Surg Clin North Am* 1980;**60**:27–40.

include electrolyte disturbance, acid-base imbalance, acute volume depletion and alterations in autonomic tone.

Wound complications

Haematoma

Wound haematoma is almost always caused by imperfect haemostasis. Haematoma produces elevation and discolouration of wound edges, discomfort and swelling. At times, blood leaks through skin sutures. Small haematomas resolve but increase the incidence of wound infection. Treatment consists of gentle evacuation of clots under sterile conditions. Neck haematomas following operations on the thyroid and parathyroid may compress the trachea and need urgent evacuation.

Seroma

This is a serous fluid collection beneath the wound. Seromas often follow operations that involve elevation of skin flaps. Seroma delays wound healing and increases the risk of wound infection. A seroma may be gently expressed or evacuated by needle aspiration.

Infection

Wound infection has undergone a change in nomenclature and the term surgical site infection (SSI) is now used. SSIs can be classified as (a) incisional or (b) organ space. Incisional SSIs are further classified as superficial or deep.

Risks of SSI can be considered as patient-related or procedure-related. The most important factor during the procedure is the degree of contamination (see Table 14.3).

Patient-related risk factors

Patient-related factors that increase risk of SSI include:

- comorbidity
- malnutrition or obesity
- smoking
- steroid use.

Prophylactic antibiotics effectively reduce the rate of postoperative infection. One pre-incisional dose is usually sufficient, although a second dose is advised during surgery lasting more than 3–4 hours. Prolonged antibiotic therapy should be avoided because of the cost and the increased likelihood of colonization and infection with antibiotic-resistant bacteria. Indeed, not all operations require the use of prophylactic antibiotics. In a meta-analysis of the use of antibiotics in hernia surgery, the incidence of infection after groin hernia repair was 3% in the placebo group and 1.5% in the antibiotic group. The number of patients that need to be treated with antibiotics to prevent one wound infection was 74, leading the authors to conclude that routine use of antibiotics as prophylaxis in groin hernia surgery is not warranted.

Dehiscence and incisional hernia

Dehiscence of the wound is most often seen in abdominal surgical procedures. Systemic risk factors are old age, diabetes mellitus, uraemia, immunosuppression, jaundice, hypoalbuminaemia, cancer and obesity. Local risk factors are poor surgical technique of wound closure, raised intra-abdominal pressure due to obstructive airway disease and infection.

Wound dehiscence is commonly seen between the fifth and eighth postoperative day. The discharge of serosanguinous fluid is often the first warning of a disruption. In some cases, sudden dehiscence may occur on coughing or straining. Patients with wound dehiscence should be returned to the theatre and the wound repaired.

Incisional hernia occurs in approximately 10% of laparotomy incisions; one important risk factor is the individual surgeon's technique and attention to detail; studies have shown no differences in the complication rate between different suture materials or between continuous and interrupted closure techniques but marked individual differences in wound complication rates between surgeons. A continuous mass (all-layer) closure with slowly absorbable monofilament suture has been found to be the optimal technique.

Anastomotic leakage

Anastomotic leak is perhaps the most feared complication after intestinal surgery. Mortality varies widely in reported series from 6 to 25% and the spectrum of effects of anastomotic leakage is equally wide, from peri-anastomotic abscess (treated simply by percutaneous drainage) to dramatic postoperative peritonitis with profound haemodynamic instability. Indeed, even the definition of anastomotic leakage can be quite elusive; Bruce *et al.* performed a systematic review of studies measuring the incidence of anastomotic leaks after gastrointestinal surgery and in the 97 studies reviewed, there were a total of 56 separate definitions of anastomotic leak. A leak may be defined by the need for reoperation, clinical findings, or by radiological criteria, making comparisons between studies difficult or impossible.

A large number of patients ultimately found to have an anastomotic leak do not have a dramatic presentation with enteric content appearing through the wound or with peritonitis but have a more insidious presentation, often with low-grade fever, prolonged ileus or failure to thrive. In these patients, making the diagnosis may be much more difficult as the clinical course is often similar to other postoperative infectious complications. Radiological imaging is usually required; even then, the diagnosis may be elusive or at least uncertain. CT scanning appears to be far more helpful than contrast enema in imaging patients with potential leaks. Contrast enemas may be falsely negative and are not technically possible to examine other than left-sided colorectal anastomoses. However, CT scan can also be falsely negative and if leak is suspected, contrast enema may complement cross-sectional imaging. Higher leak rates are typically reported for low pelvic anastomoses or anastomoses to the anal canal. Anastomotic leakage after surgery for colorectal cancer is an independent predictor of diminished overall and cancer-specific survival, aside from the immediate clinical consequences.

Risk factors predisposing to anastomotic leakage include malnutrition, weight loss, alcohol intake, lengthy operative times, peritoneal contamination, and blood transfusions.

Due to the increased anastomotic leak rate of low colorectal and colo- (or ileo-) anal anastomoses, a proximally diverting stoma is usually constructed for patients having low anterior resection or ileoanal pouch operations. There is some argument as to whether the stoma reduces the leakage rate; however, it certainly protects the patient from the worst septic consequences of pelvic anastomotic leak.

Postoperative adhesions

Adhesions after abdominal surgery are abnormal attachments between tissues or organs. Mechanical trauma to peritoneal surfaces, infection, ischaemia or the presence of bile, blood or foreign materials in the abdominal cavity such as glove powder, gauze fluff, sutures, and prosthetic mesh is a potent cause of adhesions. After laparotomy, almost 95% of patients are shown to have adhesions at subsequent surgery; after major gynaecological surgery, the incidence is 60% to 90%. Although the majority of adhesions are asymptomatic, intestinal obstruction and strangulation, chronic pain and infertility may result from adhesions. Approximately 1% of surgical admissions and 3% of laparotomies are estimated to be due to intestinal obstruction from adhesions. In a review of 11 separate studies, adhesions were found to be the most common pathology in patients with chronic pelvic pain and analysis of three studies examining the effect of adhesiolysis on chronic pelvic pain indicated significant benefits in 80%. It is estimated that 15% to 20% of cases of infertility in women are considered to be secondary to adhesions. Future surgical procedures are associated with increased morbidity, as adhesions result in more bleeding, longer laparotomies and increased iatrogenic injury to the bowel. Postoperative adhesions are the largest single cause of small bowel obstruction and account for 65% to 75% of cases. The type of primary abdominal operation is known to influence the development of intra-abdominal adhesions, with operations below the transverse mesocolon being particularly risky. A retrospective review of patients undergoing total or subtotal colectomy from 1985 to 1994 found that 18% of patients developed SBO caused by adhesions. The risk of adhesional SBO was 11% at 1 year, increasing to 30% at 10 years after surgery. A SBO rate of 25% has been reported in long-term follow up of patients after formation of an ileal pouch and this study concurs with others which have shown a cumulative probability of SBO 10 years after ileal pouch–anal anastomosis of 22%. The Surgical and Clinical Adhesions Research (SCAR) study used a national linked patient dataset to investigate the burden of disease caused by postoperative adhesions. The initial cohort comprised over 12 000 patients undergo-

ing lower abdominal surgery; over the following 10 years, patients were readmitted a mean of 2.2 times and 7.3% of readmissions were directly related to adhesions. Readmissions varied according to the site of surgery, with index procedures on colon, rectum and small intestine having the highest number of adhesion-related readmissions. Fully 40% of all readmissions were categorized as possibly related to adhesions. The first 25% of readmissions were in the first year; however, readmissions continued to occur steadily during the 10-year follow-up with no decline with time.

After a single adhesive SBO, recurrence rates are high; 53% after an initial episode and 85% after second, third or later episodes. Up to one-third of cases of adhesional SBO will require operative treatment and the risk of inadvertent bowel perforation during such reoperations has been recorded as 19%, increasing morbidity and hospital stay. Independent risk factors for these bowel injuries included obesity, increasing age and three or more previous laparotomies. The mortality in the group of patients who sustain enterotomies in this fashion is approximately 13%.

Cost

The economic burden of adhesions is enormous; in a recent study from the UK, mean (SD) length of stay was 16.3 days (11.0 days) for surgical treatment and 7.0 days (4.6 days) for conservative treatment of adhesive SBO. In-patient mortality was 9.8% for the surgical group and 7.2% for the conservative group. Total treatment cost per admission for adhesional SBO was almost £5000 for surgically treated admissions and £1600 for conservatively treated admissions.

Litigation

Although adhesions have been called 'an inevitable blight…as easily controlled as the weather,' litigation not uncommonly occurs as a result of adhesions and their surgical therapy. The commonest cause of litigation is delay in diagnosis (leading to gangrene and perforation of small bowel with its consequent morbidity), visceral injury during adhesiolysis, chronic pain and infertility.

Prevention strategies

Although patients should be warned that adhesion formation is almost invariable after laparotomy, several precautions may be taken to limit their impact. Powdered gloves should not be used; peritoneal defects and the pelvic floor should be left open as these rapidly reperitonealize and the omentum may be interposed between bowel and the laparotomy wound or wrapped around anastomoses. As adhesions are more likely after intra-abdominal complications, meticulous surgical technique should be used. Various pharmacological interventions have been tried to reduce the impact of postoperative adhesions. In a randomized trial, the severity of postoperative adhesions was reduced after placement of a bioresorbable membrane during the primary surgery. Although use of such agents has not been shown to lead to any adverse outcomes, neither do they appear to reduce the requirement for surgical adhesiolysis for intestinal obstruction. Nevertheless, large-scale, prospective, patient-masked, controlled trials are ongoing.

Fever

Fever is common in the postoperative period and it has diverse causes. Tissue trauma during surgery, with systemic release of pyrogenic substances, may be a major cause of early postoperative fever. Other non-infectious causes of early postoperative fever include drug hypersensitivity (including anaesthetic agents) and transfusion reactions.

Fever within 48 hours after surgery is usually caused by atelectasis. Lung re-expansion causes the body temperature to return to normal. When fever appears after the second postoperative day, the differential diagnosis includes venous access site phlebitis, pneumonia and urinary tract infection.

Patients without an infection are rarely febrile after the fifth postoperative day. The onset of fever this late would suggest a wound infection or, less often, anastomotic leakage and intra-abdominal abscess. Bacterial pneumonias are often precipitated by perioperative aspiration or early postoperative atelectasis and consequently tend to occur within the first week of surgery.

Urinary tract infections may appear at any time. They occur almost exclusively in patients with bladder catheterization or a previous history of urinary tract manipulation. Thrombophlebitis and pulmonary embolism are important causes of postoperative fever, which may occur either early or late.

Urinary retention

Urinary retention is common, especially after pelvic or perineal operations or operations under spinal/ epidural anaesthesia and may require temporary catheterization. In a male patient if a catheter cannot be passed, a suprapubic cystotomy may be needed.

Postoperative delirium and cognitive impairment

Delirium, or acute confusional state, is a clinical syndrome characterized by acute disruption of attention and cognition and it is associated with increased morbidity and mortality, longer hospital stays, higher costs and poor functional recovery and frequently leads to increases in dependency on carers after discharge.

Hypoxia must be excluded by either oximetry or blood gas estimation. A review of the anaesthetic chart or recovery room notes may reveal the cause. In most cases, of course, no cause is found. Management involves:

- the correction of metabolic disturbances
- elimination or reduction of all non-essential medication
- the presence of family members to provide emotional support
- hypnotics, e.g. chloral hydrate (250–1000 mg orally at bed time) if sleep disturbance is severe or a short course of low-dose neuroleptic (oral or intramuscular haloperidol).

Lesser degrees of postoperative cognitive dysfunction, characterized by impairment of memory and concentration, are common after major surgery in the elderly and symptoms may persist for months or years.

Venous thromboembolism

The pathophysiology of venous thromboembolism (VTE) involves three factors (Virchow's triad):

- damage to the vessel wall
- slowing down of blood flow
- an increase in coagulability.

Clinical risk factors include the following: increasing age; prolonged immobility, stroke or paralysis; previous thrombotic disease; cancer and its treatment; major surgery (particularly operations involving the abdomen, pelvis and lower extremities); trauma (especially fractures of the pelvis, hip or leg); obesity; varicose veins; cardiac dysfunction; indwelling central venous catheters; inflammatory bowel disease; nephrotic syndrome; and pregnancy or oestrogen use. For surgical patients, the incidence of VTE is affected by the pre-existing factors just listed and by factors related to the procedure itself, including the site, technique and duration of the procedure, the type of anaesthetic, the presence of infection and the degree of postoperative immobilization.

Graded compression elastic stockings (ES) reduce the incidence of leg deep venous thrombosis (DVT). Intermittent pneumatic compression (IPC) is an attractive method of prophylaxis because there is no risk of haemorrhagic complications. In trials comparing IPC with prophylactic heparin, both agents produced similar reductions in DVT.

All surgical patients should be assessed for risk of VTE and appropriate prophylaxis established.

Postoperative nausea and vomiting and ileus

Fear of postoperative nausea and vomiting (PONV) is a leading concern for patients about to undergo surgery. PONV is unpleasant and increases the risk of aspiration pneumonia; it is the leading cause of unexpected admission following planned day surgery. Several factors contribute to the aetiology of postoperative nausea and vomiting:

- individual susceptibility
- use of opioids in the perioperative period
- gastrointestinal procedures
- duration of surgery
- intra- or postoperative hypoxaemia.

The incidence of postoperative vomiting may be reduced by preoperative administration of ondansetron, a 5-HT3 receptor antagonist.

Minimizing harm to patients: communication skills

In industrialized countries, major complications are reported to occur in 3–16% of inpatient surgical procedures, with permanent disability or death rates of approximately 0.4–0.8%. In England and Wales, 129 419 incidents relating to surgical specialties were reported to the NPSA's Reporting and Learning System in 2007 with the degrees of harm shown in Table 14.4.

Table 14.4 Degrees of harm reported to the NPSA's Reporting and Learning System in 2007

Degree of harm	Number of reported incidents
No harm	90 368
Low harm	29 929
Moderate harm	7 746
Severe harm	1 105
Death	271

Evidence such as this suggests that adverse events resulting from error happen at unacceptably high rates in surgical patients and that ineffective or insufficient communication among team members contributes in the majority of instances. Indeed, communication failure is thought to be the leading cause of inadvertent patient harm. Within the surgical team, hierarchy, or power distance, frequently inhibits people from speaking up. Effective leaders flatten the hierarchy, create familiarity and make it feel safe to speak up and participate. Communication failure can lead to inefficiency, team tension, resource waste, delay, patient inconvenience and procedural error leading to patient harm. Efforts must be made to improve teamworking and communication as it is recognized that passage of information, at time of handover or when discussing individual patients, can be very poor.

Several recent initiatives are contributing to improving team work and communication within surgery; in June 2008, the World Health Organization (WHO) launched a Global Patient Safety Challenge, 'Safe Surgery Saves Lives', to reduce the number of surgical deaths across the world. The goal of the initiative is to strengthen the commitment of clinical staff to address safety issues within the surgical setting. This includes improving anaesthetic safety practices, ensuring correct site surgery, avoiding surgical site infections and improving communication within the team. A core set of safety checks has been identified in the form of a WHO Surgical Safety Checklist for use in any operating theatre environment. The checklist is a tool for the relevant clinical teams to improve the safety of surgery by reducing deaths and complications. In a study of the checklist in nearly 8000 surgical patients, the rate of death was 1.5% before the checklist was introduced and declined to 0.8% afterward ($P = 0.003$). Inpatient complications occurred in 11.0% of patients at baseline and in 7.0% after introduction of the checklist ($P < 0.001$).

Briefings, although standard practice in aviation, the military and law enforcement, have been uncommon in clinical medicine. Spending a few minutes at the beginning of a shift can get everyone at the same start point, avoid surprises and positively affect how the team works together.

The junior surgeon is constantly involved in passage of information about patients. Information comes from the patient, nursing and other staff and is passed between doctors of varying grades and experience. Often advice or guidance needs to be sought from more senior clinicians; communication then needs to occur effectively back from the consultant, through the team to the nursing staff, patient and relatives!

The NHS National Patient Safety Agency (http://www.npsa.nhs.uk) advocates the use of 'situation-background-assessment-recommendation' (SBAR) as a mechanism to frame professional conversation about patients. Originally used in the military and aviation industries, SBAR was developed for healthcare by Dr M Leonard and colleagues from Kaiser Permanente in Colorado, USA. In one healthcare setting, the incidence of harm to patients fell by 50% after implementing SBAR.

SBAR enables clarification of what information should be communicated between members of the team, and how. It can also develop teamwork and foster a culture of patient safety. The tool consists of standardized prompt questions within four sections, to ensure that staff are sharing concise and focused information. It allows staff to communicate assertively and effectively, reducing the need for repetition. SBAR helps staff anticipate the information needed by colleagues and encourages assessment skills. Using SBAR prompts staff to formulate information with the right level of detail.

SBAR can be used to shape communication at any stage of the patient's journey, from the content of a GP's referral, telephone contact between a nurse and a doctor, between a junior and a consultant, between peers at every level and through to communicating discharge back to a GP. When SBAR is used in a clinical setting, staff can make a recommendation which ensures that the reason for the communication is clear. This is particularly important in situations where staff may be uncomfortable about making a recommendation, e.g. those who are inexperienced or who need to communicate to a senior. The use of SBAR prevents the (inef-fective) process of communication known as 'hinting and hoping'.

SBAR

S: Situation

- Identify yourself and the site/unit you are calling from
- Identify the patient by name and the reason for your report
- Describe your concern.

First, describe the specific situation about which you are calling, including the patient's name, consultant, patient location and vital signs.

B: Background

- Give the patient's reason for admission
- Explain significant medical history
- You then inform the consultant of the patient's background: admitting diagnosis, date of admission, prior procedures, current medications, allergies, pertinent laboratory results and other relevant diagnostic results. For this, you need to have collected information from the patient's chart, flow sheets and progress notes.

A: Assessment

- Vital signs
- Clinical impressions, concerns.

You need to think critically when informing the person you want to communicate with of your assessment of the situation. This means that you have considered what might be the underlying reason for your patient's condition. Not only have you reviewed your findings from your assessment, you have also consolidated these with other objective indicators, such as laboratory results.

R: Recommendation

- Explain what you need – be specific about request and time frame
- Make suggestions
- Clarify expectations.

Finally, what is your recommendation? That is, what would you like to happen by the end of the conversation with the physician? Any order that is given on the phone needs to be repeated back to ensure accuracy. Incorporating SBAR may seem simple, but it takes considerable training. It can be very difficult to change the way people communicate, particularly with senior staff.

Further patient safety factors

When mistakes occur, they are sometimes viewed as episodes of personal failure, with the predictable result that these events are minimized and not openly discussed. Human factors science tells us that even skilled, experienced doctors will make mistakes. Effective communication that creates a well-understood plan of care greatly reduces the chances of inevitable errors becoming consequential and injuring patients. However, there has to be a robust system within the surgical department to identify poor outcomes and analyse them in a non-judgemental way in order for lessons to be learned. This is a vital component of a department's quality improvement programme and is usually achieved by regular morbidity and mortality meetings.

The Confidential Reporting System in Surgery (CORESS; http://www.coress.org.uk) is maintained by the Association of Surgeons of Great Britain and Ireland. The purpose of CORESS is to promote safety in surgical practice. Any surgeon or surgical trainee, irrespective of specialty, can submit reports, online and in confidence, to CORESS. Any safety-related incident involving yourself, other people, your hospital or other organizations that you deal with can be reported. When all identifiable data have been removed, the report is reviewed by experts in the appropriate specialty. If useful lessons can be learned an unidentifiable version may be published in the surgical literature.

Conclusion

All surgeons will treat patients who develop complications; however, recent evidence has proven that attention to detail and adherence to evidence-based best practice can significantly reduce complications. As part of the 'Better Colectomy Project' a panel of colorectal and general surgeons evaluated a set of 37 evidence-based practices that they felt were the most pertinent to the evaluation and management of a patient undergoing a colorectal resection. Fifteen of these practices were classified as 'key processes' for the prevention of complications. Nineteen per cent of the patients analysed experienced complications, of

which 82% involved postoperative infection. Nonadherence to the key processes significantly predicted the occurrence of a complication ($P = 0.002$) and each additional process missed increased the odds of a postoperative complication by 60%. It therefore seems that compliance with perioperative best practices will reduce complication rates significantly. Recognition of risk factors and appropriate perioperative management can therefore reduce the likelihood of complications and expert perioperative care can considerably reduce their impact.

It remains the surgeon's duty (and privilege) to look after patients he or she has operated on. Adverse events occurring due to failure of communication or systems within departments are potentially avoidable and we must all work together to see them eliminated. Junior surgeons are often responsible for a very wide range of hospital specialties at night and accurate communication between teams of doctors is particularly important at times of shift changes.

Further reading

Annane D et al. Effect of treatment with low doses of hydrocortisone and fludrocortisone on mortality in patients with septic shock. JAMA 2002;**288**:862–871.

Arriaga AF et al. The Better Colectomy Project: association of evidence-based best-practice adherence rates to outcomes in colorectal surgery. Ann Surg 2009;**250**(4):507–513.

Bennett-Guerrero E et al. Comparison of P-POSSUM risk-adjusted mortality rates after surgery between patients in the USA and the UK. Br J Surg 2003;**90**(12):1593–1598.

Bernard GR et al. Efficacy and safety of recombinant human activated protein C for severe sepsis. N Engl J Med 2001;**344**:699–709.

Bruce J et al. Systematic review of the definition and measurement of anastomotic leak after gastrointestinal surgery. Br J Surg 2001;**88**(9):1157–1168.

Ellis H et al. Adhesion-related hospital readmissions after abdominal and pelvic surgery: a retrospective cohort study. Lancet 1999;**353**:1476–1480.

Hebert PC et al. A multicenter, randomized, controlled clinical trial of transfusion requirements in critical care. Transfusion Requirements in Critical Care Investigators, Canadian Critical Care Trials Group. N Engl J Med 1999;**340**(6):409–417.

Mangano DT et al. Effect of atenolol on mortality and cardiovascular morbidity after noncardiac surgery.

Multicentre Study of Perioperative Ischaemia Research Group. *N Engl J Med* 1996;**335**:1713–1720.

Poldermans D *et al*. The effect of bisoprolol on perioperative mortality and myocardial infarction in high-risk patients undergoing vascular surgery. *N Engl J Med* 1999;**341**:1789–1794.

Van Den Berghe G *et al*. Intensive insulin therapy in the critically ill patients. *N Engl J Med* 2001;**345**(19):1359–1367.

Williamson LM *et al*. Serious hazards of transfusion (SHOT) initiative: analysis of the first two annual reports. *BMJ* 1999;**319**(7201):16–19.

Chapter 15

Management of sepsis

Mark J. Midwinter

Introduction

Severe sepsis and septic shock are common and account for 3% of hospital admissions and 10% of admissions to critical care units. In critically ill patients, sepsis remains the most common cause of mortality. Mortality rates approaching 40% are seen in patients with severe sepsis and up to 80% for patients with septic shock and multi-organ dysfunction syndrome (MODS). It is estimated that approximately 1400 people worldwide die of sepsis every day and 37 000 die of sepsis every year in the UK. There is evidence to suggest that the incidence of severe sepsis is increasing, with a prediction that the number of severe sepsis cases is set to grow at a rate of 1.5% per annum, adding an additional 1 million cases per year in the USA alone by 2020. Sepsis is thought to account for 40% of total ICU expenditure.

Spearheaded by the ESICM (European Society of Intensive Care Medicine), ISF (International Sepsis Forum) and SCCM (Society of Critical Care Medicine), the Surviving Sepsis Campaign® is aimed at improving the diagnosis, survival and management of patients with sepsis by addressing the challenges associated with it.

The Surviving Sepsis® programme aims to:

- increase awareness, understanding, and knowledge
- change perceptions and behaviour
- increase the pace of change in patterns of care
- influence public policy
- define standards of care in severe sepsis
- reduce the mortality associated with sepsis by 25% over the next 5 years
- working with the relevant stakeholders, the Surviving Sepsis Campaign's® mission is to

improve the management of sepsis through targeted initiatives.

The initial presentation of severe sepsis is often non-specific. The pathophysiology and optimal management of both the systemic inflammatory response syndrome (SIRS) and sepsis are still being intensively studied in hopes of developing improved therapies; however, the structured, protocol-driven approach to the septic patient has been shown to reduce mortality. In a study of 101 consecutive adult patients with severe sepsis or septic shock on medical or surgical wards in the UK, compliance with 6-hour and 24-hour sepsis care bundles adapted from the Surviving Sepsis Campaign® guidelines was evaluated. The rate of compliance with the 6-hour sepsis bundle was 52% and, compared with the compliant group, the non-compliant group had a more than two-fold increase in hospital mortality (49% versus 23%).

Definitions

In order to facilitate the adoption of universal definitions two major consensus conferences have been held to define terms used in SIRS and sepsis.

The first in 1992 was a consensus conference of the American College of Chest Physicians and the American Society of Critical Care Medicine. This led to the publication of definitions of the systemic inflammatory response syndrome (SIRS) and sepsis syndromes (Table 15.1). These definitions have been adopted worldwide and provide a universal language through which clinicians can discuss, research and improve outcomes in one of the most significant entities affecting critically ill patients.

At the second conference in 2001 several North American and European intensive care societies

Fundamentals of Surgical Practice, Third Edition, ed. Andrew N. Kingsnorth and Douglas M. Bowley.
Published by Cambridge University Press. © Cambridge University Press 2011.

Table 15.1 Definitions of SIRS and sepsis

Condition	Definition
Systemic inflammatory response syndrome	Two or more of: Core temperature >38 °C or <36 °C Heart rate >90 beats/min Respiratory rate >20 breaths/min or $PaCO_2$ <4.26 kPa or mechanically ventilated Leukocyte count >12 000/μl or <4000/μl
Sepsis	SIRS + suspected or confirmed infection
Severe sepsis	Sepsis + organ dysfunction, hypotension or hypoperfusion
Septic shock	Sepsis and refractory hypotension and perfusion abnormalities

Table 15.2 Danger-associated molecular patterns

Category	Examples
Pathogen-associated molecular patterns (PAMP)	Gram-negative and -positive bacteria Lipopolysaccharide, lipopeptides, lipoteichoic acid Bacterial DNA and RNA
Alarmins	Products of cell death DNA and RNA Heat shock protein S100 proteins Adenosine Fibrinogen

agreed to revisit the definitions for sepsis and related conditions. It was agreed that while the concepts of sepsis, severe sepsis and septic shock remain useful to clinicians and researchers these definitions did not allow precise staging or prognostication of the host response to infection. While SIRS remains a useful concept, the diagnostic criteria for SIRS published in 1992 are overly sensitive and non-specific. The idea of a staging system based on four separate characteristics was developed. This was designated by the acronym PIRO (P for predisposition indicating pre-existing comorbidity that would reduce survival; I for the insult or infection, recognizing some are more lethal than others; R for response to the infective challenge including SIRS; and O for organ or system failure).

Pathophysiology

The causes of SIRS and sepsis are multifactorial. While SIRS may or may not be a result of an infective organism, sepsis can result from virtually any infectious agent. A recent model of the initiators of the inflammatory response recognizes danger-associated molecular patterns (DAMP) which include exogenous pathogen-associated molecular patterns (PAMP) and endogenous alarmins (Table 15.2). Pattern recognition receptors (PRR) recognize both PAMP and alarmins triggering inflammatory mediators. In the past it was considered the final common pathway in both SIRS and sepsis was the result of an exaggerated inflammatory response to an insult or organism. This led to the view that strategies that could blunt the hyper-

inflammatory response would be potential therapies. Inflammatory mediators such as tumour necrosis factor alpha (TNF-alpha) and cytokines (interleukins IL-1, IL-6, IL-8) have been implicated in perpetuating this response and observations from animal models suggested inhibition of these mediators improved survival. This led to a series of clinical trials to block TNF or IL-1 which failed to show dramatic improvement in outcomes. It is now considered that there is heterogeneity in this patient group, with some showing enhanced inflammatory response and others a blunted response. Indeed a single patient may exhibit both during the course of the disease. Studies have shown intensive care patients have a reduced production of TNF and IL-6 in response to endotoxin. It has been found that T-lymphocytes from patients with severe burns and sepsis fail to proliferate with mitogenic stimulation and do not produce IL-1 or IL-12. While all these mediators clearly have an immunomodulatory role, the notion that they cause uncontrolled inflammation is now therefore being challenged. Thus, the concept of an inappropriate inflammatory response to an insult or infection and a compromised immune system (at least in some patients) is emerging.

It has become increasingly clear that the situation in SIRS and sepsis is even more complex than described above, with interactions with the coagulation system and vascular endothelium being central to processes of inflammation, in particular through activation of protein C. There is also evidence to suggest the complement and kallikrein-kinin systems are also implicated. Dysfunction of these systems and endothelial cell failure may be implicated in the development of SIRS and sepsis. Pro-inflammatory cytokines stimulate liver production of a wide range of proteins called the acute-phase proteins, such as C-reactive protein (CRP), serum amyloid P (SAP), plasminogen activator inhibitor 1 (PAI-1) and procalcitonin. Many of these proteins have antimicrobial properties and CRP is used clinically to diagnose inflammation. Biologically CRP acts as an opsinin, enhancing phagocytosis of bacteria by neutrophils.

Central to the pathophysiology of sepsis is the disorder of the microcirculation. Much work has been carried out examining the effects on the microcirculation. Vasoregulatory dysfunction with impaired flow and microaggregation lead to local hypoxia, ischaemia and impaired cellular respiration. Endothelium can synthesize inflammatory mediators as well as being a target for other mediators, in addition to reacting through the coagulation and complement systems. Activated endothelium produces IL-1, IL-6, IL-8 and colony stimulating factor (CSF). During acute inflammatory states tissue factor is expressed and normal anticoagulant mechanisms are countered by inhibition of the protein C pathway. Nitric oxide (NO) is produced in the endothelium in an activated state to above the normal background concentration, leading to vasodilatation, increased vascular permeability and mitochondrial anergy.

The potential result of these events is the progression to single or multi-organ dysfunction and then organ failure. Multi-organ dysfunction syndrome (MODS) is characterized by the sequential failure of organs. The term dysfunction rather than failure is considered more appropriate since the process starts with derangement of function and then progresses to failure. The mortality rate is high and increases with the number of organs involved: 30% when one organ fails and increases to 100% when four organs fail.

Tissue hypoxia has traditionally been considered the underlying mechanism for developing MODS, be it as a result of hypoxaemia or hypoperfusion. An emerging concept is that NO overproduction with reactive oxygen species (ROS) and reactive nitrogen species (RNS) from polymorphonuclear neutrophils leads to mitochondrial dysfunction, decreased ATP levels and organ failure. For the development of MODS multiple insults are usually required. A 'first hit' primes the immune/inflammatory response, and a 'second hit' leads to further critical deterioration and organ dysfunction. Many hypotheses have been suggested as mechanisms for this and in reality all probably contribute in a cumulative multi-faceted response. Injury stimulates mononuclear cells (particularly macrophages) to produce excessive cytokines. Humoral and cellular cascades are then activated,

Table 15.3 Non-infectious causes of SIRS

Acute mesenteric ischaemia
Autoimmune disorders
Burns
Dehydration
Drug reaction
Electrical injuries
Haemorrhagic shock
Intestinal perforation
Myocardial infarction
Acute pancreatitis
Substance abuse (e.g. cocaine and amphetamines)
Major surgical procedures
Transfusion reactions
Upper gastrointestinal bleeding
Vasculitis

causing systemic effects. Endothelial cell ischaemia, followed by reperfusion, results in the release of toxic free radicals, with the microvascular injury contributing to the inflammatory response. TNF and IL-1 change the endothelial cell from a non-inflammatory to a pro-inflammatory state. Pro-inflammatory endothelial cells can activate the extrinsic clotting pathway and promote leukocyte adherence, resulting in focal microvascular thrombosis and further leukocyte-mediated endothelial injury. Loss of the intestinal mucosal barrier leads to systemic spread of bacteria or endotoxin, a process termed bacterial translocation. Once in the circulation, the bacteria or endotoxins further stimulate an inflammatory reaction. The relative contribution of each of these responses to MODS is still debated.

It has been shown that genetic polymorphisms exist to some cytokines and inflammatory mediators described above. When these polymorphisms are functional it has been shown that differing cytokine responses can result. This differing response raises the possibility of genetic predisposition to an excess mortality from sepsis in some individuals. Polymorphisms have been described for TNF, IL-1b, IL-1ra and IL-10. The precise roles of these genetic variations on outcome from sepsis have yet to be defined.

Diagnosis

Crucial to implementation of timely treatment is rapid diagnosis. It is trivial to apply the criteria for the diagnosis of SIRS listed in Table 15.1. Causes need to be diligently sought and infective foci, if present, located. It must be considered that the cause of the SIRS may be non-infectious (Table 15.3) and require different management strategies to infectious causes.

It is of great importance therefore to be able to differentiate those patients with infective causes from those with non-infectious causes. Clinical evaluation is combined with imaging to help locate and define potential sources of infection. Direct culture of body fluids (blood, urine, sputum, CSF, pleural or ascitic), tissues or direct drainage of collections such as abscesses is used to determine the infectious agent and guide appropriate therapy. The hunt for biochemical markers to indicate an infective source has been sought but without clinically applicable success to date.

Treatment

Significant research into the pathophysiology and treatment of sepsis is slowly leading to improved outcomes in afflicted patients. The evidence-based recommendations for the treatment of severe sepsis were summarized in a recent consensus publication (2008). This 'Surviving Sepsis Campaign®' is being adopted globally.

Their recommendations are summarized below; the major components of treating sepsis are:

- resuscitation
- antibiotics
- source (infection) control
- supportive care.

The Sepsis Six represent a group of six simple tasks which can be performed easily by non-specialist staff within the first hour of severe sepsis developing. These tasks are the crucial first steps toward the completion of the severe sepsis resuscitation bundle. Their application requires no specialist training, yet the Sepsis Six can have a major impact on whether or not the patient survives:

- give high flow oxygen
- take blood cultures
- give IV antibiotics
- start IV fluid resuscitation
- check haemoglobin and lactate
- measure accurate hourly urine output.

The Survive Sepsis Campaign® has developed two severe sepsis bundles; the resuscitation bundle is a combined evidence-based goal that must be completed within 6 hours for patients with severe sepsis, septic shock and/or lactate >4 mmol/l.

Resuscitation bundle

Bundle element 1

Measure serum lactate.

Bundle element 2

Obtain blood cultures prior to antibiotic administration.

Bundle element 3

Deliver broad-spectrum antibiotic within 3 hours of ED admission and within 1 hour of non-ED admission.

Bundle element 4

Treat hypotension and/or elevated lactate with fluids.

1. Deliver an initial minimum of 20 ml/kg of crystalloid or an equivalent.
2. Administer vasopressors for hypotension not responding to initial fluid resuscitation to maintain mean arterial pressure (MAP) >65 mmHg.

Bundle element 5

In the event of persistent hypotension despite fluid resuscitation (septic shock) and/or lactate >4 mmol/l maintain adequate central venous pressure and central venous oxygen saturation.

1. Achieve a central venous pressure (CVP) of >8 mmHg.
2. Achieve a central venous oxygen saturation ($ScvO_2$) > 70% or mixed venous oxygen saturation (SvO_2) > 65%.

Sepsis management bundle

Bundle element 1

Administer low-dose steroids for septic shock in accordance with a standardized ICU policy. (Policy is often that patients who require vasopressors despite fluid replacement should be given hydrocortisone 200–300 mg/day in 3 or 4 divided doses (or continuous infusion) for 7 days.) If not administered, document why the patient did not qualify for low-dose steroids based upon the standardized protocol.

Bundle element 2

Administer recombinant human activated protein C (rhAPC) in accordance with a standardized ICU policy. If not administered, document why the patient did not qualify for rhAPC.

Bundle element 3

Maintain adequate glycaemic control (initiate insulin therapy when blood glucose levels exceed 10 mmol/l) with a goal blood glucose approximating 8 mmol/l.

Bundle element 4

Prevent excessive inspiratory plateau pressures on mechanically ventilated patients.

Controlling the source of infection is a critical part of the sepsis treatment and a surgeon is often very useful in helping to accomplish source control. This includes catheter removal, tissue debridement, abscess drainage and laparotomy for perforated viscus. Red blood cell transfusions should be administered to achieve target haemoglobin between 7 and 9 g/dl.

It should be noted that the use of recombinant human activated protein C (rhAPC) in severe sepsis came from the results of the PROWESS and ADDRESS trials. There still remains some controversy about the use of rhAPC. There may be benefit in patients with high risk of death (APACHE $\geq$25 or MODS) but not in patients with low risk of death (APACHE <25 or single organ failure). Patients who had major surgery within the preceding 12 hours were excluded in the trials.

While these guidelines were written for sepsis, they translate well to the prevention and treatment of MODS. Prevention of MODS may be achieved by early resuscitation and control of the source of sepsis. Once established, treatment of MODS involves supportive care. The definition and discussion of support of failing organs is the realm of critical care and is further discussed in Chapter 13.

As discussed, the role of surgery for sepsis is focused primarily on source control. One area of sur-gical development is the adoption of a 'damage control' philosophy for these patients where the surgical intent is abbreviated to deal with source control, minimizing operating time, to allow for physiological correction prior to any more prolonged definitive surgical procedure such as anastomoses. This surgical approach is accepted for severe trauma patients and is gaining acceptance as an approach in complex septic surgical patients.

Summary

Sepsis and SIRS result from complex pathophysiological processes with many interacting systems which are continuing to be elucidated. Immune-modulation therapies, despite promising in vitro and in vivo results, have failed to deliver major benefit in clinical trials. Treatment of these patients is based on resuscitation therapies, source (infection) control, antibiotics and supportive care. Tissue and organ blood flow and oxygenation is critical to the successful management of such patients.

Further reading

Castellheim A, Brekke O-L, Espevik T, Mollnes TE. Innate immune response to danger signals in systemic inflammatory response syndrome and sepsis. *Scand J Immunol* 2009;**69**:479–491.

Dellinger RP, Levy MM, Carlet JM, Bion J *et al.* Surviving Sepsis Campaign: International guidelines for management of severe sepsis and septic shock: *Intensive Care Med* 2008;**34**:17–60.

Gao F, Melody T, Daniels DF, Giles S, Fox S. The impact of compliance with 6-hour and 24-hour sepsis bundles on hospital mortality in patients with severe sepsis: a prospective observational study. *Crit Care* 2005;**9**(6): R764–770.

Levy MM, Fink MP, Marshall JC, Abraham E *et al.* 2001 SCCM/ESICM/ACCP/ATS/SIS International Sepsis Definitions Conference. *Crit Care Med* 2003;**31**(4): 1250–1256. Survive Sepsis website: http://www. survivesepsis.org.

Chapter

16

Assessment and early treatment of patients with trauma

Ross Davenport and Nigel Tai

Introduction

Trauma continues to be a leading cause of death and disability worldwide, and exceeds all other cause mortality combined in persons under the age of 36 years old. Globally each day 300 000 people are severely injured, with 10 000 trauma deaths. In the UK over 17 000 people die each year from accident or injury, with approximately ten times as many incapacitated or permanently disabled. The socio-economic burden to the country as a whole is difficult to quantify although estimates for trauma care in the USA are in the region of $500 billion per annum. The caveat to this is the cost of quality adjusted life years (QALYs) for injured people, which are among the cheapest in healthcare. Trauma patients are often young, fit and healthy with good potential to return to a normal life providing they receive high-quality timely intervention to enable optimal outcome from injury.

Severely injured patients have 20% higher in-hospital mortality in England and Wales (E&W) than the USA and there has been a plateau in trauma outcomes since 1994. The 2007 NCEPOD report of the management of severely injured patients reported that 52% of trauma patients receive substandard care and there may be upwards of 3000 preventable deaths in E&W annually.

One model for the organization of trauma services is to provide a regional network, with specialist major trauma centres at the hub. This has to be integrated with pre-hospital care providers and all other acute hospitals in the region as patients with major injuries would bypass the nearest available hospital facilities and be taken to specialist centres. Organization of trauma care in this way has been shown to improve outcomes and reduce preventable death from trauma by up to 15–25%. Regionalization of trauma care in

some countries (e.g. USA) is well-established but it has not yet been instituted nationwide in the UK. Trauma care in London was regionalized in April 2010 and a UK national scheme is proposed within the next few years.

Trauma surgery requires rapid decision-making with good technical ability and leadership skills. Involvement of a trauma surgeon begins at the point of injury and finishes when recovery is complete. The so called 'chain of survival' is founded in pre-hospital care and continues through resuscitation, surgery, critical care and rehabilitation. Successful outcomes from trauma are dependent on good teamwork, rapid recognition of problems, early intervention and constant re-evaluation.

Over the past 20 years advances in trauma care such as 'damage control surgery', improved resuscitation strategies and the use of interventional radiology have revolutionized the management of the severely injured.

Clinicians providing trauma care must fully appreciate the relationship between mechanism of trauma, injury pattern, pathophysiological response and importance of timely treatment in order to produce optimal outcomes from major trauma. It is impossible to provide a detailed overview of every aspect of trauma surgery in a single chapter and therefore we will provide some general principles of management with a focus on key treatments for common injury patterns.

Injury prevention and trauma epidemiology

Up to 50% of deaths occur at the scene from non-survivable CNS or great vessel injury. In most cases

Fundamentals of Surgical Practice, Third Edition, ed. Andrew N. Kingsnorth and Douglas M. Bowley.
Published by Cambridge University Press. © Cambridge University Press 2011.

injury prevention is the only mechanism by which this percentage can be reduced. Legislation is often required to bring about behavioural change with respect to preventative strategies but has proved extremely effective in reducing injury on the road, in the home and at the workplace; e.g.

- hard hats and machine safety on building sites
- control of firearms
- drink-driving campaigns
- seat belts
- airbags
- cycle lanes (cycle helmets remain voluntary in the UK)
- traffic-calming measures.

Trauma is still overwhelmingly a disease of young people and, in particular, males under the age of 40 years. As the population ages, the number of elderly people injured is set to rise; older patients have more comorbidity but less physiological reserve; therefore they often require prolonged critical care intervention.

Despite improvements in management, death from major trauma still follows a trimodal distribution.

- Immediate (minutes) – death from catastrophic injury to the central nervous system (CNS) or great vessels often at the scene of the accident/injury.
- Early (hours) – death from uncontrolled haemorrhage, e.g. major pelvic fracture with rupture of pelvic vessels or hypoxia, e.g. tension pneumothorax.
- Late (weeks) – patients who survive the initial injury insult are at risk of developing sepsis, acute lung injury, renal insufficiency and multi-organ failure due to the complex pathophysiological responses to trauma.

Injury mechanism

Blunt injury in the form of road traffic collisions (RTCs) and falls or jumps from height account for the majority of the trauma workload in the UK. Penetrating injury (gun or knife crime) is only responsible for 4% of trauma in this country although a large geographical divide exists, with rates exceeding 25% in some inner cities.

Eliciting the history of the accident or injury from the patient or bystanders is an essential part of recognizing the possible injury pattern. The magnitude and direction of force sustained by the patient is a help-

ful guide to likely injury severity. Markers of severe trauma include:

- death of other occupants in same vehicle
- ejection from vehicle
- marked intrusion into the passenger compartment of the vehicle
- fall from height (>5 metres)
- fall under a train.

Certain mechanisms of trauma are associated with typical injury patterns. A motorcyclist involved in a RTC hit from the left-hand side may present with fractured ribs and fractured left hemi-pelvis. In this example the trauma surgeon must seek to actively exclude abdominal injury, e.g. splenic rupture which, from this pattern of injury, is highly probable.

Blunt trauma

The extent of tissue injury due to blunt trauma from external compression, crush or deceleration forces is usually far greater than that from penetrating injury. Blunt trauma often involves the transfer of massive force to the body and results in multi-system injury which elicits a huge inflammatory response. Abdominal viscera are at particular risk of injury from blunt trauma as there is little protection from the bony skeleton. Clues to internal organ injury may be evident from skin marking such as the seat belt sign (Figure 16.1). Deceleration forces lead to shearing which causes viscera and vascular pedicles to tear, especially at relatively fixed points of attachment, e.g. mesenteric vasculature and descending thoracic aorta.

Penetrating injury

Gunshot wounds can be divided into either high or low energy transfer – the majority of injuries in civilian practice are from small-calibre low-velocity weapons, e.g. pistols and air guns. Low-velocity projectiles such as shotgun pellets and pistol bullets can follow an unpredictable course through the body and will often take the path of least resistance. Direct injury occurs to structures in the trajectory of the projectile. Projectiles from high-energy weapon systems, e.g. rifles and close-range shotguns, dissipate energy into the surrounding tissues, causing massive disruption to viscera. This process, known as cavitation, can suck in debris and clothing, leading to widespread contamination and associated infection. Entry and exit wounds are not always related linearly – one should maintain

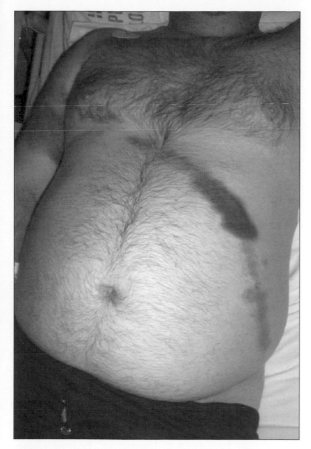

Figure 16.1 Seat belt sign.

a high index of suspicion that other body cavities may have been breached.

Knife injury is associated with low energy transfer, but direct damage to solid abdominal organs or major truncal or limb vasculature can result in catastrophic haemorrhage or cardiac tamponade. The size of knife is an unreliable guide to depth of penetration and there is no benefit in routinely exploring wounds in the emergency department (ED). Patients with life-threatening injuries following penetrating trauma should be transferred to hospital for immediate assessment as a significant proportion will require surgical intervention, e.g. intercostal chest tube drainage or haemorrhage control.

Blast injury

Trauma from detonation of explosives has the capacity to cause life-threatening multi-system injuries in one or more casualties. The mechanism of injury may be both blunt and penetrating although blast trauma produces unique effects on specific organs, e.g. blast lung, ruptured tympanic membrane. Pathophysiology of blast injury is typically divided into

- primary – shock front from blast damages air-filled structures, e.g. lung, ear, bowel
- secondary – objects energized by explosion impact upon the body, i.e. shrapnel penetration
- tertiary – high-energy explosions may cause buildings to collapse or people to be thrown through the air, e.g. blunt injury, traumatic amputations
- quaternary – burns, exposure to toxic components of explosive material or environment.

Injury severity scoring

Injury severity can be measured by extent of either anatomical injury or physiological derangement. The limitation of both methods is they are unable to accurately define the extent of overall tissue trauma or take into account the patient's physiological age, i.e. premorbid state. The most widely used anatomical scoring system is the Injury Severity Score (ISS) based on the Abbreviated Injury Scale (AIS). Injuries in each body region, e.g. chest, head/neck etc., are scored using AIS from 1 (minor) to 6 (non-survivable). The three highest scores are then squared to give the ISS; severe injury is defined by an ISS >15.

The main limitation of ISS is that it cannot be calculated in the acute phase of trauma care and does not take into account multiple injuries within the same body region, e.g. unilateral humeral fracture has the same AIS (3) as bilateral femoral fractures. GCS and the Revised Trauma Score (RTS) are the most widely used physiological scoring systems. RTS utilizes respiratory rate, systolic BP and GCS to calculate a score from 0 to 12, with lower scores associated with higher mortality.

The Trauma and ISS (TRISS) score is a combination of ISS, RTS and patient age and is a method by which trauma specialists have attempted to predict survival. TRISS is limited for the reasons discussed above and hence a very crude measure as it does not provide any information of functional outcome. Undoubtedly, a patient's predetermined genetic response to trauma affects individual outcome. Ongoing research suggests the prediction of outcome after trauma may be improved using a panel of plasma biomarkers for injury severity.

Metabolic response to trauma

The acute physiological or stress response to trauma is a complex interplay of neuroendocrine, metabolic and inflammatory changes to maintain homeostasis. Local and systemic effects are necessary to promote wound healing and tissue regeneration but, in excess, these responses can cause harm, e.g. acute lung injury and multiple organ dysfunction. In the early stages of injury the 'fight or flight' reaction predominates; central to this is the hypothalamic-pituitary-adrenal axis with activation of the sympathetic nervous system and the acute phase inflammatory response which leads to:

- increased catabolism to mobilize energy resources
- activation of the immune and coagulation systems
- haemodynamic changes to preserve cardiovascular homeostasis.

The latter phase is characterized by increased metabolic rate, protein catabolism, reductions in lean body mass and immunosuppression.

Neuroendocrine

Trauma induces release of both adrenocorticotrophin hormone (ACTH) via nociceptive stimuli (injured tissue) and vasopressin from the pituitary. Plasma levels of these hormones are directly related to the extent of injury but severe trauma diminishes the cortisol response from the adrenal cortex, possibly as a consequence of adrenal hypoperfusion. Hypovolaemia, e.g. haemorrhage, specifically activates the renin-angiotensin-aldosterone axis to promote retention of sodium and water to maintain blood pressure. Hypothalamic activation of the sympathetic nervous system by hypovolaemia and tissue damage promotes release of catecholamines from the adrenal medulla. Adrenaline, noradrenaline and dopamine within the circulation cause tachycardia, an elevation in blood pressure and peripheral vasoconstriction to support the cardiovascular system and maintain blood flow to vital organs, e.g. brain and kidney. A prolonged and excessive sympathetic response as a result of severe injury and hypovolaemia will result in end organ hypoperfusion, giving rise to hepatic insufficiency and acute renal failure. Adrenaline has additional effects on other hormones to effect mobilization of energy substrates. α-Adrenergic inhibition of insulin release from the pancreas and β-adrenergic-mediated glucagon secretion significantly elevate plasma glucose. In combination with growth hormone acting via insulin-like growth factors glucose is preferentially taken up by neurons at this time of relative glucose shortage.

Metabolic

Trauma produces a profound catabolic response to mobilize energy substrates from the breakdown of carbohydrate, fat and protein (late). The metabolic response to major trauma includes:

- increased hepatic glycogenolysis and glucogenesis
- reduced glucose utilization by skeletal muscle secondary to catecholamine-mediated suppression of insulin release and increased intracellular insulin resistance
- conversion of triglycerides by lipolysis to free fatty acids and glycerol (substrate for hepatic gluconeogenesis)
- skeletal muscle breakdown (release of amino acids for gluconeogenesis)
- increased whole body turnover of protein – negative nitrogen balance.

Inflammatory

Inflammation is critical to wound healing and survival but an overwhelming response in the face of severe trauma with systemic activation of the immune system may become self-destructive. Trauma causes local non-specific activation of the 'innate' immune response to recruit white blood cells and macrophages with activation of the complement system at the site of injury. Cytokines such as interleukin-6 cause hepatocytes to release acute-phase proteins such as fibrinogen and C-reactive protein which together with other pro-inflammatory mediators (TNF-alpha, IL-1, interferon and prostaglandins) define the immune response. Circulating immunosuppressive factors, e.g. suppressor T cells, attempt to keep the inflammatory process in check since overflow of cytokines into the systemic circulation is an important factor in the systemic inflammatory response syndrome (SIRS).

Multiple organ failure (MOF) is an extreme form of SIRS and despite advances in critical care remains the leading cause of late death in trauma. Following injury patients develop a hyper-inflammatory response, which is directly related to degree of shock, extent of tissue injury and host factors. A low-level SIRS response permits recovery but if the injury load is extensive an augmented SIRS effect can precipitate early MOF. Additionally any delayed

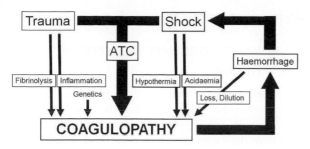

Figure 16.2 Multi-factorial drivers of trauma-induced coagulopathy; from Hess *et al.* 2008.

immunosuppressive factors which keep SIRS at bay which escape the normal negative feedback loops will result in severe immunosuppression and infection. The precise mechanism by which the immune balance is regulated and why trauma disrupts the equilibrium to predispose to sepsis and MOF is unknown. Current hypotheses include impaired mitochondrial function in severe shock; reperfusion injury with release of free radicals; hypoperfusion of the gut allowing bacterial translocation and immunosuppression following massive blood transfusion.

Trauma-induced coagulopathy

Our understanding of trauma-induced coagulopathy (TIC) has changed dramatically in recent years and continues to evolve rapidly. TIC aetiology is multi-factorial (Figure 16.2) and more complex than the classic description of clotting factor loss (bleeding or consumption), dilution or dysfunction (hypothermia and/or acidaemia). Numerous studies have demonstrated an acute traumatic coagulopathy (ATC) present at admission in nearly 25% of trauma patients prior to the administration of significant volumes of fluid. ATC appears to be an endogenous coagulopathy initiated by hypoperfusion and tissue injury. Patients with ATC are four times more likely to die compared with non-coagulopathic patients.

Analysis of data from patients receiving massive blood transfusion (>10 units PRBC in 24 hours) from combat hospitals in Iraq and Afghanistan has changed trauma resuscitation recommendations. These data suggest that for patients with exsanguination who require massive transfusion a high plasma to RBC ratio (<1:1.4) is independently associated with improved survival to hospital discharge.

These recent recommendations have been called Damage Control Resuscitation (DCR) and begin in the ED and continue until normovolaemia and haemostasis have been achieved. DCR is defined as:

- maintaining systolic BP below 90 mmHg until haemorrhage control is achieved
- transfusing PRBC (un-cross-matched type O until type-specific blood is available) and thawed fresh frozen plasma (FFP) as primary resuscitation fluids – aiming for a near equal ratio to correct hypovolaemia and promote haemostasis.

The pre-hospital phase and the trauma team

The majority of pre-hospital trauma care continues to be provided by paramedic-trained ambulance crews in a 'scoop and run' approach. On-scene treatment is kept to a minimum and the patient is rapidly transferred to the nearest hospital. Increasing numbers of air ambulances are being deployed in both urban and rural locations to enable a trained pre-hospital care doctor to be transported to the scene. The primary advantage of this strategy is definitive airway management, e.g. endotracheal (ET) intubation, and the ability to temporarily control some life-threatening events. Whatever approach is employed the time spent on scene must be kept to an absolute minimum. Definitive treatment of injuries can only be accomplished within a hospital setting. The concept of a 'golden hour' in the initial stage of trauma care is a useful reminder for clinicians of the need to expedite diagnosis and treatment of life-threatening injuries.

Prior to arrival of any severely injured trauma patient at hospital the pre-hospital care team must notify the ED in the receiving hospital. If the patient is exsanguinating this pre-alert should be a trigger for activation of the in-hospital massive transfusion protocol to ensure blood and clotting products are immediately available on the patient's arrival. Patients who fulfil criteria for activation of a trauma team must be met by a fully assembled trauma team consisting of (but not limited to):

- team leader
- doctor with advanced airway skills, e.g. anaesthetist
- general surgeon
- orthopaedic surgeon
- nurse
- radiographer.

Senior clinicians should be involved from the outset to ensure life-threatening conditions are identified early and definitive care is initiated as a priority. Trauma team training through moulage-based scenarios facilitates an organized team structure. The Advanced Trauma Life Support (ATLS®) course has long been the mainstay of trauma team training around the world but similar European courses are now available. Each member of the team should be assigned a specific role to ensure horizontal patient management – tasks are performed simultaneously by multiple personnel. Meticulous record-keeping is essential to document all injuries and treatment.

History-taking is (because of the context) difficult in major trauma, but the minimum background information should be obtained from the patient or a bystander; this has been called an AMPLE history: Allergies, Medications, Past medical history/Pregnancy, Last meal, Events leading up to injury.

Initial assessment of the trauma patient

The trauma team should be assembled prior to arrival of the patient in the resuscitation room and predefined roles allocated. The pre-hospital care team should provide a structured but concise handover including mechanism of injury, vital signs and interventions performed. The initial assessment termed a primary survey (as defined by ATLS®) must be completed as a priority to enable rapid treatment of all life-threatening injuries. All patients should be assessed in the same way utilizing the ABCDE approach:

- Airway with cervical spine control
- Breathing
- Circulation and haemorrhage control
- Disability
- Exposure.

The team leader must oversee, co-ordinate and direct the team to ensure injuries are identified as soon as possible and treatment is implemented. Following an intervention or deterioration in the patient's condition it is essential to repeat the primary survey starting from A.

Primary survey

A: airway management with cervical spine control

Management of the airway with cervical spine immobilization is the first priority for all trauma patients. A conscious, talking patient is, by definition, able to maintain their own airway whereas those who present with a reduced conscious level are unable to speak or are at risk of airway injury and may require:

Basic techniques

- Supplementary oxygen
- Clearing of the airway – suctioning, chin lift, jaw thrust
- Simple adjuncts, e.g. oro- or naso-pharyngeal airway.

Advanced airway techniques (definitive airway)

- Endotracheal (ET) intubation
- Surgical airway – needle or surgical cricothyroidotomy.

All self-ventilating patients with major injury should receive high-flow oxygen via a non-rebreathing mask with reservoir to achieve an inspired oxygen concentration of around 85%. Specific indications for ET intubation include those detailed below – the cervical collar can be removed prior to intubation but manual inline stabilization must be maintained at all times.

Indications for endotracheal intubation:

- failure of basic techniques to maintain a patent airway
- threatened airway, e.g. patient with reduced conscious level, facial burns
- poor respiratory function requiring artificial means of ventilation, e.g. lung contusions.

The potential for cervical spine injury should be considered in all patients except a select number exposed to penetrating trauma only. A well-fitted cervical collar should be fitted at the scene or on arrival in the ED to fully immobilize the cervical spine. Sand bags on either side of the head and secured to the patient will achieve three-point immobilization and must be maintained until injury is excluded.

B: breathing

One in four of trauma deaths are due to chest injury; therefore assessment of breathing requires a rapid but comprehensive examination of the thorax and global tissue oxygenation. It should be remembered the pleural cavity reaches 2.5 cm above the medial third of the clavicle and descends to the twelfth rib posteriorly. Chest X-ray (CXR) forms an adjunct to the primary survey but clinical examination should not be delayed. The following life-threatening injuries must be identified and treated immediately:

- airway obstruction
- massive haemothorax – thoracostomy with intercostal chest drainage (ICD)
- tension pneumothorax – needle decompression or thoracostomy with ICD
- open pneumothorax (sucking wound) – apply three-sided flap dressing; or sealing of wound and ipsilateral thoracostomy with ICD
- cardiac tamponade – thoracotomy or sub-diaphragmatic incision to open pericardium
- flail chest – supportive ventilation and analgesia.

Observe

- Colour of the patient (cyanosis)
- Distension of neck veins (obstructive cause of shock)
- Confusion or agitation (hypoventilation will reduce cerebral oxygenation)
- Elevated respiratory rate
- Chest wall asymmetry (may indicate pneumothorax or rib fractures with flail segment)
- Pulse oximetry – useful adjunct but unreliable in cold or vasoconstricted patients.

Palpate

- Palpate thorax for any pain, crepitus or deformity indicative of bony injury
- Tracheal deviation (late sign of tension pneumothorax).

Percuss

- Hyper-resonance – sign of pneumothorax but is often not audible at a trauma call.

Listen

- Laboured breathing (respiratory compromise)
- Stridor (obstructed airway)
- Assess adequacy and equality of air entry to both lungs by auscultation.

C: cardiovascular status and haemorrhage control

Approximately 40% of patients with major injuries who reach hospital alive subsequently die from uncontrolled bleeding. Life-threatening haemorrhage must be identified at the outset of trauma resuscitation. Military practitioners are taught to use a <C>ABC approach to ensure rapid control of catastrophic external bleeding as the first priority, e.g. application of pressure to the bleeding point, limb tourniquets and topical haemostatic dressings. In civilian trauma care catastrophic external haemorrhage is rare (1–3%). Successful outcomes after severe internal haemorrhage are dependent on prompt diagnosis and haemorrhage control by either radiological or surgical intervention, e.g. angio-embolization (AE) of pelvic vasculature or ligation of damaged vessels.

Pathophysiology of shock

Shock may be defined as inadequate tissue perfusion and oxygenation. The first step in managing shock is to appreciate its presence and then determine the likely cause. In the context of trauma, shock aetiology can be divided into haemorrhagic and non-haemorrhagic.

Causes of shock

- Haemorrhage
- Cardiogenic

  · cardiac tamponade
  · blunt cardiac injury
  · myocardial infarction

- Tension pneumothorax
- Neurogenic – loss of sympathetic tone from thoracic spinal cord injury
- Sepsis – may arise 24–48 hours following injury as a result of systemic and inappropriate activation of inflammation (see Chapter 4)
- Anaphylaxis
- NB: isolated brain injury does not cause shock.

Haemorrhage is the most common cause of shock in trauma. Blood loss leads to a progressive compensatory response of vasoconstriction. Blood is diverted from the cutaneous, muscle and visceral vasculature to preserve blood flow to the brain, kidneys and heart. Endogenous catecholamines increase peripheral vascular resistance with associated contraction of blood volume in the venous system. Cardiac output is maintained in the early stages by a rise in heart rate but as the compensatory mechanisms fail and intravascular volume continues to be lost then blood pressure will begin to fall. Cells deprived of oxygen switch to anaerobic metabolism and produce lactic acid, leading to a metabolic acidosis. Prolonged hypoperfusion damages the cell membrane architecture, leading to fluid shift, swelling of the cell and eventual cell death.

The degree of circulatory shock is often difficult to determine as age, comorbidities and premorbid medication may mask true physiology. Young people are able to compensate far longer and may not demonstrate hypotension until 30–40% of circulating volume has been lost, at which point a precipitous fall in blood pressure will occur. Anti-hypertensive medication will limit the ability of an elderly person to mount a tachycardia or initiate vasoconstriction. Clinical diagnosis is essential to the early recognition of shock and the following physiological changes are a rough stepwise approximation for the degree of shock:

- sweaty and clammy skin
- increased pulse pressure
- elevated respiratory rate
- tachycardia (a heart rate of 80–90 in a young fit person is a relative tachycardia)
- altered mental status (anxious, confused)
- hypotension
- bradycardia, pallor and lethargy are late signs of haemorrhagic shock and indicate imminent cardiac arrest.

Source of haemorrhage

Life-threatening blood loss may be external or concealed. Common sites for major internal haemorrhage include:

- thorax – each hemithorax can accommodate 2–3 litres of blood
- abdomen – solid organ injury or mesenteric vessel rupture
- pelvis – the retroperitoneum can accommodate the entire circulating volume, e.g. pelvic fracture with associated vascular injury
- limbs – long bone fractures, e.g. femur (1–2 litres of blood).

Investigations

Recognition of haemorrhagic shock can be very difficult. Some investigations can help determine the degree of shock and likely source of haemorrhage:

- lactate and base deficit – (tissue hypoperfusion)

- haemoglobin and haematocrit – (unreliable indicators of blood loss)
- CXR – (haemothorax)
- pelvic X-ray (PXR) – (open book and vertical shear type fracture)
- focused assessment with sonography in trauma (FAST) – (free fluid is intraperitoneal haemorrhage until proved otherwise).

Resuscitation

Initial treatment of severe shock is directed towards restoring end organ perfusion and securing haemorrhage control. Multiple large-bore intravenous access must be obtained as soon as possible:

- 14-gauge cannula in both antecubital fossa
- rapid infusion catheter can be inserted into the internal jugular, subclavian or femoral veins.

Traditional ATLS® protocols advocated that fluid resuscitation should be with large volumes of crystalloid solutions. This approach is now known to be associated with a transient rise in BP which may dislodge clots, precipitate a dilutional coagulopathy and reduce the patient's core temperature. Current recommendation is to give fluid boluses of 250 ml of crystalloid in patients without immediate life-threatening signs of shock to assess level of responsiveness:

1. Responder = fluid bolus leads to sustained improvement in haemodynamic parameters
2. Transient responder = pulse rate and BP improve after fluid boluses but then deteriorate
3. Non-responder = fluid boluses have no effect and blood transfusion is required.

Resuscitation targets are controversial; for penetrating disease it is reasonable to aim at a systolic BP which is associated with cerebration or between 70 and 90 mmHg until haemostasis is achieved (permissive or hypotensive resuscitation). Although the evidence base is weaker for bluntly injured patients with shock, a similar approach is justified (at least until definitive haemorrhage control is achieved). In the context of traumatic brain injury (TBI), the threshold for permissive hypotension should be higher in order to prevent cerebral hypoperfusion (a systolic BP of least 100 mmHg should be maintained).

Haemorrhage control

Following diagnosis of life-threatening shock and identification of the source of bleeding it is vital to gain haemorrhage control. There should be no delay in order to 'resuscitate the patient before theatre' since no amount of resuscitation will arrest exsanguination. Haemorrhage control can be achieved in the following ways:

- splintage – stabilize the pelvic ring with a fabric pelvic binder or splint fashioned from a bed sheet to reduce the potential volume of the pelvis and tamponade any further; splint fractured long bones and apply traction, e.g. femoral fracture
- surgery – vessel repair or ligation; organ repair or resection; temporary packing for tamponade, e.g. complex liver laceration
- interventional radiology – angiographic embolization, e.g. internal iliac artery in pelvic fracture.

D: neurological disability

Traumatic brain injury (TBI) is the most common cause of early mortality following severe injury, accounting for two out of every five trauma deaths. A rapid assessment of the CNS must be performed with early imaging of the brain and spinal cord to identify any injury. Intracerebral haematoma (ICH) must be evacuated within 4 hours to ensure optimal outcomes from TBI. Shock, hypoxia, alcohol and drugs can mask underlying CNS pathology. TBI and spinal cord injury (SCI) must be excluded before attributing an abnormal neurological examination to alcohol or drug intoxication.

Conscious level

A reduced level of consciousness at any point after injury is a predictor of TBI. Conscious level is determined by the Alert Voice Pain Unresponsive Scale (AVPU) or Glasgow Coma Scale (GCS) systems and the highest level should be recorded (Table 16.1). The best motor score is the most reliable predictor of outcome.

Pupillary response

Assess both pupils for size, equality and reactivity. A unilateral, dilated and non-reactive pupil suggests mass effect within the skull compressing the third cranial nerve. An urgent CT scan of the brain is required.

Neurological examination

A brief screening examination to check for hemiparesis/hemiplegia and the presence of reduced sensation

Table 16.1 Neurological scoring systems

A: AVPU provides a brief neurological assessment	
A	Alert
V	Responds to verbal stimuli only
P	Responds to painful stimuli only
U	Unresponsive

B: GCS is the sum of the best eye, motor and verbal responses	
Motor response (M)	
Spontaneous	6
Localizes to pain	5
Withdraws from pain	4
Abnormal flexion	3
Abnormal extension	2
No response	1
Verbal response (V)	
Oriented	5
Confused	4
Inappropriate words	3
Incomprehensible sounds	2
None	1
Eye-opening response (E)	
Spontaneous	4
Eyes open to speech	3
Eyes open to pain	2
No eye-opening	1

should form part of the primary survey. Limb weakness or altered sensation is indicative of either TBI or SCI and must be investigated as a priority. In patients complaining of neck or back pain a more detailed neurological evaluation must be performed including rectal tone reflex.

E: exposure of the patient with environmental control

A vital part of the primary survey is full external examination of the patient. This mandates removal of the patient's clothing and log rolls to examine the back of the patient. Temperature control is important and, typically, an external warm air heating device will be placed over the patient to maintain normothermia.

Initial imaging and further examination

X-ray

As part of the primary survey an antero-posterior (AP) CXR and pelvic X-ray should be performed as they may detect life-threatening injuries and can aid identification of concealed haemorrhage. X-ray imaging of the cervical spine in the initial evaluation

Table 16.2 Zone of neck injuries

Zone	Anatomical borders	Structures at risk of injury	Surgical exposure
I	Clavicles to cricoid cartilage	Vertebral and proximal carotid arteries Lung Trachea Oesophagus Spinal cord and major cervical nerve trunks Thoracic duct	May require clavicle resection or median sternotomy
II	Cricoid cartilage to angle of mandible	Jugular veins Vertebral and common carotid arteries Internal and external carotid arteries Trachea and larynx Oesophagus Spinal cord	Easily accessible
III	Angle of mandible to base of skull	Distal internal carotid arteries Jugular veins Pharynx	May require disarticulation of the mandible or resection of the skull base

remains controversial. Lateral, AP and odontoid peg views are time-consuming, cannot be completed in the resuscitation room and are unable to reliably exclude injury. Modern protocols for assessment of patients with major injury and the possibility of cervical spinal injury include CT scan with coronal and sagittal reconstruction.

Focused assessment with sonography in trauma (FAST)

In recent years FAST has replaced diagnostic peritoneal lavage (DPL) for the assessment of intra-abdominal injury. FAST is an abbreviated ultrasound examination with the sole purpose of identifying the presence of free fluid, i.e. blood, using four windows: perisplenic, perihepatic, pelvic and pericardial (for identification of tamponade). FAST is not a reliable modality for identifying specific injuries and does not replace the need for a subsequent (more sensitive and specific) CT scan of the torso. Accuracy is excellent for patients with hypotension but FAST cannot be used to evaluate retroperitoneal injury, e.g. pelvic haematoma. It is operator-dependent and good views are not possible in obese patients or in the presence of extensive surgical emphysema. In the shocked patient FAST examination may permit cavitary triage, i.e. which body cavity requires immediate exploration for haemorrhage control, but a normal FAST scan does not exclude injury.

Secondary and tertiary surveys

The patient must be completely undressed to look for concealed injuries, e.g. perineum, axilla and posterior scalp. A formal secondary survey examination should be performed once all life-threatening injuries have been treated. The aim of this systematic assessment is to identify and record all wounds, fractures and organ injury. At this stage antibiotic prophylaxis and tetanus vaccination should be addressed. Missed injuries are present in up to 50% of patients following major trauma and may lead to long-term functional deficit with associated medical litigation. All patients should therefore receive a tertiary survey within 24 hours of admission. This assessment should be undertaken by an experienced trauma nurse or clinician and must include a comprehensive review of the medical notes, appraisal of all investigations and a complete head-to-toe examination.

Traumatic brain injury (see Chapter 12)

Neck injury

The neck is relatively exposed and contains numerous vital structures; therefore it is at particular risk from penetrating injury (Table 16.2). Blunt neck trauma is rare, but injury to the cervical spine must be excluded as it can be equally life-threatening. Blunt cerebrovascular injury (BCVI) has a 30% mortality rate. Initial resuscitation should follow the ATLS® approach and ET intubation must be considered early. A surgical airway is rarely required unless there is obvious open injury to the upper airway. The risk of concomitant chest injury, e.g. pneumothorax, is high especially in penetrating trauma. Immediate exploration of neck wounds is mandated if hard signs are present (evidence of active bleeding or airway injury). Inflating the balloon of a Foley catheter in the track of a neck wound may tamponade bleeding. Haemorrhage from subclavian vessels is notoriously difficult to control – AE and endovascular stent grafts may be viable alternatives to open ligation or repair. CT angiography (CTA) is replacing angiography as the imaging modality of choice for all neck injuries which do not require immediate exploration but may miss BCVI. A full neurological examination should be performed to check for injury to the CNS or peripheral nerves which transverse the cervical region. Patients with clinical signs indicative of aerodigestive injury, e.g. haematemesis, dysphagia, subcutaneous emphysema, should undergo formal endoscopic evaluation. Good wound toilet and antibiotic cover is essential for all oropharyngeal injury.

Spine and spinal cord trauma (see Chapter 17)

Thoracic trauma

Thoracic injury is common and present in up to 50% of polytrauma patients. Chest injury is a contributory factor in 25–50% of trauma deaths. Mortality from chest trauma is the result of:

- hypoxia
- hypoventilation
- haemorrhage
- cardiac tamponade.

Securing a patent airway is the first priority and may require early ET intubation. Thoracic injuries can evolve rapidly; therefore continual re-assessment and evaluation is vital particularly if the patient's condition deteriorates. A supine CXR is required in all trauma patients but must not delay resuscitation. CT scan with contrast is the imaging modality of choice to evaluate all thoracic injury in non-shocked patients. Hypotensive patients with chest trauma require rapid surgical intervention for haemorrhage control but 90% of thoracic injuries can be managed non-operatively, e.g. artificial ventilation and/or intercostal chest drainage.

Rib fractures, flail and pulmonary contusions

The most frequent injury to the thoracic cage is rib fracture, which may also be a marker of underlying damage to truncal viscera:

- laceration of an intercostal artery (all ribs)
- great vessel injury in the neck or mediastinum (fracture of ribs 1–3 suggests high-energy impact as protected by bony architecture of upper limb)
- lung injury, e.g. pulmonary contusion (ribs 4–9)
- splenic or liver injury (lower ribs).

Pulmonary contusion is the commonest potentially lethal thoracic injury. Blunt force to the thorax disrupts the microvasculature of the lung parenchyma, resulting in multiple areas of haemorrhage, which compromises ventilation. Management includes oxygenation, supportive ventilation and fluid restriction but can be complicated by post-traumatic acute respiratory distress syndrome (ARDS).

Rib fractures alone are associated with significant morbidity as a result of pain on respiratory motion. The elderly, patients with underlying lung pathology or those with multiple rib fractures are at risk of developing atelectasis, lower respiratory tract infection and hypoxia. Flail chest is a life-threatening thoracic injury and occurs when two or more consecutive ribs are fractured in two or more places. The fracture pattern can severely compromise the normal mechanics of respiration (paradoxical motion) as the flail segment is no longer in bony continuity with the rest of the thoracic skeleton. Underlying pulmonary contusions are common and in combination with pain from rib fractures flail chest can result in profound hypoxia requiring artificial ventilation.

Rib fracture management includes:

- chest physiotherapy and high-quality analgesia – instigate early to prevent complications
- polypharmacy, e.g. non-steroidal anti-inflammatory drugs (NSAIDs), intravenous opiate patient-controlled analgesia (PCA) and anti-neuropathic medication
- epidural analgesia for patients requiring critical care – facilitates early mobility and intensive respiratory physiotherapy
- selective intercostal nerve blockade may be indicated in patients with refractory pain.

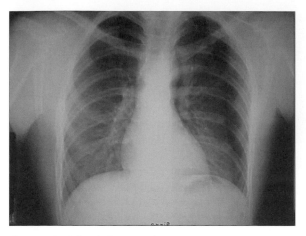

Figure 16.3 Life-sided pneumothorax.

Pneumothorax

A pneumothorax is defined as the presence of air in the potential space between visceral and parietal pleura within the thoracic cavity which leads to collapse of the underlying lung. The air can come from an injury to the lung or through a wound in the chest wall. Simple pneumothoraces can usually be diagnosed on CXR but small or anterior collections may be missed (Figure 16.3). The natural history of 'occult' pneumothoraces only detectable on CT scan is unknown – most require ICD particularly if the patient is to be placed on positive pressure ventilation.

If a 'one way valve' forms and air continues to accumulate within the pleural space but cannot escape, pressure within the pleural space increases and a tension pneumothorax will develop. The mediastinum is displaced to the opposite hemithorax, venous return falls and if left untreated the patient will rapidly deteriorate with progressive respiratory compromise until cardiac arrest occurs. Tension pneumothorax is a clinical diagnosis – do not wait for the CXR. Clinical signs include:

* agitated, dyspnoeic patient
* hyperinflated hemithorax with decreased respiratory movements
* decreased/absent breath sounds
* tracheal shift (very late sign).

Initial treatment of tension pneumothorax is thoracic needle decompression – insertion of a large-bore cannula over the second rib into the intercostal space at the mid-clavicular line. Needle decompression is a temporizing measure and should be immediately followed by insertion of an ICD.

Intercostal chest drainage

ICD is a simple technique (Figure 16.4) although the potential for iatrogenic injury is significant; a good appreciation of thoracic anatomy will minimize risks. Sterile gloves and gown should be worn. A single dose of a broad-spectrum antibiotic given intravenously has been shown in a randomized, controlled trial to significantly reduce the risk of post-insertion infection. Continued pneumothorax, massive bubbling from the chest drain and failure to maintain saturations may reflect disruption to a major bronchus. If a second chest drain and continuous low-pressure high-volume suction fail to expedite lung re-inflation a cardiothoracic opinion should be sought.

Haemothorax

A haemothorax results from damage to:

* intercostal vessels
* lung parenchyma
* thoracic spine fracture
* major mediastinal vessel.

CXR will only detect a haemothorax with volume greater than 300–500 ml blood (Figure 16.5). ICD is definitive treatment in the vast majority of cases as bleeding is usually self-limiting. A massive haemothorax (>1500 ml) or large-volume continuous blood loss into the ICD may indicate injury to a major vessel. Shock with evidence of haemothorax is an indication for urgent thoracotomy to achieve control haemorrhage.

Blunt aortic injury

Massive deceleration forces, e.g. high-speed RTCs, may be associated with injury to the proximal descending thoracic aorta. Only 10–20% of patients with blunt aortic injury (BAI) reach hospital alive. A widened mediastinum is one of 20 diagnostic clues on a CXR for BAI but 1–2% of patients with aortic injury will have a normal mediastinum. CT angiography is now the gold standard investigation with an extremely high negative predictive value and may be used alone to rule out

Patient positioned supine with arm abducted – palpate fifth intercostal space in the midaxillary line

Prepare the skin then infiltrate local anaesthetic (over the 6th rib to avoid damage to the neurovascular bundle) into the skin, subcutaneous tissues and parietal pleura

Incise through skin and subcutaneous tissues then bluntly dissect with the long forceps to split the intercostal muscles and pierce the pleura (hiss of air may be audible or gush of blood seen)

Sweep any adherent lung away with a finger before inserting a large calibre ICD (32 or 36 Fr) using the long forceps (aim Apically for Air or Basally for Blood)

Connect ICD to tubing and attach to underwater seal (check drain is swinging)

Suture ICD in place and perform check CXR to confirm correct position of ICD and lung re-expansion

Figure 16.4 Intercostal chest drain insertion (skills box).

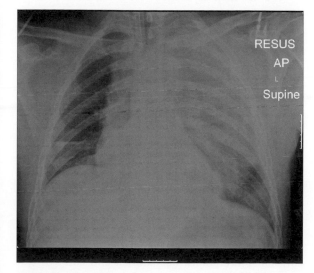

RESUS
AP
L
Supine

Figure 16.5 Haemothorax.

BAI. Thoracic endovascular aortic repair (TEVAR) has replaced open repair as the treatment of choice, with significantly lower operative mortality, paraplegia and renal failure (Figure 16.6).

Penetrating chest trauma

The majority of penetrating thoracic injury can be managed without surgical intervention; however, damage to major intrathoracic vessels or the heart is associated with mortality >70%. Initial resuscitation should follow ATLS® principles of ABC. Patients in extremis after penetrating chest injury may require a resuscitative thoracotomy (RT) in the ED. RT is rarely indicated for patients who present after blunt trauma. Indications for RT in patients are listed below but the procedure should only be performed by an appropriately trained trauma specialist:

265

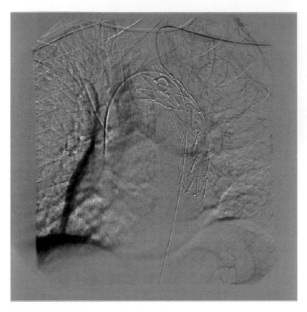

Figure 16.6 Thoracic endovascular aortic repair.

- witnessed loss of cardiac output in the ED
- patient arrives in cardiac arrest but signs of life are present (spontaneous movements, pupillary response or spontaneous respirations)
- vital signs documented at scene but deteriorates to cardiac arrest no longer than 5 minutes prior to arrival.

Access to the thorax is achieved via left anterolateral or bilateral anterolateral (clamshell) incisions with the primary aim to:

- relieve tamponade by opening the pericardium
- control myocardial haemorrhage (finger, skin clips or suture)
- clamp pulmonary hilum to control haemorrhage from root of lung injuries
- perform internal cardiac massage and/or defibrillation.

Other thoracic trauma

Traumatic diaphragmatic injury

- Blunt injury can produce large radial tears (left more common than right due to position of liver)
- Penetrating trauma produces small perforations
- CXR clues include raised hemidiaphragm and abdominal visceral herniation
- Small injuries may be missed on CT scan
- Treatment is direct surgical repair via laparotomy

Blunt myocardial injury

- Majority of cases are asymptomatic but can cause arrhythmias and conduction abnormalities
- If ECG is abnormal echocardiogram is indicated
- Cardiac enzymes are unreliable markers in the context of widespread tissue injury
- Arrhythmias should be managed as per standard ACLS® guidelines

Abdominal trauma
Blunt injury

- RTCs are the commonest cause of blunt abdominal trauma
- Typical injury patterns are associated with specific trauma, e.g. rapid deceleration from a fall from height – ruptured duodenum or pancreatic injury
- Blunt abdominal trauma is often a feature of polytrauma, which may complicate initial assessment but half of patients with intraperitoneal injury have no external signs
- Non-operative management of solid organ injury is possible in the stable patient with high-quality diagnostic imaging (CT scan) and serial abdominal examination.

Penetrating injury

- Haemodynamic instability requires early surgical intervention
- The vast majority of GSWs to the abdomen are associated with intraperitoneal injury and require exploration and repair
- Stab wounds in stable patients with normal repeated abdominal evaluation may be managed non-operatively but visceral protrusion requires early laparotomy
- Multi-cavity injury must be excluded in all junctional zone wounds (e.g. neck, costal margin and buttock creases)

Assessment

Initial evaluation and resuscitation must follow the principles of ATLS®. Fully expose and systematically examine the abdomen – pay careful attention to the flanks, back, buttocks and perineum, looking for any abrasions, lacerations, haematoma and entry or exit wounds.

Table 16.3 Management strategy for abdominal trauma

Key questions	Key information	Key interventions
Is there intraperitoneal bleeding and is it ongoing?	1. Mechanism of injury 2. Clinical evidence of shock 3. Response to initial resuscitation 4. FAST scan 5. CT scan (if stable)	A. Active bleeding ≫ laparotomy B. No active bleeding[a] ≫ close observation

Is there intraperitoneal or retroperitoneal contamination?	1. Mechanism of injury
	2. Clinical examination
	3. CT scan (if stable)
	4. Amylase (for pancreatic injury)
		A. Hollow organ injury likely ≫ Laparotomy
		B. Equivocal evidence ≫ Close observation on high-dependency unit + laparotomy if:
		    peritonitis
		    fever
		    raised white cell count

Is there retroperitoneal bleeding and is it ongoing?	1. Mechanism of injury 2. Clinical evidence of pelvic fracture and X-ray 3. Evidence of shock 4. Response to initial resuscitation 5. FAST scan (to rule out intraperitoneal cause) 6. CT scan (if stable)	1. Evidence of pelvic fracture and shock ≫ pelvic splint 2. Proceed to angio suite if no free fluid on FAST scan 3. Involve orthopaedic surgeons early for definite fixation

[a] No ongoing fluid requirements with normal pulse and blood pressure. No rise in base deficit or lactate and stable haemoglobin levels. No blush or active bleed on CT scan.

- The abdomen extends anteriorly from below the nipples between the posterior axillary lines to the groin skin crease and posteriorly from the tips of scapulas to the inferior gluteal folds
- Look for evidence of haemorrhagic shock
- Signs of peritoneal irritation (blood or rupture of a hollow viscus) may be slow to develop or absent, e.g. reduced conscious level, spinal cord injury
- Retroperitoneal haemorrhage from renal or vascular injury is unlikely to be detected on clinical examination or FAST
- Digital rectal examination is mandatory
- Markers for intra-abdominal injury include the seat belt sign, lower rib fractures, lumbar spine injury.

Investigations

Diagnostic imaging should not delay operative intervention and is not warranted in patients with evidence of ongoing haemorrhage who require immediate surgery. Laboratory tests other than markers of shock (base deficit, lactate) and blood cross-match are of little value in the acute phase. DPL has been replaced by FAST as the triage investigation of choice in shocked patients as it is non-invasive and rapid. CT scan remains the gold standard for evaluation of all abdominal injuries in stable patients but may miss small diaphragmatic or pancreatic injuries. In the stable penetrating trauma patient laparoscopy can be used to assess integrity of the peritoneum and evaluate/repair the diaphragm but it is not routinely used in most trauma centres. All intra-abdominal organs should be inspected to exclude injury at laparoscopy with a very low threshold for conversion to formal laparotomy. Table 16.3 details an algorithm for the investigation and management of abdominal trauma.

Probing the wound has no benefit, is likely to dislodge clots and may lead to further damage. Lighting and exposure in the ED is often inadequate and therefore the full extent of the wound track cannot be visualized. Organs, nerves and vessels that lie in close proximity to the cavity cannot be protected or moved out of the way and may be injured.

Trauma laparotomy

Indications

- Abdominal injury with signs of ongoing haemorrhage
- Gunshot wound of the abdomen
- Hollow viscus injury detected on CT or with signs of peritonism
- Protrusion of viscera through penetrating abdominal wound

Table 16.4 Stages of damage control (DC) surgery adapted from Johnson *et al.* (2001)

DC 0 'Ground Zero' recognition	Pre-hospital triage and rapid transport Resuscitation Oxygen, Blood, DECISION
Part I Operating theatre	Control haemorrhage (temporary packing with angio-embolization may be more appropriate) Control contamination Intra-abdominal packing Temporary closure – laparostomy
Part II: ICU	Re-warming Correct coagulopathy Maximize haemodynamics Ventilatory support Re-examination
Part III Operating theatre	Pack removal Definitive repairs Closure

Damage control surgery

Major abdominal injury (particularly with abdominal major vascular injury) may be associated with exsanguination, severe shock and a profound physiological derangement with hypothermia, progressive acidosis and a clinically obvious coagulopathy (the so-called lethal triad). A traditional surgical approach of 'early total care' requires prolonged operative time and in the presence of the lethal triad is associated with high mortality. For over 20 years trauma surgeons have favoured damage control surgery (DCS) as a deliberate strategy to stage the operative care of a patient with life-threatening injuries. DCS is an approach to the operation of a patient with massive injury that favours decision-making based on the patient's physiological status rather than the anatomical pattern of injury. Primary surgery is as quick and simple as possible with the goal of stopping bleeding and controlling contamination to allow critical care to be instituted as soon as possible. The anatomical disruption is restored at later operations once the patient's physiology has been stabilized (Table 16.4). Absolute indications for DCS in a patient with major injury include hypothermia (<34°C), acidosis (pH <7.2), shock and coagulopathy; however, the more experienced surgeon attempts to recognize an appropriate patient before hypothermia, acidosis and coagulopathy become clinically apparent. Principles of DCS are applicable to management of all major trauma, e.g. pelvic, thoracic and extremities.

Damage control laparotomy

- Communicate with operating team and anaesthetist – let them know DCS intentions and the need for simultaneous aggressive blood and clotting factor resuscitation
- Rapidly prepare patient from neck to knees positioned supine with arms out on boards
- Ensure two large-bore suckers are available and large packs are ready and opened
- Midline incision from xiphisternum to pubis
- Once inside the abdomen there may be extensive bleeding; therefore use quadrant packing to temporarily control haemorrhage (Figure 16.7)

  - Right upper quadrant – place a hand over dome of liver and pull it forwards – pack over hand above the liver (pack the sub-hepatic area to form a sandwich)
  - Left upper quadrant – place a hand above the spleen, pull it gently forward then pack over your hand and medially
  - Left and right paracolic gutters
  - Pelvis

- Remove packs starting in the quadrant with the least amount of bleeding
- Explore abdomen systematically to evaluate all organs
- Visceral rotation may be necessary to assess an expanding retroperitoneal haematoma
- Bowel can safely be left in non-continuity, i.e. staple either side of an injury to rapidly control contamination
- Abdominal compartment syndrome (ACS) is likely following severe shock in polytrauma – temporarily close abdomen with laparostomy especially if re-look procedure to remove packs is mandated.

Solid organ injury

- Injury to the liver, spleen or kidney in the non-shocked patient can be managed non-operatively – repeated examination with close observation is mandated to elicit any signs of intra-abdominal bleeding and/or peritonism from missed hollow viscus injury
- Patients not suitable for conservative management are those with a CT scan demonstrating evidence

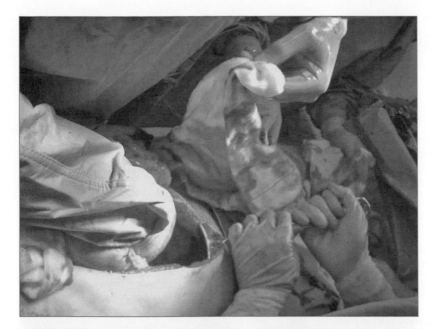

Figure 16.7 Quadrant packing of the abdomen for temporary haemorrhage control.

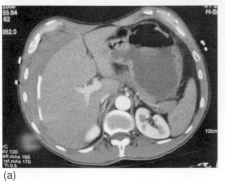

(a)

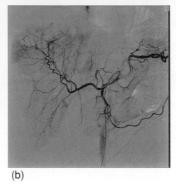

(b)

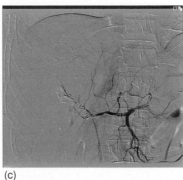

(c)

Figure 16.8 (a) Complex liver injury with contrast blush on CT scan indicating active haemorrhage. (b and c) Selective angio-embolization of hepatic artery.

of ongoing bleeding, e.g. contrast blush from hepatic artery (Figure 16.8a)

- Angio-embolization (AE) has an important role in treating haemodynamically stable patients with active haemorrhage from solid organ injury (Figure 16.8b and c) and may facilitate haemorrhage control in complex hepatic injuries following temporary packing of the liver at DCS
- Splenic conservation with AE or splenic repair is controversial although advocated in young children to prevent post-splenectomy morbidity
- All shocked patients with free abdominal fluid on FAST require an emergency laparotomy for haemorrhage control

Hollow organ injury (GI tract and pancreas)

- The duodenum and pancreas are often injured following falls from height or compression of the seatbelt against the vertebral column in high-speed RTC
- Most pancreatic injuries can be managed with drainage alone
- The lesser sac should always be explored if the stomach is injured in order to evaluate the posterior gastric wall
- The small intestine can be managed by simple repair or resection
- The safest approach to colonic injuries is exteriorization, particularly in cases where the

Table 16.5 Pelvic fracture patterns

Type	Injury pattern	Mechanism	Associated injuries
AP compression	Disruption of ligamentous complex +/− bony injury	Motorcycle RTC Fall from height Direct crush	Neurological Vascular[a]
Lateral compression	Internal rotation of hemipelvis	Side impact RTC	Genito-urinary
Vertical shear	Vertical displacement across anterior and posterior aspects	Fall from height landing on lower limbs	Major pelvic instability Vascular

[a] Disruption of the posterior venous complex and internal iliac artery.

viability of the bowel is in doubt and/or significant contamination has occurred

- Be wary of retroperitoneal colonic injuries which are easily missed in blunt abdominal trauma.

Pelvic trauma

Pelvic trauma ranges from the relatively minor pubic rami fractures common in the elderly to exsanguinating complex pelvic disruption with mortality rates up to 55%. The importance of an exemplary multidisciplinary team working to gain rapid haemorrhage control cannot be emphasized enough. Pelvic fracture can be classified according to vector of force and further subdivided according to extent of bony displacement graded I–III (Table 16.5).

Assessment

Pelvic fracture must be considered in the context of major trauma with shock. Physical examination in the obtunded patient may be negative but markers of pelvic injury include:

- pelvic/hip pain
- blood at the urethral meatus
- scrotal haematoma
- high-riding prostate on digital rectal examination
- perineal laceration (suggestive of open pelvic fracture).

Pelvic X-ray should be performed as part of the primary survey and in the hypotensive patient FAST is of benefit to guide subsequent management, i.e. laparotomy or AE (Figure 16.9).

Management

Patients with clinically suspected pelvic injury should have some form of external compression (pelvic binder

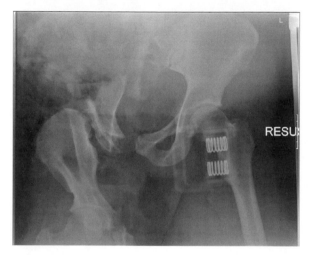

Figure 16.9 Vertical sheer pelvic fracture.

or rolled-up sheet tied around pelvis) applied as soon as possible to close the potential space of the pelvis. If the patient arrives in shock, recent evidence suggests that resuscitation should be with blood and plasma rather than crystalloid solutions. All patients with labile BP require emergency angiographic evaluation with or without AE. Patients presenting in refractory shock should be taken to the operating theatre first for packing of the extraperitoneal space to tamponade bleeding prior to angiography. Stabilization of the bony pelvic injury is a secondary priority but early definitive fixation is associated with improved functional outcome. Treatment options include simple bed-rest with traction, external fixation or more complex internal pelvic reconstruction. Open pelvic fractures and those involving the rectum or urogenital structures require extensive wound debridement and faecal diversion (colostomy).

Urological injury

Haematuria is an important sign marker of urological trauma but can arise from anywhere along the genitourinary (GU). Most injuries to the kidney are minor following blunt trauma to the loin and nearly all can be managed conservatively. Major pelvic trauma is associated with GU injuries because of the close anatomical relationship between the urethra, bladder and bony pelvis.

Renal

- Suspected injury should be investigated by CT with intravenous contrast – assess any damage to the renal vessels and evaluate function of contralateral kidney
- Hypotensive patients with suspected renal haemorrhage or pedicle injuries should undergo surgical exploration or AE
- Avulsed kidneys usually need to be removed but occasionally can be salvaged.

Lower GU tract

Suspected bladder rupture should be confirmed with CT cystogram or may be evident at laparotomy. All intraperitoneal bladder injuries should be repaired with simple suturing but extraperitoneal rupture can be managed with urethral catheterization and repeat cystogram at day 10 to confirm healing. Urethral trauma is far more common in men due to the length of the urethra. In suspected cases of urethral injury following pelvic fracture a single attempt at catheterization by an experienced clinician is reasonable. Failure to pass a urethral catheter mandates a retrograde urethrogram and supra-pubic catheterization. Anterior injuries can often be managed with simple stenting of the urethra by a Foley catheter but posterior injury usually requires delayed complex reconstruction.

Extremity trauma

It is beyond the scope of this chapter to describe in detail the assessment and management of all extremity trauma (see Chapter 23). The principles of orthopaedic and vascular surgery are applicable to limb injury and in certain cases damage control surgery principles may be appropriate, e.g. immediate amputation rather than prolonged attempts at limb salvage.

Assessment

Initial resuscitation should always begin ABC; however, major vascular injury to the extremities can result in rapid exsanguination and any external bleeding must be promptly controlled. Once the primary survey has been completed and all life-threatening conditions have been addressed attention should focus on limb-threatening injuries (in order of importance):

- closed vascular injury, i.e. without external haemorrhage*
- compartment syndrome
- open fracture
- joint injury
- neurological injury.

*Blood loss from closed bony injury can be considerable, particularly in polytrauma, e.g. femur (1–2 l), tibia (500 ml – 1 l)

The secondary survey examination must identify all non-life-threatening injuries – the mechanism of trauma is a guide to likely patterns of injury, e.g. calcaneal fracture after fall from height. Extremity assessment should be systematic:

- close inspection for any evidence of deformity, swelling, open fracture or soft tissue issue
- palpation of all long bones, major joints, hands and feet observing for pain, crepitus and abnormal range of movement
- screening neurological examination of all limb myotomes and dermatomes
- vascular integrity of each limb – capillary refill, audible bruit, palpation of pulses with/without hand-held Doppler.

Plain X-ray is the first-line investigation for all suspected skeletal limb trauma. CT has an important role in the evaluation of joint injury, complex fracture morphology and associated injuries such as vascular disruption. CTA is a useful tool to assess proximal arterial injury but may miss intimal flaps and partial tears. Digital subtraction angiography remains the gold standard for assessment of all extremity arterial injuries.

Vascular injury

Blunt injury can disrupt vessels directly after a crush or indirectly after disruption to tissues injured at some distance from the point of impact. Fractures of long bones and joint dislocations may impinge bone ends onto the vessel, e.g. popliteal artery. Penetrating

271

Table 16.6 Clinical signs associated with a vascular injury

Hard signs	Soft signs
Pulseless, cold, pale limb Expanding haematoma Palpable thrill or audible bruit Active bleeding	History of active bleeding Penetrating injury in close proximity to a major vessel Non-expanding haematoma Peripheral nerve deficit

injuries may cause partial or complete injury, depending on missile trajectory. Vascular trauma can be classified as:

- vessel disruption

  - partial – may present with expanding or pulsatile haematoma (false aneurysm) but ischaemia not usually present as channel for blood flow maintained
  - complete – usually present with haemorrhage which decreases as the vessel goes into spasm and a clot develops

- intimal injury – risk of intimal flap formation, thrombosis, dissection and distal ischaemia
- arteriovenous fistula formation – may present late after penetrating injury.

Diagnosis can be difficult and requires a high degree of suspicion and careful evaluation. The clinical features associated with vascular injury are divided into 'hard' signs and 'soft' signs (Table 16.6). Hard signs indicate vascular injury that requires attention; soft signs are suggestive of vascular injury and mandate further evaluation.

A management algorithm for vascular injuries is described in Figure 16.10 but direct pressure is the safest and most effective way to temporarily control external bleeding. Emergency tourniquet use has been shown to stop bleeding in major limb trauma in the military combat setting but benefits of use in civilian practice remain to be proven. In the haemodynamically stable, interventional radiology may be used to control bleeding by endovascular stent graft or AE. The underlying principle of surgical exploration is proximal and distal control prior to vascular repair using:

- direct lateral suture
- vein patch angioplasty
- end to end anastomosis
- interposition graft
- vascular bypass.

Compartment syndrome

Injury to the soft tissues results in inflammatory oedema – swelling within a myofascial compartment can lead to compartment syndrome. Elevation of myofascial compartment pressure above capillary pressure causes ischaemia and muscle necrosis. Common sites include the lower leg, forearm, foot and hand. In all tibial and forearm fractures, burns, crush injury and reperfusion of ischaemic muscle the trauma surgeon must maintain a high index of suspicion for compartment syndrome, particularly in patients with a reduced level of consciousness. Signs and symptoms of compartment syndrome are:

- pain out of proportion to the injury
- pain on passive stretching of the muscles involved
- tense swollen limb
- reduced sensation or power in nerves that traverse the compartment (weakness and paralysis are late signs)
- compartment pressure >35–40 mmHg is diagnostic.

Urgent fasciotomy should be performed to release all myofascial compartments – compartment syndrome is a time-dependent condition, therefore if the diagnosis is in doubt proceed to surgical exploration.

Soft tissue and fracture management

Wounds should be adequately irrigated, with removal of all contaminants and devitalized or necrotic tissue. Open fractures require thorough debridement and should be stabilized with external fixation within 6 hours of injury – antibiotic prophylaxis and anti-tetanus vaccination are essential. Contaminated wounds or where tissue viability is in doubt should be left open for relook surgery at 48 hours. Definitive wound closure should be achieved within 5 days but may require plastic reconstruction where extensive tissue loss has occurred. Degloving trauma may cause deep tractional injuries to neurovascular structures with widespread damage to the muscle; therefore monitor closely for compartment syndrome. In cases of complete or partial traumatic amputation early multidisciplinary involvement is required from senior personnel to assess limb salvageability. Major limb fractures may be associated with fat embolism whereby globules of fat are dislodged from the marrow and released into circulation as a result of either the primary injury or operative intervention. A clinical

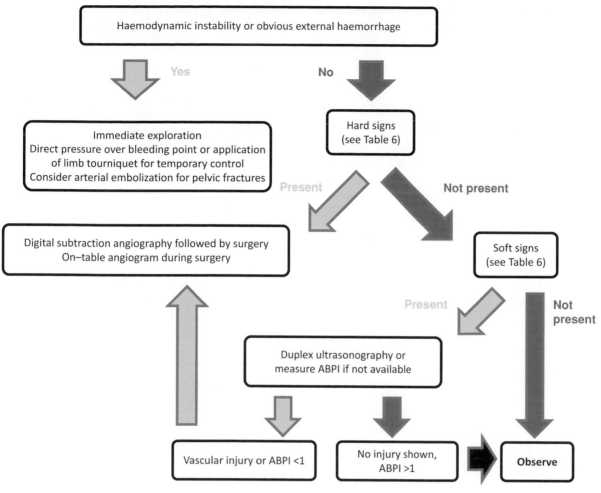

Figure 16.10 Algorithm for management of vascular trauma (ABPI: ankle-brachial pressure index).

scenario similar to ARDS may develop requiring supportive ventilatory therapy.

Peripheral nerve injury

Nerve damage is broadly classified into three forms.

- Neurapraxia (bruising) is the mildest injury type and does not involve loss of nerve continuity. Functional loss is transient.
- Axonotmesis is complete disruption of the axon and myelin sheath but preservation of the surrounding mesenchymal structures. Axon and myelin degeneration occur distal to the point of injury, causing complete denervation. Prognosis for functional recovery is good but slow – uninjured mesenchymal structures provide a framework for axonal regrowth (1 mm/day).

- Neurotmesis is complete division or destruction of a nerve. Functional loss is complete and recovery will not occur without surgical intervention (nerve grafting) as a result of scarring and loss of the mesenchymal framework.

Crush syndrome

Traumatic rhadomyolysis or crush syndrome, first described in the London Blitz, occurs following significant muscle injury, e.g. prolonged entrapment. Release of nephrotoxic myoglobin as a result of direct muscle injury, ischaemia and necrosis can give rise to hypovolaemia, metabolic acidosis, hyperkalaemia, hypocalcaemia and disseminated intravascular coagulation. Pre-emptive aggressive fluid therapy, correction of electrolytes and early renal replacement therapy is the mainstay of treatment. Alkalization of the urine with sodium bicarbonate to reduce precipitation of myoglobin in the renal tubules is indicated in most patients.

Burns (see Chapter 29)

Triage and major incidents

Triage is a process by which management of multiple patients is prioritized and mandated when resource demand cannot match resource provision, e.g. mass casualty events (major incidents). The principles of triage are:

- threat to life – does the patient require immediate intervention?
- salvageability – is the patient likely to die despite optimal care?
- resource utility – time, personnel, equipment, blood etc.

Triage must be completed rapidly at scene with additional triage by a senior trauma specialist upon arrival at hospital – it is a dynamic process and represents how the patient is at the current time. A commonly used system for civilian practice in the advent of a major incident is:

P1 Immediate priority – patient likely to die without immediate intervention (RED)

P2 Intermediate priority – severely injured but interventions can wait a few hours (YELLOW)

P3 Delayed priority – minor injuries only, e.g. walking wounded (GREEN)

P4 Deceased (BLACK).

All hospitals in the UK by law must have a 24-hour major incident plan which details how the institution will operate during a mass casualty event. It outlines pre-defined roles for personnel, triage protocol, communication systems, patient tracking/documentation and patient-transfer arrangements. It is incumbent on everyone involved in trauma care to read their own hospital's major incident plan – do not wait until an incident has been declared.

Further reading

American College of Surgeons. *Advanced Trauma Life Support Program for Doctors: TLS*. 8th edn. Chicago, 2008.

Baker S, O'Neill B, Haddon W Jr, Long WB. The Injury Severity Score: a method for describing patients with multiple injuries and evaluating emergency care. *J Trauma* 1974;**14**:187–196.

Baker C *et al*. Epidemiology of trauma deaths. *Am J Surg* 1980;**140**(1):144–150.

Bickell WH *et al*. Immediate vs delayed fluid resuscitation for hypotensive patients with penetrating torso injuries. *NEJM* 1994;**331**(17):1105–1109.

Borgman M *et al*. The ratio of blood products transfused affects mortality in patients receiving massive transfusions at a combat support hospital. *J Trauma* 2007;**63**:805–813.

Brohi K. Trauma specialist centres. *Ann R Coll Surg Eng (Suppl)* 2007;**89**:252–253.

Brohi K, Cohen M, Davenport R. Acute coagulopathy of trauma: mechanism, identification and effect. *Curr Opin Crit Care* 2007;**13**:680–685.

Dutton RP, Mackenzie CF, Scalea TM. Hypotensive resuscitation during active haemorrhage: impact on hospital mortality. *J Trauma* 2002;**52**(2):374–380.

Geeraerts T *et al*. Clinical review: initial management of blunt pelvic trauma patients with haemodynamic instability. *Crit Care* 2007;**11**:204.

Gonzalez EA, Moore FA, Holcomb JB. Fresh frozen plasma should be given earlier to patients requiring massive transfusion. *J Trauma* 2007;**62**:112–119.

Hess J *et al*. The coagulopathy of trauma: a review of mechanisms. *J Trauma* 2008;**65**:748–754.

Hoffman JR *et al*. Validity of a set of clinical criterion to rule out injury to the cervical spine in patients with blunt trauma. National Emergency X-radiography Utilization Study group. *N Engl J Med* 2000;**343**(2):94–99.

Johnson JW *et al*. Evolution in damage control for exsanguinating penetrating abdominal injury. *J Trauma* 2001;**51**:261–271.

Myers J. Focussed assessment with sonography in trauma (FAST): the truth about USS in blunt trauma. *J Trauma* 2007;**62**:S28.

Neschis D, Scalea T, Flinn W, Griffith B. Blunt aortic injury. *N Engl J Med* 2008;**359**:1708–1716.

Nicholson AA. Vascular radiology in trauma. *Cardiovasc Intervent Radiol* 2004;**27**:105–120.

Sauaia A *et al*. Epidemiology of trauma deaths: a reassessment. *J Trauma* 1995;**38**:185–193.

Shanmuganathan K. Multi-detector row CT imaging of blunt abdominal trauma. *Semin Ultrasound CT MR* 2004;**25**:180–204.

Stiell IG *et al*. The Canadian C-spine rule for radiography in alert stable trauma patients. *JAMA* 2001;**286**(15): 1841–1844.

The CRASH trial Collaborators: effect of intravenous corticosteroids on death within 14 days in 10008 adults with clinically significant head injury (MRC CRASH trial): a randomized placebo-controlled trial. *Lancet* 2004;**364**:1291–1292.

Trauma: Who cares? A report of the National Confidential Enquiry into Patient Outcome and Death, 2007.

Triage, assessment, investigation and early management of head injury in infants, children and adults, NICE Clinical Guideline (2007). http://guidance.nice.org.uk/CG56.

World Health Organization. Injury: a leading cause of the global burden of disease. http://whqlibdoc.who.int/publications/2002/9241562323.pdf.2000. www.east.org www.trauma.org.

Chapter

17

Fundamentals of the central nervous system

James Palmer and Anant Kamat

Anatomy

Scalp

The scalp is extremely vascular with blood supply coming from the external carotid arteries; anteriorly from the superficial temporal arteries which are branches of the maxillary arteries and posteriorly the occipital arteries. Since these vessels enter the scalp from the base upwards towards the vertex and since the supply is very good, provided the location of these supplying vessels is borne in mind, scalp incisions can be made almost anywhere with impunity without devascularizing the scalp. The layers of the scalp can be remembered by a mnemonic:

S *s*kin
C *s*ubcutaneous tissue
A the *a*poneurosis (galea)
L *l*oose areola tissue (the scalp is reflected back by dissecting this layer)
P *p*ericranium (periosteum).

When suturing a scalp wound absorbable sutures are used to close the galea and then clips or sutures in the skin. As all the significant vessels lie within the subcutaneous tissue this two-layer closure tamponades the vessels and can control all scalp edge bleeding.

Skull

The skull is a complex series of connected bones. In the neonate the vault bones are only loosely attached at sutures and these join with cartilagenous fusion at 18 months. The skull reaches 90% of its adult size at approximately 7 years, and maximum size at puberty; the suture lines can be seen on skull radiographs throughout life but tend gradually to obliterate with advancing age. The skull varies in thickness in differing areas, being thickest in the parieto-occipital area and thinnest in the temporal area just above the mandibular articulation. It is divided into three fossae – anterior, middle and posterior (Figure 17.1). There are a number of foramina though which pass specific structures (Table 17.1).

Table 17.1 Foramina of the skull

Foramen	Structures passing through
Optic	Optic nerve, ophthalmic artery
Superior orbital fissure	Occulomotor nerve, trochlear nerve, abducens nerve, trigeminal nerve (ophthalmic division V1)
Foramen rotundum	Trigeminal nerve (maxillary division, V2)
Foramen ovale	Trigeminal nerve (mandibular division, V2), lesser petrosal nerve
Foramen spinosum	Middle meningeal artery, meningeal branch of mandibular nerve
Foramen lacerum	Carotid artery enters into side above closed inferior portion
Carotid canal	Carotid artery, sympathetic plexus
Stylomastoid	Facial nerve (exit)
Internal acoustic meatus	Facial nerve, cochlear nerve, superior and inferior vestibular nerves, labyrinthine artery and vein
Jugular foramen	Glossopharyngeal nerves, vagus nerve, accessory nerve, sigmoid sinus, inferior petrosal sinus
Foramen magnum	Spinal cord, hypoglossal nerve, vertebral arteries, spinal arteries, cervical accessory nerve

Fundamentals of Surgical Practice, Third Edition, ed. Andrew N. Kingsnorth and Douglas M. Bowley.
Published by Cambridge University Press. © Cambridge University Press 2011.

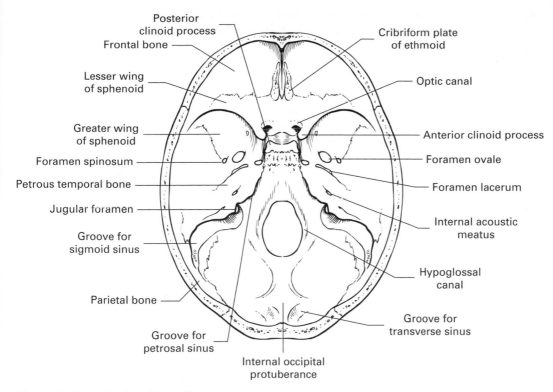

Figure 17.1 Internal surface of the skull base.

Brain

The brain is composed of neurons, neuroglia and blood vessels.

Neurons

Each neuron is composed of a cell body, dendrites, which are short non-myelinated processes, and one or more axons whose length varies from a few millimetres to over 1 m. Neurons may be unipolar, bipolar or multipolar; the first two are primarily afferent and convey sensory information from receptor endings to the central nervous system (CNS). The majority of neurons in the CNS are of the multipolar type. In the peripheral nervous system (PNS), axons are ensheathed by neurilemmal cells which form myelin in myelinated axons, although unmyelinated axons have a sheath but no myelin. The myelinated axon has regular gaps in the myelin called nodes of Ranvier. In the CNS, axons may be myelinated or unmyelinated, and some neurons, such as those in the anterior horn cell of the spinal cord, have very long axons.

In both the CNS and autonomic nervous system, axons make contact with a neuron, a dendrite or another axon through a synapse. At most synapses a nervous impulse is chemically mediated and is due to the release of a specific transmitting substance stored in the axonal ending and thus transmission is unidirectional. Synapses may be excitatory or inhibitory. There are many synaptic substances within the brain (central transmitters), the best known being dopamine, noradrenaline, adrenaline, serotonin, acetylcholine and gamma-aminobutyric acid (GABA). Excitation of a neuron gives rise to a propagated action potential which travels along the axon by a wave of depolarization at constant speed. In myelinated fibres, conduction is faster since depolarization jumps from one node of Ranvier to the next (saltatory conduction). All this depends on the permeability of the cell membrane to sodium and potassium, and the sodium-potassium pump.

Neuroglia

Neuroglia are cells which neither form synapses nor conduct impulses. Oligodendrocytes predominate in the white matter and play the same role as the neurilemmal cells in the PNS. Astrocytes are larger and stellate in form and though extremely numerous much remains to be learnt regarding their influence on neuronal activity. Microglia are derived from mononuclear cells which migrate from blood vessels and can become macrophagic in response to brain injury or disease. Ependymal cells are ciliated and line the ventricles and the central canal of the spinal cord. The neurilemma are described above.

Aggregations of neurons are called nuclei and collections or bundles of axons, fibre tracts.

General morphology

The brain comprises two hemispheres. At the base of these runs the brainstem containing fibre tracts running to and from the brain to the rest of the body as well as the nuclei of the cranial nerves (III–XII inclusive); the cerebellum is attached to the posterior aspect of the brainstem.

The cerebral hemispheres are separated in the midline by the fold of dura called the falx at the bottom of which lies the major hemispheric connection the corpus callosum. For descriptive reasons the brain is divided into four lobes which must not be thought of as discrete or isolated from one another. The surface of the brain is convoluted, with the hollows called sulci and the ridges, gyri. Two main sulci and two small ones help divide the brain into these four lobes; the Rolandic (central) sulcus lies approximately half way between the anterior and posterior poles of the hemisphere and on the lateral aspect of the hemisphere runs obliquely forward to meet the Sylvian fissure; one of the small ones is the preoccipital notch about 5 cm in front of the occipital pole laterally and the other is the parietopital sulcus, which lies mainly medially. The four lobes are thus:

- frontal lobe: area above the Sylvian fissure and anterior to the Rolandic sulcus
- temporal lobe: area below the fissure and anterior to a line joining the pre-occipital notch and the parieto-occipital sulcus
- parietal lobe: area posterior to the Rolandic gyrus above the Sylvian fissure
- occipital lobe: posterior part of the brain.

The cerebrum consists essentially of cortex, which is grey matter containing neurons, and deep to this is the white matter consisting mainly of fibre tracts. Deeper still is further grey matter of the thalamus and hypothalamus and beside the thalamus there are the basal ganglia. The cortex consists of differing types of neurons and is organized differently in differing areas. The white matter consists of commissural fibres connecting the two hemispheres (corpus callosum being the greatest), association fibres between gyri and projection fibres, the largest of the latter being the corona radiata lying close to the lateral ventricle which lower down becomes the internal capsule through which run fibres going to and away from the cortex.

There is some localization of function within the cerebrum, with some areas having a predominant function:

- precentral gyrus – voluntary movement
- post central gyrus – somatic sensation
- prefrontal cortex – control of intellect and personality
- inferior and medial frontal cortex – visceral and emotional activity
- medial temporal cortex – memory and smell
- inferior frontal gyrus, superior temporal gyrus and part of the parietal lobe – speech functions (in a right-handed person these are on the left of the brain and in left-handed people, dominance can be either right or left, and thus approximately 95% of people are left hemisphere dominant for speech)
- occipital lobe, in particular in and around the calcarine fissure – vision
- thalamus – animal behaviour
- hypothalamus – control of autonomic nervous system and anterior pituitary gland and also makes antidiuretic hormone (ADH), which passes down to the posterior pituitary gland.

Clinical examination

Conscious level

The examination of the conscious level is integral to any surgical assessment. Many vague terms can be used to describe the state of consciousness, which is very difficult to define and communicate to other clinicians. A coma scale is therefore used to describe the conscious level. The Alert Voice Pain Unresponsive (AVPU) Scale is found in the ATLS® System (Table 17.2). We recommend that surgeons should not use the AVPU system but use the Glasgow Coma Scale (GCS, Table 17.3) as the same stimuli need to be utilized for both assessments.

Table 17.2 The AVPU Scale

A	Alert
V	Responds to verbal stimuli
P	Responds to painful stimuli
U	Unresponsive

Table 17.3 The Glasgow Coma Scale

Eye opening	
E4	Spontaneous
E3	To speech
E2	To pain
E1	None
Verbal response	
V5	Orientated
V4	Confused
V3	Words
V2	Sounds
V1	None
Motor response	
M6	Obeys commands
M5	Localizes to a painful stimulus
M4	Normal flexion to pain
M3	Abnormal flexion to pain
M2	Extending to pain
M1	None

The examination starts with asking the patient to open their eyes (if not spontaneously open) and to lift up their arms. Asking the patient where they are and what day it is establishes all of the verbal response criteria. If the patient failed to obey commands then a painful stimulus is applied to determine the eye-opening and motor response. The site of the painful response in the initial assessment should be upward thumb pressure in the supraorbital groove. The neural pathway is through the trigeminal nerve and to the brain and not via spinal nerves and the spinal cord.

It has become common practice to summate the scores of the GCS into a score out of 15, with a GCS of 8 or less indicating a severe head injury. It is more meaningful to indicate the separate parts of the scale such as E1V2M5. Continuous regular recording of the GCS is essential to monitor progress or decline.

Two abnormal postures of the patient can be seen in the patient with brain injury. The first is where the upper limbs are flexed due to damage of fibres in the subcortical cerebral white matter and basal grey matter, the 'decorticate posture'. The second is where the upper limbs are extended, where there is a preponderance of damage to the afferent fibres of the upper brainstem, the 'decerebrate posture'. The painful stimulus can demonstrate these postures early after injury. The postures usually do not become spontaneous until some hours after injury.

Higher cerebral function

If the patient can talk then an assessment of higher functions is undertaken. The patient may not be able to obey commands because of a receptive dysphasia; there may be difficulty constructing a sentence because of expressive dysphasia. Disorders of naming of objects (nominal dysphasia), recognizing objects (agnosia), reading (dyslexia), writing (dysgraphia) and serial 7s (dyscalculia) are all malfunctions of the dominant hemisphere that can be easily assessed. Disorders of drawing two intersecting pentagons (constructional apraxia) and dressing (dressing apraxia) are malfunctions of the non-dominant hemisphere.

Memory disturbance

The surgeon will frequently meet a patient with a mild or moderate head injury. It has been shown that post-traumatic amnesia (PTA) can indicate the severity of the brain injury. Assessing this amnesia is quite difficult. Asking the patient for the first event that followed the injury, such as getting into the ambulance, assesses antegrade amnesia. The memory for the last event before the injury is retrograde amnesia. To determine PTA the examiner needs to establish whether the patient has continuous short-term memory, by asking a series of verifiable questions of the day's activities such as 'what did you eat for breakfast and lunch, who came to see you today, what have you been watching on TV?' PTA is therefore quite difficult to assess in the A & E department. The Galveston Orientation and Amnesia Test (GOAT) can be used in a structured way to assess PTA.

Cranial nerves

I (olfactory) nerve

The fibres originate from the olfactory cells lying in the upper nasal mucus membrane. These are collected together and pass through the cribiform plate of the ethmoidal bone and end in the olfactory bulb. They are the organs of smell and recognition of finer tastes. They can be tested by presenting a variety of smells, one at a time, to the patient and closing the other nostril. Lack of smell (anosmia) can occur after head injury as the movement of the frontal lobe of the brain can disrupt the fine nerve fibres passing through the cribiform plate.

II (optic) nerve

The fibres of the II nerve originate in the ganglion layer of the retina which converge on the optic disc and then pierce the retina, choroid and sclera to form the optic nerves. The nerve is pierced by the central retinal artery and vein 12 mm from the sclera. It runs through the muscle cone and then through the optic foramen. Once inside the skull, the nerve runs obliquely and medially to join its fellow nerve from the opposite side to form the optic chiasm lying just under the hypothalamus. In the chiasm, fibres from the nasal half of the retina, including the nasal half of the macula, cross the midline and join with the temporal fibres from the opposite retina and macula to form the optic tract, which runs through the brain to the occipital cortex. Visual acuity can be grossly checked using newspaper print or the Jaeger book of different text sizes. Ideally acuity should be tested with the Snellen chart at 6 m from the patient. Visual fields are tested in each eye sequentially and then both eyes together. Lesions of the optic pathway lead to different impairments of the visual fields: optic nerve unilateral blindness (trauma); optic chiasm bitemporal hemianopia (pituitary tumour, craniopharyngioma); optic tract homonymous hemianopia (tumour). Bilateral damage to the visual cortex can lead to reduced vision uniformly distributed in the visual field with preserved pupil reflex (cortical blindness).

Ophthalmoscopy in a surgical examination is essentially looking for the presence or absence of papilloedema. The optic disc is swollen and elevated with a blurred margin and streaks radiating from the disc. Veins are enlarged due to stasis and small haemorrhages may appear along the disc margin. It normally takes about 24 h for raised intracranial pressure (ICP) to develop papilloedema. Open subarachnoid spaces must be present for papilloedema to be present. A classic surgical eye examination is optic atrophy in one eye (from direct compression) and papilloedema in the other eye (from raised ICP) can be seen with large slowly growing tumours in the anterior fossa.

III (oculomotor), IV (trochlear) and VI (abducens) nerves

In a patient with a low GCS pen-torch assessment of pupils is a vital early part of the surgical examination; an abnormality could indicate a level of urgency that curtails further detailed examination. A dilated pupil can indicate pressure on the III nerve along its course. Arising from the nucleus in the floor of the aqueduct of Sylvius in the midbrain the III nerve runs between the superior cerebellar and posterior cerebral arteries and then forwards alongside the free edge of the tentorium to run in the lateral wall of the cavernous sinus. In brain herniation such as following head injury the medial part of the temporal lobe (the uncus) squeezes into the gap between the medulla and the free edge of the tentorium, compressing the nerve. A complete paralysis of the III nerve leads to ptosis, external strabismus due to the unopposed action of the lateral rectus and superior oblique, dilatation of the pupil and loss of accommodation and reaction to light. The route of the pupillary reflex is via optic nerve, optic chiasm, optic tract, Edinger Westphal nucleus in the brainstem, and oculomotor nerve making a synapse in the ciliary ganglion. Horner's syndrome (unilateral miosis, ptosis, decreased sweat production and conjunctival vasodilatation) is a result of decreased sympathetic innervation such as infarction of the medulla oblongata, or apical lung tumour.

The VI nerve nucleus is in the pons; the fibres emerge at the junction of the pons and the medulla. It has a long extracerebral course up the clivus and enters the lateral wall of the cavernous sinus. The IV nerve (trochlear) nucleus lies in the midbrain at the level of the caudate colliculus, fibres cross the midline and the nerve leaves the posterior side of the brainstem and continues around it to the front where it enters the cavernous sinus innervating the superior oblique muscle. Examination of occular movements is achieved by asking the patient to follow the finger, which is moved in the shape of an H. Loss of lateral movement of the eye indicates a VI nerve palsy and induces a diplopia. A VI nerve palsy can be what is termed a 'false localizing sign' as raised intracranial pressure without direct nerve compression can cause impairment of nerve function. A IV nerve defect requires careful observation of the adducted eye when looking down; for example if you ask the patient to look to the left and downward the left eye looks downward innervated by the III nerve; the right eye does not look downward if there is a IV nerve palsy.

V (trigeminal) nerve

The fibres of the sensory root arise from cells of the trigeminal ganglion, which lies near the apex of the petrous temporal bone. The central fibres pass to the pons and the peripheral fibres are divided into three main nerves – ophthalmic and maxillary (which are wholly sensory) and mandibular (which is a mixed motor and sensory nerve). V1 (ophthalmic) runs in the lateral wall of the cavernous sinus and divides into three branches which all run through the superior orbital fissure. It supplies sensation to the eyeball, conjunctiva, part of the mucus membranes of the nose and skin of the nose, eyelids and scalp from the frontal region as far posteriorly as the lambdoid suture. V2 (maxillary) runs through the lateral wall of the cavernous sinus, leaves the skull through the foramen rotundum, and then passes through the pterygopalatine fossa and enters the orbit through the inferior orbital fissure (as the infraorbital nerve). It supplies sensation to the lower side of the nose, lower eyelid, skin and mucus membrane of the cheek, and upper lip as well as the inside of the upper mouth and upper teeth. V3 (mandibular) leaves the skull through the foramen ovale. The motor root supplies the muscles of mastication as well as the tensor palati and tensor tympani. The sensory root supplies the teeth and gums of the mandible, lower lip, anterior two-thirds of the tongue, and floor of the mouth. The chorda tympani nerve of the 7th nerve hitches a lift in the lingual branch of the mandibular nerve to supply taste to the anterior two-thirds of the tongue. Examination of facial sensation should include the cornea and usually just requires light touch only. Facial sensation is a function of the V nerve (trigeminal) through three subdivisions: V1 forehead, V2 cheek, V3 mandible. The masseter is innervated through motor fibres within the nerve. Deficits of trigeminal nerve function can be due to tumours in the region of the petrous apex such as meningioma or schwannoma of the nerve itself.

VII (facial) nerve

This nerve possesses a motor and sensory root. The sensory root is the chorda tympani mentioned above. The motor root supplies the muscles of the face (facial expression), the scalp, buccinator, stapedius, stylohyoid, posterior belly of the digastric and the platysma. The motor nucleus lies in the pons and the sensory nucleus in the medulla. The two roots join and emerge from the pons and run through the cerebellopontine angle close to the 8th nerve and into the internal auditory meatus. The nerve then runs a tortuous course through the petrous bone and is close to the tympanic antrum before leaving the skull through the stylomastoid foramen. Thereafter, the nerve runs through the

parotid gland and divides into branches to supply the muscles listed above.

Paralysis may occur from central or peripheral lesions. In central cerebral lesions the lower part of the face is particularly affected and the upper part of the forehead may be relatively spared. Peripheral paralysis affects the whole face. The nerve is very vulnerable to a variety of pathological processes due to its long tortuous course through the cerebellopontine angle, petrous bone and skull base, and the parotid gland. It behoves any surgeon operating in this area to study and learn the detailed anatomy in order to attempt the preservation of facial expression.

VIII (auditory) nerve

The VIII nerve is a sensory nerve comprising two sets of fibres: one forms the vestibular nerve, which relays information on the position of the head with respect to gravity from the semicircular canals in the petrous bone; and the other the cochlear nerve, which relays hearing from the cochlear. Both nuclei lie within the pons.

Vestibular function is part of the overall function of balance and it is not surprising that there are many complicated relays between the vestibular nucleus, cerebellum, 3rd, 4th and 6th nerve nuclei, and the spinal cord. If total damage occurs to one nerve or the semicircular canals, the opposite side can function quite well, but problems occur when there is partial damage and then imbalance between the two sides resulting in vertigo and ataxia.

Auditory function is complex and has two main components – the transmission of sound across the middle ear (tympanic cavity) to the tympanic membrane and the conversion of these transmissions by the cochlear into nerve impulses; thus two main types of deafness or partial hearing loss may occur – conduction (mechanical) or sensorineural. Using a tuning fork, a clinical assessment can be carried to establish which is better heard by the patient – air or bone conduction – remembering that the norm is for air to be better than bone conduction. Detailed assessment of hearing is carried out by audiometry.

Disease processes in the middle ear can lead to hearing loss as well as 7th nerve damage. Disease processes in the petrous bone such as infections, neoplasms and fractures from head injuries can cause hearing deficit as can lesions in the intracranial cerebellopontine angle such as acoustic neuromas.

IX (glossopharyngeal) nerve

This is a mixed motor and sensory nerve. The sensory part supplies fibres to the pharynx and tonsil and both sensation and taste to the posterior one-third of the tongue. The motor fibres supply the stylopharyngeus muscle and the secretomotor fibres to the parotid gland. The nuclei are in the medulla and the nerve leaves this to exit the skull through the anterior part of the jugular foramen.

X (vagus) nerve

This is a mixed motor and sensory nerve and has probably the most extensive distribution of any nerve in the body. The nuclei are within the medulla and the nerve leaves this to exit the skull through the jugular foramen. It then runs down the neck within the carotid sheath lying between the internal jugular vein and internal carotid artery proximally and the internal jugular vein and common carotid artery distally. Thereafter the course is different for each side. On the right, the nerve crosses the subclavian artery and thence into the superior mediastinum; then it passes behind the right main bronchus and behind the oesophagus and picks up some fibres from the left vagus and runs through the diaphragm as the posterior vagal trunk. On the left, the nerve enters the mediastinum between the left common carotid and subclavian arteries. It crosses the root of the left lung and forms the anterior vagal trunk with some fibres from the right vagus and enters the abdomen as the anterior vagal nerve on the front of the oesophagus.

Both nerves give branches off during their course; in the neck they supply the muscles of the soft palate (except the tensor palati) and the pharynx. They also supply sensation to the mucus membrane of the larynx. The recurrent laryngeal nerve has a different course on each side, on the right going round the subclavian artery and on the left around the arch of the aorta; it supplies the muscles of the larynx except the cricothyroid, in particular those muscles moving the vocal cords, and paralysis leads to dysphonia. It is particularly at risk in neck surgery of the thyroid and parathyroid glands as well as anterior vertebral column surgery.

The vagus supplies the heart, stomach, first part of the duodenum, liver and kidneys. Due to its wide distribution, detailed knowledge of its anatomy is necessary for neurosurgeons, eye nose throat (ENT) surgeons, faciomaxillary surgeons and cardiothoracic and abdominal surgeons.

XI (accessory) nerve

The XI nerve is unusual in having a small cranial root and a much larger spinal root. The latter is formed from anterior horn cells as far down as the 5th cervical nerve. The fibres coalesce and run upwards through the foramen magnum and then leave the skull again through the jugular foramen. It supplies the sternomastoid and trapezius muscles.

XII (hypoglossal) nerve

This is the motor nerve of the tongue. The nucleus lies in the floor of the 4th ventricle and the fibres emerge as rootlets and pass through the anterior condylar foramen. It passes behind the internal carotid artery, then in front of the vagus nerve and enters the tongue on top of the hyoglossus muscle. Due to its course, it is particularly vulnerable to pathology and more particularly surgery in this region. Paralysis leads to failure to protrude the tongue on that side and the tongue deviates to that side as a result of unopposed action of the contralateral muscles.

The term bulbar palsy is used to describe malfunction of the lower cranial nerves from the IX to XII and is of the lower neuron type; it may be bilateral or unilateral. Pseudobulbar palsy is used to describe malfunction of these nerves when the lesion is higher and is of the upper motor neuron type.

Cerebral arteries

Arterial blood is delivered to the brain through four main arteries: the two internal carotid arteries and the two vertebral arteries. The internal carotid artery enters the skull through the carotid canal in the petrous temporal bone and then passes through the cavernous sinus to emerge through the dura close to the anterior clinoid process and as it does so it gives off the ophthalmic artery which supplies the structures off the orbit, including the central retinal artery. Thereafter the internal carotid artery forms part of the circle of Willis.

The two vertebral arteries arise from the subclavian arteries. On each side the artery ascends to run through the foramina transversaria of the upper six cervical vertebrae, then runs across the lateral mass of

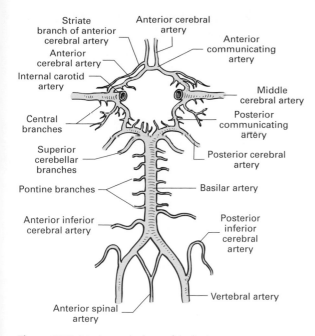

Figure 17.2 Arteries on the base of the brain.

the atlas into the vertebral canal and through the foramen magnum. The anterior and posterior spinal arteries are given off, as is the posterior inferior cerebellar artery, before the two vertebral arteries join to form the basilar artery.

The circle of Willis is a ring of arteries at the base of the brain formed in the front by the internal carotid arteries bifurcating to give the middle cerebral arteries, and the anterior cerebral arteries which are joined by a channel, the anterior communicating artery, which has very variable configurations (Figure 17.2). The internal carotid arteries before their bifurcation give off the posterior communicating artery, which runs backwards to join the posterior cerebral artery, which is formed by the bifurcation of the basilar artery.

The middle cerebral artery through its branches supplies the lateral hemisphere above and below the Sylvian fissure (Figure 17.3). The anterior cerebral artery supplies the medial aspect of the hemisphere as far back as the occipital lobe, which is supplied by the posterior cerebral artery, as is the medial aspect of the temporal lobe. Deep structures are supplied by perforating arteries from the circle of Willis. Although the arteries anastomose on the surface of the brain, once they enter the brain substance they become terminal (end arteries).

Cerebral veins

The vast majority of venous drainage of the brain is through the sagittal sinuses (Figures 17.4 and 17.5: the superior, and the straight, which is the continuation of the inferior), which join together at the confluence of sinuses inside the inion. There the lateral sinuses are formed and run around the posterior fossa to become the sigmoid sinuses, which become the internal jugular veins to leave the skull and run through the neck in the carotid sheath. There are no valves in the sinuses.

There is no lymphatic drainage of the brain, although the scalp and face do have lymphatic drainage initially to superficial lymph glands (parotid, mastoid, submental and occipital) and thence into the deep cervical glands.

Pituitary gland

The normal pituitary gland is situated at the base of the brain and connected to it by the pituitary stalk, which runs from the hypothalamus. It measures $12 \times 9 \times 6$ mm and lies within the sella turcica of the skull base. It is surrounded by pituitary capsule, which is similar to dura mater, and the superior surface (diaphragma sellae) has an opening through which the stalk runs; in approximately 20% of people the diaphragma sellae is deficient and only arachnoid covers the gland at this point.

Autonomic nervous system

As elsewhere in the body, the autonomic nervous system is composed of two parts which often have opposing action – the sympathetic and parasympathetic systems. The outflow for the sympathetic system to the head is from the upper (usually T1 and T2) spinal cord segments and the nerves relay in the superior cervical ganglion and thereafter the nerve fibres hitch a lift in or around several structures, the most important of which is around the internal carotid artery.

In the eye, the pupillary and ciliary muscles are controlled by the sympathetic system, which produces pupillary dilatation and accommodation for distant vision, and by the parasympathetic, which produces pupillary constriction and accommodation for near vision; the origin of the parasympathetic fibres is from the Edinger–Westphal nucleus in the midbrain. The lacrimal gland produces tears under the control of the parasympathetic from the facial nucleus in the pons. The salivary glands are controlled by the sympathetic

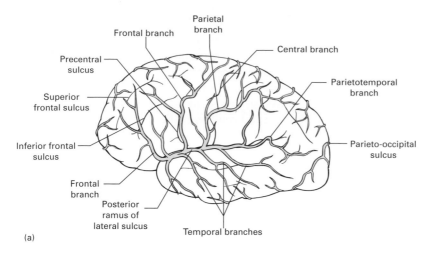

(a)

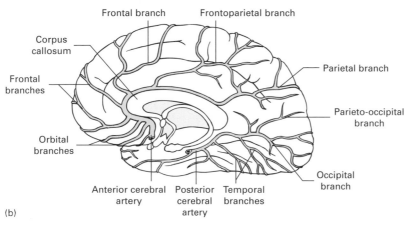

(b)

Figure 17.3 (a) Arteries of the superolateral surface of the left cerebral hemisphere and (b) of the medial and tentorial surfaces.

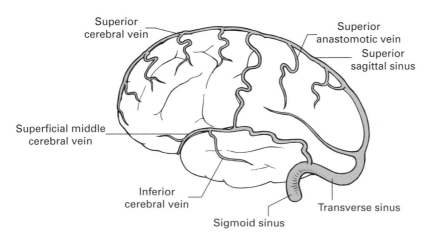

Figure 17.4 Veins of the superolateral surface of the hemisphere.

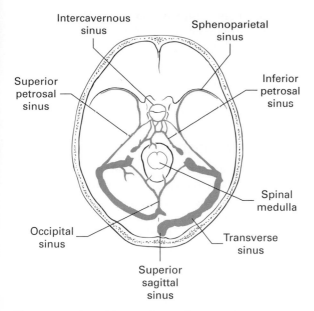

Intercavernous sinus

Sphenoparietal sinus

Superior petrosal sinus

Inferior petrosal sinus

Spinal medulla

Occipital sinus

Transverse sinus

Superior sagittal sinus

Figure 17.5 Floor of the cranial cavity, illustrating the main venous sinuses.

and the parasympathetic from salivary nuclei of the facial and glossopharyngeal nuclei in the pons and medulla.

Spinal cord

The spinal cord begins at the foramen magnum as the continuation of the medulla oblongata and runs down the vertebral canal to finish opposite the 1st lumbar vertebra in the adult. As it finishes it tapers as the conus medullaris and then a fibrous cord, the filum terminale, runs down further to the lower sacral canal. Since the spinal cord is shorter than the vertebral column, the neural segments do not correspond to the bony segments.

The grey matter is central and H-shaped and is larger in the cervical and lumbar areas. This is surrounded by columns of myelinated nerve fibres – anterior, lateral and posterior. The main columns are laterally the corticospinal dealing with voluntary movement and superficial to these are the lateral spinothalamic, which deal with pain; posteriorly the dorsal columns deal with sensation. The anterior grey matter (anterior horns) is almost exclusively efferent whilst the posterior horns are afferent and have a number of connections and relays with the incoming afferent fibres. The spinal nerve roots are posterior (afferent), entering the spinal cord close to the poster-

ior horns, and anterior (efferent), emerging from the spinal cord close to the anterior horns. The cell bodies of the posterior root fibres are in the dorsal root ganglion outside the spinal cord and those of the anterior root mainly arise in the anterior horn. The two roots join mechanically together to form the spinal nerve, one to each side, which emerges from the vertebral column through the intervertebral foramina. The spinal nerve then immediately divides into the posterior ramus, which supplies the skin and muscles of the back, and the anterior ramus, which supplies the anterior body wall, limbs and other appendages.

The segmental arrangement of the spinal cord and spinal nerves is preserved in the thoracic regions, although for the limbs there is complicated crossing over and linking in plexi, for the arm the brachial plexus and for the buttocks and legs the lumbosacral plexus. A myotome is the muscle tissue supplied by a single spinal motor root and the dermatome is the area of skin which sends sensory information inwards through a single spinal sensory root.

Neurophysiology

Cerebrospinal fluid

Each day 500 ml of cerebrospinal fluid (CSF) is secreted, mostly by the choroids plexus within the lateral, the 3rd and 4th ventricles. Very little appears to change the production rate of CSF other than quite markedly raised intracranial pressure, which reduces it. The CSF flows from the lateral ventricles through the foramina of Munro into the 3rd ventricle and thence down the aqueduct of Sylvius situated in the midbrain and upper pons. Once in the 4th ventricle, a very small amount passes down the central canal of the spinal cord but the vast majority flows out through the lateral foramina of Luschka and the central foramen of Magendie. Thereafter the CSF can flow down the subarachnoid space in the spine or pass upwards; eventually all CSF passes upward in the subarachnoid spaces around the midbrain and thence over the cerebral hemispheres and particularly to the parasagittal areas. It is reabsorbed into the blood stream through the arachnoid villi which protrude into the great venous sinuses, the superior sagittal sinus in particular.

Hydrocephalus

Hydrocephalus is an increase in CSF volume usually resulting from impaired absorption. Excess CSF production occurs only from a rare neoplasm, choroid plexus papilloma. Obstruction to the passage of CSF within the brain or within the subarachnoid spaces leads to an obstructive hydrocephalus; causes of this are a mass lesion or meningitis from bacteria or blood. Failure of absorption of CSF leads to a communicating hydrocephalus; causes include infection, subarachnoid haemorrhage or carcinomatous meningitis. As hydrocephalus develops the ventricles dilate and CSF permeates into the periventricular white matter, leading to raised intracranial pressure. In young children the head size increases and the anterior fontanelle is tense, and there can be impaired upward gaze leading to the 'setting sun' appearance of the eyes. In the neonate and young child, the skull may expand if the sutures between the skull bones give way (suture diastasis) and for this reason the monitoring process for children includes plotting of measurements of skull circumference on appropriate percentile charts. Acutely developing hydrocephalus can lead to impaired consciousness and vomiting; gradual onset leads to dementia, gait ataxia and incontinence.

Two main patterns are seen on computerized tomography (CT) or magnetic resonance (MR) imaging: one is where all the ventricles are dilated, which suggests a communicating hydrocephalus; the second is where the 4th ventricle remains a normal size with dilatation of the lateral and 3rd ventricle, which suggests obstructive hydrocephalus, most commonly at the level of the aqueduct of Sylvius, aqueduct stenosis.

Specimens of CSF can be obtained by lumbar puncture, or by a burr hole and tapping the lateral ventricle with a brain cannula. If there is any suspicion of a mass lesion, a brain scan should be performed first, since a lumbar puncture in the presence of a mass lesion and/or raised intracranial pressure is dangerous and may lead to sudden brain displacements; a burr hole is much safer since CSF is drained above any mass lesion and displacements are much less likely to occur.

Any causative mass lesion should be excised if possible. If such resection does not settle the hydrocephalus or if there is no causative mass lesion, surgical CSF diversion is required. This diversion can be temporary by placing a ventricular drain through a frontal burr hole and CSF is collected into a measuring chamber. For aqueduct stenosis the treatment of choice is an endoscopic third ventriculostomy where the floor of the third ventricle is directly visualized and punctured. Most patients will require a perma-nent CSF shunt, which is implanted subcutaneously between one of the lateral ventricles and the peritoneal cavity. These shunt systems use a valve to regulate the flow of CSF to prevent over-drainage; many of these valves have components that prevent siphoning of the CSF and can be programmable by utilizing a magnet over the valve rested on the scalp.

Cerebral circulation

The brain accounts for only 2% of the total body weight yet its blood flow represents 15% of the resting cardiac output and it uses 20% of the oxygen used by the whole body at rest. Cerebral blood flow (CBF) has been studied by the passage of biochemically inert gases (e.g. nitrous oxide, krypton and xenon) through the brain. The value for a normal conscious human at rest is 50–60 ml of blood/100 g brain tissue per min. Each day the brain requires about 1000 litres of blood in order to obtain 71 litres of oxygen. Cessation of blood flow causes unconsciousness within 5–10 s.

The brain can regulate the blood flow in accordance with its metabolic need. The cerebral vasculature can adjust to changes in arterial blood pressure, keeping the flow constant within certain limits; this is called cerebrovascular autoregulation. The CBF is autoregulated within certain parameters:

- CBF is maintained at systemic mean arterial pressures between 60 and 150 mmHg. Below systemic blood pressures of 60 mmHg, CBF lessens such that if the pressure falls rapidly to 20 mmHg, CBF virtually ceases. Slower falls under controlled conditions, such as hypotensive anaesthesia, can be tolerated to 40 mmHg before CBF starts to lessen. When the systemic arterial pressure is raised, CBF remains constant until 150 mmHg, when an increase occurs, often described as breakthrough of autoregulation. In chronically hypertensive patients, this limit may be higher at around 170 mmHg.
- Arterial blood gases have a major influence on CBF. CBF and cerebral blood volume increases when the arterial $PaCO_2$ is raised due to dilatation of pial arterioles. When the arterial PaO_2 falls, CBF starts to rise.

When CBF falls to 25–30 ml/100 g per min, neurological dysfunction occurs, leading to cellular chemical events culminating in neuronal death. Some areas are particularly sensitive, including not only the deep nuclei but also the boundary areas of the cortex where the distal branches of the major vessels of the circle of Willis meet and as a consequence the circulation and perfusion are less resistant to falling CBF (these areas may infarct, giving rise to the so-called boundary zone lesions/infarcts). These changes have major implications not only for intracranial pathological processes such as stroke, head injury and neoplasia, but also for systemic processes such as shock and severe respiratory dysfunction. Therefore, it is imperative to attempt to normalize blood pressure and arterial blood gases and reduce raised intracranial pressure (ICP) when it occurs.

The difference between the arterial pressure and the intracranial pressure is the cerebral perfusion pressure (CPP). In patients where autoregulation is impaired such as after head injury falls in the CPP will lead to cerebral ischaemia and infarction. It is currently recommended to keep the CPP above 70 mmHg following severe head injury. Often the intracranial pressure after head injury can be in the region of 30 mmHg; it therefore follows that the mean arterial blood pressure (MABP) should be maintained at around 100 mmHg until the intracranial pressure can be directly measured.

Investigations

At the outset it must be stated that the clinical history and clinical examination are the most important clues to the underlying pathology of any patient with suspected disease of the nervous system. A tentative clinical diagnosis can frequently be made and then, if necessary, taken further by special investigations.

Imaging

Radiographs

Plain radiographs of the skull, face and vertebral column can yield important data. Their use is becoming more limited as CT becomes more widely available. Radiographs of the facial skeleton can also be useful, although CT scanning probably yields more information. Radiographs of the vertebral column can be useful in suspected spinal injuries, spondylosis, metastatic and primary neoplasms and spinal infection. Chest radiographs are mandatory for any suspected intracranial mass lesion, in particular looking for possible bronchogenic carcinoma.

CT scanning

CT scanning uses ionizing radiation; scintillation detectors measure and a computer localizes the absorption characteristics at all points within a planar cross section (the thickness of each varying from 1 to 10 mm). Absorption is expressed on the Hounsfield scale between +400 (bone), 0 (water) and −1000 (air), and the images are viewed on a grey scale between black and white. CT is good at detecting mass lesions, particularly if these are enhanced by giving the patient an intravenous injection of iodinated contrast medium before a second scan. An unenhanced scan is good at detecting blood, bone anatomy and pathology. The main disadvantage of CT is the relatively high dose of ionizing radiation needed and if possible repetitive scans should be kept to a minimum.

Magnetic resonance imaging

MR imaging has rapidly become the primary tool for investigation of the CNS. MR is based on the fact that a nucleus can have one of two magnetic spins with differing energy levels. The nucleus will preferentially hold the lower energy state but can be changed to the higher state through a radiofrequency pulse which, once withdrawn, allows the nucleus to relax and give off the absorbed energy. It is the relaxation time of giving up this energy that is the basis of MR. The unit of magnetic field strength is the tesla; the MR scanning magnets into which the patient is inserted are 0.5–3.0 tesla.

MR contrast is due to how water in different tissues responds to magnetic disturbance. There are two main types of sequence, T1 and T2, that are used in imaging and gadolinium is used as a contrast medium. Water is seen as black on T1 and white on T2 images. Intrinsic brain tumours can be seen on the T1 scan as areas with lower density than surrounding brain; gadolinium enhancement in these tumours suggests malignancy. T2 images can show the extent of brain oedema around the tumour. The various pathologies in the CNS have differing characteristics on the images.

MR can also determine the chemical content of the tissue through a technique of nuclear magnetic resonance (NMR) spectroscopy; by determining areas of higher glucose metabolism functional MR can define areas of the brain such as the speech centres, which can help in surgical planning.

Myelography

Myelography today is only used when there is no access to an MR scanner or if the patient suffers from claustrophobia and is unable to enter the scanner. A non-ionic iodine-containing substance is injected into the subarachnoid space, usually by lumbar puncture, and the patient lies on a tilting table which is used to run the dye up and down the spine.

Angiography

This technique is used to demonstrate the blood vessels, in particular the arteries. In adults it is performed under local anaesthesia. A non-ionic iodine-containing medium is injected into the arteries. It is usual to catheterize the femoral artery and advance the catheter retrogradely up the aorta, placing its tip in the carotid and vertebral arteries in the neck, at the skull base or even within the branches of the circle of Willis. The images are computer-enhanced, which reduces the amount of iodine required and produces better images (digital subtraction angiography (DSA)) unobscured by overlying bone. Angiography is used to determine the cause of intracerebral haemorrhage and to assess the blood supply of mass lesions. For examination of the carotid and vertebral arteries in the neck for suspected atheroma, it is now considered safer to use the non-invasive technique of Doppler duplex ultrasound.

The interventional neuroradiologist now has the technology of microcatheters that can be manipulated up the carotid or vertebral arteries to most locations in the brain. Detachable coils can be fed up the catheters into aneurysms, packing them internally; stents can be passed that expand and hold open narrowed vessels; substances that harden (e.g. Onyx) can be injected in liquid form. These techniques are rapidly changing the therapies available to CNS vascular pathology. In tandem with these developments diagnostic angiography obtained by MRI or CT is now able to produce images very close to conventional angiography.

Neurophysiological investigations

The two commonest techniques are the electroencephalogram (EEG) and nerve conduction studies. EEG is used in the investigation of epilepsy and suspected brain damage after hypoxia and drug poisoning. Nerve conduction is used to confirm and localize disease of peripheral nerves and, in particular, is used in suspected compression neuropathies before attempting surgical release.

Traumatic brain injury

Pathology

Death from head injury in the UK has an incidence of 6–10 per 100 000 population each year. Head injuries can occur in isolation or with multiple traumas. They result either from deceleration of the head, for example in road traffic collisions, or acceleration, for example in assaults. The head may come into contact with an object, resulting in damage to the scalp and/or skull, or the body may decelerate/accelerate without direct contact to the head. Since the brain is soft and jelly-like, there is inertia between it and the skull and it oscillates and is often forced against the skull several times along the line of force. Penetrating missile injuries are unusual in the UK but common in some countries and in war zones; they cause impact damage, as above, but also focal damage along the missile tract within the brain.

Lesions are classified as primary if they occur at the time of injury and secondary if as a result of complications. Primary lesions may be:

- intracerebral haemorrhages: these may be single or multiple and vary in size from large to petechiae
- localized areas of contusion; these (like a bruise elsewhere on the body) are softened swollen brain with haemorrhages and occur maximally in the temporal, frontal and occipital lobes; the term contre-coup contusion is used to describe the oscillation of the brain whereby it is contused at the opposite pole from the impact
- laceration and diffuse axonal injury: lacerations occur either from an open direct penetration or within a closed injury and can occur anywhere on the cerebral cortical surface or even in the corpus callosum; in diffuse axonal injury (DAI) there is widespread damage to the white matter of the cerebral hemispheres and fibre tracts within the brainstem.

Secondary lesions include:

- oedema: around contusions and lacerations this adds to the local mass effect and there is an increase in brain tissue water and increased permeability of blood vessels; there may be diffuse brain swelling, which is thought to be most probably due to vascular engorgement, although if the brain becomes hypoxic there may be cytotoxic oedema as well

- displacement of brain and internal herniations: under the falx or the undersurface of the temporal lobe being forced into the tentorial opening leading to compression of the midbrain
- surface haematomas: subdural or extradural; the former arise from tearing of surface veins or the cerebral cortical substance and tend to spread over the cerebral hemisphere. Extradural haematomas result from either tearing of one of the meningeal vessels or from a fracture site; in either event the dura is stripped from the overlying bone for some surrounding distance and the haematoma develops in the potential space. Most frequently, extradural haematomas occur in the middle fossa, but can occur in the anterior or posterior fossae. Both subdural and extradural haematomas lead to secondary displacement and compression of the underlying brain.

The compounding effects of poor pulmonary gaseous exchange and falling systemic blood pressure upon an already damaged and deranged brain can never be overestimated (see above).

Clinical features

Neurological deficits

Focal or generalized neurological deficits can occur from either the primary or secondary injuries. Their nature varies depending on the site and severity of brain damage. These may include limb disturbance with weakness, dyspraxia and sensory loss. Eye movement disorders may occur from damage to the III, IV and VI nerves or to the midbrain. I nerve damage can occur and is irrecoverable if total and bilateral. Ataxia of the trunk with balance and gait disturbance is common after severe injuries.

Some of the most serious deficits are cognitive and speech disorders. Speech disorders may include dysphasia and dysarthria. Cognitive disorders can be severe and distressing, yet are often not appreciated in the early phases after a head injury. They include reduction of short-term memory, learning and ability to retrieve new information and logical thought. Personality changes can also occur and are often best recognized by relatives and friends.

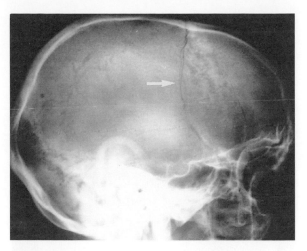

Figure 17.6 Lateral skull radiograph showing linear fracture (arrow) of a 45-year-old man with blow to the head.

Management

The acute management of traumatic brain injury (TBI) can be divided temporally and logistically into three phases:

- scene of the incident
- emergency department
- (if required) inpatient admission and care.

The scene of the incident is attended by the Ambulance Service, whose paramedics are trained in resuscitation. Any unconscious patient requires immobilization of the neck in a firm collar during retrieval back to the emergency department. The airway needs protection if the patient is still unconscious.

At the emergency department, patients can be triaged into major, moderate and mild injuries. Approximately 80% of TBI is classified as mild (GCS 14–15), 10% moderate (GCS 9–13) and 10% severe (GCS 3–8).

The key element of managing a patient with a head injury is the ABC of trauma care to ensure airway patency, adequate breathing and circulation. Following that attention is given to the exclusion of intracranial mass lesions that cause the secondary injuries as described above. Patients who have a decreased conscious level after head trauma have a high risk of an intracranial mass lesion and most of these patients will require a CT scan to exclude. The presence of a skull fracture also greatly increases the risk of an intracranial mass lesion and if an X-ray demonstrates a fracture then a CT must follow in most cases (Figures 17.6 and 17.7).

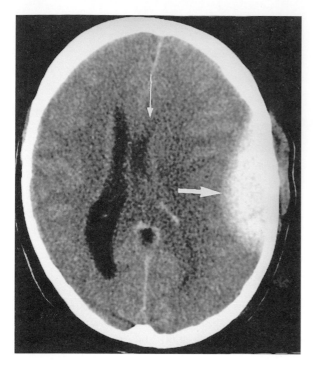

Figure 17.7 CT scan of the same patient as in Figure 17.6 showing extradural haematoma (large arrow). Note also severe shift of the brain (thin arrow).

Small children, in particular, are vulnerable and a full GCS assessment is often difficult to achieve, and the vast majority of these should be admitted.

If alcohol is detected, care must be taken in assessing the patient and any confusion or reduction of GCS must not be exclusively attributed to the alcohol. Patients with medical conditions that might have a bearing upon their response to a head injury should also be admitted, for example diabetes mellitus, epilepsy, respiratory and cardiac conditions and also patients who are taking anticoagulants or corticosteroids.

Observations, including the GCS, should be performed half-hourly and any decline in the GCS and the development of neurological deficits or both should alert the clinician to a complication and a cause should be immediately sought. Investigations including an urgent CT scan should be performed.

Patients in coma after TBI present major problems and immediate attention must be given to the establishment and maintenance of their airway and the maintenance of normal cardiovascular status. The upper airway must be protected, if necessary by endotracheal intubation. Adequate gaseous exchange must

be checked by arterial blood gas analysis and, if abnormal, reasons sought and the necessity for artificial ventilatory support considered. The cardiovascular status must be checked by measuring blood pressure, pulse volume and heart rate. The patient must be checked for other injuries by using the log-roll procedure and full frontal and posterior examination carried out. After resuscitation, a GCS score is derived and note taken of any injuries about the head, face and neck. Any suspected areas about the body must be radiographed and the cervical collar should not be removed until injury has been excluded.

Indications for CT scanning of the head after TBI:

- GCS ≤ 8
- focal neurological signs
- post-traumatic epileptic fit
- penetrating injury.

Following this, the nearest neurosurgical department should be contacted; if no CT scanner is available, the neurosurgical department should be contacted as soon as possible.

If transfer to a distant neurosurgical department is deemed necessary, the patient should be stabilized with respect to his pulmonary and cardiovascular status as quickly as possible before being transported by ambulance and accompanied by an anaesthetist.

Analgesia

The control of pain from injuries outwith the brain can be difficult, since opiates depress the level of consciousness and lead to pupillary constriction. Codeine, as a milder opiate, can be given but if there is severe pain, morphine may be required and its use agreed between surgeons and anaesthetists.

Post-traumatic epilepsy

Epilepsy can occur early after head injury. Whilst it is important to prevent further seizures, it must be appreciated that intravenous anticonvulsants (e.g. phenytoin and diazepam) not only may make neurological assessment more difficult, but can induce apnoea as well as cardiac dysrhythmias, and an anaesthetist with full resuscitation equipment must be present when the drug is administered. Post-traumatic epilepsy requires treatment but there is no need for routine prophylactic anticonvulsants simply because the patient has suffered a head injury. Patients at greatest risk for this complication have penetrating brain injuries, with the dura being breached, long PTA, intracranial haematomas and early post-traumatic epilepsy. In the UK, such patients should not drive a motor vehicle until they have reported themselves to the Chief Medical Officer and to the Driving and Vehicle Licensing Authority (DVLA), who may suspend them from driving for between 6 and 12 months, or longer if they have epilepsy or neurological deficits.

CSF leak

CSF fistulae may occur through the nose or ear. In these cases prophylactic antibiotics are not currently recommended but vigilant observation and investigation of all potential pyrexia are essential. CSF rhinorrhoea requires investigation and possibly repair by a neurosurgeon, as does persisting CSF otorrhoea.

Surgery for trauma

Scalp lacerations

The scalp is very vascular and patients can lose large volumes of blood from extensive lacerations. In an emergency situation, a pressure dressing can be applied. After assessment and/or resuscitation, a scalp laceration requires exploration and any rough irregular edges with possible skin damage require debridement. The wound is then sutured, preferably in two layers with absorbable sutures to the galea and sutures to the skin; if done properly, haemostasis will be achieved. Skin sutures can be removed after 5 days. If there is loss of scalp, this requires urgent surgery by a neurosurgeon or a plastic surgeon.

Burr holes

Only liquid haematomas can effectively be removed though burr holes, and therefore this form of surgery is only suitable for a fluid chronic subdural haematoma. However, burr holes are the starting point for a craniectomy or craniotomy (see below). A burr hole is performed by making a linear 4 cm long incision down to the pericranium, which is then scraped to each side. A Hudson brace with a perforator is then used to drill as far as the dura. The perforator is changed for a conical or spherical burr which enlarges the hole to about 15 mm. The exposed dura is then incised in a cruciate fashion to expose the brain.

Craniectomy and craniotomy

Ideally, it is better to perform a craniotomy, although for the less experienced surgeon a craniectomy can be life-saving for the patient. For a craniotomy, four burr holes are drilled at the corners of a square with sides at least 6–8 cm in length. Three of the four burr holes are connected with a saw and the fourth side is broken to keep the pericranium and/or temporalis muscle intact, thereby rendering the bone flap osteoplastic such that the bone will survive.

A craniectomy is performed by drilling a burr hole and then, with a bone rongeur, nibbling bone away to give sufficient exposure (the minimum being at least 5 cm in diameter); adequate exposure is vital and bone defects can always be repaired at a later date. An extradural haematoma is immediately encountered if the burr hole is in the right place; this will be solid and requires suction removal. The dura should be opened if a subdural haematoma is also suspected. The cause of the haematoma needs to be sought; if it is from the skull fracture this requires smearing with bone wax, but if it is from a tear of a branch of the middle meningeal artery, diathermy is required. The exposed dura must then be hitched, by interrupted sutures, over the bone edge to the pericranium to prevent further stripping of the dura and further extradural haematoma formation. A suction drain must be inserted and left for at least 24 h postoperatively.

Depressed skull fracture

Compound depressed skull fractures require a CT scan and need to be fully explored by a neurosurgeon, since bone fragments or other solid objects may be driven into the brain and lead to subsequent brain abscess. Simple depressed fractures require elevation only if they are significant and in a cosmetically important area. In the child under 3 years of age, considerable remodelling of the skull is possible and only severe depressions require elevation.

Missile injuries

Penetrating missile injuries demand particular neurosurgical expertise.

Rehabilitation

Any patient who suffers a head injury requires rehabilitation, although in the case of minor injuries the patient may require advice rather than major rehabilitation. A head injury with a PTA (post-traumatic amnesia) of 1 h may take 1–2 months, but often less, for full recovery. Whilst it is important to get the patient back to his former life-style, it is also important to ensure he is fully recovered before so doing. Headaches are a frequent problem and are variable in intensity and duration but usually subside after a few months; if they continue, a CT scan is required to check for chronic lesions such as a subdural haematoma or hydrocephalus.

Patients with longer PTA and those with neurological deficits need longer to recover and may have continuing cognitive problems that require assessment by a clinical neuropsychologist. Those with severe problems require the services of a fully trained rehabilitation team, which will include a neurosurgeon, rehabilitation expert, physiotherapist, occupational therapist, speech therapist and neuropsychologist or, in the case of children of school age, an educational psychologist. The CNS is slow to repair and reorganize and 2 years is the usual time span for maximal recovery to take place. Relatives are particularly important since they often have to bear the heavy burden of a difficult patient in the home environment and they need support; they can also often make useful contributions in rehabilitation.

Brain death

As a result of resuscitation and intensive care, patients who are deeply comatose and unresponsive may be maintained on artificial ventilation. In these circumstances if brain death is diagnosed it is appropriate to withdraw ventilatory support.

For a diagnosis of brain death to be made, all of the following must coexist:

- Patient is deeply comatose and there is no suspicion that this is due to narcotics, hypnotics or neuroleptic drugs. There should be no hypothermia (core body temperature must be $\geq 35°C$). There should be no major metabolic or endocrine disturbance and the serum glucose and electrolytes should be normal or nearly normal.
- Patient is maintained on a ventilator because spontaneous respiration had become inadequate or ceased. Neuromuscular blocking drugs should not be present, or if they have been used they should have been stopped at least 24 h previously.
- There should be no doubt that the patient's condition is due to irremediable brain damage and the reason for this has been fully established.

Tests to confirm brain death must be performed as a set closely together in time as follows:

- brainstem reflexes are absent:
  - pupils are fixed and dilated and do not respond to light
  - no corneal reflex
  - no eye movements when 20 ml of ice cold water is slowly perfused through each external auditory meatus
- no motor response can be elicited in any area of the body by painful stimuli
- no gag reflex in response to bronchial stimulation by passing a catheter down the trachea
- no respiratory movements occur on stopping the ventilator for 10 min. Samples can be checked both pre- and post-ventilatory arrest to confirm that the CO_2 has risen to levels which would drive respiration.

The tests should be carried out by two doctors who have both been registered for at least 5 years.

Transplantation/organ donation

Currently potential recipients for cadaveric organ donation exceed potential donors, particularly with respect to kidneys, heart, liver and pancreas. It is incumbent on the treating doctors to raise this issue with the relatives and it is also possible that the patient may carry a donor card or have expressed premorbid wishes. If consent is possible, the transplant team should be informed and will make the necessary arrangements; it must be made absolutely clear to relatives that the treating team and transplant team are completely separate.

Spinal injuries

In the UK, the great majority of spinal injuries are closed and occur from the indirect effect of violence applied to the vertebral column. In military practice open and compound from penetration by missiles of various sorts are found. The distributions of spinal injuries are as follows: 10% occur in the cervical region, 10% in the upper thoracic, 50% in the lower thoracic and 30% in the lumbar. Approximately 50% are the result of road traffic incidents, 30% from industrial incidents and most of the remainder from sport or falls. Approximately 75% occur in patients under 40 years and 80% are males.

The effects can most easily be described by considering spinal cord and vertebral column injury separately, although clearly these are intertwined.

Spinal cord injury

Spinal concussion is the transient loss of neurological function which may recover quickly and fully, and is similar to minor concussion of the brain. Spinal contusion involves swelling and haemorrhages in the spinal cord and very quickly there may be a central necrosis. The myelin sheaths are broken up, the axons are ruptured and neurons degenerate. Eventually the swelling subsides; some neural tissues may recover but those that have died are replaced by gliosis. An occasional late complication is the development of a syrinx (cyst) within the cord.

If injury is severe, there is an immediate and total loss of function at the level of the contusion and in the distal cord. Paralysis is complete and flaccid and there is total sensory loss. The bladder ceases to function. It is generally agreed that if there is no return of function within the first 48 h after injury, then the lesion is a complete functional transection and there will be no subsequent return of functions running up and down the spinal cord. If the lesion is partial and if there is some distal function remaining or returning, the neurological deficits are variable from one case to the next, as is the extent of recovery.

Spinal shock is the term used to describe the early phase lasting several weeks after injury; muscles are flaccid and there is also paralysis of the bladder and intestinal tract. As spinal shock wears off, distal spinal cord function returns but is shut off from the brain. Spinal cord reflexes return, the major one being the mass reflex, which is where limbs reflexively withdraw on stimulation, the rectum and bladder evacuate and there is profuse sweating.

Cervical spinal cord injuries bring particular problems dependent on the level of injury. The lower the lesion in the cervical spinal cord, the more arm function is preserved, remembering that the main neurological supply to the arm is between C5 and T1. The higher the lesion, the greater the problems with respiration, since if the injury is at C4 or above not only are the intercostal muscles paralysed but so are the diaphragm muscles due to loss of the phrenic nerve innervation, and the patient can only survive by artificial ventilation or by electrical pulsed stimulation of the phrenic nerves.

Vertebral column injury

The types of vertebral column injury are many and only a brief account is given here. One important concept to grasp is the difference between a stable injury which will not displace further and an unstable injury which may displace further and cause further neurological damage.

The upper two cervical vertebrae are more complex and different from those lower down the neck. Three main types of fracture occur:

- Jefferson fracture involves the ring of the atlas and is usually a stable fracture
- hangman's fracture involves both sides of the neural arch of the axis, thus separating the arch from the body
- the dens (odontoid) may fracture at variable distances from the body of the axis, which is unstable and may lead to avascular necrosis of the dens above the fracture line.

In the cervical spine, fracture dislocations may occur as well as compression (burst) fractures. Dislocations can also occur when the facet joints dislocate unilaterally or bilaterally. All these injuries should be regarded as unstable and require some form of fixation.

It must also be appreciated that patients with pre-existing cervical spondylosis are less tolerant of acute flexion or hyperextension and the osteophytes may contuse the spinal cord without there necessarily being a vertebral column injury.

Thoracolumbar injuries are usually due to violent hyperextension or vertical compression when a heavy object falls on the shoulders. If the posterior ligaments remain intact, there may only be a crush (compression) fracture of the vertebral body.

Management

At the scene of the incident, great care must be taken to avoid causing further damage, particularly to the spinal cord. In the case of suspected cervical spinal injuries, ideally a hard collar should be applied but if none is available, manual in-line immobilization should be applied. The patient must be kept flat and moved in a straight position onto a stretcher, which requires four people.

On arrival in hospital, the same precautions must continue. Plain radiography may be performed; however, CT is now the screening modality of choice. Any suspected unstable cervical spinal injury requires immobilization using a suitable hard collar. If the cervical spine is mal-aligned skull traction using Gardner–Wells forceps may be required; these can be applied to the skull above the ears in the under 60s, and exert a pull of at least 3–5 kg weight. In the past decade there has been a thrust to give large doses of methyl-prednisolone early in an attempt to diminish some of the spinal cord damage; the evidence for the efficacy of this is limited.

Conservative measures

- The patient must be given details of his injury and any prognosis; maintaining his morale is of paramount importance.
- Skin care is critical particularly in those patients with sensory loss. The prevention of bedsores is a real challenge to the nursing staff, who may be helped by turning beds, such as the Stryker frame, or motorized beds that constantly change position.
- Respiratory care is essential though the intensity depends on the level of the lesion. Upper cervical lesions will require ventilatory support, though all patients require regular chest physiotherapy.
- The bladder requires drainage to prevent back-flow, urinary damage and infection. In the long term for lesions above the conus medullaris, reflex bladder action may return stimulated by manual compression or by implanted electrodes. If there is no reflex bladder action, the bladder can be drained by an indwelling catheter or by teaching the patient self-catheterization. Renal function must be carefully and regularly monitored.
- Joints rapidly deteriorate if not moved passively and gently and the prevention of contractures is vital.
- Blood pressure must be watched since patients with severe high lesions develop orthostatic hypotension. G-suits can be used when attempting to elevate the patient beyond the horizontal.
- Deep venous thrombosis must be carefully looked for since not only is the muscle pump inefficient or non-existent but pain is also diminished or lost and as a result the patient may not complain of calf or thigh pain.
- The gastrointestinal tract may not function normally in the early phases and there may even be a paralytic ileus and thus parenteral nutrition may be necessary. Thereafter, nutritional requirements must be carefully assessed.
- Further displacement may occur at the fracture/dislocation site and further plain radiology is essential to monitor this area.
- Sexual and reproductive function may be possible even in patients with quite severe neurological deficits, although details of treatment are for specialists in spinal injuries.

Surgery for spinal injury

The role of surgery is relatively limited and the indications few; some of the techniques are quite complex. The indications for possible surgery are:

- Further deterioration in an incomplete lesion requires urgent radiography in the form of CT or MR scanning. If there is evidence of cord compression from the impingement of bone or disc fragments or an extradural haematoma, then urgent decompression by the appropriate route is indicated.
- Unstable injuries require fixation after they have been reduced. This is mostly by internal fixation, but in some cases of cervical injury, a skull halo and body fixation may be used. The vertebral column is slow to heal and any external fixation may be required for 3–6 months.

In the UK, it is usual to transfer the patient to a regional spinal injuries unit where there are facilities for acute care, rehabilitation and long-term follow-up.

Spinal cord compression

The spinal cord lies within the vertebral canal from the foramen magnum to approximately the first lumbar vertebra, and thereafter continues as the nerve roots of the cauda equina. It is surrounded by the three meningeal layers of dura, arachnoid and pia. There is very little spare room within the vertebral canal and space-occupying pathological processes soon lead to spinal cord compression. To some extent the symptomatology depends on the vertebral level, the layer of meninges containing the pathological process and the speed of onset of compression – the faster the onset, the poorer the prognosis for recovery even with expeditious treatment, and the converse applies for slowly compressing lesions.

In the cervical region, compression expresses itself as sensory and motor symptoms and signs of

numbness and weakness in the upper limbs, which may be flaccid or spastic depending on the level, and weakness of the trunk and lower limbs, which will have increased tone or even spasticity. If vertebrae are involved in the pathological process, there is often neck pain (or referred interscapular pain), but intradural lesions are often painless.

In the thoracic region if the bone is involved, there is often pain in the spine and girdle pain around the chest wall in the distribution of the appropriate intercostal nerve, unilaterally or bilaterally. The arms are unaffected but the legs develop weakness and increased tone, and there is usually a sensory level in the trunk and lower limbs distal to the affected level. Bladder function is often compromised.

In the lumbar region there is a motor and sensory paraparesis with bladder dysfunction, depending on the level of cord or cauda equina compression.

Neurological dysfunction of the bladder (the neurogenic bladder) is particularly important to recognize. In the early phases, there is failure fully to empty the bladder such that the bladder enlarges, eventually building up back pressure on the ureters and kidneys. Finally, the patient goes into urinary retention which is often painless due to the involvement of the sensory pathways. In the male, neurogenic bladder is accompanied by failure of penile erection and ejaculation.

Causes of spinal cord compression

Vertebral column

Malignancy may be secondary or primary. Metastases occur most commonly in the thoracic spine and may weaken the bone, leading to collapse. Malignant tissue may also spread into the extradural space as well as into the paraspinal tissues. The single commonest primary site is bronchogenic carcinoma but other sites are carcinomas of breast, prostate and kidney. Less commonly, other primary malignancies may metastasize to the spine. Malignancies from the reticuloendothelial system and blood-forming tissues also occur, either as part of widespread disease or starting primarily in the spine; these include myeloma (Figure 17.8), Hodgkin's and non-Hodgkin's lymphoma and reticulosarcoma.

Primary neoplasms occur in the spine and are similar to those occurring in bones elsewhere in the body such as osteogenic sarcoma, osteoclastoma, chondroma and chrondrosarcoma. In children, Ewing's sarcoma may occur in the vertebrae and neuroblastoma within the extradural space. In patients with osteo-

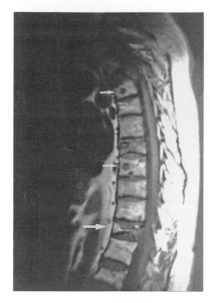

Figure 17.8
Magnetic resonance scan of the thoracic spine in a 60-year-old man with a pathological collapse fracture of vertebra (large arrow) and multiple vertebral body lesions (small arrow). The diagnosis was found by needle biopsy to be multiple myeloma.

porosis, particularly in postmenopausal women, collapse fractures can occur spontaneously or with minimal trauma (pathological fractures). Such fractures may be single or multiple. Osteomalacia can also lead to pathological fractures.

The spine can be infected by tuberculosis or pyogenic bacteria such as staphylococci. As the infection takes hold, the bone is weakened although the intervertebral disc is more resistant (Figures 17.9 and 17.10). Pus may be formed and the abscess spreads both inwards into the extradural space and outwards into the paraspinal tissues.

A small proportion of defective intervertebral discs may protrude centrally and cause spinal cord or cauda equina compression, often fairly acutely, although more chronic compression may develop from osteophytes in spondylosis of the spine.

Intradural lesions

Intradural lesions may be either in the subdural space but extrinsic to the spinal cord, or intrinsic within the spinal cord. The commonest subdural extrinsic neoplasms are meningiomas and neurofibromas; the latter may also grow through an intervertebral canal and enlarge outside the spine (dumb-bell tumour). The commonest intrinsic neoplasms are ependymomas and astrocytomas and both can compress and destroy the spinal cord from within outwards. Rarely, subdural pyogenic abscesses may form in the subdural space and can spread for quite long distances within the vertebral canal.

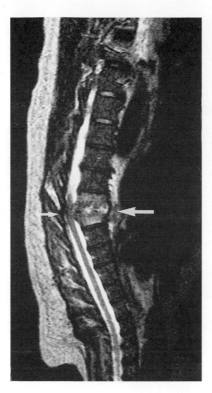

Figure 17.9
Magnetic resonance scan of the thoracic spine in a 40-year-old man showing collapse with abnormal signals of two contiguous vertebrae in mid-thoracic region (large arrow). Note some preservation of intervertebral disc. Note also spinal cord compression (small arrow).

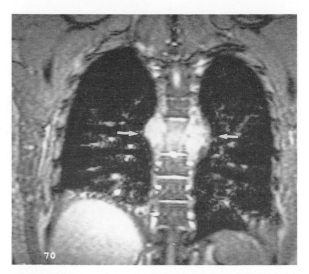

Figure 17.10 Same case as Figure 17.8 with coronal images. Note paravertebral mass (arrows). The patient was explored and an abscess found with osteomyelitis due to *Staphylococcus aureus*.

Investigations

Recognition of acute spinal cord compression demands real urgency. Often patients have been previously well but primary malignancies elsewhere should be suspected. However, even if there is an antecedent proven malignancy elsewhere in the body, it is unwise to assume that cord compression is due to metastasis since there may be an alternative unrelated process in the spine.

Radiological tests play a key part in the investigation. Plain radiographs of the spine should be performed looking for destruction of bone and paraspinal masses. At the same time, a chest radiograph is mandatory to look for bronchogenic carcinoma. The spine must be imaged by MRI of the whole spine, or if this is not available then by myelography and CT of any areas of myelographic block or indentation.

Management

Emergency referral to a neurosurgeon is essential for consideration of decompression of the cord compression, usually by laminectomy and excision or drainage of the pathological process. The patient should have an indwelling urinary catheter inserted for free drainage of urine. In the case of metastasis, partial excision is all that can be effected, although this does have the additional merit of yielding a histological tissue diagnosis. If the cord compression is incomplete, needle biopsy of the spine can be performed under radiological guidance. Instability of the spine is treated by instrumented fixation with products now specifically designed for all parts of the spine. The treatment thereafter of a metastasis is usually radiotherapy of the affected portions of the spine and treatment of the primary malignancy. Abscesses require drainage and in the case of the thoracic spine this is usually performed through a thoracotomy and an anterolateral approach to the spine.

The general care of patients with neurological deficits is as for patients with spinal injuries (see above), although special treatments may be necessary and obviously the prognosis will depend on various factors outlined above.

Intracranial neoplasms

Cerebral neoplasms may be primary or secondary (metastasis). In the latter case, they may occur in patients already diagnosed as suffering from malignancy elsewhere in the body or may be the first manifestation of malignancy from an initially occult primary neoplasm. Primary neoplasms may be classified as benign or malignant: benign intracranial

neoplasms have some of the same histological hallmarks as benign neoplasms elsewhere in the body, although their mass effect may kill the patient; malignant primary intracranial neoplasms invade and spread into the brain locally and may metastasize through the CSF pathways but only extremely rarely do they metastasize outwith the CNS. Another description that is used is extrinsic, that is within the skull but not part of the CNS, or intrinsic, that is within the skull and deriving from the CNS. Knowledge of the amazing variety of primary neoplasms is only essential to the neurosurgeon, although a few common types are mentioned below.

In the young child without fusion of the sutures, gradually expanding lesions, with or without accompanying hydrocephalus, may lead to enlargement of the head, but the skull of the older child and adult cannot expand.

In discussing pathophysiology it is simplest to subdivide neoplasms into those that occur above and those that occur below the tentorium in the posterior fossa.

Supratentorial neoplasms

The supratentorial site is the most common location for adult brain tumours. Tumours occur in about six persons per 100 000 per year; epilepsy is the presenting feature in about 30%. The effects of an expanding space-occupying lesion may lead to raised intracranial pressure or cerebral or cranial nerve dysfunction. Most neoplasms, whether benign or malignant, are surrounded by local swelling of the brain which is seen on CT as a pale area with a high water content; this has the effect of compounding the mass volume effect of the lesion, often by 2–3 times. Focal neurological defects can occur and usually steadily deteriorate; the type of defect depends on its site. As the lesion enlarges, the brain may be pushed aside and displaced and other more remote areas of the brain may be compressed against the skull and/or dural partitions such as the falx or tentorium. Eventually, raised ICP occurs since the compensating mechanisms, such as squeezing CSF outside the skull, often fail quite quickly. In the chronic phase, the patient complains of headache which is often worse in the morning; fundoscopy may reveal papilloedema and in severe cases retinal haemorrhages. With higher levels of ICP, CBF is reduced, the midbrain and thalamus are compressed and there is a steadily decreasing level of consciousness.

Infratentorial neoplasms

The infratentorial site is the most common location for childhood brain tumours. Hydrocephalus is very common and is usually of the obstructive type since the passage of CSF through the Sylvian aqueduct or exit from the fourth ventricle or both is held up. If the process is slow, the ventricles can enlarge and cause cognitive defects without necessarily leading to raised ICP; if there is more rapid expansion, raised ICP with papilloedema may ensue. Focal neurological defects may occur depending on the site of the lesion and there is often concomitant truncal ataxia with disorders of balance and gait.

Investigations

A careful clinical history and examination of the patient may suggest a mass lesion and give a clue to its site. A brain scan is then performed with contrast enhancement – iodine for CT and gadolinium for MRI. MRI is a little more sensitive and can show small multiple metastases better and has become the investigation of choice. Thallium single photon emission computed tomography (SPECT) scanning can show increased metabolism in malignant tumours; positron emission tomography (PET) scanning will become more widely available. A CT of the chest and abdomen is indicated to determine the primary source of disease when a metastatic tumour is suspected.

Management

The two main goals are to remove the lesion and to preserve neurological function; sometimes these are incompatible and the neurosurgeon has to settle for the latter as the prime goal even if this means only partially excising lesions. Dexamethasone is used to treat the associated brain swelling, which reduces ICP and can reverse deficits of neurological function. If there is hydrocephalus, this can be controlled by either excising the lesion or draining the ventricles by a temporary external ventricular drain through a frontal burr hole or permanently with a ventriculoperitoneal shunt.

Benign primary neoplasms

Other than pituitary adenomas (see below), the commonest benign neoplasm is a meningioma which is a neoplasm of arachnoid cells arising from the inner surface of the dura mater or the arachnoid granulations. The commonest sites are parafalcine, over the

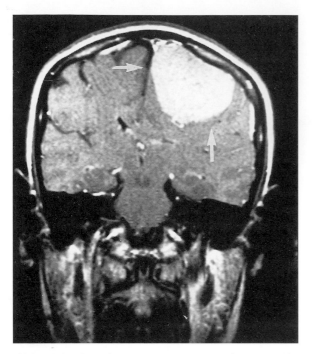

Figure 17.11 Coronal magnetic resonance scan of a 45-year-old woman showing large meningioma (arrows). Note the distortion of the brain, in particular the midline.

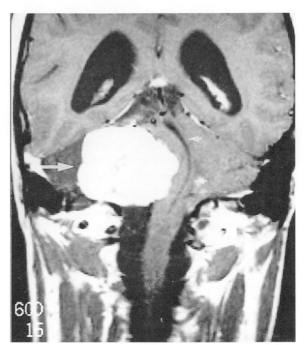

Figure 17.12 Coronal magnetic resonance scan of a 25-year-old man showing large acoustic neuroma (large arrow). Note also the distortion of the brainstem and fourth ventricle (small arrows).

convexity of the cerebral hemispheres (Figure 17.11), the tentorium and skull base. Treatment is by surgical excision, which should be total but may be subtotal, particularly in the case of meningiomata involving the skull base. Residual tumour following surgery may remain sessile but stereotactic radiosurgery has become the treatment of choice when the tumour shows signs of enlargement.

Acoustic neuromas, or more accurately vestibular schwannomas, arise on the vestibular portion of the VIII nerve and expand in the cerebellopontine angle (Figure 17.12). They have a variable growth potential and may be of variable size. They can occur in association with Type 2 neurofibromatosis, where they may be bilateral. When small, they may be detected by sensorineuronal nerve deafness on audiometry. Treatment is by surgical excision either through the posterior fossa or through the labyrinth or by stereotactic radiosurgery. Even with large lesions, preservation of the facial nerve is now possible in most patients.

Malignant primary neoplasms

Gliomas are neoplasms that arise from the glial cells of the brain. The commonest are the astrocytomas,

which may occur at any site (Figure 17.13). They show variable degrees of malignancy and are graded into four types. The grade I and II tumours are called low grade. Grade III tumours are called anaplastic astrocytoma and the most malignant of all is the glioblastoma multiforme (grade IV) which has tumour necrosis. Low-grade neoplasms undergo surgery and no radiotherapy if they have symptoms and surgery can be completed with low risk of deficit. Maximally resective surgery and radiotherapy are used for high-grade tumours unless resection would cause too great a risk of deficit when a needle biopsy is used. Surgery is commonly guided by image guidance and biopsies by stereotactic techniques. Adjuvant chemotherapy can also be used but effects on survival are small; local wafers of carmustine are now used intraoperatively for some indications. The results for the more malignant grades are poor, with few cures. In children, a subset called juvenile astrocytoma which occurs principally in the cerebellum is virtually benign and, although total excision is preferable, subtotal excisions can often preserve good quality of life for up to 30 years.

The main other type of glioma is an oligodendroglioma, which has a propensity to haemorrhage.

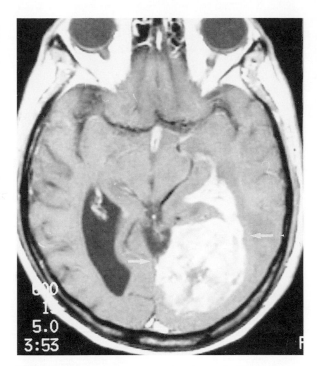

Figure 17.13 Magnetic resonance basal scan of a 60-year-old man with large parieto-occipital glioma (arrows). Note combination of mass effect and brain replacement.

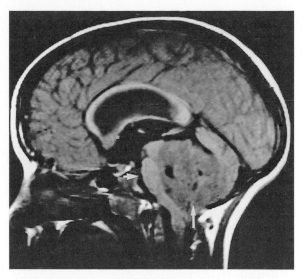

Figure 17.14 Magnetic resonance sagittal scan of a 9-year-old boy with large medulloblastoma of the vermis cerebelli (large arrow). Note also the compression of the brainstem (small arrow).

In immunosuppressed patients (e.g. transplanted patients on immunosuppressive therapy) or immuno-compromised patients (e.g. HIV-positive patients) lymphomas can occur; these are usually non-Hodgkin lymphomas which can be B cell, T cell or mixed and are usually highly malignant.

Primitive neurectodermal tumours (PNET) occur principally in childhood. The commonest were previously called medulloblastomas (Figure 17.14), but since they contain elements from both ependymomas and medulloblastomas, though in variable proportions, they have been renamed. They are thought to be embryonic tumours. They can be highly malignant and can seed through the CSF pathways. Treatment is by as radical excision as possible followed by radiotherapy to the whole neuraxis, including the spinal cord, in an attempt to sterilize the CSF pathways. They are radiosensitive and chemotherapy is also used. The 5-year survival rate is approximately 50% and the cure rate is 25%. Ependymomas occur close to the lining ependyma of the CSF pathways and within the spinal cord and conus medullaris and treatment is by surgical excision, followed by radiotherapy.

Secondary neoplasms

Almost any primary malignant neoplasm outwith the CNS may metastasize to the brain; however, the commonest primary sites are the breast and lung. Other sites which metastasize to the brain are renal, melanoma, prostate, stomach, testis and ovary. The metastases may be solitary or multiple or can be widespread within the CSF pathways leading to carcinomatous meningitis and hydrocephalus. A single metastasis can be excised, giving symptomatic relief, and thereafter the treatment is as for the primary site and metastases elsewhere. Not infrequently, a cerebral metastasis appears without any obvious primary malignancy being found elsewhere in the body for some time. Multiple metastases are considered inoperable. Dexamethasone has a beneficial effect in dealing with pressure effects. Stereotactic radiosurgery is a developing treatment for metastases.

Pituitary gland

This is an endocrine gland in two parts: the adenohypophysis and neurohypophysis. The anterior pituitary secretes six hormones:

- growth hormone (GH) is essential for skeletal growth in the pre-pubertal child and in the adult for regeneration of tissues and its release is controlled by the opposing hypothalamic hormones of somatostatin (inhibition) and growth hormone releasing hormone (GRH)

- prolactin (PRL) is necessary for lactation but it is also released in the normal male and its action here is uncertain; production and release is controlled by a variety of factors and inhibition is under the control of dopamine
- adrenocorticotrophic hormone (ACTH) controls the release of corticosteroids from the adrenal gland
- thyroid stimulating hormone (TSH) has an effect on the thyroid gland and is controlled by thyrotrophic releasing hormone (TRH)
- the gonadotrophins – luteinizing (LH) and follicular stimulating (FSH) – have an effect on the gonads to control sexual characteristics, ovulation and spermatogenesis.

The posterior pituitary releases antidiuretic hormone (ADH), which is involved in the control of osmoregulation through an effect on the kidneys.

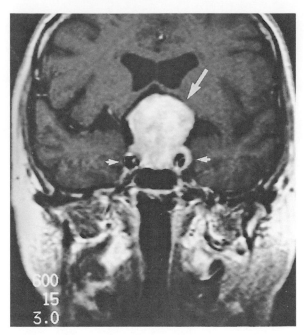

Figure 17.15 Magnetic resonance coronal scan of a 65-year-old woman with a large pituitary adenoma (large arrow). Note also the compression of the brainstem (small arrows).

Adenomas

Pituitary neoplasms are virtually all benign adenomas. They arise from cells producing one or more of the anterior hormones, from cells producing partially formed hormones or from inactive cells. They cause symptoms through endocrinological effects, pressure mass effects on the optic nerves and chiasm which lie above the pituitary or in the case of very large adenomas on the cerebral structures such as the hypothalamus (Figure 17.15).

Excess GH leads to acromegaly in the adult and gigantism in the pre-pubertal child. Acromegaly is characterized by overgrowth of hands, feet and the facial skeleton and distortion of other parts of the skeleton, leading to progressive osteoarthritis. Internally, it leads particularly to visceromegaly and insulin-resistant diabetes mellitus.

Prolactinomas in premenopausal women lead to amenorrhoea, infertility and galactorrhoea and in men to impotence and loss of secondary male sexual characteristics.

ACTH adenomas lead to Cushing's disease. Cushing's syndrome involves loss of elastic tissue in the body, with easy bruising of the skin, increased deposition of fat, myopathy and systemic hypertension. The syndrome can be due to one of three causes: a pituitary adenoma (Cushing's disease), an adenoma or carcinoma of the adrenal cortex, or oat-cell carcinoma of the bronchus leading to ectopic ACTH production.

Gonadotrophinomas lead to similar problems as prolactinomas without galactorrhoea. Thyrotrophinomas lead to secondary hyperthyroidism.

It is important to realize that a hypersecretory adenoma may compress the pituitary gland, leading to anterior hypopituitarism of other hormones. Anterior hypopituitarism leads eventually to deficiencies in all the pituitary hormones and the attendant effects on the target endocrine glands such that there is hypothyroidism, amenorrhoea or early menopause, infertility or loss of secondary sexual characteristics and loss of the cortisol response to physical stress. The onset may be insidious and may not be easily recognized.

Investigations

Investigation of patients with suspected adenomas is by a full endocrinological biochemical assessment, testing the visual acuity and fields and an MR scan.

Management

The two main aims of treatment are to normalize endocrine function and remove pressure mass effects.

These can be effected by surgical excision, radiotherapy or hormone/antihormone therapy or by combinations of these. When surgical excision is employed, this is performed in over 90% of patients by the trans-sphenoidal route; basically, this involves going behind the nose, through the vomer and into the sphenoid air sinus and then cutting a bone window in the sellar floor and thence into the sella and excising the adenoma and leaving the pituitary gland behind. Occasionally, for very large adenomas, a frontal craniotomy is performed and the adenoma approached from above within the cranial cavity. Radiotherapy can be given to the sella, particularly in the case of inadequately excised adenomas, and over a number of years will usually eliminate the adenoma but at the expense of also killing most of the normal gland as well.

Antihormones are also used – for acromegaly, this is with somatostatin given by injection or occasionally a dopamine-agonist, bromocriptine. The latter, given by tablet or capsule, is much more effective in reducing excess PRL, has no obvious teratogenic effect and can be maintained through pregnancy. More recent analogues, for example cabergoline, only need to be taken every 3 days. In the case of Cushing's disease, the preferred option is surgery since this is a fatal disease and the antagonist metyrapone is effective for a limited period only.

Replacement hormones are given, except for PRL deficiency:

- GH is replaced in children by injection until they have grown sufficiently and recent trials suggest adults may also benefit
- TSH deficiency is replaced using thyroxine
- ACTH deficiency is replaced by hydrocortisone, which is required twice daily for ordinary life, but if the patient has an intercurrent illness or undergoes surgery for lesions elsewhere in the body, it is absolutely essential that the dose is at least doubled whilst the physical stress lasts, and if the patient cannot take or absorb oral fluids then hydrocortisone must be given parenterally; the patient must also carry a blue steroid card with him at all times
- ADH deficiency is replaced with the synthetic drug 1-deamino-8D-arginine vasopressin (DDAVP), which can be given orally, by nasal inhalation or by injection.

Intracranial vascular disease

Stroke and transient ischaemic attacks

The management of these conditions consumes about 5% of health service hospital costs within the UK. Stroke is not a diagnosis as such but is merely a description of a symptom complex ending in a cerebral infarct or haemorrhage as a result of a variety of vascular diseases.

A transient ischaemic attack (TIA) is a sudden-onset episode of focal neurological deficit due to inadequate blood supply to the brain which resolves within 24 h and leaves no residual deficit. The majority occur in the internal carotid artery territory, although they can occur in the vertebrobasilar territory as well. Following TIA 5–10% of patients will have a stroke in each year after the event; the risk is highest in the first few days and weeks. Most TIAs are embolic and due to disease in the carotid arteries or heart. Such patients require urgent investigation of the heart by electrocardiogram and possibly echocardiography and of the carotid arteries by Doppler/duplex ultrasound and of the brain by CT scanning. If there is a carotid stenosis of >70%, then consideration needs to be given to carotid endarterectomy.

Of strokes, 85% are due to thromboembolic disease and 15% to haemorrhage (5% secondary to subarachnoid haemorrhage and 10% to intracerebral haemorrhage); the clinical distinction between occlusive and haemorrhagic stroke is often extremely difficult and CT scanning is required. The vast majority of strokes are treated medically but intracranial aneurysms, arteriovenous malformations and a small number of intracranial haemorrhages without obvious structural abnormality are treated surgically.

The risk factors for stroke include increasing systemic hypertension, cardiac disease, diabetes mellitus and smoking. Hypertension is the most important risk factor and lowering blood pressure to the norm corrected for the patient's age is essential; in the non-urgent surgical case, referral should be made to a physician and surgery delayed until the blood pressure is controlled; in the emergency case it is essential to discuss the problem with the anaesthetist, who will try and stabilize the situation during induction and maintenance of anaesthesia, although it must also be appreciated that sudden lowering of blood pressure can be dangerous.

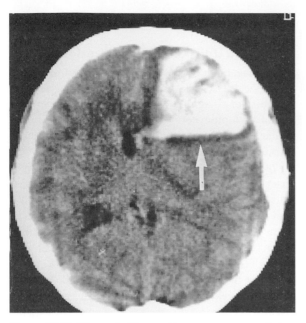

Figure 17.16 CT scan of a 30-year-old woman on uncontrolled warfarin. Note the large frontal spontaneous intracerebral haematoma (arrow).

Intracranial haemorrhage

Spontaneous intracranial haemorrhage may occur within the brain substance or subarachnoid space, and less commonly in the subdural space. The commonest cause is rupture of an intracranial aneurysm; rarer causes are rupture of a cerebral arteriovenous malformation, haemorrhage from a neoplasm or a bleeding diathesis (most commonly iatrogenically induced by the anticoagulant warfarin; Figure 17.16).

The patient complains of a sudden very severe headache the like of which they have never experienced before. They may then lose consciousness (coma-producing haemorrhage) or remain unwell without going into coma (non-coma producing); approximately 20% die immediately or very soon after the haemorrhage. The survivors develop meningism due to the blood passing into the spinal subarachnoid space; meningism causes painful stiffness of the neck and lumbar region, which worsens with movement, and must not be confused with spinal pathology (see Chapter 20). Patients may develop neurological deficit either from the site of the aneurysm (e.g. a 3rd nerve palsy from an aneurysm of the internal carotid artery) or from ischaemia resulting from spasm of the major vessels and/or narrowing or occlusion of more distal vessels within the cerebral substance.

The diagnosis of a subarachnoid haemorrhage (SAH) is confirmed by the finding of blood on CT brain scan provided the scan is completed within 48 h of the ictus. If the scan is negative then a lumbar puncture is indicated but this is best left to longer than 6 h after the ictus if the patient's condition allows. SAH is confirmed by the finding of uniformal blood staining or xanthochromia. Thereafter, referral should be made to a neurosurgeon, who will then obtain cerebral angiography of all four major vessels (both internal carotid and both vertebral arteries) to ascertain the cause of the haemorrhage.

Aneurysms are true aneurysms. They are nearly always situated at junctions of the major vessels of the circle of Willis, most commonly the anterior communicating complex, the internal carotid close to the junction with the posterior communicating artery and the trifurcation of the middle cerebral artery (Figures 17.17 and 17.18). If they occur in the young, they are thought to be congenital and they may also be familial. The majority occur from 40 years onwards and these are thought to arise from a slight pre-existing weakness of the arterial wall which is then further weakened by atheroma and/or systemic hypertension. Once rupture has occurred, there is a propensity for further rupture and treatment is directed towards early obliteration of the aneurysm by inserting coils inside the aneurysmal sac and inducing clotting by interventional radiology or if this is not possible by craniotomy and placing of a spring clip across the neck, thus excluding the aneurysm from the circulation.

Arteriovenous malformations

Arteriovenous malformations (AVM) can occur anywhere in the cerebral substance. The majority are mainly capillary in structure and they all have arteriovenous shunts, leading in some to increasing demands for blood and as a result further enlargement (Figure 17.19). They cause problems in three main ways: haemorrhage, epilepsy and cerebral steal whereby blood is diverted from normal areas of brain to feed the AVM and thus causes neurological deficits. There is usually no normal neural tissue within an AVM and treatment is by surgical excision, embolization by interventional radiology and/or stereotactic radiosurgery.

Occasionally, intracranial haematomas without an obvious structural aetiology require evacuation; this

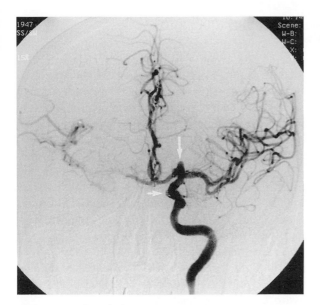

Figure 17.17 Digital subtraction angiogram anterior projection in 40-year-old woman with subarachnoid haemorrhage showing an aneurysm of bifurcation of internal carotid artery (large arrow) and posterior communicating aneurysm (small arrow).

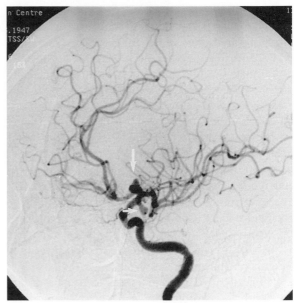

Figure 17.18 As for Figure 17.17 but lateral projection.

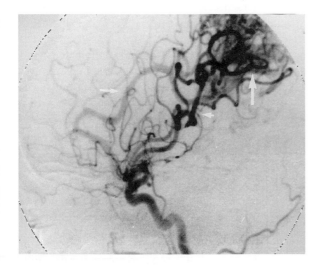

Figure 17.19 Lateral digital subtraction angiogram of a 38-year-old woman with subarachnoid and intracerebral haemorrhage showing arteriovenous malformation (large arrow). Note the enlarged feeding artery (smallest arrow) and cerebral steal with filling of contralateral artery (middle-sized arrow).

particularly applies to haematomas of the cerebellum. The patient on warfarin presents particular problems and haemorrhage usually occurs as a result of an elevated international normalized ratio (INR). If evacuation of the haematoma is thought necessary, warfarin must be temporarily stopped and in an emergency

situation actually reversed. Thrombolysis for myocardial infarct or stroke can lead to intracerebral haemorrhage; emergency surgery is preceded by the administration of aprotinin to reverse the thrombolytic state.

CNS infections

The CNS is particularly sensitive to infection and the infective agents can be bacterial, viral and fungal or agents such as prions (small-chain deoxyribose nucleic acid (DNA) fragments) which are the suspected causative agents in Creutzfeldt–Jakob disease. Bacteria and fungi cause meningitis or brain abscess, viruses lead to encephalitis and prions to spongiform encephalopathies.

Meningitis

Acute bacterial meningitis

This is an acute infection of the subarachnoid space which invokes an inflammatory reaction from the meninges. Bacteria gain access to the CSF pathways through a variety of routes such as through the sinuses, if the dura has been breached such as through a CSF fistula, or most commonly indirectly through the bloodstream. The common infecting organisms vary at different stages of life: in neonates Gram-negative bacilli such as *E. coli*, in children *Haemophilus influenzae*, in adults pneumococcus or meningococcus. In immunocompromised patients, for example those on immune suppressing therapy and those with HIV infection, the bacteria may be opportunistic; that is, they are usually commensal elsewhere in the body of a healthy patient and thus harmless, but in these patients somehow they gain access to the CSF and grow. In this context, it should be realized that one of the commonest causes of death in a patient with HIV infection is intracranial infection, with the commonest bacterium being *Listeria monocytogenes*.

A purulent exudate forms in the basal cisterns and the brain becomes oedematous and ischaemic. The process of acute inflammation in the subarachnoid space can lead to an external obstructive hydrocephalus. Infarction of the brain can occur as the inflammation leads to an arteritis or venous thrombophlebitis.

Clinically, meningitis manifests as fever, headache, neck stiffness, photophobia and a deteriorating level of consciousness. A transient petechial skin rash can occur in meningococcal meningitis. Seizures and cranial nerve signs including deafness can develop. Focal neurological deficits can occur, usually from focal ischaemia or the development of an abscess.

Diagnosis is suspected clinically and confirmation is by examination of the CSF by lumbar puncture. If there is focal neurological deficit, decreased conscious level or papilloedema, it is essential to perform a CT brain scan first to look for any space-occupying lesion. The CSF must be taken immediately to microbiology, where a white cell count will be performed together with a Gram-stained film (Gram +ve cocci, pneumococcus; Gram +ve bacilli, haemophilus; Gram −ve intra- and extracellular cocci, meningococcus). A raised white cell count in the CSF is diagnostic (100–10 000 cells/mm^3); the glucose is reduced; the causative organisms can only be correctly identified by culture. Further investigations are then needed to determine the source of the infection, for example chest X-ray, sinus X-ray, skull X-ray.

The main mode of treatment is with antibiotics, which should be started immediately after diagnosis. Antibiotics must penetrate the blood–brain barrier, be in appropriate doses, and the causal organism must be sensitive. Benzylpenicillin, cefotaxime and gentamicin are the most commonly used drugs. Treatment is continued until the patient is asymptomatic and a follow-up lumbar puncture shows resolution of the white cell count; the minimum period should be at least 10 days.

Tuberculous meningitis

Tuberculosis involves the CNS in 10% of infected patients. Following a bacteraemia, foci of infection can lodge in the meninges, cerebral or spinal tissue or choroid plexus. The basal meninges are most severely affected and hydrocephalus is common. The illness is progressive over months with a dementia. In the CSF a lymphocyte pleocytosis is present, the CSF protein is elevated, and the CSF glucose is usually significantly lowered compared to the blood glucose. Microscopy using a Ziehl Neelsen stain can reveal the acid-fast bacilli; CSF culture confirms the diagnosis but takes many weeks; most laboratories have polymerase chain reaction (PCR) tests available to detect the bacterial DNA. Treatment is with antibiotics, usually including isoniazid, rifampicin and pyrizinamide; steroids may be used if the conscious level is deteriorating and hydrocephalus may need CSF drainage.

Viral meningitis

CNS involvement in viral infection can occur through massive viraemia or along peripheral nerves. The infection can not only lead to meningitis but also cause encephalitis, cerebritis or myelitis. Infection of the motor neurons and spinal nerves is poliomyelitis and of the dorsal root ganglia radiculitis. The commonest causal organisms are enteroviruses, mumps virus or herpes simplex. The meningeal phase of infection with headache, photophobia and drowsiness usually lasts about 7–10 days. CSF cell count is elevated and if obtained early can contain the virus. Treatment is for the symptoms apart from severe herpes simplex meningitis, where acyclovir is used.

Abscess

Intracerebral abscess can occur either as a result of haematogenous emboli of bacteria with, for example, congenital heart disease or bronchiectasis, or by direct spread from the nose and paranasal sinuses or from the middle ear and mastoid cavities (Figure 17.20), through compound depressed fractures or infected dental caries. In either event the bacteria grow and initially lead to an area of septic encephalitis. Thereafter, the centre liquefies and the surrounding brain reacts by forming a gliotic capsule and thus a true abscess develops. In direct spread from sinusitis or mastoiditis, the bacteria spread either intracranially through a hole in the dura or by retrograde spread

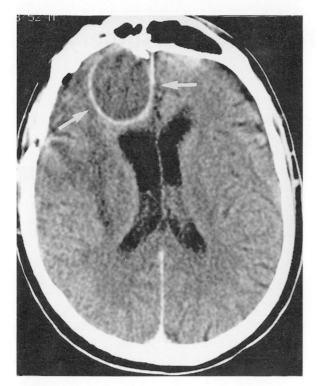

Figure 17.20 CT scan of a 40-year-old-man who 8 years previously had a head injury with fracture of the frontal bone. Note the frontal intracerebral abscess (arrows).

along a draining emissary vein and the commonest sites are in the frontal or temporal lobes. Also direct spread can lead to extradural or subdural abscess formation; occasionally the bone is involved and develops osteomyelitis.

Clinically, an abscess is suspected in a patient with symptoms and signs of raised intracranial pressure, focal neurological deficit and only occasionally fevers. Systemic signs of infection can often be absent. An infectious source may or may not be apparent. Diagnosis is by CT scanning (although MR is able to show multiple lesions not seen on CT) and lumbar puncture is contraindicated. Emergency referral should be made to a neurosurgeon, who in the majority of cases will perform a burr hole and aspirate the pus for microbiological analysis. Treatment is by appropri-

ate antibiotics and abscess drainage. The infectious source must be found and dealt with early to prevent further abscesses forming. Persistent abscesses may require excision by craniotomy particularly those in the cerebellum. Intracerebral and subdural empyema are accompanied by a very high incidence of epilepsy and anticonvulsants are usually necessary. The patient must be informed that he should report himself to the DVLA before recommencing driving.

Creutzfeldt–Jakob disease

This is one of the prion diseases characterized by the accumulation of a modified cell membrane protein within the central nervous system. The infective agent is resistant to heat and radiation and therefore is potentially transmissible through contaminated surgical instruments. Creutzfeldt–Jakob disease (CJD) has an incidence of 1 in 1 million and presents with rapidly progressive myoclonus, ataxia and dementia. The new variant form vCJD presents in younger patients with a slower time course and has been linked to bovine spongiform encephalopathy (BSE). Other prion diseases include Gestmann Straussler syndrome, similar to CJD, and kuru, spread by cannibalism in Papua New Guinea.

Further reading

Apuzzo MLJ (ed). *Brain Surgery: Complications, Avoidance and Management*. Churchill Livingstone, 1993.

Crockard A, Hayward R, Hoff JT (eds). *Neurosurgery: The Scientific Basis of Clincal Practice*. Blackwell Scientific, 1992.

Findlay G, Owen R (eds). *Surgery of the Spine*. Blackwell Scientific, 1992.

Lindsay KW, Bone I (eds). *Neurology and Neurosurgery Illustrated*. Churchill Livingstone, 1997.

Palmer JD (ed). *Manual of Neurosurgery*. Churchill Livingstone, 1996.

Russell DS, Rubinstein LJ. *Pathology of Tumours of the Nervous System*. Edward Arnold, 1989.

Schmidek HH, Sweet WH (eds). *Operative Neurosurgical Techniques: Indications, Methods and Results*. WB Saunders, 1995.

Chapter

18

John K.S. Woo and Walter W.K. King

Fundamentals of head and neck surgery

Inflammatory disorders of the ear, nose, sinuses and throat

The ear

Preauricular sinus

Preauricular sinus is a common congenital condition; there is no requirement for treatment unless it becomes infected (Figure 18.1). It may then present with pain, swelling and discharge. If seen at an early stage, infected preauricular sinus may be controlled with antibiotics. If a patient presents with a preauricular abscess, incision and drainage together with antibiotic will then become necessary. The site of incision should be through the sinus opening so as to minimize branching of the sinus tract. This is particularly important with recurrent preauricular abscesses. Abscess formation or recurrent infections are indications that the sinus tract should be excised. It is important that all tracts connected to the sinus should be excised to prevent recurrence. If in doubt, any soft tissue adherent to the tract should be excised as deep as the temporalis fascia.

Auricular haematoma

The pinna, because of its exposed and protruding position, is frequently traumatized. Blunt injury may lead to formation of an auricular haematoma. The haematoma typically forms in the subperichondrial plane. If treatment is delayed, the haematoma may dissect along the subperichondrial plane and result in unsightly deformity. Thus auricular haematoma needs to be evacuated promptly and a pressure dressing applied to conform with the shape of the pinna by means of through and through stitches.

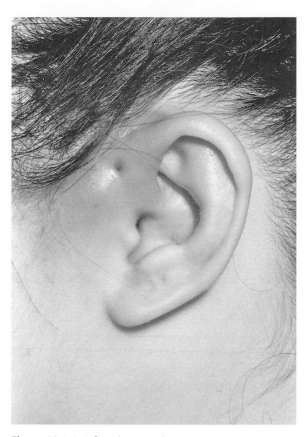

Figure 18.1 An infected preauricular sinus.

Auricular perichondritis

Perichondritis may complicate any external ear trauma. It is a serious condition and needs to be treated with full respect. Once developed, perichondritis rapidly spreads to involve the whole pinna, sparing only the ear lobule (as the lobule has no cartilage). The patient will have severe pain and itchiness in the affected ear. Initial antibiotic treatment

---

Fundamentals of Surgical Practice, Third Edition, ed. Andrew N. Kingsnorth and Douglas M. Bowley.
Published by Cambridge University Press. © Cambridge University Press 2011.

should be given intravenously covering both Gram-positive and Gram-negative organisms (especially pseudomonas). Patients presenting early may be treated orally with a combination of cloxacillin and ciprofloxacin. Patients presenting late or when prompt response to oral antibiotics is not observed should be given intravenous antibiotics. A second-generation cephalosporin together with an aminoglycoside is a good combination. Further antibiotic treatment should be guided by the result of culture and sensitivity tests. Antibiotics should be given until all signs of infection have subsided and this may often involve several weeks of treatment. If an abscess develops during therapy, this should be incised and drained immediately and the cavity irrigated with aminoglycoside solution to treat or prevent pseudomonas infection. Once it becomes clean, the cavity should be closed by a pressure dressing applied to conform with the contour of the pinna. Some deformity is often inevitable; however, with prompt and proper treatment a cauliflower ear should be avoidable.

Otitis externa

Otitis externa is a very common ear condition. It usually occurs following minor (often self-inflicted) trauma to the external auditory canal. Treatment is usually straightforward with local toilet and topical medications. In severe cases, the external canal should be packed with an otowick or ribbon gauze impregnated with a steroid-containing antibiotic cream. The dressing should be changed daily or as required by the condition. When the condition becomes recurrent or is resistant to treatment, an underlying cause should be excluded. Conditions such as diabetes mellitus and a chronic dermatosis may need to be treated simultaneously. In chronic otitis externa, especially when topical antibiotics have been used for a prolonged period, fungal infection (Figure 18.1) is not uncommon and should be treated with an antifungal agent. Occasionally, stenosis of the external auditory canal may be the cause and needs to be treated surgically.

Necrotizing otitis externa

Necrotizing otitis externa is also known as 'malignant otitis externa'. It is not that the condition may become malignant, but because of the occasional fatal outcome. This typically occurs in an elderly patient who is diabetic or is immunocompromised for other reasons. There is usually a long history of ear discharge and otalgia is frequently present and pronounced. The

causative organism is almost always pseudomonas. The clinical features of 'necrotizing otitis externa' are often misleading in the early phase of the disease. However, the response to treatment is usually poor. Ear examination often shows exuberant granulation tissue. A biopsy should be taken for microbiological work-up and for histological examination to exclude malignancy. Infection and the necrotizing process may spread to involve the temporal bone, causing osteomyelitis. The first indication is often facial nerve palsy. In advanced disease, the jugular foramen may also be affected by osteomyelitis, resulting in ninth, tenth and eleventh cranial nerves palsies. Thrombosis of the internal jugular vein and retrograde cavernous sinus thrombosis may also occur.

If the condition is suspected, the patient should be treated vigorously with intravenous antibiotics. A combination of a second-generation cephalosporin, an aminoglycoside and metronidazole should be used. This combination should adequately cover the common Gram-positive, Gram-negative (including pseudomonas) and anaerobic bacteria. Computer tomography scanning of the temporal bone should be performed to delineate the extent of the disease. In diabetic patients, the control of blood sugar level plays an important role. Hyperbaric oxygen therapy has been used in the more severe cases with good results. Surgical treatment of this condition is purely secondary. The traditional mastoidectomy is rarely useful as the disease does not spread through the mastoid air cells. However, aggressive debridement of surrounding necrotic soft tissues and drainage of secondary local abscesses are important.

Acute otitis media

Acute otitis media most commonly occurs in paediatric patients less than 6–7 years old. It typically occurs, following an upper respiratory tract infection, as an ascending infection through the Eustachian tube. The natural course of acute otitis media follows four stages:

- hyperaemic
- inflammatory
- suppurative
- resolution.

In the hyperemic phase, the patient has otalgia without hearing loss and otoscopy reveals a hyperaemic eardrum. The inflammatory phase is characterized by increasing otalgia and hearing loss. Fever is usually present in this phase. Otoscopy reveals a hyperaemic eardrum and middle ear effusion. The disease reaches a climax at the suppurative phase. The patient often becomes irritable because of intense otalgia and hyperpyrexia is frequently present. Otoscopy reveals pus collecting behind a bulging and intensely hyperaemic eardrum. The eardrum is now under severe tension and may rupture spontaneously. Once the eardrum ruptures, the condition enters the resolution phase. All the symptoms, especially otalgia, resolve rapidly.

The natural course of acute otitis media may be altered by therapy. The underlying upper respiratory tract infection will need to be treated. Nasal decongestants are useful to reduce the oedema of the Eustachian tube. A second-generation cephalosporin is a logical choice for initial antibiotic therapy. Acute otitis media usually settles quickly with oral antibiotics; however, if the eardrum becomes perforated in the course of treatment, antibiotic eardrops such as sofradex may be added to enhance treatment results. If the facial nerve canal is dehiscent, facial nerve palsy may very rarely complicate the condition. If this occurs, myringotomy is indicated to hasten resolution of the suppurative phase and recovery of the facial nerve.

Chronic suppurative otitis media

Chronic suppurative otitis media (CSOM) is the commonest form of chronic otitis media. Clinically it is characterized by otorrhoea and conduction hearing loss of variable severity. Otoscopy reveals a perforated eardrum. The condition is classified into the safe (tubotympanic) and unsafe (atticoantral) variety depending on the likelihood of coexisting cholesteatoma.

The safe variety is CSOM without cholesteatoma. It can be further classified into active or inactive depending on whether there is infection or not. Safe inactive CSOM can be managed either conservatively or surgically. Safe active CSOM should be treated initially conservatively to control the infection. A tympanoplasty procedure should then be performed to prevent recurrent infection.

The unsafe variety is CSOM with cholesteatoma (Figure 18.2). The presence of cholesteatoma is usually obvious on otoscopy. Occasionally, cholesteatoma may be more difficult to diagnose. If otoscopy reveals granulation tissue, aural polyps or middle ear infection that is resistant to conservative treatment, cholesteatoma should be excluded. Traditionally, in the presence of a marginal perforation or a deep retraction pocket, CSOM is considered potentially unsafe. However

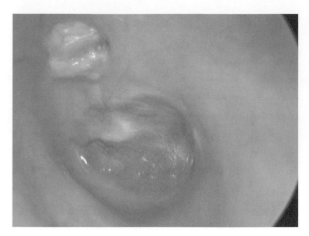

Figure 18.2 Chronic suppurative otitis media with cholesteatoma (note the attic defect above the eardrum).

with modern endoscopic equipment and computerized tomography, assessment of the middle ear is much more accurate than before. Diagnostic uncertainty occurs only rarely. The treatment of unsafe SCOM is surgical as cholesteatoma can cause serious complications that may be fatal. The type of surgical procedure to employ is controversial. The classic radical mastoidectomy, modified radical mastoidectomy or the 'combined approach tympanoplasty' may be chosen depending on the extent of cholesteatoma and more importantly on the experience of the surgeon. Whatever the procedure chosen, the aim of the surgery is to remove all the disease and to give the patient a dry and functioning ear.

The nose and sinuses

Rhinitis

'Rhinitis' is a non-specific term meaning inflammation of the nasal mucosa. The multifactorial aetiology and overlapping symptomatology makes 'rhinitis' difficult to classify. To date, the classification proposed by the 'International Rhinitis Management Working Group' in 1994 is the most comprehensive one although it is still far from being universally accepted. Management is dependent on the underlying cause, the commonest cause being allergy. Superimposed infection is not uncommon and should be treated accordingly.

Sinusitis

Sinusitis is a better-defined clinical condition. The pathogenesis of sinusitis is better understood nowadays since the importance of mucous transportation has been realized. Bilateral sinusitis is not uncommon although unilateral cases are more frequent. Its symptoms are better appreciated at four levels.

1. Specific primary symptoms of sinusitis are unusual as the sinuses serve no important function. However, if the involved sinus becomes totally blocked, local pain and tenderness may occur as tension develops within the sinus.
2. Secondary symptoms develop as entrapped and infected secretions overflow from the involved sinus. The patient may then present with mucopurulent rhinorrhoea.
3. Tertiary symptoms develop as the mucopus collects around the Eustachian tube, causing middle ear dysfunction.
4. Quaternary symptoms develop if a totally obstructed sinus also becomes infected or develops into a mucocele. Under these situations, progressive tension will develop and may decompress itself along a line of weakness where the neurovascular bundles pass through the involved sinuses. Patients may then present with orbital or intracranial complications.

Acute sinusitis

This commonly follows an upper respiratory tract infection and presents acutely with fever, local pain and tenderness over the involved sinus. Nasal symptoms may not be prominent. Nasal endoscopy reveals local congestion and pus may be seen streaming down from the diseased sinus. A pus swab should be taken for microbiological work-up and meanwhile the patient should be treated symptomatically with an analgesic and antipyretic. A 2-week course of antibiotics with coverage for Gram-positive and Gram-negative organisms should be started immediately. The regime may need to be revised if clinical progress is slow or as determined by culture and sensitivity results. Most acute sinusitis resolves with conservative treatment.

Chronic sinusitis

This usually presents with chronic nasal congestion and recurrent mucopurulent rhinorrhoea (level 2 symptoms). There is usually an underlying cause such as nasal polyposis, a septal deviation, an abnormal middle turbinate, etc. The presence of any condition which obstructs mucous transportation out of the sinus will lead to recurrent infection and sinusi-

tis becomes chronic. Therefore, surgery is frequently required as a definitive procedure. Functional endoscopic sinus surgery (Stammberger 1991) (FESS), which aims at re-establishing normal mucous transportation, is now a well-established operation for this condition. When considering any patient for FESS, coronal CT of the sinuses must be done so that the full extent of disease and any variation in sinus anatomy are known to the surgeon.

The throat

Tonsillitis

Acute tonsillitis is a very common condition in children. Clinically it is characterized by acute sore throat and fever. It is usually part of an upper respiratory tract infection and mostly viral in origin. On examination, the tonsils are usually enlarged and erythematous. Treatment is mainly symptomatic. Isolated follicular tonsillitis is less common and is frequently due to streptococcal infection. On examination, the tonsils are usually slightly enlarged with a rough surface. The roughness is due to the presence of numerous follicles. Treatment should include an antibiotic. Exudative tonsillitis is much less common and usually means a more severe infection. A blood sample must be taken from the patient for haematological evaluation to exclude infectious mononucleosis. If an antibiotic is needed, as in patients with hyperpyrexia, ampicillin should be avoided. Membranous tonsillitis is extremely rare but potentially serious. In a developing country, consider diphtheria. In a developed country, a haematological malignancy should be excluded. It is not uncommon for patients who have had tonsillectomy to present with sore throat; in these instances, lingual tonsillitis should be excluded by a mirror examination.

Quinsy

Acute tonsillitis may sometimes be complicated by abscess formation. Quinsy, which is peritonsillar abscess, commonly follows partially treated acute tonsillitis. Patients with quinsy present with severe unilateral sore throat. Some degree of trismus will be present due to irritation of the pterigoid muscles by the abscess. Examination will reveal a unilateral tonsillar swelling with red hot mucosa. There will usually be fever as well. The diagnosis is confirmed when pus is obtained by fine-needle aspiration. The pus should be sent for microbiological work-up. The treatment should consist of high-dose intravenous penicillin and

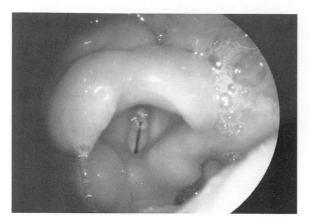

Figure 18.3 Acute supraglottitis (note the whole supraglottitis is swollen, sparing only the vocal cord).

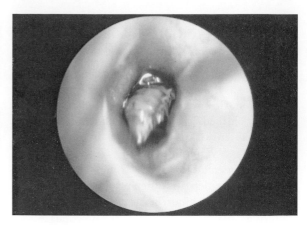

Figure 18.4 Cockroach in the external auditory canal.

incision and drainage of the abscess. If progress is slow, metronidazole should be added or antibiotics modified according to culture and sensitivity results. Sometimes the incision site may need to be opened again with a pair of sinus forceps to ensure no recollection of pus. Patients with quinsy may need an interval tonsillectomy if there is a previous history of quinsy or recurrent tonsillitis. A single attack of quinsy is considered only as a relative indication for interval tonsillectomy.

Acute supraglottitis

'Acute epiglottitis' is a misnomer and 'acute supraglottitis' (Figure 18.3) should be used instead. Anatomically, there is no boundary to separate the epiglottis from the rest of the supraglottis. Therefore the whole supraglottis will inevitably be involved by an inflammatory or infective process. Previously it was believed that this condition affected only paediatric patients. However, supraglottitis affecting adults has been reported increasingly in the literature. In children, the condition usually presents with airway obstruction. Adult patients usually present with sudden severe sore throat. Respiratory distress may occasionally be the presenting symptoms. Children suspected to have the condition should be taken to the operating theatre immediately for direct laryngoscopy under general anaesthesia. Both the anaesthetist and the surgeon should be experienced in dealing with the paediatric airway. If the diagnosis is confirmed, endotracheal intubation should be performed and the patient should be observed in the intensive care unit. In adult patients without respiratory dis-

tress, the diagnosis should be confirmed by mirror examination or flexible laryngoscopy. Carefully performed, these examinations will not precipitate airway obstruction. It is safer to have a correct diagnosis by a gentle examination. In adult patients with respiratory distress, they should be treated in a similar way to children. Adult patients with supraglottitis and stable airway should be observed in the intensive care unit where facilities and expertise for endotracheal intubation are readily available. A tracheostomy can be avoided in most cases as prolonged intubation is unlikely. In paediatric patients, the commonest pathogen identified is *Haemophilus influenzae* type b. In adults the pathogens are more variable, including various streptococcal species, anaerobes as well as *Haemophilus influenzae* type b. The choice of antibiotics should be guided by the prevalence of pathogens and may vary between hospitals. In general, a second-generation cephalosporin is recommended.

Foreign bodies in the ear, nose and throat

Aural foreign bodies

A foreign body in the ear typically entraps in the external auditory canal. Diagnosis is usually straightforward. Foreign bodies may be classified as living insects, vegetable or inorganic materials. A living insect in the external auditory canal (Figure 18.4) is most disturbing. It should first be killed with a non-irritant eardrop such as olive oil, paraffin oil or cooking oil. The insect should then be removed by suction or by fine forceps. Vegetable foreign bodies are best removed by curettage and suction. Syringing is contraindicated as the foreign body may swell and subsequent removal is more difficult. Inorganic foreign bodies if diagnosed early may be removed with forceps, suction, syringing or curettage depending on their shape. Inorganic foreign bodies, being inert, can be left in the external canal for a long time with minimal symptoms. These long-standing foreign bodies can sometimes become very adherent to the canal skin and may require general anaesthesia for their removal. For young children or mentally deranged individuals in general, whenever a foreign body is found in one ear, the other ear and perhaps the nostrils should also be checked. Simultaneous multiple foreign bodies may rarely be present. Multiple attempts at removing any foreign body in an uncooperative patient are inadvisable as tympanic membrane perforation and ossicular chain injury may occur. Under these circumstances, general anaesthesia may be warranted.

Nasal foreign bodies

Nasal foreign bodies occur almost exclusively in young children and mentally deranged individuals. Live insects enter the nose extremely rarely probably due to the nasal airflow, high humidity and heat inside the nose. Thus common nasal foreign bodies are either vegetable or inorganic matter. Most foreign bodies present as such and diagnosis is simple. Vegetable foreign bodies are irritant to the nose and induce a strong local reaction. In the absence of a definite history, they usually present with unilateral obstruction and foul-smelling nasal discharge for weeks or months that respond poorly to conservative treatment. Inorganic nasal foreign bodies, being inert, may present as rhinoliths with non-specific nasal symptoms for years. Whenever the diagnosis is in doubt, nasendoscopy should be performed. Nasal foreign bodies should always be removed with a blunt hook. The hook should be lubricated with K-Y jelly and passed to the upside of the foreign body. The movement of the hook should always be towards the floor and the front of the nose in order to avoid pushing the foreign body further backward. Multiple attempts should be avoided, especially in struggling patients, otherwise the foreign body may be dislodged and inhaled. General anaesthesia should be used instead.

Button battery nasal foreign body (Tong *et al.* 1992) (Figure 18.5) deserves special mention because significant damage can be done if the battery is left *in*

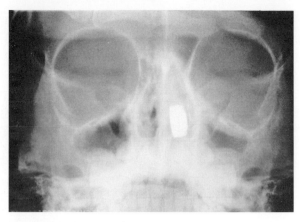

Figure 18.5 Plain X-ray of the nose showing a button battery in the left nasal fossa.

situ for any length of time. As a result of the contour of the nose, the poles of a button battery will fit tightly between the septum and the turbinates. Four types of injury may occur resulting in serious morbidity. Mechanical injury may occur due to the tight mucosal contact. Electrical injury may arise as the battery is short-circuited by contact with the moist nasal mucosa. Electrochemical injury may occur as electric current passes through the mucosa, causing electrolysis. Chemical injury may occur due to leakage of chemical from the battery. Maximum damage usually occurs to the nose on the side in contact with the negative pole and the most significant damage occurs as a result of chemical injury. In order to avoid serious injury such as septal perforation or alar collapse, this type of foreign body should be removed without any delay. A course of antibiotics should always be used after removal and a case can be made for the addition of a short course of systemic steroids.

For selected children with a nasal foreign body, it is worth attempting the 'parent's kiss' technique. The child is held and the parent blows firmly into the child's mouth while occluding the unaffected nostril. This can be surprisingly effective and avoids general anaesthesia in a proportion of cases.

Ingested foreign bodies

As a result of their eating habits, ingested foreign bodies are extremely common in some populations, especially the Chinese. The presentation varies depending on whether the patient can give a clear history. Thus in prelingual children and in mentally retarded patients, the presentation may be refusal to feed or

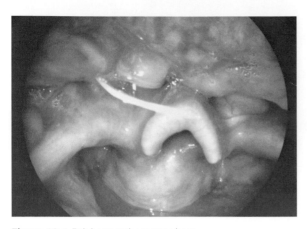

Figure 18.6 Fish bone in the tongue base.

vomiting, or presentation with a complication such as a neck abscess. Otherwise patients always present with foreign body sensation immediately following the episode of foreign body ingestion. The commonest foreign body ingested is a fish bone (Figure 18.6). Others include meat bones and skeletons of shrimps and lobsters, etc. The commonest metallic foreign body is a coin. A careful history is very useful both in making a diagnosis and in localization of the foreign body. Symptoms that lateralize to one side and localize at a site at or higher than the cricoid are usually very accurate. Symptoms that migrate downward are pathognomonic of an ingested foreign body.

There will be hardly any physical signs in uncomplicated cases. Therefore the purpose of physical examination is to confirm or exclude the presence of any foreign body. Larger and blunter foreign bodies, e.g. coins or meat bones, tend to be trapped by the narrowest part of the upper aero-digestive tract at the cricopharyngeus. Smaller and sharp foreign bodies such as a fish bone may be impacted anywhere from the tonsils or tongue base to any level of the oesophagus. Most of the impacted foreign bodies will be found on clinical examination with a tongue depressor or a laryngeal mirror. When no foreign body is found, a direct flexible pharyngolaryngoscopy should be performed. This gives a better and dynamic view of the hypopharynx as the patients are instructed to phonate and swallow. Most ingested foreign bodies can be removed by simple means with a pair of Tilly's forceps or with flexible laryngoscopy. Oesophagoscopy may occasionally be required to remove foreign bodies. Rigid oesophagoscopy gives a better view of the cervical oesophagus while flexible oesophagoscopy is preferred below the thoracic inlet.

The usefulness of a plain lateral X-ray of the neck depends on the type of foreign body and the site of impaction. Thick bones such as meat bones are radio-opaque and will readily be picked up by a plain X-ray. Similarly, metallic foreign bodies such as coins will be clearly shown on plain X-rays. Most fish bones are radiolucent and therefore can easily be missed by plain X-rays. When foreign bodies are impacted above the cricopharyngeus, radiological investigations will not be as accurate as clinical examination. Foreign bodies impacted below the thoracic inlet are difficult to demonstrate on plain X-rays as the view will inevitably be overlapped by the vertebrae and the thoracic skeleton. The cervical oesophagus is the only segment of the upper digestive tract where plain X-rays are reliable enough to be clinically useful. Complications of 'ingested foreign bodies' may arise as a result of impaction or passage of the foreign bodies. They can also be iatrogenic from attempts to remove the foreign bodies. These include perforation of the pharynx or oesophagus (Figure 18.7), retropharyngeal or mediastinal abscesses.

Epistaxis

Epistaxis is an extremely common complaint; it is estimated that up to 60% of people will experience at least one episode in their lifetime, with 6% requiring medical attention. The underlying cause should be sought whenever possible in order to apply treatment logically. In the majority of cases, however, the bleeding is idiopathic. When a cause can be identified, epistaxis is usually secondary to nasal trauma, a local nasal pathology, a blood vessel abnormality or a blood dyscrasia.

Isolated mild epistaxis probably requires no specific treatment. However, if this happens in an adult patient, a careful examination of the nose and nasopharynx should be performed, so that a tumour will not be missed. For patients with recurrent epistaxis, the primary cause, if identified, should be treated. Systemic causes should be treated medically and local causes controlled with local measures. The commonest local cause is self-inflicted injury to some engorged vessels in the Little's area. Chemical cautery of the vessels in the Little's area under topical anaesthesia is a useful measure. Sometimes if the bleeding is more profuse, electrocautery should be used instead.

considered in three steps: identification of the bleeding source, surgery for local control of bleeding and arterial ligation .

Identification of the bleeding source

Although the cause of epistaxis may not be found, the site of bleeding should not be difficult to identify. Nowadays with modern endoscopes and the necessary accessories the nose can be adequately examined even in the presence of active bleeding. When the source of bleeding is found, a more logical approach to management can be planned.

Surgery for local control of bleeding

This part in the management of epistaxis has largely been neglected. In fact, there is a lot to be done for local control if the source of bleeding can be localized. Most bleeding vessels inside the nose are less than 1 mm in size and should easily be controlled with diathermy. Occasionally, a septal spur may need to be removed before the bleeding point becomes accessible. If the bleeding point is in the nasopharynx or at the back of the nasal septum, a combined approach to the nasopharynx may be employed.

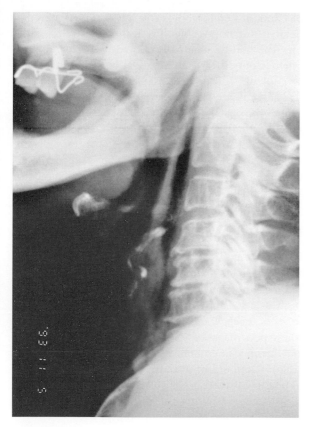

Figure 18.7 Plain X-ray of the neck showing free gas in the retropharyngeal space due to perforation of the oesophagus after oesophagoscopy.

Arterial ligation

Arterial ligation, although not cause-specific, is an effective means of epistaxis control and should be considered when rapid control of epistaxis is critical, other methods to control the bleeding have failed or there is recurrent severe epistaxis. The aim of arterial ligation for the control of epistaxis is to lower the perfusion pressure so that bleeding will stop or may be stopped more easily by local measures.

For patients with severe epistaxis, the initial management aims to control the bleeding. Attempts should be made to stop anterior nasal bleeding with an anterior nasal pack, while for posterior bleeding balloon tamponade is more effective. When balloon tamponade is used, the pressure should be adjusted to the minimum required to arrest the bleeding. When nasal packs are used for more than 48 hours, it is advisable to give prophylactic antibiotics. It is only in the most unusual situation that surgery may be required to stop bleeding or to prevent recurrent epistaxis.

Surgical treatment for epistaxis is controversial, with many options being available. The controversy relates more to the timing and type of surgical intervention than how to perform a particular operation. In general surgical intervention is indicated when there is continuous bleeding despite adequate conservative management, there is re-bleeding immediately after nasal packs are removed or there is frequent and significant rebleeding. Surgical intervention can be logically

In general, the more distal the site of ligation the more effective the procedure as the development of anastomotic channels will be less likely. The decision to ligate an individual artery or a combination of arteries will depend on whether the site of bleeding is identified or not. A clear understanding of the principle of arterial ligation and the blood supply of the nose is necessary. When the bleeding is from the roof of the nose, the ethmoidal arteries should be dealt with first. On the other hand, when the bleeding is from the lower part of the nasal fossa or the lateral nasal wall, the maxillary or the external carotid artery should be ligated. When the bleeding is profuse and the source is poorly localized a combination of arteries from both systems may need to be ligated.

The external carotid artery can be ligated in the neck close to its origin. This approach has the advantage of being a simple procedure. The external carotid is identified by demonstrating at least two of its branches. It is then doubly ligated in continuity with O silk distal to its lingual branch. Although complications are rare, blindness may occur if the ophthalmic artery originates from the middle meningeal branch of the external carotid artery.

The tributaries of the maxillary artery to the nose begin in the pterygopalatine fossa. This can be approached transantrally and is the ideal site to ligate the maxillary artery and its branches to the nose. As the main trunk of the maxillary artery comes from a deeper aspect than its branches, it can occasionally be missed. The infra-orbital branch may be mistaken for the main trunk of the maxillary artery. Complications are uncommon, although isolated cases of total ophthalmoplegia have been reported in the literature.

The internal carotid system contributes much less to the nasal blood supply than the external carotid. The anterior and posterior ethmoidal arteries, both being derived from the ophthalmic artery, are conveniently reached in the orbit. The anterior ethmoidal artery is the larger of the two and contributes more to the blood supply of the nose. In many instances, only the anterior ethmoidal artery requires ligation. The ethmoidal vessels perforate the medial orbital wall into the anterior and posterior ethmoidal canal respectively at or close to the fronto-ethmoidal suture. The anterior ethmoidal artery will be encountered at a distance about 1.5–2 cm from the lacrimal fossa. The posterior ethmoidal artery will be encountered about 0.5–1 cm further back. The anterior ethmoidal artery can be absent in as high as 14% of cadaver dissections unilaterally and 2.5% bilaterally. This is especially important to bear in mind if both the anterior and posterior ethmoidal arteries are to be clipped. The optic nerve may then be mistaken for the posterior ethmoidal artery and mistakenly clipping this will result in blindness in the affected eye.

Transnasal endoscopic ligation

Endoscopic endonasal surgery is gaining popularity. Transnasal endoscopic ligation of the sphenopalatine artery has been reported with good results for epistaxis control. This is particularly useful for the prevention of recurrent epistaxis. In patients with active profuse bleeding, any endoscopic surgery will be extremely difficult if not impossible. The technique itself is simple. The middle meatus is cleared by performing an uncinectomy, and the ethmoidal bulla is removed if prominent. The natural maxillary ostium is identified and enlarged if necessary so as to allow visualization of the posterior antral wall. A convenient vertical mucosal incision is made just in front of the imaginary medial projection of the posterior antral wall. The sphenopalatine artery should then be easily identified and clipped as it passes medially from the sphenopalatine foramen.

Hereditary haemorrhagic telangiectasia

Epistaxis requiring surgery in most patients arises from arterial bleeding. However, in the case of hereditary haemorrhagic telangiectasia epistaxis is due to both arterial and capillary bleeding. Results of any form of therapy, including arterial ligation, are poor. These patients usually require a combination of arterial ligation (or embolization) together with local control. It is important to cause as little mucosal damage as possible as there is almost always a need for repeated local therapy. A number of lasers have proved useful in the management of this condition.

Infection of the deep neck spaces

Surgical anatomy

The deep neck spaces are potential spaces bounded between fascial planes of the deep cervical fascia. Anatomically there are three layers of deep cervical fascia: the superficial (investing) layer, the middle (visceral) layer and the deep (prevertebral) layer. Conceptually, it is helpful to visualize these fascial layers as forming three concentric tubes. The superficial layer forms the outermost tube and splits to enclose the major salivary glands, the sternomastoid, trapezius and the strap muscles. The middle layer forms the visceral tube to enclose the larynx, trachea, oesophagus and thyroid glands. The deep layer forms the innermost tube that encloses the vertebral column, the prevertebral and paraspinous muscles. All the three layers of deep fascia contribute to form the carotid sheath as it traverses through the different layers. Thus, sepsis of the deep neck spaces can spread along the carotid sheath from one compartment to another and eventually to the mediastinum.

It is important to refer to a standard anatomy text-book for a detailed relationship of these fascial planes as this knowledge is crucial to the management of deep-neck-space infections.

Deep-neck-space infections in general

Deep-neck-space infection is relatively rare nowadays when most of the primary infections of the upper aero-digestive tract can be adequately treated with modern antibiotics. However, when treatment of the primary infection is delayed or in patients who are immune compromised, this possibility should not be overlooked. Infection of the deep neck spaces is dangerous as progression of the infection can be very rapid. Thus these infections should be diagnosed and treated promptly otherwise fatal complications may occur. The first step of such diagnosis should be clinical. There are usually symptoms and signs of a preceding upper aero-digestive tract infection that rapidly worsens. The patient is often febrile and septic. If the infection is picked up early at the cellulitic stage, a full sepsis work-up should be done followed by prompt broad-spectrum intravenous antibiotic covering both aerobes and anaerobes. This is necessary as the common pathogens causing such infections include both aerobes and anaerobes; Gram-positive as well as Gram-negative organisms. These include beta-haemolytic streptococci, anaerobic streptococci, *Streptococcus viridans*, *Staphylococcus aureus*, *Klebsiella pneumoniae*, *Bacteroides* species and *Haemophilus* species. Unless quick clinical improvement is evident, abscess formation should be suspected. With abscess formation, the involved part of the neck often becomes tense, tender, hot and erythematous. Contrast-enhanced computer tomography, if available, should be performed immediately to confirm both the diagnosis and the anatomic extent of the abscess. Deep-neck-space abscesses should be surgically explored and drained to avoid serious and potentially fatal complications such as airway obstruction, mediastinitis, internal jugular vein thrombosis and necrotizing fasciitis.

Ludwig's angina

Ludwig's angina (Figure 18.8) is the most commonly encountered deep-neck-space infection. It refers to infection of the floor of the mouth. The origin of infection typically arises from bacterial dental sepsis. The progression of the infection is usually very rapid, so in

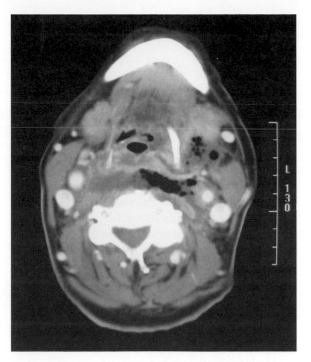

Figure 18.8 Ludwig's Angina with parapharyngeal and retropharyngeal abscesses.

most cases by the time of diagnosis the whole floor of the mouth is inflamed. If the origin of the infection is from the root of the molar or premolar that extends below the mylohyoid line, both the sublingual and submaxillary spaces will be involved. Although rare, Ludwig's angina has been reported to follow piercings of the lingual frenulum.

Patients usually present with fever, marked sore throat and odynophagia. In severe cases, dysphagia and stridor may be present. The cardinal features include marked pain, erythema and firm swelling of the floor of the mouth. The tongue is often pushed upward and backward. The patient as a whole presents with severe malaise and signs of sepsis.

Once the diagnosis is made, sepsis work-up and broad-spectrum intravenous antibiotics with aerobic and anaerobe coverage should be used immediately. The airway should be closely monitored and preparation for surgical drainage should be planned in case the patient's condition deteriorates. If surgical drainage is deemed necessary, the anaesthesiologist and surgeon should be prepared to control a difficult airway and fibreoptic intubation or urgent tracheostomy may be necessary. The result of treatment is usually good;

however, a dental consultation should always be made before discharge.

Parapharyngeal abscess

Parapharyngeal abscesses developed *de novo* are extremely rare. Most such cases are secondary to severe tonsillitis, quinsy or a penetrating ingested foreign body. As the carotid sheath passes through this space into the anterior mediastinum, infection can spread quickly along the carotid sheath, resulting in mediastinitis. Thus, irrespective of the primary cause, any parapharyngeal abscess is potentially fatal if not promptly and adequately treated with intravenous antibiotics and surgical drainage. As the parapharyngeal space is relatively deep, a small abscess in this situation may only be picked up by a contrast-enhanced computerized tomography (CT) scan. The latter is also useful to rule out extension of the abscess into other deep neck spaces such as the retropharyngeal space and the mediastinum (Figure 18.8).

Retropharyngeal abscess

Because of its deep position, sepsis and abscess formation of the retropharyngeal space is relatively rare compared to other forms of deep-neck-space infections. It may develop following suppurative upper respiratory tract infections, a penetrating injury such as impaction of a sharp ingested foreign body or tuberculous infection involving the cervical vertebra. Retropharyngeal abscess, which used to affect children predominantly, is being increasingly observed in adults. Retropharyngeal abscess poses a diagnostic challenge for the primary care clinicians because of its rarity and variable presentation depending on the primary cause.

In most cases, clinical features of a concurrent upper respiratory tract infection such as sore throat, cough and fever are very common. However, presence of odynophagia, dysphagia, neck pain and neck stiffness should raise the suspicion of retropharyngeal abscess. Retropharyngeal abscess secondary to a penetrating ingested foreign body should be suspected in patients who have developed a fever and have persistent symptoms. Retropharyngeal abscess secondary to a tuberculous infection involving and breaking through the prevertebral fascia of the cervical vertebra is extremely rare nowadays. The presentation of such an abscess is usually subtle with vague neck pain and stiffness. When the abscess eventually bursts through the middle visceral layers of the deep cervical

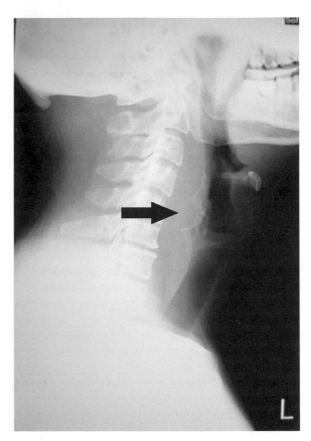

Figure 18.9 Lateral neck X-ray showing retropharyngeal soft tissue thickening.

fascia, a painless fluctuant lateral neck swelling, often referred to as a cold abscess, may appear. However, the clinical picture can become acute if the 'cold' abscess becomes 'hot' with secondary bacterial infection.

Diagnosis requires a high index of suspicion. A simple lateral neck X-ray (Figure 18.9) is a very useful initial investigation that is readily available. If the retropharyngeal soft tissue is greater than one and a half times the width of the corresponding vertebral body, it should be considered abnormal. Such a finding, if associated with free gas, is indicative of a retropharyngeal abscess secondary to a penetrating foreign body. If radiolucent spots are shown over the cervical vertebral body, tuberculous abscess needs to be excluded.

Head and neck tumours

Successful management of head and neck tumours requires early detection, correct histological diagnosis and a thorough understanding of the biological behaviour of the tumour. For malignant lesions, a multidisciplinary approach provides the best care. A head and neck tumour conference (MDT) involving the head and neck surgeon, otolaryngologist, plastic surgeon, neurosurgeon, oncologist, radiotherapist, radiologist and pathologist offers the best environment for interdisciplinary review and interaction.

Skin

The skin is the largest organ of the body. The head and neck region, being largely exposed and susceptible to the carcinogenic effect of sunlight (ultraviolet light A and B), is the site of most skin cancers.

Seborrheic keratoses

These are benign superficial, brown-black hyperkeratotic skin lesions that are commonly present on the sun-exposed face as multiple raised, thickened,waxy plaques of variable sizes that may resemble a mole or even a melanoma. Treatment is by electrosurgery and curettage. Occasionally, excisional biopsy is warranted to exclude melanoma.

Actinic keratoses (solar keratoses)

These are small, erythematous, scaly macules commonly found on the sun-exposed face. Biopsy shows hyperkeratoses and parakeratoses with dysplasia in the epidermis. About 5% of the lesions may progress to squamous cell carcinoma. Treatment is preferably by cryosurgery or excision.

Cutaneous horn

The clinical term 'cutaneous horn' is a hard, horn-like growth that may develop from the base of an actinic keratosis, seborrheic keratoses (benign superficial, brown-black hyperkeratotic lesions) or squamous cell carcinoma. Therefore, nodular growth in the base of a cutaneous horn usually represents squamous cell carcinoma (Figure 18.10). Treatment is by surgical excision.

Bowen's disease

Bowen's disease is squamous cell carcinoma *in situ* (cytological atypia confined to epidermis). This commonly presents as a circumscribed scaling erythema-

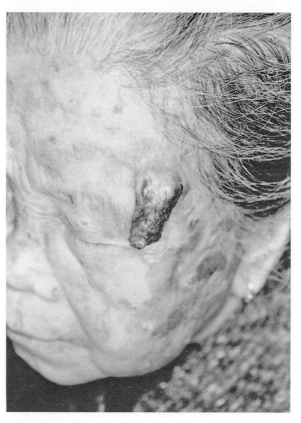

Figure 18.10 Cutaneous horn with squamous cell carcinoma in the base.

tous patch. About 10% develop into invasive squamous cell carcinoma and therefore should be surgically excised.

Lentigo maligna melanoma (Hutchinson's freckle)

This commonly appears as a pigmented patch on the face with distinct borders. This is melanoma *in situ* (Clark's Level I). The treatment is surgical excision with clear margin.

Keratoacanothma

This is a common, rapidly enlarging nodular skin growth with central keratinous crater that occurs mainly on sun-exposed areas in the elderly. Excisional biopsy is required to distinguish it from squamous cell carcinoma.

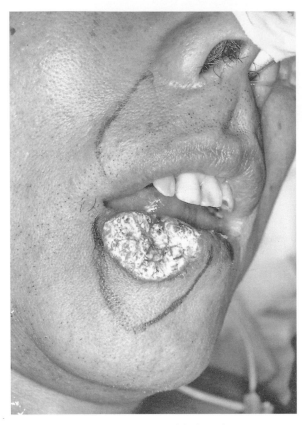

Figure 18.11 Verrucous carcinoma of the lower lip.

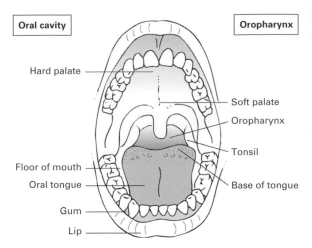

Figure 18.12 Anatomic sites of the oral cavity and oropharynx.

Skin cancer

For basal cell carcinoma, squamous cell carcinoma and melanoma, see Chapter 29.

Merkel cell carcinoma

This is an uncommon neuroendocrine tumour occurring in the face and neck of elderly patients. It is an aggressive dermal nerve cell tumour that has a propensity for regional and distant metastasis. Treatment is wide surgical excision with consideration for regional lymph node dissection or sentinel node biopsy. Postoperative radiotherapy can also be considered.

Scalp

The scalp has five anatomic layers: skin, subcutaneous layer, galea (aponeurosis), subgaleal layer and periosteum. All of the above tumours can occur in the scalp, especially if the scalp has long-standing sun exposure as a result of alopecia. In addition, carcinoma of skin appendages may arise from the scalp.

Oral cavity and oropharynx

Anatomy

The oral cavity extends from the lips to the junction of the hard and soft palate above and to the circumvallate papillae of the tongue below and consists of six anatomic sites: lip, buccal mucosa, gum, floor of the mouth, hard palate and anterior two-thirds of the tongue (oral tongue). The oropharynx consists of the faucial arch (Waldeyer's ring), which includes the soft palate, uvula, tonsillar pillar, tonsillar fossa and tonsil, base of tongue and posterior pharyngeal wall (Figure 18.12).

History

Strong predisposing factors for squamous cell carcinoma of the oral cavity and the upper aerodigestive tract include smoking and drinking of alcoholic beverages and the carcinogenic effects of these are additive. Other observed predisposing factors to oral cavity cancer include continuous trauma by ill-fitting dentures or sharp teeth, chewing of betel nuts or tobacco and regular use of alcohol-containing mouth washes.

Physical examination

The entire oral cavity should be thoroughly inspected with a good light and a tongue depressor, paying attention to mucosal abnormalities arising from the various anatomic sites. The tonsils should be inspected. The oral tongue and base of the tongue should be palpated and bimanual examination should be done for the floor of the mouth and submandibular glands. The neck should be palpated systematically to look for enlarged lymph nodes, bearing in mind that oral cavity and oropharyngeal tumours tend to metastasize to submental, submandibular and upper jugular or jugulodigastric lymph nodes before spreading to lower level lymph nodes (mid and lower jugular lymph nodes).

Diagnostic tests and procedures

Ultrasound examination of the neck is performed to detect nodal metastases. For a complex mucosal tumour or neck mass, computed tomography (CT) or magnetic resonance imaging (MRI) will be more useful for clinical staging and treatment planning. High-resolution CT with three-dimensional views is useful in delineating the local extent of the tumour in relationship to adjacent vascular and other important structures. Incisional or punch biopsy of mucosal lesions is usually required for diagnosis. Excisional biopsy is done for small lesions. Fine-needle aspiration (FNA) for cytology is routinely done for palpable neck nodes. This is usually carried out with a 21 or 23 gauge needle with the aspirated contents placed on a glass slide to make a smear or injected directly into 50% alcohol for examination by a cytopathologist. Excisional biopsy of a suspected malignant cervical node should be avoided unless lymphoma is suspected or when the primary remains unknown after a diligent search that includes panendoscopy (nasopharyngolaryngoscopy, oesophagoscopy and bronchoscopy), CT or MRI and examination under general anaesthesia. A positron emission tomographic (PET) scan is very useful in detecting distant metastasis, recurrent cancer and in the search for an unknown primary with metastatic cervical lymph nodes. Panendoscopy is recommended for proven squamous cell carcinoma of the oral cavity, oropharynx, larynx, hypopharynx and oesophagus in order to exclude a concurrent second primary occurring at a different site that is caused by the same predisposing factors of smoking and drinking of alcohol.

Erythroplakia

Erythroplakia is defined as a red, erythematous, granular mucosal plaque or lesion that bleeds easily and is likely to represent the earliest sign of asymptomatic cancer. On biopsy, approximately 60% of erythroplakia contain *in situ* or invasive squamous cell carcinoma.

Leukoplakia

This is a clinical term which refers to any white plaque or patch of oral mucosa. Histology may reveal a wide variety of lesions ranging from inflammation, lichen planus dysplasia to microinvasive cancer. Those with dysplasia can be considered to be premalignant. Leukoplakia should be biopsied and those mucosa and submucosa showing dysplasia excised with a cold knife or carbon dioxide laser.

Squamous cell carcinoma

Squamous cell carcinoma is the commonest (90%) malignancy of the upper aerodigestive tract (others are lymphoma, adenocarcinoma arising from minor salivary glands and sarcoma). It presents typically as a painful ulcerative lesion or mass and has a propensity to metastasize to cervical lymph nodes as tumour volume increases.

The TNM staging of oral cavity and oropharyngeal tumours is by size of primary tumour:

- T1: tumour <2 cm
- T2 tumour <4 cm
- T3 tumour >4 cm
- T4 tumour >4 cm and with deep invasion to involve antrum, pterygoid muscles, root of tongue or skin of neck

and extent of cervical nodal involvement:

- N0: no clinically positive node
- N1: single positive node <3 cm
- N2: positive node >3 cm but <6 cm, or multiple positive nodes, or bilateral/contralateral nodes
- N3: positive node >6 cm.

Treatment

Treatment of early disease (T1 and early T2) by either surgery or radiation gives equivalent survival rates. However, most lesions are conveniently treated by surgery, which is generally preferred by patients. Advanced disease (late T2, T3, T4 or clinically positive neck node) is best treated by surgery followed by postoperative radiotherapy.

The aim of surgical treatment is excision of the primary tumour with a 1–2 cm margin, with tumour clearance confirmed by frozen section. For access to posteriorly located tumours, a lower cheek flap or mandibular swing (median mandibulotomy) may be required. Reconstruction of the surgical defect after

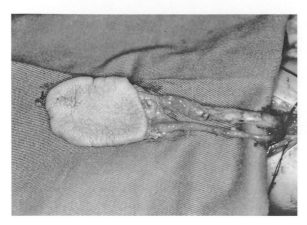

Figure 18.13 Free forearm flap based on the radial artery.

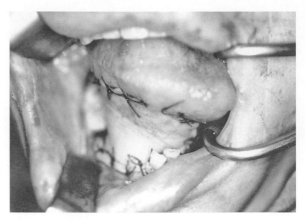

Figure 18.14 Reconstruction of a surgical defect of the floor of the mouth by free forearm flap.

resection of a large tumour may require a latissimus dorsi myocutaneous flap, pectoralis major myocutaneous flap or a free forearm flap with microvascular anatomosis of the radial artery and forearm vein to the recipient neck vessels (Figures 18.13 and 18.14). Surgical treatment of clinically positive neck nodes requires comprehensive neck dissection in the form of radical neck dissection or modified radical neck dissection. Radical neck dissection is en bloc removal of lymph-node-bearing tissues in the submental, submandibular, upper jugular, mid jugular, lower jugular and posterior triangle region along with the submandibular gland, internal jugular vein stern ocleidomastoid muscle and the spinal accessory nerve.

Modified radical neck dissection differs from radical neck dissection in that the spinal accessory nerve is preserved to maximize shoulder function. The use of selective neck dissection in the form of supraomohyoid neck dissection (en bloc removal of submental, sub-mandibular, upper and mid jugular node-bearing tissues) is limited to the management of a clinically negative neck, and confirmation of microscopic disease on frozen section generally requires conversion to a comprehensive neck dissection. Selective neck dissection is also suitable for the management of neck node metastasis arising from well-differentiated thyroid cancer. The complication rate of radical neck dissection, even in the previously irradiated neck, is low and may include wound haematoma, wound infection, flap necrosis and, rarely, carotid artery rupture. When a myocutaneous or free flap is used for the reconstruction of an oral cavity defect, orocutaneous fistula and partial or complete flap necrosis may occur.

Induction chemotherapy with 5-fluorouracil and cis-platinum may make surgical resection of a locally advanced tumour possible; concurrent chemotherapy and radiotherapy may also be of benefit for a locally advanced tumour. Typical 5-year survival rates for early disease (stages I and II) are 60–80% and for advanced disease (stages III and IV) 20–40%.

Minor salivary gland tumours

These tumours arise from the mucosal minor salivary glands distributed throughout the upper aerodigestive tracts. The majority of these minor salivary gland tumours are malignant and occur predominantly in the oral cavity. Adenoid cystic carcinomas make up over one-third of the minor salivary carcinomas. Other carcinomas include adenocarcinoma and mucoepidermoid carcinoma. These tumours have a low rate of cervical lymph node involvement but a high rate of distant metastasis. Their 5-year cure rates following surgical resection are typically lower than for a squamous carcinoma of the same site.

Nasopharynx

Anatomy

The nasopharynx serves as a conduit for air and nasal and paranasal sinus secretion, and is lined by squamous, respiratory and transitional epithelium. It lies above the level of the soft palate and posterior to the choana (Figure 18.15). The lateral wall consists of the Eustachian tube opening, the lateral pharyngeal recess (fossa of Rosenmuller) and the cartilaginous medial end of the Eustachian tube (torus tubarius). The

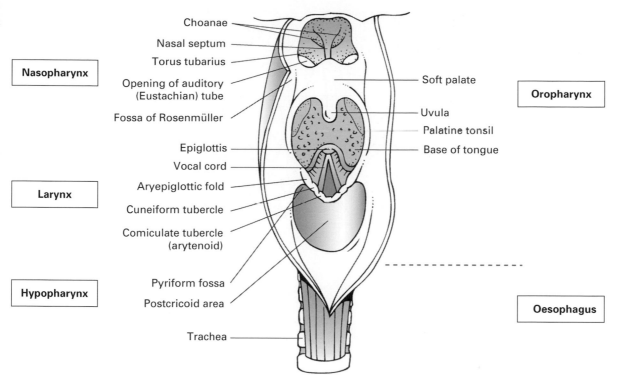

Figure 18.15 Anatomic sites of the nasopharynx, oropharynx, hypopharynx and larynx.

fossa of Rosenmüller is a cleft-like pouch lined by the pharyngobasilar fascia and it extends to the parapharyngeal space within which runs the internal carotid artery, internal jugular vein, cranial nerves IX–XII and the sympathetic nerve (Figure 18.16).

Nasopharyngeal cancer

The first sign of nasopharyngeal carcinoma is often an enlarged metastatic cervical node in the posterior triangle. Common local signs and symptoms include nasal (blood-stained discharge, obstruction), aural (serous otitis media, tinnitis, conductive hearing loss) and neurological symptoms (diplopia due to abducen nerve paralysis). Diagnosis is by flexible fibreoptic nasopharyngoscopy and biopsy. Elevated blood levels of antibodies to Epstein-Barr virus capsid antigen (IgA-VCA) and early antigen (IgA-EA) are often seen. CT and MRI are useful in staging the disease and in detection of recurrence. Radiation is the first-line treatment for nasopharyngeal carcinomas of all stages because of the radiosensitivity of undifferentiated carcinoma. For recurrent disease after radiotherapy, surgical resection of the nasopharynx by the transoropalatal, mandibular swing or maxilla swing approach is a well established surgical salvage procedure that is preferred over re-irradiation, which is associated with complications including radiation myelitis, encephalopathy, cranial nerve palsy, otitis media, hearing loss, trismus, cataract formation and osteoradionerosis of the maxilla and mandible. For recurrent disease limited to the neck, radical neck dissection provides excellent control of the neck disease.

Juvenile nasopharyngeal angiofibroma

This is a benign but locally destructive vascular tumour of the nasopharynx occurring exclusively in boys. Surgical resection is facilitated by maxilla or mandibular swing.

Larynx and hypopharynx

Anatomy

The larynx consists of three single cartilages (epiglottis, thyroid cartilage and cricoid cartilage) and three smaller paired cartilages (cuneiform, corniculate and arytenoid cartilages). The larynx can be divided into

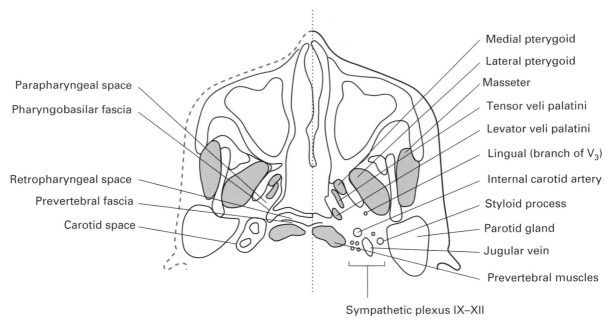

Parapharyngeal space

Pharyngobasilar fascia

Retropharyngeal space

Prevertebral fascia

Carotid space

Medial pterygoid

Lateral pterygoid

Masseter

Tensor veli palatini

Levator veli palatini

Lingual (branch of V_3)

Internal carotid artery

Styloid process

Parotid gland

Jugular vein

Prevertebral muscles

Sympathetic plexus IX–XII

Figure 18.16 Parapharyngeal space at the level of the nasopharynx.

three sub-sites; the supraglottic larynx consists of the epiglottis, aryepiglottic folds, arytenoids and ventricular bands (false cords); the glottic larynx consists of true vocal cords; and the subglottic larynx is the region below the glottis bounded by the cricoid cartilage (Figure 18.15).

The recurrent laryngeal nerve innervates the vocal cord muscle and dysfunction results in hoarseness. The internal branch of the superior laryngeal nerve provides laryngeal and hypopharyngeal mucosal sensation and dysfunction may cause aspiration. The external branch of the superior laryngeal nerve innervates the cricothyroid muscle, which is the tensor of the vocal cord, and injury leads to a weak voice.

The hypopharynx extends from the level of the hyoid bone to the level of the cricoid cartilage. It encompasses the pyriform sinus, the postcricoid area (posterior surface of the larynx) and the lower posterior pharyngeal wall. The cervical oesophagus is below the hypopharynx (Figure 18.15).

Clinical evaluation

Vocal cord polyps and tumours may cause hoarseness. Large laryngeal tumours and infraglottic tumours cause airway obstruction. Hypopharyngeal tumours frequently cause dysphagia or pain on swallowing. Following examination of the neck and oral cav-

ity, the larynx and upper portion of the hypopharynx are best examined by mirror examination (indirect laryngoscopy) and direct laryngoscopy by flexible fibreoptic nasopharyngolaryngoscopy, which is done as an outpatient procedure. For more complete examination of the hypopharynx, direct laryngoscopy with a rigid laryngoscope under general anaesthesia is required.

Panendoscopy

The term 'panendoscopy' means examination of the entire upper aerodigestive tract including the pharynx, larynx, oesophagus, trachea and bronchus with a combination of flexible and rigid laryngoscope, bronchoscope and oesophagoscope. Panendoscopy is essential in delineating the extent of deep-seated tumours, in the detection of a synchronous second primary and in searching for an unknown primary causing cervical nodal metastasis. Panendoscopy is recommended as part of the initial evaluation for proven squamous cell cancer of the head and neck when a second primary needs to be excluded.

Second primary

The risk of multiple primary tumours in the head and neck area is higher than elsewhere because of

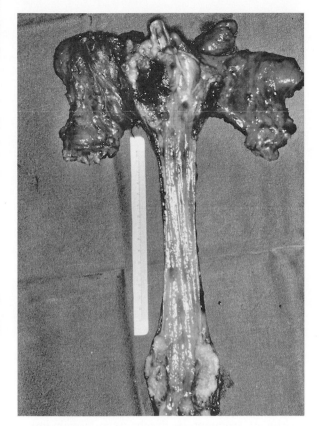

Figure 18.17 Patient with obstructing pyriform fossa squamous cell carcinoma requiring pharyngolaryngoesophagectomy and bilateral neck dissections. Surgical specimen revealed a synchronous oesophageal second primary.

the field cancerization theory related to susceptibility of head and neck mucosa to common carcinogens (smoking and alcohol intake). Of 573 patients with squamous cell carcinoma of head and neck (lung cancer excluded) observed over a $4\frac{1}{2}$-year period, 2.4% had multiple second primary carcinoma (69% with synchronous primary tumours) and 63% of all second primary tumours occurred in the oesophagus (Figure 18.17).

Laryngeal papilloma

The juvenile form is believed to be acquired during birth from maternal vaginal warts. The condition does not manifest, however, until months or years later when significant papillomata develop. In general, those who present early usually present with airway obstruction, while older children usually present with progressive hoarseness. Treatment is extremely difficult and frequent recurrence is a rule rather than

an exception. At laryngoscopy, there is usually extensive involvement of the whole larynx; simultaneous tracheal and pharyngeal involvement by the papillomata is not uncommon. Repeated CO_2 laser therapy offers the best control of the disease. In severe cases, antiviral therapy including interferon therapy may be tried. Although the effectiveness of treatment is unpredictable, spontaneous regression of the papilloma may occur at any age.

The adult form typically presents with progressive hoarseness and laryngoscopy, and reveals either a solitary papilloma or multiple but discrete papillomata. These usually affect the true cord. Histologically, they are squamous papilloma and should be considered a premalignant lesion. The papilloma should be removed for histological evaluation and the base of the lesion treated with a CO_2 laser. The patient should refrain from smoking and be closely followed-up for recurrence.

Laryngeal and hypopharyngeal cancer

Over 90% of these malignancies are squamous cell carcinoma. The remaining malignancies arise from minor salivary gland or from supporting tissue, such as fibrosarcoma, chondrosarcoma or rhabdomyosarcoma. Early-stage squamous cell carcinoma of the larynx is usually treated by external radiation. Early or intermediate-stage supraglottic laryngeal carcinoma can be treated by conservation surgery (supraglottic subtotal laryngectomy) and localized glottic carcinoma can be treated by hemi-laryngectomy. When there is cord fixation or extension of disease into the hypopharynx or when hypopharynx cancer causes fixation of the hemi-larynx, total laryngectomy is usually required. Hypopharyngeal cancer requires partial or total pharyngectomy in addition to laryngectomy. Reconstruction of the pharyngeal defect is by regional myocutaneous flap (based on the latissimus dorsi or the pectoralis major muscle), free forearm flap (Figure 18.13), free jejunal segment or gastric pull-up. Extrathoracic gastric pull-up or colon interposition is required to reconstruct the oesophagus when total oesophagectomy is carried out for upper cervical oesophageal disease (Figure 18.17). Voice rehabilitation is by learning oesophageal speech, use of an electrolarynx, or by creation of a tracheo-oesophageal fistula for insertion of a Blom-Singer prosthesis. Advanced-stage laryngeal/hypopharyngeal cancer often requires concommitant neck dissection for a clinically positive neck followed by postoperative radiotherapy. Induction chemotherapy with 5-fluorouracil and cis-platinum in selected patients may allow preservation of the larynx since complete response to chemotherapy may allow the patient to proceed to radiotherapy without undergoing surgery.

Tracheostomy

Tracheostomy is indicated for airway control after major oropharyngeal surgery, especially when the mandible continuity is disrupted, and in severe maxillofacial trauma to prevent aspiration of blood. A transverse skin incision is preferred. With retraction of the thyroid isthmus upward, the pretracheal fascia is incised in order for a transverse incision to be made between the second and third tracheal rings. Initial tracheostomy care includes humidification and frequent suctioning. The tracheostomy tube is usually changed after the first 5 days when the track in the subcutaneous tissue is established.

Cricothyroidotomy

In an urgent situation, a cricothyroidotomy allows quick access to the airway by insertion of a small-size tracheostomy tube through the cricothyroid membrane into the trachea. To avoid subglottic stenosis, a formal tracheostomy should be performed within 24 hours.

Paranasal sinuses

Of paranasal sinus tumours, 80% occur in the maxillary sinus with the rest arising from the ethmoid, frontal and sphenoid sinuses. The maxillary sinuses are lined by ciliated columnar epithelium and the majority of the malignant epithelial neoplasms are squamous cell carcinoma. Oral signs and symptoms appear early while nasal obstruction and bloody nasal discharge are late symptoms. Invasion of the orbit is associated with ocular signs, including unilateral proptosis and diplopia. Anterior extension leads to facial asymmetry and deformity. Extension of tumour posteriorly leads to destruction of the pterygoid plates and invasion of the infratemporal fossa. There may be unilateral deafness and facial palsy. Both axial and coronal CT scans are required to define the extent of the paranasal tumour since extension of tumour to adjacent sinuses and structures is common due to delay in presentation and in diagnosis.

Localized tumour can be successfully treated by subtotal maxillectomy, including the orbital floor, hard palate and lower pterygoid plates. Rehabilitation with dental prosthesis is required. For cancer extending to or arising from the ethmoid sinus, a craniofacial resection is required safely to resect the roof of the ethmoid sinus, i.e. the cribriform plate. For extensive malignant tumours not amenable to curative surgical resection, palliation by combined chemotherapy and external radiotherapy may give useful control of the disease. Regional metastasis is uncommon at presentation and distant metastases are rare.

Neck masses

History

Age group is important. Congenital lesions are more likely to occur in children, whereas in the adult persistent cervical lymphadenopathy represents malignancy until proven otherwise. Inflammatory lesions may have a history of recent onset, rapid increase in size and pain. Tuberculosis is associated with fever and night sweats, whereas upper aerodigestive malignancy is usually associated with chronic intake of alcoholic products and smoking, and there may be symptoms of hoarseness, haemoptysis, dysphagia and weight loss.

Physical examination

A complete head and neck examination and a general examination should be carried out. The emphasis of the latter is the detection of peripheral lymphadenopathy, hepatosplenomegaly and abdominal mass. Initial head and neck examination includes examination of the oral cavity and oropharynx by direct inspection. The neck is palpated to note the location, size, consistency, mobility, surface topography and tenderness of the mass. Associated lymphadenopathy or thyromegaly is noted.

Investigations

If an inflammatory cause is considered, a complete blood count and sedimentation rate are obtained. In patients who are at risk of developing nasopharyngeal carcinoma, blood levels of IgA-VCA and IgA-EA are determined. When the neck mass is consistent with lymphadenopathy, flexible fibreoptic nasopharyngolaryngoscopy is carried out to look for a possible head and neck primary. Any suspicious mucosal lesions should be biopsied. FNA can be carried out on all neck masses, including salivary gland tumours. Exceptions are pulsatile masses with bruit which may represent a high-flow carotid body tumour, arteriovenous malformation and haemangioma. The aspirate is sent for cytology and, for suspected inflammatory lesions, it is also sent for Gram stain and Ziehl Nissen stain for acid-fast bacilli and DNA for mycobacterium. Plain X-ray is not used in the routine evaluation of a neck mass unless para-oesophageal abscess is suspected. The neck mass is best studied by an ultrasound examination, which can confirm the anatomic location of the mass, its composition (cystic or solid) and relationship to adjacent structures as well as associated lymphadenopathy in the neck. More sophisticated imaging such as CT scan, MRI and digital angiography are indicated in the evaluation of a complex mass or a suspected vascular lesion. The diagnosis of a haemangioma can also be established by red blood cell (RBC) scintigraphy, using sodium pertechnetate radioisotope.

The long list of differential diagnosis for neck mass can be simplified by considering four major categories:

- congenital
- inflammatory (viral, bacterial, fungal, granulomatous)
- neoplastic (benign, malignant)
- miscellaneous (Zenker's diverticulum).

Congenital masses

Common congenital neck masses include thyroglossal duct cyst, branchial cyst, cystic hygroma, teratoma (mostly in infants) and haemangioma.

Thyroglossal duct cyst

A thyroglossal duct cyst originates from the epithelial remnants of the thyroglossal tract and therefore is typically located in the midline between the isthmus of the thyroid gland and the foramen caecum of the tongue base. It can be at, below or above the level of the hyoid bone. The typical thyroglossal duct cyst moves with swallowing and protrusion of the tongue because of its adherence to the hyoid bone and adjacent strap muscles. It may or may not have a ductal connection to the tongue base. Ultrasound examination is useful in ruling out ectopic thyroid and in confirming the presence of a normal thyroid gland in the lower neck. Treatment is by Sistrunk's operation (excision of entire cyst with a small central segment of hyoid bone and any ductal connection to the tongue base). Small thy-

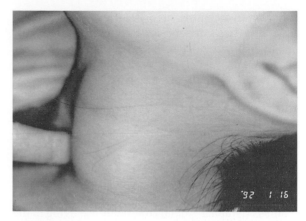

Figure 18.18 Large second branchial cyst.

roglossal duct cysts with no history of infection can be observed as the risk of malignant change is well under 1%.

Branchial cyst

During the fifth embryonic week, the branchial apparatus, which is phylogenetically related to the primitive gill slits, develops into five paired mesodermic arches separated by four pairs of invaginations of ectoderm and endoderm known respectively as branchial clefts and pouches. Each branchial arch develops into cartilage, artery, nerve and muscles. Branchial anomalies in the form of a cyst, sinus (communicates to the viscera or skin) or fistula (communicates to both skin and viscera) can form from vestigial remnants of branchial pouches and clefts. Branchial anomalies are lined by squamous epithelium or respiratory epithelium or both. First branchial anomalies are rare and are of two types. A type I lesion is usually postauricular in location (commonly mistaken as a postauricular sebaceous cyst) and represents a duplication of both membranous and cartilagenous portions of the external auditory canal. A type II lesion typically presents as a cyst or sinus in the preauricular or upper neck with the fistula tract intimately related to the parotid gland and the facial nerve. Second branchial anomalies commonly present as a cyst in mid-neck (Figure 18.18). It may course between the external and internal carotid arteries and may reach the tonsillar fossa. Third branchial lesions are uncommon. They present lower in the neck and may track posterior to the internal carotid artery to exit near the pyriform fossa. In children, an inflamed third branchial cyst may present clinically as acute thyroiditis.

Differential diagnosis of a branchial cyst includes nodal metastasis of papillary carcinoma of thyroid or squamous carcinoma with cystic change and other inflammatory mass. Ultrasound examination and CT scan are useful to help differentiate branchial cyst anomalies from other conditions. Treatment of branchial anomalies is surgical excision. Surgical treatment of type II first branchial anomalies requires facial nerve dissection.

Cystic hygroma

These are congenital malformations of lymphatic channels (lymphangioma) commonly occurring in the posterior neck. They are usually present at birth. They may be cystic or cavernous and the cavernous form tends to infiltrate diffusely adjacent tissues and structures. Surgical resection should be considered in childhood.

Teratomas and dermoid cysts

These are developmental cysts composed of trigeminal components foreign to the site of origin. In the head and neck region, true teratomas tend to arise from embryonic tissue near the primitive streak and notochord. According to Batsakis, teratomas include dermoid cysts and related cystic lesions (epidermoid or epidermal cyst, teratoid cyst and teratoma of the neck). Epidermoid cysts are lined by simple squamous epithelium, dermoid cysts are an epithelial-lined cavity with skin appendages, and teratoid cysts may contain squamous epithelium or ciliated respiratory epithelium. Dermoid cysts of the floor of the mouth may present in the mid-line submental area. Teratomas of the neck are commonly present at birth and the mass effect may be associated with respiratory distress and dysphagia. Therefore, surgical excision is always indicated. Malignant teratoma of the neck is rare.

Haemangioma

In the head and neck area, haemangioma typically present as diffuse, soft, subcutaneous masses that may gradually increase in size over many years. Unless localized, haemangioma is best treated conservatively once the diagnosis has been confirmed by ultrasound, CT scan or RBC scan. Haemangioma of skin (port-wine stain) can be treated by pulsed dye laser. Nodular or deep haemangioma can be treated by pulsed dye laser (585–590 nm) and/or long pulsed Nd:YAG laser

(1064 nm) in multiple treatment sessions. Radiation should not be used for the treatment of haemangioma.

Inflammatory masses

Inflammatory neck masses include lymphadenitis of viral, bacterial, fungal and granulomatous aetiology as well as bacterial abscesses of the neck.

- In viral lymphadenitis, pharyngitis or tonsillitis have associated cervical nodal enlargement that is usually self-limiting, <1.5 cm in size and resolves in 2 weeks.
- Infectious mononucleosis due to Epstein-Barr virus usually causes pharyngitis and cervical lymphadenopathy in older children and young adults. Monospot (heterophile agglutination) test is positive.
- Bacterial lymphadenitis: in children, streptococcal tonsillitis is commonly associated with cervical lymphadenitis. Peritonsillar abscess, odontogenic infections or bacterial lymphadenitis can lead to neck abscesses.
- Ludwig's angina is gangrenous cellulitis and abscess of the submandibular region that can progress to mediastinitis, empyema and death. Common causes are mandibular molar infection, floor of mouth perforation and extension of a peritonsillar abscess. Treatment is antibiotics and emergency surgical drainage.

Granulomatous lymphadenitis

In areas such as Asia where tuberculosis (TB) is largely still endemic, patients with scrofula or cervicofacial myobacterial infections commonly present with multiple tender, matted, posterior or supraclavicular lymph nodes that may progress to form 'cold abscesses'. Less than 10% of patients with scrofula have associated extranodal TB. When FNA of the involved cervical node fails to yield acid-fast bacilli on Ziehl Nissen stain, incisional or excisional biopsy is required for diagnosis. A longer course of drug treatment than for pulmonary disease is usually required. Actinomycosis may cause persistent facial-cervical abscess and draining sinuses. It is caused by a bacterium with microaerophilic and anaerobic growth requirements. Typical sulphur granules (branching filaments with calcium phosphate) may be microscopically demonstrated. Cat-scratch disease is due to a cat scratch or bite. The cervical lymphadenitis is associated with a small rod-shaped bacillus. No specific treatment is required.

Neoplasms

Neoplasms can be benign or malignant. Malignant lesions can be primary or metastatic.

Benign neoplasms

These include thyroid tumours, salivary gland tumours and soft tissue tumours (e.g. lipoma). Madelung's disease (multiple symmetrical lipomatosis) is a rare disease of unknown aetiology. Rarer benign tumours include paraganglioma, carotid body tumour, schwannoma (solitary encapsulated nerve tumour) and neurofibroma (non-encapsulated, usually multiple).

Von Recklinghausen's disease is an inherited autosomal dominant trait. Affected patients have cafe-au-lait spots neurofibroma of the skin (multiple neurofibromatosis) and Lisch nodules (pigmented iris hamartomas). Acoustic neuroma and other tumours of the central nervous system can occur. Carotid body tumours arise from the paraganglion cells of the carotid body located at the bifurcation of the carotid artery. They are usually benign, firm, slow growing masses that may occur bilaterally. The tumour may involve adjacent cranial nerves. Surgical excision by an experienced surgeon is recommended.

Fibromatosis

This is a group of aggressive fibroblastic proliferative lesions that are benign but locally infiltrative. The term fibromatosis is generally preferred over extra-abdominal desmoid.

Malignant neoplasms

Malignant causes of lymph node enlargement may be due to primary involvement by lymphoma or secondary involvement by head and neck primary (upper aerodigestive squamous cell carcinoma, salivary gland carcinoma and thyroid gland carcinoma) as well as by infraclavicular primary (breast, lung, stomach, colon, kidney and ovary). Ultrasound is useful in differentiating lymphoma and cervical metastatic lymph node.

Rarely, malignancy may arise from extranodal soft tissues of the neck (e.g. sarcoma and dermatofibrosarcoma protruberans).

Miscellaneous

Miscellaneous neck masses that may be palpable include *Zenker's diverticulum,* which is a herniation of pharyngeal mucosa through a weakness between the inferior constrictor muscle and the cricopharyngeous muscle. Symptoms include regurgitation of undigested food and dysphagia. Treatment is by surgical repair.

Kikuchi's disease

This is a self-limiting necrotizing lymphadenitis, possibly of autoimmune basis. Patient presents typically with non-tender, persistent cervical lymphadenopathy. Excision biopsy of the enlarged lymph node is required for diagnosis. Some patients may have associated lupus erythematosis; therefore, serology for antinuclear antibody and rheumatoid factor should be obtained.

Salivary gland disease

Salivary gland inflammation

Acute parotitis causing diffuse enlargement of the parotid gland may be due to viral infection (e.g. mumps) or bacterial infection. Submandibular sialadenitis is usually associated with obstruction of Wharton's duct by calculi. *Staphylococcus aureus* and *Streptococcus viridans* are the main pathogens. Intravenous antibiotic is required for the treatment of acute bacterial parotitis. Mycobacterial infection may also involve the parotid gland, causing nodular enlargement. Chronic recurrent enlargement of bilateral parotid gland is seen in Sjogren's syndrome, which is usually associated with keratoconjunctivitis sicca, xerostomia (dry mouth) and rheumatoid arthritis. Benign lymphoepithelial lesions and lymphoma may arise in a parotid gland affected by long-standing Sjogren's syndrome.

Salivary gland tumours

Benign and malignant salivary gland tumours can arise from the parotid gland, submandibular gland and rarely the sublingual gland. They typically present as a parotid or submandibular mass. Approximately 10% of parotid and 50% of submandibular gland tumours are malignant. Both ultrasound and FNA are useful in delineating the nature of the salivary gland lesions. A CT scan may be required to evaluate a complex mass such as deep lobe tumours and invasive tumours.

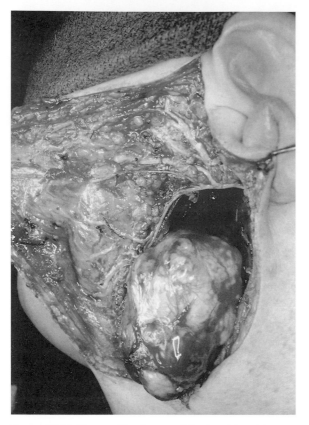

Figure 18.19 Pleomorphic adenoma of the deep lobe of the parotid gland being dissected out of the parapharyngeal space.

When the facial nerve or its major branches are scarified, a nerve graft is desirable. Radical neck dissection is necessary in the presence of clinically evident cervical nodal metastasis. Prognosis is dependent on the size and grade of the malignant tumour. For high-grade tumours, postoperative radiotherapy is recommended.

Parapharyngeal space tumours

The parapharyngeal space (lateral pharyngeal space) is a pyramid-shaped loose fascial plane around the pharynx between the skull base and the hyoid bone (Figures 18.16 and 18.19). Tumours of the parapharyngeal space can present as an upper neck mass or submucosal oropharyngeal mass. They may be salivary gland tumours, neurogenic tumours, carotid body tumours, vascular tumours, lymphomas or miscellaneous soft-tissue tumours (e.g. lipoma). Treatment is surgical excision by the transcervical or parotidectomy approach.

Further reading

Beall J, Scholl P, Jafek B. Total ophthalmoplegia after internal maxillary artery ligation. *Arch Otolaryngol* 1985;**111**(10):696–698.

Brucher J. Origin of the ophthalmic artery from the middle meningeal artery. *Radiology* 1969;**93**(1):51–52.

Choy ATK, Van Hasselt CA, Chisholm EM, Williams SR, King WWK, Li AKC. Multiple primary cancers in Hong Kong Chinese Patients with squamous cell cancer of the head and neck. *Cancer* 1992;**20**:815–820.

Cox GJ, Vinayak BC. Deep neck space infection. In Bleach N, Milford C, van Hasselt CA (eds). *Operative Otolaryngology*. Blackwell Scientific, 1997; 462–468.

Endicott JN, Seper J. Deep neck infections and postoperative infections. In Mandell GL, Brook I (eds). *Atlas of Infectious Diseases: Volume IV – Upper Respiratory and Head and Neck Infections*. Churchill Livingstone, 1995; 10.1–10.15.

Hughes GB. Inflammatory disorder. In Hughes GB (ed.) *Textbook of Clinical Otology*. Georg Thieme, 1985; section V.

Kanski JJ. *Clinical Ophthalmology*. 3rd edn. Butterworth-Heinemann, 1994; 1–150.

King WWK. Head and neck cancer. *J HK Coll Radiol* 1998;**1**(2):88–93.

King WWK, Ku PKM, Mok CO, Teo PML. Nasopharyngectomy in the treatment of recurrent

Common benign tumours are pleomorphic adenoma and Warthin's tumour (papillary cystadenoma lymphomatosum). Pleomorphic adenoma is usually rubbery firm in consistency and may recur if not excised with an adequate margin. Warthin's tumour may be bilateral and tends to occur in the elderly. Malignant salivary gland tumours include mucoepidermoid carcinoma, adenoid cystic carcinoma, acinic cell carcinoma, adenocarcinoma, undifferentiated carcinoma, squamous cell carcinoma and lymphoma. Metastases to the parotid gland can originate from the scalp, cheek, nasopharynx and oral cavity. Superficial parotidectomy via a preauricular incision is the recommended minimal surgical procedure. Open incisional biopsy should be avoided due to the concern for facial nerve damage and unsightly scarring. When malignancy is confirmed by intraoperative frozen section, total parotidectomy and sampling of the jugulodigastric lymph node are recommended. The facial nerve is preserved unless directly involved by the tumour.

nasopharyngeal carcinoma : a twelve year experience. *Head Neck* 2000;**5**:215–222.

King WWK, Li AKC. Nasopharyngeal cancer. In Morris PJ, Wood WC (eds). *Oxford Textbook of Surgery*. 2nd edn, vol. 3. Oxford University Press, 2000; 2925–2937.

King WWK, Teo PML, Li AKC. Patterns of failure after radical neck dissection for recurrent nasopharyngeal carcinoma. *Am J Surg* 1992;**164**: 599–602.

Maran AGD. Infections of the pharynx. In Maran AGD (ed). *Logan Turner's Diseases of the Nose, Throat and Ear*. Butler & Tanner, 1988; section 2.3.

McGuirt WF. Neck mass: patient examination and differential diagnosis. In Cummings CW, Fredrickson JM, Harker LA, Krause CJ, Schiller DE (eds). *Otolaryngology – Head and Neck Surgery*, vol 2. CV Mosby, 1986.

Shaheen OH. Thesis for the Master of Surgery. University of London, 1967.

Shaw CB, Wax MK, Wetmore SJ. Epistaxis: a comparison of treatment. *Otolaryngol Head Neck Surg* 1993;**109**: 60–65.

Soo KC, Spiro RH, King W, Harvey W, Strong EW. Squamous carcinoma of gums. *Am J Surg* 1988;**156**: 281–285.

Stammberger H. Secretion transportation. In Stammberger H (ed). *Functional Endoscopic Sinus Surgery*. B.C. Decker, 1991; Chapter 2.

The International Rhinitis Management Working Group. International Consensus Report on the Diagnosis and Management of Rhinitis. *Eur J Allergy Clin Immunol* 1994;**49**(19):Supplement.

Tong MCF, van Hasselt CA, Woo JKS. The hazards of button batteries in the nose. *J Otolaryngol* 1992;**21**(6): 458–460.

Tong MCF, Woo JKS, Sham CL, van Hasselt CA. Ingested foreign bodies – a contemporary management approach. *J Laryngol Otol* 1995;**109**:965–970.

Walters DAK, Ahuja AT, Evans RM, Chick W, King WWK, Metrewel C, Li AKC. Role of ultrasound in the management of thyroid nodules. *Am J Surg* 1992;**164**: 654–657.

Woo JKS, van Hasselt CA. Acute epiglottitis: a misnomer. *Otolaryngol Head Neck Surg* 1994;**111**: 538–539.

Woo JKS. Surgery for epistaxis. In Bleach N, Milford C, van Hasselt CA (eds). *Operative Otolaryngology*. Blackwell Scientific, 1997a; 256–262.

Woo JKS. Nasopharyngoscopy. In Bleach N, Milford C, van Hasselt CA (eds). *Operative Otolaryngology*. Blackwell Scientific, 1997b; 265–268.

Fundamentals of thoracic surgery

Richard S. Steyn and Deborah Harrington

Surgical anatomy

Tracheobronchial tree

The bony skeleton of the larynx consists of the hyoid bone superiorly, and the thyroid and cricoid cartilages, from which the trachea is suspended. The thickened edge of the cricovocal membrane forms the cricovocal ligament, which is covered with mucous membrane and thus forms the vocal fold (cord). The vocal cord is responsible not only for phonation, but also for protection of the tracheobronchial tree from food and fluids during deglutition. The nerve supply of the vocal cords is largely by the recurrent laryngeal nerves, which originate from the vagus nerve within the thorax. On the right side the recurrent laryngeal nerve originates in the root of the neck, hooks around the right subclavian artery and ascends to the larynx between the trachea and oesophagus. On the left it originates at the level of the aortic arch in the thorax, hooks around the ligamentum arteriosum, and ascends to the right of the aortic arch, again between the trachea and oesophagus. Thus the left recurrent laryngeal nerve in particular is susceptible to involvement by mediastinal pathology.

The laryngeal prominence (Adam's apple) is formed by the junction of the two laminae of the thyroid cartilage. Below this is the cricoid cartilage, and between the two is the cricothyroid membrane which is the landmark used for emergency cricothyroidotomy or more commonly, the insertion of a minitracheostomy (Figure 19.1).

The trachea is held open by C-shaped rings of cartilage with a flat posterior membranous portion. Posterior to the membranous trachea is the oesophagus. The trachea bifurcates to form the left and right

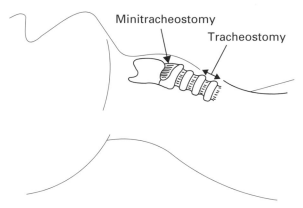

Figure 19.1 Pharynx showing cricothyroid membrane for minitracheostomy.

main bronchi at the level of the manubrio-sternal joint (angle of Louis) or lower edge of the fourth thoracic vertebra.

The tracheobronchial tree is lined by ciliated epithelium containing mucus-secreting glands. This lining is damaged by smoking, causing deficient cilia and tenacious mucus, resulting in a chronic 'smoker's cough'.

The right lung is divided into three lobes by the oblique (major) and horizontal (minor) fissures, forming the upper, middle and lower lobes. The left lung is divided into upper and lower lobes by the oblique fissure. Each lobe is divided further into bronchopulmonary segments, which are served by their own segmental bronchus (Figure 19.2).

The lungs receive a blood supply from the bronchial arteries, which are direct branches from the descending aorta. Lymphatic drainage is via segmental, hilar and then mediastinal lymph nodes on each side and ultimately to the scalene nodes (Figure 19.3).

Fundamentals of Surgical Practice, Third Edition, ed. Andrew N. Kingsnorth and Douglas M. Bowley.
Published by Cambridge University Press. © Cambridge University Press 2011.

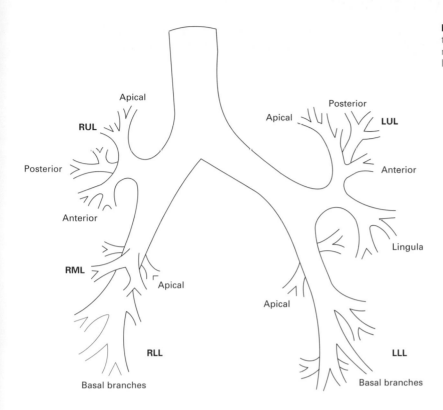

Figure 19.2 Anatomy of the bronchial tree. RUL: right upper lobe; RML: right middle lobe; RLL: right lower lobe; LUL: left upper lobe; LLL: left lower lobe.

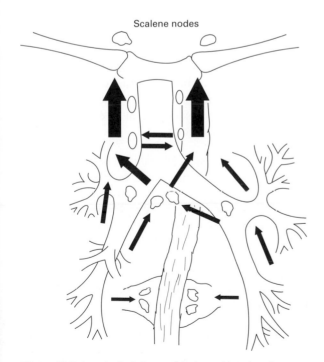

Figure 19.3 Lymphatic drainage of the lungs. Note there is more crossover from the left to right than right to left side.

Pleural space

The pleural space is a potential space formed between the visceral and parietal pleura. The pleura secretes and absorbs approximately 600 ml of pleural fluid each day, but if there is increased production or decreased reabsorption, a pleural effusion results.

Mediastinum

The mediastinum is the space between the two pleural cavities. It is divided into three compartments, anterior, middle and posterior. Certain tumours are characteristically found in one or other compartment, for example thymomas anteriorly and neurofibromas posteriorly (Figure 19.4).

Oesophagus

The oesophagus is situated between the pharynx and the stomach, and has three components, cervical, thoracic and abdominal. In the thorax it lies posterior to the trachea until the bifurcation. The aortic arch then crosses it from right to left, and anteriorly to posteriorly. Spontaneous ruptures of the oesophagus tend

331

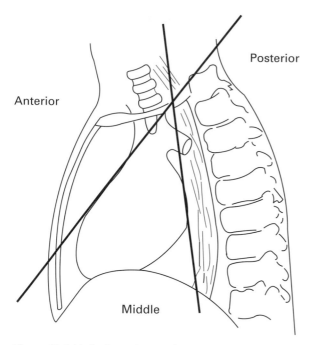

Anterior

Posterior

Middle

Figure 19.4 Mediastinum showing divisions.

to occur in the lower thoracic oesophagus, generally towards the left side. The entrance to the short abdominal oesophagus is formed by the crurae, originating from the diaphragm. Weakness in these may result in either sliding or paraoesophageal hiatus hernia formation.

Vagus and phrenic nerves

The phrenic nerves course anteriorly to the lung roots on either side, then run along the pericardium towards the diaphragm. The left phrenic is situated more anteriorly than the right. The vagus nerves are posterior structures, passing behind the lung hilum on each side, then down the oesophagus to the stomach.

Diaphragm

The diaphragm is the muscle separating the thorax from the abdomen, and is vital for normal respiration. It is an inverted J shape in sagittal section, being higher anteriorly than posteriorly, important when considering pleural aspiration and drainage. Most of the diaphragm is innervated by the phrenic nerves, with some peripheral nerve supply from the intercostal nerves. During inspiration the diaphragm contracts and moves down into the abdomen, and during expiration, which is passive, it relaxes and rises back

up into the thorax. A paralysed diaphragm appears higher than normal on a chest X-ray. Eventration of the diaphragm is caused by deficient muscle with a stretched fibrous portion and may also lead to a raised diaphragm on chest X-ray. Congenital diaphragmatic hernias usually present in the neonate, but occasionally are not discovered until adulthood. Morgagni hernias are situated anteriorly, and Bochdalek hernias posteriorly.

History and examination

A number of symptoms and signs are typical of respiratory disease and should be specifically looked for during history taking and physical examination of a patient with suspected chest disease.

Symptoms

Cough –– A persistent cough in a person who does not normally cough or an increased cough in a smoker should be regarded as suspicious. Sputum production is also important. Yellow or green sputum implies infection, which if recurrent should be investigated. Red or dark brown sputum implies haemoptysis (coughing up blood) and should always be further investigated.

Dyspnoea –– Shortness of breath may be cardiac or respiratory in origin. A careful history of other associated features, such as cough or wheeze, or chest pain and orthopnoea may help to distinguish between the two. An assessment of the patient's functional capacity or exercise tolerance is important in establishing the severity of their symptoms.

Wheeze or noisy breathing implies airway obstruction –– This may involve small airways, for example in asthma, or larger airways, where it may cause stridor, for example due to obstruction caused by tumour or foreign body.

Chest pain –– Constant chest pain or pleuritic pain suggests chest wall involvement of a disease process. Chest pain on exertion is more suggestive of ischaemic heart disease.

Constitutional symptoms –– Symptoms such as weight loss, reduced appetite, fevers and night sweats are all important indicators of respiratory disease and may be either infective or malignant in origin.

Table 19.1 Differences between exudative effusion and transudate.

	Exudate	Transudate
Colour	Dark yellow	Pale yellow
Pleural fluid/serum protein ratio	>0.5	<0.5
Pleural fluid/serum LDH ratio	>0.6	<0.6
LDH	>200 U	<200 U

Note: LDH – Lactic dehydrogenase.

Signs

Inspection –– Cyanosis, respiratory rate, use of accessory muscles, nicotine staining and finger clubbing are all important physical signs elicited on visual inspection. In addition, chest wall deformities and scars from previous surgery may also be important.

Palpation –– The position of the trachea should be confirmed. It is important to palpate for cervical lymphadenopathy, and any areas of bony tenderness. Any lumps or bumps should also be palpated.

Percussion –– The normal chest is resonant to percussion. Dullness implies pleural effusion or consolidation. Hyper-resonance may be found in severe emphysema or pneumothorax.

Auscultation should reveal vesicular breath sounds –– Added sounds include crackles and wheezes. Reduced air entry may be due to effusion, consolidation or pneumothorax.

Investigations

Routine blood tests of patients with chest disease should include a full blood count, clotting screen, urea and electrolytes, liver function tests and erythrocyte sedimentation rate (ESR) or C reactive protein (CRP). Anaemia may occur due to haemoptysis or chronic disease. Raised white cell count, ESR or CRP may suggest infection or inflammation. Hyponatraemia may be caused by infection or malignancy, as can altered liver function. Hypercalcaemia should also be excluded.

Sputum should be examined for cytology and microbiology including the presence of acid-alcohol-fast bacilli and culture for tuberculosis.

Pleural fluid should be subjected to biochemical, microbiological and cytological examination. Biochemistry will reveal whether the fluid has high protein content and is therefore an exudate, or low protein content and therefore a transudate. Differences between exudates and transudates are shown in Table 19.1. Typically exudates are caused by infection or malignancy and transudates by heart failure.

All patients suspected of chest disease should have a chest radiograph. This should be systematically examined, e.g. Airways, Breathing (lungs), Circulation (blood vessels and heart), Densities (bones and skeleton), Extras (soft tissues, breast shadows, air under diaphragm, foreign bodies, lines, drains and tubes).

Most patients will then go on to have a computed tomographic (CT) scan of the chest and upper abdomen to further characterize abnormalities such as masses and mediastinal lymph nodes. These studies are usually contrast-enhanced in order to differentiate vascular structures. They can also be used as guidance for the performance of biopsies of lung, mediastinal and chest wall masses.

Magnetic resonance imaging (MRI) scans do not often add much more information than CT scans but may be useful in diagnosing vascular or neurological involvement, for example with posterior mediastinal masses or the thoracic inlet.

Ultrasound is useful for distinguishing between pleural effusion and lung consolidation or collapse. It can be used to mark or guide a suitable site for aspiration or intercostal drain insertion particularly if an effusion is small or loculated.

Flexible bronchoscopy is usually performed by respiratory physicians with the patient awake or lightly sedated. It is used for the investigation of proximal bronchial diseases and haemoptysis. Bronchial washings, brushings and biopsies can be taken, and samples sent for cytological and microbiological analysis. Transbronchial biopsies may be taken of lung tissue or lymph node masses. Recently endobronchial ultrasound has been developed as an adjunct to bronchoscopy, and can be used to examine and biopsy mediastinal lymph nodes, particularly useful in the staging of lung cancer.

Positron emission tomography (PET) scans have also now become widespread in their use in the investigation and staging of lung cancer and solitary pulmonary nodules. Tissues with a high metabolic rate, such as tumours, preferentially take up glucose. An intravenous injection of the positron-emitting 18-FDG (18F-fluorodeoxyglucose) is used which then causes metabolically active tissues to light up on the whole-body PET scan. However, not all malignancies

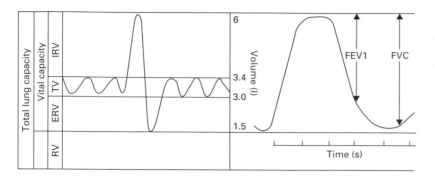

Figure 19.5 Basic spirometry. RV: residual volume; ERV: expiratory reserve volume; TV: tidal volume; IRV: inspiratory reserve volume; FEV1: forced expiratory capacity in 1 s; FVC: forced vital capacity.

are PET-positive and infection and inflammation can also sometimes light up on PET.

Pulmonary function tests should always be performed before contemplating lung resection (Figure 19.5). This may only involve basic spirometry testing in fit patients but in borderline cases, full lung function tests including an estimate of lung diffusion capacity and reversibility to bronchodilators should be performed. Pulmonary exercise testing, for example either a shuttle or a 6-minute walk test, is also useful to assess a patient's fitness for surgery. A quantitative ventilation-perfusion scan can be used to estimate the relative functional contribution of each area of lung, and thus whether resection is appropriate.

Thoracic surgical procedures

Intercostal drains

Intercostal (chest) drains are placed to drain the pleural cavity of air and fluid. Ideally a drain placed apically is best positioned to drain air and a basal drain is positioned to drain fluid. Small Seldinger drains are now frequently used by more and more physicians; however, it is important to be able to safely perform a conventional intercostal drain insertion using an open technique. The following description of intercostal drain insertion assumes an awake patient with the procedure performed under local anaesthetic. Firstly the patient should be consented for the procedure, and adequate analgesia and or premedication administered. The safest position to insert a chest drain without an operation is in the so called triangle of safety. This is through the lateral chest wall, posterior to the lateral border of pectoralis major, anterior to the lateral border of latissimus dorsi, and superior to a line drawn across the axilla horizontal to the nipple. You should avoid the mid-axillary line to prevent damage to the long thoracic nerve. The patient

should therefore be positioned appropriately, usually upright with the arm on the side of the drain held behind the head. It is important to have adequate assistance and preparation for the procedure as described. The insertion should be performed under strict aseptic conditions to prevent introduction of infection. The drain insertion site is anaesthetized, bearing in mind that the most painful layers are the skin and pleura. The aspiration of air or fluid should be confirmed prior to drain insertion. An incision is made in the skin, and blunt dissection using a curved forcep is used to traverse the muscles and parietal pleural layer. The incision should be over the top of a rib to avoid damage to the neurovascular bundle. A finger should be inserted into the pleural space to ensure its patency and the lack of adhesions. The drain may then be inserted. A trocar may only be used to aid direction, once the space is made, but should not be used to make the incision in the pleura. The drain is then secured in position, and a mattress suture placed for use on drain removal. The drain is then connected to an underwater seal which acts as a one-way valve. High-volume low-pressure suction may be applied to the bottle, usually set at around 20 cmH$_2$0 (2.5 kPa), or just above the normal range of pressure found in the pleural space. There are a number of commercially available drainage bottles ranging from the simple single-chamber underwater seal, to the three-bottle systems (Figure 19.6). which incorporate a bottle to collect fluid, a bottle to regulate suction pressure, and a bottle to act as a safety valve between the system and the suction source.

As a general rule, a chest X-ray should always be performed after drain insertion, to confirm position, and after drain removal, to confirm absence of a pneumothorax. Also, it is a safe general rule to never clamp a chest drain apart from during drain bottle changes and after a pneumonectomy, which will be considered separately later in this chapter.

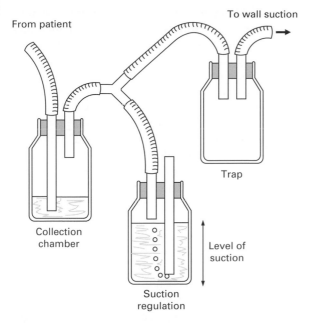

Figure 19.6 Three-bottle system of underwater sealed drainage.

Rigid bronchoscopy

Rigid bronchoscopy is performed under general anaesthetic, and respiration is maintained using a Venturi jet ventilator attached to the bronchoscope. It is performed prior to all pulmonary surgery, to assess the airways and aspirate any secretions. A flexible bronchoscope may also be passed down the rigid instrument. It is the procedure of choice for assessment of massive haemoptysis, foreign body removal, biopsies, stent insertion and laser treatment of endobronchial lesions.

Posterolateral thoracotomy

This is the standard incision used for most thoracic operations. The patient is under general anaesthetic, usually with single lung ventilation via a double lumen endotracheal tube, so that the upper lung may be isolated and collapsed. The patient is placed in the lateral decubitus position and secured in position. The landmarks for the incision are a fingerbreadth below the inferior angle of the scapula, continuing anteriorly horizontally, and posteriorly to a point halfway between the vertebrae and the medial border of the scapula. The latissimus dorsi muscle is cut and serratus anterior may be cut or spared depending upon the size of the incision. The chest is entered usually through the fifth intercostal space although this depends upon

the site of the pathology. The posterior end of the rib is usually divided and a small piece of rib removed to allow easy spreading and so the cut ends of the ribs do not rub together. At the end of the procedure, the ribs are held together with absorbable pericostal sutures, and each layer is then closed separately with absorbable sutures.

An alternative muscle-sparing incision uses retractors to pull the latissimus and serratus muscles apart rather than cutting them, and may result in less postoperative pain but gives less good access.

Anterior thoracotomy

This incision gives access to the anterior mediastinum. It is the incision most often used in trauma cases, and can also be used to obtain lung biopsies in ventilated patients who cannot tolerate single lung ventilation. The patient remains in the supine position, and the incision curves under the breast or nipple along the line of the rib. The chest should be entered via the fourth or fifth intercostal space.

Clamshell incision

An anterior thoracotomy can be continued across the lower end of the sternum to the opposite side, and thus gives excellent access to the whole chest, particularly useful in trauma cases. The xiphisternum can usually be cut with heavy scissors, and it is important to tie off both internal thoracic arteries. Two abdominal retractors can then be placed, one on each side.

Median sternotomy

This is the incision of choice for most cardiac surgery and also for surgery of the anterior mediastinum and some bilateral pulmonary surgery. A midline incision is performed, and the sternum divided with a saw. At the end of the procedure the sternum is reapproximated using wires. This incision is generally less painful than a lateral thoracotomy.

Video-assisted thoracoscopic surgery (VATS)

VATS surgery is generally less painful than a thoracotomy due to lack of rib spreading and less muscle damage. The patient is still prepared and positioned as for a thoracotomy, however, as conversion to an open procedure is always a possibility. The first port is generally introduced in the mid-axillary line in the sixth or seventh interspace after passing a finger into the chest to ensure there are no adhesions present. The camera is then introduced and other ports placed as necessary under vision. The ports are usually placed in an arc pointing to the expected pathology, so the surgeon works forwards, and instrument clashes are avoided. VATS is now the method of choice for management of spontaneous pneumothorax, pleural effusions and lung and pleural biopsies. Pulmonary resections can also be performed. The main disadvantage is the inability to palpate lesions, for example small pulmonary nodules, and this may necessitate conversion to open surgery.

Cervical mediastinoscopy

This procedure is performed under general anaesthetic with the patient positioned supine, but with the neck extended and a roll placed under the shoulders. It is used to biopsy mediastinal masses. A transverse cervical incision is made above the sternal notch, and a combination of sharp and blunt dissection is used down to the trachea. A finger is then inserted to sweep any adhesions away. The mediastinoscope is then inserted, allowing inspection and biopsy of paratracheal lymph nodes and anterior mediastinal masses. There is a small but significant risk (<1%) of major haemorrhage during this procedure and the patient should therefore always be consented for median sternotomy.

Anterior mediastinotomy

Also known as the Chamberlain procedure, this incision allows the inspection and biopsy of anterior mediastinal structures. It is a small anterior thoracotomy, usually through the second intercostal space, but lateral to the internal thoracic artery.

Pulmonary resections

Pulmonary lobectomy is the standard operation for lung cancer. It can be performed if the tumour is confined to the lobe in question, without mediastinal lymph node spread, and the patient is fit enough for the procedure. It involves the identification, ligation and division of the appropriate pulmonary arterial, venous and bronchial branches. It is, however, still a large operation, with mortality rates around 2% even in experienced centres.

Pneumonectomy is the removal of a lung, usually performed for a large or centrally placed tumour which is inoperable by lobectomy. It is, however, a significantly bigger operation with much higher mortality rates of 8–10%. It is therefore important to adequately assess the patient preoperatively to ensure that their lung function is adequate and they will be able to tolerate a pneumonectomy. At the end of the procedure it is common practice to place a drain which is clamped and released once every hour, to check for postoperative haemorrhage. This is usually removed on the first postoperative day, thus allowing the space to gradually fill with fluid. Over time the mediastinum shifts to the operated side, and the fluid gradually becomes more jelly-like in consistency.

An anatomical segmentectomy is a smaller lung resection, of a bronchopulmonary segment, but still requiring identification and division of individual vessels and bronchi.

A wedge resection is a non-anatomical resection of lung tissue using a stapling device. It is performed for biopsy or because a patient is unable to tolerate a bigger anatomical resection.

Complications of thoracic surgery

Apart from the usual complications after any surgery, for example bleeding, wound infection and thromboembolism, there are a number of complications relatively specific to thoracic surgery.

A posterolateral thoracotomy is a painful incision, and thus adequate postoperative analgesia is vital. There are many techniques now available including epidurals, paravertebral and intercostal blocks, as well as the traditional opiate-based intravenous analgesia. A small proportion of patients will experience long-term post-thoracotomy neuralgia and they are probably best managed in conjunction with a pain specialist.

One of the main reasons for good postoperative pain control is the avoidance of sputum retention. Compliance with chest physiotherapy is also vital, and some patients with increased amounts or tenacious sputum, particularly recent smokers, will benefit from the insertion of a minitracheostomy to aid suctioning and bronchial toilet. This is inserted using a Seldinger technique through the cricothyroid membrane.

The aim of these techniques is to prevent lobar and pulmonary collapse. Once a bronchus becomes blocked, the lung beyond it loses aeration and collapses. This leads to infection and mediastinal shift and can rapidly result in respiratory failure in a postoperative patient. Once collapse has occurred a bronchoscopy is usually required in order to aspirate secretions and re-expand the lung.

Arrhythmias are relatively common after thoracic surgery. There are a number of reasons including hypoxia, mediastinal shift and manipulation or opening of the pericardium. The most common arrhythmia is atrial fibrillation, which is now most often treated after correction of any electrolyte imbalance by the administration of oral amiodarone. In some circumstances digoxin or beta-blockers are preferred.

One of the most serious complications following pulmonary surgery is a bronchopleural fistula. This is a breakdown of the bronchial stump anastomosis, due to either infection, tumour regrowth or faulty technique. If an intercostal drain is still in position this will manifest as a large airleak. The most important bronchopleural fistula occurs after a pneumonectomy, when the pneumonectomy space then also becomes infected. Characteristically the patient coughs up copious amounts of serous 'space' fluid and a chest X-ray reveals a drop in the fluid level. Emergency management involves placing the patient with the pneumonectomy space dependent and inserting an intercostal drain to empty the space. After early stump breakdown it may be possible to repair the defect, but in the presence of sepsis it may be necessary to perform formal drainage with a rib resection first. Muscle or omental flaps may also be required to help close the defect.

Surgical emphysema

Surgical emphysema occurs when air is driven into the tissues. It usually follows injury or operation when there is a space, with an air leak into it, for example a pneumothorax, and a communication through the chest wall. Air is driven out into the tissues as the patient coughs.

In the vast majority of cases it is a benign condition but it can track up into the head and neck, and around the eyelids so the patient cannot see, which becomes disconcerting. It can also track around the larynx, causing changes to the voice, and very rarely respiratory obstruction. In most cases it can be treated by the insertion of an intercostal drain on the side of the air leak. The emphysema usually takes several days to subside, however, and the patient should be reassured. Very occasionally if surgical emphysema is particularly severe respiratory compromise can occur

due to restriction of chest wall movement. The skin will become very tense. This is called tension surgical emphysema. If chest drainage does not give relief then stab incisions may be made into the anterior chest wall through the subcutaneous fascia to release some of the air.

Common thoracic surgical conditions

Infection

Empyema

Empyema denotes the collection of pus in a cavity, which is usually taken to be the pleural cavity as this is the most common site. Empyema necessitans develops when pus points through the chest wall due to an untreated empyema.

Empyemas generally evolve in three phases:

1. Exudative: the fluid is thin and contains bacteria and polymorphonuclear cells.
2. Fibropurulent: the fluid is thicker with a turbid appearance and contains some fibrin.
3. Organizing: thick pus with a rind of fibroblasts surrounding both the lung and pleural cavity.

The aetiology of empyema is most commonly an effusion following pneumonia, but it may also be due to a ruptured lung abscess, subphrenic abscess, post-traumatic infected haemothorax, oesophageal perforation, or postoperatively after cardiothoracic surgery.

Physical signs include fever and sweats along with those of a pleural effusion. A chest X-ray demonstrates the presence of a pleural effusion. Empyema is confirmed by the aspiration of pus from the pleural cavity. A CT scan should be performed to assess loculations of fluid and whether there is a cortex of fibrinous material around the lung. Treatment involves the institution of appropriate antibiotics and drainage of the pleural space. In the exudative phase, it is usually possible to drain the empyema by a simple intercostal tube, the insertion of which may be radiologically guided for accurate placement. Once the fibropurulent stage is reached, however, an operation to drain the pleural space is probably required. This may be possible via a VATS technique, involving the breakdown of loculations, aspiration of fluid and exudate, re-expansion of the lung and the placement of intercostal drains.

When the empyema has become organized and the lung is trapped by a fibrin shell the most commonly performed procedure is a formal thoracotomy and decortication, which is a major operation. The fibrin layer is painstakingly peeled off the lung and the chest wall, allowing the lung to fully re-expand. Two or three large-bore intercostal drains are then placed at the end of the procedure. The major risks of the operation include blood loss, which may be considerable, and large air leak due to damage to the underlying lung. In patients who are deemed unfit for such a major procedure, a less invasive alternative is to perform a rib resection and tube thoracostomy, thus allowing long-term drainage of the pleural space. If there is a large residual space, and the patient is fit enough, this may be filled with either a muscle or omental flap. Another alternative is a thoracoplasty, a rarely used technique today. This was originally developed for the treatment of tuberculosis, and involves collapsing the chest wall by rib removal to obliterate the space. It produces a severe chest deformity, however, and often long-term pain as a result.

Bronchiectasis

This is an inflammatory condition of the lobar bronchi, which become dilated and chronically infected. It usually follows a childhood infection, of which pertussis (whooping cough) used to be the most common. Patients have a persistent cough with large amounts of purulent sputum expectorated each morning and sometimes haemoptysis. Treatment includes postural drainage and managing episodes of acute infection with antibiotics. High-resolution CT scans are able to delineate the bronchiectatic areas which can be surgically excised if limited to localized areas, often the middle lobe. More generalized disease requires lifelong medical management.

Lung abscess

A lung abscess is a mass of infected lung tissue which usually contains a cavity and necrotic material. Causes are aspiration, often in alcoholics or under general anaesthesia, post-pneumonic, common in immunosuppressed patients and diabetics, and secondary to regional or distal sepsis, stenosis, or an aspirated foreign body.

Clinical presentation is with foul sputum and an opacity or cavity on chest X-ray. Management is based upon appropriate antibiotic therapy and ensuring free drainage through the bronchial tree. This may involve bronchoscopy to exclude obstructing lesions. Occasionally surgical de-roofing and drainage or resection may be required.

Table 19.2 World Health Organization histologic classification of lung cancer.

Dysplasia/carcinoma *in situ*
Squamous cell carcinoma
Small cell carcinoma
  1. Oat cell carcinoma
  2. Intermediastinal cell type
  3. Combined oat cell carcinoma

Adenocarcinoma
  1. Acinar adenocarcinoma
  2. Papillary adenocarcinoma
  3. Bronchioalveolar carcinoma
  4. Solid carcinoma with mucus formation

Large cell carcinoma variations
  1. Giant cell carcinoma
  2. Clear cell carcinoma

Adenosquamous carcinoma
Carcinoid tumours
Bronchial gland carcinoma
  1. Adenoid cystic carcinoma
  2. Mucoepidermal carcinoma
  3. Others

Lung cancer

Primary bronchogenic carcinoma remains the leading cause of cancer deaths in males and its incidence is still rising in females. The majority of cases, although not all, are due to tobacco smoking. Overall 5-year survival remains dismal at around 10%; however, certain select patient subgroups have a much better prognosis. For practical purposes, bronchogenic carcinoma is divided into small cell and non-small cell carcinoma. The WHO histological classification of lung cancer is shown in Table 19.2.

Small cell carcinoma

Small cell cancers tend to occur centrally and grow rapidly. They metastasize early via the bloodstream and are rarely amenable to surgical resection, but do usually show some response to chemotherapy. They account for approximately 20% of cases of lung cancer overall. Surgical involvement is usually limited to diagnostic purposes only, but if found at an early stage small tumours can be removed with a conventional lung resection, followed by adjuvant chemotherapy postoperatively.

Non-small cell carcinoma

Non-small cell cancers make up the remainder of primary lung cancers. They are mainly divided into squamous cell carcinomas and adenocarcinomas. Squamous cell cancers tend to occur centrally and metastasize via the bloodstream relatively late, whereas adenocarcinomas tend to occur more peripherally but have a great tendency to metastasize earlier. Both types of tumour initially spread via the lymphatic system. The staging of lung cancer involves an assessment of the primary lesion (T), lymph node involvement (N), and presence of distal metastases (M). Lung cancer staging has recently undergone a revision with several changes from the previous system. The new staging system is shown in Table 20.3.

The preferred method of treatment for non-small cell lung cancer is surgical excision. However, this depends upon resectability – the staging of the tumour (can the surgeon remove the tumour) and operability – the fitness of the patient (can the patient survive the operation required). Generally, tumours should be confined to the lung with no spread to mediastinal lymph nodes, although there are certain exceptions to this, including some tumours invading the chest wall, and some upper lobe tumours involving only a single mediastinal lymph node. Also, spread to the mediastinal nodes should be histologically confirmed before denying a patient potentially curative surgery. Some fit patients with locally advanced disease not amenable to surgery can benefit from downstaging chemotherapy and/or radiotherapy with the object of restaging and allowing subsequent resection. The fitness of the patient also plays a huge role. A tumour may be technically resectable by a pneumonectomy but the patient's lung function may prohibit this. Thus both accurate staging and a thorough assessment of the patient are vital. Following lung resection, patients with large tumours or those found to have histological confirmation of lymph node involvement at operation are usually offered adjuvant chemotherapy. Results after lung resection for early lung cancer can offer survival rates as high as 70% at 5 years, although this is significantly reduced by lymph node spread.

Secondary lung tumours

The lung is a common site for tumour metastasis, and these are often multiple, in which case the role of the thoracic surgeon is usually confined to that of diagnosis. However, in certain circumstances pulmonary metastatectomy is becoming an increasingly performed operation. Some tumours have a predilection for metastasis to the lung and these are often either isolated or few in number. If the primary tumour has been well controlled, and there is no evidence of other organ metastases, particularly if there is a significant disease-free interval, then it is worth performing

metastatectomy. Examples of such tumours include colorectal cancer, renal cell carcinoma and osteosarcoma. These often occur in young patients and are therefore treated aggressively with the aim of resecting all the pulmonary lesions but preserving as much lung tissue as possible.

Malignant pleural effusion

The presence of a malignant pleural effusion signifies incurable disease. Treatment should therefore be aimed at symptomatic relief. They often appear insidiously and patients typically present with increasing dyspnoea with or without an unproductive cough. Patients who have recurrent effusions with a reasonable level of fitness and who are expected to live at least a few months should be offered thoracoscopic drainage with biopsy and talc pleurodesis, for both diagnosis and symptomatic relief. Patients who are not fit enough for surgery may still benefit from talc pleurodesis instilled via an intercostal drain. Pleurodesis only works if the lung is able to re-expand and thus is in contact with the chest wall. If the lung is trapped by tumour and unable to expand, a long-term drain or indwelling pleural catheter may be required.

Pleural tumours

Primary malignant pleural mesothelioma is unfortunately becoming more common due to its association with prior asbestos exposure. Even though asbestos has now largely been removed from industry, the lag time of 20 to 30 years prior to mesothelioma development means there is still some way to go yet before the expected peak in the number of cases. Patients usually present with increasing shortness of breath, often caused by effusion, and local chest pain. Diagnosis is usually by either thoracoscopic or open pleural biopsy. Unfortunately the prognosis in patients with mesothelioma is extremely poor. Very few patients are amenable to surgery and overall results are disappointing.

Spontaneous pneumothorax

Spontaneous pneumothoraces may be divided into primary and secondary categories.

Primary pneumothoraces tend to occur in young thin adults, more often in males than females, and are usually due to the rupture of a bleb at the apex of the upper lobe. Their aetiology remains uncertain; however, they are more common in smokers, and are particularly prevalent at times of change in barometric pressure. They may follow minor infection with patchy fibrosis and resultant contraction of the lung surface. There is also an association with Marfan's syndrome, and in women at the onset of menses (catamenial pneumothorax).

The clinical presentation of a spontaneous pneumothorax is usually the sudden onset of pleuritic chest pain and shortness of breath. This is confirmed by either reduced or absent breath sounds on the affected side, and confirmed by a chest X-ray.

If the pneumothorax has a less than 2 cm rim of air on a chest X-ray and is not causing respiratory compromise it may simply be observed. If larger than this or the patient is breathless, current guidelines state that aspiration should be performed. If this is not successful or the pneumothorax is large, an intercostal drain should be placed.

After a first spontaneous pneumothorax there is a 20% chance of a further episode, but this increases to 70% after a second episode and up to 90% after a third episode. Spontaneous pneumothorax is rarely fatal, but takes up a considerable number of hospital beds and time off work for an otherwise young and healthy population. The indications for definitive surgical treatment are: tension pneumothorax, haemopneumothorax, unresolving airleak or failure of the lung to re-expand after a first-time pneumothorax (>5 days), two ipsilateral pneumothoraces, or bilateral pneumothoraces. In addition, certain groups of patients require surgery after a single episode, for example people working in the aviation industry, divers and those travelling to remote areas with unpredictable medical services.

Surgery for primary pneumothorax is usually performed by video-assisted thoracoscopic (VATS) techniques, and involves two main components. Firstly, the lung is examined for blebs, which are usually apparent at the upper lobe apex. This area is then excised using an endoscopic stapler. Even if a bleb is not identified, most thoracic surgeons recommend still stapling the lung apex. The second component of the procedure is to perform a parietal pleurectomy. The parietal pleura is stripped from the chest wall, predominantly over the apex and upper chest, with the aim of creating a raw surface area for the re-expanded lung to adhere to. Either one or two intercostal drains are placed at the end of the procedure, and these are removed usu-

ally after approximately 48 hours. The introduction of VATS techniques has allowed a much swifter recovery time postoperatively, with success rates generally over 95%. Operative risks still include bleeding, conversion to open thoracotomy and postoperative pain due to intercostal neuralgia, however.

Spontaneous haemopneumothorax is a relatively uncommon condition but life-threatening if undiagnosed. Usually an apical adhesion is torn as the lung deflates, and this continues to bleed, often with hidden blood loss inside the chest. Any chest X-ray in a patient with a spontaneous pneumothorax but also with a fluid level should always undergo intercostal drain insertion, and the diagnosis of haemopneumothorax be considered. Treatment consists of an emergency thoracotomy with evacuation of haematoma and haemostasis of the bleeding point.

Secondary pneumothoraces tend to occur in older patients, and are due to underlying lung disease. This is usually emphysema with multiple bullae within the lung tissue, and the pneumothorax is caused by rupture of one of them. Other causes include pneumonia, malignancy, *Pneumocystis carinii* infection, granulomas and lymphangioleiomyomatosis. A CT scan is often helpful in planning the management of these patients, in particular with regard to the condition of the underlying lung. Generally patients are more likely to be managed conservatively, depending upon their fitness for surgery. An operation for secondary pneumothorax is more likely to be via a full thoracotomy as opposed to VATS techniques due to the complexity of the underlying disease process. In older patients pleurodesis is usually achieved by instilling sterilized talc into the pleural cavity. This acts as an irritant and allows the lung to adhere to the chest wall. Talc pleurodesis may also be performed at the bedside via an intercostal drain in patients considered unfit for a major operation.

Thoracic trauma

Fifty per cent of fatalities due to trauma have significant thoracic injuries. However, most thoracic injuries can be managed conservatively with admission to hospital for analgesia and possible intercostal drain insertion, and only around 5% require operative intervention.

There are six complications of thoracic trauma which can be rapidly fatal:

Airway obstruction. Re-establishing a patent airway is the number one priority. This may require either endotracheal intubation or rarely an emergency surgical airway.

Tension pneumothorax results in lung collapse, mediastinal shift to the contralateral side and severe haemodynamic compromise. Emergency treatment consists of the placement of a large-bore cannula into the second intercostal space anteriorly, in the mid-clavicular line, on the affected side. This should be followed by the insertion of an intercostal drain.

Open pneumothorax is usually easily recognized, and should be controlled initially by placement of a pad taped on three sides or a proprietary chest-seal dressing depending upon availability, again followed by the insertion of an intercostal drain.

Massive haemothorax presents with shock and hypoxia. Initial management consists of fluid resuscitation and intercostal drainage, but may require emergency thoracotomy in the event of continued bleeding.

Flail chest is defined by the fracture of two or more ribs in two or more places. This causes inefficient respiration due to instability of the chest wall and paradoxical movement. Primary treatment consists of adequate analgesia, for example a thoracic epidural or intercostal nerve blocks, and physiotherapy. Positive pressure ventilation may be required. Occasionally fixation is performed either because the instability is so great, or because there are other indications for operation.

Cardiac tamponade should be suspected in a shocked patient who fails to respond to fluid resuscitation. The usual signs of hypotension, muffled heart sounds and raised jugular venous pressure (Beck's triad) are easily masked in a busy emergency unit, and therefore diagnosis relies upon a high index of suspicion. Diagnosis is by trans-thoracic echocardiography or surgical exploration. Pericardiocentesis should only be performed in the trauma setting if there is an inevitable delay to surgical exploration and release of tamponade. Pericardiocentesis should never delay surgery as in trauma pericardiocentesis may be negative, in the presence of tamponade, due to blood clots. The technique for pericardiocentesis involves placing the needle 2 cm inferior to the xiphoid process, slightly to the left of the midline, at an angle of 45° heading towards the left shoulder.

Other serious thoracic sequelae of trauma include:

Traumatic aortic disruption, which usually occurs just distal to the left subclavian artery where the relatively mobile aortic arch becomes fixed at the descending aorta. This is due to a rapid deceleration injury and is often immediately fatal. Only a small percentage of survivors reach hospital, due to containment of the rupture by the aortic adventitia, which may itself rupture at a later date. A non-specific sign is mediastinal widening on chest X-ray, but diagnosis is now achieved in the vast majority of cases by contrast-enhanced CT scanning. Management options include either operative repair or, increasingly more commonly, endovascular stent placement, depending upon the other injuries of the patient and local expertise. Pending assessment heart rate and blood pressure should be managed to avoid tachycardia and hypertension.

Tracheobronchial rupture occurs in the lower main trachea or major bronchi, also usually as the result of a deceleration injury. There will be a pneumothorax with potentially a massive air-leak on the side involved, and possibly also haemoptysis. Surgical exploration and repair are required.

Oesophageal rupture is relatively uncommon as a result of trauma but may occur as a result of penetrating injury, or compression of the chest with a closed glottis. Treatment is usually by surgical repair.

Diaphragmatic rupture is generally due to abdominal compression and usually occurs on the left side, due to the relative protection of the right side afforded by the liver. It is often associated with abdominal injuries and therefore generally best repaired via laparotomy. It can be missed on CT scan and can sometimes present late as eventration of the diaphragm on chest X-ray. Diagnosis by thoracoscopy may then be required.

Pulmonary contusions are common after thoracic trauma. They do not require specific treatment other than respiratory support, which may include positive pressure ventilation.

Myocardial contusion may affect the right ventricle, which lies directly behind the sternum. Diagnosis is by transthoracic echocardiography and inotropic support may sometimes be required. Sternal fractures indicate significant injury and associated myocardial contusion should be excluded. They rarely require fixation.

Rib fractures are common after thoracic trauma. Treatment consists of adequate analgesia and physiotherapy. Fractures of the first or second rib indicate significant trauma, and other major injury needs to be excluded.

Emergency thoracotomy following thoracic trauma

There are relatively few indications for emergency thoracotomy following thoracic trauma, but the general surgeon and emergency room physician need to be aware of them and be able to perform emergency thoracotomy as it can be life-saving. Often specialist cardiothoracic surgical assistance is not immediately at hand, and temporizing measures need to be taken until further assistance can be obtained.

Indications for emergency thoracotomy include cardiac tamponade, exsanguinating intrathoracic haemorrhage, massive airleak and cardiac arrest, with witnessed signs of life at the scene of the incident. Thoracotomy for penetrating chest trauma has a higher chance of success than blunt trauma.

The operative approach taken depends upon the individual skills of the operator, available equipment and likely injuries. In most circumstances the initial incision will be a left anterior thoracotomy, through the fourth or fifth intercostal space, which may easily be converted into a bilateral clamshell incision for further exposure. Alternatively a median sternotomy can be performed if the appropriate technical expertise and equipment are available. It is important to note that the pericardium should be widely opened to inspect the heart and perform adequate internal cardiac massage.

Further reading

Goldstraw P, Crowley J, Chansky K *et al.* The IASLC Lung Cancer Staging Project: proposals for the revision of the TNM Stage groupings in the forthcoming (seventh) edition of the TNM classification of malignant tumours. *J Thorac Oncol* 2007;**2**:706–714.

Henry M, Arnold T, Harvey J. BTS guidelines for the management of spontaneous pneumothorax. *Thorax* 2003;**58**(Suppl II):ii39–ii52.

Laws D, Neville E, Duffy J. BTS guidelines for the insertion of a chest drain. *Thorax* 2003;**58**(Suppl II): ii53–ii59.

Maskell NA, Butland RJA. BTS guidelines for the investigation of a unilateral pleural effusion in adults. *Thorax* 2003;**58**(Suppl II):ii8–ii17.

McMinn RMH. *Last's Anatomy*. 9th edn. Churchill Livingstone, 1994.

Patterson GA, Cooper JD, Deslauriers J *et al. Pearson's Thoracic and Esophageal Surgery*. Churchill Livingstone Elsevier, 2008.

Chapter

20

Oesophago-gastric surgery

Tim Wheatley

Anatomy

Oesophagus

The oesophagus is 25 cm long, extending from the pharynx to the cardia. It lies in the posterior mediastinum, and is traditionally divided into upper, middle and lower thirds. The upper third is closely related anteriorly to the trachea, down to the carina. The middle third extends from the carina to approximately 7 cm above the diaphragmatic hiatus, and is related anteriorly to the pericardium. The lower third extends through the hiatus to include a short segment of intra-abdominal oesophagus, and is related (in the thorax) to the left atrium. The oesophagus receives its blood supply via direct branches from the aorta, and branches from other organs such as thyroid, trachea and stomach. Venous drainage is via the azygos and hemiazygos veins. The vagus nerves lie closely applied to the surface of the oesophagus, and it must be remembered that the right recurrent laryngeal branch arises in the upper thorax, passing around the subclavian artery, and the left recurrent laryngeal branch passes around the ductus arteriosus. These branches can be injured during surgery on the upper oesophagus. The oesophageal hiatus is surrounded by the crura, pillars of diaphragmatic muscle that help contribute to the lower oesophageal sphincter. A hiatus hernia involves herniation of the proximal stomach through this area, and can predispose to gastro-oesophageal reflux. Giant hiatus hernia can occur where most, or all, of the stomach herniates into the thoracic cavity.

Stomach

The normal stomach is impalpable with the fundus lying underneath the left diaphragm. The body of a

stomach distended secondary to gastric outlet obstruction may be visible and palpable and a succussion splash may be heard from it. Gastric masses are rarely palpable and if at this stage they represent a malignant process, they will invariably be inoperable. The stomach has a rich blood supply which comprises the left gastric artery from the coeliac axis, the right gastric artery from the common hepatic artery, the right gastroepiploic artery from the gastroduodenal branch of the hepatic artery, the left gastroepiploic artery from the splenic artery and the short gastric arteries from the splenic artery. When the stomach is used as a conduit in the chest following oesophagectomy, the left gastric, left gastroepiploic and short gastric arteries are divided and the organ suffers no ischaemic damage. Corresponding veins drain into the portal venous system and the lymphatic drainage follows perigastric glands and thence to groups around the spleen, aorta, retropancreatic, suprapancreatic and subpyloric zones.

Investigations

Some of the investigations that can be used in the investigation of oesophago-gastric conditions are described below. These do not replace a carefully taken history, but do provide a very useful adjunct to clinical examination, and it is important to understand the uses and limitations of the various techniques.

Endoscopy

Upper GI endoscopy is a vital investigation for imaging the upper GI tract, and is sometimes referred to as OGD (oesophago-gastro-duodenoscopy). Using flexible endoscopes it is possible to directly visualize the oesophagus, stomach and duodenum to check for mucosal abnormality and obtain biopsies. Modern video-endoscopes project the image onto a

Fundamentals of Surgical Practice, Third Edition, ed. Andrew N. Kingsnorth and Douglas M. Bowley.
Published by Cambridge University Press. © Cambridge University Press 2011.

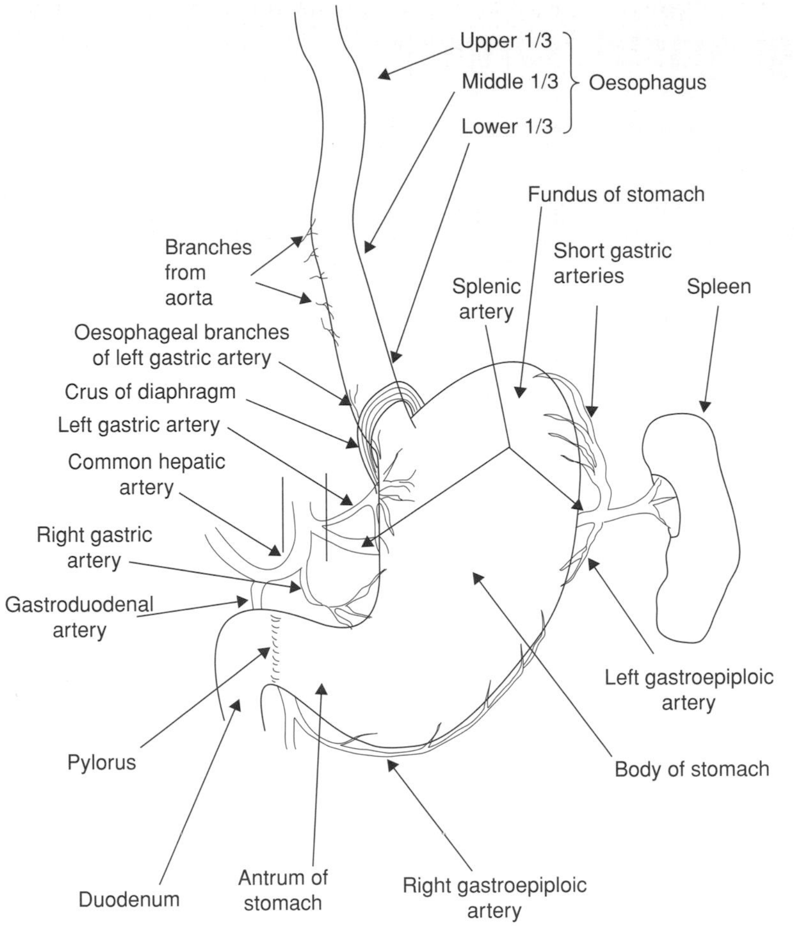

Figure 20.1 Anatomy of the oesophagus and the stomach.

monitor, allowing easier use, more accurate diagnosis and the ability to record photographic and video images. Endoscopy is not only diagnostic, but interventional as well, and has become first-line treatment for many causes of upper GI bleeding. Oesophageal strictures can be dilated, obstructing cancers can be stented and polyps and early cancers can be resected. Most endoscopy can be performed using simple anaesthetic throat spray, but sedation (and occasionally general anaesthesia) is required for some patients and procedures. Rigid oesophagoscopy performed under general anaesthesia may rarely be required for removal of foreign bodies. Morbidity and mortality are rare but include bleeding and perforation – which are more common with interventional techniques.

Contrast radiology

Endoscopy has become the common, first-line investigation for symptoms of dysphagia and dyspepsia, but contrast studies still have a role in some cases of dysphagia, defining anatomy of complex strictures and hiatus herniae, and illustrating perforations and anastomotic leaks. Barium is the contrast medium most commonly used, but less viscous agents (Gastromiro, Gastrografin) are preferable in suspected perforation or leak, as barium may cause a severe reaction in such situations. Oesophageal and gastro-oesophageal junction (GOJ) pathology would be visualized by a barium swallow, gastric pathology by a barium meal.

Endoscopic ultrasound (EUS)

The use of high-frequency sound waves (frequencies of 1–5 MHz) to image soft tissues is safe, effective and widely available. Small ultrasound probes at the end of a flexible endoscope are used to provide images of oesophageal and gastric wall structure as well as local lymph nodes. Radial EUS probes are used widely for T and N staging (see Malignancy) of oesophago-gastric

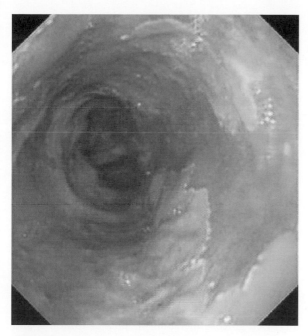

Figure 20.2 Endoscopic view of Barrett's mucosa in the distal oesophagus.

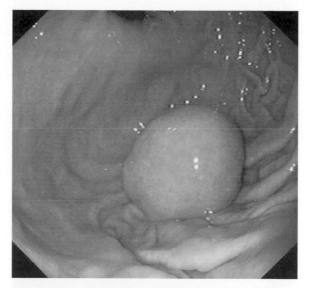

Figure 20.3 Endoscopic view of a gastrointestinal stromal tumour (GIST) in the stomach.

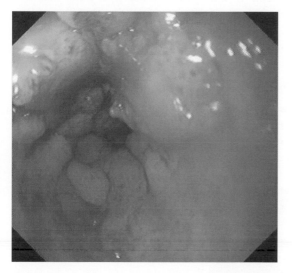

Figure 20.4 Endoscopic view of an oesophageal cancer.

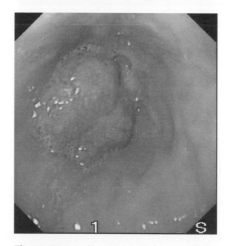

Figure 20.5 Endoscopic view of an oesophageal cancer causing obstruction.

tumours, and linear probes can be used to provide EUS-guided biopsy of oesophageal and gastric lymph nodes.

Computed tomography (CT)

CT scanning relies on multiple X-ray images taken as 'slices' and reconfigured under computer control to display cross-sectional images of the body. Early scanners were slow and resolution was poor for structures measuring less than 1 cm, but newer scanners are much quicker, using spiral scanning techniques, and provide greatly improved resolution. It is relatively straightforward with current technology to create computerized 3D images to allow easier appreciation of anatomy. CT scans of solid organs, such as the liver, spleen and pancreas, are useful for both benign and malignant lesions; and staging of oesophago-gastric cancers relies heavily on CT scans of the chest, abdomen and pelvis. CT scanning is much less operator-dependent than ultrasound, and does not

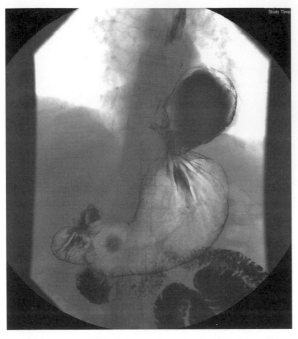

Figure 20.6 Barium meal showing hiatus hernia with fundus and proximal body of the stomach lying above the diaphragm.

require real-time images for accurate interpretation. As with ultrasound it is possible to perform interventional procedures (biopsy, drain insertion) under CT guidance.

Positron emission tomography (PET)

PET imaging utilizes a gamma camera to detect radio-nuclides, such as 18F-fluorodeoxyglucose (FDG), which are produced in a cyclotron and have a very

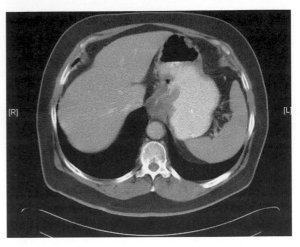

Figure 20.7 Computed tomography (CT) scan demonstrating a large cancer of the gastro-oesophageal junction.

short half-life. FDG uptake is high in tissues with increased glucose metabolism, such as tumours, and FDG PET scanning is becoming commonplace for staging oesophageal cancers, in spite of the logistic problems inherent with producing the radio-nuclides. PET scanning is often combined with CT scanning (PET-CT) and has proved very accurate at detecting metastatic disease not seen on other modalities.

Oesophageal function tests

Oesophageal motility and acid exposure can be measured very accurately to provide useful information on oesophageal disorders. Most surgeons would insist on oesophageal function studies being performed

Figure 20.8 Endoscopic ultrasound (EUS) view of a T3N1 oesophageal cancer.

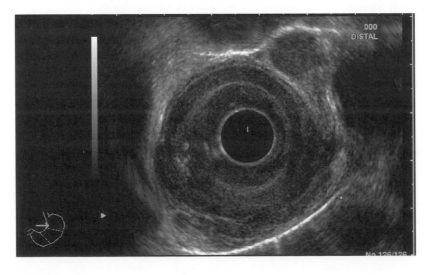

before considering a patient for anti-reflux surgery. These investigations are performed by trained individuals and require careful interpretation by a specialist.

Manometry

Intra-oesophageal pressure readings are measured using catheters with multiple fluid-filled channels, or miniature pressure transducers. Manometry is commonly performed in a laboratory over a very short time period. It is possible to carry out 24-hour ambulatory assessments, which may be combined with pH studies, for a more representative view of motility. Primary peristalsis is initiated by swallowing and progresses from the pharynx, terminating in relaxation of the lower oesophageal sphincter. Secondary peristalsis is initiated by distension of the oesophagus (e.g. by food bolus) and progresses in a similar fashion. Tertiary contractions do not result in peristaltic waves, and occur as isolated, sporadic events. Motility disorders include: achalasia, where failure of both normal peristaltic activity and relaxation of the lower oesophageal sphincter results in dysphagia and a dilated oesophagus proximal to the gastro-oesophageal junction; and diffuse oesophageal spasm, where isolated high-pressure contractions cause chest pain. A low-pressure lower oesophageal sphincter is commonly seen in gastro-oesophageal reflux disease.

pH monitoring

Intra-oesophageal pH is measured with a transducer positioned 5 cm above the manometrically determined lower oesophageal sphincter. Ambulatory readings are taken over a 24- or 48-hour period, and correlated with symptoms recorded by the patient. Normally the pH is less than 4 for no more than 4% of a 24-hour period, but with significant reflux the percentage is much higher. Some patients have a normal percentage of pH <4, but very good correlation between reflux episodes and symptoms, which often indicates significant reflux. Others have pH <4 for more than 4% of the period measured, but no correlation with symptoms, suggesting reflux is an incidental finding. It is important that pH studies are interpreted carefully, and correlated with the patient's history.

Impedance monitoring

This technique detects fluid regurgitation into the oesophagus, rather than the presence of acid. As such it can be very useful at demonstrating 'volume' reflux,

Table 20.1 Causes of upper GI bleeding, and relative frequency

35%	Peptic ulcer
25%	No cause found
19%	Oesophageal cause – oesophagitis, varices, Mallory-Weiss
11%	Gastric erosions
6%	Rare causes – vascular malformation, Dieulafoy lesion, haemobilia, aorto-duodenal fistula
4%	Malignancy

particularly when the refluxate is not acidic. The results need more careful interpretation than pH studies, but can be very useful in patients with atypical symptoms, normal pH studies in the presence of good history, and following failed anti-reflux surgery.

OG emergencies

Upper GI bleeding

Bleeding from the upper GI tract places a high demand on medical services, because of both the number of admissions to hospital and the often complex, multidisciplinary approach required to treat those with significant bleeds. In the 1990s the incidence of upper GI bleeding was 103 cases per 100 000 population, and the in-patient mortality was 14%. One-quarter of those presenting to hospital with a bleed are over 80 years old, which is a significant contributory factor to this high mortality rate. About a third of all bleeds are due to peptic ulcers, with a variety of other causes listed in Table 20.1.

The majority of patients present with overt bleeding in the form of haematemesis and/or melaena, or more rarely with fresh bleeding per rectum. Haematemesis may produce fresh blood, as commonly seen with varices, or altered blood (coffee grounds) from a slowly bleeding ulcer. Melaena occurs when blood is partially digested during passage through the GI tract, resulting in a black, liquid stool with an unmistakable, foul smell. The passage of fresh blood per rectum from an upper GI source is a very worrying feature, as it implies a significant bleed causing rapid transit through the gut without time for melaena to form.

Some patients present with covert bleeding and are investigated for collapse or anaemia. In time it becomes obvious that they are bleeding, either by the

Table 20.2 Rockall scoring system for upper GI bleeding

Age	<60 yrs 0	60–79 yrs 1	>80 yrs 2
Shock	None 0	Systolic BP >100 Pulse >100 1	Systolic BP <100 2
Comorbidity	None 0	Major comorbidity (ischaemic heart disease etc.) 1	Renal or hepatic failure Disseminated malignancy 2
Endoscopic diagnosis	No lesion, or Mallory-Weiss 0	All other lesions 1	Upper GI cancer 2
Stigmata of recent haemorrhage	None 0		Blood in upper GI tract, adherent clot, visible vessel, active bleeding 2

Total score ≤3 → predicted low mortality.
Total score ≥8 → predicted high mortality.

appearance of overt bleeding or as a result of endoscopic investigation.

The initial management of patients with bleeding is resuscitation appropriate to the severity of their condition. Most patients have a minor episode of bleeding and are never haemodynamically compromised by it, but others lose a lot of blood relatively quickly and require prompt resuscitation. Patients who have lost a lot of blood will be tachycardic initially, and hypotensive as blood loss increases. Tachypnoea develops as oxygen delivery decreases, and at the same time conscious level is affected, leading to restlessness, irritability, drowsiness and even unconsciousness. Oxygen supplementation is often required, and intravenous fluid replacement must start immediately in patients who are compromised. It is important to remember that many patients take beta-blockers regularly, so will not show a tachycardia, and that younger people can maintain their blood pressure well with significant blood loss so tachycardia is an important sign. Whether the intravenous fluid used is crystalloid or colloid is less important than the amount given, and it is important to have good venous access (two large-bore cannulae). If a lot of blood has been lost the best resuscitation fluid is blood, even O-negative if there is no time for a cross-match. A clotting screen must always be performed on patients with bleeding, and those who require active resuscitation benefit from central venous pressure monitoring and urethral catheterization with hourly urine output measurement.

Once patients have been stabilized the next step is diagnosing the cause of the bleeding, so that definitive treatment can be started. The single most important investigation for upper GI bleeding is endoscopy, and hospitals require 24-hour access to endoscopy facilities. Ideally all patients with a bleed should have an endoscopy performed within 24 hours of admission irrespective of the severity of the bleed and this needs to be done by an experienced endoscopist. Endoscopy should provide a diagnosis of the cause of the bleeding, and may allow treatment. Endoscopic findings, combined with clinical features, can be used in scoring systems to predict patients at high risk of both further bleeding, and poor prognosis (Table 20.2).

Endoscopic management of upper GI bleeding employs a variety of different techniques to arrest bleeding. Oesophageal varices have traditionally been injected with ethanolamine or sodium tetradecyl sulphate (STD); currently elastic bands are used to ligate varices using devices attached to flexible endoscopes. Results from variceal banding are generally better than injection sclerotherapy, especially as banding devices have become easier to use. Bleeding peptic ulcers can be treated by injection, coagulation or clips. Injection therapy has been tried with many different agents: adrenaline, alcohol, STD, tissue glue and fibrin are the commonly used ones. Coagulation can be achieved with diathermy (bipolar, monopolar or argon beam), laser energy or heat probe. All coagulation techniques rely on heating tissue, though they differ in how that heat is generated. Clipping devices are available that allow small metal clips to be delivered down the working channel of flexible endoscopes.

Endoscopic management of bleeding is accepted as first-line treatment in patients who are stable enough to tolerate it. It has been shown to decrease transfusion requirements, reduce the likelihood of re-bleeding, and decrease the need for surgery (Sung *et al.* 2007). Whether it decreases the mortality rate from bleeding is less certain. If endoscopic treatment fails the options for further treatment depend on the individual circumstances. If varices re-bleed after banding, then repeat banding should be performed. If primary control of variceal bleeding cannot be achieved then balloon tamponade with a Sengstaken-Blakemore or Minnesota tube should be attempted. These tubes have a large, distal balloon which is inflated in the stomach, and pulled back to lodge at the gastro-oesophageal junction. The more proximal oesophageal ballon is then inflated, thus compressing the cardia and distal oesophagus to tamponade varices. If this fails then trans-jugular intrahepatic portal-systemic shunting (TIPSS) will lower the portal venous pressure, and is very useful for preventing re-bleeding and stopping primary bleeding. If TIPSS is unavailable or unsuccessful then surgery with oesophageal transection using a circular staple gun is an option, but these days is rarely required. For bleeding ulcers the choice is more straightforward: if bleeding cannot be controlled at the first endoscopy then surgery is necessary, and if the patient re-bleeds then it may be worth trying further endoscopic treatment, but surgery is often more appropriate.

Surgery for bleeding ulcers has one main aim – to secure haemostasis. The bleeding point must first be displayed adequately, and a good preoperative endoscopy is invaluable for identifying the anatomical location of the bleed. A gastrotomy or duodenotomy is performed depending on where the lesion is, and the bleeding point is controlled by under-running the area with multiple sutures. If the lesion is a gastric ulcer then a biopsy must be taken, because of the risk of malignancy, and it may be possible to excise the ulcer and close the resulting gastric defect. It is usually unnecessary to perform a definitive anti-ulcer operation as an emergency, as medical management for peptic ulcers is currently preferable.

The successful management of upper GI bleeding requires close cooperation between physicians, endoscopists and surgeons, and benefits from clear, local guidelines outlining management pathways. Although the majority of patients presenting with bleeds will settle with minimal treatment, the 10–20% who do not need early, co-ordinated management to minimize mortality rates.

Perforated viscus

The oesophagus, stomach and duodenum can all suffer from perforation, and by far the commonest cause of an upper GI perforation is a peptic ulcer in either the stomach or duodenum.

Perforated peptic ulcer

Complications of peptic ulcer disease are now much less common than 20 years ago due to improved medical management (see Peptic ulcer, below), but perforations still imply a mortality of approximately 10% (higher in older patients) (Hermansson *et al.* 2009). The well-recognized risk factors for developing a perforated ulcer are long-term non-steroidal anti-inflammatory drug (NSAID) use and *Helicobacter pylori* infection.

The usual presentation is a sudden onset of severe epigastric pain, followed quickly by signs of peritonitis. Patients with perforated ulcers will lie still with a 'rigid abdomen', are often pale and clammy, and may show hypotension, tachycardia, tachypnoea and pyrexia. Breathing will be shallow as well as rapid because of peritonitis. Sometimes in elderly patients and those taking steroids the early symptoms may be mild or absent. The initial peritonitis is chemical due to the presence of gastric and/or duodenal fluid in the peritoneal cavity, but within hours a bacterial peritonitis supervenes. Delays in appropriate treatment being started result in higher mortality and morbidity – after 24 hours the mortality rate has increased by seven times.

The diagnosis is made on clinical grounds, and supported by the presence of free gas seen under the diaphragm on an erect chest X-ray, but it must be remembered that 20–30% of perforations do not show free gas. If the diagnosis is in doubt a left lateral, decubitus abdominal X-ray may show free gas more clearly against the liver, and contrast studies with water-soluble agents can confirm an ongoing leak from a perforation. Ultrasound and CT examinations may show free intraperitoneal fluid, and/or localized collections in late presentations, but are not part of the usual work-up of this condition.

The management of perforated ulcers includes initial resuscitation, treatment of the perforation and treatment of the ulcer. Resuscitation and optimization requires intravenous fluids and antibiotics, urethral catheterization to aid accurate fluid balance, nasogastric drainage, oxygen by facemask and prompt, adequate analgesia (usually opiates). A variety of options are available for treating the perforation and are classified as conservative or surgical.

Conservative treatment relies on the fact that perforations have a tendency to seal themselves (up to 50% are sealed at the time of presentation) and seeks to provide conditions for spontaneous healing to occur and persist, while also dealing with intra-abdominal sepsis. IV fluids, antibiotics and acid anti-secretory drugs (H_2 blockers or proton pump inhibitors) are given, and patients are kept under close review. Contrast studies are helpful here to confirm sealed leaks, and ultrasound/CT scanning will show collections, which may then be drained percutaneously. A low threshold to revert to surgical management is important for those patients who deteriorate or fail to improve.

Surgical treatment has two main aims: to close the perforation, and to deal with intra-abdominal sepsis. Surgery used also to include definitive treatment for the ulcer in the form of vagotomy and pyloroplasty, partial gastrectomy or other anti-ulcer procedures. With current medical management being so effective, it is unusual to perform such procedures, unless the ulcer is too large to close adequately or the ulcer has failed to respond to maximum medical treatment already. The majority of surgeons will deal with perforations at laparotomy, though it is possible to obtain similar results with a laparoscopic approach in certain cases. At laparotomy the perforation must first be identified, sometimes requiring exploration of the lesser sac to see the posterior wall of the stomach. Once the perforation has been found it may be closed by interrupted sutures, but if this is not possible a patch of omentum is sutured over the defect, taking care not to render the omentum ischaemic. Even after suture closure an omental patch should be performed as additional security. If the ulcer is in the stomach then a biopsy from its edge must be taken to exclude the possibility of malignancy. Thorough peritoneal lavage is performed, and there is no benefit in using solutions containing antibiotics or antiseptics compared to sterile water or normal saline. Whether to leave a drain in the abdomen is contentious, as it may be linked to increased morbidity, but many surgeons do drain the peritoneum after laparotomy.

Once the perforation has been successfully dealt with, the peptic ulcer must be treated with full medical management as described below. This will include eradication of *H. pylori* if present, stopping NSAIDs as appropriate (or switching to alternative analgesia) and a healing course of anti-secretory medication.

Perforated oesophagus

The oesophagus may rupture spontaneously during vomiting (Boerhaave syndrome), but by far the commonest cause of perforation is iatrogenic. Instrumentation of the oesophagus is increasingly common, at both diagnostic endoscopy and therapeutic intervention for strictures, achalasia and even endoscopic resections. The perforation rate varies from around 0.001% for diagnostic, flexible endoscopy, up to 5% for balloon dilatation for achalasia.

Patients complain of pain, which they can localize quite accurately to the level of the perforation. Surgical emphysema may develop within a few hours of perforation, as well as a high temperature. A history of recent oesophageal intubation or vomiting raises suspicion, and a perforation can be confirmed by plain chest X-ray, contrast swallow or sometimes repeat endoscopy. Prompt diagnosis and treatment are crucial to reducing mortality, which may be as high as 50%. Conservative management with antibiotics, parenteral nutrition and percutaneous drainage may be suitable for small, uncomplicated perforations in an otherwise healthy oesophagus. Larger perforations, and those with associated oesophageal pathology (e.g. cancer), benefit from early intervention, to either repair or resect the affected oesophagus. If surgery is indicated it is best performed within the first 12 hours following perforation, before mediastinal sepsis is established.

Oesophageal foreign body/bolus obstruction

Foreign bodies (coins, batteries, anything small enough to swallow) and food bolus (usually poorly chewed meat) can impact in the oesophagus, causing both dysphagia and/or odynophagia. The site of impaction may coincide with existing pathology, such as a tumour or peptic stricture, or at anatomically narrow areas, such as the cricopharyngeus or the gastro-oesophageal junction. The history is usually diagnostic, except in young children; plain X-ray films and contrast swallow may help to confirm and localize the problem. Anti-spasmodics (Buscopan) may encourage passage of the obstructing object, but more commonly oesophagoscopy is required. Flexible endoscopes can be used to push food boluses into the stomach, and various grasping devices and baskets are available to retrieve objects. Rigid oesophagoscopy under general anaesthesia is sometimes required to enable larger graspers to be used on more awkward objects. If there has been any suggestion of dysphagia prior to the episode of obstruction or evidence of oesophageal pathology at the time of endoscopic management, then an early, repeat endoscopy must be arranged to exclude an underlying condition, such as a tumour or peptic stricture, which will require further treatment.

OG malignancy

Oesophageal carcinoma

Cancer of the oesophagus has an incidence of 5–10 cases per 100 000 people in Western countries, but this varies widely throughout the rest of the world, and may get as high as 150–200 per 100 000 in parts of China and Iran. Worryingly, the incidence is increasing sharply, especially for tumours of the distal third of the oesophagus, and at the gastro-oesophageal junction. Men are twice as likely to be affected as women, and people in their 60s and 70s are at highest risk. Aetiological factors are multiple, but oesophagitis is a common link, while smoking, alcohol ingestion and nitrosamines in foodstuffs have all been implicated. Metaplasia of normal squamous epithelium to columnar (Barrett's oesophagus) is a significant risk factor for adenocarcinoma, and as Barrett's is linked to gastro-oesophageal reflux disease (GORD) the increasing incidence of GORD may partly explain the rise in number of oesophageal cancer cases.

The commonest presentation of oesophageal cancer is dysphagia, which is progressive. Initially patients notice that certain solid foods stick as they swallow, then they become unable to swallow solids and rely on soft, sloppy foods, then they can only tolerate liquids, until eventually complete dysphagia develops and they cannot even swallow their own saliva. Dysphagia is a very distressing symptom, and is invariably linked with weight loss, which worsens as dysphagia progresses. Tiredness and lethargy develop, linked both to the gradual starvation and to anaemia from chronic low-grade blood loss. Occasionally patients are diagnosed during investigation for anaemia, at endoscopy for other upper GI symptoms and from screening programmes for Barrett's oesophagus.

Barium swallow may show features of a malignant stricture, or an irregular mucosa, but endoscopy is essential for visualization of the tumour and obtaining biopsies for histological diagnosis. Once a cancer has been confirmed further management depends on the patient's suitability for surgery, the stage of the cancer and, of course, the patient's wishes. Surgical resection of oesophageal cancer is a major undertaking and carries a mortality rate of 5–10% (lower in specialized centres), and significant comorbidity, especially cardiorespiratory, increases this to unacceptable levels. If patients are fit enough for surgery then they will undergo staging investigations, otherwise they will require palliative care to control symptoms. Palliation of dysphagia can been achieved by physical methods such as dilatation, alcohol injection, laser re-canalization and stenting, the latter two being the commonest methods employed currently. Stenting was revolutionized by the introduction of self-expanding metal stents (SEMS) that are introduced on a small-diameter trocar over a guide-wire placed across the cancer, and then deployed to expand to a much larger diameter over a period of 12–24 hours. SEMS are best used in patients with at least dysphagia to solids as they grip better in a relatively tight stricture, and are not without morbidity and mortality. They may block either with impacted food boluses or with tumour overgrowth/ingrowth, and repeat endoscopic interventions are then required. Short-course (5–10 days) radiotherapy has a role in palliating some patients' dysphagia, but can initially make symptoms worse before they improve due to tissue oedema.

Staging of oesophageal cancer must be performed preoperatively to identify patients who have tumours that are suitable for resection. The current TNM (Tumour, Nodes, Metastases) staging classification for oesophageal cancer is shown in Table 20.3. A variety of investigations are required to produce an accurate preoperative stage; these include CT scanning, PET scanning, endoscopic ultrasound (EUS) and laparoscopy. CT scanning is good at detecting metastatic disease, particularly in the liver and lungs, but rarely detects peritoneal disease. It is not good at predicting T or N stage, but may show extension of a bulky tumour into adjacent structures (T4). PET scanning is more sensitive than CT alone at detecting metastatic disease. EUS is good at predicting T stage, and is now the investigation of choice for this aspect of staging. EUS is also better than CT at predicting lymph node

Table 20.3 TNM staging classification for oesophageal cancer

Tx – primary tumour not assessable	Nx – regional nodes not assessable
T0 – no primary tumour	N0 – no regional nodes involved
Tis – carcinoma *in situ*	N1 – regional nodes involved
T1 – tumour invading lamina propria/submucosa	
T2 – tumour invading muscularis propria	Mx – metastasis not assessable
T3 – tumour invading adventitia	M0 – no distant metastasis
T4 – tumour invading adjacent structures	M1 – distant metastasis

involvement, and it is possible to perform fine-needle aspiration of suspicious nodes with the right equipment. Laparoscopy is useful with distal oesophageal tumours to detect metastatic disease that could be missed at CT, such as peritoneal and omental seedlings and small liver metastases.

Tumours are suitable for resection if preoperative staging suggests no more than T3 disease, N0 or N1 lymph node status, and no distant metastases – i.e. T3 N1 M0 or better. Unfortunately only 20–25% of patients who present with oesophageal cancer are suitable for resection, mainly because the presenting symptom, dysphagia, often occurs late in the disease process. Recent studies in the UK, Holland and America have suggested survival benefits in certain patients receiving neoadjuvant chemotherapy, and current practice in the UK is to offer this to patients with T2 and T3 tumours. Patients with T1 tumours are offered surgery alone. A variety of operations are available and a variety of different organs can be used to replace the resected oesophagus. The most commonly used organ for reconstruction is the stomach, which is mobilized at laparotomy by dividing the left and short gastric vessels, but preserving the gastro-epiploic arcade along its greater curve. Excising the lesser curve and gastro-oesophageal junction provides a gastric tube that can be brought up to anastomose to the cervical oesophagus in most people. Colon and jejunum have been used instead if the stomach is not suitable or fails. Mobilization of the stomach may be combined with a right thoracotomy and resection of the mid/distal oesophagus (Ivor-Lewis procedure), a left sided thoraco-abdominal approach for tumours of the cardia, a right thoracotomy and cervical incision for resection of the majority of the oesophagus (three-stage, McKeown procedure) or just a cervical incision along with a trans-hiatal dissection to perform a sub-total oesophagectomy without need for a thoracotomy. Interest in minimally invasive techniques is growing, but there remain significant problems due to the complexity of this approach, and no clear benefits have been demonstrated. As experience grows it is likely that minimally invasive oesophagectomy (MIO) will have a widespread role in managing oesophageal cancer, but the optimum technique has yet to be identified.

Significant complications from oesophagectomy include respiratory problems related to thoracotomy, myocardial infarction and arrhythmias, anastomotic leak, chylothorax from thoracic duct injury, anastomotic stricture, recurrent laryngeal nerve palsy and death.

Survival rates from oesophageal cancer are low, due to the aggressive nature of the disease and its tendency to present at an advanced stage. Of patients who undergo surgery, the 5-year survival rate is 20%, and the overall 5-year survival rate for all comers is no more than 5%.

Gastric carcinoma

Gastric carcinoma has an incidence of 10–20 cases per 100 000 people in the UK and USA, a rate that has fallen from 35 per 100 000 in the 1920s. As with oesophageal cancer, the site of cancers is changing, with a decrease in the number of distal tumours, and an increase in the number of proximal tumours. Men are 2.5 times more likely to develop gastric cancer than women, and over three-quarters of patients are 65 years or older. Chronic gastritis, leading to metaplasia, has been implicated in the aetiology, as seen in patients with pernicious anaemia. Recently the gastritis associated with *Helicobacter pylori* infection has been linked with gastric cancer, increasing the risk by up to six times. The exact role of *H. pylori* remains unclear though, as eradication treatment may increase the incidence of more proximal cancers. Other risk factors include smoking, a diet lacking in fresh fruit and vegetables and having a first-degree relative with gastric cancer.

The main, and often only, symptom of an early gastric cancer is dyspepsia. As the cancer becomes more advanced symptoms include anorexia, weight loss, vomiting and anaemia. Unfortunately dyspepsia is a very common symptom, and is often treated by patients and doctors alike with a variety of ant-acid

Table 20.4 Referral guidelines for suspected upper GI cancers (patients with dyspepsia)

Patient >55 yrs old, with dyspepsia:	continuous onset within 12 months
Dyspepsia with alarm symptoms:	weight loss anaemia anorexia
Dyspepsia with risk factors:	pernicious anaemia previous surgery for peptic ulcer atrophic gastritis intestinal metaplasia first-degree relative with gastric cancer

Table 20.5 TNM staging classification for gastric cancer

Tx – primary tumour not assessable	Nx – regional nodes not assessable
T0 – no primary tumour	N0 – no regional nodes involved
Tis – carcinoma *in situ*	N1– 1–6 nodes involved
T1 – tumour invading lamina propria/submucosa	N2– 7–15 nodes involved
T2 – tumour invading muscularis propria/ subserosa	N3– >15 nodes involved
T3 – tumour penetrating serosa	
T4 – tumour invading adjacent structures	Mx – metastasis not assessable M0 – no distant metastasis M1 – distant metastasis

therapies. Guidelines have been produced to encourage referral of patients with dyspepsia who are at risk, and these are shown in Table 20.4. Even so, it is uncommon to see early gastric cancers and it is often the case that when advanced cancers are diagnosed patients have often had a long history of dyspepsia prior to diagnosis.

Although barium studies have been used to investigate dyspepsia and diagnose gastric cancer, the investigation of choice is endoscopy, which allows visualization of the mucosa, and diagnostic biopsy. Early cancers may be missed on barium examinations, and subtle changes are more easily seen at endoscopy, especially if dye-spraying techniques are used to accentuate mucosal abnormalities. Once a cancer has been diagnosed, staging investigations are required to enable an appropriate treatment plan to be discussed with the patient. The current TNM staging system is shown in Table 20.5. Staging investigations include CT scanning, EUS and laparoscopy, in a similar fashion to oesophageal cancer. CT scanning provides good information about metastatic disease, detecting up to 80% of liver metastases, but is unreliable at predicting T stage (other than T4). Laparoscopy is advocated for all patients in whom a potentially curative gastric resection is contemplated, as it is highly accurate at detecting peritoneal disease and malignant ascites.

The mainstay of treatment for gastric cancer is surgery, which may be curative or palliative. Patients fit enough to withstand surgery, and who have localized disease on preoperative staging, should undergo a potentially curative resection. Tumours in the distal 1/3 of the stomach can be resected with a sub-total gastrectomy, preserving a pouch of proximal stomach that is vascularized by the short gastric vessels. Intestinal continuity is restored with a gastro-jejunostomy, either as a loop or as a Roux-en-Y reconstruction. Tumours

of the proximal 2/3 require total gastrectomy, with a jejunal anastomosis onto the distal oesophagus. Some surgeons will create a pouch in the jejunum to act as a neo-stomach, but whether they improve nutrition significantly is unproven. Recently there has been much debate as to the extent of the lymphadenectomy that should be performed with a gastrectomy. The Japanese experience is that radical lymph node dissection to remove not only the lymph nodes immediately adjacent to the cancer (N1 nodes) but also those along the arterial supply to the stomach (N2 nodes) increases the survival rate. Such a radical resection (a D2 lymphadenectomy) has been compared in Western centres with the lesser procedure of just removing N1 nodes (D1 lymphadenectomy), and no survival benefit has been shown. However, as expertise in performing D2 resections has increased, so the mortality rate associated with surgery has decreased, and D2 resection is now recommended in specialist centres. Mortality rates from gastrectomy are 5–10%, with sub-total procedures being safer than total and specialist, high-volume centres achieving better results as with oesophageal resection. Specific complications include anastomotic leak, duodenal stump leak and respiratory infections. Achieving adequate nutritional input can be difficult for many patients, and general advice to eat 'small amounts, more frequently' may need to be combined with expert dietetic input. After total gastrectomy vitamin B12 is not absorbed due to lack of intrinsic factor and parenteral supplementation must be given indefinitely.

Five-year survival after gastrectomy for cancer in Western centres has been 35–45%, some 20% worse than equivalent-stage disease treated in Japan. The centralization of cancer surgery to specialized centres has started to improve these figures, but there is still significant room for improvement.

Surgery may be required for palliation of gastric outlet obstruction caused by large cancers, or for persistent bleeding. Gastro-jejunostomy has been the operation of choice for obstructing tumours, and may be performed laparoscopically. Increasingly, SEMS have been used to stent such tumours, and may yet become as widely used as in oesophageal obstruction.

Neoadjuvant chemotherapy is currently offered to patients in the UK with resectable cancers (other than early gastric cancers), following recent evidence which shows a definite survival advantage.

Cancer of the gastro-oesophageal junction (GOJ)

Cancers of the oesophagus and stomach are becoming more common at the GOJ, and this form of the disease presents its own particular problems. One issue is whether to treat such cancers as gastric or oesophageal, with important implications for chemotherapy and surgical approach. The Siewert classification describes three types of tumour depending on their anatomical situation:

Type I – cancer centred 1–5 cm above the GOJ

Type II – cancer centred at the GOJ (from 1 cm above to 2 cm below)

Type III – cancer centred 2–5 cm below the GOJ.

In reality it is often difficult to accurately allocate a GOJ tumour to one of these types, and a degree of flexibility is required in management decisions. It is hoped that a revised TNM staging system for oesophageal and gastric cancer will incorporate the difficulty raised by GOJ tumours.

For the purposes of resection, Type I should be managed by oesophago-gastrectomy, Type III by total gastrectomy and Type II by whichever of the two approaches seems more appropriate.

Other OG conditions

Peptic ulcer

The management of peptic ulcer disease has changed dramatically in the last 20 years as the aetiology of peptic ulceration has become more clearly understood and more powerful and effective medical treatment

has evolved. At the same time there has been a dramatic decrease in both elective and emergency surgery for peptic ulceration. Aetiological factors in peptic ulceration include *Helicobacter pylori* infection, non-steroidal anti-inflammatory drug (NSAID) ingestion, smoking, renal failure, liver disease and Zollinger-Ellison syndrome. *H. pylori* is by far the most important and adequate management of *H. pylori* is the mainstay of modern ulcer therapy. *H. pylori* is a spiral, Gram-negative bacterium which is spread by direct contact, and infects up to 60% of the population, though only 5–10% of those infected develop ulceration. *H. pylori* causes increased gastrin levels, a rise in gastric acid production and also has a direct effect on gastric and duodenal mucosa. NSAIDs have both a localized and systemic effect on gastric and duodenal mucosa, which seems to be through their inhibition of cyclooxygenase enzyme (particularly COX-1). Newer NSAIDs are specific for the COX-2 enzyme and are less ulcerogenic.

Patients with ulcers have a variety of symptoms, including epigastric pain, anorexia, vomiting and weight loss. Epigastric pain may be relieved by food or associated with anorexia, and radiates through to the back. Some patients are asymptomatic. Examination is often unremarkable, except for melaena when there has been bleeding, or a succussion splash with gastric outlet obstruction. The best diagnostic investigation is upper GI endoscopy, which allows visualization of ulcers as well as gastric biopsy. All patients with peptic ulceration must be investigated for *H. pylori* by serology, breath testing, CLO (campylobacter-like organism) test or histology. The last two are performed on biopsies taken at endoscopy and are the most accurate. All gastric ulcers must be biopsied from their margin to exclude the possibility of malignancy.

Treatment depends on the presumed causal factor. If *H. pylori* is identified it must be eradicated. If NSAIDs are being used they should be stopped if at all possible and alternative analgesia used. If neither *H. pylori* is identified nor NSAIDs are being used then the initial presumption should be a false-negative result from the *H. pylori* test, and eradication prescribed – other causes of ulceration are extremely rare. Eradication of *H. pylori* is achieved by a combination of antibiotics in conjunction with an anti-secretory agent – a common combination would be a proton pump inhibitor (PPI), with clarithromycin and amoxycillin, or metronidazole. This 'triple therapy' would be given for 1 week, and followed by continuing anti-secretory therapy for 8–12 weeks to heal the ulcer, which must also be prescribed for NSAID-induced ulcers.

If ulcers fail to heal then repeat testing for *H. pylori* must be performed, and this is most effective by CLO test and histology at repeat endoscopy. Persistent infection must be treated before alternative diagnoses are sought, and a different combination of antibiotics over a 2-week period is recommended. NSAID ingestion must be re-assessed, and malignancy excluded with endoscopic biopsies. In the absence of other causes Zollinger-Ellison (ZE) syndrome must be considered, where gastrin-secreting tumours result in high gastric acidity and resistant peptic ulceration. Serum gastrin levels must be measured to diagnose ZE syndrome and the possibility of multiple endocrine neoplasia (MEN) considered.

Surgery for peptic ulcer disease is now much less common than it used to be. Elective surgery is extremely rare, and consists of acid-reducing procedures (vagotomy, selective vagotomy, antrectomy) and gastric resections. Complications from these operations were common, and recurrent ulceration was well recognized. It is still occasionally necessary to perform elective surgery for resistant ulcer disease, but only after all medical treatment has been tried thoroughly. Emergency surgery for complications is still common, but less common than 20 years ago. The treatment of bleeding ulcers and perforations has been described already (see Upper GI bleeding and Perforated viscus). Gastric outlet obstruction may result from scarring and fibrosis secondary to ulceration in the pyloric region and duodenum, and this often requires surgical intervention. Balloon dilatation at endoscopy is a good first-line treatment, but may result in perforation requiring surgery. Operative treatment of gastric outlet obstruction includes pyloroplasty, gastro-enterostomy and distal gastrectomy.

Gastro-oesophageal reflux disease (GORD)

Gastro-oesophageal reflux occurs when gastric contents pass retrograde through the gastro-oesophageal junction into the oesophagus. Everybody experiences episodes of reflux, but in 10–40% of the population of the UK this occurs frequently enough to significantly impair their quality of life. The incidence of this problem seems to be increasing, though it is hard to accurately measure just how many people are affected. What is clear is that it is a highly significant problem accounting for a large number of

attendances at both primary and secondary care, and requiring a large amount of money for therapeutic measures (mainly anti-secretory agent prescriptions). There are a number of mechanisms which help to prevent GORD, including a lower oesophageal 'sphincter', the diaphragmatic crura at the hiatus, and the presence of a short segment of distal oesophagus within the abdominal compartment. Some patients with GORD have a hiatus hernia, but it must be realized that the presence of a hiatus hernia does not imply reflux (most hernias are asymptomatic for GORD), and that having reflux does not imply the presence of a hiatus hernia (30–90% of reflux patients have a hernia).

Symptoms are variable; 'heartburn' is common with retrosternal burning and discomfort, regurgitation of food and acid into the mouth is unpleasant, and dysphagia to both solids and liquids can occur. Symptoms are worse when lying down or bending over, and waking at night choking is described. Respiratory disease may be worsened by nocturnal aspiration and teeth may be eroded by gastric acid. Clinical examination is unremarkable and the diagnosis is most often obtained from history alone.

The majority of reflux responds to lifestyle adjustments and medical treatment. Losing weight, stopping smoking and avoiding spicy foods and alcohol help some people, but most require some form of acid reduction therapy with either H_2 antagonists or PPIs. Surgical intervention is only considered in cases that do not respond to medical therapy, and sometimes when patients request surgery as an alternative to life-long medication. Some patients have only a partial response to high doses of PPIs, and others have relief of the acid-related problems but still have a large volume of gastric fluid regurgitating into their oropharynx.

Before considering surgery the oesophagus must be investigated to prove the diagnosis of GORD and show motility disorders and anatomical variants. Endoscopy with distal oesophageal biopsies should be performed, as well as manometry and 24-hour pH studies (see Oesophageal function tests).

There are many types of anti-reflux operations, but most include some form of fundoplication. The principles of a fundoplication procedure include reducing hiatus hernia if present, restoring a length of intra-abdominal oesophagus and repairing the diaphragmatic hiatus. The commonest anti-reflux procedure is the Nissen fundoplication, which involves a 360° wrap of the gastric fundus around the distal oesophagus.

Various partial fundoplications exist with either anterior or posterior wrapping of the fundus over 180° or 270°. The development of laparoscopic surgery has renewed enthusiasm for anti-reflux surgery, as it can be performed without the need for a painful laparotomy or thoracotomy. The results from well-selected patients are good, with 85–95% reporting cure or significant improvement of reflux. Patients must know that certain complications occur with anti-reflux surgery: dysphagia affects at least 30% immediately postoperatively, but this resolves over the first 3 months; gas-bloat affects up to 30%, where inability to belch air from the stomach causes gastric distension. Persistent dysphagia can be treated with endoscopic balloon dilatation.

There is a well-described link between GORD and Barrett's oesophagus, and between Barrett's and oesophageal cancer (see Oesophageal cancer). It would seem logical that a mechanical solution to reflux as provided by surgery would help prevent progression of Barrett's, but so far there is no evidence to support this theory. Anti-reflux surgery is not indicated as treatment for Barrett's oesophagus alone.

Hiatus hernia

A hiatus hernia exists when part or all of the stomach protrudes through the diaphragmatic hiatus to lie above the diaphragm within the chest. The true incidence of hiatus hernia is unknown as many are likely to be asymptomatic, but the presence of a small hiatus hernia at upper GI endoscopy is a common finding. A classification of hiatus hernia is shown in Table 20.6, but this correlates poorly with symptoms or management. 'Small' hiatus herniae, with no more than a few centimetres of stomach above the hiatus, are common, and may predispose to symptoms of GORD (see above), but are also likely to be asymptomatic and identified only as incidental findings at OGD. 'Large' or 'giant' hiatus herniae are rare and though they may also be asymptomatic or associated with GORD they do have the potential for more serious problems. A hiatus hernia may be deemed 'large' when at least 25–50% of the stomach lies within it, and probably corresponds to Types III and IV (Table 20.6). In addition to the heartburn and regurgitation symptoms of GORD, such large hernias may lead to dysphagia and dyspnoea from decreased lung capacity. The potential for gastric volvulus exists, presenting with chest pain and/or upper GI bleeding. Gastric necrosis is reported, but

Table 20.6 A classification of hiatus herniae

Type I 'sliding': GOJ moves up into chest, along with proximal stomach
Type II 'rolling': GOJ remains below diaphragm, while proximal stomach 'rolls' into chest
Type III 'mixed': combination of Type I and II, although GOJ is always above the diaphragm
Type IV involves other viscus, such as spleen or colon

probably much rarer than the 30% incidence quoted by Belsey in 1967. Nonetheless, a patient with a large, symptomatic hiatus hernia should be offered surgical reduction and repair, both to improve quality of life and reduce risk of mortality.

Surgical repair may be performed via laparotomy or thoracotomy, but a laparoscopic approach is most commonly favoured. The principles of surgery involve careful reduction of the hernial contents into the abdomen; dissection and excision of the hernial sac (peritoneum); repair of the hiatal defect by suturing the crus of the diaphragm; and some form of gastropexy and/or fundoplication. The hiatal repair may be reinforced with some type of mesh, but the risk of erosion into the oesophagus of a synthetic mesh is very real, and if necessary some form of non-synthetic biomesh should be considered. Patients with large, symptomatic herniae are often elderly, and the surgery can be technically very difficult, so the decision to operate must be very carefully considered by both surgeon and patient.

Small hiatus herniae do not warrant surgical intervention, unless as part of the management of GORD as described previously.

Further reading

Allum WH *et al.* Guidelines for the management of oesophageal and gastric cancer. *Gut* 2002;**50**(suppl V):v1–v23.

Cai W, Watson DI, Lally CJ *et al.* Ten year clinical outcome of a prospective randomised clinical trial of laparoscopic Nissen versus anterior (180 degree) partial fundoplication. *Br J Surg* 2008;**95**:1501–1505.

Di Franco F, Lamb PJ, Karat D, Hayes N, Griffin SM. Iatrogenic perforation of localised oesophageal cancer. *Br J Surg* 2008;**95**:837–839.

Enns RA, Gagnon YM, Barkun AN *et al.* Validation of the Rockall scoring system for outcomes from non-variceal upper gastrointestinal bleeding in a Canadian setting. *World J Gastroenterol* 2006;**12**(48):7779–7785.

Gemmill EH, McCulloch P. Systematic review of minimally invasive resection for gastro-oesophageal cancer. *Br J Surg* 2007;**94**:1461–1467.

Griffin SM, Raimes SA. *A Companion To Specialist Surgical Practice: Oesophagogastric Surgery*. 3rd edn. Elsevier Saunders, 2006.

Hermansson M, Ekedahl A, Ranstam J, Zilling T. Decreasing incidence of peptic ulcer complications after the introduction of the proton pump inhibitors, a study of the Swedish population from 1974–2002. *BMC Gastroenterol* 2009;**9**(25):13 pp.

Kiss J. Surgical treatment of oesophageal perforation. *Br J Surg* 2008;**95**:805–806.

Lunevicius R, Morkevicius M. Systematic review comparing laparoscopic and open repair for perforated peptic ulcer. *Br J Surg* 2005;**92**:1195–1207.

Pearson FG *et al*. *Esophageal Surgery*. 2nd edn. Churchill Livingstone, 2002.

Shaheen NJ, Richter JE. Barrett's oesophagus. *Lancet* 2009;**373**:850–861.

Sujendran V, Wheeler J, Baron R *et al*. Effect of neoadjuvant chemotherapy on circumferential margin positivity and its impact on prognosis in patients with resectable oesophageal cancer. *Br J Surg* 2008;**95**: 191–194.

Sung JJY, Tsoi KKF, Lai LH *et al*. Endoscopic clipping versus injection and thermocoagulation in the treatment of non-variceal upper gastrointestinal bleeding: a meta-analysis. *Gut* 2007;**56**:1364–1373.

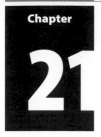

Chapter 21

Fundamentals of hepatobiliary and pancreatic surgery

Mark Duxbury and Rowan Parks

Liver

Segmental anatomy, blood supply and physiology

The adult human liver accounts for approximately 2% of body mass. Couinaud (1957) divided the liver into eight functionally independent segments. The middle hepatic vein divides the liver into a left hemiliver (segment 1 (caudate) and segments 2–4) and right hemiliver (segments 5–8). This 'principal' plane corresponds to an imaginary line joining the inferior vena cava and the gallbladder fossa. The right hepatic vein divides the right hemiliver into an anterior sector (segments 5, 8) and posterior sector (segments 6, 7). The left hepatic vein separates segment 2 (left lateral sector) from segments 3 and 4 (left medial sector). The portal vein divides the liver into upper and lower segments. Left and right portal vein branches project into the centre of each segment. Portal blood flow represents 65% of total liver perfusion but 50% of liver oxygen delivery, the remaining 50% being delivered via the hepatic artery.

The liver is a critical organ for detoxification as well as carbohydrate, protein and lipid metabolism. In addition to bile secretion, important functions include glycogen storage, haemoglobin degradation, plasma protein synthesis (including coagulation factors I (fibrinogen), II (prothrombin), V, VII, IX, X and XI, protein C and S), hormone production (insulin-like growth factor, thrombopoietin), vitamin and mineral storage (vitamin A, D, B12, iron, copper). The liver also has important immunological functions.

Disorders of the liver

Liver tumours

Liver tumours may be benign or malignant and can be divided into cystic or solid lesions.

Liver cysts

Liver cysts are a common incidental finding in patients undergoing abdominal imaging. Features suggestive of a simple cyst include a thin regular wall, unilocularity, no surrounding tissue response and uniform cyst density. While usually asymptomatic, larger cysts can cause abdominal pain and may require treatment. Aspiration is typically followed by recurrence, and surgical deroofing may be required, which can be performed laparoscopically.

Congenital polycystic disease is an autosomal dominant multi-organ disorder, often involving the pancreas and kidney, which results from abnormalities of ductal plate fusion. The appearances can be dramatic but liver function is usually remarkably well preserved. Pain may indicate haemorrhage into a cyst. Surgical deroofing may be considered, although outcomes are less favourable than for simple cysts and surgical resection or occasionally liver transplantation may be required.

Benign solid liver tumours

Haemangioma

Haemangioma is the commonest liver lesion and is usually asymptomatic, being identified incidentally on abdominal imaging. Haemangiomata are of mesenchymal origin and probably represent a congenital,

Fundamentals of Surgical Practice, Third Edition, ed. Andrew N. Kingsnorth and Douglas M. Bowley.
Published by Cambridge University Press. © Cambridge University Press 2011.

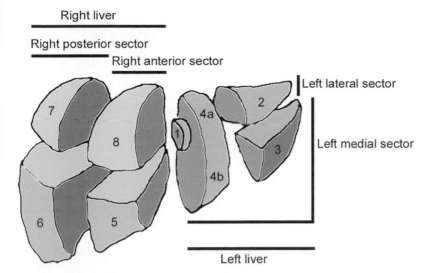

Figure 21.1 Segmental and sectoral liver anatomy.

hamartomatous proliferation of vascular endothelial cells. They consist of abnormal plexi of vessels. Small lesions may present a diagnostic challenge. Once diagnosed, small lesions require no further treatment and have no malignant potential. Haemangiomata are often multiple and occasionally reach a large size. Surgical resection of such 'giant' symptomatic haemangioma may be required. Biopsy should be avoided because of the risk of bleeding.

Hepatic adenoma

This rare benign tumour usually appears well-defined and vascular on axial imaging. Development in an otherwise normal liver is typical. Association with oral contraceptive use is recognized and regression on withdrawal of treatment is reported. Adenomata are regarded as having malignant potential and also pose a risk of haemorrhage. Owing to these risks, once diagnosed, resection is usually advisable in fit patients. The presence of more than 10 adenomata is referred to as adenomatosis.

Focal nodular hyperplasia (FNH)

FNH usually affects middle aged females with an otherwise normal liver. This unusual benign process may be difficult to differentiate from other liver lesions. The lesion contains hepatocytes and Kupffer cells which take up sulphur colloid sometimes allowing differentiation from adenoma or malignant tumours by nuclear medicine. Central scarring is a classic but variable finding. FNH is not believed to have malignant potential although malignancy may co-exist. Management

remains controversial and ranges from conservatism to resection, which should be performed if the diagnosis is not certain.

Biliary hamartoma (Von Meyenburg complex)

Biliary hamartomata are benign developmental abnormalities of the liver occurring in over 5% of the population. They are of clinical interest due to the frequency of their submission for intraoperative frozen section to differentiate them from metastases. They are usually less than 5 mm in diameter and multiple lesions are common. Microscopic features include bile ductules with enlarged lumina, inflammatory infiltrate and fibrosis. No treatment is required.

A summary of benign solid tumours of the adult liver lesions is shown in Table 21.1. Most are very rare and will not be detailed further here.

Malignant liver tumours

Hepatocellular carcinoma

Hepatocellular carcinoma (HCC) is one of the commonest malignant tumours worldwide with an estimated 10^6 people dying from the disease annually; however, it is relatively rare in the West. The incidence varies between 5 per 100 000 in the UK and 70–80 per 100 000 in parts of Africa and Asia. Most cases are associated with viral hepatitis (hepatitis B and C) and 80% of patients develop HCC on a background of cirrhosis. Patients with defined risk factors for HCC (e.g. haemochromatosis, hepatitis) should undergo ultrasonographic surveillance. Diagnosis is often made late

Table 21.1 Benign solid tumours of the adult liver

Hepatocellular origin
  Hepatocellular adenoma
  Hepatocellular hyperplasia:
    Focal nodular hyperplasia
    Nodular regenerative hyperplasia
    Regenerative nodule
    Dysplastic nodules

Cholangiocellular origin
  Biliary hamartoma
  Biliary adenoma
  Biliary cystadenoma
  Congenital hepatic fibrosis

Mesenchymal origin
  Vascular
    Haemangioma
    Adult haemangioendothelioma
    Peliosis hepatis
    Hereditary haemorrhagic telangiectasia
  Lymphangioma
  Adipose
    Focal fatty changes
    Lipoma
    Angiomyolipoma
    Myelolipoma
  Smooth muscle
    Leiomyoma
    Fibroma
  Mesothelioma

Mixed epithelial and mesenchymal
  Mesenchymal hamartoma
  Teratoma
  Inflammatory pseudotumour

Heterotopic tissue
  Adrenal rests
  Pancreatic heterotopia

Table 21.2 Childs scoring system

	Points		
	1	2	3
INR	<1.7	1.7–2.3	>2.3
Albumin, g/l	>35	28–35	<28
Bilirubin, μM	<35	35–51	>51
Ascites	None	Slight	Moderate to severe
Encephalopathy	None	Slight	Moderate to severe
Childs grade	A: 5–6 points	B: 7–9 points	C: 10–15 points

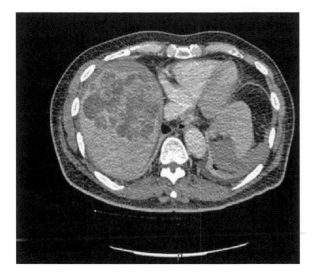

Figure 21.2 Large hepatocellular carcinoma within right liver.

as patients are commonly asymptomatic until tumour haemorrhage or multifocal disease develops. Presentation may be with pain, ascites, jaundice and cachexia. The diagnosis of HCC is supported by a high serum alpha-fetoprotein (AFP). Axial imaging (CT, MRI) is usually able to identify HCC.

Small lesions can be difficult to differentiate from benign lesions, e.g. haemangioma or adenoma, although improved scanners and modern contrast agents have increased diagnostic accuracy. Percutaneous biopsy should generally be avoided as it may jeopardize a potential curative resection by increasing the risk of tumour seeding.

Patients with otherwise normal liver or mild cirrhosis (Childs grade A) may be suitable for resection in a specialist unit but only 10–20% of patients with HCC are amenable to surgical resection. It must be appreciated that patients with Childs grade A cirrhosis still have a significant risk of perioperative mor-

bidity and mortality. Patients with moderate or severe liver dysfunction (Childs grade B or C) (Table 21.2) require a different approach, including consideration for transplantation. Transplantation assessment may be pursued if the patient fits defined criteria, e.g. Milan criteria (solitary lesion ≤5 cm or ≤3 lesions with diameter ≤3 cm, no major vessel invasion, and no extrahepatic involvement), although the criteria for patient selection are currently being revised and extended.

Unresectable tumours may be amenable to ablation (radiofrequency, ethanol injection, cryotherapy, microwave). Another alternative is transarterial chemoembolization (TACE). Transfemoral arterial access is established and a catheter advanced into hepatic artery branches, usually via the coeliac axis. Following subselective catheterization of the tumour arterial supply, chemotherapeutic and embolizing

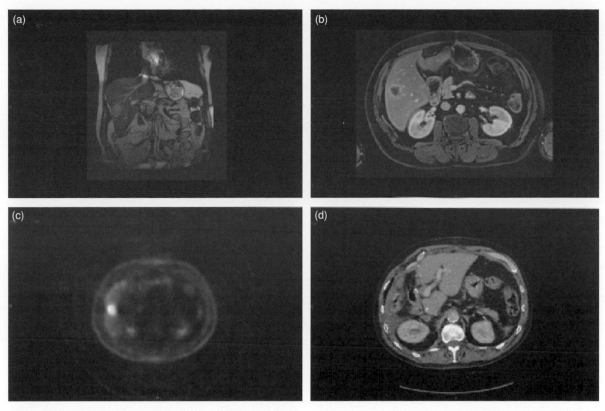

Figure 21.3 Colorectal liver metastasis: (a) coronal MRI; (b) axial MRI; (c) FDG-avid lesion on PET; (d) following curative right hepatectomy.

agents are delivered to the tumour. The technique can be repeated, based on clinical and radiological response. Novel approaches for the treatment of unresectable HCC are under evaluation. The tyrosine kinase inhibitor sorafenib has been shown to double the lifespan of late stage HCC patients.

Liver metastases

Liver metastases are the commonest form of malignant liver tumour in the UK. Most metastases arise from primary tumours of the gastrointestinal tract, breast, lung and kidney.

Colorectal metastases are considered in more detail as they are one of the few liver metastases that respond relatively well to surgical treatment. Up to 50% of colorectal cancer patients develop metastases and without treatment almost all will die from their disease within 1 year. Colorectal liver metastases can now be resected with low mortality (<5%) and an overall 5-year survival rate of 30–50%. To achieve these results, careful patient selection and preparation is required. Improved detection and more comprehensive follow-up of colorectal cancer patients may

increase the number of potential operative candidates. Detection of a suspicious lesion will prompt further assessment and imaging with CT and MRI as well as PET to exclude extrahepatic metastases, which would generally preclude resection. The effect of follow-up on colorectal cancer patient outcome is being assessed by a range of studies (e.g. FACS trial).

Extending resectability

Patients with a single small lesion and favourable anatomical location have the best outcomes following resectional surgery; however, several recent advances have increased the indications for surgical resection. Three-dimensional CT reconstruction and volumetry allows preoperative planning and estimation of the future liver remnant volume. These techniques also allow a preoperative 'virtual liver resection' to be performed. New neoadjuvant chemotherapy options designed to 'down-size' previously unresectable tumours prior to surgery have emerged. Contralateral portal vein embolization allows hypertrophy of the future liver remnant to be induced, permitting more extensive resection. Two-staged liver resections

361

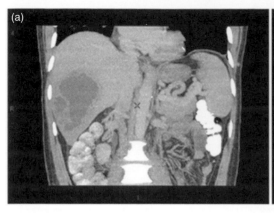
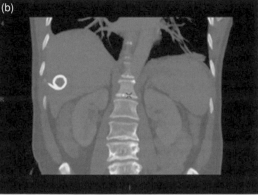

Figure 21.4 (a) Right-sided liver abscess and (b) following percutaneous drain placement.

can also be undertaken and re-resection of hepatic recurrences results in comparable outcomes. These techniques have all increased the options for management of complex presentations.

Provided that patients avoid infective complications and the liver remnant functions satisfactorily, regeneration occurs and normal liver volume is complete within a few weeks. Ablation of non-resectable tumours is possible and this approach may be used in conjunction with resection. The results for resecting non-colorectal metastases are more variable and will require further evaluation in carefully selected patients.

Laparoscopic liver surgery has become more widely adopted in recent years for resection of both benign and malignant liver lesions. Oncological results and perioperative morbidity appear to be acceptable in experienced centres. The minimally invasive approach offers potential advantages in terms of postoperative pain, length of hospital stay and return to work, although enhanced recovery programmes have improved some of these parameters following open surgery.

Other primary malignant tumours of the liver

Intrahepatic cholangiocarcinoma is an unusual type of liver tumour that arises from the intrahepatic biliary tree. This tumour has a strong propensity to invade along ducts but may have a mass-forming component. Surgical resection is the only potentially curative therapeutic modality, although this is rarely possible. Other rare malignant tumours of the liver include angiosarcoma, which is associated with historical use of the contrast agent thorotrast (containing thorium dioxide), haemangioendothelioma and cystadenocarcinoma, which is a slow-growing tumour that arises through transformation of an initially benign biliary cystadenoma.

Surgical liver infections

Pyogenic liver abscess

Liver abscesses may occur due to biliary sepsis or other intra-abdominal infection such as diverticulitis or appendicitis that causes portal venous microbial dissemination. Although a gastrointestinal tract source should be sought, the cause is often not identified. The incidence of liver abscess is increased in the immunocompromised patient. Common organisms include *Streptococcus milleri*, *Streptococcus faecalis*, *Klebsiella*, *Escherichia coli* and *Proteus*. Mixed organisms are commonly isolated. Treatment generally involves drainage of the abscess under image guidance and long-course (∼6–8 weeks) antibiotics targeted on the basis of microbiological culture of aspirated pus or blood. Occasionally tumours that have undergone necrosis may become infected and atypical appearances should raise this concern.

Amoebic liver abscess

Entamoeba histolytica is the causative organism and is endemic in many areas of the world. Presentation is usually with dysentery. Isolation of *E. histolytica* from the abscess or stool confirms the diagnosis. Aspiration or drainage and metronidazole is the treatment of choice.

Hydatid disease of the liver

Echinococcus granulosus is the causative tapeworm. Carnivores such as dogs are the definitive host,

Table 21.3 Causes of portal hypertension

Prehepatic
Congenital
Atresia of portal vein (PV)
Acquired
Portal vein thrombosis
tumour, trauma, sepsis
Extrinsic compression of PV
pancreatic / biliary cancer
Increased flow
Hypersplenism
Arteriovenous fistula
Intrahepatic
Cirrhosis
Schistosomiasis
Posthepatic
Budd-Chiari
Constrictive pericarditis

while intermediate hosts are usually sheep and cattle. Humans are 'accidental' hosts. Abdominal discomfort is common. The cyst may rupture, resulting in an acute abdomen. Imaging classically demonstrates a floating membrane within the cyst, which commonly contains daughter cysts and may become calcified. The diagnosis is supported by serological detection of hydatid antigen. Medical treatment is with mebendazole or albendazole. Surgical resection may be required if medical therapy fails. At operation, contamination of the peritoneal cavity with cyst contents must be avoided.

Portal hypertension and ascites

Portal hypertension is present if the portal venous pressure exceeds 12 mmHg and can be classified into prehepatic, hepatic and posthepatic causes. Alcoholic cirrhosis remains the commonest cause in the West.

Consequences and management of portal hypertension

Bleeding from sites of portosystemic communication, e.g. oesophageal or anorectal varices, is a problem that may be encountered by the surgeon. Bleeding from oesophago-gastric varices is covered in Chapter 20. Patients found to have oesophageal varices are usually offered secondary prevention. Medical therapeutic options include beta antagonists, endoscopic banding and, less commonly, injection sclerotherapy followed by surveillance endoscopy. Splenic vein thrombosis may lead to left-sided portal hypertension and isolated gastric varices. Gastric varices are not as amenable to endotherapy as oesophageal varices and surgical intervention, e.g. variceal underrunning, gas-

tric devascularization, splenectomy or creation of a portosystemic shunt, may be required for persistent bleeding. Anorectal varices are common in those with portal hypertension but rarely cause major haemorrhage. Treatment with balloon tamponade and endoscopic thrombin injection or embolization using interventional radiology may rarely be required. Occasionally, surgical ligation is indicated.

Ascites is another troublesome feature of portal hypertension. Ascites is usually managed medically with a low-sodium diet and diuretics, although paracentesis may be useful to relieve tense ascites. Failure of medical therapy may warrant consideration of portal-systemic shunting. This is usually performed as a transjugular intrahepatic portosystemic shunt (TIPSS) procedure, which involves creation and stenting of a fistula between the portal and hepatic venous systems. Shunts between the peritoneal cavity and systemic venous system have also been in use for over 30 years and can provide relief from refractory ascites but complications are common, including infection, blockage, disseminated intravascular coagulation and encephalopathy. Surgical portosystemic shunts, which may be classified as total or partial and selective or non-selective, are now rarely performed except transiently during liver transplantation. Surgical intervention in patients with portal hypertension is challenging as multiple dilated thin-walled veins are encountered, making surgery risky and technically demanding. These vessels respond poorly to diathermy and suture is usually the preferred technique for their control.

Liver trauma

The liver is second only to the spleen as the most frequently injured intra-abdominal organ. Decisions regarding the management of liver injury require involvement of an experienced surgical team and commonly liaison with a specialist hepatobiliary unit.

Classification of liver injury (see Table 21.4) aids communication and may guide therapy. Management has tended away from initial operative treatment, with more emphasis now on conservative management and interventional radiological management if required, e.g. embolization. Extensive liver injuries may still require laparotomy for packing to allow patient stabilization and transfer to a specialist unit. Intrahepatic haematoma, biloma, necrosis or haemobilia may require specialist management.

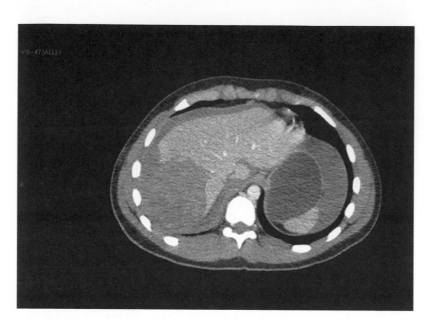

Figure 21.5 Liver haematoma following non-penetrating trauma.

Table 21.4 Liver injury scale

Grade	Type of injury	Extent of injury
1	Haematoma	Subcapsular, <10% surface area
	Laceration	Capsular tear, <1 cm depth
2	Haematoma	Subcapsular, 10% to 50% surface area
		Intraparenchymal <10 cm diameter
	Laceration	Capsular tear 1–3 cm depth, <10 cm length
3	Haematoma	Subcapsular, >50% surface area of ruptured subcapsular or parenchymal haematoma; intraparenchymal haematoma >10 cm or expanding
	Laceration	>3 cm depth
4	Laceration	Parenchymal disruption involving 25% to 75% hepatic lobe or 1–3 segments
5	Laceration	Parenchymal disruption involving >75% of hepatic lobe or > three segments within single lobe
	Vascular	Juxtahepatic venous injuries
6	Vascular	Hepatic avulsion

Jaundice, gallstones and disorders of the biliary tree

Biliary anatomy and physiology

The common hepatic duct is formed by the union of right and left hepatic ducts. It continues approximately 2 cm inferiorly, becoming the common bile duct which is formed by the union of the common hepatic duct and the cystic duct which communicates with the gallbladder. The common bile duct is about 7.5 cm long and consists of a supraduodenal portion, a retroduodenal portion, an infraduodenal portion and an intraduodenal portion which terminates at the ampulla of Vater, surrounded by the sphincter of Oddi.

Bile is produced by hepatocytes and consists of water, cholesterol, bile pigments, bile acids (glycocholic and taurocholic acid), phospholipids (mostly lecithin), bicarbonate and other ions. The gallbladder is a reservoir for bile and secretion is stimulated at meal times by the release of cholecystokinin (CCK) from the duodenum as acidic gastric contents enter its lumen. CCK causes relaxation of the sphincter of Oddi. The bile acids, cholic and chenodeoxycholic acid, emulsify lipids and help solubilize cholesterol by forming micelles. Bile acids and phospholipids form the outer layer of the micelle, the lipid-soluble core contains cholesterol. Each day 20–30 g of bile acids secreted in the bile are actively reabsorbed in the ileum, a process known as the enterohepatic circulation. Disruption of the cyclical process due to terminal ileitis or following ileal resection can predispose to stone formation.

Biliary pathology

Congenital structural abnormalities of the gallbladder (e.g. Phrygian cap) are well recognized. Congenital absence is also reported. Even more common are

Table 21.5 Classification of jaundice

Prehepatic
  Congenital
    Haemolysis, e.g. hereditary spherocytosis
  Acquired
    Haemolysis
    Abnormal/artificial heart valves
    Hypersplenism

Hepatic
  Congenital
    Inborn errors of metabolism
    Wilson's disease
  Acquired
    Acute hepatitis
    Alcohol, drugs
    Infection/sepsis
    Cirrhosis
    Neoplasia

Posthepatic
  Congenital
    Biliary atresia
  Acquired
    Choledocholithiasis
    Neoplasia, e.g. cholangiocarcinoma
    Biliary stricture, e.g. primary sclerosing cholangitis
    Pancreatic cancer
    Portal lymphadenopathy
    Trematode infestation
    Right heart failure

variations in biliary anatomy, which can prove a hazard for surgeons undertaking cholecystectomy. It is estimated that more than 25% of patients have atypical biliary anatomy. Specific congenital abnormalities of the biliary tree are covered in Chapter 14.

Jaundice

Hyperbilirubinaemia occurs when the serum bilirubin concentration exceeds its normal upper limit of 17 μmol/l; however, jaundice is only clinically detectable at levels of 30–50 μmol/l when yellow discolouration of skin, sclera and other tissues can be detected. Jaundice can be classified into prehepatic (excessive destruction of red blood cells), hepatic (failure to remove bilirubin from the bloodstream) and posthepatic or cholestatic (obstruction of bile flow from the liver) causes.

Clinical assessment

Patients are often presented to the surgeon when a diagnosis of posthepatic (obstructive) jaundice has been made. It remains important to consider other causes of jaundice, and obtaining an appropriate history including occupation, travel, drug use, alcohol intake, transfusion of blood products, contact with jaundiced individuals and sexual history will identify risk factors for hepatic causes of jaundice. Weight loss may indicate a malignant aetiology whereas pain, fever and rigors may suggest gallstones.

Signs of chronic liver disease, e.g. palmar erythema, clubbing, bruising, spider naevi, gynaecomastia and evidence of portosystemic shunting in the anterior abdominal wall such as caput medusa, should be sought. It remains worth bearing in mind Courvoisier's rule, which states that the finding of a palpable gallbladder in the presence of jaundice suggests that gallstones are not the cause, raising the possibility of malignancy. Exceptions to this rule can occur in patients with a coexisting gallbladder empyema.

Additional features of cholestasis such as pruritus, dark urine and pale stools may be elicited. The liver conjugates bilirubin, resulting in a water-soluble compound. If biliary obstruction occurs, conjugated bilirubin accumulates in the blood and is excreted by the kidneys, darkening the urine. Urinary urobilinogen, a product of bacterial decomposition of bilirubin in the gut, is reduced. Reduced bile flow into the duodenum results in fewer bile faecal pigments and pale stools. Pruritus occurs due to elevated levels of bile acids.

Investigation

In posthepatic cholestasis, liver function tests exhibit a characteristic pattern with a more significant rise in alkaline phosphatase concentration compared to transaminase levels, whereas in hepatic jaundice the transaminases are usually grossly elevated. Serum albumin may be decreased in long-standing disease. Absence of bile leads to malabsorption of fat-soluble vitamins such as vitamin K. The prothrombin time, often expressed as the international normalized ratio (INR), may therefore be prolonged.

Abdominal ultrasonography is sensitive for detecting gallbladder calculi and intra/extrahepatic biliary dilatation; however, it is less sensitive for identifying ductal gallstones. Ultrasonography may also demonstrate liver tumours, ascites and portal lymphadenopathy; however, the pancreas is often poorly visualized. If malignancy is suspected, axial imaging in the form of CT thorax and abdomen is indicated and will provide useful staging information.

Magnetic resonance cholangiopancreatography (MRCP) is a non-invasive method of evaluating the biliary tract and has replaced endoscopic retrograde cholangiopancreatography (ERCP) as a diagnostic tool, the latter being associated with complications such as pancreatitis, bleeding and perforation. ERCP is now predominantly performed with therapeutic rather than diagnostic intent.

Prompt investigation of the jaundiced patient is important as the management strategy is very dependent on the likely diagnosis established from these initial investigations.

Gallstones

Gallstones are classified according to their constituents into cholesterol, mixed and pigment stones. Ninety per cent of gallstones are mixed, containing cholesterol, calcium salts including bilirubinate, phosphates, carbonate and proteins. Gallstones form as a result of abnormalities in metabolism, infection and bile stasis. Imbalance in the cholesterol solubilization system, i.e. increased cholesterol levels or low bile acid levels, lead to cholesterol crystal precipitation, which acts as a nidus around which gallstones can form. Lithogenic bile also results when excess bile pigments are present due to excessive breakdown of haemoglobin in haemolysis. Pigment stones are darker in colour than cholesterol stones. Pigment stones often form in the intrahepatic ducts.

Gallstones are common in an increasingly obese Western population. Over the age of 70 years approximately 20–30% of the population are estimated to have gallstones. Gallstones are twice as common in women as in men. Some populations, e.g. Native Americans, have a high prevalence of gallstones. Other predisposing factors include terminal ileal disease (causes interruption of the enterohepatic circulation), oral contraceptive use and, in the oriental population, intrahepatic chlonorchiasis (*C. sinensis*), which predisposes to intrahepatic pigmented cholelithiasis. Gallstones are a common incidental finding on investigation and asymptomatic stones must be differentiated from truly symptomatic stones. The majority of individuals with gallstones remain asymptomatic, although complications may supervene in 20–30%.

Management of gallstones and their sequelae

Laparoscopic cholecystectomy is the treatment of choice for symptomatic gallstones. Routine administration of antibiotics at laparoscopic cholecystectomy is unnecessary in patients at low risk of postoperative infection. Rates of conversion to open surgery are approximately 5%. There is no evidence to support intervention for the 70–80% of patients with

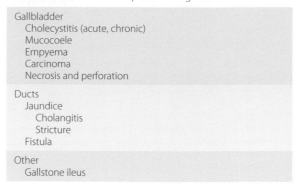

Table 21.6 Common complications of gallstones

Gallbladder
Cholecystitis (acute, chronic)
Mucocoele
Empyema
Carcinoma
Necrosis and perforation
Ducts
Jaundice
Cholangitis
Stricture
Fistula
Other
Gallstone ileus

asymptomatic gallstones. Patients found incidentally to have gallstones may request surgery although these patients should be treated with caution as at least 5% of all patients who undergo cholecystectomy are troubled by persistent symptoms postoperatively. 'Post-cholecystectomy syndrome' more often reflects the continuation of preoperative non-gallbladder-related symptoms, rather than being a specific cholecystectomy-induced condition. Cystic duct stump neuroma is reported to cause symptoms in a small minority of post-cholecystectomy patients and is reported to respond to excision.

Acute cholecystitis

Acute cholecystitis usually presents with right upper quadrant pain and systemic features of an inflammatory response. Episodes of biliary colic, which are not associated with a systemic inflammatory response, may have preceded the attack. The pain is usually constant when present and may radiate to the back, sides or shoulder tip. Movement may exacerbate the pain. Fatty food intolerance is a suggestive but very nonspecific feature of gallstone disease. Examination may reveal signs of sepsis and jaundice may occur if choledocholithiasis is present. Deep palpation in the right upper quadrant during inspiration leads to pain and an arrest of inspiration (Murphy's sign). A thickened inflamed gallbladder wall with pericholecystic fluid may be demonstrated by transabdominal ultrasound.

When systemic upset is mild, cholecystitis can be treated supportively. Intravenous fluid and antibiotic therapy are generally indicated together with adequate analgesia. Many centres support a strategy of early cholecystectomy for patients with acute cholecystitis. Cholecystectomy performed within the first 36 hours of an episode may actually be

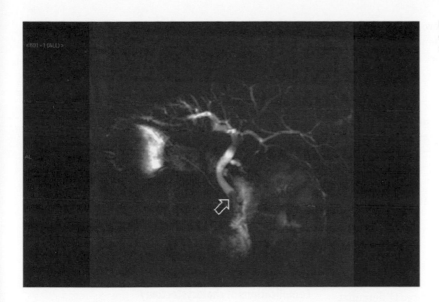

Figure 21.6 MRCP showing choledocholithiasis (arrow indicates stone).

facilitated by pericholecystic oedema. This approach avoids a second admission, although some series report a higher rate of conversion to an open technique. Urgent surgery is required for patients with more profound systemic upset, signs of peritonitis from gallbladder perforation or those suspected of having a gangrenous gallbladder or empyema. Occasionally, frail patients with a gallbladder empyema may be treated with a radiologically placed percutaneous cholecystostomy drainage catheter with good results. Non-surgical management of gallstones, e.g. with pharmaceutical dissolution or shockwave lithotripsy, has proven largely unsuccessful. Recurrence rates are high if the gallbladder is not removed although there may be no alternative in patients unfit for anaesthesia and surgery.

Patients found to have common duct stones can be safely treated by laparoscopic exploration or postoperative ERCP. Correction of coagulopathy is often required (vitamin K initially). In frail patients, unfit for general anaesthesia and surgery, endoscopic biliary sphincterotomy may be used as definitive treatment for choledocholithiasis, as residual gallbladder stones infrequently cause problems in this population. However, fit patients should be offered cholecystectomy. Some centres prefer to offer patients combined cholecystectomy and laparoscopic duct clearance either using a transcystic approach or following choledochotomy. The latter technique is usually best avoided in patients with a duct of 8 mm or less due to the risk of stricture formation.

Chronic cholecystitis

The gallbladder can develop chronic inflammatory changes which include cholesterolosis (strawberry gallbladder), cholesterol polyposis and cholecystitis glandularis proliferans. Mural calcification may occur. The association of calcific cholecystitis (porcelain gallbladder) with carcinoma remains controversial. Many series report low rates of associated malignancy although certain patterns of calcification, particularly intramucosal, may reflect a higher risk group. Symptoms should prompt cholecystectomy.

Cholangitis

Bacterial infection of the biliary tract is a surgical emergency that usually occurs in an obstructed system. Presentation is typically with jaundice, pain and fever (usually with rigors), known as Charcot's triad. Presentation with additional hypotension and mental status changes is known as Reynolds' pentad. It should be noted that these classic features may be absent and are not required for diagnosis. Treatment includes resuscitation and administration of intravenous antibiotics. Arrangements should be made for urgent endoscopic or percutaneous biliary drainage. Choledocholithiasis is a common cause of cholangitis and this can often be addressed at ERCP.

Gallbladder polyps

Gallbladder polyps that develop in a chronically inflamed gallbladder may require cholecystectomy if they are large (>1 cm) or demonstrate an increase in size on serial imaging. Cholesterol polyps have no malignant potential although adenomatous polyps require cholecystectomy, because of the risk of transformation.

Gallbladder mucocele

This develops when the gallbladder neck is obstructed by a stone (or tumour) but the contents do not become infected. The gallbladder fills with mucus secreted by the gallbladder mucosa. Bile is reabsorbed leaving clear mucus. A mass may be palpable on examination. The treatment for a stone-related mucocoele is cholecystectomy.

Mirizzi's syndrome

This occurs when there is compression of the common hepatic duct by a stone impacted in Hartmann's pouch, occasionally leading to jaundice. Differentiating Mirizzi syndrome from proximal cholangiocarcinoma or carcinoma of the gallbladder may be problematic both radiologically and at operation. A fistula may be present resulting in a defect in the bile duct wall which if encountered during surgery will require hepaticojejunostomy.

Biliary fistula and gallstone ileus

Gallstone ileus results from the formation of a cholecystoenteric fistula. Gallstones may pass directly into the bowel. If a larger stone passes into the small intestine it may impact at the ileocaecal junction, causing mechanical obstruction. The patient typically presents with obstructive symptoms. A calcified stone may be seen in the right lower quadrant and aerobilia may be appreciated on plain abdominal radiography. Treatment usually involves enterolithotomy. Controversy exists regarding the merits of concurrent cholecystectomy. Cholecystectomy is probably desirable if this can be achieved safely although dense pericholecystic adhesions and deranged patient physiology commonly conspire against this approach.

Acalculus cholecystitis

Inflammation of the gallbladder can occur in the absence of stones and may result in a clinical presentation similar to that of calculous cholecystitis. The process may be acute or chronic. Acute acalculous cholecystitis is usually seen in patients who have suffered major trauma, burns, sepsis or have undergone extensive surgery. Gallbladder necrosis and perforation can occur.

Atypical biliary pain

Pain suggestive of biliary colic in the absence of gallstones affects a small proportion of patients. Gallbladder dyskinesia, in which gallbladder contraction is poorly coordinated, is a difficult diagnosis to establish but may respond to cholecystectomy. Isotope-based estimation of gallbladder ejection is occasionally helpful.

Sphincter of Oddi dysfunction is a recognized cause of atypical biliary pain and can be associated with liver function test abnormalities and biliary dilatation. ERCP with biliary manometry may demonstrate high sphincter pressures and endoscopic sphincterotomy may provide symptomatic relief. In some cases surgical sphincteroplasty is necessary.

Complications of cholecystectomy

Standard general complications include haemorrhage and infection. Failure of a patient to follow the usual post-cholecystectomy course should prompt concern that a complication has occurred. The development of abnormal liver function tests or abdominal pain postoperatively requires urgent evaluation. Retained ductal stones are relatively common. Small stones pass without symptoms or further intervention, but larger stones are usually removed at postoperative ERCP. Bile leakage or bile duct injury is fortunately an uncommon but troublesome complication of cholecystectomy.

Bile leakage may be due to inadequate securing of the cystic duct stump or accidental division of an unrecognized segmental bile duct. Inadvertent injury to the common hepatic or common bile duct can be sustained as a result of traction or diathermy. Bile duct injury occurs in 0.1–0.2% of laparoscopic cholecystectomies, a rate similar to that from historical open cholecystectomy series. Misidentification of the biliary anatomy may result in excision of the extrahepatic bile duct and a major bile duct injury. In the absence of biliary peritonitis, an ERCP may identify the site of leakage and allow placement of a biliary stent; however, patients with biliary peritonitis will require surgical intervention. Bile leakage from a slipped clip may be managed by laparoscopic washout and re-application of the clip, but if a bile duct injury is suspected at operation, drains should be placed in the sub-hepatic area and the patient urgently transferred to a specialist hepatobiliary unit for definitive management, as data indicate that repair by the injuring surgeon leads to poorer outcomes. Simple suture of duct injuries produces poor results and most injuries will require biliary reconstruction by a specialist surgeon. Failure to identify complications promptly and manage them appropriately is a source of considerable patient dissatisfaction and litigation. Iatrogenic biliary injury may be associated with long term impaired quality of life and shortening of life expectancy.

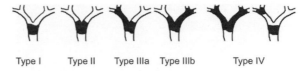

Figure 21.7 The Bismuth Corlette classification of cholangiocarcinoma.

Biliary tract tumours

Management of malignant biliary obstruction

Management of patients with obstructive jaundice due to a suspected malignancy depends on the site of biliary obstruction and bilirubin concentration. Patients with potentially resectable disease causing distal biliary obstruction may be considered for prompt surgical resection without preoperative biliary drainage. However, those with significant hyperbilirubinaemia (bilirubin > 250–300 μmol/l) or with proximal biliary obstruction requiring hepatic resection should undergo preoperative biliary drainage. Unfortunately, the majority of patients with malignant biliary obstruction have advanced disease and definitive biliary stenting remains an effective palliative treatment modality. ERCP is preferable for distal biliary obstruction, whereas biliary obstruction due to a proximal lesion, e.g. hilar cholangiocarcinoma, may be more easily managed by percutaneous transhepatic cholangiography (PTC). Biliary brushings for cytological examination can be obtained and a plastic or metal stent can be placed as definitive treatment of the biliary obstruction. Occasionally, a combined PTC/ERCP (rendezvous) procedure is required for effective biliary decompression.

Gallbladder cancer

Adenocarcinoma of the gallbladder is a highly aggressive malignancy. Although rare in the West, gallbladder carcinoma is common in parts of India. Histological examination of cholecystectomy specimens reveals gallbladder carcinoma in approximately 1% of Western series. Adenocarcinoma is usual although squamous and mixed tumours are occasionally identified. Gallstones are present in 90% of cases. The disease is more common in females. Spread is initially by direct invasion through the gallbladder wall into the serosa and liver as well as via the lymphatics and neighbouring vasculature. Differentiation from extensive inflammation may be difficult at operation. Man-

agement depends upon disease stage. Patients found to have an intramucosal tumour on pathological assessment following cholecystectomy require no further treatment. More extensive invasion mandates gallbladder bed resection and lymphadenectomy. Excision of laparoscopic port sites may be difficult to achieve with certainty, is of unproven benefit and is not universally practised. For patients with tumours that have invaded the serosa, prognosis is poor, with a median survival of approximately 1 year. Unfortunately, patients who present with jaundice due to gallbladder cancer cannot be cured by surgical resection and palliation by endoscopic or percutaneous stent insertion is indicated.

Cholangiocarcinoma

Cholangiocarcinoma usually presents with painless obstructive jaundice. Lesions are classified according to the Bismuth Corlette system.

Elderly patients are usually affected although patients with primary sclerosing cholangitis may develop cholangiocarcinoma at an earlier age. The tumour may arise at any site within the biliary tree, but most often arises at the biliary confluence (Klatskin tumour) before invading along ducts and into liver parenchyma.

Ultrasound usually demonstrates intrahepatic biliary dilatation and may reveal metastases. Magnetic resonance cholangiography will demonstrate the stricture and complete staging should include CT imaging of the thorax and abdomen. Surgery represents the only curative modality but is only possible in a minority of patients. Biliary stenting at PTC may be followed by laparoscopy to confirm the absence of peritoneal disease if radical surgery is proposed. Resection is necessarily wide, usually requiring an extended right or left hepatectomy. As an adjunct, preoperative portal vein embolization may be used to promote hypertrophy of the future liver remnant. Despite R0 resection, 5-year survival rates remain poor.

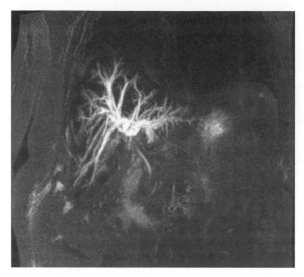

Figure 21.8 MRCP demonstrating hilar cholangiocarcinoma.

Pancreas

Surgical anatomy and physiology

The pancreas consists of a head, neck, body and tail. The gland lies retroperitoneally, behind the stomach and lesser sac with the head of the gland within the 'C' of the duodenum overlying the inferior vena cava, L2 vertebra and medial aorta. Posterior to the neck lies the superior mesenteric vessels. Behind the neck, the splenic vein joins the superior mesenteric vein to form the portal vein.

The functions of the pancreas are divided into endocrine and exocrine. The exocrine pancreas secretes alkaline bicarbonate-rich fluid in response to secretin, released from the duodenum following ingestion of a meal. Cholecystokinin, also produced by the duodenum, promotes enzyme secretion. Pancreatic protein synthesis occurs at a high rate. Proteolytic enzymes are synthesized as proenzymes preventing pancreatic autodigestion and pancreatitis.

The islets represent the endocrine portion of the pancreas. Within the islets, pancreatic alpha cells produce glucagon, beta cells produce insulin and amylin, delta cells produce somatostatin, PP cells produce pancreatic polypeptide and epsilon cells produce ghrelin. Insulin inhibits alpha cells, promotes glucose transfer into cells and activates glycogen formation. Glucagon inhibits beta cells and delta cells and causes glycogen to be broken down into glucose in the liver. Somatostatin inhibits alpha and beta cells. Ghrelin plays a role in appetite regulation.

Anatomical abnormalities of the pancreas may occur and reflect the organ's embryogenesis. Ectopic pancreas is commonly seen, particularly in the duodenum at endoscopy. An annular pancreas may result in duodenal obstruction. Pancreas divisum results from failure of the embryological dorsal and ventral ducts to fuse and produce the usual single duct configuration.

Acute pancreatitis

Acute pancreatitis is an acute inflammatory process of the pancreas with variable involvement of surrounding tissues and distant organ systems. In the UK, 20–40 per 100 000 cases occur per year. The overall mortality rate for acute pancreatitis remains approximately 10%. A diagnosis of acute pancreatitis requires two of the following features: (1) abdominal pain strongly suggestive of acute pancreatitis, (2) serum amylase and/or lipase at least three times greater than the upper limit of normal and (3) characteristic findings on transabdominal ultrasound or contrast-enhanced abdominal computed tomography.

Aetiology

The most common causes of acute pancreatitis remain gallstones and alcohol, and therefore a history suggestive of biliary colic or high alcohol intake should be sought. In Western populations, these two aetiologies account for >85% of cases. In Eastern cultures, gallstones are the commonest cause. Among children, trauma is the commonest cause of acute pancreatitis.

Clinical presentation

Patients typically present with severe epigastric pain radiating to the back. Vomiting is a common feature. Presentation and diagnosis within 24–48 hours of onset is usual but atypical presentations can make diagnosis difficult. Examination commonly reveals signs of dehydration and upper abdominal tenderness. Grey-Turner's sign (haemorrhagic flank discolouration) and Cullen's sign (haemorrhagic umbilical discolouration) may be present in severe cases. Clinical examination in the first 24 hours of admission, although specific, lacks sensitivity and hence is unreliable and should be supported by objective measures.

A peak in serum amylase may only be sustained for 12–24 hours. Early or late presentation may result in the amylase peak being missed. In addition, patients with a depleted acinar cell mass, e.g. those with chronic

Table 21.7 Cause of acute pancreatitis

Gallstone
Alcohol
Trauma
Steroids
Viral: mumps (paramyxovirus), EBV, VZV
Autoimmune: PAN, SLE
Hypercalcaemia, hyperlipidaemia/hypertriglyceridaemia and
   hypothermia
ERCP
Drugs – sulfonamides, azathioprine, NSAIDS, diuretics
   (frusemide and thiazides), didanosine
Pancreas divisum
Abnormal biliopancreatic duct junction
Carcinoma of the head of pancreas, paraneoplastic in other
   cancers
Cystic fibrosis
Scorpion and snake bite
Ascaris
Chinese liver fluke
Ischaemia, e.g. from bypass surgery
Pregnancy
Marathon running
Idiopathic

Table 21.8 SIRS

Heart rate > 90 min^{-1}
Temperature $< 36\,°C$ or $> 38\,°C$
WCC < 4 or $> 12 \times 10^9$/l (or the presence of greater than
   10% immature neutrophils)
RR > 20 or PaCO$_2$ < 4.3 kPa
SIRS + infection = sepsis

Table 21.9 APACHE II and approximate mortality rate from acute pancreatitis

APACHE II score	Mortality rate
Up to 9	5%
10–15	15%
16 or more	>33%

pancreatitis, may develop a relatively low amylase peak. Hypertriglyceridaemia may also lead to false negative amylase results. The serum amylase is neither a marker of clinical severity of pancreatitis, nor is its serial measurement indicative of the patient's physiological progress. Although amylase is widely available and provides acceptable accuracy, where lipase is available it is preferred for the diagnosis of acute pancreatitis. The differential diagnosis for hyperamylasaemia includes cholangitis, perforated peptic ulcer, mesenteric ischaemia, small bowel obstruction, acute cholecystitis, ectopic pregnancy and salpingitis.

Classification of severity

The Atlanta symposium attempted to form a global consensus and universally applicable classification system for acute pancreatitis. The definition of severity was based on the development of local or systemic complications. However, this system of classifying acute pancreatitis is currently being redrafted, taking into account a recent shift in emphasis towards defining severity by means of organ dysfunction and need for subsequent intervention rather than simply applying established scoring systems to define disease severity.

Systemic effects of acute pancreatitis include the systemic inflammatory response syndrome (SIRS), diagnosed if two or more of the criteria given in Table 21.8 are present.

SIRS due to a suspected or proven infection is called sepsis. Evidence of organ dysfunction should be sought. Respiratory compromise may occur due to adult respiratory distress syndrome (ARDS), which is characterized by acute onset bilateral infiltrates on chest radiography, without evidence of left ventricular failure (or pulmonary artery wedge pressure <18 mmHg if pulmonary artery catheterization is performed) and PaO$_2$:FiO$_2$ <27.

Potential risk factors for severity and markers of organ dysfunction that should be evaluated include age, comorbidity, body mass index, haematocrit, chest radiographic abnormalities and the APACHE II (Acute Physiology, Age and Chronic Health Evaluation II) score. APACHE II is a composite score derived from age, chronic health and dysfunction of the cardiovascular, respiratory, liver and renal systems. Although relatively cumbersome, APACHE II is the only one of the commonly used scoring systems that can be fully calculated on admission. Serum C-reactive peptide levels (>150 μM) have been shown to reflect disease severity although rises in CRP have a delayed onset and are most predictive at 48–72 hours after disease onset.

The course of acute pancreatitis is divided into an initial early phase (weeks 1–2), during which severity is defined by organ dysfunction persisting for more than 48 hours or by death. A second phase follows, during which severity is defined not only by persisting organ failure or death but also by complications that develop within the pancreatic parenchyma or peripancreatic tissues. As the need for intervention in the first phase is determined primarily by organ dysfunction, clinical parameters are central to classifying severity and determining treatment.

In the second phase, the need for treatment depends on symptoms and/or complications of necrotizing pancreatitis. The type of treatment will be determined by the abnormal morphological features of the pancreatic and peripancreatic region. The revised Atlanta definitions aim to establish a more coherent imaging-based classification of pancreatic collections and necrosis. Two types of acute pancreatitis are recognized: (1) interstitial oedematous pancreatitis and (2) necrotizing pancreatitis, the latter having three forms: (i) pancreatic parenchymal necrosis alone, (ii) peripancreatic necrosis alone, (iii) pancreatic and peripancreatic necrosis.

Patients should undergo US examination to exclude cholelithiasis within 24 hours of admission. In suspected severe cases, contrast-enhanced CT to assess pancreatic perfusion/necrosis should be performed in the first week, or if there are clinical signs of deterioration. The Balthazar CT severity scoring system is the sum of a CT-based inflammation/collection score and a necrosis score. The accuracy of MRI-based assessment has been reported to be comparable to that of CT. The presence of 30% necrosis is an additional marker of the most severe cases and should prompt discussion with or referral to a specialist pancreatic surgery unit.

Treatment

Patients with mild acute pancreatitis can be treated conservatively with intravenous fluids and analgesia, although management must be revised based on clinical progress. Rapid recovery is usual. Where gallstone aetiology is confirmed, early cholecystectomy on the index admission or within 2 weeks is recommended. Choledocholithiasis may require ERCP. Patients with severe gallstone pancreatitis benefit from early (<72 hours) ERCP and sphincterotomy. Duct stones should be cleared or adequate biliary drainage effected.

Patients with severe disease warrant high-dependency or intensive care unit admission. Complications are common and mortality rates remain around 20%. Given there is no specific treatment that reverses acute pancreatitis, complications must be detected early and addressed promptly. In addition to general resuscitative measures, adequate monitoring with goal-directed fluid management and cardiorespiratory support, patients require adequate analgesia.

Maintaining nutrition is critical during this catabolic process and naso-enteric feeding is preferable to parenteral nutrition.

The value of antibiotic prophylaxis in acute pancreatitis remains a topic of debate. Although some early meta-analyses supported the role of prophylactic antibiotics, more recent meta-analyses do not support routine antibiotic administration. However, if antibiotics are used, current guidelines recommend limiting the duration of prophylaxis to 7–14 days. Treatment should not be continued beyond that time without microbiological evidence of infection.

Infected collections require drainage. The recommended treatment for infected necrosis is appropriately timed debridement. Radiologically guided placement of percutaneous drains is now a key component of the management of these patients to address sepsis.

Then under general anaesthesia, the radiologically placed drain track can be dilated and a modified nephroscope passed to allow minimally invasive debridement of necrotic tissue from the retroperitoneum (videoscopic assisted retroperitoneal debridement, VARD, or minimally invasive retroperitoneal pancreatic necrosectomy, MIRP). Alternative approaches include laparoscopic debridement, endoscopic transgastric debridement and open surgical debridement. Minimal access techniques offer the potential benefit of minimizing the physiological insult inflicted on the patient.

Chronic pancreatitis

Excessive alcohol accounts for over 70% of causes of chronic pancreatitis, but the condition may develop due to congenital abnormalities of pancreatic enzyme function, e.g. cationic trypsinogen mutation. Gallstone disease, sphincter of Oddi dysfunction, therapeutic drugs and autoimmune disease account for a proportion of cases of chronic pancreatitis. Cystic fibrosis is the most common cause of chronic pancreatitis in children.

Chronic pancreatitis results in glandular atrophy with impairment of exocrine and endocrine function. Risk factors for pancreatitis need to be addressed. Patients should be advised to abstain from alcohol. IgG4 levels may be elevated in patients with autoimmune sclerosing chronic pancreatitis, who may respond to steroid therapy.

In addition to addressing exocrine and endocrine pancreatic insufficiency, pain can be a significant

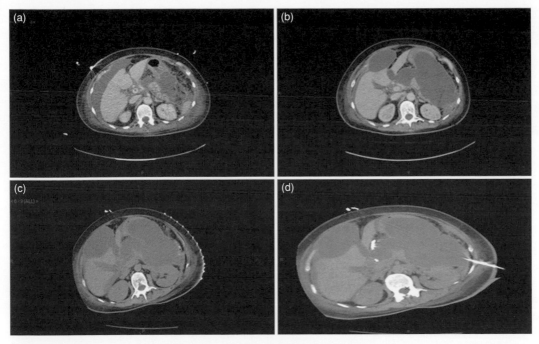

Figure 21.9 (a, b) Peripancreatic collection at two levels (note trace of gas); (c) during preparation for CT-guided percutaneous drainage and (d) following drain placement.

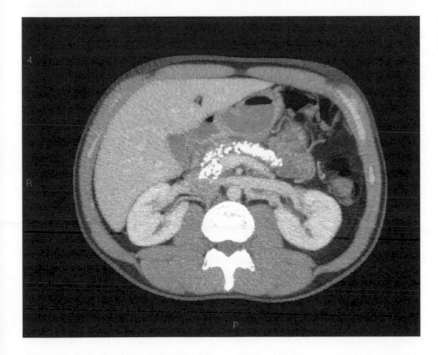

Figure 21.10 Pancreatic calcification secondary to chronic alcohol-related pancreatitis.

management problem. Patients are often opiate-dependent. On imaging, a proportion of patients will have pancreatic duct dilatation and this group may derive benefit from a surgical pancreatic drainage procedure (pancreaticojejunostomy), whereas those with an inflammatory mass may benefit from local-ized resection (pancreaticoduodenectomy if head of gland involved or distal pancreatectomy if tail of gland

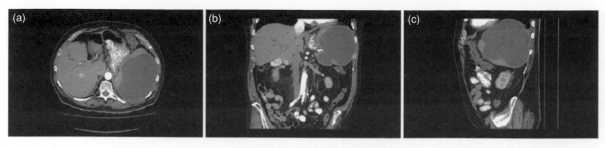

Figure 21.11 Pancreatic pseudocyst: (a) axial, (b) coronal and (c) saggital sections.

involved). Percutaneous and thoracoscopic neuroablation techniques may also be of use.

Pancreatic pseudocyst

A pseudocyst is a collection of fluid, often within the omental bursa, which, although often cystic in appearance, is lined by granulation and/or fibrous tissue and hence cannot be regarded as a true cyst. Classically, a pseudocyst of over 6 cm persisting for more than 6 weeks is unlikely to resolve spontaneously and will probably require a drainage procedure. Drainage can be performed endoscopically, laparoscopically or at open operation. The pseudocyst is usually anastomosed to the stomach (cyst-gastrostomy) or small bowel (cyst-jejunostomy) to allow decompression and resolution. Smaller cysts are generally managed conservatively.

Pancreatic cancer

Pancreatic cancer is among the deadliest types of cancer. Ninety-five per cent of pancreatic cancer is ductal adenocarcinoma. This malignancy is associated with factors such as smoking and a high-fat diet, and is more common in the African American population. Chronic pancreatitis appears to predispose to pancreatic cancer. The origin of pancreatic cancer remains unclear although precursor lesions known as pancreatic intraepithelial neoplasia (PanIN) may be evidence of a dysplasia to carcinoma sequence. A small proportion of cases are associated with a family history and genetic risk factors have been identified, e.g. mutations in SPINK1 and CFTR in hereditary pancreatitis, STK11 in Peutz-Jeghers syndrome, BRCA1 and 2 in hereditary breast and ovarian cancer, hereditary non-polyposis colorectal cancer and mutations in the CDKN2A in familial atypical multiple mole melanoma and pancreatic cancer.

Presentation is usually late due to a significant asymptomatic phase. Features include obstructive jaundice, weight loss, new-onset diabetes and back pain, an ominous symptom which often indicates locally advanced unresectable disease. Uncommon presentations include pancreatitis, thrombophlebitis and acanthosis nigricans. Gastric outlet obstruction and cachexia often develop.

Abdominal findings may be minimal but can include a palpable gallbladder (see Courvoisier's rule) and pancreatic mass. Metastatic liver involvement and ascites may also be detectable. Liver function tests may show an obstructive pattern (high alkaline phosphatase, minimal transaminase rise). Anaemia from duodenal bleeding may be present. Abdominal ultrasonography will usually confirm biliary dilatation and may confirm liver metastases. In 50–60% of patients the head of the pancreas will be visible to ultrasound and a tumour may be identified; however, bowel gas commonly obscures views of the pancreas and CT of abdomen and thorax is usually indicated, certainly if resection is being considered. CT will demonstrate vascular involvement (superior mesenteric vessels and portal vein). While venous resection is possible with some long-term survivors, arterial involvement indicates irresectability. The use of endoscopic ultrasound and MRI is increasing.

Surgical intervention may be with curative or palliative intent. In 10–20% of patients, carcinoma of the pancreatic head can be resected by means of a Whipple's pancreaticoduodenectomy. This is major surgery which should be performed in specialist units. The procedure involves removal of the pancreatic head, duodenum, distal stomach (unless a pylorus preserving procedure is performed), common bile duct and gallbladder, together with immediately associated lymphoid tissue. Reconstruction may be complicated by anastomotic leakage, particularly from the pancreaticojejunostomy. Five-year survival rates remain poor

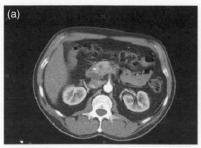
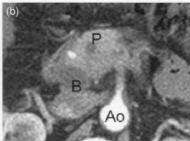
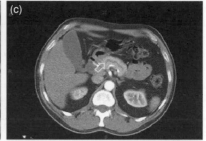

Figure 21.12 Head of pancreas tumour (a), and magnified view (b), causing pancreatic (P) and bile (B) duct dilatation. Ao, aorta. (c) Arrow indicates dilated pancreatic duct.

(5–10%), although series from Japan report rates of 30–40% for small (<2 cm) tumours. Radical lymphadenectomy has not been shown to improve outcome and is not recommended. Left-sided and pancreatic body adenocarcinoma is rarely resectable due to late presentation, but may be amenable to distal or total pancreatectomy.

Patients with unresectable disease but with a potential life expectancy of over 6 months may benefit from surgical bypass (Roux en Y hepaticojejunostomy and gastrojejunostomy) to palliate jaundice and prevent symptoms of gastric outlet obstruction; however, the majority of patients undergo palliative biliary stenting. If late gastric outlet obstruction develops, endoscopic duodenal stenting is growing in popularity as a palliative intervention. Coeliac axis neuroablation with 20 ml 50% ethanol can also be performed intraoperatively or under CT or endoscopic ultrasound guidance.

Chemotherapy (e.g. gemcitabine) is often offered postoperatively for completely excised (R0) disease as well as for microscopically positive margins (R1). Interest is also growing in neoadjuvant chemotherapy. Following the ESPAC1 trial, radiotherapy has not been widely used in the UK although this is also being reconsidered. Palliative chemotherapy offers a small benefit in terms of survival and quality of life. Earlier detection of this disease is a key to improving outcomes. K-ras gene mutations can be detected in duodenal juice of pancreatic cancer patients and similar approaches may form the basis of screening tests. As our understanding of the genetics and cell biology of pancreatic cancer improves, new avenues likely to yield useful new therapeutic agents will open. Novel agents such as tyrosine kinase inhibitors show promise and are progressing through clinical evaluation.

Ampullary adenocarcinoma

These tumours arise from the area around the ampulla in the second part of the duodenum and have a slightly more favourable prognosis than true pancreatic ductal adenocarcinoma. This tumour is common in those with APC gene mutation (familial polyposis). Radical treatment typically involves pancreaticoduodenectomy. Five-year survival rates exceed those for pancreatic ductal adenocarcinoma.

Pancreatic neuroendocrine tumours

Pancreatic neuroendocrine tumours can be classified as functional and non-functional depending on whether they produce hormones. Patients present with a wide range of symptoms, including peptic ulcers, diabetes, diarrhoea, abnormal blood glucose levels and skin rashes. Insulinoma and gastrinoma are the most common functioning neuroendocrine tumours. Insulinoma produces hypoglycaemic symptoms and affects women more commonly than men. The tumours are usually small and in 90% of cases are benign. Once located, surgical enucleation is effective and 90% of patients require no further treatment.

In Zollinger-Ellison syndrome, increased levels of gastrin are produced by a gastrinoma, usually of the pancreas or duodenum, causing the stomach to produce excess hydrochloric acid and refractory peptic ulceration. Twenty-five per cent of patients with gastrinomas have multiple endocrine neoplasia type I (MEN I). MEN I patients typically have tumours of the pituitary and parathyroids in addition to tumours of the pancreas.

Glucagonoma can produce a necrolytic migratory erythema of the skin. Two-thirds of patients with glucagonoma may develop diabetes. Surgical resection may be curative. Chemotherapy including streptozocin, fluorouracil, dacarbazine and octreotide may also help some patients. Unfortunately, approximately 50% of patients die within 5 years of diagnosis. VIPomas secrete vasoactive intestinal polypeptide, producing a syndrome of watery diarrhoea, hypokalaemia and hypochlorhydia. Somatostatinoma is extremely rare and, because of the regulatory role of somatostatin over other hormones, symptoms are variable and include diabetes, gallstones, diarrhoea and constipation.

Cystic pancreatic neoplasms

The differential diagnosis of a cystic pancreatic lesion includes benign lesions such as pseudocyst and serous cystadenoma. These must be differentiated from mucinous cystic neoplasia (MCN) of the pancreas. These are unusual lesions and their management remains controversial.

Mucinous cystic tumours of the pancreas predominate in the body and tail of the pancreas and have a strong female predilection. MCNs are the most common pancreatic cystic neoplasm (45–50%). They are often multiloculated and result from mucus hypersecretion by the abnormal duct lining. The cysts contain viscous material, which can also be haemorrhagic. MCNs are generally regarded as at least having malignant potential. Patients fit for surgery are usually offered resection. Although clinical outcome varies with gene expression profiling, survival rates are better than for pancreatic ductal adenocarcinoma.

Intraductal papillary mucinous neoplasm (IPMN)

IPMN is a non-cystic neoplasm that produces abundant mucin, which may be encountered emerging from the ampulla at ERCP. If untreated, IPMN appears to follow the dysplasia-carcinoma sequence undergoing malignant transformation. Given the low mortality rate associated with pancreatic resection (1–2% in specialist centres) an aggressive approach can be justified. Four patterns of IPMN are recognized: (1) diffuse main duct ectasia, (2) segmental main duct ectasia, (3) side branch ectasia, (4) multifocal cysts with pancreatic duct communication. Thorough preoperative assessment is essential. EUS and FNA, often with estimation of fluid carcinoembryonic antigen (CEA), may be a helpful adjunct to axial imaging. The application and extent of resection remains contro-versial. Branch duct tumours have a better prognosis than main duct tumours. Branch duct tumours often involve the head/uncinate and in fit patients may be treated by pancreaticoduodenectomy. Diffuse disease may require total pancreatectomy, while side branch disease may be managed by limited resection with intraoperative frozen section or observation.

Pancreatic lymphoma

Lymphoma may be suspected in a patient with a pancreatic mass and lymphadenopathy at distant sites. Although rare, the diagnosis of lymphoma should be confirmed and treated with chemotherapy.

Pancreaticoduodenal trauma

Injury to the pancreas and duodenum is frequently misdiagnosed and is often difficult to detect radiologically or at laparotomy. Initial suspicion based on the mechanism of injury is vital. In addition to axial imaging, pancreatography (MRCP or ERCP) may help define the injury. Where duct disruption or devitalization has occurred, pancreatic resection with Roux en Y reconstruction by a specialist surgeon may be required.

Further reading

Al Ghnaniem R, Benjamin IS, Patel AG. Meta-analysis suggests antibiotic prophylaxis is not warranted in low-risk patients undergoing laparoscopic cholecystectomy. *Br J Surg* 2003;**90**(3):365–366.

Belghiti J, Pateron D, Panis Y, Vilgrain V, Flejou JF, Benhamou JP *et al.* Resection of presumed benign liver tumours. *Br J Surg* 1993;**80**(3):380–383.

Connor S, Garden OJ. Bile duct injury in the era of laparoscopic cholecystectomy. *Br J Surg* 2006;**93**(2): 158–168.

Cunningham JD, Fong Y, Shriver C, Melendez J, Marx WL, Blumgart LH. One hundred consecutive hepatic resections. Blood loss, transfusion, and operative technique. *Arch Surg* 1994;**129**(10):1050–1056.

Flum DR, Cheadle A, Prela C, Dellinger EP, Chan L. Bile duct injury during cholecystectomy and survival in medicare beneficiaries. *JAMA* 2003;**290**(16):2168–2173.

Hart PA, Bechtold ML, Marshall JB, Choudhary A, Puli SR, Roy PK. Prophylactic antibiotics in necrotizing pancreatitis: a meta-analysis. *South Med J* 2008;**101**(11):1126–1131.

Jalan R, Hayes PC. UK guidelines on the management of variceal haemorrhage in cirrhotic patients. British

Society of Gastroenterology. *Gut* 2000;**46** (Suppl 3–4): III1–III15.

Mazzaferro V, Regalia E, Doci R, Andreola S, Pulvirenti A, Bozzetti F *et al*. Liver transplantation for the treatment of small hepatocellular carcinomas in patients with cirrhosis. *N Engl J Med* 1996;**334**(11):693–699.

Nathanson LK, O'Rourke NA, Martin IJ, Fielding GA, Cowen AE, Roberts RK *et al*. Postoperative ERCP versus laparoscopic choledochotomy for clearance of selected bile duct calculi: a randomized trial. *Ann Surg* 2005;**242**(2):188–192.

Neoptolemos JP, Dunn JA, Stocken DD, Almond J, Link K, Beger H *et al*. Adjuvant chemoradiotherapy and chemotherapy in resectable pancreatic cancer: a randomised controlled trial. *Lancet* 2001;**358**(9293): 1576–1585.

Papi C, Catarci M, D'Ambrosio L, Gili L, Koch M, Grassi GB *et al*. Timing of cholecystectomy for acute calculous cholecystitis: a meta-analysis. *Am J Gastroenterol* 2004;**99**(1):147–155.

Schindl MJ, Redhead DN, Fearon KC, Garden OJ, Wigmore SJ. The value of residual liver volume as a predictor of hepatic dysfunction and infection after major liver resection. *Gut* 2005; **54**(2): 289–296.

Terminology of nodular hepatocellular lesions. International Working Party. *Hepatology* 1995;**22**(3):983–993.

UK guidelines for the management of acute pancreatitis. *Gut* 2005;**54**(Suppl 3):iii1–iii9.

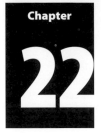

Fundamentals of endocrine surgery

Peter Cant

Introduction

Endocrine surgery involves the treatment of diseases affecting endocrine organs or networks to achieve hormonal or anti-hormonal effects in the body. Since these organs are anatomically and physiologically diverse, lesions are often managed by surgical location rather than by generic endocrine surgeons. For example, upper gastrointestinal surgeons may treat pancreatic lesions, adrenal lesions may be resected by urologists and ENT surgeons may operate on the thyroid and parathyroids. This requires exemplary multidisciplinary interaction with endocrinologists, radiologists and pathologists, together with other essential members of the team.

Endocrine surgery has common principles and themes. Incongruities in homeostatic positive and negative feedback mechanisms produce systematic abnormalities, which can then be localized anatomically. Endocrine surgeons must deal with duality; physiology and morphology; function and form; over-activity and tumour formation.

A number of fascinating endocrine diseases, such as the MEN syndromes, are very rare indeed and have a status that belies their incidence; however, the principles of management are fundamental to endocrine surgery.

Thyroid

Introduction

Goitres are very common and are defined clinically as any enlargement or change in consistency of the thyroid gland. Examination by ultrasound will show about 40% of middle-aged females to have nodular change in their thyroids. The thyroid produces hormones that influence metabolism; normal euthyroid control is maintained by thyroid stimulating hormone (TSH) from the pituitary. Alterations and diseases can produce over-activity (toxicity or hyperthyroidism) or under-activity (myxoedema or hypothyroidism). Surgery may be indicated for reduction of function in an overactive gland or removal of thyroid tissue in cases of excessive size of the gland or neoplasia.

Presentation

Patients present commonly with either changes in the form of the thyroid gland (a goitre or a lump in the neck) or changes in function of the thyroid gland, or a combination of these. History, examination and special investigations focus on these elements of form and function. The most common surgical presentation is that of a mass in the neck, followed by symptoms of compression such as dysphagia or choking. Surgeons are less frequently referred cases of toxicity and increasingly changes noted coincidentally on cross-sectional imaging are coming forward.

History

Theoretically, an enlarging thyroid mass can compress or invade neighbouring structures. In the neck these could be:

- the trachea, leading to difficulty in breathing
- the oesophagus, leading to difficulty swallowing
- nervous structures, leading to changes in the voice
- the venous system, leading to sensations of choking, fullness and pressure
- cosmetic concern.

Symptoms may be non-specific and do not predict compression or pathology with any degree of accuracy. Obstruction to the extra-thoracic upper airway should give symptoms of stridor with difficulties on

Fundamentals of Surgical Practice, Third Edition, ed. Andrew N. Kingsnorth and Douglas M. Bowley.
Published by Cambridge University Press. © Cambridge University Press 2011.

inspiration rather than wheeze or bronchospasm. Voice changes can be very significant if due to recurrent laryngeal nerve palsy secondary to malignant infiltration from a thyroid carcinoma, but this is very rare, whilst voice change secondary to environmental effects is very common. Difficulty swallowing will focus on solids, and cosmetic concerns are perceptual.

The most indicative symptom is that of choking, a feeling of tightness or fullness in the neck, especially when lying flat or extending the arms above the head. Lesions of the thyroid are not normally painful.

Familial factors include cancers of the thyroid and autoimmune thyroid disease. A history of irradiation has significance, but risk of thyroid cancer is not influenced by the size, duration or pain of a mass, and cancers are found in patients at opposite ends of the age range.

Clinical features

Changes in function are challenging to diagnose clinically, but are accurately determined biochemically. Features of toxicity and myxoedema are sought but estimation of thyroid stimulating hormone (TSH) is an excellent screen. A high TSH indicates hypothyroidism, but a TSH at the lower limit is less specific and estimation of thyroxine levels is required. Alterations in function are best controlled preoperatively since they have profound effects on anaesthesia. Toxicity has an effect akin to sensitizing catecholamine receptors, leading to clinical features of sweating, tachycardia, increased pulse pressure and anxiety. Hypothyroidism slows metabolism, including clearance of drugs.

Classically, the thyroid is examined from behind with the fingers palpating the trachea bilaterally, medial to the sternomastoid muscles, low in the neck, whilst asking the patient to swallow. The normal thyroid lies in the central fascial compartment of the neck, which moves with the muscles of deglutition. Consequently a thyroid mass will move with swallowing, as will any other lesion attached to the thyroid, lying within this compartment or attached structures within it. Examples include laryngocoeles, pharyngeal lesions, central lymph nodes and thyroglossal duct remnants.

The thyroid is usually impalpable, except in the young and thin. What is palpable through the normal gland is the trachea, which is ringed with cartilage. Palpation of lateral tracheal rings is indicative that the ipsilateral thyroid lobe is normal.

Natural history of the thyroid

The thyroid originates as a down-growth from the pharyngeal pouches along the thyroglossal tract from the base of the tongue at the foramen caecum to its final situation bilaterally alongside the larynx and trachea. With the thyroid come parafollicular 'C cells' which are diffusely distributed within the gland. The parafollicular cells are vestigial. The thyroid traps iodine to form thyroxine via an active transport system in the follicular cell membrane to form iodothyronines. Once formed the thyroid hormones are stored in the colloid of the follicles bound to thyroglobulin for subsequent release. The whole process together with growth of the cells is orchestrated by TSH.

With the passage of time, the thyroid tends to enlarge and become nodular. The aetiology of nodular goitre is not defined. Conceptually, metabolic demand varies throughout life. Putative cyclical changes lead to growth of follicles and development of hyperplastic and adenomatous nodules, colloid sequestration and microcyst formation, followed by atrophy, connective tissue and vessels partitioning the gland into nodules. The nodules have a peripheral blood supply; they can necrose centrally due to ischaemia, forming 'pseudo' cysts which can bleed and enlarge rapidly. Females, who are more prone to metabolic variation with menstruation and child-bearing, exhibit more nodular change than men, the process increasing in prevalence with age.

Most goitres submitted for pathological examination surgically show these features and are labelled multinodular goitre (MNG). The goitre itself can be smooth, nodular or frankly bossilated, and consequently can be labelled synonymously as simple, colloid, non-endemic, or a number of other terms for the same process. Other labels such as endemic, iodine deficiency, Derbyshire neck and physiological goitre imply aetiology, but all refer to variations of the same process. With this background the clinical nomenclature of goitre can be explained (Figure 22.1). A single nodule occurs in an otherwise normal and impalpable thyroid. A multinodular goitre is bilaterally palpable, even if individual nodules are not discernible. A dominant nodule is a harder, larger, tender or otherwise notable lump in a MNG.

The nodular change leads to an increase in thyroid mass, much of which is inactive, but commonly is associated with a suppressed TSH although thyroxine levels remain within normal limits. This is not a disease

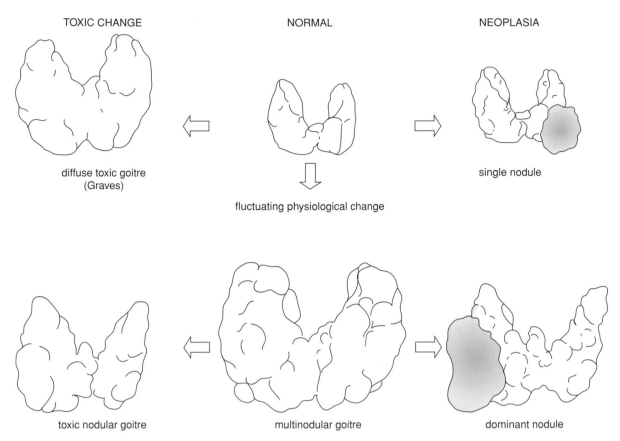

TOXIC CHANGE   NORMAL   NEOPLASIA

diffuse toxic goitre
(Graves)

fluctuating physiological change

single nodule

toxic nodular goitre   multinodular goitre   dominant nodule

Figure 22.1 The clinical nomenclature of goitres.

or a premalignant change, but equally does not protect against the development of neoplasia. It is unsurprising therefore that about 30% of thyroid malignancies occur in MNG, that being the prevalence of nodular change in the population.

Thyroid diseases and disorders

Other changes do represent diseases of the thyroid. Antibodies have a profound influence on the form and function of the gland. The Graves auto-antibodies influence the TSH receptor complex on the follicular cell, producing a range of changes from stimulation and growth to inhibition, atrophy and destruction. This can result in a diffusely enlarged overactive thyroid with an amplified blood flow, or similar changes in an existing MNG, where the functional tissue between the nodules is predominantly overactive and toxic. Individual nodules can also become overactive and autonomous, the toxic nodular goitre or Plummer's disease (Figure 22.1).

Table 22.1 Clinical goitre and malignancy risk

Clinical goitre	Risk of malignancy
MNG	0.4% to 2%
Dominant nodule in MNG	1% to 4%
Single nodule	8% to 16%

Neoplastic change

In MNG, the nodules are polyclonal and not neoplastic. Follicular adenomas and carcinomas are monoclonal and tend to produce focal masses in the thyroid. These occur with nearly equal frequency in normal thyroids and those exhibiting nodular change. In a normal thyroid this presents clinically as a single nodule and in a pre-existing MNG as a dominant nodule (Figure 22.1). Consequently the clinical differentiation into these groups has pathological and surgical significance.

Investigations

Thyroid function tests are routine and clearly define over- and under-activity. Estimation of thyroid peroxidase is useful in thyroiditis.

Ultrasound

Modern high-frequency ultrasound is the initial investigation of choice for suspected changes in thyroid morphology. Expert interpretation of these images can determine not only the size of the gland, but the size and features of any nodules. The margins, vascularity, orientation and calcifications have predictive value, and autoimmune changes, cystic degeneration and nodal abnormalities can be evaluated. These features are predictive of pathological changes but cannot determine histology.

Cytology

Fine-needle aspiration for cytology is best performed under US control to optimize appropriate sampling and specimen quality. Used in conjunction with ultrasound it can determine risk of malignancy and therefore the indications for surgery.

Some neoplastic changes are reliably diagnosed by cytology. These changes need to be sufficiently different from normal thyroid cell morphology to be diagnostic, such as medullary carcinoma, anaplastic carcinoma and some papillary cancers. Unfortunately follicular carcinomas are too similar to normal follicular cells. There are differences in terms of cellularity and paucity of colloid, but these are not sufficiently specific to be reliable. The differentiation here depends on the features of capsular and vascular invasion available only on specimen histology.

Thyroid isotope scan

Thyroid isotope scan has a very limited role in the nodular thyroid. Technetium 99m pertechnate is taken up by normal thyroid cells. Neoplastic cells are less functional, and should be 'colder', but so are many thyroid nodules and cysts, and small cold or hot lesions can be masked by adjacent tissues.

CT and MR

CT scan of the thyroid, although anatomically revealing, has a tendency to exaggerate the surgical significance of goitre, since the examination is performed supine, often with the arms abducted and the neck flexed. It does provide documentation of aspects such as tracheal compression and sub-sternal extension, but these often bear little relevance to function of the upper airway or surgical hazard. Cross-sectional imaging is very useful to stage malignancies.

Respiratory function testing has no proven value in estimating the severity of tracheal compression from goitre; however, flow volume loops, a maximum inspiratory–expiratory manoeuvre, can be useful in assessing preoperative fitness and anticipating postoperative problems but cannot be used to estimate the risk of tracheomalacia and airway collapse or to anticipate success of surgery in relieving symptoms.

Preoperative vocal cord checks play a prominent part in many clinical governance policies but add very little to practical management except in cases where there is a voice change or previous thyroid surgery.

Surgery of the thyroid

The surgical procedure matches the indication for surgery;

- diagnosis: to remove a thyroid lesion to determine its histology
- treatment of cancer: to remove and stage thyroid malignancy
- mass reduction: to reduce function in a toxic goitre or reduce size where enlarged and compressive.

Where a suitably secure diagnosis of a nodule cannot be made, an ipsilateral lobectomy is appropriate. There is little indication for less than a thyroid lobectomy as the complication rate is minimal in competent hands and subtotal removal has little advantage. The problem may not be resolved with a partial removal and repeat operation to remove the remnant is fraught with hazard.

For thyroid cancer, the operation is at least a total thyroidectomy. There are sophisticated debates for less in small well-differentiated tumours, but these are exceptions.

For mass reduction, be this for toxicity or compression, enough thyroid tissue needs to be removed to resolve the problem. For toxicity this will be a total or near total thyroidectomy, but for nodular change often a lobectomy on the largest side will suffice.

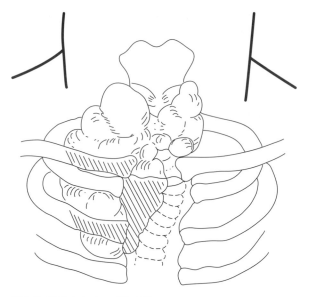

Figure 22.2 Sub-sternal thyroid.

Thyrotoxicosis is treated initially with antithyroid drugs and, if relapsing, with radioactive iodine or surgery. Surgery is now an unpopular choice, the preferences being for I^{131} unless there are specific indications such as large goitre, pregnancy or social difficulties with isolation. It is mandatory that any candidate for surgery be euthyroid for anaesthetic, control being medical with addition of Lugol's iodine or beta-blockers as indicated.

Subacute and chronic thyroiditis attacking other elements of the follicular cell leads to a variety of morphologies, including the shrunken firm uncomfortable gland of Hashimoto's disease (lymphocytic thyroiditis). Infection is rare.

Retro-sternal goitre

The space in the central compartment of the neck is limited and expansion of the thyroid can occur through the thoracic inlet into the superior mediastinum. A gland which extends below the clavicles is by definition retro-sternal. If, however, the majority of the gland is below the clavicles, the thyroid is said to be sub-sternal (Figure 22.2). Chest X-ray will show retro-sternal extension, and this can be defined more specifically with CT scan if required. A retro-sternal goitre can trap the contents of the thoracic inlet, thyroid corking. Retro-sternal extension is not an absolute indication for surgery, but the thyroid is unlikely to shrink and with age the axial skeleton shortens and the goitre will extend deeper.

Operative surgery

The thyroid is usually removed under general anaesthetic with guarded airway. Regional and local anaesthesia have been used but are a specialist taste. The standard approach is via a transverse cervical incision placed in a suitable skin crease to allow access to the superior pole, which in young people can be high in the neck. A sub-platysmal pocket is fashioned to allow mobility inside the neck, enabling separation of the strap muscles, the sternohyoid and sternothyroid, in the midline from laryngeal cartilage to the sternal notch.

The thyroid is vascular, and removal of a lobe is accomplished with control of the ipsilateral superior and inferior thyroid arteries. The thyroid capsule is thin and can be separated from the strap muscles in a bloodless plane perforated by variable veins to the internal jugular laterally. The superior pole is mobilized under vision to divide the superior thyroid artery and veins and protect the closely applied external branch of the superior laryngeal nerve. The gland can then be rotated medially to allow access to and identification of the recurrent nerve and division of the inferior thyroid artery. The inferior thyroid artery is a branch of the thyrocervical trunk off the subclavian artery, and runs behind the carotid bundle to enter the thyroid at the mid to lower pole posteriorly. Ligation of this artery on the thyroid capsule may protect the parathyroid glands, but forceful rotation of the gland to access it may also stretch the recurrent nerve. Consequently when bleeding is a problem, control can be achieved laterally by ligation of the vessel in continuity (without division) where the risk to the recurrent nerve is least.

Identification and protection of the recurrent laryngeal nerve and the parathyroid glands allows division of the tough vascular ligament that holds the medial aspect of the lobe to the side of the trachea below the cricothyroid muscle of the larynx. This fibrous band (the ligament of Berry) cannot be divided without control of the multiple small vessels within it, and this is done with care and avoiding monopolar diathermy owing to the proximity of the nerve.

The lobe can then be removed off the trachea to which it is loosely connected, the isthmus being divided and the variable inferior veins ligated.

Drainage is not usually required. Most retrosternal goitres can be removed cervically, especially with the aid of an ultrasonic scalpel. Very rarely a sternotomy is needed to deliver the mediastinal component.

Complications and consequences of surgery

Early concerns relate to bleeding and airway obstruction. Both are fortunately rare, about 2% of cases in most series, but can prove disastrous if not managed appropriately. Most bleeding is early and is recognized as an increase in drainage or swelling, either on the table or in recovery.

Of more concern is late secondary bleeding, when the patient is back on the ward, where the problem is progressive airway obstruction due to laryngotracheal oedema. The treatment here is not to remove the skin sutures, but to get the patient rapidly back into an operating theatre or ICU where suction, lighting, equipment and support are available to re-establish a patent airway before surgical correction of the problem.

Removal of part of the thyroid reduces the size of the organ and hypothyroidism can result if there is inadequate functional reserve. Stimulation by TSH is trophic to the gland and consequently replacement may not be required in time.

Voice changes are fortunately quite uncommon, but this may relate to their subtlety. Damage to the recurrent laryngeal nerve is evident immediately with an immobile cord, but clinically there may be little change. Slight huskiness of the voice may be noted. Bilateral cord palsy is more profound with risk to the airway, voice change and inability to cough. Damage to the external branch of the superior laryngeal nerve is often only noted in the trained voice as failure of projection. This nerve tenses the cricothyroideus and compensates for fatigue of the cords in singing or public speaking. The voice may also change due to scarring around the larynx, which is not really preventable.

Parathyroid damage is common, but not usually evident clinically. The glands are actively protected during surgery but the blood supply is often from the inferior thyroid artery and division of this, or even mobilization of the glands, may damage them. With unilateral procedures, compensation is the rule, but with total thyroidectomy, especially with nodal dissection, calcium supplementation may be required.

Seroma and infection are infrequent, as are hypertrophic and keloid scars. More common problems include numbness due to severance of cutaneous nerves and bulging of the cervical flap due to division of the platysma.

Thyroid cancer

Thyroid cancer is unusual without being rare, the spectrum being from the treatable well differentiated to the aggressive and rapidly fatal.

Papillary and follicular cancers are well differentiated, the tumours retaining much of the functionality of thyroid cells. Consequently these tumours often take up iodine, secrete thyroglobulin (TG) and are stimulated by TSH. These features determine the surgical approach.

Papillary cancers are the commonest form (60%), with a biphasic age distribution. The lesion tends to spread to lymph nodes rather than metastasize distantly and can be multicentric. Variants include follicular and tall cell variant with a poorer prognosis. Radiation exposure predisposes to this form of cancer.

Follicular cancers have a poorer prognosis, and can spread distantly to lungs and bones. The differentiation between follicular adenoma and follicular cancer is dependent on capsular invasion. Microinvasive cancer penetrates the capsule without evidence of lymphatic or vascular invasion and has a better prognosis than frankly invasive follicular cancer.

These tumours are treated by total thyroidectomy. The rationale is to remove as much thyroid tissue as feasible surgically to enable ablation of the remainder with radioactive iodine, I^{131}. With functional thyroid tissue removed, any remaining cells which take up iodine can be maximally stimulated by TSH by allowing the patient to become hypothyroid. Consequently, tumour cells which take up iodine less avidly than normal cells can be destroyed. The tumour cells may also secrete thyroglobulin (TG), and in the absence of any normal thyroid a rising level of TG serves as a marker for recurrent disease. Lastly, long-term TSH suppression with thyroxine has an endocrine holding effect on the tumour.

For regional metastases, nodal dissection is appropriate. This includes the nodes in the central compartment, together with those laterally as indicated by size and pathology.

The prognosis for these tumours is determined, unusually, by age and sex, being superior in the young and in females. Staging systems include standard TNM but also unique systems such as MACIS, which embodies the concept that prognosis is not determined by nodal metastases so long as the tumour is completely removed.

Poorly differentiated thyroid cancer, the anaplastic form, is fortunately uncommon, occurs in the older age groups, and is rapidly progressive despite therapy.

Medullary cancer, which, although of the thyroid, originates from the parafollicular C cells, is a fascinating tumour and unique in many ways. Medullary carcinomas occur in familial and sporadic forms; these two forms need to be separated if possible because of the genetic implications. The cancer is aggressive and avidly spreads to lymph nodes, often wide of the primary. The treatment is total thyroidectomy and extensive nodal dissection, often extending into the mediastinum, surgery offering the best chance of success. The tumour does have endocrine markers, calcitonin and CEA, which can be useful monitors of progress. The familial form is associated with the MEN syndromes.

Other malignancies include secondaries and lymphomas.

Thyroglossal duct remnants

Embryological remnants of thyroid descent from the region of the tongue are the cause of thyroglossal duct cysts. These are lined by respiratory epithelium, are sensitive to viruses that attack these tissues and can present in the adult with sudden enlargement and inflammation. Thyroid follicular cells are sparse in these lesions, and consequently they are negative on isotope scan. They recur following aspiration and are best excised. The cyst needs to be removed with the central portion of the hyoid bone to which it is embryologically attached and via which the duct can extend to the base of the tongue (Sistrunk procedure). Nondescent of the thyroid is rare but is found as a lingual thyroid. A pyramidal lobe is a remnant in the midline at the thyroid isthmus.

Parathyroid

Introduction

Hyperparathyroidism is defined as a raised level of serum parathyroid hormone (PTH). This can be due to hypocalcaemia and an increased demand for calcium (secondary hyperparathyroidism), which is an appropriate homeostatic endocrine feedback mechanism. Primary hyperparathyroidism, however, is autonomous and inappropriate. Adenomas or hyperplasia of the parathyroid glands (PTG) produce excessive PTH and an increased serum calcium load.

Presentation

Surgically, hyperparathyroidism presents with hypercalcaemia. It is unusual to find advanced secondary disease today and since most blood auto-analysers have a dedicated calcium channel the condition is milder and detected earlier. In primary care raised serum calcium is commonly due to hyperparathyroidism, but in a hospital setting the most common cause of hypercalcaemia is malignancy. Other causes include renal failure, fractures and immobility, thiazide diuretics, vitamin D toxicity and bowel disease, which have to be excluded.

The clinical features are non-specific. The commonest feature is fatigue, but inquiry is made of muscle pain and weakness, bone disease such as osteoporosis or fractures, ulcers and pancreatitis, renal stones, hypertension and heart disease, psychological problems, familial traits and cancers. A parathyroid mass in the neck is uncommon, as is a coincidental finding of a mass on imaging.

The natural history of the disease

Asymptomatic hypercalcaemia is surprisingly common, and many of these are due to primary hyperparathyroidism. The incidence increases with age and is more common in females. Males with hyperparathyroidism tend to have more renal stone disease, even though renal stones are not often due to hyperparathyroidism. Untreated mild asymptomatic disease is often indolent; there is, however, a statistically increased risk of death, mainly due to heart disease and cancer, which is reversed with parathyroidectomy. For patients who become symptomatic, surgery is the only curative therapy. Conservative management is a strategy for the infirm, the undecided and patients with borderline asymptomatic hyperparathyroidism. There is a strong familial association with the MEN syndromes.

Historically patients presented with severe bone (osteitis fibrosa cystica and Brown tumours) and renal changes (nephrocalcinosis and nephrolithiasis). Progression to hypercalcaemic crisis (dysequilibrium syndrome) is unusual and presents with anorexia, nausea and vomiting and polyuria, leading to hypotension, collapse, cardiac changes, confusion and oliguria secondary to rapidly rising serum calcium. The condition is more common in parathyroid carcinoma and treatment is with fluid resuscitation, saline diuresis, osteoclast inhibitors and parathyroidectomy.

The parathyroid gland is unusual because the secretory product, PTH, is tightly regulated in a direct feedback loop by the cation it controls, calcium sensors on cell membranes of parathyroid cells responding to ionized calcium. PTH exerts its influence through specific receptors in peripheral target tissues. In the kidneys and bone, production of cyclic AMP reduces calcium excretion and regulates bone remodelling. Indirectly PTH influences intestinal absorption via vitamin D, by increasing the conversion of renal 25-hydroxyvitamin D3 (calcifediol) to 1,25-dihydroxyvitamin D3 (calcitriol).

Investigation

The condition is diagnosed biochemically, a contemporaneous and sustained hypercalcaemia in the presence of a raised or unsuppressed level of parathyroid hormone. Very few conditions mimic this state, the most important being benign familial hypocalciuric hypercalcaemia, a congenital condition affecting the tubules of the kidneys. This is differentiated on the basis of a low 24-hour urinary calcium secretion. Historically the situation was not always as straightforward. The parathyroid hormone assay was non-specific, being focused on fragments of the 84 amino acid chain, which lead to confusion in malignant states. Parathyroid related proteins, PTHrP, secreted by tumours and leading to malignant hypercalcaemia, were indistinguishable. Consequently complex investigations were carried out to determine calcium secretion and renal tubular activity and the diagnosis was less secure. Whole molecule assay has resolved these issues.

Once diagnosed biochemically, localization anatomically is advantageous. A modern approach, localization leads to less invasive surgery; although it is likely that the success rates are very similar to bilateral exploration in experienced hands.

Radioisotope scans using, for example, technetium Tc 99m sestamibi localizes the offending gland in 80% of cases. The isotope targets metabolically active tissues with high levels of mitochondrial uptake, as found for example in the heart and thyroid. A subtraction technique is used, the activity being washed out of the thyroid more rapidly than the parathyroid glands, showing as a persistent hot spot. SPECT (single parti-

cle emission CT) is complementary, providing three-dimensional anatomical information.

Ultrasound is useful; the abnormal parathyroid gland can be seen on most occasions and when concordant with isotope scans is nearly 100% accurate. More importantly the condition of the thyroid gland can be evaluated. A parathyroidectomy in the presence of a multi-nodular goitre is challenging.

Surgery

Experience in this operation is advantageous. The orthodox cases are easily resolved, but knowledge of the variations is invaluable. A bloodless field using bipolar diathermy and optical aids improves visualization of the glands. Some surgeons favour methylene blue as a localizing dye. Conventionally both sides are explored and all four glands are identified. Frozen section intraoperatively can help decision-making if more than one enlarged gland is found, and avoids confusion with lymph nodes. The half-life of PTH is short, a few minutes only, and intraoperative PTH assay can confirm successful removal of the source.

The embryology of the PTG has surgical relevance here. The lower PTG arises from the third pharyngeal pouch, paradoxically superior to the upper PTG which comes from the fourth pouch. The lower glands therefore descend past the upper and can be ectopic, anywhere from the base of the skull to the mediastinum. Usually, however, the superior gland lies superior to the inferior thyroid artery and lateral to the recurrent laryngeal nerve. The inferior gland is more variable and lies medial to the nerve and inferior to the artery (Figure 22.3). Minimally invasive approaches focus on localized glands, often with small incisions and endoscopic techniques. Success rates are as good as bilateral exploration in appropriately selected cases.

The surgical pathology of primary hyperparathyroidism shows that about 85% are due to a single adenoma, 13% due to hyperplasia or the presence of more than one abnormal gland and 2% are carcinomas.

Complications and consequences of surgery

Success following surgery (normocalcaemia) should be over 95%, with some centres reporting levels of 98%. PTH does not always return to normal immediately and relief of symptoms is far less predictable. Clearly established bone and renal damage is irreversible, as is hypertension. However, improvements in fatigue, muscle weakness and mental function are relatively

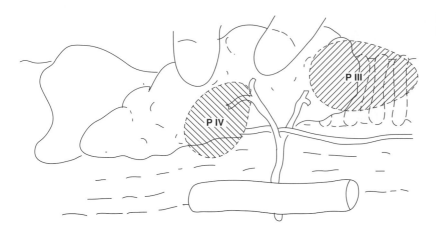

Figure 22.3 Anatomical relationships of the parathyroid gland.

encouraging and the prevention of consequences such as progressive stone disease is worthwhile.

Hypocalcaemia perioperatively is common but not always symptomatic, occurring usually within 24 hours of surgery. The calcium check the day after surgery is diagnostic; the first symptom is usually perioral numbness. Asymptomatic hypocalcaemia does not require treatment, since the trigger to PTG recovery is low serum ionized calcium, but once symptoms develop, intravenous calcium gluconate may be necessary to augment oral calcium and vitamin D therapy. Calcium chlorine intravenously is dangerous and best avoided owing to its high degree of ionization.

Prediction of postoperative hypocalcaemia is difficult. High preoperative levels of calcium, bone disease and high levels of alkaline phosphatase (hungry bones) can be warning features.

More problematic is persistent postoperative hypoparathyroidism. If suspected intraoperatively (bilateral, reoperative and total parathyroidectomies) autotransplantation into muscle or cryopreservation can restore functional tissue. Persistent or recurrent hyperparathyroidism is difficult to treat. Accurate anatomical localization is mandatory before surgery and all localization tests should be used together with careful review of the operative and pathological details. Selective venous sampling is particularly valuable. Performed angiographically, samples of blood are taken under image control, from the veins around the thyroid. Raised levels of PTH are found adjacent to functional parathyroid tissue, usually determining the side of the lesion and sometimes the level in the neck.

Carcinoma of the parathyroid is found in about 2% of primary hyperparathyroid patients, the alerting features being severe hypercalcaemia, very high levels of PTH and a palpable neck lump. Treatment is surgical, typically a very fibrotic lesion being removed widely. Pathologically the differentiation from benign parathyroid disease is difficult. Nodal and distant metastases occur and calcium and PTH are markers of recurrence.

Tertiary hyperparathyroidism

Although secondary hyperparathyroidism is physiological and appropriate to chronically low calcium, in chronic renal failure parathyroid hyperplasia can in time become autonomous. The calcium levels rise, the parathyroid glands do not respond to ionized calcium and the levels of PTH remain elevated. This is uncontrolled secondary or tertiary HPT and clearly involves all the parathyroid glands.

Before kidney transplantation, parathyroidectomy is indicated when medical therapy fails to control hypercalcaemia, and there is progressive bone damage or calciphylaxis (extraskeletal calcification). After transplantation the main indication is persistent or symptomatic hypercalcaemia, which if severe can damage the transplant.

The operation is usually subtotal parathyroidectomy or total parathyroidectomy with autotransplantation or cryopreservation. With removal of all four glands, hypoparathyroidism is problematic except in patients on dialysis who are not candidates for transplantation.

Adrenal

The adrenal gland functions as two separate endocrine organs, the outer layers of the cortex and the inner medulla, which is neuroendocrine in origin. The cortex secretes corticosteroids (the most important being cortisol), mineralocorticoids (aldosterone) and sex steroids. The medulla secretes catecholamines. Anatomically the two suprarenal glands lie retroperitoneally applied to the superior pole of the kidney, on the crura of the diaphragm.

Incidentalomas

An incidental adrenal tumour, discovered during investigation for other symptoms, may also be called adrenalomas. Any endocrine activity (although not obviously overt by nature of the clinical presentation) is unknown, as is whether it is benign or malignant, and, if malignant, primary or secondary. Such tumours are quite frequent (about 4%), and most are non-functioning cortical adenomas, but other findings include nodular hyperplasia, cysts, myelolipomas, ganglioneuromas, carcinomas and pheochromocytomas.

Investigations include baseline hormonal evaluation (metanephrines, dexamethasone suppression test and serum potassium monitoring). Imaging with CT and MRI is not completely specific, but some lesions can be reliably diagnosed (e.g. myelolipomas) and treated conservatively; imaging can also help to exclude a primary tumour elsewhere. Aspiration cytology is rarely useful.

Malignant and functional lesions are treated appropriately; the remainder are managed according to size criteria. Large tumours are more likely to be malignant and lesions less than 2–3 cm can be watched. The size criterion is not due to malignant transformation of small adenomas, it is because malignant neoplasms select themselves for growth and the adrenal is not in an anatomical location which is easy to examine. It must be pointed out, however, that size alone is not a guarantee of benignity and minimally invasive surgery is now very safe, so there is a move to more resections.

Adrenocorticoid carcinoma

These very rare and very malignant adrenal tumours can present in three ways.

- an overt hypersecretion syndrome, hypercortisolism, virilization and mixed (60%)
- a mass, often painful, compressive and very large in the flank (30%)
- an incidentaloma (10%).

Adrenocorticoid carcinoma can occur in children; early detection and surgery offer the best prospects of success.

Functional diseases of the adrenal

Cushing's syndrome

All conditions resulting in chronic glucocorticoid excess are eponymously called Cushing's syndrome. Cushing's *disease* relates to hypercortisolism due to a pituitary microadenoma.

Clinical presentation

The course is insidious with centripetal obesity and buffalo hump, oligo-amenorrhoea in females, muscular atrophy and skin changes with striae and bruising. The appearance is well known, since the commonest cause of Cushing's syndrome is iatrogenic steroid administration. Other causes are:

1. ACTH dependent (production of ACTH or ACTH-like substances)

   · pituitary (70%), adenomas and microadenomas
   · ectopic (10%), from malignant lung, pancreas, thymus, medullary thyroid and carcinoid tumours

2. ACTH independent

   · functional adrenal adenomas or adenocarcinomas, and primary adrenal hyperplasia.

The investigation of Cushing's syndrome is by exclusion: serum cortisol estimation and low-dose dexamethasone suppression. Suppression of ACTH by a small 1 mg dose of dexamethasone causes suppression of plasma cortisol and a normal urinary free cortisol and rules out Cushing's syndrome.

Failure to suppress indicates the need for further testing; direct measure of plasma ACTH and high dose dexamethasone suppression.

- Adrenal tumours will produce high un-suppressible levels of cortisol, and have low levels of ACTH due to negative pituitary feedback.
- On the other hand, pituitary causes will have normal or elevated ACTH levels, but cortisol will usually be suppressed.
- Ectopic sources from tumours will have elevated ACTH and will not show suppression of cortisol

owing to maximal stimulation of the adrenal by the ectopic hormone.

On the basis of these results localization tests are performed on the adrenal and pituitary.

Pituitary-dependent Cushing's syndrome (70%) is best treated by tumour removal with transphenoidal microsurgery, but this is not always possible or successful. Consequently bilateral adrenalectomy may be indicated. Ectopic sources are extirpated if possible and adrenal causes are subject to unilateral adrenalectomy.

Removal of a benign adrenal adenoma results in a gradual disappearance of the signs over 12 months and long-term survival. Bilateral adrenalectomy for pituitary Cushing's is less successful, and secondary pituitary tumours (Nelson syndrome) may occur.

Hyperaldosteronism

Conn's syndrome or primary hyperaldosteronism is one of five surgically remediable causes of hypertension (the others are Cushing's syndrome, phaeochromocytoma, renal artery stenosis and coarctation of the aorta).

The clinical features of Conn's syndrome are very non-specific, moderate hypertension and features compatible with low potassium such as muscle weakness or cramps. The disease is usually due to a functional adenoma of the adrenal, but may be caused by bilateral adrenal hyperplasia or rarely glucocorticoid suppressible hyperaldosteronism or carcinoma.

Aldosterone normally controls blood pressure via the renin angiotensin system. Renin is released from the afferent glomerular arteriole in response to decreases in intravascular volume, enabling angiotensinogen cleavage and conversion to angiotensinogen II, which activates cells in the zona glomerulosa of the adrenal to secrete aldosterone. This mechanism is amplified by a high serum potassium, low sodium and ACTH. Aldosterone acts on the distal renal tubules to retain sodium in exchange for potassium and hydrogen ions to restore plasma volume.

The complexity of the physiology and variability of pathology means that reliable diagnosis is challenging. In a patient with hypertension and hypokalaemia, a raised level of plasma aldosterone and a suppressed level of plasma renin activity are virtually diagnostic. However, tests are often equivocal, diuretics can produce hypokalaemia and antihypertensives can affect renin angiotensin regulation; so other complex investigations may be required.

In patients with a confirmed diagnosis, localization tests are indicated. CT scans can show a lesion, but, if equivocal, isotope scanning or venous sampling studies can help.

Patients with a unilateral aldosteronoma are candidates for surgery, which normalizes the renin aldosterone system in most cases, and reverses hypertension in 40 to 80%. The results are best in young females with a short duration of hypertension.

Phaeochromocytoma

Tumours of the adrenal medulla are characterized by the production of catecholamines and subsequent hypertension.

Presentation

Even today, phaeochromocytoma presents commonly at autopsy with sudden death syndromes due to cardiomyopathy or vascular accident. This may also become apparent in hospital following relatively minor interventions with intravenous contrast or operations in the unsuspected. The classic clinical features of sweating, palpitations, headache and hypertension are not consistent; if anything this tumour is characterized by its variability. Phaeochromocytoma has been called the 10% tumour, so termed for the incidence of malignancy, extra-adrenal location, multifocality and occurrence in children. It is notable for the association with the MEN and other syndromes.

Symptoms of phaeochromocytoma are due to the hormone soup excreted by these tumours, not just adrenaline but noradrenaline, dopamine and other amines. Non-functional tumours are uncommon. These amines exert α-adrenergic effects on the cardiovascular system, notably extreme vasoconstriction, causing hypertension, which leads to near total inhibition of the renin angiotensinogen system and the body adjusts by shrinking the plasma volume.

Diagnosis depends on measurement of plasma or urinary catecholamines or the breakdown products, notably metanephrines. Stimulation tests are problematic and suppression tests unreliable, and none is specific for malignancy. Localization for surgery with CT scan will define the 90% of tumours in one adrenal gland, but may fail to identify paraganglionomas. MRI is more accurate here and MIBG scans are likewise useful in searching for metastases and multiple tumours.

Preoperative management has led to major improvements in outcomes, mainly due to re-expansion of the plasma volume preoperatively, which minimizes the postoperative hypotension which occurs on removal of the tumour. The standard is an α-blocker, such as phenoxybenzamine (10 mg to 160 mg BD) for at least a week, and until there is nasal stuffiness and warm well-perfused extremities with postural hypotension. Beta-blockade may be necessary for arrhythmias but is problematic for two reasons. In the absence of α-blockade it can lead to severe and refractory hypertension, and in the presence of α-blockade it limits the ability of the body to increase cardiac output by increasing the heart rate in response to hypotension or hypovolaemia.

The diagnosis is suspected in patients with symptoms, or those with associated family histories of hyperparathyroidism or medullary carcinoma of the thyroid.

Paragangliomas are also called chemodectomas and glomus tumours. These neuroendocrine tumours contain neurosecretory granules although only a few have evidence of over-secretion. They are related to phaeochromocytomas and can occur in MEN syndromes.

Surgery of the adrenals

Operative management and technique is critical for phaeochromocytomas. Operative monitoring and blood pressure control are anaesthetic specialities, as is blood pressure control postoperatively when the source of catecholamines has been removed. The adrenals are supplied variably by branches of three arteries, the inferior phrenic, the renal and the aorta. However, there is only one vein on each side, a short right adrenal vein into the vena cava and a longer left into the renal vein. Surgically the adrenal vein should be ligated as soon as feasible in phaechromocytomas, but this is difficult given the approaches to the gland. Most operations are now done laparoscopically.

Gastrointestinal

Pancreas

The pancreas is a mixed endocrine and exocrine gland and the most prominent site for endocrine tumours in the gastrointestinal system.

Insulinomas

These small, rare tumours are sometimes part of a genetic process and, as such, can be associated with a diverse array of hormone products and consequent symptoms and signs. Patients with insulinomas are best managed in specialist centres.

Isolated insulinomas produce insulin outwith the normal regulatory pathways, a classic endocrine feedback loop regulated by levels of glucose. Beta cells produce proinsulin in response to stimulation, releasing C peptide in equal quantities to insulin. Insulinomas do not respond to the negative feedback of a low level of glucose (non-suppressible) and continue to produce insulin and C peptide.

Presentation

The signs and symptoms are not based just on low levels of glucose, but can be grouped into neurological, cardiovascular and gastrointestinal manifestations. Hypoglycaemia produces changes from apathy to coma, and also stimulates catecholamines, causing tachycardia and palpitations. This can be associated with hunger, obesity, nausea and vomiting, not unlike the profile of hypoglycaemia, with 'dumping syndrome' following gastrectomy.

The diagnosis is that of hypoglycaemia, for which there are many causes, mainly those which occur after eating (postprandial) or those which occur with fasting or exercise. It is the latter which occur in insulinomas, but with other causes such as alcoholism or other sources of underproduction of glucose. Definition of the diagnostic criteria is useful (Whipple's triad):

- signs and symptoms of hypoglycaemia occurring with fasting or exercise
- low blood glucose levels at the time of symptoms
- symptoms resolved by administration of glucose.

Confirmation is made by demonstration of an inappropriately high level of insulin at a time of severe hypoglycaemia (insulin-glucose ratio) and to achieve this, fasting for up to 3 days may be necessary. Further testing of proinsulin and C peptide can be helpful, especially in distinguishing factitious self-administration of insulin as a cause.

Localization of these small tumours (90% are less than 2 cm) is problematic. Ultrasound and most cross-sectional imaging is unreliable and venous sampling is invasive. These are essential for reoperative cases but for initial operations intraoperative ultrasound may be most helpful. Operative strategies depend on situation and risk of malignancy (about 10%). Enucleation is the approach for single lesions, but multiple and malignant lesions may require partial or even total pancreatectomy.

Gastrinomas

The history here is iconic, the syndrome of Zollinger and Ellison being described before gastrin was identified.

Presentations vary, the clues being:

- peptic ulcers refractory to maximum therapy
- diarrhoea in a patient with peptic ulcer disease
- recurrent ulcers after cure and maintenance or adequate ulcer surgery
- jejunal ulcers, atypical and multiple ulcers
- hypertrophic gastric mucosa, with jejunitis and hypersecretion.

The effects are due to excessive secretion of gastrin, a trophic hormone secreted by the G cells of the antrum of the stomach in response to high pH (low acid). As is typical for endocrine disease, gastrinomas are unresponsive to stomach acid, usually because they are separated from the stomach content, which suppresses normal G cells. Consequently the diagnosis is made by finding hypergastrinaemia in the serum with high gastric acid secretion and a positive secretin stimulation test.

These tumours are elusive, often multiple and associated with the familial syndromes. There is no standard protocol for localization. Endoscopy, ultrasound of the liver and pancreas, cross-sectional imaging, isotope scanning and venous sampling may all be relevant depending on the management plan, which may be medical or surgical.

Medical therapy is now the first line since omeprazole blocks the secretion mechanism, allowing time for investigation and not precipitant surgery for symptom control. The lesion(s) are indolent; however, 60% are malignant. For sporadic gastrinoma, surgery is preferred, since the lesion is usually single, localizable and resection is often curative. Familial gastrinoma is more complex, with other tumours complicating the picture, multiple gastrinomas which are difficult to find and the surgery being more aggressive; omeprazole is often a better option.

The operative strategy involves adequate exposure of the duodenum and pancreas and associated nodal drainage. Nodal metastases are often the source of persistent symptoms. Metastatic disease, complete resection of the tumour and tumour size are predictors of survival and follow-up is life-long.

Rare pancreatic endocrine tumours

Gastrinomas and insulinomas are the most common functional pancreatic islet cell tumours (about 90%). The remainder are very rare indeed and include somatostatinomas, glucagonomas and VIPomas. These often have associated symptom complexes or may present as malignant masses. The principles remain the same; endocrine diagnosis, localization and aggressive surgical ablation.

Carcinoid

Carcinoid tumours are rare lesions of endodermal origin, derived from the enterochromafin cell; they can be found anywhere from the bronchus to the anus. The WHO has recently reclassified carcinoids as part of the spectrum of neuroendocrine tumours.

Presentation is variable and diagnosis based on a clinical suspicion is unusual.

The tumours are APUDomas (amine precursor uptake decarboxylase) and behave differently depending on site of origin. About 70% are found in the gastrointestinal tract, where they can cause obstruction due to stenosis, bleeding or pain. The tumours secrete many different hormones, neuropeptides and neurotransmitters, but serotonin classically produces the rare syndrome of flushing, diarrhoea and cardiac fibrosis, and may be responsible for the local fibrotic response. Carcinoid syndrome is uncommon and usually associated with small bowel tumours. The presence of the syndrome suggests metastatic disease owing to first-pass inactivation of the hormones by the liver.

If suspected the diagnosis is made on the basis of 24-hour 5-HIAA estimation in the urine and serum serotonin levels. The lesions are not easy to see endoscopically, being submucosal, but strictures can be visualized on contrast studies. MIBG scan can detect metastases of the liver and bronchial carcinoids can be detected on chest X-ray and CT.

Prognosis is dependent on site and stage; bronchial and hind gut tumours tend to be benign, but foregut carcinoids and those of the thymus are often malignant. Small tumours (<15 mm) and somatostatin receptor positivity are favourable features.

Table 22.2 Multiple endocrine neoplasia

Characteristic	MEN 1	MEN 2A	MEN 2B	FMTC
Gene	MEN1 gene	RET	RET	RET
Pancreas	Insulinoma, gastrinoma, vipoma			
Pituitary adenoma	yes			
Parathyroid	90%	20%		
Medullary carcinoma		Nearly 100%	100%	100%
Phaeochromocytoma		40–50%	50%	
Eponym and phenotype	Wermer's syndrome	Sipple syndrome	Marfanoid and neuromas	

Resection of the primary and the liver metastases is the first treatment, even if only debulking. Somatostatin analogues, cyto-embolization and interferon-alpha are options.

Multiple endocrine neoplasia

Multiple endocrine neoplasia (MEN) is a syndrome when two or more endocrine tumour types occur in a patient due to a causative mutation or hereditary transmission.

These are distinct clinical entities, characterized by hyperplastic, adenomatous and neoplastic change (Table 22.2).

MEN 1

MEN 1 is a syndrome characterized by the development of endocrine lesions in the parathyroid, pancreas and pituitary. Carcinoids and thyroid tumours can occur. The condition is inherited as a genetically defined autosomal dominant, and many cases come from recognized kindreds. Clinically it manifests in the adult, and serum calcium screening is valuable, leading to focused investigations of pancreas and pituitary.

The parathyroid disease can be hyperplasia or multiple adenomas and surgical removal of at least three and a half glands is recommended; recurrence is common. Pancreatic tumours occur in about 70%, often multiple. Many of the tumours secrete 'non functional' substances such as pancreatic polypeptide, and this can serve as a useful tumour marker.

Anterior pituitary tumours can secrete prolactin or growth hormone (acromegally).

MEN 2

These syndromes consist of at least three separate subgroups, MEN 2A, MEN2b and familial medullary carcinoma (only). Caused by mutations in the RET proto-oncogene, the inheritance is autosomal dominant and penetrance is about 70%.

MEN 2A

Virtually all cases develop medullary carcinoma of the thyroid, often early in life, with about 50% developing phaeochromocytomas, often bilaterally.

Glandular hyperplasia begins with the C cells, and progresses to malignancy, typically bilateral and multicentric. Calcitonin screening can alert to change in the young, enabling total thyroidectomy to prevent MTC.

MEN 2B

Parathyroid hyperplasia is not a feature; MEN 2B is characterized by aggressive medullary carcinomas and the phenotypic features of ganglioneuromas which can occur in the gut, causing symptoms. Surgery is required in infancy often to prevent MTC. The patient should be screened for phaeochromocytomas before surgery on the thyroid because of the operative risk of catecholamine release.

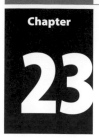

Chapter

23

Fundamentals of the breast

Steven D. Heys

Basic biology

Anatomy of the breast

Embryology

The breast is a modified sweat gland which originates from the ectodermal layer of the embryo between the fifth and sixth week of gestation. It arises from the 'milk lines', which are two ridges of ectodermal thickening, running from the axilla to the groin. Although most of the 'milk line' eventually disappears, a prominent ridge remains in the pectoral area to form the breast. The ectoderm in this area subsequently grows into the underlying mesoderm as a series (15–20) of buds. These ectodermal buds, which are initially solid, eventually form the lactiferous ducts and their associated alveoli. The adjacent mesenchyme develops into the surrounding adipose and connective tissues. During the final two months of gestation, the ducts become canalized and a 'mammary pit' is formed in the ectoderm. The lactiferous ducts subsequently communicate with the mammary pit.

Gross anatomy

Morphological features

The breast is situated within the subcutaneous tissue of the anterolateral chest wall. It extends from the second to the sixth rib and from the edge of the sternum to the mid-axillary line, overlying the pectoralis major, serratus anterior, upper part of the rectus sheath and external oblique muscles. The breast extends in a supero-lateral direction along the border of the pectoralis major muscle, through the foramen of Langer in the deep fascia of the axilla, to lie close to the pectoral group of axillary lymph nodes. This is termed the axillary tail of Spence. The breast is separated from the muscles it overlies by the deep fascia. However,

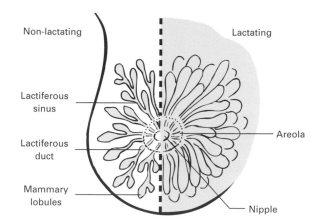

Figure 23.1 Anatomy of the breast and chest wall. Permission from *Essential Clinical Anatomy*, Williams & Wilkins, Baltimore.

between the breast and the deep fascia is the retro-mammary space, which contains loose areolar tissue. Supporting connective tissue strands pass between the dermal layer of the skin and the underlying breast. They are well developed in the upper aspect of the breast and are referred to as the suspensory ligaments of Cooper.

The nipple usually lies at the level of the fourth intercostal space and 15 to 20 lactiferous ducts open on to its surface through small openings. Surrounding the nipple is the areola, which is made up of pigmented skin and subcutaneous tissue in which lie smooth muscle fibres. The epithelium contains sweat glands, sebaceous glands and accessory mammary glandular tissue.

Arterial supply and venous drainage

The blood supply to the breast is from the perforating branches of the internal thoracic artery (lateral edge of the sternum), the lateral thoracic artery and the

Fundamentals of Surgical Practice, Third Edition, ed. Andrew N. Kingsnorth and Douglas M. Bowley.
Published by Cambridge University Press. © Cambridge University Press 2011.

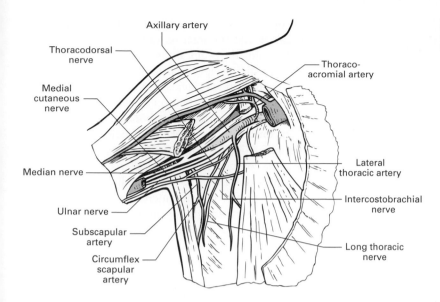

Figure 23.2 Anatomy of axilla. Permission from *Gray's Anatomy*, 35th edn. 1973, Churchill Livingston, p. 648.

pectoral branch of the acromiothoracic artery (the latter two derived from the axillary artery). In addition, there is also a variable blood supply from perforating branches of the intercostal arteries and from the subscapular artery. The venous drainage is through veins corresponding to the arterial supply.

Lymphatic drainage

The lymphatic drainage of the breast is predominantly through lymph vessels which are located in the interlobular connective tissues. These lymph vessels communicate with the cutaneous and subcutaneous lymphatic plexuses, the subareolar plexus of Sappey, and a plexus lying beneath the breast on the deep fascia covering the pectoralis major muscle. It has been estimated that approximately 75% of the lymph drainage of the breast is to the axillary groups of lymph nodes. These are the anterior (or pectoral nodes), which are situated along the lateral thoracic vessels, the posterior (or subscapular nodes), which are on the subscapular vessels, the central group of lymph nodes lying within the axilla, and the apical group sited at the apex of the axilla (Figure 23.3). In addition, there can be a few nodes situated between the pectoralis major and minor muscles (Rotter's nodes).

These lymph nodes can be subdivided anatomically, depending on their relationship to the pectoralis minor muscle: level I – nodes lying below the muscle; level II – nodes lying behind the muscle; and level

III – nodes above the muscle in the apex of the axilla. The lymphatic drainage from the apical nodes is to the supraclavicular and lower cervical groups of nodes, but there are also connections between the supraclavicular and infraclavicular nodes. However, it is also recognized that 25% of the lymph drainage of the breast (medial aspect) is to the internal thoracic nodes and, in

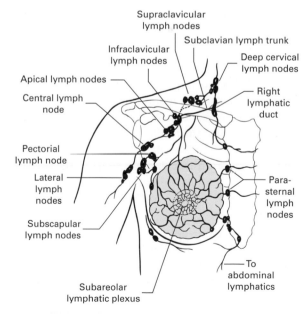

Figure 23.3 Lymphatic drainage of the breast. Permission from *Essential Clinical Anatomy*, Williams & Wilkins, Baltimore.

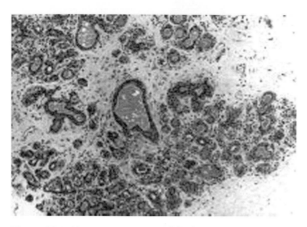

Figure 23.4 Microscopic anatomy of the breast.
Permission from *Atlas of Human Histology*, ed M.S.H. di Fiore. Lea and Febiger, Philadephia, p. 245.

addition, some lymphatic drainage is through the lymphatics of the anterior abdominal wall and also possibly via lymphatic connections to the opposite breast.

Microscopic anatomy –– The breast is composed of glandular elements, fibrous and fat tissues. The glandular part of the breast consists of between 15 and 20 lobes. A lobe has approximately 30 lobules, which terminate in the acini (10 to 100). The acini are separated from each other by the intralobular connective tissue and the lobules are separated from each other by fine connective tissue. Light microscopic examination of an acinus demonstrates that it is composed of two cell types; the secretory epithelial cell and the contractile myoepithelial cell. The terminal duct and the acini of a lobule are termed the 'terminal duct–lobular unit'. These ducts unite to form subsegmental and segmental ducts, which in turn drain into the lactiferous ducts and sinuses. The lactiferous ducts (15 to 20) pass towards the nipple and areola, where they undergo dilatation to form the lactiferous sinuses. The sinuses open onto the surface of the nipple through separate ductular orifices.

Anatomy of the axilla

Structure

The axilla is a pyramidal space with an apex, base (or floor) and four walls – anterior, posterior, medial and lateral. The apex is bordered by the outer border of the first rib, the posterior surface of the middle third of the clavicle and the upper border of the scapula. The base of the axilla is formed by skin and deep fascia, the axillary fascia. The anterior wall is made up of the pectoralis major, the pectoralis minor and subclavius muscles, and the clavipectoral fascia (lying between the lower border of subclavius and upper border of pectoralis minor). The extension of the clavipectoral fascia, running from the lower border of the pectoralis minor muscle to the floor of the axilla, is termed the suspensory ligament of the axilla. The posterior wall of the axilla comprises the subscapularis, teres major and latissimus dorsi muscles. The medial wall is formed by the first five ribs, the intercostal muscles and the overlying serratus anterior muscle. The lateral wall is the intertubercular sulcus of the humerus, the coracobrachialis and biceps muscles. The structures passing through the axilla are important and include blood vessels, nerves, lymphatic vessels and lymph nodes (see Lymphatic drainage, above), areolar tissue and fat.

Neuro-vascular contents

The axillary artery and vein, together with the brachial plexus of nerves, run from the apex of the axilla along its lateral wall into the upper arm. Two important nerves running through the axilla are the long thoracic and the thoracodorsal nerves. The long thoracic nerve lies along the posterior aspect of the medial wall of the axilla and supplies the serratus anterior muscle. The thoracodorsal is joined by the thoracodorsal vessels on the anterior surface of subscapularis and supplies motor fibres to the latissimus dorsi muscle. The intercostobrachial nerve (lateral cutaneous branch of the second intercostal nerve) traverses the axilla and supplies the skin of the floor of the axilla and inner aspect of the upper arm, communicating with the posterior brachial cutaneous branch of the radial nerve. A second intercostobrachial nerve, also supplying the axilla and medial aspect of the arm, is commonly given off from the lateral cutaneous branch of the third intercostal nerve and other variations can also exist.

Congenital abnormalities of the breast

A variety of congenital anomalies of the breast may occur.

Types of abnormalities
Supernumerary nipples and breasts

Accessory nipples can be found anywhere along the 'milk line', from the axilla to the groin, but most often are found below the normal breast. Accessory breasts (with or without nipples) may also occur along the 'milk line' but are usually found in the axilla and this is termed polymastia.

Congenital inversion of the nipple

This arises because the mammary pit fails to become evaginated to form the nipple. This may spontaneously correct itself during pregnancy or by traction on the nipple.

Other abnormalities

These include amastia (congenital absence of a breast) or breast hypoplasia, both with a variable degree of underdevelopment of the pectoral muscles. Less commonly, this may be found in association with other defects of the ribs, upper limb and hands, and this is known as Poland's syndrome.

Physiological changes in the female breast

Thelarche

As menarche approaches, under the influence of the activation of the hypothalamic-pituitary-ovarian axis, the breast begins to develop (called thelarche). There is an initial development of the 'breast bud', which is a small nodule of breast tissue, located under the nipple, and gradually starts to increase in size under the influence of oestrogen. There is also a thickening and darkening of the areola with a more prominent nipple and this becomes more evident as development progresses, which can take between 2 and 5 years to become complete.

Menstrual cycle

Changes occur in the breast in a cyclical fashion during the menstrual cycle. After cessation of menstruation there is proliferation of ductal and ductular cells. Subsequently, in the second phase of the menstrual cycle, there is proliferation of the terminal duct structures, in association with increased mitosis in the basal epithelial cells and stromal cell proliferation. In addition, the stroma of the lobules becomes oedematous during this phase. However, towards the end of the cycle there is a reduction in cell numbers through the process of apoptosis. These changes are dependent on the stimulatory effects of oestrogens and progestogens.

Pregnancy and lactation

Marked changes occur in the breast during pregnancy under the influence of a variety of hormones, e.g. oestrogens, progestogens, prolactin, insulin, growth hormone and chorionic gonadotrophins. There is an increase in the number and size of lobules and an increase in the number of acini within each lobule. During the third trimester, secretory vacuoles of lipid material appear in the epithelial cells, and are the precursor of milk production. Following birth, milk is secreted by the epithelial cells into the ductules, mainly under the influence of prolactin. Once breast feeding has ceased, these changes regress, with atrophy of the gland, hyalinization of the lobules and reduction in the size of the ducts, occurring over approximately 3 months.

Involution changes

From the age of approximately 35 onwards, progressive involutional changes occur in the female breast. There is a gradual involution of breast glandular elements, especially lobules, a thickening of the basal lamina of the acini, a reduction in the amount of inter- and intralobular connective tissue but with an increase in the amount of fat within the breast. In some women there may be almost total disappearance of the lobules as ageing progresses.

Diagnostic modalities used in the assessment of breast disease

The key to the diagnosis of breast disease is 'triple assessment', which comprises clinical examination, imaging and fine-needle aspiration cytology (FNAC). In some centres FNAC is not used and a needle biopsy may be used instead.

Clinical assessment

A thorough history is necessary in all women presenting with breast disease. Careful details about the presenting breast complaint (lump, pain, nipple discharge, etc.) should be taken and, in addition, the following points should be carefully noted as a 'picture' is built up of the patient:

(i) Past history: this should focus on the risk factors that are known for breast cancer and include age at menarche and menopause, parity, age at first full-term pregnancy, breast feeding, usage of oral contraceptives and/or hormone replacement

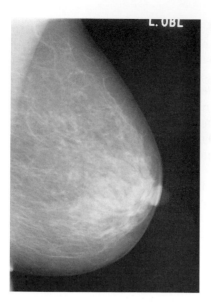

Figure 23.5
Normal
mammogram.

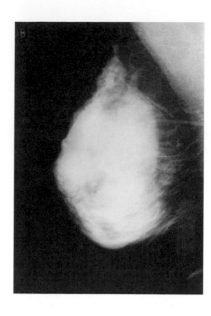

Figure 23.6
Mammogram
showing dense
breast tissue.

therapy, previous history of breast disease and type (if known), alcohol consumption.

(ii) Family history: relatives (in particular first-degree) with breast cancer, ovarian cancer or family members with any type of cancer (ages of onset and relationship). This aspect is discussed in more detail later in this chapter

Clinical examination of the breast must be carried out as follows. First, as in all clinical examination, a general inspection of the breast is carried out with the patient sitting and with their arms elevated and on their hips. With the patient reclining at 45 degrees (arms behind head) both the breasts (quadrants and tail) are palpated using the flat of the hand in a systemic and organized way. The axilla is examined and lymph node status ascertained; the supraclavicular area is palpated for lymphadenopathy (examiner standing behind the patient). There are many variations with respect to breast examination techniques but the key is a systemic approach and a thorough examination of these areas.

Although clinical examination is crucial it does have some limitations. For example, an experienced clinician will only diagnose that a person has cancer in eight out of ten patients who actually have breast cancer and who are presenting to a symptomatic breast clinic. Therefore, other modalities are clearly necessary to confirm or establish the nature of breast symptoms and/or lesions in addition to clinical examination.

Imaging

Mammography

Mammography (soft tissue radiography) involves having two radiographs taken of the breast – cranio-caudal and medio-lateral oblique views of each breast. If an abnormality is found, to delineate this further the radiologist requires additional views to be taken of the abnormal breast, e.g. magnification views, cone views focusing on a particular area or there may be a need for a true lateral or extended cranio-caudal view of the breast. The total X-ray dose is usually less than 1 mSv. This technique is most useful when the breasts contain less dense glandular tissues and are composed predominantly of fat (Figure 23.5). Therefore, in younger women (with dense glandular elements in the breasts) it is less accurate and reliable (Figure 23.6). In general, mammography is reserved for women over the age of 35 years but should be carried out in younger women if there is a good clinical indication (e.g. suspicion of cancer, or a strong family history as part of a screening programme, as discussed later).

The mammographic features of malignancy include: (i) microcalcification, comprising multiple particles of irregular size and density (see Figures 23.7 and 23.8 for examples of benign and malignant microcalcification); (ii) an opacity with characteristically irregular, ill-defined or spiculated margins, which is usually dense (Figure 23.9); and (iii) an area of distortion of the normal breast architecture or an asymmetrical difference between breasts, which may

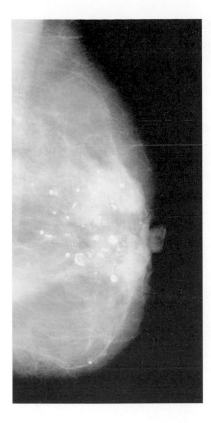

Figure 23.7
Mammogram demonstrating benign microcalcification.

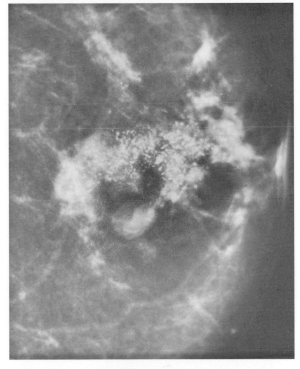

Figure 23.8 Mammographic appearances of microcalcification associated with malignancy.

be an indication of a breast cancer (Figure 23.10); in contrast, benign lesions are often smooth or lobulated and have normal density or a 'halo' around them. For example, the appearances of a breast cyst are shown in Figure 23.11. In some patients, axillary lymph nodes may also be visible, whilst in others thickening (oedema) and retraction of the skin of the breast can be seen. The sensitivity of mammography ranges from 75% to 90%, whilst its specificity varies from 70% to 85%.

Ultrasonography

Breast ultrasound is being used with increasing frequency in clinical practice. It is most useful in distinguishing solid from cystic lesions (Figure 23.11), in imaging the dense breast tissue in young women (e.g. under the age of 35 years) and it may also be helpful when mammography has been performed and has not been diagnostic.

The classic appearance of a benign lesion is of a smooth outline, oval shape and with acoustic enhancement. In contrast, a malignant lesion has an irregular outline, an interrupted breast architecture and acoustic shadowing. As with most ultrasound investigations,

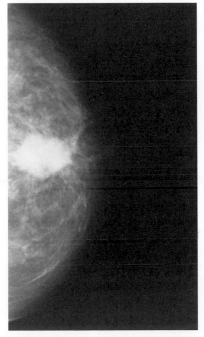

Figure 23.9
Characteristic appearances of a breast cancer on mammography.

397

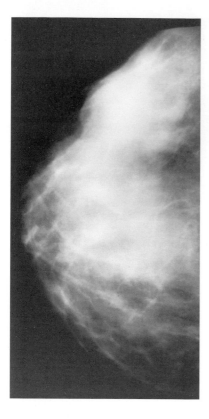

Figure 23.10 Mammographic appearances of a breast cancer showing increased density and architectural changes.

Magnetic resonance mammography

Magnetic resonance mammography (MRM) can have a sensitivity of between 88% and 100% but with a specificity ranging from as low as 37% to 97%, which limits the widespread clinical use. The main indications for use are:

- in patients with suspected local recurrence
- the detection of multifocal disease within the breast and many have adopted the policy of undertaking an MRM on all patients with invasive lobular cancer due to the increased risk of further disease in either breast
- assessing the response of a breast cancer to primary chemotherapy
- used in screening women at high risk of developing breast cancer (see later in chapter)
- Detection of leakage from breast implants.

Fine-needle aspiration cytology (FNAC)

After clinical examination and imaging procedures have been carried out and a 'lump' has been documented a definitive diagnosis is required. The latter can be established by carrying out fine-needle aspiration cytology (FNAC), obviating the need for a formal biopsy (requiring surgery) or a core or TruCut biopsy (which can be uncomfortable for the patient).

FNAC is performed using a standard (10 ml) syringe and needle (21G); a special gun containing the

breast ultrasound is operator-dependent and the sensitivity varies from 70% to 90%, with a specificity of approximately 80% to 95%.

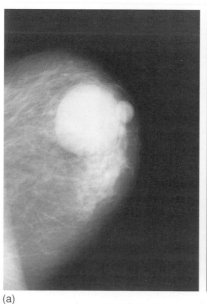

(a)

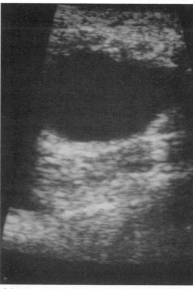

(b)

Figure 23.11 (a) Mammographic appearances of a breast cyst; (b) Ultrasonographic appearances of a breast cyst.

Table 23.1 Fine needle aspiration cytology scoring system

C0	No epithelial cells present
C1	Scanty benign epithelial cells
C2	Benign epithelial cells
C3	Atypical cells
C4	Cells which are highly suspicious of cancer
C5	Definitely malignant cells

syringe may be used. The needle is inserted into the palpable lump and suction is applied to the syringe in order to aspirate material into the needle. Multiple passes are made into the lump, in a range of directions, in order to obtain as representative an aspirate as possible. The needle is then withdrawn from the lump and the contents of the needle spread out onto microscope slides, with some being dried in air and others put into a fixative solution. The cells can then be stained (e.g. Giemsa, Papanicolaou, haematoxylin and eosin) prior to microscopic examination. Many major centres have a cytologist present at the breast clinic who will examine and report on the breast aspirates whilst the patient is at the clinic and an immediate report is provided. The scoring system used for reporting the results of FNAC is shown in Table 23.1. The sensitivity of FNAC is approximately 95% (ranging from 80% to 99%), with a specificity of 98% (ranging from 95% to 99%) (Figures 23.12 and 23.13).

If a lesion in the breast has been detected on either mammography or ultrasonography (but is not clinically detectable) then cytological examination of the lesion can still be made. This is carried out either stereotactically using mammographic-guided FNA or by ultrasound-guided FNA. In some specialized centres facilities also exist for MRM-guided FNAC and core biopsies to be undertaken.

Established centres using triple assessment (clinical examination, imaging (mammography, ultrasonography) and FNAC) report a sensitivity of >95%, specificity of >96% and a predictive value of >97%, with this approach. However, in some patients it is still not possible to make a definitive diagnosis despite use of triple assessment and in these cases a biopsy will be required for histological examination.

Breast biopsy

Needle biopsy –– Breast biopsy can be performed under local anaesthesia by using a 'TruCut' needle or a 'drill' type needle which removes a core of tissue. Both

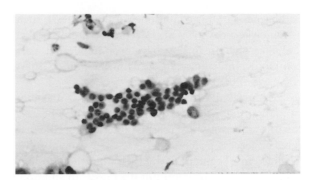

Figure 23.12 Benign cells obtained using FNAC.

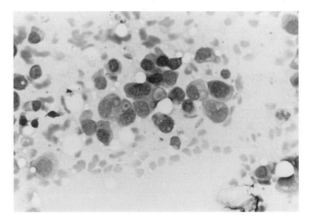

Figure 23.13 Malignant cells obtained using FNAC.

of these techniques can be uncomfortable and lead to bruising. However, they allow an assessment of tumour type and grade of tumour to be determined.

Operative biopsy –– Operative biopsy (incisional or excisional) can be performed under a local or general anaesthetic. The skin incision should be made circumferentially (Langer's lines) and not radially as this can result in hypertrophic scarring. Generally, the diagnosis of breast cancer is made without the need to recourse to operative biopsy.

Benign breast disorders

Infections

Non-lactating breast

Infections in non-lactating breasts usually occur in the periareolar region as periductal mastitis, typically in premenopausal women. The precise aetiology is unknown but smoking is thought to play a role in the pathogenesis of this condition. Various bacteria, such as *Staphylococcus pyogenes*, streptococci, enterococci and anaerobic organisms, have been implicated. Less commonly, infections can occur in the more peripheral parts of the breast.

Periductal mastitis usually presents as a tender swelling in the periareolar region. There may be erythema of the overlying and surrounding skin, and features of abscess formation. These changes tend to be localized to a segment of the breast but the infection may spread to involve most of the breast. In addition, there may also be a discharge from the nipple and/or nipple retraction. Systemic manifestations of sepsis (fever, leucocytosis, systemic upset) may be present.

With localized infection, and in the absence of an obvious abscess, the treatment is systemic antibiotic therapy. If a collection of pus is present (confirmed clinically, ultrasonographically) this should be aspirated with under ultrasound control usually; this can be repeated. However, if this is unsuccessful or the abscess is multi-loculated and it is not possible to remove all the pus, then surgical incision and drainage of the abscess under general anaesthesia is required. Although the infective episode resolves with treatment recurrent infections/abscesses occur in many patients. A mammary duct fistula may develop (usually as a result of surgical intervention) and will require definitive treatment (see later). It should also be noted that inflammatory cancers of the breast can present in a similar way with a comparable clinical appearance to sepsis and inflammation, and biopsies of the abscess cavity may be required for definitive histological examination.

Lactating breast

Infections may occur during lactation. The organisms most commonly involved are *Staphylococcus pyogenes* and *epidermidis* and more rarely other organisms such as enterococci. The bacteria may originate from the mother or the child and access to the breast parenchyma through a break in the skin of the nipple is believed to occur. Engorgement of the breast with milk and stasis are thought to be predisposing factors. The clinical features and treatment of these infections are the same as those already described above. Treatment consists of adequate pain relief, continuation of breast feeding (or expression of milk) if the patient wishes, and then drainage/antibiotic therapy as explained previously.

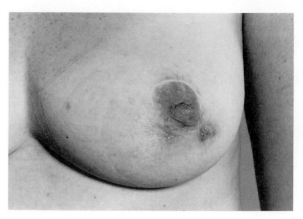

Figure 23.14 Example of a mammary duct fistula.

Other infections

Other, uncommon acute and chronic infections and inflammatory processes can also affect the breast and axilla. These include tuberculosis, actinomycosis, fungal infections, chronic granulomatous mastitis, pilonidal sinus disease, and the spread of infections from the chest wall. Although rare, they do occur and should be considered.

Mammary duct fistula

A mammary duct fistula is an abnormal connection between the skin (usually periareolar) and a major breast duct (usually subareolar). As already discussed, the commonest cause is periductal mastitis, with the fistula typically arising after an abscess has formed and discharged spontaneously or as a result of surgical intervention. Others have suggested that an inverted nipple with obstruction of the duct by debris and keratin may also be an important factor.

Clinically, the condition usually presents as a discharging area(s) in the breast in the vicinity of the areola; recurrent (and sometimes common) episodes of infection involving the fistula are not uncommon and can be a major problem for patients and cause much morbidity (Figure 23.14). Treatment of this condition requires excision of the whole fistula tract, and adjacent area of scar tissue, with healing either by secondary intention or by primary closure under antibiotic cover. However, in some patients the fistula can recur and then more radical surgery (e.g. subareolar excision of all the ducts) is required.

Mammary duct ectasia

There has been much debate as to the relationship between periductal mastitis and mammary duct ectasia, which is defined as a dilatation of the ducts. The duct diameter is normally between 0.5 and 1 mm and if greater than 1 mm is considered to be dilated. Although it has often been held that periductal mastitis and duct ectasia are variants of the same pathological process, with the former possibly resulting in the latter, the two conditions are probably different.

Periductal mastitis occurs in young premenopausal women whilst mammary duct ectasia occurs more commonly in peri- and postmenopausal females, with approximately 40% of women aged 50 years having duct ectasia. Histological examination shows there is dilatation of ducts filled with inspissated breast secretions and lipid-filled macrophages. In some patients, there may be squamous metaplasia of the lactiferous ducts and fibrous tissue formation. The aetiology of this is unclear but some have shown an association between cigarette smoking and duct ectasia, with the severity being also associated with the length of smoking. Why this might occur is not clear but it has been postulated that the high levels of nicotine and some metabolites in the duct fluid, or other tobacco-related products, may lead to damage, metaplasia of the duct epithelial cells and duct dilatation.

Clinically, mammary duct ectasia presents as nipple discharge, often affecting multiple ducts. The discharge varies in colour from clear to black, and in many of the cases it contains blood (microscopic or macroscopic). It is often thick and white. The patients may also have varying degrees of nipple retraction. If treatment is required (for symptomatic control or diagnostic uncertainty), and as multiple ducts are likely to be involved, subareolar duct excision should be carried out.

Nipple discharge

Nipple discharge is relatively common in the female population and is the third commonest cause of referral to a specialist breast clinic. However, it has been estimated that less than 10% of cancers are associated with breast nipple discharge.

Nipple discharge can be categorized into several types – clear or watery, milky, serous, multicoloured or blood-stained. In addition, the discharge may come from a single or from multiple ducts. The most common causes of the different types of nipple discharge

Table 23.2

Usual underlying cause	Nipple discharge characteristics
Benign breast change	Unilateral or bilateral, multiple ducts, yellow or green colour
Abscess/infection	Purulent discharge
Duct ectasia	Unilateral or bilateral, multiple ducts, green or white colour and may have a thick creamy consistency
Hyperprolactinaemia	White, milky discharge, usually bilateral and multiple ducts
Intraduct papilloma or malignancy (DCIS or invasive disease)	Solitary duct, blood or blood-stained discharge
Pregnancy/lactation/post lactation for up to 2 years	Milky discharge, bilateral, multiple ducts
Drug-induced (antidepressants, phenothiazines, antihypertensives)	Unilateral or bilateral, usually yellow, green or clear and does not contain blood

are shown in Table 23.2. However, in a very small number of cases of watery or serous discharge coming from a single duct, an underlying cancer may be found. In a small number of women with prolonged, profuse, bilateral milky discharge abnormal serum prolactin levels may suggest a prolactinoma of the pituitary gland.

After clinical examination of the breast various investigations are undertaken. The discharge should be tested for the presence of blood (e.g. Labstix testing) and examined microscopically for the presence of malignant cells. All patients over the age of 35 years should also have mammography; ultrasound examination of the breast may reveal the presence of dilated lactiferous ducts, particularly those close to the nipple and areola. In some patients, if there is discharge from a single duct, a ductogram (injection of contrast material into the duct) may demonstrate an intraduct papilloma, carcinoma or duct ectasia. In some centres ductoscopy is carried out although this is not used generally in clinical practice.

In many women in whom no underlying cause for the discharge has been found, the discharge may resolve, be intermittent and/or of small amount which does not concern the patient (see Figure 23.15 for management). However, if there is a large amount of discharge, if it comes from a single duct or tests suggest underlying pathology (e.g. prominent red blood

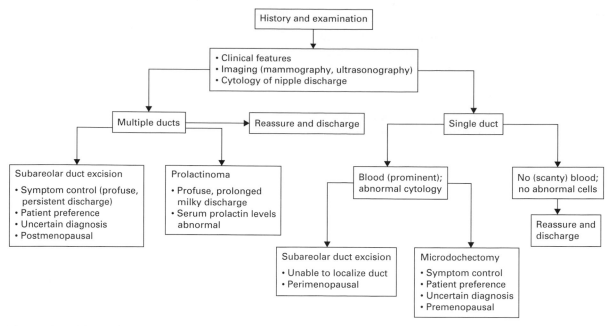

Figure 23.15 Scheme of management for patients with nipple discharge.

cell content, atypical or malignant cells), then the duct should be removed surgically (microdochectomy). In older women or those not intending to conceive and breast feed, if the duct cannot be identified or the discharge comes from several ducts, then subareolar central duct excision is undertaken through a circumareolar incision.

Nipple retraction (inversion)

The terms nipple retraction and inversion have come to be used interchangeably. However, nipple inversion is most often used when the whole of the nipple is permanently pulled inwards, whilst nipple retraction is used to describe variable degrees (usually intermittent) of the nipple being pulled inwards.

Congenital nipple inversion (of variable degree) occurs in up to one-fifth of all women. This is usually of no clinical significance unless it interferes with breast feeding. The woman may present because of the cosmetic deformity. However, two of the most common causes of nipple retraction are mammary duct ectasia and periductal mastitis. Clinically, this manifests as a transverse depression in the nipple which progresses to complete retraction (there may also be an associated nipple discharge). This process may be intermittent in its early stages and can be present in both breasts.

Nipple retraction may also occur in patients with breast cancer. In the latter this is unilateral and there may be an associated breast lump, with or without a nipple discharge (often blood-stained).

Investigations of patients with nipple retraction include mammography and, if appropriate, ultrasonography to determine whether there is an underlying tumour present. However, in the absence of malignancy, and in the majority of women, reassurance only is required. In young women and in those seeking cosmesis, surgical correction with eversion of the nipple may be carried out. However, this may cause damage to the underlying ducts and can interfere with attempts at breast feeding subsequently.

Nipple and areola skin disorders

The skin of the nipples may become involved with dermatitis and/or eczematous skin disorders. These often affect both nipples, the typical skin changes being erythema and scaliness. However, these must be differentiated from Paget's disease of the breast (see later).

The glands of Montgomery (large sebaceous glands opening on to the areola) may become blocked, with the formation of a lump in the areola. This can be removed, if necessary.

Mastalgia

Breast pain is one of the commonest symptoms in patients attending a specialist breast clinic, occurring in up to 50% of patients. Furthermore, up to two-thirds of women will experience breast pain during their lifetime. In some women, this may be of a minor nature occurring infrequently, but in others this may be severe pain which can interfere with daily activities and have a major impact on quality of life. Breast pain is commonly categorized into two main types – cyclical and non-cyclical. Whilst breast pain is considered as a benign condition, pain alone may be the presenting symptom in up to 1 in 10 patients with breast cancer.

Cyclical mastalgia

Cyclical mastalgia usually affects younger women, with the median age being 35 years. The mastalgia is related to the menstrual cycle and is commonly described as a fullness, heaviness, discomfort or pain (of varying degrees of severity), felt particularly for the few days prior to the onset of menstruation. The mastalgia is often described as occurring in the upper and outer quadrant of the breast and may be bilateral. In some cases the pain/discomfort may be referred to the upper arm or axilla. The mastalgia usually abates after the onset of menstruation, only to return as the menstrual cycle progresses. Physical examination may reveal no overt clinical abnormality apart from some tenderness. Examination, on the other hand, may demonstrate associated breast nodularity (localized, diffuse, uni- or bilateral).

Non-cyclical mastalgia

Non-cyclical mastalgia is less common and occurs in an older age group of women and is not related to the menstrual cycle. It may occur intermittently, although in some patients it can be continuous. This type of pain is usually felt in the medial aspect of the breast and also in the peri-areolar regions; it may resolve spontaneously. In addition to pain and discomfort arising in the breast, non-cyclical mastalgia may also arise from the musculoskeletal system, for example Tietz's syndrome (pain arising from the costochondral areas).

Pathogenesis

The relationship of cyclical mastalgia to the menstrual cycle has suggested that there may be a hormonal basis for the symptom complex, for example, abnormal lev-els of gonadotrophins, oestrogens, prolactin or inflammatory cytokines. However, to date, no consistent abnormalities in circulating levels of these hormones have been demonstrated. An alternative explanation, therefore, is that there is an increased sensitivity to circulating hormones, possibly at the level of the hormone receptors within the breast tissues. Other suggestions for the cause of mastalgia have included increased water retention and electrolyte imbalances within the breast tissues, an increased dietary intake of saturated fats or deficiencies of vitamins (e.g. B1, B6 and E), and increased levels of anxiety and depression have been reported in some studies.

In addition, the intake of methylxanthines has been suggested to be an important 'trigger' mechanism, although the precise reasons for this remain unclear. Previously, interest had focused on alterations in essential fatty acids, in particular gamma-linolenic acid, in patients with mastalgia. For example, some studies had shown that patients with mastalgia have low circulating levels of gamma-linolenic acid. Furthermore, women with severe cyclical breast pain appeared to have low plasma levels of the metabolites of gamma-linolenic acid, although it is unclear whether this represents a dietary deficiency or some abnormality in metabolism. Although some of these mechanisms may also be important in the aetiology of non-cyclical mastalgia, this is less well understood although some have suggested that there may be an anatomical abnormality underlying this. For example, one study indicated that non-cyclical mastalgia was related to duct ectasia, and in particular to an increased diameter of the mammary ducts, but other explanations have not been forthcoming.

Management

Investigations

A careful history should be taken from patients with mastalgia (a pain diary will help to differentiate cyclical from the non-cyclical variety) and a careful examination carried out (in up to 10% of patients with breast cancer, pain is the presenting symptom). Investigations that may be required are breast imaging (mammography and/or breast ultrasound), FNAC or core biopsy.

Treatment

One of the most important aspects of therapy in patients with mastalgia is reassurance, with approximately two-thirds of patients requiring no other forms of therapy. General measures include good supporting bras, use of sports bras during exercise and some patients find a soft bra for sleeping in will help and simple analgesics may also provide some degree of relief.

However, when treatment is required then a variety of substances are available, not all of which have been shown to be effective in randomized controlled trials. These are each discussed in more detail below.

Dietary modification –– One small study has shown that reducing substantially the dietary fat intake resulted in a significant improvement in breast tenderness but others have not found this to be of benefit. Certain foods (e.g. caffeine) are also considered as possible triggers of mastalgia, and it may be worth reducing intake.

Gamma-linolenic acid –– Trials have shown that gamma-linolenic acid can be effective in reducing breast pain and tenderness. In patients with cyclical mastalgia up to 60% appear to benefit, whereas only approximately 40% of those with non-cyclical mastalgia will have some relief of pain. Patient compliance is excellent and side effects are minimal (occasionally patients may experience mild gastrointestinal symptoms). It was previously recommended that up to 320 mg per day should be given for at least 4 months as it may take this long to achieve the maximum benefit. However, a recent meta-analysis has questioned the value of gamma-linolenic acid and suggested that it may not offer any benefit over placebo.

Danazol –– This is a synthetic steroid derived from ethisterone. It binds with a marked affinity to androgen receptors, with less affinity for progesterone and oestrogen receptors. Randomized controlled studies have also shown that danazol can significantly reduce breast pain and tenderness if given in doses of 100 mg to 200 mg twice daily for 3 to 6 months. However, although this is an effective therapy (80% with cyclical and 40% with non-cyclical mastalgia experience relief of symptoms), androgenic side-effects (e.g. hirsutism, acne, deepening of the voice), weight gain, headache and nausea are relatively common. These side-effects may occur in up to 30% of patients.

Bromocriptine –– This is a dopamine agonist which stimulates dopamine receptors and lowers circulating levels of prolactin (by inhibiting pituitary secre-

tion). Randomized controlled studies have demonstrated that bromocriptine (5 mg/day) is beneficial, with up to 55% of patients with cyclical and 30% with non-cyclical mastalgia gaining significant relief. Unfortunately, side-effects (e.g. nausea, headache, postural hypotension, constipation) occur in up to one-third of patients and can be treatment-limiting.

Tamoxifen –– The anti-oestrogen tamoxifen also reduces breast pain and tenderness. However, although metaanalysis has shown it to be a very effective treatment, its product licence does not include the treatment of mastalgia. A more recent development has been the use of topical 4-hydroxytamoxifen gel, which, when used daily for 4 months, can improve mastalgia.

Goserelin –– This is a synthetic analogue of naturally occurring luteinizing hormone releasing hormone (LHRH). When given over a long period it causes an inhibition of pituitary LH secretion, leading to falls in serum testosterone levels in men and serum oestradiol in women. Although it may result in significant improvements in breast symptoms in up to 90% of women with cyclical mastalgia, the side effects (headaches, hot flushes, loss of libido, vaginal dryness) are treatment-limiting.

Other treatments –– A variety of other agents have been used in the treatment of mastalgia, including topical non-steroidal anti-inflammatory creams, injection of steroids and local anaesthetics at the site of tenderness, oral pyridoxine, diuretics and progestogens. However, the efficacy of these in general clinical practice remains to be proven but they may be of value in selected patients although the mechanisms of action remain unclear.

Surgery –– Surgical treatment for mastalgia is rarely indicated. However, very occasionally the mastalgia may be refractory to all forms of therapy and may be very incapacitating for the patient. In these rare instances, and with assistance from a psychologist, surgery may be indicated but with the awareness that pain may not resolve after surgery.

Tietze's syndrome

This was described almost 100 years ago and may be occasionally present in patients being referred to a breast clinic with 'mastalgia'. It is thought to be an inflammation of the costal cartilage, possibly related to physical activity, but which presents with pain and tenderness over the affected area which is usually aggravated by movement, coughing or sneezing. This will usually resolve spontaneously although non-steroidal anti-inflammatory drugs can provide symptomatic relief.

Fibroadenomas

Fibroadenomas are the commonest benign tumours to arise in the breast and are most often seen in women under the age of 35 years. They comprise approximately 10% of symptomatic breast lumps and may be multiple in up to one-fifth of patients. In older women, particularly after the menopause, they are quite uncommon. In the latter age group they can undergo involution and become calcified. Large, rapidly growing fibroadenomas may occur in girls and young women.

Clinically, fibroadenomas are smooth, well-circumscribed, mobile lumps and in a few patients they can be multiple. Their size can vary, ranging from less than 1 cm to more than 10 cm in diameter. Those greater than 5 cm in diameter are termed 'giant fibroadenomas' (which are more common in non-Caucasians).

Fibroadenomas are derived from the intralobular stroma and are composed of both fibrous and glandular elements. Histologically, there is an abundant fibroblastic stroma which surrounds glandular and cystic cavities lined by an epithelium (pericanalicular type) or there is a more active proliferation of the connective tissue stroma with a resultant compression of the glandular spaces (intracanalicular type). The epithelium in a fibroadenoma may be hormonally sensitive and result in an increase in size during the menstrual cycle, pregnancy and lactation. There is a consensus that they are not associated with an increased risk of malignancy except when a fibroadenoma is found with atypical hyperplastic changes.

The diagnosis is confirmed by imaging (ultrasound and/or mammography) and FNAC. It has been recommended that fibroadenomas of greater than 4 cm in size should be removed. This is carried out through a circumferential incision, under general (or local) anaesthesia. However, if triple assessment confirms the diagnosis the fibroadenoma may be left alone (approximately 20% of fibroadenomas will regress with time) depending on patient preference. However, if it enlarges in size or causes symptoms, it should be removed.

Breast cysts

Breast cysts are a common cause of referral to a specialized breast clinic, with up to 7% of all women presenting with a palpable cyst at some time during their life. The true incidence of cysts amongst the general population has been estimated to be as high as 20%. Cysts most commonly present in the 35–50-year age group as a lump (circumscribed, smooth, mobile) with a variable degree of discomfort or pain; up to 30% of such women will have multiple cysts. The aetiology of breast cysts is poorly understood. Although hormones have been implicated no consistent differences in hormonal levels in women with cysts have been identified.

A breast cyst arises from a breast lobule and on microscopy is found to be lined by either a flattened epithelium (simple cysts) or by columnar secretory epithelium (apocrine cysts). Biochemically the contents of these two types of cysts are different. For example, simple cysts have high sodium and low potassium concentrations, with a sodium:potassium ratio of greater than 4 and a pH of less than 7.4. However, apocrine cysts have low sodium and high potassium concentrations, with a sodium:potassium ratio of less than 4 and a pH of greater than 7.4. The fluid from these cysts also contains a range of hormones, enzymes and growth factors.

The diagnosis of a cyst is confirmed by triple assessment. Mammography typically shows a well-defined opacity, although this may be difficult to demonstrate in dense breasts (Figure 23.11a). Ultrasound examination, however, usually confirms that the lesion is a cyst (Figure 23.11b). Fine-needle aspiration cytology usually reveals straw-coloured fluid (sometimes bluish-green or brown). The fluid is not normally sent for cytological assessment. However, if the cyst is blood-stained the fluid should be sent for cytological examination to exclude malignant cells and the presence of an intracystic growth. Following aspiration of a cyst the breast must be carefully examined to ensure that there has been complete resolution of the lump. If there is a residual palpable lump then this should undergo FNAC in case there is an underlying cancer.

Many surgeons will re-examine the breast 6 to 8 weeks later to determine whether the cyst has re-accumulated. If so, it may be aspirated on a second and possibly third occasion. Although the management of cysts which repeatedly re-fill is debatable, it is probably best to excise them for therapeutic reasons as well as to exclude an underlying malignancy. Some authors have

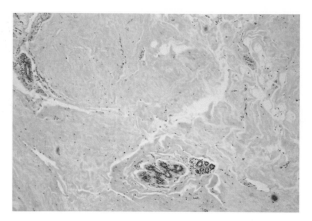

Figure 23.16 Histological appearances seen in fibrocystic disease – fibrous obliteration of the normal breast parenchyma (×50).

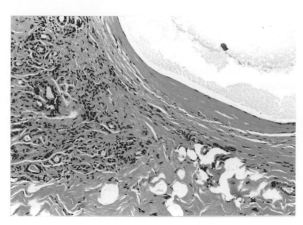

Figure 23.17 Histological appearances of fibrocystic disease – cyst formation, fibrosis and sclerosing adenosis (×150).

reported an increased tendency for cysts to repeatedly re-fill when associated with an underlying malignancy. The management of patients with multiple cysts also poses problems, as they may require repeated aspirations. A 3-month course of danazol may reduce the number and subsequent rate of cyst formation. However, the side-effects of danazol (see above) must be taken into account when prescribing this form of therapy.

There is a continuing debate as to whether breast cysts are associated with an increased risk of developing breast cancer. Some studies have suggested that those with multiple, bilateral and apocrine cysts are at most risk. Other long-term studies have failed to demonstrate any link to subsequent development of malignancy.

Galactocoele –– This is a benign lesion which usually occurs under the areola in women who are pregnant or lactating. Clinically, the lesion is a smooth, well-defined lump and can become quite large. FNAC will result in the aspiration of milky fluid (can be inspissated) with resolution of the lump.

Mammary dysplasia

General

The aetiology of mammary dysplasia (also termed fibrocystic disease, fibroadenosis, cystic mastopathy) is poorly defined but it is thought to arise as a result of a disordered proliferation and involution of breast tissues that occurs as part of the normal cyclical physiological process during the reproductive years (see Physiological changes). Thus, it tends to occur in

women in the 25–45-years age group and presents clinically as mastalgia, breast lump or nodularity, particularly in the second part of the menstrual cycle. Microscopy of breast tissues reveals a variety of pathophysiological changes (Figures 23.16 and 23.17); these are discussed in more detail below.

Micro-architectural changes

Adenosis

Adenosis is associated with an increase in acini and glandular tissue. There may be an increase in the myoepithelial component and in the connective tissue of the lobule.

Sclerosing adenosis

This is characterized by prominent intralobular fibrosis and proliferation of small ductules or acini. The fibrosis may be extensive, resulting in dense spiculated strands with prominent architectural distortion of the normal breast pattern. Complex sclerosing lesions are variants of this but are associated with prominent epithelial hyperplasia. In addition, there may be an increase in the myoepithelial component. As a result of the accumulation of dense fibrous tissue these lesions may be difficult to differentiate clinically and mammographically from breast cancers.

Epitheliosis

This is characterized by hyperplasia of the epithelium lining the terminal ducts and acini. The proliferation of epithelium may result in a solid mass with obliteration of the ducts or it may take the form of epithelial projections which grow into the ducts (ductal papillomatosis). The morphological appearance of the epithelial cells can vary and different degrees of atypia may be seen. A variant is atypical lobular hyperplasia, which is characterized by hyperplasia of the terminal duct and acini; this has some of the features of lobular carcinoma *in situ*. The importance of this lies in the increased risk of the subsequent development of breast cancer (see later).

Fibrosis (sclerosis)

There is a substantial increase in the content of dense fibrous tissue, with loss of elastic tissue, fat and epithelial elements.

Cyst formation

Numerous cysts (macro or micro) may also develop and this is discussed in more detail in the appropriate section above.

Fat necrosis

Fat necrosis of the breast occurs most commonly in obese and postmenopausal women and comprises 3% of all benign lesions. The aetiology is thought to be most commonly trauma-induced but is also related to radiotherapy, surgery (e.g. breast reduction), infections, warfarin therapy, together with idiopathic causes. Within the tissue there is saponification, cell death, inflammation and then fibrosis occurs as recovery takes place.

Frequently, patients give a history of trauma to the breast and complain of a subsequent breast lump. Alternatively there may be several small regular or irregular lumps. The lump(s) may be difficult to differentiate (clinically and mammographically) from a breast cancer as it can be hard, be associated with skin tethering and show varying inflammatory changes in the overlying skin of the breast. Macroscopically, the tissue is yellow in colour and haemorrhagic; microscopically there is necrosis of fat, scar formation and infiltration with polymorphs, macrophages and giant cells. Triple assessment is required to diagnose this condition and although FNAC may be helpful, biopsy may sometimes be necessary to obtain a definitive diagnosis.

Mondor's disease

This is characterized by thrombophlebitis of the superficial veins of the breast but the aetiology is unknown. Clinically, this presents as taught, firm, subcutaneous bands with associated skin dimpling and retraction. The clinical features usually resolve spontaneously but if there is associated discomfort, non-steroidal anti-inflammatory drugs may be helpful.

Gynaecomastia

Gynaecomastia is defined as enlargement of the male breast which is benign. This can occur unilaterally or bilaterally and can range from a minimal increase of the breast plate beneath the areola to resembling the female breast. Microscopically, there is proliferation in the dense connective tissue and hyperplasia of the ductal lining cells resulting in the formation of a multi-layered epithelium.

The essence of development of gynaecomastia is an increased effect of oestrogens or a decreased effect of androgens because the breast tissue contains receptors for androgens, oestrogen and progesterone. Stimulation of these receptors results in the physiological effects as described above. Under normal circumstances, the interstial cells of Ledig in the testis produce the majority of testosterone, with only a small amount being produced by the adrenal cortex. Both circulating testosterone and androstenedione (produced by the adrenal cortex) can be converted by the enzyme aromatase which is found in peripheral tissues (see later in this chapter) to oestrodiol and oestrone, respectively. Another consideration is the effects that elevated levels of prolactin have in reducing androgen levels through the hypothalamic/pituitary axis. Whilst levels of hormones may be different it has also been postulated that there may be, in some patients, an alteration in the sensitivity of hormonal receptors in the breast tissue.

Gynaecomastia may be physiological when it occurs in neonates (trans-placental passage of maternal hormones), in boys aged between 14 and 18 (there is a rise in oestrogen levels preceding the normal rise in testosterone), and in older individuals due to a fall in testosterone levels and perhaps compounded by increasing obesity.

Reduced levels of androgens, causing gynaecomastia, occur in the following:

- post orchidectomy, chemical castration, testicular torsion
- primary hypogonadism, e.g. after mumps, trauma
- Kleinfelters syndrome
- conditions which produce high prolactin levels.

Elevated levels of oestrogens can be found in:

- production by tumours, e.g. increased aromatase enzyme, production of oestrogen itself
- Sertoli cell tumour
- adrenal tumours producing feminization syndromes
- exogenous oestrogen administration.

Other causes include renal failure, thyrotoxicosis and cirrhosis and a variety of drugs (e.g. spironolactone, digoxin, anti-hypertensives, ranitidine and some proton pump inhibitors, anti-androgens, etc.)

A thorough history and examination of the breasts and axillae, chest, testes and abdomen should be performed in all patients. Mammography and FNAC may also be performed. Further investigations may include liver function tests and measurement of serum androgen, oestrogen and prolactin levels and a chest radiograph. Abdominal and testicular ultrasound examinations may also be required.

If there is an underlying cause for the gynaecomastia treatment of this will usually result in resolution of the gynaecomastia. However, in the absence of any demonstrable cause, and particularly in young patients, reassurance is frequently all that is required as the condition tends to be self-limiting. If the gynaecomastia persists and/or the patient is concerned by the appearance then either liposuction or surgical excision of the breast tissue, sometimes with concomitant excision of excess redundant skin, may be indicated.

Carcinoma of the breast

Introduction

Breast cancer accounts for approximately 31% of all malignancies occurring in the female population in industrialized Western societies and 18% of deaths in women due to malignant disease. In the UK there are approaching 45 000 patients newly diagnosed with breast cancer per annum. Thus, at least 1 in 9 women will develop breast cancer during their lifetime and the incidence has been rising. Breast cancer rarely occurs in women under the age of 25 years. Thereafter, the incidence increases steadily. After the menopause there is again a steady increase in the incidence of breast cancer, although this is less rapid than before (Figure 23.18) and the latest figures suggest that in women in their 50s this is decreasing. This is possibly related to decreasing use of HRT. It is interesting to

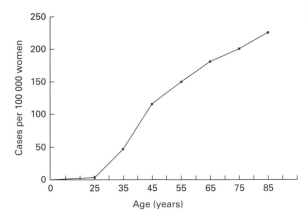

Figure 23.18 Incidence of breast cancer and age of diagnosis.

note that more than 500 000 people are living in the UK at the present time having been diagnosed with breast cancer and more than 78% will survive for at least 5 years.

Risk factors for breast cancer

Genetic factors

It has been estimated that approximately 5% of patients under the age of 50 years with breast cancer have a genetic predisposition to developing breast cancer. For example, the breast cancer (BRCA1) gene, which is found on the long arm of chromosome 17 and is implicated in approximately 4% of all breast cancers, has been cloned. It has been found that mutations in this gene are associated with a high risk (up to 85%) of developing breast cancer before the age of 80 years and up to 65% risk of developing ovarian cancer by age 80. Furthermore, approximately one-half of these cases will occur before the age of 50. A second breast cancer gene, BRCA2, which has been identified on the long arm of chromosome 13 is also associated with a risk of up to 85% of developing breast cancer but a lower risk of up to 30% of developing ovarian cancer. A wide range of mutations of these genes have been described which alter the estimated risk, although some populations exhibit the phenomenon of 'founder effect' where only a few specific mutations are found, e.g. Ashkenazi Jews. Mutations in BRCA1 and 2 are thought to be associated with 4% of breast cancers. These mutations can also occur in the tumour tissue of the sporadic form of breast cancer. In the inherited type of breast cancer other genetic defects have been established.

For example, there is either a mutation or loss of heterozygosity of the Tp53 tumour-suppressor gene on

Table 23.3 The increased risk of breast cancer occurring in patients with certain types of benign breast disease

Type of benign breast disease	Risk of developing breast cancer
Sclerosing adenosis	1.5–2 ×
Papilloma (one)	1.5–2 ×
Moderate hyperplasia but there is no cellular atypia	1.5–2 ×
Atypical ductal hyperplasia	4–5 ×
Atypical lobular hyperplasia	4–5 ×

Table 23.4 Age-standardized incidence of breast cancer amongst different countries

Country	Incidence
England	54.0
Scotland	59.6
USA	77.8
Sweden	60.7
Yugoslavia	37.7
Japan	19.7

Data are for 100 000 of the population, taken from the 1980s.

the short arm of chromosome 17. This event occurs in the Li-Fraumeni syndrome, where young-onset soft tissue sarcomas, other types of epithelial tumours and childhood adreno-cortical tumours occur in members of affected families, with a high risk of breast cancer – 50% of female mutation carriers will develop breast cancer before age 50. Another type of genetically determined breast cancer is the Lynch type II syndrome (autosomal dominant with high penetrance), where there is a high incidence of breast and ovarian cancers. (NB: Lynch syndrome type II is no longer thought to be associated with high risk for breast cancer although recent studies suggest that there may be a small increase in risk of breast cancer with mutations in hMLH1.) Mutations in other genes, such as PTEN on chromosome 10 in Cowden's syndrome, have been associated with an increased risk of breast cancer. The earlier the age of onset of the breast cancer, and the more close relatives who are affected, the more likely it is that there is a genetic susceptibility to the disease.

There is increasing evidence to suggest that lower penetrance genes may contribute to an increased genetic risk for breast cancer, which may be cumulative depending on the number of these genes inherited by an individual.

Benign breast disease

The relationship between benign breast disease and the subsequent development of breast cancer has been a matter of debate for some time. It appears that most benign conditions of the breast probably do not increase the risk of developing breast cancer (e.g. fibrocystic disease, cysts, fibroadenomas). However, there are some benign conditions which do increase the risk, in some instances substantially; these are listed in Table 23.3.

Geographical factors

There is a difference in the incidence in breast cancer between different countries and this is illustrated in Table 23.4. The reasons for these differences are unclear. However, although genetic aspects are important, environmental factors play a key role. For example, the incidence of breast cancer in the daughters of immigrants who arrive from countries with a low prevalence approaches the high level found in the established indigenous population.

Hormonal factors

Data have accumulated from different epidemiological studies that a prolonged exposure to oestrogens may increase the risk of subsequently developing breast cancer. Therefore, the following have been shown to increase the relative risks of developing breast cancer: early menarche, delayed menopause, late age of birth of first child and nulliparity.

The possible relationship of the oral contraceptive pill to breast cancer has also been considered and discussed in detail. A recent large study (involving more than 150 000 women) found that there was a small increase in the number of cancers diagnosed in women when taking the contraceptive pill and during the 10 years after stopping its usage. However, after this 10-year period there was no increased risk of developing breast cancer. Other studies have found that it is the prolonged use of the oral contraceptive pill prior to the first pregnancy which is most likely to predispose to breast cancer.

Recent studies have demonstrated that hormone replacement therapy (HRT) may possibly predispose to breast cancer. For example, it has been shown in a recent metanalysis from the USA that an exposure of 5 to 10 years to HRT was associated with an increased risk of breast cancer in those women with a family history of breast cancer. Furthermore, an analysis from the UK also suggested that 5 years of HRT resulted in an increase in an individual's risk of developing breast cancer. Furthermore, a recent study from the UK (the million women study) has suggested that the risk of developing breast cancer was dependent on the type of preparation used. For example, after 10 years of combined oestrogen/progesterone HRT there would be expected to be an excess of 19 cases of breast cancer per 1000 compared to women who had not used HRT, and for oestrogen only HRT there would be only 5 extra cases per 1000.

The most recent data suggest that there is a fall in breast cancer incidence in women in their 50s and a substantial reduction in the prescribing of HRT, thus further suggesting this as a causal factor.

Ionizing radiation

An increased risk of breast cancer occurs as a result of exposure to ionizing radiation. For example, in survivors of atomic bomb explosions, in patients who have received multiple and high-dosage chest radiographs and in women who have received radiotherapy which has included the breast there is an increased risk of breast cancer. This risk is most apparent if the exposure to the radiation occurred in those under 30 years of age.

Of particular concern has been the risks that might be associated with the use of radiation (mammography) in screening populations for breast cancer. However, it has been estimated that if two million women above the age of 50 years received a low-dose mammogram (mean radiation dose of 0.15 cGy), there would be one excess breast cancer per year in the population after a latent period of 10 years.

In clinical practice, perhaps the most common groups of patients who have been exposed to ionizing radiation and have an increased risk of breast cancer are those who have been treated with supradiaphragmatic radiotherapy for Hodgkin's disease.

Healthy life-style

Obesity

Obesity is associated with an increased risk of breast cancer in postmenopausal women, the mechanisms of which may be hormonal. It has been demonstrated that obese women metabolize androstenedione (from the adrenal gland) into oestrogen in adipocytes and a range of other growth factors are produced by metabolically active fat cells. The circulating levels of oestrone are higher in obese postmenopausal women than non-obese individuals. In premenopausal women obesity may be associated with a reduced risk of breast cancer, although the reasons for this difference are unclear.

Diet

Attention has focused on the role of dietary fat in the pathogenesis of breast cancer. Animal studies have shown that the total fat consumption and, more importantly, the composition of fats in the diet are important in the development of breast cancer. In studies in man, close correlations between the per-capita consumption of fat and breast cancer mortality rates have been demonstrated. However, when individuals are considered the association is lacking. There is no well-established relationship between dietary fat consumption and an individual person's risk of developing breast cancer.

Anti-oxidant nutrients (e.g. fruit, greens) may be important in protecting against the development of breast cancer. These molecules protect against reactive oxygen species which can damage DNA within the cell. Examples of these substances are vitamins A, C and E and selenium. Other dietary substances which may be important in causing breast cancer are the heterocyclic amines (found in charbroiled foods) and plant oestrogens (soy products).

Exercise

Physical activity, especially in the teenage and young adult years, may protect against breast cancer in both pre- and postmenopausal women. From available data the protective effect requires 4 hours of strenuous exercise per week. One explanation for this has been the exercise-induced delay in the onset of the menarche and the reduction in the number of menstrual cycles.

Alcohol

Alcohol consumption increases the risk of breast cancer. An intake of more than 2 units of alcohol per day has been found to be associated with a significant increase in the risk of breast cancer when compared with people who do not consume alcohol and the effect is thought to be dose-dependent. This may be because of a hormonal effect – alcohol consumption results in increased circulating levels of oestrone and oestradiol.

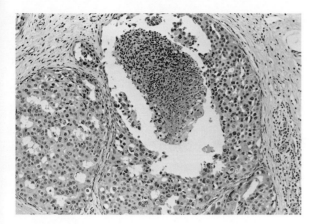

Figure 23.19 An example of ductal carcinoma *in situ* – high-grade DCIS with comedo necrosis distending and filling terminal ducts. Note the cellular pleomorphism and well-defined cell borders (×150).

Cigarette smoking

There is controversy regarding the role of smoking in the aetiology of breast cancer. Although some studies have suggested there is an increased risk (possibly due to carcinogens in smoke) others have shown a reduced risk (possibly due to decreased circulating levels of oestrogens). There is no convincing evidence that smoking causes breast cancer although a small number of studies have indicated there may be a very weak link.

Breast cancer: pathological types

Non-invasive breast cancer

There are two main types of non-invasive breast carcinoma: ductal carcinoma *in situ* (DCIS) and lobular carcinoma *in situ* (LCIS). Of these, DCIS is the more common histological type.

Ductal carcinoma *in situ*

DCIS is characterized by an abnormal proliferation of breast epithelial cells lying within the duct but not penetrating the basement membrane (Figure 23.19). Different types of DCIS can be recognized histologically: (i) comedo (characteristic central necrosis), (ii) cribriform (sieve-like appearance), (iii) papillary or micropapillary (the epithelium forms projections into the ducts) and (iv) solid (sheets of cells fill the duct system). Different types of DCIS may be found in the same breast, but the comedo type is recognized as the most aggressive biologically. DCIS may also arise in several areas of the breast and the risks of this

occurring are related to the size of the detected DCIS. For example, one study reported that if the area of DCIS was less than 2.5 cm, DCIS was found in other areas of the same breast in less than 15% of cases and there was no evidence of microinvasion by tumour cells.

However, if the DCIS was greater than 2.5 cm, then almost one-half of these patients had other areas of DCIS within the same breast and, furthermore, in over 40% of these cases there was evidence of microinvasion, with 4% having lymph node metastases. In addition, there is also a risk of patients with DCIS subsequently developing invasive cancer. Although different estimates of this risk have been reported, approximately 2% of these patients are likely to develop invasive breast cancer each year.

Clinically, DCIS may present as:

- an incidental finding on a mammogram (localized, widespread, or multifocal microcalcifications, of variable density and branching pattern) (Figure 23.8)
- a soft tissue mass
- a blood-stained (or less commonly serous) nipple discharge
- a palpable mass (uncommon)
- or it may occur in association with Paget's disease of the nipple.

The treatment of DCIS is controversial, with trials currently evaluating several treatment regimens. If mastectomy is performed, there is a 98% 5-year survival rate. However, this is probably over-treatment in many cases and more conservative surgery for the treatment of a circumscribed area of DCIS (excising the area of DCIS only) has also been carried out.

This approach, however, is associated with a recurrence of DCIS in up to 20% of cases, particularly with the comedo-type DCIS. The role of radiotherapy in preventing local recurrence following conservative surgery remains unclear and is currently being evaluated. In practice the van Nuys prognostic index is used to predict the risk of recurrence, which is a numerical value obtained from the four most important predictors of recurrence – size of DCIS, distance from the margin, pathological nuclear grade and patient's age. Based on this determination of an increased likelihood of recurrence radiotherapy is recommended. As regards tamoxifen, then this may reduce the risk of a subsequent invasive cancer developing but the benefits are less if radiotherapy is being given.

Table 23.5 Frequency of invasive breast cancers

Type	Frequency (% of total)
Invasive ductal carcinoma	75–80
Invasive lobular carcinoma	<5
Tubular carcinomas	<5
Medullary carcinomas	<5
Mucinous carcinomas	<5
Inflammatory breast cancer	2–5

It is usually recommended that, if the area of DCIS is extensive (>4 cm), or if there are multiple sites of DCIS within the same breast, mastectomy should be performed. Axillary surgery is not necessary for DCIS, but some surgeons will undertake a sentinel node biopsy if the DCIS is more extensive or high grade on core biopsy in view of the possibility of finding invasion when the lesion is removed.

Lobular carcinoma *in situ*

LCIS is less common than DCIS and has no characteristic clinical or radiological features. It is not associated with microcalcification (although very rarely microcalcification has been reported). Pathological examination is characterized by a proliferation of cells in the terminal ducts and/or acini. LCIS can be both multicentric and bilateral (30%). It has been estimated that up to 1% of patients per annum will develop invasive cancer, but this may be in either breast (in contrast with DCIS) and histologically this may be either lobular or ductular carcinoma.

Following the diagnosis of LCIS in a breast biopsy the treatment is contentious. Small incidental findings (pathological assessment) are of doubtful clinical relevance. However, most commonly the patients are monitored by regular clinical examination and mammography (e.g. at yearly intervals). However, very anxious patients and especially those with evidence of multicentricity may wish to consider the option of bilateral mastectomy with or without reconstruction.

Invasive breast cancer

The commonly occurring invasive cancers and their relative frequencies are listed in Table 23.5 and are discussed in more detail below.

Invasive ductal carcinoma

The most commonly occurring type of breast cancer is the invasive ductal carcinoma of no special type (75%

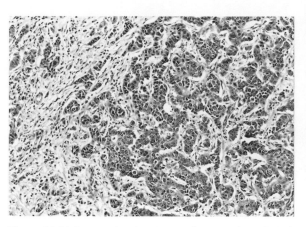

Figure 23.20 Invasive ductal carcinoma of no special type (×250).

to 80% of all cases). Histologically, the tumour cells can be arranged in groups or cords and can also form gland-like structures set in a dense fibrous stroma, which gives the tumour a hard consistency (scirrhous tumour) (Figure 23.20).

The degree of aggressiveness of these tumours is variable and can be determined from the cytological and histological appearance of the tumour cells. Bloom and Richardson developed a grading system (1 to 3) for these tumours which was based on three characteristics: (i) the formation of tubules, (ii) the degree of nuclear pleomorphism, and (iii) the mitotic rate. Tumour grade is an independent prognostic factor, with grade 3 tumours having the worst prognosis, and grade 1 tumours having the best outcome.

Invasive lobular carcinoma

Invasive lobular carcinoma occurs much less frequently, comprising less than 5% of all breast cancers. Histologically, there are strands of tumour cells which infiltrate into the surrounding stromal tissues; typically these are one cell in width ('Indian filing'). Tumour cells may also be found in concentric rings around normal ducts (Figure 23.21). However, in some cases it can be difficult to differentiate between an invasive ductal and an invasive lobular cancer. Furthermore, both of these types may co-exist in the same tumour. This tumour can be multicentric within the same breast and is bilateral in up to 20% of patients.

Tubular carcinoma

Tubular carcinomas are usually small and well-differentiated tumours. Histologically, they are characterized by the tumour cells being arranged into well-differentiated tubular structures.

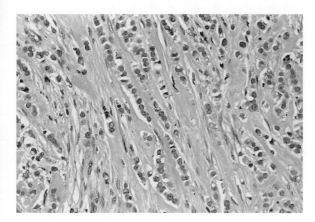

Figure 23.21 Invasive lobular carcinoma, with 'Indian filing' (×125).

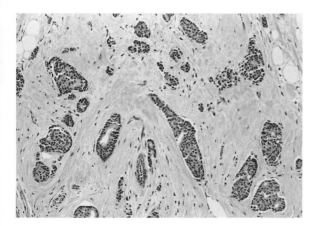

Figure 23.22 Tubular carcinoma (×150).

The tumour cells have a low mitotic rate and there is little nuclear pleomorphism. The stromal tissue is also very dense and can be found within the tubular structures (Figure 23.22). Patients with this type of tumour generally have an excellent prognosis as it usually remains confined to the breast and rarely metastasizes, either regionally or more distally.

Medullary carcinoma

Medullary carcinomas constitute less than 5% of all breast cancers. They have a well-defined margin and are soft. Histologically, they are characterized by a marked lymphocytic infiltration, high cellularity and have less fibrous tissue than is seen in other histological types of breast cancer. They are less commonly associated with axillary gland metastases than are invasive ductal cancers. Even if the axillary lymph glands do contain tumour the prognosis is still better than for the invasive ductal tumour type.

Table 23.6 The Nottingham Prognostic Index (NPI)

- NPI = 0.2 × tumour size (cm) + lymph node status (1–3 according to stage A–C) + tumour grade (I–III).
- An NPI of less than or equal to 3.4 is good prognosis, 3.41–5.4 is moderate prognosis, and greater than 5.4 is a poor prognosis. Patients in the good prognostic group have a 15-year survival of 85%, but patients with an NPI of equal to or less than 2.4 have a 15-year survival of 94%.

Mucinous carcinoma

Mucinous tumours comprise less than 5% of all breast cancers. They tend to occur in the older population and are believed to be more slowly growing than other types, rarely metastasizing to the regional lymph nodes. Histologically, there are large areas of mucin in the tumour. The tumour cells themselves can be seen to lie within pools of mucin forming small islands of cells or gland-like structures. This type of tumour is also associated with a good prognosis.

Inflammatory breast cancer

Inflammatory breast cancer occurs in approximately 2% to 5% of patients with malignant lesions in the breast. It is recognized clinically by redness of the skin and signs of inflammation of the breast, often with peau d'orange of the skin. The histological findings may be non-specific, but the characteristic feature is invasion of the dermal lymphatics by malignant cells and tissue oedema and a variable degree of infiltration of the breast by inflammatory cells. It is biologically more aggressive than the other tumour types and is associated with a worse prognosis.

Prognostic factors in breast cancer

Prognostic factors relating to the degree of tumour spread and its biological behaviour have been identified (Table 23.6). These factors determine the outcome (disease recurrence) and survival for the patient and are discussed in more detail below.

Tumour size –– This is an important prognostic indicator. Generally, the larger the tumour clinically the worse the prognosis, with tumours less than 0.5 cm having an excellent prognosis and those greater than 4 cm a poor outcome. Tumours less than 1 cm have a good prognosis but in 15% of these patients there is histological evidence of lymph node involvement with tumour.

Tumour type –– Invasive ductal carcinomas of no special type have a worse prognosis than certain tumours

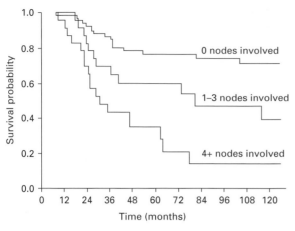

Figure 23.23 Relationship of lymph node status to survival in patients with breast cancer.

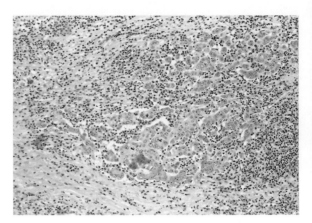

Figure 23.24 Ductal carcinoma infiltrating into a lymph node, pleomorphic cells in a lymphoid background (×150).

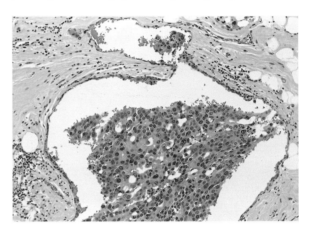

Figure 23.25 Invasive ductal carcinoma invading into vascular lymphatic spaces (×250).

of a special type (e.g. tubular, mucinous or medullary cancers).

Tumour grade -- Tumours can be graded (1 to 3) using the Bloom and Richardson classification (tubule formation, mitotic rate and nuclear pleomorphism) as already described.

Cell kinetics -- Cell proliferation has been shown to be a prognostic indicator. Those tumours with enhanced rates of mitosis, increased percentage of cells in the S phase of the cell cycle and with tumour cells showing the greatest expression of the Ki67 nuclear antigen (expressed by proliferating cells) have a poorer prognosis.

Lymph node status -- This has been shown to be the single most important prognostic indicator (Figure 23.23). If there is no lymph node involvement by tumour patients have an 85% 5-year survival. However, if there is lymph node involvement then the 5-year survival is reduced to 65%. Furthermore, this reduction in survival is related to the number of lymph nodes being involved – the greater the number the poorer the survival (Figure 23.24).

Lymphatic or vascular invasion -- Invasion of the lymphatic system or blood vessels (Figure 23.25) has also been shown to be a poor prognostic indicator.

Hormone receptor status -- Oestrogen receptor (OR) status has been shown to be a prognostic indicator, with 50–75% of tumours being oestrogen receptor positive. Those patients whose tumours strongly express OR receptors have a survival advantage, when com-

pared with patients who have no OR expression. Progesterone receptors (PR) depend on a satisfactory OR pathway for their presence, which correlates, therefore, with OR status. However, there is some evidence to suggest that the presence of both OR and PR expression is associated with a better prognosis than OR expression alone.

Her2 status -- Approximately 25% of breast cancers over-express the gene for human epidermal growth factor receptor 2, HER2. This will lead to increased tumour cell growth and proliferation with a resultant poorer prognosis. The over-expression of the HER2 gene is an independent predictor of a poorer prognosis (see later).

Other prognostic indicators -- A variety of other possible prognostic indicators are currently being evaluated. These include the expression of other growth

Table 23.7 Staging of breast cancer

TNM system	
Primary tumour – (T)	
TX	Primary tumour cannot be assessed
T0	No evidence of primary tumour
TIS	Carcinoma *in situ*, Paget's disease
T1	Tumour <2 cm in greatest dimension
T1a	<0.5 cm in greatest dimension
T1b	<0.5 cm but <1.0 cm in greatest dimension
T1c	>1 cm but ≤2.0 cm in greatest dimension
T2	Tumour >2 cm but <5 cm in greatest dimension
T3	Tumour >5 cm in greatest dimension
T4	Tumour of any size with direct extension to the skin or chest wall
T4a	Extension to chest wall
T4b	Oedema, or ulceration of the skin of the breast or satellite skin nodules confined to the same breast
T4c	Both T4a and T4b
T4d	Inflammatory carcinoma (diffuse browny induration of the skin, with an erysipeloid edge, often with no underlying palpable mass)
Regional lymph nodes – (N)	
NX	Regional lymph nodes cannot be assessed
N0	No regional node metastases
N1	Mobile homolateral axillary nodes
N1a	Nodes not considered to contain tumour
N1b	Nodes considered to contain tumour
N2	Homolateral axillary nodes fixed to each other or to adjacent structures
N3	Metastases to ipsilateral internal mammary nodes
Distant metastases – (M)	
MX	Presence of distant metastases cannot be assessed
M0	No distant metastases
M1	Distant metastases (includes metastases to supraclavicular lymph nodes)

Table 23.8 Staging of breast cancer UICC staging

Stage	Corresponding TNM
0	Tis, N0, M0
I	T1, N0, M0
II	T1, N1, M0; T2, N0–1, M0
III	Any T, N2–3, M0; T3, any N, M0
IV	Any T, any N, M1

Lymph node stage is given a value of 1 (no nodes affected), 2 (up to three glands involved with tumour) or 3 (more than three glands involved). Tumour grade is given a value of 1 (for a grade I tumour), 2 (grade II), or 3 (grade III tumour).

The resultant numerical score means that patients can then be placed into one of three prognostic groups:

- 3.4 – good prognosis (>80% 10-year survival)
- 3.4 to 5.4 – a moderate prognosis (70% 10-year survival)
- 5.4 – a poor prognosis (less than 50% 10-year survival).

Staging of breast cancer

Several staging systems have been developed for use in patients with breast cancer. However, the TNM system is the one which is most frequently used and is given in Table 23.7. This is a clinical staging system and the measurements of tumour size and lymph node status are established on clinical examination. In pathological staging, the prefix 'p' must be added in front of the T or N. Another commonly used staging system is that advocated by the UICC. The correlation of this with the TNM system is shown in Table 23.8.

Clinical features

The majority of women present with a breast lump, which is confirmed on examination. In two-thirds of patients it is in the upper outer quadrant of the breast and characteristically is well defined, hard and with an irregular surface. The lump may be fixed to the skin or to the underlying chest wall and retraction or dimpling of the skin may be seen. The skin of the breast must be carefully examined for the presence of erythema, which may indicate an inflammatory cancer (see above). Locally advanced cancers are characterized by oedema, skin infiltration, satellite skin nodules, ulceration, fixity to the chest wall and/or large fixed axillary nodes (N2) (Figure 23.27). Some patients may

factor receptors, expression of cell adhesion molecules, expression of oncogenes and products and mutations of wild type suppressor genes (e.g. p53). These are listed in Table 23.6.

Prognostic indices –– Combinations of these prognostic indicators have been developed using statistical modelling techniques in an attempt to improve prognostic information. One such example is the Nottingham Prognostic Index (NPI), which takes into account the tumour size, tumour grade and lymph node staging. This allows the identification of the likelihood of survival of patients with breast cancer and is derived from the following simple formula which includes the three key prognostic factors in breast cancer:

$$NPI = 0.2 \times \text{tumour size (in cm)} + \text{lymph node stage} + \text{tumour grade}$$

also have oedema of the ipsilateral arm. However, not all cancers have these features and occasionally some may be difficult to differentiate clinically from benign tumours such as fibroadenomas. Other breast cancers may present as a diffuse nodularity, with no localized lump being found, and up to 10% of patients with breast cancer may present with pain as the predominant complaint.

The nipple should also be carefully examined for the presence of distortion or inversion. A nipple discharge may be present. This often contains blood and emanates from one duct. However, a variety of other nipple discharges (clear, coloured) may be present (see above). The presence of a scaly, erythematous nipple should raise the suspicion of Paget's disease of the nipple (see later).

Less commonly, patients may present with features of regional tumour spread (e.g. involved and enlarged axillary lymph nodes). Alternatively, metastatic disease in distant sites may be responsible for symptoms, e.g. breathlessness (intra-thoracic metastases), bone pain and pathological fractures, jaundice and abdominal pain (liver metastases), ascites (intra-abdominal metastases), neurological symptoms (intra-cerebral metastases), difficulty in walking (spinal cord compression), etc.

Diagnosis

Triple assessment

The investigations that are used to establish the diagnosis of breast cancer include mammography, ultrasonography of the breast, FNAC and biopsy. These have all been discussed earlier in this chapter.

Staging investigations

All patients should have a full blood count, urea and electrolytes (including serum calcium), liver function tests (bilirubin, transaminase, alkaline phosphatase and gamma glutamyl peptidase) and a chest radiograph performed. In patients with small tumours (T1–2, N0), and in the absence of suggestive clinical features, further imaging to detect metastatic disease (bone scans, abdominal ultrasound) has been shown to be unnecessary, as they have a very low incidence of detecting metastases. However, in patients with larger or more advanced tumours or if abnormalities have been detected on the basic staging investigations then further appropriate imaging investigations are more likely to show detectable metastatic disease and these

can be undertaken (e.g. isotope bone scans, abdominal ultrasound, CT scans of thorax and/or brain). There are no tumour markers with such sensitivity and specificity to recommend for routine clinical use.

Treatment

General

Treatment of breast cancer requires a multidisciplinary approach with input from several specialties which include the surgeon, radiotherapist and medical oncologist, cytologist and pathologist, radiologist, nurse counsellor and psychologist. The patient and partner should also be given the opportunity to participate and make informed choices (if they wish) in the decision-making processes, following full discussion and provision of appropriate information.

The principles of treatment of a patient with a palpable breast cancer comprise the following:

- management of the lesion in the breast (to achieve local control of disease)
- treatment of possible regional metastases in the tumour-draining lymph nodes (to obtain regional control of disease and to determine prognostic outcome and possible adjuvant therapy
- treatment of possible occult micrometastatic disease (e.g. grade 3 tumours, nodal invasion) where there may be a requirement for adjuvant therapies.

Primary breast tumour

Treatment of the primary breast tumour

The treatments initially advocated for breast cancer were based on the belief that cancer cells spread in a centrifugal pattern – from the tumour to the regional draining lymph nodes and then sequentially to the vascular system and distant metastatic sites. Thus, it was recommended that a radical mastectomy (which includes removing the pectoralis major muscle) should be undertaken. However, in the 1920s and 1930s this approach was challenged and surgeons began to realize that less radical surgery was associated with good results. Indeed, Geoffrey Keynes in the UK had treated early breast cancers by local excision of the tumour and implantation of a radioactive source (radium seeds) at the site of the excised tumour 'bed'.

Randomized controlled trials (both Europe and the USA) evaluated more precisely the role of breast-conservation surgery versus mastectomy in the treatment of patients with breast cancer. It was demonstrated that if the clinical size of the tumour was 2 cm or less then wide local excision of the tumour or a 'quadrantectomy' (for tumours 2 to 4 cm), in conjunction with radiotherapy given to the breast in the post-operative period, could be carried out safely. When this approach was compared with patients undergoing mastectomy there were no differences in survival between the two groups of patients.

Therefore, the principle of such surgical treatment is to excise the tumour with a clear margin of normal breast around the periphery of the tumour. The extent of the size of the margin excites much debate and discussion but current guidelines state that there must be at least 1 mm of clear margin, although some surgeons routinely try to obtain wider clear margins. All patients undergoing breast-conservation surgery will receive adjuvant radiotherapy (4500 to 5000 cGy) to the breast to reduce the risk of local recurrence, which is increased following breast-conservation surgery when compared with mastectomy – up to 1% ('recurrent disease') of patients per annum on a cumulative basis for the first 10 years; 0.5%, thereafter, will have local recurrence of disease.

However, a number of clinical and pathological features have been identified which are considered to be contraindications to breast conservation because they are associated with a much higher risk of local recurrence of disease. Therefore, contraindications to breast-conserving surgery would be:

- tumours with a clinical size of greater than 4 cm
- incomplete excision of tumour with margins of the resected specimen involved by tumour
- extensive associated DCIS
- multiple primary tumours in the breast.

Patients must be suitable for radiotherapy to the affected breast after surgery and the presence of co-existing skin, respiratory and cardiac disease may preclude this (see later).

The patient's own wishes must also be taken into consideration when planning treatment.

Patients who undergo mastectomy do not receive adjuvant radiotherapy to the chest wall unless they are considered to be at a high risk of chest wall recurrence. This is the subject of debate at present but there is agreement that patients with tumours 5 cm in size or more and who have four or more lymph nodes involved with tumour do have a much higher risk of chest wall recurrence and they should have radiother-

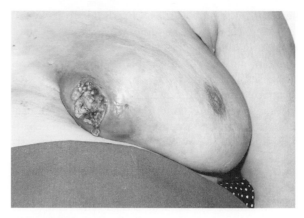

Figure 23.26 Locally advanced carcinoma of the breast with associated skin ulceration.

apy after mastectomy. However, there are differences of opinion and some radiotherapists will treat women with smaller tumours and a lesser degree of nodal involvement. However, randomized clinical trials are currently trying to answer this question definitively.

Locally advanced breast cancer (LABC)

LABC occurs in up to 15% of patients presenting with breast cancer (Figure 23.26). LABC can be defined as:

(i) presence of a large tumour (>5 cm: T3)
(ii) fixation of the tumour to the chest wall, skin oedema (peau d'orange) or infiltration, with or without ulceration (T4)
(iii) large, fixed or matted axillary lymph nodes (N2)
(iv) inflammatory carcinoma (localized or generalized induration of the breast, oedema and erythema of the skin, especially in the lower half of the breast (T4d)).

If these patients undergo surgical resection of the tumour, approximately 50% of patients will develop a local recurrence of disease and the 5-year survival is very low (<10%), with most patients dying from metastatic disease. Therefore, combination chemotherapy is given primarily (neoadjuvant chemotherapy) with the aim of destroying micrometastatic disease and destaging the primary tumour. This may enable breast-conserving surgery to be undertaken subsequently. Although different regimens have been used, most of these contain anthracyclins (epirubicin, doxorubicin), which have been shown to be the most active chemotherapeutic agents against breast cancer cells. More recently the taxanes group of agents, e.g. docetaxel, paclitaxel, has been shown to be at least as active as doxorubicin and to be active even against tumours which are resistant to anthraclins.

Using this approach, complete and partial clinical responses (UICC criteria) can usually be obtained in approximately 70% to 80% of all patients – the smaller the initial tumour the higher the clinical and pathological response rates. Following neoadjuvant chemotherapy surgery is undertaken (breast-conservation surgery or mastectomy). Complete destruction of all tumour cells in the breast occurs in up to 15% of cases; the remaining patients have varying numbers of residual tumour cells.

Radiotherapy is given to the breast (or chest wall) and lymph draining areas approximately 4 weeks after surgery. Using this approach, survival rates have ranged from 35% to 65% at 5 years although randomized trials have not shown that neoadjuvant chemotherapy has a better effect than adjuvant chemotherapy which is given after surgery. However, recent studies have suggested that although tumours can be downstaged and thus enable breast-conservation surgery to be carried out rather than mastectomy, there may be a slightly higher risk of local disease recurrence in these patients.

Impalpable lesions

If an impalpable abnormality is detected in the breast which is shown to be malignant on FNAC or core biopsy (stereotactically, ultrasound-guided or guided by magnetic resonance mammography) further treatment is necessary. In the first instance, the lesion is removed in order to obtain a histological diagnosis and assessment, in particular whether this is an *in situ* or an invasive cancer. Pre-operative localization of the abnormality is carried out by inserting a wire into the lesion under mammographic or ultrasound control. If a lesion is not visible on mammography or ultrasound but is seen on MRM, then it is possible to insert a metal coil into the tumour using MRM guidance and then localize the coil which is at the tumour site stereotactically! This will enable the lesion to be accurately found and removed at operation. The excised tissue is oriented and is then X-rayed to ensure that the abnormality (e.g. opacity, microcalcification) has been removed. The breast specimen is inked and sent fresh to the pathology department, where 3 mm thick slices are cut which are then X-rayed again so that paraffin sections can be cut of abnormal areas for histopathological examination.

The extent of, or need for, further surgery will depend on whether this is an *in situ* cancer or an invasive tumour. Small invasive lesions, particularly if of low grade, carry a very good prognosis and a local excision and breast-conservation surgery may be all that is required. However, if the lesion is larger or there is multi-focal disease then consideration should be given to mastectomy because of the increased risk of recurrent malignancy or the subsequent development of further invasive cancers in the residual breast (as discussed previously).

Axillary lymph nodes
General principles

The lymphatic drainage of the breast has already been described in some detail (see previous section).

Clinical assessment of the axillary node status as to whether or not they contain tumour cells is most unreliable – in some studies less than 60% of involved nodes are clinically detectable. Radiological imaging procedures (mammography and ultrasound) do not reliably detect tumour-involved lymph nodes. Although magnetic resonance imaging and positron emission tomography have shown some promise they are not used in routine preoperative assessment of the axilla. Therefore, some form of axillary surgery to remove the lymph nodes and examine them histologically is the only way, at present, of accurately determining whether they are involved with tumour. This is essential for two reasons:

- to provide prognostic information about the disease and its spread because lymph node involvement is a surrogate marker for the likelihood of distant micrometastatic spread and hence determines the need for adjuvant therapies
- if there is lymph node involvement with tumour then regional control of disease must be obtained to prevent the progression of disease within the axilla and the involvement/destruction of major structures within the axilla.

What should be done to the axilla with these two points in mind is always the subject of hot debate amongst breast specialists as there are different approaches that can be taken, e.g. sentinel lymph node biopsy, axillary sample, axillary clearance. These are each described in more detail below and then finally a suggested plan for axillary management is given which is being used with increasing frequency in many breast cancer treatment units.

Sentinel lymph node biopsy

Recently, the use of sentinel node biopsy has gained widespread acceptance and increasing usage in the management of patients with breast cancer. The theoretical basis of this technique is that the malignant cells will disseminate in an orderly fashion to the axillary nodes, spreading first to the 'sentinel' lymph node (which may be more than one node). Therefore, by removing this lymph node for histological examination a representative view of the state of axillary nodal involvement can be achieved with the minimum of disruption to the axilla itself and hence the potential for less morbidity subsequently. One consideration for both the surgeons and patients is that in about 3% of patients the tumour bypasses the sentinel nodes and spreads to other lymph nodes in the axilla.

There are different techniques which are available to localize the sentinel node and again these have been the subject of much discussion. However, usually the patient is given an injection of a radiocolloid prior to surgery in the periareolar region and in addition, after induction of anaesthesia, a subdermal injection of a vital blue dye (e.g. patent blue) is given to the patient in the periareolar area, which binds to albumin and is carried in the lymphatics, so that the sentinel lymph node can be detected by one or both of these methods. This increases the likelihood of finding and removing the sentinel node. One major concern is the possible anaphylactic reactions to the blue dye which is reported to occur in 1 in 100 patients and which can be of a severe nature. Minor reactions include a bluish tinge to the patient's skin and urine which is of a temporary nature.

At the time of surgery, the sentinel node can then be localized using a probe to detect the radioactively labelled colloid which has accumulated in it and the site marked. Through a small incision the sentinel node(s) are located and if the blue dye has also been used, this will give a further visual identification of the lymphatics and the sentinel node(s). The sentinel node can be found in more than 95% of cases by surgeons experienced with this technique.

Once the sentinel node is removed it is usual to then wait for the pathologist to carry out a standard histological examination with formalin-fixed paraffin-embedded material. This means a delay of several days to know the patients' axillary status and therefore alternative techniques have been used to try to determine the patients' axillary status whilst they are still anaesthetized so that further surgery (axillary clearance if the node is involved with tumour) can be undertaken immediately if necessary.

- 'Frozen sections' or imprint cytology have been used and, if there is evidence of metastatic tumour in the node, an axillary clearance can be carried out immediately. However, this is not routinely used.
- A more recent development which has been stimulating much interest has been the use of real-time polymerase chain reaction (RT-PCR) to detect the gene expression of two markers which are found in breast tissue but not normal lymph nodes – these are mammaglobulin and cytokeratin 19. This can be performed whilst the patient is anaesthetized by analysing the sentinel node; the detection of these markers is taken as an indication of metastatic disease in the axillary node and this technique should detect metastases greater than 0.2 mm. However, further studies are required to confirm the sensitivity and specificity etc. before this is used in routine clinical practice.

Axillary sample

This involves the removal of four lymph nodes (confirmed at operation) from the proximal anterior/pectoral and central group of draining lymph nodes in the axilla. This has been shown to provide an accurate assessment of the nodal status of the axilla. Some surgeons, however, have had difficulty in identifying the required number of lymph nodes and have questioned whether sampling is an adequate procedure to stage the axilla, but nevertheless the procedure is in widespread use with satisfactory long-term results.

The main indications for its use would be:

- if patients are thought likely to be node-negative but facilities do not exist for sentinel lymph node biopsy to be carried out
- after a patient has had neoadjuvant chemotherapy prior to surgery and is thought to be node-negative because the impact of chemotherapy on patterns of lymphatic drainage is unclear.

If the sampled nodes contain malignant cells, then radiotherapy to the axilla and supraclavicular areas (4500 cGy) is given. The internal thoracic group of lymph nodes should also be considered. It has been estimated that approximately 90% of women with internal thoracic node involvement also have axillary nodes involved with tumour. If there is a strong possibility of tumour spread to the internal mammary group of lymph nodes (e.g. from tumours in the medial aspect of the breast), these nodes can also be irradiated.

Axillary dissection and clearance

An alternative approach to axillary node sampling is dissection of the axilla to various anatomical levels, as outlined below.

Level one –– Removal of lymph nodes lateral to the inferior border of the pectoralis minor muscle.

Level two –– Removal of level one lymph nodes and those behind and in front of pectoralis minor muscle.

Neither a level one nor two dissection of the axilla is an adequate therapeutic manoeuvre on its own. For example, if level one nodes are involved there is a 10% chance of further nodal involvement at levels two or three; if level two nodes are involved there is a 50% chance of level three nodes being involved with tumour. Radiotherapy to the axilla, therefore, is also required in patients with involved lymph nodes and who have undergone level one or two dissections. The likelihood of lymphoedema is significantly increased with irradiation of the axilla following axillary dissection.

Level three (clearance) –– This is the preferred of these procedures and is the removal of all the axillary lymphatic tissue and is better called axillary clearance. In order to achieve this, division or removal of the pectoralis minor muscle allows better access to the upper aspect of the axilla. The axillary contents (fat, fascia, lymphatic tissue) are cleared, from the apex (outer border of the first rib), below and medial to the axillary vein. The brachial plexus, the major axillary vessels, the long thoracic nerve and the thoracodorsal vessels and nerve are preserved during dissection. With a thorough axillary clearance no further treatment of the axilla is required, irrespective of whether there is involvement of the lymph nodes by tumour. Radiotherapy to the axilla following a clearance is associated with up to 30% incidence of lymphoedema. However, this does not result in a substantial improvement in regional disease control. Axillary surgery is not recommended for DCIS or minimal cancers.

Morbidity of axillary treatment

Axillary surgery and radiotherapy are associated with a recognized morbidity. During surgery, there is the risk of damage to nerves, most commonly the intercostobrachial nerve – not infrequently cut and result-

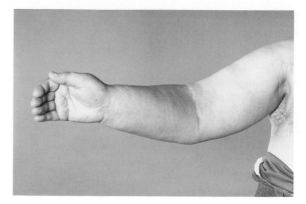

Figure 23.27 An example of lymphoedema of the arm following axillary clearance (Level 3).

ing in anaesthesia and/or paraesthesia of axilla and inner aspect of upper arm. The long thoracic and thoracodorsal nerves may also be damaged on occasions. Furthermore, wound seromas or infections may occur in up to 5% of patients. Radiotherapy may also be associated with nerve damage, and more rarely a brachial plexopathy. Both radiotherapy and surgery are associated with some reduction in the range of movements at the shoulder joint (particularly in elderly patients). Fewer than 10% of patients will develop lymphoedema (variable degree) following radiotherapy or a level two or three axillary dissection (Figure 23.27).

Suggested plan for management of the axilla

Therefore, whilst there are many ways to manage the axilla, how should we put this together for the management of patients with breast cancer in routine clinical practice? It is possible to put together a rational management plan and the following is used in many breast centres in clinical practice:

- all patients with a diagnosis of breast cancer should have their axilla subjected to ultrasound scanning to determine whether axillary lymph nodes are visualized and whether they are likely to be involved with tumour (note the limitations of this as described above)
- if there are ultrasonically suspicious lymph nodes then ultrasound-guided FNAC is carried out in an attempt to determine whether tumour cells are present
- if tumour cells are present, these patients will have an axillary clearance for their axillary treatment and will not undergo a sentinel lymph node procedure as we already know that tumour is in the axilla

- if tumour cells are not detected they will undergo a sentinel lymph node biopsy; if this does not contain tumour then no further treatment is required to the axilla
- if tumour cells are detected then the patient must undergo further axillary treatment, which at present may be either a surgical axillary clearance or alternatively radiotherapy to the axilla.

Breast reconstruction

Breast reconstruction aims to reverse the deformity of the breast and chest wall following breast surgery for cancer. This not only requires the creation of a new 'breast mound' but may also involve the creation of a nipple areola/complex and/or a symmetrization procedure on the opposite breast to try to ensure that the natural breast matches as closely as possible the reconstructed breast.

Therefore the following must be considered to achieve this:

- adequate skin of good quality is available for the new breast (e.g. from skin left after mastectomy, by tissue expansion or by the import of 'new' skin)
- adequate 'filling' to provide the 'volume' of the new breast (e.g. by using a prosthesis or fat and muscle tissue as part of a myocutaneous flap)
- a new nipple/areola complex (e.g. local skin flap, nipple sharing from the opposite side, tattooing or, if oncologically safe, the nipple/areola complex on the side of the mastectomy can be used as a free graft on a reconstructed breast mound).

This complex process requires a team approach, with the breast surgeon (and/or a plastic and reconstructive surgeon), the radiotherapist and medical oncologist and nurse counsellors being involved. The reconstructive surgery may be undertaken immediately at the same time as when mastectomy is undertaken or delayed until a later time, depending on the type and stage of disease and the adjuvant treatments that might be required. There does not appear to be any detrimental effects of immediate reconstruction in terms of subsequent local or systemic relapse of disease. As is clear from the principles listed above, the choice of approach will depend on the available skin on the chest wall (quality and quantity), the amount of skin, fat and muscle in other areas (back, abdomen) and the patient's own wishes. The various procedures used are outlined below.

Implant reconstruction

This is a way of providing breast volume if there is adequate skin left after, for example, skin sparing or subcutaneous mastectomy. The implant, which has an outer shell made of silicone elastomer and inner silicone gel, is inserted beneath the pectoralis major muscle at the same time as the mastectomy and is relatively simple and, although the results are not as good as some of the more complex techniques, the complications are fewer. A concern has been any potential adverse effects of silicone but a recent review of all the evidence has found that there is no evidence that patients with silicone-containing implants have an increased risk of connective tissue disorders, or have silicone toxicity or abnormalities of their immune systems.

Tissue expansion reconstruction

If there is insufficient skin left after the mastectomy, tissue expansion provides a way of obtaining an adequate quantity of good quality skin together with a new breast 'volume' to make the new breast. However, this technique is not suitable for patients with larger breasts or if they have radiotherapy with poorer-quality skin. The tissue expander comprises an outer shell of silicone elastomer with an inner compartment that can be filled with saline over a period of time by a filling port which is implanted subcutaneously, usually in the axilla. This is gradually filled with saline (over weeks) and results in an expansion of the overlying area of skin. The expander can then be removed and replaced with a silicone breast prosthesis. Alternatively, the expander may also be a breast prosthesis and can then be left *in situ* once the required degree of skin expansion and shape of the breast mound has been achieved.

Concern has been expressed because of the silicone content of the prosthesis and the expander and its possible association with connective tissue disorders. However, this association has not been definitively established. Complications occurring with the use of these implants include:

- infection of the prosthesis, usually necessitating removal
- formation and contraction of a fibrous capsule around the prosthesis which shrinks over time and is the commonest complication; the reasons for this are unknown but it is more likely in patients who have had radiotherapy
- rupture and leakage of silicone from the prosthesis.

More recent developments in implant technology have led to the use of implants with textured surfaces and this seems to reduce the risk of capsular contracture.

Myocutaneous transposition flaps

If the simpler forms of breast reconstruction discussed above are not suitable for the patient (e.g. lack of skin, radiation damage to skin, larger breast), then a myocutaneous flap, which provides both skin and volume, may be used to make the breast mound, with or without extra volume provided by an implant as necessary. Some of these are used as 'pedicled' flaps where the blood supply is kept intact as the flap is being used locally, or 'free' flaps where the blood supply is disconnected and the myocutaneous flap moved from a distal site to reconstruct the breast, therefore needing a microvascular anastomosis for the new blood supply. Whilst a detailed knowledge of the pros and cons of each individual flap is not necessary and beyond the scope of this chapter, it is necessary to have an outline knowledge of what each of these myocutaneous flaps is.

Latissimus dorsi flap

This is an example of a pedicled flap and involves the transfer of an ellipse of skin and latissimus muscle from the back which receives its blood supply from the thoracodorsal neurovascular pedicle. More recently an 'extended' latissimus flap procedure can be undertaken where much more muscle and subcutaneous fat is taken and used to reconstruct the breast. This gives excellent results.

Transverse rectus abdominis flap

An alternative is the TRAM flap, in which an ellipse of skin, fat and rectus muscle from the lower abdominal wall are utilized. This can remain attached to its vascular pedicle (pedicled flap), but can be a free flap (based on the deep inferior epigastric vessels), requiring a microvascular anastomosis but giving a better cosmetic result for the patient. Complications associated with this procedure include flap necrosis, infection and abdominal wall herniation.

Deep inferior epigastric perforator (DIEP) flap

This is another variety of abdominal flap which is based on the deep inferior epigastric artery by using the perforating blood vessels and avoids the need to remove the transversus rectus abdominis muscle. It is more complex, takes a longer period of time but because it retains the abdominal wall musculature then herniation should not occur.

Other flaps

It is important to be aware that myocutaneous flaps can be taken from other sites for breast reconstruction: for example, the superficial inferior epigastric artery flap, also using the abdominal wall, or the superior and inferior gluteal artery perforator flaps, which use the upper or lower buttock skin and muscle, and transverse upper gracilis flaps using the upper thigh.

Nipple-areola reconstruction

Reconstruction of the nipple and areola can be carried out at the same time as the breast mound construction or at a later date, when tissues have settled and it may be a better time to accurately site the position of the new nipple. There are a variety of techniques available for this, e.g. tissue from the other nipple (a nipple sharing graft), skin from the labia minora or upper thigh. Techniques using skin from the breast mound can also be used to create a nipple (a nipple flap procedure) and this can be carried out under local anaesthetic. The areola colour can be developed and modified by using tattooing techniques by injection of a semipermanent pigment which can be varied in tone to obtain the best match to the contralateral nipple. An alternative and very simple technique to this, which gives excellent cosmesis, is to use a prosthetic nipple (either already made or made in the hospital by taking a mould from the contralateral nipple) which 'sticks' to the skin and is removable.

Surgery to the contralateral breast

An integral part of breast reconstruction is to consider the contralateral breast when attempting to 'match' the two sides. For example, in patients with a ptotic contralateral breast, surgery to correct this and thus achieve symmetry may also be required, or in patients with a large contralateral breast then breast reduction may be necessary to achieve the best symmetry possible.

Adjuvant therapy

Following definitive surgical therapy of the primary breast cancer adjuvant therapy may be considered necessary to deal with suspected occult micrometastases.

This may take the form of either chemotherapy or hormonal therapy; in some patients both forms of treatment may be used.

Adjuvant chemotherapy

There is well-documented evidence that the administration of chemotherapy (two or more agents) will improve survival (overall and disease-free), albeit in a small group of women. These effects are greatest in women who are younger than 50 years of age and particularly in patients who have lymph node involvement by tumour.

Initially, combination chemotherapy comprising cyclophosphamide, methotrexate and 5-fluorouracil (CMF) was given at monthly intervals for 6 months and this was shown to be beneficial in reducing disease recurrence and increasing overall survival. In recent years, the Early Breast Cancer Trialists Collaborative group has carried out an overview to examine all these studies. The key points to emerge from this overview are that:

(a) patients with tumour involving lymph nodes in the axilla gain more benefit than those whose axillary nodes are not involved by tumour; however, there is still a significant but smaller benefit in the latter category of patients;

(b) an anthracycline-containing regimen also reduces the risk of death when compared with combination chemotherapy regimens which do not contain an anthracycline such as doxorubicin.

Whilst there are different combination chemotherapy regimens in usage throughout the world, one which is commonly used is six cycles of 5-fluorouracil, doxorubicin (or epirubicin) and cyclophosphamide given to patients at 21-day intervals. There have been several trials evaluating other combinations of chemotherapeutic agents, particularly the taxanes (paclitaxel and docetaxel), with evidence now emerging that there can be a significant benefit, albeit a higher toxicity, therefore limiting use to a very fit patient population.

Hormone therapy

The history of endocrine treatment for breast cancer dates back over 100 years, with two key individuals, first Schinzinger in Germany, and then Beatson in Scotland, suggesting that there was an association between hormones produced by the ovaries and breast cancer cell proliferation. They reported that in small numbers of selected patients bilateral oophorectomy could result in a temporary regression of breast cancer, thereby beginning the study of endocrine treatment in breast cancer.

It is important to remember that whilst the ovaries are the key source of oestrogens in premenopausal women there is another mechanism of production of oestrogens both in postmenopausal women and in men. The key to this is the aromatase enzyme which is found in the adrenals, muscle, skin, adipose tissue and often in breast cancer cells and which will convert circulating androgens (synthesized by the adrenals) into oestrogens.

Over the next 100 years knowledge of the effects of oestrogens on breast cancer cell growth has become better understood and the key role of the oestrogen receptors (present in 50–75% of breast cancers) has become clearer. The oestrogen receptor is located in the nucleus and after combining with oestrogen then binds to specific DNA sites, called oestrogen response elements, and gene activation ensues with subsequent production of RNA and key proteins which then leads to cellular proliferation and growth. Further details of this complex system, if required, can be found in standard texts.

Therefore, endocrine treatments are designed to interfere with either the production of oestrogens or the function of the oestrogen receptor and these are described below.

Drug treatment

Tamoxifen

Adjuvant hormonal therapy with tamoxifen (20 mg daily), an oestrogen receptor blocker but which also has partial agonist activity, has also been shown to improve time to disease recurrence and overall survival. The greatest effect is seen in postmenopausal women and in those in whom the tumours are oestrogen receptor positive. However, beneficial effects are seen in younger women, and those whose tumours are oestrogen receptor negative, but progesterone receptor positive, will also benefit from tamoxifen therapy.

The annual odds of death in women taking tamoxifen is reduced by approximately 17% (a 6% absolute improvement in survival at 10 years) and it is recommended for 5 years duration. Of concern have been the possible side effects of long-term tamoxifen use, in particular the risk of endometrial cancer. In addition, tamoxifen may reduce the risks of the development of a contralateral breast cancer by up to 30% although this benefit is less pronounced with time. Other side effects of tamoxifen include vaginal dryness, loss of libido and hot flushes and retinal damage.

Aromatase inhibitors

Studies have demonstrated the efficacy of aromatase inhibitors (AIs), which inhibit the aromatase enzyme system which is the main source of oestrogen in postmenopausal women, in the adjuvant treatment of breast cancer. There are currently three main ones in general clinical use: exemestane, letrozole and anastrozole. They have important biochemical differences which are beyond the requirements for this chapter, but they have similar side effects, most notably resulting in an increased risk of osteoporotic fracture and joint pains (guidelines have been published for monitoring bone density during treatment and are available elsewhere), but fewer hot flushes and without the endometrial effects of tamoxifen.

Trials which have compared the AIs with tamoxifen for 5 years are the ATAC trial (anastrozole versus tamoxifen) and the BIG 1–98 trial (letrozole versus tamoxifen) and both showed a significant risk of disease recurrence by using an AI, although a beneficial effect on overall survival has not been shown to date, but this would take more time to become evident.

An alternative approach using an AI has been termed the 'Switch' strategy where patients who have not relapsed after 2–3 years of tamoxifen (therefore endocrine sensitive) have received a further treatment with an AI to make a total of 5 years therapy. When this approach was compared in two randomized trials with 5 years of only tamoxifen (ITA and ABSCG8/ARN05), there were benefits of the Switch strategy in terms of an increased disease-free survival time.

Given these data then how are we to decide which adjuvant endocrine treatment should be given to patients? It is clear that premenopausal patients only receive tamoxifen, but should all postmenopausal patients receive AIs in view of the demonstrated benefits? Some have argued that they should and therefore do treat these patients with AIs, but others have tried to develop more 'tailored' therapy based on the likelihood of disease relapse. This has meant that AI-containing regimens have been given to patients judged to be most likely to develop a disease recurrence. One example of such a tailored protocol based on the risk of disease relapse is that used in Scotland:

- low risk – tamoxifen only
- intermediate risk – 'Switch' regimen
- higher risk – AI for 5 years.

However, the most recent NICE guidelines are at variance with this and have suggested that if the patients are not in the low-risk group then they should have an aromatase inhibitor if postmenopausal.

Ovarian ablation

Ovarian ablation has also been shown to improve survival in premenopausal women. The reduction in the annual odds of death is 25% (a 10% reduction in the risk of death after 5 years), which is comparable to that demonstrated from the use of chemotherapy. Ovarian ablation may be achieved by radiotherapy, surgery and more recently by using luteinizing hormone releasing hormone (LHRH) agonists and has been used in premenopausal women with aggressive disease in addition to chemotherapy and when a decision has been made to give an AI in view of its possible benefits. However, there is still a lack of clear data about how and what benefit is conferred by oophorectomy in addition to current management protocols.

Trastuzumab

An exciting development has been the understanding of the function of the HER receptor which is found on the surface of breast cancer cells and is over-expressed in approximately 20–30% of breast cancers. The presence of this receptor is determined by standard routine immunohistochemistry, and, if the results are equivocal, then fluorescent *in situ* hybridization (FISH) is a definitive, but expensive and complex, sensitive molecular biological method for determining whether the gene for this receptor is over-amplified.

Patients who are receiving adjuvant chemotherapy have been shown to benefit from additional treatment with a monoclonal antibody called trastuzumab which is directed against the HER2 receptor, with a 40–50% increase in disease-free survival. The major side effect is cardiotoxicity, with congestive cardiac failure of varying degrees occurring in up to 4% of patients treated in this way.

Metastatic breast cancer

Patients with metastatic disease may present because of symptoms caused by the metastatic deposits. However, up to one-half of patients who present with a loco-regional recurrence of disease have demonstrable metastatic disease either at the time of presentation or shortly thereafter. Once metastatic breast cancer has been diagnosed the mean survival of these patients is approximately 18 to 24 months. However, if metastases are limited to bone only, survival on treatment may extend to several years. Thus, the primary aim of any treatment is to palliate and improve the quality of life.

Treatments for such patients can be divided into (i) those aimed primarily at control of symptoms (e.g. general supportive care; relief of debilitating, disabling and distressing symptoms; management of pathological fractures; correction of disorders of body functions, etc.) and (ii) treatment to retard the growth of the tumour. These latter treatments are either chemotherapy or hormonal therapy.

Chemotherapy

Chemotherapy is associated with side effects which can impair the patient's quality of life and a considered decision must be made as to which patients are most likely to gain benefit (and what these benefits are) from chemotherapy. Patients who are most likely to benefit are those with a good performance status, metastatic disease in one or only a few sites and previous beneficial response to hormonal therapy.

It is currently recommended that if patients have had treatment with an anthracycline already the sequence of chemotherapeutic agents used should be as follows:

first line – docetaxel (as a single agent)
second line – capcetibine or vinorelbine (as a single agent)
third line – whichever of the above two was not used as second-line therapy.

The response rates to these regimens vary and the median time to disease relapse is only 6 to 10 months. Following further relapse of disease, other chemotherapeutic regimens may be tried but the response rates are low. A small group of women (up to 20% in some series) have a prolonged (5 year) survival benefit with palliative chemotherapy.

Hormonal therapy

Hormone therapy has the advantage of less-severe side effects than chemotherapy. Hormone therapy would be indicated in patients who were unfit for chemotherapy and also in those with disease present in multiple sites and with bone metastases. Responses

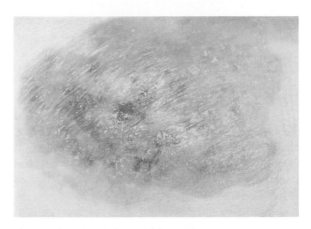

Figure 23.28 Paget's disease of the nipple.

to hormonal therapy have been reported in up to 60% of patients whose tumours have a high level of oestrogen receptors. Response rates are unlikely in oestrogen receptor negative tumours or in patients with hepatic metastases. If patients have been taking tamoxifen as adjuvant therapy before the development of metastatic disease then only 20% to 30% will respond to second-line hormonal manipulation, for example using medroxyprogesterone or aromatase inhibitors. It is also important to remember that even if patients demonstrate no response to first-line hormonal therapy, 20% will respond to second-line hormonal treatment. A further 10% to 15% may show a response to third-line hormonal treatment. In premenopausal women ovarian ablation (e.g. oophorectomy or radiation-induced menopause, LHRH agonists) is tried initially. Following relapse, aromatase inhibitors (e.g. aminoglutethamide, 4-hydroxyandrostenedione) or progestagens (e.g. medroxyprogesterone acetate) can be tried. Postmenopausal women are treated with anti-oestrogens or other hormonal treatments (see above). Bisphosphonates are also given if bone metastases are present.

Paget's disease of the nipple

Paget's disease of the nipple was first described over 200 years ago by Sir James Paget. Clinically, this is recognized by reddening, excoriation and/or scaling of the skin of the nipple with or without a nipple discharge (Figure 23.28). These appearances may resemble eczema or dermatitis but are unilateral. This is associated with an underlying intraduct carcinoma and up to one-half of the patients have a palpable lump. If there is a palpable lump present then up to 90% of this group of patients will have an invasive cancer present. In the absence of a palpable lump up to one-third of patients will have an invasive cancer.

Histologically, Paget's cells are located in the epidermis of the nipple. Morphologically, these cells are large and rounded, with vacuolated cytoplasm and pleomorphic hyperchromatic nuclei. Their origin is unclear but it is believed that they have migrated from the underlying cancer through the mammary ducts or, alternatively, they are malignant cells that have arisen in the skin of the nipple.

The treatment of Paget's disease has been controversial. If local excision and breast-conserving surgery only is carried out, then tumour recurrence may occur in up to 40% of patients. Therefore, some surgeons advocate mastectomy and axillary surgery.

Phylloides tumour of the breast

Phylloides tumours (previously called 'cystosarcoma phylloides') account for up to 1% of all breast neoplasms. Although they can be found in any age group the median age is 45 years and they present clinically as a discrete lump in the breast which is very similar, if not identical, to a fibroadenoma. In terms of investigations, the appearances on mammography and ultrasonography may be similar to a fibroadenoma although the phylloides tumour may be more dense, have cystic areas and be lobulated. FNAC and core biopsy are required and these may or may not confirm the diagnosis of a phylloides tumour.

Macroscopically, they range in size from a few millimetres to up to several centimetres in diameter; when cut they demonstrate cystic cavities associated with fronds of tissue projecting into them. Microscopically, they have two distinct components; an epithelial component which covers the fronds of tissue and a stromal component. The stromal component is more cellular than that seen in a fibroadenoma. Furthermore, the cells may show mitoses, have marked nuclear pleomorphism and may have an infiltrative border. The histological appearances may resemble a sarcoma and biologically the tumour may behave either as a benign lesion (85%) or as a malignant growth (15%). In the latter situation, it is the stromal component which is malignant and they metastasize via the bloodstream to lungs and bone. Spread to regional tumour-draining lymph nodes rarely occurs with phylloides tumours.

It may be difficult to determine the likely behaviour of a phylloides tumour. However, factors which are considered to be important are the number of mitoses per 10 high-power microscopic fields ($\times 400$); 0–4 mitoses being benign, 5–9 potentially malignant and 10 or more malignant. Benign lesions are treated conservatively whilst those with features of a sarcoma are treated by a mastectomy. Treatment of the lesion is usually wide local excision with clear margins and then careful follow-up for local recurrence of disease, which has been estimated to occur in up to 10–20% of patients who have benign lesions and in up to 30% or more of those with malignant phylloides tumours, usually within 2 years.

If the tumour recurs further local excision or mastectomy will be required. Unfortunately, when the tumour recurs it tends to be biologically more aggressive, with the tumour cells having a higher mitotic rate. The tumours are not radio- or chemo-sensitive and there are no trials to indicate the value of such treatments as adjuvants.

Breast cancer in the elderly

The incidence of breast cancer continues to rise through life, with 40% of all cases occurring in patients older than 70 years. A small number of these patients, because of concurrent disease, will be unfit for any form of locoregional therapy other than letrozole, which is more effective than tamoxifen in this situation. With letrozole as the sole therapy it has been shown that approximately one-half of the tumours will show a reduction in size and of these up to 50% will be complete responses (6 to 12 months of treatment may be required). However, approximately 50% of those tumours which initially responded may relapse within 2 years, with tumour growth then occurring. It should also be noted that if the tumours are oestrogen receptor negative they are unlikely to respond to letrozole (or other anti-oestrogen therapies) and oestrogen receptor status should be established before commencing therapy. If the patients are hormone receptor negative then palliative radiotherapy may be used in attempting to obtain locoregional control of disease.

However, in general, therefore, it is recommended that older patients should be treated along the same principles as outlined previously but taking into account their general health and life expectancy and the impact that these have on all the treatments proposed. Stage for stage the results of therapy in women over 65 years are comparable to those in younger women. However, population-based audit shows that the prognosis in women over 80 years is worse than in younger age groups.

Bilateral breast cancers

A second primary cancer in the opposite breast may be found either at the time of the initial presentation (synchronous tumour, 0.5% to 2%) or more commonly at a subsequent date (metachronous cancer, 3% to 9%). A woman who has a primary breast cancer has a four- to six-fold risk of developing a cancer in the opposite breast. Other risk factors for the development of a cancer in the opposite breast include lobular carcinoma *in situ* and multifocal disease.

The prognosis for patients with bilateral breast cancers depends on the staging of the tumours and treatment should be appropriate for the disease stage. Patients who have a genetic predisposition (mutations of the putative breast cancer gene(s) and associated genomic abnormalities (e.g. loss of heterozygosity of the p53 suppressor gene)) are at very high risk of developing bilateral breast cancers. In these patients, consideration may be given as to whether prophylactic mastectomy (with or without reconstruction) should be undertaken.

Breast cancer related to pregnancy

Breast cancer presenting during pregnancy or lactation occurs in up to 3 in 10 000 pregnancies, and overall is less than 2% of all breast cancers. Although initially it was believed that the prognosis was worse in pregnancy, more recent studies have suggested that when considering non-pregnant patients with similar disease characteristics and stage, there may be little difference in survival, although others still suggest pregnancy is an independent factor of poorer survival. Breast cancers arising in pregnant women, compared to non-pregnant women, are:

- larger and at a more advanced stage
- more likely to be histological grade 3 (up to 75%)
- more likely to have lymph node involvement (50–70%)
- more likely to be oestrogen receptor negative.

In terms of investigations that pregnant women may undergo, although mammography and chest X-rays are usually avoided, with appropriate protection for the fetus mammography can be carried out, mini-

mizing fetal risk. For staging purposes, CT and MRI of the abdomen are usually avoided because of possible teratogenic effects, but ultrasound and modified isotope bone-scanning techniques can be carried out, minimizing risks to the fetus.

The treatment of the breast cancer should be as for non-pregnant women but with some modifications due to the effects of radiotherapy and chemotherapy and their potential for fetal damage. The surgical treatment of the breast itself (conservation or mastectomy) can be carried out safely, with some studies suggesting a slightly increased risk of intrauterine growth retardation and low birth weight. Similarly, axillary surgery in the form of sample or clearance may be carried out; sentinel node biopsy is usually avoided as its safety is not clear at present.

If the patient requires adjuvant radiotherapy this is usually not given until after the fetus has been delivered as the risks of fetal damage are higher, although some do advocate radiotherapy with appropriate fetal protection. Chemotherapy is given, if indicated, after the first trimester has passed (period of organ formation and greatest risk of damage). At least two studies have indicated that doxorubicin-based chemotherapy given during the second and third trimesters of pregnancy is safe with no increased risk of malformations or fetal death, but there was an increased risk of premature labour and the fetus being small. Currently, anti-oestrogen therapy and trastuzumab are not given during pregnancy because of unknown risks. There are no data to suggest that termination of the pregnancy has any effect on subsequent survival from breast cancer.

Patients presenting with locally advanced breast cancer and who would normally be treated with neoadjuvant chemotherapy pose a difficult problem. If the pregnancy is in the first trimester consideration has to be given to terminating the pregnancy prior to starting chemotherapy. However, this requires a multidisciplinary approach between the surgeon, obstetrician, medical oncologist, psychologist and the patient and her partner.

As regards the risks of a subsequent pregnancy in a patient who has been successfully treated for breast cancer, current advice is that there is no evidence of an increased risk of disease recurrence and interestingly there is a suggestion that survival might be enhanced. However, it is commonly recommended that women wait for 2 to 3 years after treatment before a pregnancy as this is the time of higher risk of disease recurrence.

Breast cancer in the male

Cancer of the male breast accounts for 0.5% to 1% of all breast cancers and less than 1% of all male malignancies. Only 5% of male breast cancers occur before the age of 40 years and the median age of presentation is 68 years (older than that of the female population who develop breast cancer). The aetiology of male breast cancer has not been elucidated but there are risk factors which may predispose to the development of breast cancer. These include increased levels of oestrogens either in the circulation or in the breast tissue (Kleinfelter's syndrome, treatment with oestrogens for prostatic cancer), increased prolactin levels, exposure to ionizing radiation, genetic predisposition and occupational risk factors (steel and news printing workers). Also, an increased incidence of breast cancer in males has been shown to occur in families who have a BRCA2 mutation on chromosome 13q.

The clinical presentation is usually a lump, most commonly centrally placed or in the upper outer quadrant. Up to 20% of patients may have nipple discharge, which can be either serous or sero-sanguineous. Histologically, invasive ductal carcinomas of no special type comprise the majority of cancers, as in the female population. All histological types of cancer may be found with the exception of lobular cancer, which occurs less frequently. In approximately 80% of tumours, there are oestrogen or progesterone receptors present. The reported 5-year survival for male patients with breast cancer has ranged from 36% to 75%, but when the patient's age, tumour stage, lymph node and hormonal status are taken into account the survival is comparable with that of female patients.

Treatment is as described for female breast cancer. Control of locoregional disease (with surgery and radiotherapy) is important. In addition, systemic therapy is required for overt or occult micro-metastatic disease and this may involve either hormone or chemotherapy.

Screening for breast cancer

The general principles for cancer screening have been discussed elsewhere in this book but there are commonly three situations where individuals who have been identified as having an increased risk of breast cancer on the basis of age, family history and previous radiation exposure are screened for breast cancer and these are outlined below.

NHS breast screening programme

In 1988 a UK National Health Service breast screening programme was introduced with the aim of reducing breast cancer mortality following initial studies which had reported that this would be the result. Whilst there has been debate as to the results from many subsequent studies, a WHO expert review panel has indicated that there is a significant reduction in breast cancer mortality if women aged between 50 and 69 years undergo mammographic screening.

The NHS breast screening programme invites women aged between 50 and 70 years to attend a specialist screening facility. There are 85 in the UK, which may be located in hospitals or other types of facility, with each serving a defined population, and these are subjected to very detailed audit and quality assurance procedures. Women are invited to undergo mammography every 3 years (two views taken are craniocaudal and mediolateral) on the basis of which GP practice a person is registered with. Women aged above 70 years can have this mammogram but must initiate this themselves as they are not routinely invited. It is anticipated that by 2012 all women aged between 47 and 73 will be invited to attend for screening in the NHS programme.

After the initial mammogram has been carried out, between 7 and 10% of women are recalled for further investigations. These may include further mammographic examinations, ultrasound assessment and FNAC. Additional diagnostic procedures may be required after these assessments to establish the nature of the abnormality detected in the breast and approximately six individuals are identified with cancer per 1000 women screened.

This process requires a multidisciplinary team composed of radiologists, surgeons, cytologists and pathologists who are specifically trained and experienced in the diagnosis and treatment of breast disease. The cancers detected through breast screening are smaller and at an earlier stage than the tumours of those patients who attend symptomatic breast clinics, and the 5-year survival of a patient diagnosed with an invasive cancer by breast screening is 90%.

Screening after radiotherapy for Hodgkin's lymphoma

It has been recognized that up to 1 in 3 women who have received supradiaphragmatic (mantle) radiotherapy (includes part of the breast) for Hodgkin's disease will develop breast cancer. The risk is dependent on a series of factors: age at which treatment was given, time since treatment, and the dose and size of the area that was treated. It seems that women are most at risk if they were treated at or under the age of 35 and from 8 years after treatment. Given these facts the guidelines state that:

- if patients were treated under the age of 16, surveillance should start at 20 years of age
- if patients were treated between 16 and 35 years of age, then surveillance should start 8 years later.

In terms of the type of surveillance programme recommended, then:

- if patients are less than 30 years of age – annual MRI of the breasts
- if they are between 20 and 50 years of age then annual mammaography supplemented by MRI scanning of the breast if required because of the increased density of the breast tissue
- when patients are over 50 years of age they then receive 3-yearly breast mammography.

Screening for individuals depending on family history of breast cancer

This is a rapidly changing area and currently three genes have been identified as predisposing to breast cancer, as discussed earlier in this chapter. However, the key is the family history and in all patients attending a breast clinic and/or diagnosed with breast cancer a detailed history focusing on first- and second-degree relatives should be taken. A first-degree relative is a parent, sibling or child and a second-degree relative is a grandparent, aunt/uncle or nephew/niece.

Most familial types of breast cancer are due to mutations in genes which are more common but which have a lower penetrance. The magnitude of this is dependent on several factors. For example, the relative risk if the mother had the disease is 1.8, whilst with a sister it is 2.5. If both first-degree relatives were affected, the risk rises to 5.6 (approximately 40%). Further studies have shown that the relative risk for sisters of patients with bilateral disease is approximately 5.3. However, if the age of presentation of the cancer is less than 40 years of age then the relative risk increases to approximately 9 (i.e. approaches 80%).

Whilst there are several guidelines, which may rapidly change, there are a variety of protocols for clinical and mammographic surveillance, and mag-

netic resonance mammography is becoming increasingly used. The following are based on adaptations of the current guidelines and are followed in many centres, with individuals being categorized as either being at 'high', 'moderate' or 'population' risk of developing breast cancer, and form a basis for clinical practice which can be modified by different centres.

High-risk individuals

- Women who carry a mutation in a known cancer gene, e.g. BRCA1 or 2, or who are at 50% risk of inheriting a known family mutation in one of these genes
- Four or more first- and/or second-degree relatives on the same side of the family with breast or ovarian cancer, or
- One first-degree relative with breast and ovarian cancer.

Mammographic screening recommended for these individuals is every 2 years between the ages of 35 and 40 years, then annually between the ages of 40 and 50 years, and then every 18 months between 50 and 64 years, and 3-yearly thereafter.

Moderate-risk individuals

- One first-degree relative with breast cancer and less than 40 years at diagnosis, or one first-degree male relative with breast cancer at any age, or
- Two or more relatives on the same side of the family with breast cancer under 60 years at diagnosis, or a male with breast cancer of any age, but one of these relatives is first-degree, or
- Two or more relatives on the same side of the family with breast cancer diagnosed under the age of 60 years, or ovarian cancer at any age, but one of these is a first-degree relative.

Mammographic screening recommended for these individuals is the same as for the high-risk individuals but after the age of 50 years is then 3-yearly.

There are a variety of protocols for clinical and mammographic surveillance and magnetic resonance mammography is becoming increasingly used in conjunction with mammography for women at very high risk (e.g. gene mutation carriers). However, the above will form a sound basis for practice.

Chapter

24

Lower gastrointestinal surgery

Chris Cunningham

Surgical anatomy

Small bowel

The small bowel extends from the pylorus to the caecum. Disorders of the duodenum are discussed elsewhere and this chapter will be concerned with the small bowel from the duodenal–jejunal junction to the caecum. The entire small bowel is enveloped in peritoneum, the attachments or 'root' of which run from the ligament of Treitz to the terminal ileum. The upper two-fifths of the small bowel is jejunum and the distal portion is ileum but the transition point lacks clear demarcation. The arterial supply, innervation and venous and lymphatic drainage pass through the mesentery. The arterial supply arises from the superior mesenteric artery, which enters the mesentery over the superior border of the third part of the duodenum. The venous drainage returns to the superior mesenteric vein, joining the splenic vein to become the hepatic portal vein. The small bowel is rich in immune cells with Peyers patches in the submucosa and nodes within the mesentery subsequently draining to the cysterna chyli. Parasympathetic and sympathetic fibres are relayed through Auerbach plexus and parasympathetic continue through Meissner's submucosal plexus.

Visceral pain from the small bowel is relayed through sensory afferents running with the sympathetic nerves. Distension or colic causes pain in the paraumbilical region, reflecting the mid-gut embryological origin of the small bowel. Localized inflammatory conditions of the small bowel relay pain through parietal sensory innervations in the peritoneum of the abdominal wall. The primary role of the small bowel is absorption of nutrients but it also has important secretory and digestive functions. Pathology in the small bowel is frequently associated with malnutrition and dehydration.

Colon and rectum

The colon extends from the ileocaecal valve to the rectosigmoid junction. The portion proximal to the splenic flexure is derived from the mid gut and shares its blood supply with the small bowel arising from the superior mesenteric vessels dividing into the ileocaecal, right colic and middle colic vessels. The distal portion of the colon and rectum is supplied through the vessels of the hind gut arising from the inferior mesenteric vessel and appreciation of these vessels is a critical event in bowel resection and anastomosis. Venous drainage is similarly divided, with proximal colon passing to the superior mesenteric veins and the hindgut colon and rectum to the inferior mesenteric vein that drains into the splenic vein behind the pancreas. The colon is characterized by three outer longitudinal muscle bands, the taeniae coli. These bands fuse at the base of the appendix and again at the rectosigmoid junction. These bands cause shortening of the colon, creating mucosal haustrations that characterize the colonic pattern on plane radiographs. The appendices epiploica are pedunculated fat pads that arise between the taeniae and mark the sites of the vasa rectae, arteries that perforate the muscular wall of the colon and mark the sites through which diverticular disease arises. The ascending and descending colon are usually retroperitoneal whereas the caecum, transverse and sigmoid colon are on mesenteries that in certain cases may be abnormally mobile, predisposing to volvulus.

The appendix arises from the caecum and its mesentery contains an end artery from the ileocolic vessels. The appendix is rich in lymphatic tissues and

Fundamentals of Surgical Practice, Third Edition, ed. Andrew N. Kingsnorth and Douglas M. Bowley.
Published by Cambridge University Press. © Cambridge University Press 2011.

its narrow lumen is susceptible to obstruction through faecolith or lymphoid proliferation. Inflammation and subsequent thrombosis result in gangrenous perforation of appendicitis.

The rectum is usually described as 15 cm in length but at surgery it is identified as the point of transition where the longitudinal muscle coalesces to form a single outer coat. The rectum also lacks appendices epiploicae. The rectum lies in the sacral hollow passing over the levator ani muscle of the pelvic floor to continue to the anus. Blood supply arises from the superior rectal artery as a continuation of the inferior mesenteric vessel and supply is also taken from the internal iliac vessels through the middle and inferior rectal vessels. Venous drainage is both through the inferior mesenteric vessels but also laterally to the pelvic wall and a porto-systemic anastomosis is found in the haemorrhoidal vessels at the anus. Lymphatic drainage from the hindgut passes to the para-aortic nodes but drainage from the low rectum may be more diverse through both the iliac and even inguinal nodes, particularly in the face of pathology such as malignant infiltration.

The colon and rectum are important in absorbing around 1–2 litres of fluid per day and the rectum also has an important function in storing and evacuating stool. Disturbances in function will frequently result in an alteration in bowel habit, dehydration, but no direct effect on nutrition. Greater understanding of pelvic anatomy has led to improvements in rectal cancer surgery, with reduced collateral damage to pelvic nerves and improved rectal excision. This technique, known as total mesorectal excision (TME), is critical to achieving good oncological and functional outcomes after rectal excision and was popularized by Heald during the 1980s. TME consists of separate high ligation of the inferior mesenteric vessels to define the proximal limits of the lymphatic clearance, followed by rectal mobilization with sharp dissection under direct vision in the avascular plane outside the mesorectum, excising the envelope of fat containing vessels and lymphatics surrounding the rectal tube. This surgical innovation has been shown to reduce local recurrence of cancer dramatically, while maximizing the chances of sphincter-preserving surgery and preservation of pelvic nerve function.

Anorectal anatomy

As the rectum passes through the pelvic floor visceral sensation gives way to somatic innervations at the dentate line. Associated with this is the transition zone, which is thought to be important in maintaining continence by offering discrimination between, gas, liquid and solid. The inner circular muscle continues as the internal anal sphincter and remains under involuntary control, providing resting anal tone, protecting against passive incontinence. The longitudinal fibres of the rectum continue as the intersphincteric fibres and the external sphincter muscle is formed from skeletal muscle taken from the levator ani muscle. This protects against urge incontinence, raising anal squeeze pressure above rectal pressure. The levator ani comprises a complex of muscles forming a support to pelvic structures. Puborectalis is the best defined of these, passing as a sling around the anorectal junction maintaining an angle that is thought to be important in continence. Anorectal anatomy is presented in Figure 24.1.

Normal pelvic function requires the intact musculature of the pelvic floor and anal sphincter with adequate sensory and motor innervation. Pelvic floor structures are most commonly compromised in pregnancy and childbirth, with traction injuries to nerves and tears to muscles of the pelvic floor and sphincter. Surgical misadventure in the treatment of common anorectal problems such as fistulas, fissures and haemorrhoids is also an important cause. Faecal incontinence is an obvious sequel to such injuries but evacuatory problems and rectal intussusceptions may also occur and the functional impact can be significant to quality of life.

Colorectal investigations

Radiology

Imaging in lower gastrointestinal surgery has seen many advances in the last five years. Traditional contrast examinations have been largely replaced by high-resolution cross-sectional imaging. Imaging of advanced malignancy has been helped by PET-CT scanning and modifications of endoscopic ultrasound have improved staging of early disease, particularly rectal cancer. However, a basic understanding of contrast imaging is valuable and will be summarized.

Contrast enema examination

Barium enema is usually 'double-contrast' liquid barium and air introduced sequentially into the colon. Double-contrast barium enema is able to show detail of the mucosa and gives a permanent record of the

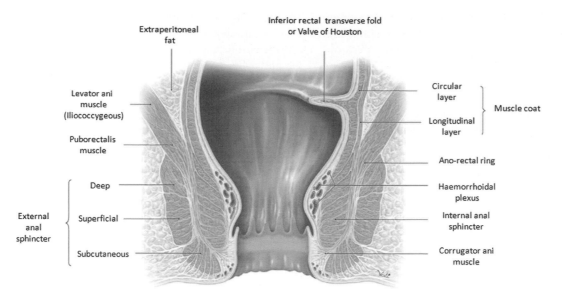

Extraperitoneal fat

Inferior rectal transverse fold or Valve of Houston

Levator ani muscle (Iliococcygeous)

Puborectalis muscle

External anal sphincter

Deep

Superficial

Subcutaneous

Circular layer

Muscle coat

Longitudinal layer

Ano-rectal ring

Haemorrhoidal plexus

Internal anal sphincter

Corrugator ani muscle

Schünke et al., Prometheus, Innere Organe, Thieme Verlag, 2005

Figure 24.1 Anorectal anatomy. Coronal section of anorectum. The three components of the external anal sphincter are considered as one functional group. The internal anal sphincter is essentially a continuum of the longitudinal muscle layer of the rectum and is important in providing resting (involuntary) tone to the anus. The external anal sphincter is closely related to the levator ani muscle offering voluntary control over continence. Kindly provided by Professor Dr med. Thilo Wedel, Institute of Anatomy, University of Kiel, Germany.

bowel examination. It is no longer recommended as the primary investigation of bowel disease but can be useful in the assessment of diverticular disease. Water-soluble contrast enemas are used to diagnose structuring in acute large bowel obstruction and to assess colorectal anastomosis for leakage, either acutely in the postoperative period or prior to closure of defunctioning ileostomy. Water-soluble contrast offers crude single-contrast detail but has the advantage of avoiding chemical peritonitis in the presence of perforation. Water-soluble contrast is frequently used to delineate the small bowel and rectum in CT scanning.

Small bowel enteroclysis, also known as small bowel enema, is mainly used to assess stricturing of inflammatory conditions such as Crohn's disease. Contrast is delivered through a naso-jejunal tube aiming for a high concentration of contrast to optimize mucosal detail. This is superior to the small bowel follow-through study, where contrast is diluted in gastric secretions, reducing resolution.

Abdominal and pelvic computed tomography

Computed tomography (CT) has transformed the assessment of emergency and elective patients in lower

gastrointestinal practice. In the acute setting, CT provides early and accurate diagnosis of bowel obstruction and helps identify those patients likely to require early surgery, as well as those for whom non-operative or palliative measures may be more appropriate, e.g. in the presence of extensive metastatic disease. In addition it has valuable application in the management of inflammatory conditions such as diverticulitis and Crohn's disease, identifying complications such as abscess formation that may be better treated with percutaneous drainage. In the elective setting, CT scanning is the cornerstone of staging in colorectal cancer, providing information on local invasion and metastatic disease affecting liver and lungs.

CT colonography

CT colonography uses computer programming to combine helical CT scans in order to create two- or three-dimensional images of the interior of a patient's colon acquired after bowel preparation and insufflation of air or carbon dioxide through the anus. These images can be rotated for different views and even combined for a complete view of the colon, which is known as 'virtual colonoscopy', as shown in Figure 24.2. The accuracy of CT colonography appears

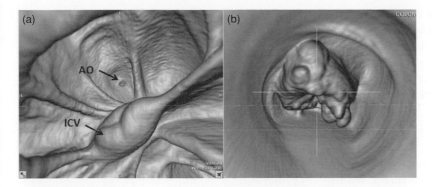

Figure 24.2 Virtual colonoscopy. 'Fly-through' reconstruction of CT pneumocolon examination showing normal caecum in A and presence of a tumour in B. Detailed anatomical view seen in the caecum with the ileocaecal valve (ICV) and appendix orifice (AO) identified. Pictures kindly provided by Dr Andrew Slater, Consultant Radiologist, Oxford Radcliffe Hospitals.

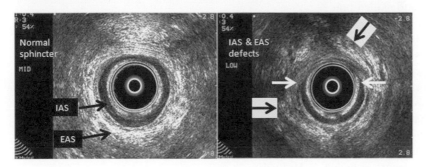

Figure 24.3 Anal ultrasound with radial probe giving axial view of sphincter. The left panel shows a normal sphincter with internal anal sphincter (IAS) and external anal sphincter (EAS) labelled. The right panel shows deficient internal sphincter between the 9 and 3 o'clock positions in the low anal canal defined by white arrows. The external sphincter has a defect between 9 and 1 o'clock defined by the black arrows. This defect is typical of an obstetric injury.

to be comparable to conventional colonoscopy for the detection of cancers and polyps greater than 10 mm. The main limitation of the technique is radiation exposure, which makes it unsuitable for young patients and those undergoing frequent surveillance examinations for a family or personal history of colorectal neoplasms. Patients in whom significant polyps are identified at CT colonography will proceed to therapeutic colonoscopy.

Magnetic resonance imaging

MRI scanning has two common applications in colorectal disease: staging of pelvic malignancy, especially rectal cancer, and assessment of pelvic floor and perineal pathology such as fistula disease or sphincter injury. Many centres use MRI to guide use of neoadjuvant treatment in rectal cancer prior to surgery. In inflammatory conditions MRI is particularly valuable in recurrent or complex anal fistula such as that of Crohn's disease. A developing role of MRI is the assessment of small bowel by MR enteroclysis. The principles are similar to CT enteroclysis but soft tissue detail is greater and, of course, radiation exposure is avoided.

Anorectal ultrasound

The widest use of anorectal ultrasound is in defining anal sphincter anatomy in the assessment of damage from surgery or obstetric injury (Figure 24.3) as well as detail of anal sepsis and fistula disease. Ultrasound is used to stage rectal tumours, where it is valuable in defining benign tumours and early-stage cancers that may be suitable for potentially curative local excision.

Anorectal physiology

Anal manometry provides objective measurement of the resting and squeeze pressure within the anal canal, giving valuable information in the management of patients with constipation and anal incontinence. Resting pressure is largely due to the internal anal sphincter; squeeze pressure is a reflection of the voluntary muscles of the anal canal (external sphincter and puborectalis). Normal resting canal pressure is 50–70 mmHg and the resting pressure in the anal canal increases from cranial to caudal, creating a 'high-pressure zone' 1 or 2 cm from the anal verge. In normal individuals, the maximum squeeze pressure is an additional 50–100% of the resting tone. The anal canal is rich in sensory receptors and when rectal distension is detected, the internal sphincter reflexly relaxes and the external sphincter contracts. This rectoanal inhibitory reflex enables rectal contents to be 'sampled' by the anal canal mucosa and facilitates discrimination between gaseous and non-gaseous contents of the rectum. The rectoanal inhibitory reflex is absent in Hirschsprung's disease.

Endoscopy

Colonoscopy provides detailed views of the colon and rectum, and enables interventions such as biopsy and polypectomy. However, it is an invasive technique, requiring bowel preparation and skilled practitioners and exposes the patient to the risks of perforation (0.06–2%) and bleeding after polypectomy (0.4–2.7%). Most colorectal cancers are assumed to have a premalignant adenomatous polyp phase; therefore colonoscopy provides the opportunity for cancer screening and prevention. The USA National Polyp Study observed a 70–90% lower than expected incidence of colorectal cancer in patients undergoing colonoscopy compared to three reference populations.

Wireless capsule endoscopy represents a major advance in the imaging of the small intestine. It is able to capture video-images of the mucosal surface of the entire length of the intestine, which can then be interpreted by an observer.

Colorectal emergencies

Obstruction

The cardinal features of gastrointestinal obstruction are abdominal distension, pain, vomiting and constipation. The exact nature of these depends on the level of obstruction within the fore, mid or hind gut. Distension and constipation are features of distal small bowel and colonic obstruction whereas early vomiting is more common in proximal obstruction. When vomiting does occur in distal obstruction it may become faeculent. Pain tends to be colicky in nature and the origin reflects the embryological origin with referral to the epigastrium, paraumbilical or low abdomen. There are two components to obstruction. The first relates to the obvious sequel of mechanical obstruction. These can be controlled and corrected with nasogastric aspiration and intravenous fluid replacement. The second relates to the development of compromised bowel which results in infarction, perforation, sepsis and ultimately multi-organ failure if surgery is not under-

Table 24.1 Indications for lower GI endoscopy

Colonoscopy	Flexible sigmoidoscopy
Dark red rectal bleeding	Bright red rectal bleeding
Iron deficiency anaemia	Left-sided abnormalities on other imaging
Change in bowel habit	Left-sided mass
Suspected inflammatory bowel disease	Population screening
Further assessment of abnormalities suspected on other imaging	
Population screening	

taken. This complication is most common in closed loop obstruction, as occurs in volvulus or in colonic obstruction in the presence of a competent ileocaecal valve preventing decompression into the small bowel. Evidence of compromised bowel is suggested by the systemic inflammatory response and mandates surgical intervention.

Volvulus

Volvulus describes the twisting of a segment of bowel around its mesentery. It is usually associated with a congenitally long mobile mesentery but may also result from twisting around band adhesions. It most commonly involves sigmoid colon, caecum or segments of small bowel affected by adhesions.

Although the incidence of sigmoid volvulus is rare in Western countries, it is one of the most common causes of emergency large-bowel surgery in other countries, particularly in Africa. In the UK, sigmoid volvulus often occurs in elderly and frail individuals who are frequently institutionalized. The clinical symptoms and signs are those of colonic obstruction, often the abdomen is hugely distended and 'drum-like' and the rectum is empty on digital examination. The diagnosis is supported by a typical X-ray appearance. In the absence of signs of peritonitis, de-torsion of the volvulus can be attempted by use of a rigid sigmoidoscope and a flatus tube; however, flexible sigmoidoscopy may be more effective. If colonic ischaemia is suspected, then prompt laparotomy is indicated. Recurrence rates after endoscopic de-torsion are high and an operative procedure is usually recommended if the patient is fit. The options are fixing the colon without resection (colopexy) or a resection with either a colostomy or an anastomosis. Simply fixing the colon without resecting the volvulus is associated with high recurrence rates and a resection is usually undertaken. The decision to anastomose or not will be taken according to the state of the patient and the skills of the operator.

Malignancy

About 15–20% of patients with primary colorectal cancer present with intestinal obstruction. Initial management is aimed at addressing fluid resuscitation and assessment for surgery depending on tumour location, comorbidity and extent of metastatic disease. Several options exist: defunctioning via formation of a proximal stoma, surgical resection with or without anastomosis and endoluminal stenting. Adequate investigation of patients at presentation by CT scan is important as disease stage, e.g. metastases or local perforation, may strongly influence decisions. In addition, a small proportion of patients with colonic obstruction will present with peritonitis from caecal perforation; the only life-saving intervention is surgery.

In the last decade self-expanding metallic stents (SEMS) have been used increasingly in the management of colonic obstruction. Initially, their use was restricted to patients with extreme comorbidity or metastatic disease in whom surgery could be avoided. However, with growing confidence these are now employed in many patients presenting with large bowel obstruction (particularly when due to more accessible left colonic tumours) as a so-called 'bridge to surgery'. Following decompression, patients can benefit from more thorough staging and laparoscopic resection, usually avoiding a stoma. Colonic stent placement comes at some cost. There is a complication rate of perforation in 2–10% of cases and a risk that stent expansion may fracture tumours, potentially upstaging disease. Large bowel obstruction arising from the right or transverse colon is usually managed by surgery. In these cases access with colonic stenting is difficult and surgical options are generally safer and easier in proximal colonic obstruction.

Concerns over potential complications of colonic stenting or lack of availability in some centres may mean that surgery is employed as first-line management of large bowel obstruction. The options for surgery include proximal diversion, resection without anastomosis and resection with primary anastomosis. Resecting the entire distended proximal colon and forming an ileo-sigmoid or ileo-rectal anastomosis is

an attractive option, but postoperative bowel function can be relatively poor. If it is decided to perform a segmental colectomy, then an on-table colonic lavage is usually undertaken. Results suggest that in a specialist environment, resection with on-table lavage and primary anastomosis can be undertaken with acceptable morbidity and mortality rates that are certainly as good as staged procedures.

Pseudo-obstruction

Colonic pseudo-obstruction is also called Ogilvie's syndrome, and mimics the appearances of obstruction (with colonic distension) although mechanical obstruction is absent. It typically occurs in patients hospitalized for other reasons, such as recent surgery, trauma or infection. It is thought to occur due to an imbalance in the autonomic supply of the colon, with over-exaggerated effects of the sympathetic nervous system.

The diagnosis rests on the exclusion of mechanical obstruction by contrast enema or flexible endoscopy. Treatment is to exclude mechanical obstruction and is then initially conservative, with attempts to correct underlying causes if possible, correction of electrolyte abnormality and avoidance of drugs that affect colonic motility, such as opiates and anti-cholinergics. Nasogastric decompression and intravenous fluids are likely to be required. Plain X-ray of the abdomen is essential to monitor the diameter of the colon, particularly the caecum. Gross distension (>12 cm) suggests imminent perforation. Colonoscopy can be therapeutic; however, some authorities recommend intravenous neostigmine (2.5 mg in 100 ml of saline over 60 min) to hasten colonic decompression. This must be given in a 'high care' hospital setting with cardiac monitoring to detect bradycardia. Surgery can be indicated in Ogilvie's syndrome, if there are signs of colonic ischaemia or perforation.

Diverticulosis

Diverticulosis coli is a common colonic condition of the elderly in Western societies; up to two-thirds of people aged over 80 years are affected; however, most are asymptomatic. Diverticulosis has been labelled a disease of Western societies, as the disorder is rare in rural Africa and Asia and highly prevalent in Europe, the USA and Australia. Colonic diverticula typically form in parallel rows between the taenia coli because of weakness of the muscle wall at the site of penetration of the vasa recta supplying the mucosa. It is thought that increased intraluminal pressure causes the mucosa to herniate through the muscle wall to create the diverticula. The underlying problem is thought to be dietary deficiency of fibre; however, there is likely to be a constitutional component perhaps related to connective tissue as some individuals appear susceptible, with complicated disease arising at an early age.

Complications of diverticular disease

Diverticulitis has been likened to appendicitis, with a diverticulum becoming obstructed by inspissated stool in its neck. The inflammatory process varies in severity from inflammation alone to pericolic abscess to free perforation of the colon with faecal peritonitis. This is graded according to the Hinchey classification.

- Stage I – diverticulitis with phlegmon or small, confined paracolic abscess
- Stage II – diverticulitis with distant (pelvic, retroperitoneal) abscess
- Stage III – diverticulitis with purulent peritonitis
- Stage IV – diverticulitis with faecal peritonitis.

Most patients present with symptoms of pain and signs of tenderness or a mass accompanied by varying degrees of systemic inflammatory response. CT scanning is regarded as the diagnostic modality of choice. Endoscopy is generally avoided due to the increased risk of perforation. Pericolic abscess may result from the perforation of a diverticulum; when identified an abscess should be drained percutaneously if possible. Diverticular disease may lead to fistulas into adjacent organs; the most common is colovesical fistula. Colovaginal fistula may also occur and is more common if the patient has had a previous hysterectomy. Diverticular disease is the commonest cause of major lower gastrointestinal (GI) bleeding (see following section). Treatment is based on confirming the diagnosis (exclusion of co-existing colonic carcinoma is sometimes difficult as the features of both conditions can appear to overlap on colonic imaging) and conservatism is generally advised for mild attacks. Treatment with antibiotics usually settles mild attacks and dietary advice is given to increase both fibre and fluid in the diet. Pericolic abscess should be treated by percutaneous drainage and patients with peritonitis or colonic fistulas are usually submitted to laparotomy and colonic resection. Whether to reconstruct intestinal continuity or leave the patient with a Hartmann's operation is dependent on the patient's general condition, the

state of the bowel (presence of infection usually precludes anastomosis) and the skill and experience of the surgeon. Recent years have seen the introduction of laparoscopy in the initial management of complicated diverticular disease. Following disease staging by CT scan, patients with significant clinical signs undergo laparoscopy. The abdomen and pelvis are irrigated and in the absence of obvious colonic defect or faecal peritonitis the conservative management is continued with antibiotics. Enthusiasts for this approach report low rates of complications and, of course, successful cases avoid bowel resection and colostomy formation. This practice is slowly being adopted in specialist colorectal surgical practice.

Lower GI haemorrhage

Lower GI haemorrhage is defined as the abnormal loss of blood from the GI tract distal to the ligament of Treitz. Bleeding can be occult, slow, moderate, or life-threatening.

Diverticular disease

Diverticular disease is the most likely cause of lower GI haemorrhage in adults and accounts for between 30% and 40% of all cases. The severity of bleeding caused by diverticular disease ranges from mild to life-threatening. The vast majority of bleeding episodes caused by diverticular disease stop spontaneously.

Inflammatory bowel disease

Inflammatory bowel disease (ulcerative colitis (UC) and Crohn's disease (CD)) is a common source of lower GI haemorrhage, usually manifesting as bloody diarrhoea. Although the risk of life-threatening GI haemorrhage is reported to be low in these disorders, it does occur and occasionally mandates emergency operation. Ischaemic colitis should also be considered in the differential diagnosis.

Arteriovenous malformations

Arteriovenous malformations, also known as vascular ectasias, angiomas and angiodysplasias, are degenerative lesions of the GI tract that occur with increasing frequency as patients age. It is estimated that up to 30% of the population older than 50 years of age have arteriovenous malformations. It is thought that colonic muscle wall contraction leads to intermittent partial obstruction of the submucosal veins and these become dilated and tortuous, resulting in incompetence of the precapillary sphincters, which results in arteriovenous communications. Arteriovenous malformations are usually multiple and occur most frequently in the ascending colon, particularly in the caecum. The caecum is the single most likely location of arteriovenous malformations because, according to Laplace's law (tension in wall = internal pressure × radius), it has the greatest wall tension. Bleeding caused by arteriovenous malformations is characteristically chronic, slow, intermittent and recurrent. Endoscopic coagulation (using argon beam diathermy) is the treatment of choice.

Neoplasia

Although bleeding commonly occurs with both benign adenomatous polyps and adenocarcinomas of the colon and rectum, large-volume bleeding is an unusual presenting sign.

Benign anorectal conditions

Colonic, anorectal and peristomal varices arise as a complication of portal hypertension and can cause painless, massive lower GI haemorrhage. Nevertheless, it is the more humble anorectal conditions that present more typically with lower GI bleeding. In a review of nearly 18 000 patients with lower GI bleeding, haemorrhoids, fissure and fistula-in-ano were the cause in 11% of patients. It is, therefore, important to examine the anorectum thoroughly early in the evaluation before proceeding to more invasive and complex diagnostic methods. Digital rectal examination, proctoscopy and sigmoidoscopy should be performed in all patients with rectal bleeding. Discovery of benign anorectal disease does not eliminate the possibility of a more proximal bleeding source, and complete colonic evaluation is recommended.

Upper GI bleeding

Approximately 10% of cases of bright red rectal blood loss result from massive, continuous, life-threatening bleeding from an upper GI source (i.e. proximal to the ligament of Treitz). Normally upper GI bleeding presents as melaena due to digestive alteration of the blood in the small intestine. When the upper GI blood loss is massive, with rapid transit of blood down the intestine, this digestive process does not have time to take place.

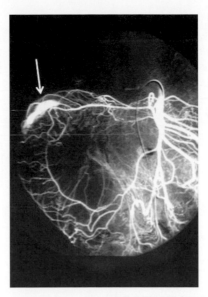

Figure 24.4
Angiogram with catheter introduced through the femoral artery and cannulating the superior mesenteric vessels. The arcade between the ileocolic vessels and middle colic vessels is demonstrated with intraluminal flush of contrast, indicated by the arrow.

Management of lower GI bleeding

Resuscitation of the patient is the priority, with airway control and provision of oxygen plus large-bore intravenous access. Blood should be taken for estimation of haemoglobin, urea, electrolytes, liver function and coagulation profile. Blood should be cross-matched and blood and products given as required. Urinary and nasogastric catheters are helpful and arterial blood gas analysis will also help to guide the resuscitative effort. The history is important and evidence should be sought of previous GI bleeding, peptic ulcer or inflammatory bowel disease, liver disease, nonsteroidal anti-inflammatories, warfarin usage or previous aortic surgery. The abdomen and anorectum must be carefully examined and bedside examination of the anal canal and rectum is mandatory. An upper GI source should be ruled out by upper GI endoscopy. Recent evidence supports the use of early colonoscopy after mechanical bowel preparation in a stable patient. Endoscopic haemostasis, either by adrenaline injection or bipolar coagulation, has been shown to reduce the requirement for surgery. In the presence of active bleeding, angiography could be traditionally used to detect haemorrhage at a rate of 0.5–1 ml/min. The technique is performed via transfemoral placement of an arterial catheter. The hallmark of a positive examination is extravasation of contrast material into the lumen of the bowel (Figure 24.4). Angiography requires the availability of a skilled radiologist and the overall sensitivity of angiography is variable, and may be as low as 40%. If a bleeding source is identified then

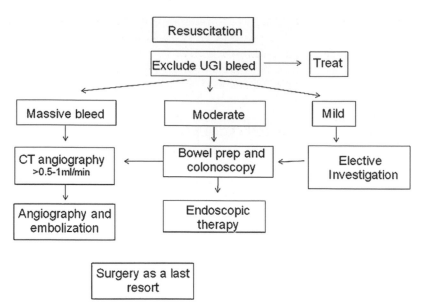

Figure 24.5 Algorithm in colonic bleeding. This algorithm provides a reasonable structure for investigation of patients presenting with colonic bleeding. Important highlights are exclusion of upper gastrointestinal source for bleeding, localization of bleeding with CT angiography and avoidance of surgery unless the patient continues to bleed in a life-threatening manner in the presence of maximum conservative efforts. CT angiography is only of value in the presence of continuing bleeding of at least 0.5–1 ml per minute.

selective transcatheter embolization of the bleeding site may be effective. Developments in cross-sectional imaging have allowed the use of CT angiography as a non-invasive preliminary investigation to localize bleeding and direct selective therapeutic angiography or surgery. Another angiographic option for control of haemorrhage is vasopressin infusion through the catheter. Vasopressin is a pituitary extract that causes arteriolar vasoconstriction and bowel wall contraction. The role of technetium-labelled red blood cell scintigraphy in lower GI haemorrhage is controversial because its accuracy in locating the precise site of haemorrhage is variable, with reports of false localization ranging from 3% to 59%. Emergency operations for acute lower GI bleeding may be required in approximately less than 5% of patients. The indications for an operation are persistent or recurrent haemorrhage leading to haemodynamic instability despite resuscitation or a high transfusion requirement. In general, patients with ongoing bleeding who have required transfusion of six or more units of blood should undergo an operation. If the bleeding site has been successfully localized by angiography then segmental resection is the treatment of choice because of its low morbidity, mortality and rebleed rate. If operation is required before accurate localization of the bleeding site has been possible, then attempts should be made intraoperatively to identify the precise site of bleeding. Blind segmental colectomy should not be performed because of its high risk of rebleeding

and associated mortality. Intraoperative colonoscopy should be undertaken; if diagnostic confusion still exists, oesophogastroduodenoscopy (OGD) should be repeated and a paediatric colonoscope used to perform on-table small bowel enteroscopy, as small intestinal sources such as arteriovenous malformations, diverticula and neoplasia account for up to 5% of all cases of severe lower GI bleeding. If the bleeding site remains unidentified, then subtotal colectomy with ileorectal anastomosis or ileostomy should be undertaken. An algorithm of management of colonic bleeding is presented in Figure 24.5.

Anorectal sepsis

Anorectal sepsis is a common feature of acute surgical emergencies all over the world. Presenting features are usually pain with fever and malaise. Perianal abscess is usually obvious, but intersphincteric abscesses may cause pain without obvious pointing of an abscess at the anal margin and examination under anaesthetic may be necessary to achieve a diagnosis. Perianal abscess is thought to arise through infection of an anal gland and anal fistula may result. Treatment of the acute infection is to relieve the abscess. Examination of the anal canal with a bi-valved speculum (Eisenhammer) with gentle pressure on the abscess may reveal evidence of an internal opening, and some surgeons routinely lay open such fistulas acutely. However, there is some evidence that simple drainage of the abscess will allow resolution of the infection without subsequent fistula formation. Pus should be sent routinely for microbiology and the abscess drained with an incision circumferential to the anal canal over the fluctuant part. Pus must be drained and the cavity irrigated. Packing with gauze should be avoided, as it is very painful to remove and impractical. The patient must be followed up carefully to identify those who require further treatment of anal fistula (see below). Anorectal sepsis may progress to become the disease eponymously credited to Professor Jean-Alfred Fournier, a Parisian dermatologist and venereologist. Fournier's gangrene is a rapidly progressive infection of the perineal soft tissue and polymicrobial cultures of anaerobes and aerobes are the rule rather than the exception. Anorectal sepsis is a common precursor for Fournier's gangrene and early aggressive treatment is associated with a reduced mortality rate. King Herod the Great of Judaea (74 BC – 4 BC) is suspected to have succumbed to Fournier's gangrene in association with diabetes mellitus, a common co-factor in the condition.

Colorectal injury

Rectal injuries usually occur in association with pelvic fractures, although impalement injuries and penetrating injuries of the abdomen or perineum from knives or gunshots can also damage the rectum. A high index of suspicion is required as these injuries can be subtle and are easily missed. In stable trauma patients where clinical suspicion exists, careful clinical examination aided by flexible endoscopic examination is vital. Initial experience with rectal injury was obtained in warfare where wounds can be severe with gross destruction and contamination plus delay from point of wounding to definitive surgical care. Experience with such wounds led to a policy of treatment based on faecal diversion with exposure, debridement and repair of the rectal wound, distal washout of the rectum and pre-sacral drainage. There is evidence that the majority of rectal injuries encountered in civilian practice do not require such an aggressive surgical approach and can be treated with simple faecal diversion alone. In impalement injuries, careful perineal debridement is necessary and sphincteric damage should ideally be assessed and managed by an expert. Defunctioning colostomy was the standard management of penetrating colonic injury from the time of World War II until 1979, when the first ran-

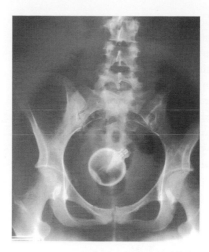

Figure 24.6
Foreign body in rectum is a common occurrence. In this instance a perfume bottle has been inserted and was removed under general anaesthesia.

domized trial was undertaken, which showed that primary repair of colonic injuries was appropriate for selected patients. A *Cochrane Database Review* from 2003 demonstrated that mortality was not significantly different between patients with penetrating colonic injury treated by primary repair or faecal diversion. However, total complications were significantly less in the primary repair group. While primary repair is appropriate for non-destructive (involvement of <50% of the bowel wall without devascularization) colon wounds in the absence of peritonitis, patients with penetrating intraperitoneal colon wounds that are destructive (involvement of >50% of the bowel wall or devascularization of a bowel segment) should undergo resection and primary anastomosis. However, if there are significant associated injuries, there has been haemodynamic instability or the patient has serious underlying comorbidity, serious consideration should still be given to the use of colostomy. Colonic injury after blunt trauma is rare and difficult to diagnose. There is little guidance in the literature to know what is the best way to manage these injuries; however, experience of treating patients with penetrating colonic injury suggests that primary repair (or resection and anastomosis) is appropriate in the absence of delay to diagnosis, severe associated injury or haemodynamic instability.

Foreign body

Human beings appear to have an inexhaustible fascination for inserting objects into their rectums (Figure 24.6). Retained rectal foreign bodies can present a challenge in management. Digital rectal examination, proctoscopy and abdominal radiography are helpful and soft or low-lying objects can be grasped and removed safely in the emergency department. However, simply grasping objects may result in upward migration toward the sigmoid. Insufflation of air with a rigid or flexible sigmoidoscope proximal to the object can break the apparent 'vacuum seal' and aid retrieval. Many innovative approaches (such as obstetric forceps) have been used, but occasionally general anaesthesia with transrectal manipulation and bimanual palpation is necessary to withdraw the foreign body. Laparoscopy may help to retrieve objects, but laparotomy and colotomy may ultimately be required.

Inflammatory bowel disease

Ulcerative colitis (UC)

UC is characterized by ulcerative inflammation of all or part of the colonic mucosa; at presentation half of patients have inflammation confined to the rectum. UC is characterized by exacerbation and remission and may be associated with extraintestinal manifestation such as arthropathy or sclerosing cholangitis.

Symptoms of UC include rectal bleeding and urgency, tenesmus and diarrhoea. Medical therapy is the mainstay of treatment and the goal is first to induce and then maintain remission of the colitis. The 5-aminosalicylic acid (5-ASA) agents are the treatment of choice for mild to moderate disease. Corticosteroids are useful agents to help induce remission in severe colitis; intravenous cyclosporine or infliximab can be used in refractory disease but if remission does not occur, then colectomy is indicated.

If medical therapy achieves remission, maintenance should be sustained with aminosalicylates, orally, topically (by enemas) or in combination. In some patients, immunomodulation may be required with azathioprine or 6-mercaptopurine.

UC can be either distal or extensive; in distal UC, the inflammation is limited to the area below the splenic flexure and is amenable to oral or topical treatment. In extensive UC, inflammation extends proximal to the splenic flexure and requires oral therapy with or without topical therapy. Disease severity is classified as mild (four stools/day, with or without blood, and no systemic signs of toxicity), moderate (4–6 stools/day with minimal signs of toxicity), or severe. The criteria that define severity were first described by Truelove and Witts.

Truelove and Witts definition of 'severe' ulcerative colitis

Bowels open >six times per 24 hours, plus any one or more of the systemic manifestations

- large amounts of rectal bleeding
- haemoglobin <10.5 g/dl
- ESR >30 mm/h
- pulse rate >90 bpm
- temperature >37.8°C.

A stool frequency of ≥8 or a C-reactive protein (CRP) of >45 on day 3 of admission predicts an 85% likelihood of requiring a colectomy during that admission. It is vital that surgeons are involved early in all patients admitted with severe colitis, as delay to surgery leads to avoidable morbidity and even mortality.

Crohn's disease

CD is a chronic transmural inflammation that may affect any part of the GI tract, from the mouth to the anus. In approximately one-third of cases, the disease is confined to the small intestine, whereas approximately one-half of patients will have involvement of both the small intestine and the colon (ileocolitis). In approximately 20% of cases, only the colon is involved. Most patients present with symptoms of abdominal pain and tenderness, chronic or nocturnal diarrhoea, rectal bleeding, weight loss and fever. Perianal disease is occasionally the dominant feature of CD.

CD evolves over time from a primarily inflammatory disease into one of two clinical patterns: stricturing (obstructive) or penetrating (fistulizing). The 5-ASA compounds are effective for establishing remission of mild to moderate CD. Budesonide, a newer corticosteroid with a lower systemic bioavailability than the older corticosteroids, is indicated for mild to moderate CD involving the ileocaecal area. Corticosteroids are used in order to induce remission and azathioprine or 6-mercaptopurine can be used in conjunction with steroids for establishing remission in patients with refractory, moderate to severe CD and as corticosteroid-sparing maintenance agents. Surveillance full blood counts must be undertaken, every 3 months, as long as patients continue azathioprine, in view of the risk of agranulocytosis. Infliximab and its newer version, adalimumab, antagonists of tumour necrosis factor, are effective in CD but must be used with care as there is a risk of anaphylaxis (infliximab contains non-human (murine) protein) and there are reports of reactivation of latent tuberculosis in patients after treatment and reports of lymphoma appearing in patients with CD who have received anti-TNF therapy.

Surgical therapy

Between 30% and 40% of patients with UC will eventually require surgery. Surgical removal of the entire colonic and rectal mucosa in UC can be curative. Surgery is required for emergency presentations, such as toxic colitis, bleeding or perforation, or for colitis refractory to optimal medical therapy. Longstanding total colitis increases the risk of carcinoma and surgery is required if there is dysplasia in the colon or rectum. Restoration of intestinal continuity after removal of the colon and rectum is by creation of a neorectum fashioned from the terminal ileum and anastomosed to the anal canal; the so-called ileal pouch operation. The primary indications for surgery in patients with CD are intestinal obstruction and septic complications, such as internal fistula or abscess. Other indications include perforation, haemorrhage, failure to thrive despite optimal medical therapy and carcinoma. One of the main principles of operating for CD is to maintain as much small bowel length as possible. Microscopic disease may be present at resection margins without compromising results and strictureplasty is preferred over resection when possible. Smoking after a surgical resection doubles the risk of recurrence and use of 5-ASA drugs also reduces the risk of recurrence after surgery. Patients with Crohn's disease often present a complex challenge particularly if they have been compromised by chronic illness and complications from previous surgery. In such circumstances the guiding principles are to control sepsis by surgical or radiological drainage and antibiotics, ensure good medical management of active disease, optimize nutritional status with parenteral nutrition if necessary and finally consider surgery when the patient is in the best possible condition.

Perianal disease in CD

CD has an association with perianal lesions, which may be primary Crohn's-associated fissures or ulcers, or secondary lesions such as tags, fistulas or rectal stricture. The perianal manifestations range from mild to severe (so-called watering-can perineum) and are usually amenable to surgical therapy. In some cases proctectomy may be required.

Colorectal cancer

Background and aetiology

Each year colorectal cancer affects 32 000 people in the UK and is responsible for around 22 000 deaths. In males it is second only to lung cancer and in females it falls third behind lung and breast cancer. In the developed world, lifetime risk for colorectal cancer is around 1:25 and this is increased by genetic predisposition and certain conditions such as chronic colitis. Colorectal cancer is mainly a disease of the elderly, with a marked rise in incidence after age 70 years; however, 10% of individuals are under age 55 years at diagnosis. In 1972, Burkitt described the relationship between diet and incidence of bowel cancer; he hypothesized that a diet rich in fibre was associated with regular bulky stools and reduced bowel carcinogenesis, perhaps by reducing exposure of colonic mucosa to dietary carcinogens. It does seem likely that the combination of high fibre and low fat may be protective against bowel cancer. Protection against colorectal carcinogenesis is also derived from dietary supplements of calcium and folate and evidence from the Nurses Health Study (North America) suggested that oestrogen in the form of hormone replacement therapy (HRT) lowers the incidence of colorectal neoplasia. There has been interest in the potential influence of non-steroidal anti-inflammatory drugs in colorectal carcinogenesis. Cyclooxygenase (COX)-2 inhibition appears to have potent effects on the colonic mucosa, increasing apoptosis and reducing cellular proliferation. It is also likely that these drugs function through COX-independent mechanisms. Impressive effects on the growth on adenomas have been described in certain polyposis syndromes and uncontrolled population studies suggest a reduction in colorectal cancer-associated mortality. These beneficial effects are mitigated by an increased incidence of major gastrointestinal bleeding; however, there is evidence that regular use of aspirin is protective against developing colorectal cancer.

Chronic inflammatory conditions often predispose to carcinogenesis and in the colon and rectum this is best demonstrated by chronic UC. The risk of developing malignancy is proportional to the duration and extent of colitis. An approximate incidence of 10% per

Table 24.2 Presentation of colorectal cancer

Site	Bleeding	Constipation or obstruction	Diarrhoea
Rectum	Bright or dark	Disturbance of bowel function common with frequent defaecation and tenesmus. Locally advanced cancers may obstruct	May be spurious due to obstruction or result from mucus production
Left colon	Dark and mixed with stool	Tendency to constipation and erratic bowel habit leading to obstruction	May be spurious due to obstruction or result from mucus production
Right colon	Usually occult resulting in anaemia	Liquid stool makes obstruction a late symptom; advanced caecal lesions cause small bowel obstruction	Large mucin-producing cancers may cause loose stools

annum after a decade of extensive colitis is often cited. However, careful surveillance for dysplasia and precursor lesions followed by colectomy can reduce this risk. Similar risks and surveillance strategies apply to Crohn's colitis. Vogelstein has proposed a model for colorectal carcinogenesis, with cancer resulting from an accumulation of somatic genetic defects manifested in the progression from small adenoma to larger adenoma and ultimately cancer. The time course to this endpoint is around 10 years but, typically, conditions which lead to familial predisposition hasten this pathway to carcinogenesis with inherited mutations in the critical cancer genes or systems which maintain the integrity of DNA replication and repair. Examples of this are seen in familial adenomatous polyposis, where an inheritable inactivating mutation in the antigen-presenting cell (APC) gene occurs, and hereditary non-polyposis colorectal cancer (HNPCC), where defects in DNA mismatch repair genes result in a high frequency of mutation. The presence of early-onset cancer, synchronous cancers or multiple polyps in a patient should prompt referral to a clinical genetics service.

Clinical presentation

Clinical presentation is determined by the site of tumour within the bowel (Table 24.2). Transient changes in bowel function are common as a result of GI infection and functional bowel disease such as irritable bowel syndrome. However, persistence of bowel symptoms for more than 6 weeks is of concern, particularly in those over 40 years of age; malignant disease should be actively excluded in this group. As a generalization, cancers of the left colon and rectum present with change in bowel habit and/or bleeding whereas right colon cancers cause anaemia and small bowel obstruction. General malaise, anorexia and weight loss and uncommon features of bowel cancer generally reflect

the presence of metastatic disease. The majority of patients with colorectal cancer are detected through outpatient investigation, but as many as 25–30% are diagnosed as emergencies, with obstruction and perforation being common features.

Screening

The UK National Bowel Cancer Screening Programme was introduced as a phased programme in 2006. This was a faecal occult blood screening test aimed at people aged between 60 and 69 years. In the pilot project, 478 250 residents of the pilot areas were invited to take part in the screening programme. Uptake (the proportion in whom a final faecal occult blood test result was available) was 56.8%. The overall rate of a positive test result was 1.9% and the rate for detecting cancer was 1.62 per 1000 people screened. Five hundred and fifty-two cancers were detected by screening; 92 (16.6%) were polyp cancers; 48% of all screen-detected cancers were Dukes stage A, and 1% had metastasized at the time of diagnosis. This suggests that the screening programme will identify early-stage neoplasia.

Outside a screening programme, most patients presenting to outpatients have no abnormality detected on clinical examination. However, an abdominal mass may be detected, particularly most commonly with caecal tumour in the right iliac fossa. Rectal examination and rigid sigmoidoscopy may detect a lesion; however, normal clinical examination does not exclude significant bowel pathology. Bowel symptoms suggestive of malignant disease are usually best investigated by direct visualization of the mucosa by means of colonoscopy. However, limited endoscopy resources coupled with increased complications from colonoscopy mean CT colonography, minimum-preparation CT colonography and even double-contrast enema may be undertaken as alternatives. When the presenting symptom is rectal bleeding alone, flexible sigmoidoscopy may be sufficient. In an emergency setting, patients present with the consequences of obstruction, perforation or bleeding. It may be impossible to distinguish bowel cancer from other pathology, particularly diverticular disease. Plain abdominal X-ray may confirm the diagnosis with dilated large bowel, and second-stage investigation with water-soluble contrast enema and CT scan should provide a definitive diagnosis and help plan appropriate management through disease staging.

Preoperative staging of colorectal cancer

Following the diagnosis of bowel cancer staging is important in determining the optimum management plan and in providing prognostic information. Three areas need to be considered.

Local invasion

This is particularly important in rectal cancer, where proximity of tumour to the circumferential margin of resection can determine the need for neoadjuvant chemoradiotherapy. In the rectum this information is obtained by MRI and/or endoluminal ultrasound to clearly define the layers of the bowel wall, surrounding mesorectal fat and the enveloping mesorectal fascia. In colon cancer, local assessment by CT scan is adequate and can provide information on invasion of adjacent structures, such as ureter or duodenum, which can assist surgical planning.

Metastatic disease

Bowel cancer most commonly spreads to the liver and lungs, and these organs should be assessed routinely before surgery. CT scan of the abdomen and chest offers the most accurate and convenient means and also provides a baseline for subsequent routine examinations.

Synchronous lesions

Adenomas are found in 20% of patients with colorectal cancer and around 3% have multiple cancers. Identifying these lesions preoperatively can dramatically alter surgical planning.

Management of early cancer

Some cancers are diagnosed at an early stage and this is best demonstrated by the finding of invasive cancer in a polyp. Endoscopic removal of the polyp is adequate treatment in many cases and this should be balanced against the risk of colonic resection. The presence of poorly differentiated cancer, lymphovascular invasion and involvement of the excised margin would suggest that resection should be undertaken. Small rectal cancers can be removed by full-thickness local excision. This is best achieved with transanal endoscopic microsurgery (TEM) using sophisticated instrumentation offering a magnified view and precise surgical technique. This is an area of increasing experience as early cancers are likely to be asymptomatic and therefore diagnosed in screening programmes.

The management of advanced cancer

The majority of bowel cancers are managed by surgical resection. The principle of surgery is to remove the primary tumour with draining lymph nodes while preserving anatomical planes around the mesentery. This is best demonstrated in the rectum where the application of this principle, 'total mesorectal excision', has resulted in a reduction in local recurrence of cancer. The main arterial supply and venous drainage are identified and divided. The bowel ends are then divided at appropriate points determined by the need to achieve an adequate margin around the cancer and leave healthy, well-vascularized normal bowel that can be sutured or approximated by stapling devices. The resulting anastomosis is critical and problems in healing lead to dehiscence or 'leak'. This commonly results in reoperation and is associated with high morbidity and mortality. In some cases where the cancer is immediately above or invading the sphincter muscle it is not possible to form an anastomosis and an abdominoperineal excision is performed. This involves the complete removal of the anus and rectum with formation of a permanent colostomy. Segmental colonic resections are usually described in a logical fashion according to the involved segment: right hemicolectomy, left hemicolectomy, sigmoid colectomy. Removal of the rectum with formation of an anastomosis is often abbreviated to 'anterior resection', indicating that the rectum surgery is performed through the anterior or abdominal route rather than perineal or posterior approach. Under some circumstances the surgeon may regard formation of an anastomosis as unsafe. This situation most often arises in emergency surgery where bowel perforation or obstruction has led to contamination of the peritoneal cavity. An anastomosis is avoided by forming a stoma, where the proximal end of the bowel is brought to the skin through a separate trephine in the abdominal wall. The resulting stoma is known as a colostomy or ileostomy depending on the origin.

The most common procedure at which a colostomy is formed is a Hartmann's resection, where sigmoid pathology is removed with the formation of an end colostomy. This colostomy can be reversed at a later date but in this generally elderly population up to 40% of patients choose not to have further surgery. If a high-risk anastomosis is formed, for example, deep in the pelvis after a low anterior resection a temporary ileostomy or colostomy may be formed to protect the downstream join in the bowel should it fail to heal. The use of a defunctioning stoma in this fashion tends to reduce the sequelae of a failed anastomosis. This type of stoma is usually a 'loop' and can be closed when the primary anastomosis has been confirmed to have healed adequately, usually after 3–4 months.

Metastatic cancer

Around 25% of patients with bowel cancer present with metastatic disease, most commonly affecting the liver. There are several treatment options depending on the extent of metastatic disease and the patient's symptoms and wishes.

In those patients with advanced metastatic disease treatment is aimed at optimizing palliation. Early use of chemotherapy has been shown to increase the quality and length of survival in metastatic colorectal cancer. However, some patients choose not to have treatment until symptoms develop. If significant symptoms can be attributed to the primary cancer within the bowel then a range of surgical options can be explored.

Surgical resection as described above for localized disease can provide effective treatment for bowel symptoms arising from bleeding or obstruction of the lumen. If patients are unfit for surgery, cancers causing obstruction can be treated with endoluminal stenting (see above). Rectal cancer symptoms such as tenesmus, bleeding, discharge or obstruction can be improved by transanal resection, radiotherapy, stoma formation or combination treatment. Localized metastatic disease, either at the time of initial presentation or following primary surgery, may be amenable to potentially curative treatment. Surgical resection of liver secondaries is associated with a 5-year survival of 20–25% in experienced centres. The population with advanced disease who may benefit from liver resection is increased by a multimodal approach using neoadjuvant chemotherapy and local treatments such as high-intensity focused ultrasound, radiofrequency and cryo-ablation, which induce tumour necrosis. Poor prognostic factors for failure of hepatic resection include large or multiple metastases, surgical clearance margin of less than 1 cm, metastases appearing within 6 months of surgery and the presence of involved lymph nodes in the primary colonic resection.

Pathology

Three gross morphological forms of colorectal cancer exist: polypoid, ulcerative and stricturing. The vast majority are adenocarcinomas. Carcinoid tumours, lymphoma, sarcoma and adenosquamous cancers are also described. The histology of adenocarcinomas is characterized further on the basis of differentiation and mucin production: well-differentiated cancers (where cells show a propensity to form glandular structures from which they were derived) and those without mucin production are associated with an improved prognosis. Histological factors such as vascular and lymphatic invasion within the tumour are also associated with poorer prognosis.

Pathological staging systems are important in determining appropriate treatment as well as standardizing populations for research and audit. For these reasons, accurate staging in colorectal cancer is vital. Pathological staging offers the definitive report but, as noted above, radiological staging in rectal cancer is an important determinant of treatment.

Pathological staging

Dukes stage is the most widely employed staging system. It lacks detail on local tumour invasion but overall provides a robust if rather crude predictor of prognosis. Dukes classification has been largely replaced by the internationally agreed Union Internationale Contre Cancer (UICC) tumour, nodes, metastases (TNM) system of classification, the principles of which are shared with many cancers. In North America, The American Joint Committee on Cancer (AJCC) system is employed. Table 24.3 summarizes these systems. TNM classification offers more detail and flexibility without becoming unduly complex. The modification to Dukes stage detailing apical lymph node involvement is a useful prognosticator: C2 is associated with a 5-year survival of 35% compared to 55% associated with C1 disease. In the TNM system, N1 or N2 may or may not involve the apical lymph node and accordingly

Table 24.3 Pathological staging of colorectal cancer

Stage	Degree of invasion	Lymph node status	Metastasis
Dukes A	Confined to bowel wall	Not involved	Absent
Dukes B	Through muscularis propria	Not involved	Absent
Dukes Cl	Any	Local lymph node(s) involved	Absent
Dukes C2	Any	Apical lymph node ± others involved	Absent
Dukes D	Any	Any	Present
Tis	*In situ* cancer, basement membrane intact	Any	Any
Tl	Into submucosa	Any	Any
T2	Into muscularis propria	Any	Any
T3	Through muscularis propria	Any	Any
T4	Breaches peritoneal surface. Includes free perforation, abscess and invasion of adjacent organ	Any	Any
NX	Any	Lymph nodes not assessed	Any
N0	Any	None	Any
Nl	Any	1–3 lymph nodes	Any
N2	Any	>3 lymph nodes	Any
MX	Any	Any	Not assessed
M0	Any	Any	Absent
Ml	Any	Any	Present
AJCC I	Submucosal or into muscularis propria	Not involved	Absent
AJCC II	Through muscularis propria	Not involved	Absent
AJCC III	Any	Involved	Absent
AJCC IV	Any	Any	Present

this useful prognostic factor is lost. The TNM staging system is also employed in preoperative clinical and radiological assessment. This is identified by prefixing a report with 'c', for example, cT3N2M0. Pathological stage is prefixed by 'p' and if neoadjuvant treatments may have changed the pathological stage the report is prefixed by 'yp'.

Non-surgical treatment of colorectal cancer

Chemotherapy and radiotherapy have well-defined roles in the treatment of colorectal cancer. They can be considered in three forms: adjuvant, neoadjuvant and palliative.

Neoadjuvant therapy

Neoadjuvant treatment is employed with the aim of reducing tumour size, thereby improving the chances of curative resection. It is employed in the treatment of rectal cancers where preoperative staging suggests the circumferential margin of the mesorectum may be threatened or involved with tumour. This group of patients receive radiotherapy as a long course: 45 Gy over 5 weeks combined with 5-FU. A complete pathological response with no cancer present in the resected specimen occurs in 10–15% of patients. Neoadjuvant chemotherapy is also used in the treatment of liver metastases, potentially reducing tumour size to improve the chances of successful surgical resection.

Short-course preoperative radiotherapy given over 1 week and followed immediately by surgical resection has been shown to reduce local recurrence in rectal cancer by about 50%. However, it is probable that only a subset of rectal cancers may benefit and ideally these can be identified by accurate preoperative staging. Radiotherapy in this context does not offer any reduction in tumour size as surgery is undertaken before tumour regression occurs.

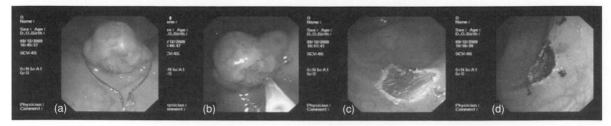

Figure 24.7 Colonic polypectomy sequence. A 10 mm snare is placed around the base of the polyp (A) and closed securely (B), allowing the complete removal using diathermy, leaving a healthy base exposing the submucosa (C). In this instance the site has been tattooed with permanent ink (D) to allow surveillance or surgical resection of the segment of bowel should the pathology be unfavourable, with malignancy or risk of recurrence.

Adjuvant therapy

Chemotherapy in the form of 5-fluorouracil (5-FU) and folinic acid increases survival in patients following potentially curative surgery. This effect is through eradication of occult metastases and offers an overall improvement in survival by approximately 5%. However, in those patients at higher risk of metastatic disease (those with lymph node involvement) this benefit may increase to 20%. Therefore, it is generally advised that adjuvant chemotherapy with 5-FU is reserved for patients with lymph node involvement. In practice, adjuvant therapy is frequently extended to younger patients with no lymph node involvement where the primary tumour shows vascular invasion, peritoneal (T4) disease or poor differentiation. However, in all patients the potential benefits of adjuvant therapy must be balanced against the risk of side effects and accordingly it tends to be employed less often in elderly patients with comorbidity, especially ischaemic heart disease.

Postoperative radiotherapy is of benefit in rectal cancer patients where the cancer is shown to have threatened the resection margin. This has some disadvantages compared to preoperative treatment in that the surgical field including the neorectum is irradiated, causing deterioration in function and increased side effects from collateral damage to other structures such as small bowel. In some respects, use of postoperative radiotherapy may be viewed as a failure of preoperative assessment to identify advanced cancers.

Palliative therapy

In patients with metastatic disease not suitable for surgical resection, chemotherapy in the form of 5-FU may be employed. In this setting increased survival can be achieved but the benefits need to be balanced against the potential side effects. More recently, irinotecan and oxaliplatin have been used at earlier stages of palliative treatment. They are generally more efficacious than 5-FU, but more expensive and with an increased incidence of adverse effects. New monoclonal biological agents such as cetuximab (epidermal growth factor receptor inhibitor) and bevacizumab (which blocks vascular endothelial growth factor A) offer exciting prospects in combination treatment. Cetuximab is effective in K-RAS wild-type colorectal cancers and this 'designer' approach, where treatment is directed by molecular profiling, will hopefully see more applications in future. Palliative radiotherapy can be targeted for symptom relief in locally advanced rectal cancer. It is also valuable in the treatment of painful bone metastases from colorectal cancer.

Screening and surveillance for colorectal cancer

As discussed above, colorectal cancer presents an ideal opportunity for asymptomatic population screening. There is a protracted premalignant phase (adenoma), which can be identified and removed endoscopically, halting the development of invasive disease (Figure 24.7). Several methods of population-based screening and surveillance of high-risk groups exist.

Population screening

Faecal occult blood testing

Cancers and large adenomas bleed into the bowel lumen and this can be detected by simple stool analysis. Various forms of faecal occult blood testing (FOBT) exist and these vary in sensitivity and specificity. Three large randomized trials in England, Denmark and the USA have demonstrated a reduction in colorectal cancer deaths with FOBT. Those with positive FOBT undergo colonoscopy. This approach leads to the earlier diagnosis of colorectal cancer and in the Nottingham (UK) trial colorectal cancer mortality was reduced by 17%.

Flexible sigmoidoscopy

Seventy per cent of cancers and adenomas occur in the rectum and sigmoid colon within reach of a flexible sigmoidoscope. A single flexible sigmoidoscopy examination between 55 and 65 years is likely to reduce the incidence of colorectal cancer through two means. First, all polyps identified at this examination are removed and with them the risk of developing into invasive disease. Second, those individuals with large, multiple or severely dysplastic adenomas undergo colonoscopy to exclude more proximal lesions. Although this screening method will detect some early cancers, the main thrust is to remove adenomas and identify the subgroup of patients at high risk who are likely to benefit from more intensive follow-up.

Colonoscopy

This provides a sensitive and specific means of examining the bowel but it is expensive and associated with a relatively high incidence of complications, which makes it unsuitable for population-based screening. However, it is the method of choice in the surveillance of high-risk individuals such as those with a genetic predisposition or chronic colitis.

Faecal DNA analysis

Extraction of DNA from stool is now feasible and some genetic abnormalities commonly found in colorectal cancer can be detected, including mutations in k-ras, APC, p53 and BAT26. This approach is likely to become more sensitive with improved techniques and ultimately may be used in combination with flexible sigmoidoscopy or non-invasive approaches such as virtual colonoscopy.

Anal cancer

Anal cancer is rare, accounting for less than 5% of large bowel cancers. Over 80% of anal cancers are squamous cell in origin; however, adenocarcinoma and malignant melanoma may occur in the anal canal. The recognition of a high incidence of squamous cell carcinoma of the anus amongst some homosexual men led to the search for an infective aetiological agent. Risk factors for anal cancer include a history of gen-

ital warts and evidence now suggests an association between human papilloma virus types 16, 18, 30, 31 and 33 and anal cancer. It is believed that anal cancer may occur due to progression of anal intraepithelial neoplasia in a manner analogous to intraepithelial carcinoma of the cervix, vulva or vagina. Anal cancer typically presents with pain and bleeding, and these symptoms are often initially disregarded or misdiagnosed. Clinicians must be most suspicious of a patient with an indolent anal ulcer or rectal bleeding who complains of persistent or severe pain. Treatment is usually by combination chemoradiotherapy using 5-FU and mitomycin C combined with high-dose external beam irradiation. Surgery is reserved for those who relapse despite oncological therapy; however, small lesions at the anal margin may still be treated by local excision only. Anal cancer spreads to inguinal lymph nodes, which should always be assessed by the clinician. Typically, inguinal nodes are included in the radiation field.

Minor anorectal conditions

Fistula-in-ano

The so-called 'cryptoglandular hypothesis' ascribes the aetiology of fistula-in-ano to the glands that sit in the intersphincteric space around the anal canal. Spread of sepsis from an infected gland leads to perianal abscess which usually presents acutely (see above). Epithelialization of the track leads to establishment of a fistula-in-ano. A classification of fistulas was done by the late Sir Alan Parks in 1976, describing four main groups:

- intersphincteric
- trans-sphincteric
- suprasphincteric
- extrasphincteric.

A full assessment of a fistula-in-ano requires the identification of the internal and external openings, the primary track, any secondary extension and any diseases complicating the situation. Extensions occur in approximately 10–15% of patients, and are more prevalent in recurrent or Crohn's fistulas. The goal of treatment of fistula-in-ano is to eradicate the fistula while maintaining continence. Up to 25% of fistulas recur, and this is usually due to sepsis missed at surgery and left untreated. MRI is effective at identifying the cause of recurrent sepsis and surgery guided by MRI can reduce further episodes of recurrence by up to 75%. The traditional way to cure fistula is to lay open the track and allow it to heal by secondary intention, thus obliterating the fistula. This offers effective treatment but damage to the sphincter muscle may result in incontinence. This is particularly apparent in the short female sphincter, which is also likely to be compromised by childbirth, and even in the presence of a bulky male sphincter laying open may result in deformity at the anal verge that can lead to leakage and difficult hygiene. There are various sphincter-preserving options for the treatment of high or complex fistulas, mucosal advancement flaps or the use of tissue glues and collagen plugs. Unfortunately none of these offers a reliable solution and all are associated with high recurrence rates. For many patients multiple surgeries and protracted uncertainty over cure mean that control of sepsis with a long-term Seton drain may be preferred.

Anal fissure

Anal fissure is a linear split in the lining of the lower half of the anal canal and may be primary, or related to other pathology, such as CD. The cause of anal fissure is unclear, but the initiating event is usually thought to be the difficult passage of a constipated stool that traumatizes the anal canal. Patients with anal fissure are likely to have high resting pressures in the anal canal and it is thought that high resting pressures in the canal lead to relative hypoperfusion and reduced tissue oxygen tensions, impairing healing. This understanding underpins the therapeutic strategy, which is based on interventions that reduce the resting pressures in the canal. However, an important subgroup of patients develop anal fissure despite normal or low pressures (e.g. it is common postpartum). Patients usually present with pain at defaecation and there may be some associated bright red bleeding. Pain results from distraction of the tear but more significantly from the presence of intense anal spasm, which can be protracted and debilitating. Visual inspection of the anus while gently everting the perianal skin is usually sufficient to make the diagnosis and further examination may be too painful in a conscious patient. Always bear in mind the possibility of other diagnoses: CD, sexually transmitted disease (e.g. syphilis and herpes simplex) and anal carcinoma. Management is based on altering two factors: the stool consistency and the resting muscle tone in the anal canal. Dietary advice to increase fluid and fibre in the diet helps and stool-softening agents such as isphagula and osmotic laxatives can be useful. In the past, resting tone in the anal canal was reduced surgically by submitting the patient to an anaesthetic and dilating the anal canal. This caused an injury to the internal sphincter and reliably reduced the resting tone but in an uncontrolled manner with an unacceptably high rate of anal incontinence. Controlled surgical sphincterotomy is still considered by many to be the 'gold standard' against which other therapies must be judged but it is associated with incontinence rates as high as 30% in females. As a consequence, 'chemical sphincterotomy' with topical glyceryl trinitrate 0.4% or dilitazem 2% is effective when used in a protracted course with stool softeners. Treatment with botulinum toxin injection provides protracted reduction in resting pressure for 8–10 weeks and is valuable in more resistant cases especially when combined with fissure excision. The majority of anal fissures heal within a few weeks and chronicity is defined by a history of 3 months. There is growing evidence that a proportion of recalcitrant fissures may be resulting from more profound anorectal dysfunction from occult rectal prolapse. This group of patients warrants specialist assessment and pelvic floor investigation. The appearances of chronic anal fissure are shown in Figure 24.8.

Haemorrhoids

Haemorrhoids, or piles, are a common complaint which patients tend to use as a 'catch-all' diagnosis to encompass a variety of anal conditions. To the colorectal surgeon, haemorrhoids refer to the symptoms that arise from the anal cushions. These cushions are three submucosal spaces filled with arteriovenous communications, which lie in the upper half of the anal canal and help to keep it 'airtight' at rest. Haemorrhoids are said to have occurred when the cushions bleed or prolapse, or both. Haemorrhoids have been arbitrarily classified as:

- first degree: bleeding alone
- second degree: prolapse on defaecation with spontaneous reduction
- third degree: prolapse on defaecation requiring manual reduction
- fourth degree: prolapse on defaecation, unable to replace.

Figure 24.8 includes examples of prolapsed and thrombosed haemorrhoids. The bleeding of haemorrhoids is classically bright red in colour and seen on the toilet paper or in the toilet pan. A rectal neoplasm

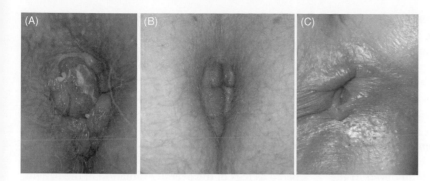

Figure 24.8 Common anal pathologies. Prolapse haemorrhoids with mucus (A) tend to cause irritation and mucus discharge as well as bleeding. The thrombosed haemorrhoid in B will cause discomfort that settles with rest and stool softeners. A chronic anal fissure is shown in C. This will typically cause severe pain immediately after defaecation and often a residual ache from sphincter spasm that may last hours as well as bright bleeding.

can produce similar bleeding and steps must be taken to exclude such a lesion. Flexible sigmoidoscopy is the investigation of choice in bright red rectal bleeding. Advice about dietary changes (to include more fibre and fluid) may be sufficient to manage some haemorrhoidal symptoms and explicit advice on defaecatory habit (i.e. avoiding straining, prolonged sitting and especially reading while on the toilet) is important. It is also important to establish whether the patient requires treatment or just reassurance that no sinister pathology is to blame. Minor symptoms can be treated effectively in outpatient treatment by the application of rubber bands or by injection of 5% phenol in almond or arachis oil as a sclerosant. A recent meta-analysis suggested that rubber-band ligation was better than sclerotherapy. Surgical haemorrhoidectomy is usually described as the Milligan–Morgan technique, with excision of the three cushions to leave a 'clover leaf' type wound in the anal canal. This is a painful operation and careful attention should be paid to the perioperative regime. Pre- and postoperative aperients, intraoperative local anaesthetic with postoperative balanced analgesia and antibiotics is thought to be the optimal regime. Skin bridges need to be preserved between the pile excision wounds to prevent anal stenosis. In 1998, Longo introduced a new surgical approach to haemorrhoids, stapled haemorrhoidectomy or procedure for prolapsed haemorrhoids (PPH). In this technique, a circumferential strip of mucosa is excised from above the dentate line by use of a stapling device. Pain is less compared to conventional surgical haemorrhoidectomy, with earlier return to the activities of daily living. Initial enthusiasm for this procedure has been tempered by reports of rare, but very serious, complications such as sepsis and anovaginal fistulation and the technique is clearly operator-dependent.

Prolapse

Rectal prolapse is a distressing condition for the patient. Approximately 50–75% of rectal prolapse patients suffer from associated anal incontinence, and the prolapse itself is socially embarrassing. The cause of rectal prolapse in adulthood is unknown; however, it is thought to begin as an internal intussusception. A typical patient will have a lax pelvic floor and a floppy, redundant sigmoid colon. Patients usually present with complaint of a lump that prolapses at defecation and either reduces spontaneously or has to be manually replaced. Incontinence and evacuatory difficulties are commonly associated. Occasionally, prolapse presents as an emergency and prolonged difficulty replacing the prolapse can lead to its strangulation. The best way to reduce an apparently irreducible prolapse is to raise the foot of the bed and coat the prolapse liberally with sugar; the osmotic effect reduces oedema and the prolapse can then be replaced. The best way to confirm the diagnosis in the outpatient setting is to ask the patient to go to the clinic toilet and demonstrate the prolapse. Colonic investigation is recommended, although very elderly patients are unsuitable for colonoscopy and minimum-preparation CT colonography alone or in combination with flexible sigmoidoscopy is sufficient.

There have been many surgical approaches described for rectal prolapse, but they can be broken down into two main types: abdominal or perineal. Initial surgical attempts were perineal; Thiersch's anal encirclement operation was described in 1891 and Delorme's mucosal sleeve resection was described in 1900. The perineal approach may also involve rectosigmoidectomy (Altemeier operation). Abdominal approaches can be open or laparoscopic and surgeons may elect to remove redundant colon or not.

Abdominal approaches have lower recurrence rates than the perineal approaches (in a major retrospective series from the University of Minnesota, the recurrence rate after abdominal procedures was 5% and 16% after perineal rectosigmoidectomy) but as the patients are often elderly and very frail a perineal operation, which avoids the morbidity of abdominal surgery, is attractive. Recent developments in our understanding of rectal prolapse have led to laparoscopic ventral mesh rectopexy offering effective treatment with low recurrence rate and acceptable morbidity even in the elderly population. This procedure also avoids constipation, which is a common accompaniment to previous abdominal procedures for rectal prolapse.

Solitary rectal ulcer syndrome (SRUS) is frequently, but not universally, associated with internal intussusception or full-thickness rectal prolapse. SRUS without full-thickness prolapse usually responds to dietary and biofeedback treatment; however, an abdominal procedure such as laparoscopic rectopexy is usually indicated if there is demonstrable rectal prolapse.

Although the majority of patients are elderly women, prolapse can occur at all ages and is not infrequent in infants under the age of 2 years. Prolapse in infancy is usually precipitated by acute diarrhoeal illness or severe coughing; however, the association of rectal prolapse in infancy and cystic fibrosis makes a sweat test mandatory.

Functional anorectal disorders

Constipation

There is a large variation in stool frequency between individuals and infrequent bowel actions in the absence of symptoms can be regarded as part of the normal spectrum of bowel function. However, constipation is a symptom that may affect a quarter of the population at some time and patients with decreased bowel frequency or impaired rectal evacuation have impaired quality of life and consume a large amount of healthcare resources.

For people with mild longstanding constipation investigations are not required, and dietary management is usually sufficient to relieve symptoms. When chronic constipation is more severe further investigation aims to determine the underlying cause. It is important to exclude endocrine causes such as hypothyroidism and metabolic derangement such as hypercalcaemia and use of constipating medications. Exclusion of sinister colorectal pathology is mandatory, although this rarely presents with chronic constipation. Further efforts focus on determining whether the constipation arises from slow transit within the colon or abnormal evacuation. Clues to the latter come from a history with no call to stool or incomplete evacuation requiring repeated visits to the toilet. Psychological morbidity, such as depression, is commonly associated with severe constipation and should be considered as part of the overall evaluation of the patient.

Use of proprietary laxatives may be of value if dietary manipulation alone is insufficient. Stimulant laxatives such as senna, bulking agents and polyethylene glycol-based laxatives (such as Movicol) may be effective in patients with idiopathic constipation and faecal impaction and many patients find benefit in changing regularly. However, for many patients laxatives do not provide sustained relief of symptoms and those with constipation predominant and those with irritable bowel syndrome may experience bloating and discomfort. Detailed dietetic assessment and advice can be of value in this group. Appropriate investigation of severe intractable constipation includes transit studies and anorectal physiology and defaecating proctography. Obstructed defaecation may result from failure to relax the puborectalis or the external sphincter during defaecation. Poor support around the rectum may also result in evacuatory difficulties from rectocele or rectal intussusception. Biofeedback therapy has become established as an effective treatment for patients with impaired evacuation, but in the face of a significant anatomical abnormality surgical correction may be considered. These treatments must be provided by experts and comprise a multidisciplinary approach.

Patients with a dilated rectum and faecal impaction (idiopathic megarectum) are usually teenagers or young adults of either sex. They have often soiled since childhood. In some the problem has a behavioural basis, whereas in others there may be subtle neuromuscular abnormalities of the gut. Constipation with faecal impaction is also seen in elderly patients, especially those in care. Poor general health, impaired mobility and inadequate toilet facilities may all contribute. Patients with idiopathic megarectum should have their bowel emptied completely before titrating an osmotic laxative. Such a laxative may be required in the long term, although behavioural treatment also seems to help some of these patients. Hirschsprung's disease should always be considered in the differential diagnosis for patients with severe intractable constipation as, although usually diagnosed and treated in infancy, the diagnosis may have been missed. Anorectal physiology is diagnostic for Hirschsprung's as the anorectal inhibitory reflex is absent.

If conservative treatment of intractable idiopathic constipation fails, then subtotal colectomy with ileorectal anastomosis may be considered; however, this has a high failure rate and is associated with significant morbidity. A colostomy may relieve symptoms but it is an unattractive option for most patients, and abdominal pain and bloating may persist. Antegrade irrigation through an appendicostomy or retrograde through rectal washouts may be acceptable. More recently sacral nerve stimulation has been shown to produce a clinical benefit for patients with idiopathic constipation with improvements in symptoms of abdominal pain and bloating, plus improvement in overall quality of life scores. Almost all patients with spinal injury experience constipation and, along with bladder control, bowel control is the function that individuals with spinal cord injury would most like to regain. All spinal-injured patients should have dedicated bowel continence regimes initiated by their carers but sacral nerve stimulation has also been shown to be of benefit in this group of patients.

Anal incontinence

Continence depends on a number of factors, notably normal anatomy and function of the internal-external anal sphincters and of the pelvic floor muscles, and normal anal-rectal sensation. Other variables that play a part in preserving continence are stool volume and consistency, intestinal transit and normal mental function. In the elderly, particularly institutionalized, and the very young, incontinence can result from faccal impaction with overflow or spurious diarrhoea. Improving bowel function and evacuation with osmotic laxatives can be effective. Pregnancy and obstetric injury are important causes of anal incontinence due to traction injuries in the pudendal nerve and injury to the pelvic floor and sphincter muscles. Around one-third of first vaginal deliveries result in sphincter damage, although two-thirds of these will be asymptomatic. An estimated 1% of vaginal deliveries result in a third-degree tear into the anal sphincter complex. Sphincter damage can also result from surgery, such as haemorrhoidectomy or internal sphincterotomy for anal fissure. Anal endosonogra-

phy enables identification of structural damage to the sphincter muscles (Figure 24.1) and anorectal physiology complements this investigation and gives valuable additional information. Anal incontinence is frequently associated with urogynaecological symptoms. Finally, incontinence may arise from organic bowel disease. This is usually apparent from the history with a change in bowel habit. Other possible causes include rectal tumours and inflammatory bowel disease.

A complete history, examination for inflammatory bowel disease, sphincter damage or faecal impaction, and correction of predisposing factors can lead to successful treatment in many patients. Loperamide reduces the force of bowel contractions and enhances absorption of water from the stool. It may also increase the resting pressure in the anal canal. It can be effective in patients with faecal urgency or leakage and the dose should be titrated to achieve control of symptoms. Dietary modification may also be helpful. Additional behavioural interventions, with bowel-focused counselling (biofeedback), including advice on resisting urgency and titrating loperamide, can lead to marked improvement in the symptoms, sometimes even when there is structural damage to the sphincter.

Sacral nerve stimulation

In patients with a weak but structurally intact sphincter it may be possible to alter sphincter and proximal bowel behaviour using the surrounding nerves and muscles. Sacral nerve stimulation is a treatment option for these patients. It involves low-level electrical stimulation applied via electrodes through the sacral foramina to the sacral nerve supply of the lower bowel and sphincters. A permanent stimulator, similar in size to a cardiac pacemaker, is located in the subcutaneous tissues just above the iliac crest. Electrical stimulation is tailored to achieve the optimum response through a wireless remote control. The UK National Institute for Health and Clinical Excellence (NICE) has studied sacral nerve stimulation and found that, in patients who had permanent implants, complete continence was achieved in up to 75% of patients, whereas up to 100% of patients experienced a decrease of 50% or more in the number of incontinence episodes. There was also evidence to suggest an improvement in the ability to defer defecation after permanent implantation. Patients also reported improvements in both disease-specific and general quality-of-life scores after the procedure. Of 266 patients receiving temporary sacral nerve stimulation, 4% (10/266) experienced an adverse event. Fifty-six per cent (149/266) went on to receive permanent implantation. Of the patients who had permanent implants, 13% (19/149) reported adverse events. These included three patients who developed infections requiring device removal, seven patients who had lead migration requiring either relocation (five cases) or removal of the device, and six patients who experienced pain after implantation.

Surgical options in incontinence

In patients with structural defects in the external anal sphincter, an overlapping repair of the sphincter will improve continence in the majority of patients, but the results tend not to be durable. It is most effective in younger women, where sphincter injury is the predominant cause of incontinence, as opposed to the elderly population with more complex aetiology. Silicone biomaterial may be injected to augment a weak internal anal sphincter and the final surgical options are reconstruction of the sphincter or permanent faecal diversion. An electronically stimulated gracilis muscle flap can be used to create a neosphincter around the anal canal and some centres implant artificial neosphincters. Both of these operations have been associated with implant-related infection and impaired evacuation. In recent years the potential role of occult rectal prolapse or intussusceptions in faecal incontinence has been proposed. Certainly, a proportion of women with incontinence improve with laparoscopic rectopexy.

Minimally invasive colorectal surgery

Laparoscopic techniques have been shown to reduce the physical impact of surgery on patients. Benefits include lesser cosmetic insults, less pain, earlier mobilization and return to normal functioning. In a randomized trial, laparoscopic colorectal surgery resulted in a significant reduction of 30-day postoperative morbidity compared to open surgery. Concerns over the oncological effectiveness appear to be unfounded. In a randomized trial from Spain can-

cer outcomes were improved in patients with lymph node involvement. This may reflect a reduced stress response to laparoscopic surgery or improved uptake of adjuvant chemotherapy in this group. In the UK, the National Institute for Health and Clinical Excellence (NICE 2006) judged that laparoscopic surgery should be the preferred option in patients undergoing elective surgery for colorectal cancer. Laparoscopic colorectal surgery is technically demanding and also requires increased resources. Its growth in the UK has been slow to date but there is an ambitious programme to encourage uptake. The advantages of laparoscopic resection should be universally available within 5 years.

Further reading

Atkin WS, Saunders BP. Surveillance guidelines after removal of colorectal adenomatous polyps. *Gut* 2002;**51**(Suppl 5):V6–V9.

Braga M, Vignali A, Gianotti L, Zuliani W, Radaelli G, Gruarin P, Dellabona P, Di Carlo V. Laparoscopic versus open colorectal surgery: a randomized trial on short-term outcome. *Ann Surg* 2002;**236**(6):759–766.

Eke N. Fournier's gangrene: a review of 1726 cases. *Br J Surg* 2000;**87**(6):718–728.

Heald RJ, Moran BJ, Ryall RD, Sexton R, MacFarlane JK. Rectal cancer: the Basingstoke experience of total mesorectal excision, 1978–1997. *Arch Surg* 1998;**133**(8): 894–899.

Kamm MA. Constipation and its management. *Br Med J* 2003b; **327**(7413): 459–460.

Kamm MA. Faecal incontinence. *Br Med J* 2003a; **327**(7427):1299–1300.

Lacy AM, Garcia-Valdecasas JC, Delgado S, Castells A, Taura P, Pique JM, Visa J. Laparoscopy-assisted colectomy versus open colectomy for treatment of non-metastatic colon cancer: a randomised trial. *Lancet* 2002;**359**(9325):2224–2229.

Stollman N, Raskin JB. Diverticular disease of the colon. *Lancet* 2004;**363**(9409):631–639.

Vernava 3rd AM, Moore BA, Longo WE, Johnson FE. Lower gastrointestinal bleeding. *Dis Colon Rectum* 1997;**40**(7):846–858.

Chapter

25

Fundamentals of the genitourinary system

Angela Cottrell and Andrew Dickinson

Urology is the study of diseases of the urinary tract and the male reproductive system. Some of the earliest operations described are urological procedures and the ancient Egyptians are known to have performed circumcision, surgical castration and cystolithotomy (open removal of bladder stones).

Functional disorders of micturition may lead to urine incontinence or urine retention. Metabolic abnormalities may result in renal stone disease. Developmental abnormalities are seen in the neonate and the developing child. Urological cancers are common and their management can affect continence, fertility and quality of life.

Despite the numerous diseases that can affect the urinary tract, the presenting symptoms are few, making accurate diagnosis dependent on the careful imaging of structural abnormalities as well as a functional assessment of voiding and renal function.

Anatomy and developmental anomalies

Kidney

Gross anatomy

The adult kidney, a paired organ, is approximately 11 cm long, weighs 150 g and lies in the retroperitoneum. Posteriorly, the upper half lies on the diaphragm with the psoas, quadratus lumborum and transversus abdominis muscles from medial to lateral on the lower half.

Anteriorly, the right kidney is covered on its medial aspect by the second part of the duodenum and the liver overlying the upper pole and hepatic flexure of the colon covering the lower part of the anterolateral aspect. The left kidney has the tail of the pancreas together with the edge of the greater curve of the stomach separated by the lesser sac on its medial aspect, the spleen lateral to this and the lower half of the kidney related to the splenic flexure of the colon. Both kidneys have the adrenal glands superomedially.

Surgical anatomy

The 11th and 12th ribs are floating ribs and related to the upper half of the kidney. They provide useful surface markings for loin incisions, which divide skin, latissimus dorsi muscle, external and then internal oblique muscles. The pleura lies in the upper part of the incision and can be punctured, causing a pneumothorax. The transversus abdominis muscle is then divided and the kidney, surrounded by the perinephric fat contained within the Gerota's fascia, lies in the retroperitoneal space (Figure 25.1). It should be noted that the pleural cavity may be deliberately opened during surgery to improve access to the upper pole of the kidney. Other common approaches to the kidney include the transabdominal route (e.g. via a subcostal incision) and also laparoscopic approaches which can be either transabdominal or retroperitoneal.

Developmental anomalies

The kidney can fail to develop from its primitive precursor, the metanephros, giving rise to a small dysplastic often cystic remnant. The ureter and trigone are normal. If renal dysplasia is bilateral, the neonate will be in renal failure (Potter's syndrome) and will die in utero.

The kidneys may fuse during embryological development. If one shifts to the other side (crossed renal ectopia), the ureter crosses the midline on its route to the bladder. If fusion occurs at the lower pole of

Fundamentals of Surgical Practice, Third Edition, ed. Andrew N. Kingsnorth and Douglas M. Bowley.
Published by Cambridge University Press. © Cambridge University Press 2011.

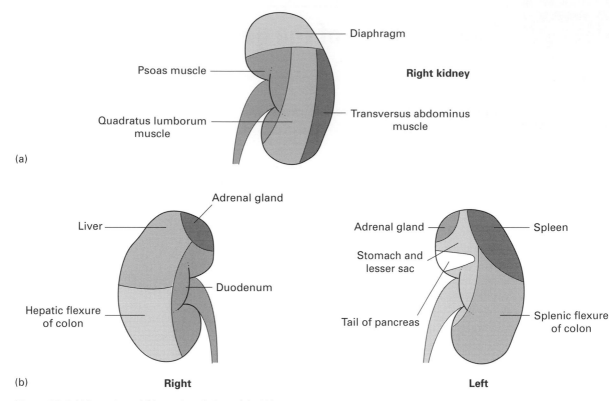

Figure 25.1 (a) Posterior and (b) anterior relations of the kidney.

each kidney, ascent into the upper retroperitoneum is impaired by the inferior mesenteric artery. Due to its shape, such a kidney is called a horseshoe kidney. It has an anomalous blood supply which makes renal or aortic surgery difficult. Similarly, if the developing kidney remains within the pelvis and fails to ascend correctly, a pelvic kidney will result.

Ureter

Surgical anatomy

The ureter is a 25 cm long muscular tube; the upper half lies in the retroperitoneum and the lower half in the pelvis. Three areas are narrow and are particularly prone to obstruction by ureteric stones:

1. the upper part at its junction with the pelvis (the pelvi-ureteric junction, PUJ)
2. the lower part as it passes through the bladder detrusor muscle (vesico-ureteric junction, VUJ)
3. at the junction of the upper and lower half as it passes over the bifurcation of the common iliac artery.

Urine is propelled down the ureter by peristalsis and this worm-like motion (vermiculation) can be demonstrated at operation by pinching the ureter gently with forceps. This can be used to distinguish the ureter from the nearby iliac vessels. The ureter passes through the bladder wall obliquely. This acts as a flutter valve so when the bladder contracts during voiding the intravesical ureter is compressed, thereby preventing reflux of urine.

Developmental anomalies

The renal pelvis divides inside the kidney to form the major and minor calyces. This division may occur early, giving rise to two ureters draining the kidney and joining at a variable distance to form a common ureter. Occasionally, such duplex ureters fail to join and each drains separately into the bladder. The ureter draining the upper part (or moiety) of the kidney passes into the lowest and medial-most aspect of the bladder. The ureters therefore cross, as they pass down to the bladder.

Bladder

Surgical anatomy

The normal adult bladder is a hollow muscular organ with a capacity of about 500 ml and lies in the bony pelvis. In the child, the shallow pelvis allows the bladder to rise up into the abdomen, making suprapubic puncture relatively easy.

Developmental anomalies

In utero, urine drains from the bladder to the placenta via the urachus along the umbilical cord. At birth the urachus closes to form a fibrous cord connecting the dome of the bladder to the umbilicus. Occasionally, it can remain patent or develop cysts that become inflamed. Occasionally, the urachal remnant can undergo malignant change.

As part of a major congenital abnormality of the lower abdominal wall musculature the bladder may open directly onto an incompletely formed abdominal wall; so-called ectopia vesicae. Previously the bladder was excised and the ureters diverted into the rectum (uretero-sigmoidostomy). With modern surgical reconstructive techniques it is now possible to close the bladder and repair the abdominal wall a few days after birth.

Prostate

Surgical anatomy

The prostate gland is rudimentary until adolescence, when it grows to about the size of a large grape and weighs about 15 g. It lies at the exit of the bladder with the urethra passing through it. Proximally lies the bladder neck, distally the external urethral sphincter. In the prostatic urethra, the ejaculatory ducts drain out at the verumontanum. This is a surgical landmark for the proximal limit of the external sphincter. Superoposteriorly lie the seminal vesicles and together with the prostate they rest on the posterior condensation of pelvic fascia (Denonvillier's fascia). Digital rectal examination allows the posterior aspect of the prostate to be palpated.

Continence mechanisms

The bladder neck or internal urinary sphincter is automatic and unlike the external urinary sphincter is not under voluntary control (Figure 25.2). For normal voiding, both these sphincters must relax. If the external sphincter is damaged it is possible to

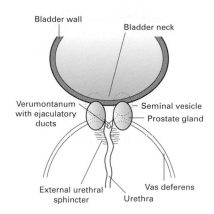

Figure 25.2 Male continence mechanism.

remain continent with the internal sphincter alone. The operation of transurethral resection of the prostate (TURP) removes the prostatic adenoma obstructing the prostate urethra, and it is common for the bladder neck and the internal sphincter to be resected as well. This leads to retrograde ejaculation following TURP.

Testis

Surgical anatomy

The normal adult testis is an ovoid sphere measuring approximately $5 \times 4 \times 3$ cm. Posterolaterally lies the epididymis, which is continued superiorly as the vas deferens. This lies in the spermatic cord together with the testicular artery, pampiniform plexus of veins, nerves and lymphatics. Around the testis lies the tunica vaginalis, a double layer of peritoneum brought down as the testis descends during embryological development from its abdominal position in the foetus.

Developmental anomalies

The testis may fail to descend completely into the scrotum, but remain either intra-abdominal or within the inguinal canal. A testis may have a strong cremasteric reflex and be retractile but such a testis can usually be brought down into the child's scrotum by gentle massage. If it cannot be brought down, it requires surgical mobilization and fixation in the scrotum (orchidopexy).

The testis lies surrounded by the tunica vaginalis. In some cases, the testis is so mobile that the free movement allows it to twist and obstruct its blood supply. Testicular torsion is acutely painful and requires prompt surgical exploration. The testis is untwisted and, if viable, returned to the scrotum and anchored with sutures to prevent a recurrence. As the testicular mobility is bilateral, the other testis should be fixed prophylactically at the same time.

Penis and urethra

Surgical anatomy

The urethra is about 20 cm long in the adult male and comprises the prostatic urethra, the membranous urethra and the penile urethra, which passes from the bulb of the penis along the shaft to the meatus. The female urethra is much shorter and is surrounded by the sphincter muscle.

Developmental anomalies

During development, the male urethra may fail to form a complete tube to the end of the glans and open onto the ventral surface of the penis. This is termed hypospadias. The foreskin is often deficient ventrally and has the appearance of a dorsal hood. As the foreskin may be used in the reconstructive surgical repair of a hypospadias, circumcision under these circumstances is contraindicated.

Urological symptoms

The three main urological symptoms are:
1. functional urinary symptoms
2. haematuria
3. pain.

Functional urinary symptoms

The micturition cycle involves two relatively discrete processes:
1. bladder filling and urine storage
2. bladder emptying.

Therefore, for descriptive purposes symptoms affecting the lower urinary tract (LUTS) can be divided into 'storage' and/or 'voiding'. The term 'prostatism' should be abandoned and terms such as bladder outflow obstruction (BOO) due to benign prostatic enlargement (BPE) should only be used when an appropriate diagnosis has been made (see Table 25.1).

Voiding symptoms

The longer urethra and the prostate gland in men make them more likely to complain of 'voiding' symptoms, whereas the shorter urethra and changes in pelvic floor musculature following childbirth means that 'storage' symptoms are more common in women.

Table 25.1 Voiding and storage symptoms

Storage symptoms	Voiding symptoms
Frequency	Hesitancy
Urgency	Reduced stream
Nocturia	Straining
Incontinence	Terminal dribble Prolonged voiding times Post-micturition dribble

However, men with BOO due to BPE will often complain of both storage and voiding symptoms. The symptoms typically have a slow, gradual onset with periods of apparent improvement due to compensatory increases in detrusor contractions developing to overcome the obstruction. The patient will find he has to pass urine more frequently during the day. Eventually he will reduce fluid intake to try and limit the need to pass urine at night. This may lead to a life dominated by having to know the location of all public conveniences since the bladder will be incompletely emptied at voiding and thereby refill quickly, reducing its effective capacity.

Acute urinary retention is the inability to pass urine associated with severe suprapubic discomfort. It may be precipitated by events such as the use of medication such as anaesthetic or anticholinergic medication, constipation or urinary tract infection. Where a triggering event is not identified the episode is described as spontaneous acute urinary retention. The patient is usually restless and agitated and catheterization is needed to relieve the obstruction.

In contrast, chronic urine retention is painless. Over a long period of time the bladder is incompletely emptied at each void and the residual volume of urine gradually increases, leading to a reduced effective storage capacity and a chronically distended bladder. The bladder becomes full more quickly and the frequency of voiding increases. Eventually the bladder never completely empties. The post-micturition dribble increases and eventually becomes continuous. This is chronic retention with overflow incontinence. Occasionally, high pressure in the chronically overfilled bladder results in damage to the kidneys. This is known as an obstructive uropathy and must be treated with catheterization of the bladder and eventually outflow surgery (usually a TURP) to relieve the high-pressure retention. A post-obstructive diuresis may occur when this pressure is relieved.

As stated above, these symptoms are most commonly due to obstruction from enlargement of the prostate gland or, rarely, failure of the bladder neck sphincter to relax and open during normal voiding. In malignant enlargement of the prostate gland, urinary symptoms may develop more quickly without episodes of remission. A urethral stricture will produce a poor urine stream, but usually the bladder empties completely, and hesitancy and nocturia are not characteristic.

LUTS are a feature in women with urethral stenosis or obstruction of the urethra by a gravid uterus or severe genital organ prolapse. Failure of the normal sphincter mechanisms to relax and open during voiding will lead to voiding symptoms. This is seen after spinal trauma and in some patients with multiple sclerosis.

Storage/filling symptoms

The normal detrusor muscle undergoes receptive relaxation to allow urine storage, without causing a rise in intravesical pressure. When the bladder capacity is reached, sensory stimuli generate a desire to void and, when socially appropriate, the detrusor muscle contracts and voiding takes place due to the rise in intravesical pressure. If the ability for receptive relaxation is lost, the sensory stimuli are produced before the bladder is full and an intense urge to void is experienced. This recurs again as the bladder refills. The urge to void can be so intense that the patient becomes incontinent. This is known as urge incontinence and often includes the triad of symptoms:

1. urgency of micturition
2. frequency of micturition
3. urge incontinence.

These symptoms are seen in detrusor overactivity, formerly called detrusor instability, which can be proven with urodynamics (UDS). This condition may be secondary to increased stimulation of the trigone, for example bladder stone, urine infection, malignant cystitis or a neurological cause such as stroke. Alternatively, if no cause for the detrusor overactivity is identified, it is termed primary detrusor overactivity. The term overactive bladder (OAB) is also used and can be defined from either UDS findings (e.g. detrusor overactivity) or symptoms (e.g. urgency).

Symptoms due to detrusor underactivity

If the bladder is chronically distended, it can lose the ability to contract during normal voiding. The sensory stimuli of the over-stretched bladder are lost and the bladder becomes a flaccid, painless storage bag. Voiding may be achieved by abdominal straining or direct suprapubic pressure. Overflow incontinence of urine may occur. This is seen in the end stages of outflow obstruction due to prostate disease or as part of an autonomic neuropathy (e.g. in a diabetic patient).

The diagnosis of detrusor underactivity (DUA) is made following formal UDS assessment, although its presence may be suspected with an appropriate history and simple flow rate measurement. It often coexists with other symptoms of BOO.

Symptoms of pelvic floor dysfunction weakness

Urine incontinence may occur when there is a sudden rise in intra-abdominal pressure (classically coughing or sneezing), so-called stress incontinence. If this is demonstrated by objective measurement (UDS), it is called urodynamic stress incontinence (USI). Although occasionally seen in men following traumatic or iatrogenic damage to the urinary sphincter, this is a symptom most commonly seen in women with damage to the muscles and/or nerves and/or connective tissue within the pelvic floor following childbirth.

Often the women will wear sanitary towels to avoid wetting their clothes, thereby coping with, but hiding, the problem. The number of times the pads become wet and need changing is a good estimate of the severity of the incontinence.

Haematuria

Haematuria is the presence of blood in the urine. If it is visible, it is called frank, or macroscopic, haematuria. Whether the blood appears at the beginning, during or the end of the urine stream gives little useful information as to the likely cause and all forms of haematuria require a full evaluation.

Classically, glomerulonephritis produces a smoky brown haematuria and at microscopy (using phase contrast) cells may be misshapen (dysmorphic).

Haematuria identified at urine microscopy is as important a sign as frank haematuria and requires an equally full investigation. Dipstick testing of urine, often performed as a screening test in asymptomatic patients, may be the first indication of haematuria, but can give false-positive results and therefore confirmation by urine microscopy may be appropriate.

Pain associated with haematuria, either when passing urine or over the renal or bladder area, suggests an inflammatory cause, for example infection or mechanical trauma from a stone. Painless macroscopic haematuria may be the first sign of a bladder or kidney cancer. Associated symptoms such as malaise, anorexia and weight loss may be present, due to disseminated disease or paraneoplastic syndrome. Haematuria following direct trauma to the renal tract will be evident from the history, but bleeding following minimal trauma should be investigated carefully as there may be some underlying pathology. Patients on anticoagulants who develop haematuria also require full investigation, as a lesion in the urinary tract may be unmasked by the anticoagulants.

Blood found in the urine of a menstruating woman may be a contaminant, but the urine should be tested again after the period has finished.

Red-coloured urine may be caused by drugs (e.g. rifampicin) and some food stuffs (e.g. beetroot). Microscopy, however, will fail to demonstrate red cells.

Haemospermia

Blood in the ejaculate (haemospermia) is usually non-sinister up to the age of 40 or 50 years. Occasionally, a cancer of the prostate or bladder may present with haemospermia.

Pain

Pain in the urinary system relates to the anatomical site fairly accurately.

Kidney and ureter

Pain and tenderness in the kidney, because of their retroperitoneal location, are felt posteriorly in the loin and renal angle. Pain from a stone passing from the renal pelvis down the ureter may be felt initially posteriorly. The pain then radiates around the loin into the iliac fossa and scrotum. Renal colic produces an intense, severe colicky type pain where the patient can find no relief by either movement or rest. In contrast, pain from a renal tumour or pyelonephritis is likely to be constant, but less intense.

Bladder and prostate gland

Acute retention of urine results in an intense pain suprapubically, with an unremitting desire to void. A similar pain can be experienced in a urinary infection, although more commonly there is severe suprapubic pain unrelieved by voiding, which itself is painful. Irritation of the trigone, either by inflammation or mechanical trauma from a stone or catheter, can cause pain referred to the urethral meatus.

Inflammation of the prostate causes a variety of urinary symptoms, which can include perineal and penile pain, as well as a dull suprapubic or ill-defined rectal discomfort. These symptoms form part of the chronic pelvic pain syndrome. This syndrome can also affect women. In a minority of cases a diagnosis of interstitial cystitis can be made (see below).

Scrotum and penis

Sudden onset of severe testicular pain associated with a dull abdominal ache is classically seen with torsion of the testis. Such pain will persist for many hours until untwisting the testis relieves the ischaemia. Inflammation of the epididymis and testis (epididymo-orchitis) has a more gradual onset, often developing over several days. The pain can become intense but signs of inflammation, swelling and redness of the scrotum are also present.

A malignant testicular tumour may cause mild pain or discomfort, but most commonly it is painless. Similarly, cystic swelling such as hydrocoele or epididymal cysts are usually painless, although once noticed by the patient they can become a constant worry and source of discomfort. The dilated pampiniform plexus of veins in a varicocoele is usually asymptomatic, but can cause discomfort.

Penile pain is relatively uncommon. Pain on erection occurs in Peyronie's disease (a fibrosis of the corpora cavernosum, resulting in a curved erection), but this is usually self-limiting.

Urological history and examination

History

The presenting symptoms should be assessed in context. The age of the patient, any past surgery or present medication will often direct the doctor towards the most likely pathologies to consider. For example, urinary infections in a child will have a different list of likely causes from those in an elderly man, a pregnant woman or an immunosuppressed transplant patient.

Presenting complaint

For most of the major symptoms ask about:

- onset
- duration
- severity.

The sudden onset of pain in renal colic or acute urine retention contrasts with the gradual build-up of pain from a renal tumour or the slow development of LUTS due to outflow obstruction. The duration of pain from renal colic will be a few hours and will recur, whereas pain from a urine infection will be persistent. Other features such as pain, haematuria or incontinence should also be established.

The severity and inconvenience to the patient of their LUTS can be best assessed by direct questions or examples:

- How many times does the patient get up at night to pass urine?
- How many times is the patient incontinent or have to change their pads?
- Does the patient take longer to pass urine than their friends of the same age?
- Are trips out of the house or holidays limited by access to a toilet?

Frequency–volume charts can be filled in by patients, to allow an objective and recordable assessment of their voiding pattern throughout the day and night.

Special questionnaires

Various useful and internationally validated scoring questionnaires have been developed to assess and monitor a patient's symptoms. They also provide a measure of quality of life (QoL), and can be used to assess the results of treatment. Such questionnaires exist for LUTS due to BPE (the International Prostate Symptom Score, IPSS), various aspects of continence (International Continence Society, ICS) and the International Index of Erectile Function (IIEF).

Social and occupational history

Occupation or past occupation

Exposure to chemical carcinogens such as 2-naphthylamine or benzidine in the chemical or rubber industries may take 20 years to induce bladder cancer. Smoking is now the commonest aetiological factor in patients with transitional cell carcinoma (TCC).

Foreign travel

A trip to Egypt or central Africa may result in exposure to *Schistosomiasis haematobium* (a trematode parasite fluke that lives in fresh water snails and parasitically in the human bladder and pelvic blood vessels) causing haematuria. Dehydration during a holiday to a hot climate may be the start of renal stone formation.

Family history

A family history of renal failure or polycystic kidney disease may reveal anxieties about kidney failure. A recent diagnosis or death from cancer of a family member or friend may provoke anxiety about non-specific symptoms. A family history of prostate cancer may be important.

Medical history

- NEUROLOGICAL DISEASES: for example Parkinson's disease, multiple sclerosis, diabetes, a stroke or back injury may cause abnormal bladder function and lead to various LUTS.
- PAST INFECTIONS (EITHER VENEREAL OR URINARY): it may indicate underlying urinary tract pathology.
- MEDICATION: diuretics may explain mild LUTS. Antihypertensives may indicate intrinsic kidney disease.

Surgical history

- CHILDHOOD problems should be asked about specifically, as the patient may forget to mention them. Recurrent urine infections as a child may suggest reflux treated by surgical re-implantation of the ureters.
- UNDESCENDED testes that have been either excised or placed in the scrotum (orchidopexy).
- ABDOMINAL or pelvic surgery can cause denervation injury to the bladder (e.g. abdomino-perineal resection of the rectum).

- URETERIC injury may occur in abdominal or gynaecological operations. Previous pelvic surgery may also result in fistulas, which can present with incontinence and/or abnormal discharge.

Obstetric history

Damage to the pelvic floor during pregnancy can lead to stress incontinence. Problems with vaginal delivery or a forceps delivery may also damage the perineum causing various LUTS.

Examination

All patients with urological symptoms must have their blood pressure measured.

Signs of dehydration such as a dry mouth and tongue may indicate renal failure or the polyuria of diabetes.

Cervical lymph nodes may be enlarged due to metastatic spread from any urological cancer.

Sit the patient up to look at the back and loins. A forgotten laminectomy scar may be seen or the vesicles of shingles identified that would explain the loin pain.

Tenderness over the kidney should be tested by gentle pressure over the renal angle.

Abdominal examination allows palpation for the kidneys and bladder – the kidneys by bimanual examination with a hand posteriorly lifting up the kidney towards the examining abdominally placed hand; the bladder by percussion over the suprapubic region. A suprapubic mass can be shown to be a bladder if it disappears when the patient is catheterized. Occasionally, an enlarged liver or spleen will be detected as an incidental finding.

Examine the foreskin to exclude a phimosis and signs of hypospadias. Palpate the scrotal contents to feel the normal features of the testis and epididymis. A cystic mass such as a hydrocoele or epididymal cyst will transilluminate, whereas a testicular mass will not. Stand the patient up to exclude an inguinal hernia and palpate the cord while the patient coughs for an impulse in a varicocoele.

Rectal examination is performed to palpate the prostate gland and identify any malignant changes in the gland. A hard lump in either or both lobes suggests a cancer and a biopsy is needed to obtain histological proof.

Investigations

Urine tests

Dipstick testing

This is a valuable test as it gives an immediate result. Urine is tested for glucose to exclude diabetes mellitus and the presence of red blood cells. The latter test is based on the peroxidase-like activity of haemoglobin and is very sensitive, although false positives are seen. Protein in the urine can also be detected and its presence suggests an inflammatory process such as infection or protein loss from a glomerular or tubular lesion (e.g. glomerulonephritis).

Microscopy and culture

A mid-stream specimen of urine (MSSU) is collected, taking precautions to minimize contamination. Microscopy also allows red blood cells to be identified. If a urine infection is present, pus cells will be seen and bacteria will grow on the culture plates. If pus cells are present without evidence of infection (sterile pyuria), tuberculosis should be considered and special stains and culture medium used. Any bacterial cultured is tested for antibiotic sensitivities, according to local protocols.

Phase contrast microscopy allows the shape of the red blood cells to be assessed. They may be abnormal (dysmorphic) in glomerular bleeding.

Urine cytology

The urine specimen is fixed in formaldehyde, centrifuged to collect the cellular sediment and this is examined microscopically after Papanicolaou staining. Neoplastic cells can be identified by their characteristic features, which include abnormal nuclear:cytoplasm ratios and ploidy status.

Molecular markers

Several new molecular markers have been developed as a means to detect bladder cancer non-invasively; using exfoliated cells from patients' voided urine and bladder washings. They generally exhibit greater sensitivity but lower specificity than urine cytology. These markers are based on the pathogenesis of bladder cancer and include telomerase, survivin, bladder tumour antigen (BTA) and nuclear matrix protein (NMP-22). They are not yet in routine clinical use, but as refinements continue, their utilization is likely to become increasingly widespread.

24-hour urine collection

Creatinine measurement

The urinary excretion of creatinine over 24 h (u) together with the urine volume (v) and plasma creatinine concentration (p) can be used to calculate the creatinine clearance (uv/p). This gives a working guide to the glomerular filtration rate (GFR), which is a surrogate for renal function. Alternatively, the renal clearance of radioisotopes can be used as a quicker, but less physiological, measure of GFR.

Stone metabolites

24-h urinary calcium, uric acid and oxalate can be measured in recurrent stone formers.

Blood tests

General tests

Malignant disease and chronic inflammation in the urinary tract may alter haemopoiesis. A measurement of haemoglobin and red blood cell parameters is essential. Renal function is estimated by serum urea and creatinine concentrations. Electrolyte concentrations, especially potassium, may be abnormal in renal failure. In metabolic or malignant bone disease, serum calcium and alkaline phosphatase will be abnormal, with high serum calcium also found in hyperparathyroidism.

Special tests

Prostate-specific antigen (PSA) is a glycoprotein, responsible for liquefying semen in vivo. As a tumour marker it is used to aid in the diagnosis and also monitor treatment of prostate cancer. It should be remembered that the 'normal range' for PSA varies with age and that PSA levels can also be affected by other conditions, such as urinary tract infection (UTI). The widespread use of PSA testing as part of a process of prostate cancer screening (particularly in the USA) has significantly reduced the proportion of patients diagnosed with advanced-stage prostate cancer. In the UK, however, the use of PSA for screening remains controversial.

The tumour markers alpha-fetoprotein (AFP), lactic dehydrogenase (LDH) and beta-human chorionic gonadotrophin (b-HCG) are used to monitor treatment of testicular germ cell tumours. An elevated AFP implies the presence of non-seminomatous elements in the tumour.

Imaging

Ultrasound scan

This versatile, non-invasive and safe technique is used widely in the investigation of the urological patient. The kidneys are scanned via the loin and the bladder is assessed transabdominally. A transrectal probe is used for prostate scanning and facilitates accurate guiding of the prostate biopsy needle. A smaller probe with higher frequency (and better image resolution) is available for very precise scanning of the testes.

Kidney

- Accurate assessment of the renal outline will identify a renal mass and distinguish between a fluid-filled cyst (probably benign) and a solid mass (possibly malignant).
- Shows the renal pelvis and any hydronephrosis or mucosal lesion (e.g. upper tract TCC).
- Shows parenchymal changes such as scarring from pyelonephritis or reflux.
- Renal stones will cast an acoustic shadow. This is especially useful for radiolucent stones.
- Guides percutaneous biopsy or placement of percutaneous drainage catheters.
- Identifies tumour thrombus in the renal vein or the inferior vena cava (IVC), especially when used in duplex mode to detect blood flow.
- May detect radiolucent stones.

Bladder

- Accurate measurement of bladder volume pre- and post-micturition. Can be used to assess post-void residual volume.
- Measures bladder wall thickness. Bladder wall hypertrophy is seen secondary to outflow obstruction and in other chronic inflammatory conditions, such as schistosomiasis.
- Bladder mucosal lesions, such as tumour, may be clearly shown although muscle invasion by bladder cancer cannot be accurately assessed.
- Dilated lower ureter often visible. Obstruction from a stone or tumour can usually be seen.

Prostate

- Transrectal ultrasound scanning of the prostate can reveal abnormal echoic areas that can indicate malignancy. A channel down the probe allows ultrasound-guided biopsy.

- In cases of infertility, transrectal ultrasound can be used to assess abnormalities such as seminal vesicle enlargement, cysts or prostatic duct calcifications which may be an obstructive cause of infertility as well as a guide to aspirate seminal vesicle fluid.

Testes

- Accurately identifies testicular masses. These are invariably malignant.
- Cysts are well demonstrated (e.g. hydrocoele and epididymal cyst).
- Varicocoeles can be shown to fill when the patient coughs.
- A swollen inflamed epididymis due to epididymitis may be difficult to differentiate from a testicular torsion clinically, but may be distinguished by ultrasound, especially if duplex (combined Doppler) mode is used to assess blood flow.

Limitations of ultrasound

- Fails to show the ureter throughout its length. Ultrasound can miss ureteric stones and tumours.
- Does not assess renal function. An obstructed but non-dilated kidney may look normal on an ultrasound scan.
- Will not detect all stones. For this reason a plain abdominal radiograph (kidney, ureter and bladder, KUB) is performed as part of a renal tract ultrasound scan to look for renal stones and bone abnormalities.

Intravenous urogram

This invasive technique, also referred to as the intravenous pyelogram (IVP), involves injection of an intravenous bolus of an iodine-based radio-opaque solution (Conray or Hypaque) and taking sequential radiographs using ionizing radiation. To obtain the best concentration of the contrast in the kidneys, the patient may be dehydrated for a few hours before the test.

A plain abdominal radiograph or 'scout' film is taken initially to identify any renal stones that may be later obscured by contrast and to assess the bony skeleton for abnormalities. Following the injection of intravenous contrast, radiographs are taken at 5 and 15 min. After a further 20 min, a further film is taken to demonstrate the KUB. Further films may be taken

if particular features need to be assessed, for example oblique films or delayed films. Finally, the patient is asked to void and a post-micturition film is taken. If there is delayed renal function due to an obstructive hydronephrosis, films at 12 or 24 h can be taken to demonstrate contrast at the level of obstruction.

Uses

- Crude assessment of renal function can demonstrate a non-functioning kidney.
- Anatomical demonstration of renal pelvis and calyces. Distortion may indicate a renal mass.
- Demonstration of hydronephrosis and the level of any obstruction.

Disadvantages

- Invasive and uses ionizing radiation.
- Can miss renal masses and does not differentiate between solid and cystic lesions.
- Limited use in renal failure, due to poor renal function or perfusion.

Computed tomography scan

In computed tomography (CT) scanning, a thin, collimated X-ray beam is directed through the patient and images are detected via a series of X-ray detectors arranged circumferentially. It provides an excellent method of staging renal, ureteric and bladder cancers. Although also used to stage prostate cancer, it remains relatively inaccurate.

Intravenous contrast can be administered to demonstrate functioning renal tissue. The timing of image acquisition, relative to the contrast injection, can be used to determine whether renal masses enhance and by measuring the relative tissue densities on the scan (Hounsfield units), fat, fluid and blood can be accurately differentiated (Figure 25.3). This allows renal lesions such as angiomyolipoma and haemangioma to be identified. CT scanning is the ideal way of demonstrating a retroperitoneal or pelvic collection of pus and oral contrast agents can be used to opacify small bowel and differentiate it from lymph nodes.

In some hospitals, CT scanning is also beginning to replace conventional intravenous urogram (IVU) in the initial diagnosis of acute loin pain, in patients with suspected renal or ureteric stones. The advantage of this technique over the IVU is that radiolucent stones may be detected that may not be seen on plain films.

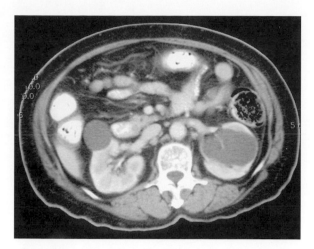

Figure 25.3 CT scan demonstrating bilateral renal cysts.

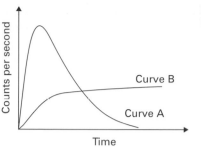

Figure 25.4
Renogram curve.

The scan is usually performed without contrast and will detect a greater proportion of calculi than plain X-rays. It involves a radiation exposure similar to a standard IVU series and is considered to be the best investigation for detecting renal and ureteric stones. If no stones are present a CT scan will often provide information about the differential diagnoses of acute abdominal pain such as a ruptured abdominal aortic aneursym.

Magnetic resonance scan

By employing a strong electromagnetic field, small magnetic changes can be stimulated in body tissues and the signal generated when the dipole is lost can be detected and measured. This non-invasive method of imaging is excellent at staging certain urological tumours, including prostate cancer. Lymph nodes can also be well demonstrated.

Using catheters

Micturating cystoureterogram

A catheter is passed into the bladder and the urine drained out. Contrast is used to fill the bladder. The catheter is removed and the patient positioned to allow radiographical screening of the KUB during voiding. This allows an assessment of ureteric reflux to be made.

Retrograde ureterogram

This is usually performed under general anaesthesia in the operating theatre. A ureteric catheter is passed, via a cystoscope, into the ureteric orifice and contrast injected directly up the ureter. Using radiographical

screening the flow of contrast into the ureter is demonstrated and any obstruction or filling defects shown.

Antegrade ureterogram

Contrast is injected via a percutaneous nephrostomy tube during radiographical screening, to demonstrate any hold-up to the free flow of contrast down the ureter.

Urethrogram

This is performed to assess a urethral stricture or, in cases of trauma, to assess rupture. Contrast is injected down a metal probe or catheter passed into the meatus and radiographs are taken.

Vasogram

This test demonstrates vasal obstruction in an infertile (azoospermic) male. Under a general anaesthetic the vas is identified either percutaneously or after a scrotal incision. A fine needle is passed into the lumen and contrast is injected antegradely. A radiograph will demonstrate contrast in the seminal vesicles if there is no obstruction.

Functional tests

Nuclear isotope renography

The compound mercaptoacetyltriglycine (MAG 3) labelled with an isotope of technetium is now the most commonly used agent for renography. An intravenous bolus is given and the uptake and rate of excretion by the kidneys are measured, by the rise and fall of radioactive activity, using a gamma camera placed posteriorly against the patient's back. In Figure 25.4, curve A shows a rapid uptake by the kidney to a maximum with a smooth decay as the isotope is excreted with the urine. Curve B shows a reduced uptake suggesting reduced renal function. However, no fall in the curve is seen. This is characteristic of an obstructed kidney,

463

where the urine containing the isotope is not excreted. Classically, this pattern is seen in a PUJ obstruction. Occasionally, urine production is poor and the isotope is excreted slowly or the calyces and renal pelvis are dilated and baggy and take a long time to fill. An intravenous diuretic is routinely given to increase urine (and isotope) excretion and determine whether the delay in excretion is due to an obstruction. The relative differential function of the kidneys can be assessed from the renogram (e.g. 60% right and 40% left). However, to assess the absolute function of each kidney, the GFR must be measured and this is not usually assessed using MAG 3. An alternative technetium-labelled compound used in evaluating renal function and obstruction is diethylenetriaminepentaacetic acid (DTPA).

Chromium ethylenediaminetetraacetic acid clearance

Ethylenediaminetetraacetic acid (EDTA) labelled with a radioactive isotope of chromium is given intravenously and measurement of blood and urine concentration gives a close approximation to the GFR. The agent is filtered at the glomerulus only, with little or no tubular secretion occurring. It therefore provides a quick and convenient test of GFR.

Dimercaptosuccinic acid renogram

This agent is both filtered and resorbed by the kidney. It has high cortical fixation and is therefore the agent of choice for renal cortical imaging in cases of acute pyelonephritis and renal scarring. A non-functioning obstructed kidney can also have its tubular function assessed by a static renogram using technetium-labelled dimercaptosuccinic acid (DMSA).

Bone scan

Radioisotope bone scanning, using technetium-99 m tracer, is the standard method for assessing potential bone metastases from prostate cancer. With widespread bone metastases, a so-called superscan image may be seen. This superscan demonstrates high uptake throughout the skeleton, with poor or absent renal excretion of the isotope. Although used particularly for patients with prostatic cancer, bladder and renal cancer can also metastasize to bone.

Urodynamics

The purpose of a UDS evaluation is to provide a pathophysiological diagnosis for a patient's voiding symp-

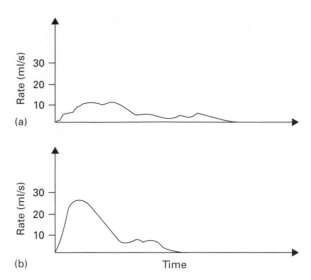

Figure 25.5 Urine flowmetry: (a) obstructed flow or poor detrusor muscle contraction and (b) non-obstructed flow.

toms. In addition, it is often possible to reproduce their symptoms at the time of performing UDS. There are various aspects to a UDS assessment, but not every patient will require all the tests.

Urine flow test

This is the simplest form of UDS assessment and provides an objective measurement of urine flow. A reduced flow may indicate outflow obstruction or poor detrusor muscle contraction. Urine is voided directly onto a motor-driven rotating disc. The change in electrical impedance induced by the stream of urine is plotted by a pen recorder previously calibrated to give a curve of rate of voiding in ml/s against time (Figure 25.5). Flow testing is usually combined with an ultrasound measurement of residual urinary volume, which is frequently elevated when flow rates are reduced. Whilst urine flow tests can identify a low flow rate in a man, it is not possible to tell whether this is due to a poorly contractile bladder or bladder outflow obstructions. Further evaluation, in the form of cystometry, can help distinguish the cause.

Cystometry and pressure flow studies

Cystometry is used to evaluate the storage phase of voiding by recording the bladder pressure during filling. Pressure flow studies record the bladder pressure during voiding thus cystometry and pressure flow studies enable a determination of the pressure–volume relationship of bladder function. To measure the bladder pressure a thin catheter is passed into the bladder and is attached to a fluid pressure transducer. To record abdominal pressure, a similar catheter attached to a second transducer is placed in the rectum and the two signals are subtracted electronically to give a pure reading of the detrusor pressure. The difference between the two is the intravesical pressure generated by the contracting bladder. The filling phase allows diagnosis of detrusor overactivity and reduced compliance, whereas the voiding phase looks at flow and detrusor pressures (p_{det}), allowing diagnosis of obstruction. The poor flow rate curve (Figure 25.5a) is most commonly seen in men with BOO due to prostatic disease. However, a poorly contracting detrusor muscle can result in a similar flow pattern. A simultaneous measurement of the flow rate plotted against intravesical pressure will demonstrate the cause of the poor flow.

Videourodynamics cystometrogram

This combines the pressure and flow measurements of a videourodynamics (VUDS) cystometrogram together with radiographical screening of contrast in the bladder during filling and voiding. The images are recorded on videotape and can be analysed after the test. The technique allows additional useful information to be obtained such as degree of bladder neck opening and descent, the presence of any vesicoureteric reflux (VUR) and the shape/calibre of the urethra.

Endoscopic examination

Cystourethroscopy

By direct visualization of the urethra and bladder, stones or tumour can be identified directly. This may be done under local anaesthesia, but with general anaesthesia therapeutic procedures can also be carried out, for example fragmentation of bladder stones or transurethral resection of bladder tumours (TURBT).

Ureteroscopy and renoscopy

Ureteroscopy is defined as upper urinary tract endoscopy (ureteroscopy) and is performed most commonly with an endoscope passed through the urethra, bladder and then directly into the ureter. Indications for ureteroscopy have broadened from diagnostic endoscopy and now include a variety of additional minimally invasive therapies. Flexible ureteroscopes are a recent development, allowing improved access to the upper ureter and kidney, but more limited therapeutic options due to their smaller size.

Endoscopic stone fragmentation, treatment of upper urinary tract urothelial malignancies, division of strictures and treatment of PUJ obstructions (PUJO) are all current treatments facilitated by contemporary ureteroscopic techniques. To achieve stone fragmentation and tissue fulguration, it is possible to use standard monopolar diathermy, various types of laser and other lithoclastic modalities. With this progression of ureteroscopic procedures from diagnostic to more complex therapeutic interventions, one would expect a proportional increase in the rate and severity of complications. However, with improved instrumentation and an evolution of surgical technique, the complication rate from most procedures has decreased significantly.

Investigation of common urological conditions

Haematuria

Macroscopic haematuria always requires investigation. However, the evaluation of patients with microscopic (or dipstick) haematuria is more controversial, but in general should be investigated in individuals over 40 years of age. A typical haematuria evaluation will include the following investigations:

- An MSSU is sent for microscopy, culture and sensitivities to demonstrate any urinary infection.
- Urine may be sent for cytology where TCC is suspected. A positive result is helpful, but malignancy is not excluded by a negative result.
- All patients must have a cystoscopy. With modern flexible cystoscopes, this can be performed under local anaesthesia and with open-access haematuria clinics it is often done at the time the patient is first seen, along with the additional imaging investigations.
- Imaging the upper tract presents some difficulties. An ultrasound scan is non-invasive and excellent at identifying a renal mass. However, urothelial lesions may be missed. An IVU will show the collecting system and ureter but is not as reliable at demonstrating a renal mass. If in doubt both tests should be performed.
- Blood tests to demonstrate a normal haemoglobin and renal function are necessary and in certain patients the PSA will be measured.

Urine outflow obstruction

- An MSSU is sent and the urine examined with a dipstick to exclude microscopic haematuria or urine tract infection.
- Flow rate is tested to determine maximum flow rate and voided volume.
- An ultrasound scan of the bladder is done to measure the post-micturition residual urine. The upper tracts should also be scanned for hydronephrosis if there is any evidence of renal failure.
- Blood tests are done for haemoglobin and of renal function. The PSA level should also be determined as a raised level may be suggestive of prostate cancer which requires further investigation. PSA may also be increased in a large, benign prostate gland.
- Plain abdominal radiograph may be taken if bladder or renal tract stones are suspected.
- A frequency–volume chart and/or IPSS questionnaire is completed.

Urinary incontinence

- A urine culture should be performed to exclude a UTI.
- Stress incontinence in women can often be demonstrated at physical examination by getting the patient to cough whilst observing the urethral meatus. This test can be quantified using the pad test: the female patient is fitted with a dry, weighed sanitary towel and then given fluid to drink and standardized exercises to perform. The pad is weighed at the end of the test to measure the urine lost.
- A frequency–volume chart is a useful tool to evaluate fluid intake, number of voids, voided volume and number of wet episodes.
- An ultrasound scan of the bladder will demonstrate whether the bladder fails to empty on voiding.
- If the incontinence is associated with urgency, then detrusor overactivity is likely and UDS may be helpful.

Urinary stones

- Ideally send the stone for biochemical analysis.
- Serum calcium is measured to identify hyperparathyroidism.

- 24-h urine collection for calcium, uric acid and oxalate should be performed in recurrent stone formers. Cystinuria should also be excluded, but is very uncommon.

Loin pain

- A plain abdominal radiograph may identify a possible stone and this should be confirmed by an IVU or CT urogram.
- Urinalysis for blood: this will usually be present if a stone is passing down the ureter.
- If the loin pain is less acute, or exposure to ionizing radiation contraindicated, an ultrasound scan of the kidney will demonstrate any hydronephrosis or renal masses.

Urinary infection

- Urine should be sent for microscopy and culture and the infection treated with appropriate antibiotics.
- It is usually appropriate to establish the likely cause of an infection. A haematuria evaluation should be performed if indicated (see above). In young girls, reflux may be a cause of recurrent UTI and a micturating cystoureterogram (MCUG) may be required.

A number of conditions that were hitherto diagnosed when patients developed symptoms are now detected as incidental findings, or during routine (or selective) screening. The two main urological conditions to which this applies are detection of early prostate cancer and the detection of asymptomatic renal tumours as incidental findings during the investigation of other conditions. The significance of this change is that the conditions are now being diagnosed at an earlier stage, which has implications for both treatment and prognosis.

Common diseases and their treatment

Kidney

Inflammation

Pyelonephritis

This is a urine infection leading to inflammation of the kidney. Clinically it is associated with a high temperature, rigors and vomiting. In recurrent cases renal scarring may occur, particularly if the infections occur in childhood.

Glomerulonephritis

Acute glomerulonephritis is the term applied to a wide range of renal disease, in which an immunological mechanism triggers inflammation and proliferation of glomerular tissue. The condition can occur following a streptococcal throat infection and may present as a sudden onset of haematuria and proteinuria. This clinical picture often is accompanied by hypertension, oedema and impaired renal function. Other types of glomerulonephritis have an unknown aetiology and are usually more gradual in onset, with slowly developing renal impairment. Microscopic haematuria can be a feature; these conditions all require expert management by nephrologists.

Stones

Stone formation occurs as a result of an imbalance between the solubility of salts and their crystallization. In the Western world, 70–80% of stones are composed of calcium oxalate. Ureteric stones form initially in a renal papilla from a small submucosal concretion. As the crystallization increases, it separates from the papilla and passes into the collecting system with the urine. Before they pass into the calyces, such stones are seldom symptomatic. Conversely, a staghorn renal calculus that fills the renal pelvis and calyces is formed within the collecting system. Such stones are often seen with urine chronically infected with *Proteus mirabilis*. This bacterium splits urea to ammonia, alkalinizes the urine and precipitates magnesium ammonia phosphate. This becomes calcified and the stone may form a complete cast of the collecting system.

Treatment

Patients with stones in the ureter usually present acutely, with severe loin pain ('renal colic'). The majority of these stones are <5 mm in diameter and will pass spontaneously. Medical treatment in the form of alpha-blockers may improve stone-passage rates. However, larger ureteric stones often require surgical intervention. Various techniques can be utilized, but ureteroscopy and fragmentation (using a laser) is the most widely used, along with ESWL in certain situations.

Small kidney stones can be fragmented by extracorporeal shock-wave lithotripsy (ESWL). The technique uses a machine to generate shock waves, which are focused through the skin and body tissues onto the dense stones, leading to fragmentation. It requires analgesia and careful monitoring afterwards to ensure the stone fragments pass down the ureter satisfactorily.

Direct access to the renal collecting system via a percutaneous tract can allow larger stones to be removed endoscopically – known as percutaneous nephrolithotomy (PCNL).

Staghorn stones represent a surgical challenge. If there is minimal renal function, then a nephrectomy may be the best way of eradicating the stone and the recurring urine infections. If renal function is good, percutaneous removal of the stone (PCNL) can be attempted. Sometimes fragments remain and these can be removed using ureteroscopy and appropriate fragmentation techniques, such as the laser (see above), or ESWL. Any remaining fragments may act as a nucleus for new stone formation and will act as a reservoir for continuing infection.

The management of patients with a ureteric stone causing obstruction and in whom the urine becomes infected represents a urological emergency. Urgent decompression of the infected and obstructed kidney is required by insertion of a percutaneous nephrostomy, or placement of a ureteric stent to 'bypass' the obstruction and allow drainage of the infected urine.

Tumour

Adenocarcinoma

Adenocarcinoma of the kidney (also known as renal cell carcinoma) is the most common type of renal tumour. It can occur at any age, but is commonest in the sixth and seventh decade. About 60% of cases occur in men. Presenting symptoms can include haematuria, loin pain or a palpable mass. However, an increasing number of renal tumours are now diagnosed as incidental findings on CT or ultrasound scan, following investigation for other conditions (Figure 25.6). Occasionally, a tumour will present with a paraneoplastic phenomena, such as thromboembolism, polycythaemia or anaemia. The primary tumour may metastasize directly to adjacent lymph nodes and the adrenal gland or distantly to the lungs and occasionally bone.

Treatment of renal cell carcinoma depends on its stage, at presentation. If the tumour is confined to the kidney, radical nephrectomy (removing the kidney, perinephric fat and adrenal gland) is frequently curative. The operation can be performed using the

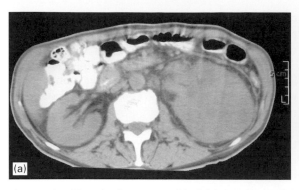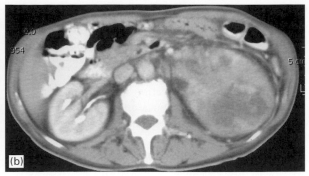

Figure 25.6 CT: renal cell carcinoma of the left kidney showing (a) pre- and (b) post-contrast images.

traditional open approach, or via a minimally invasive laparoscopic approach. In addition, small, peripherally placed tumours may be amenable to removal by partial nephrectomy or enucleation. If the cancer has spread beyond the capsule of the kidney, or has metastasized, the disease is usually incurable. The cancer does not respond to radiotherapy, although palliation from painful bony metastases can sometimes be achieved with localized irradiation. Immunotherapy, using agents such as alpha-interferon and interleukin-2, has been shown to increase median survival, but is not curative. Recently novel drugs acting as angiogenesis inhibitors (e.g. sorafenib, sunitinib, bavacizumab and temsiolimus) have been used to treat metastatic renal cell carcinoma and have been shown to increase progression-free survival.

Transitional cell carcinoma

This uncommon tumour may be associated with an existing bladder TCC. The condition may present as haematuria, 'clot colic' or be found incidentally, or during surveillance of a patient with known bladder cancer. Treatment for a localized tumour is nephroureterectomy. Metastatic disease is incurable and treated symptomatically.

Wilms' tumour

For more details refer to Chapter 30. Wilms' tumour (malignant nephroblastoma) is an uncommon tumour of young children. It usually presents as an abdominal mass in a child under the age of 5 years. The majority of cases are curable with a combination of surgery, chemotherapy and radiotherapy and it requires expert management in a paediatric oncology unit.

Trauma

For more details refer to Chapter 16.

Blunt trauma

Renal trauma is often associated with multiple injuries, particularly blunt trauma. Management should initially be aimed at resuscitation, using Advanced Trauma Life Support (ATLS®) algorithms. The vast majority of patients with isolated renal trauma can be managed conservatively and do not require surgery. Radiological evaluation (usually in the form of CT) should be performed in a patient with haematuria and hypotension, or those with significant associated injuries. Patients with microscopic haematuria and who are normotensive have a low likelihood of significant injury. Management of a damaged solitary kidney requires greater effort to preserve it. Although surgical exploration of a bleeding kidney is occasionally necessary, it is not uncommon to find the bleeding impossible to stop and nephrectomy is then required. Complications following renal trauma are rare, but include urinoma, delayed haemorrhage, arteriovenous (A-V) fistula formation and occasionally hypertension.

Penetrating trauma

A renal injury from a knife or bullet wound is more likely to require surgical exploration; however, selected, isolated penetrating renal injury can be treated conservatively.

Renal failure

Acute renal failure

This may be caused by:

- pre-renal factors (e.g. hypotension)
- renal factors (e.g. glomerulonephritis)

- post-renal factors (the clinical situation most commonly presenting to the urologist) (e.g. bilateral obstructive uropathy).

An obstruction causing a sudden complete blockage of two previously normal kidneys is uncommon (e.g. bilateral ureteric stones). The sudden presentation of anuria, dehydration and abnormal biochemistry is more often due to a chronic condition causing the long-term partial obstruction of the kidneys; for example, backpressure from a chronically distended bladder, or malignant obstruction from a carcinoma of the prostate in men, or carcinoma of the cervix in women.

Clinically, the patient is often confused and disoriented. Fluid balance is abnormal either with oedema and heart failure due to overload or dehydration from vomiting. The serum urea and creatinine will be raised and when the obstruction is released, a dramatic osmotic diuresis can occur, placing the patient in danger of dehydration unless careful fluid balance is maintained. The serum potassium may be raised and this can cause cardiac dysrhythmias and death. The potassium level must be treated urgently, either by dialysis or short-term measures such as shifting the potassium from the serum back into the cells using glucose and insulin intravenously, or calcium resonium to absorb it directly from the gut.

Patients with an obstructive cause of anuria should be catheterized to allow any urine in the bladder to be drained and any potential backpressure on the kidneys to be released. Any urine that is then produced can be measured accurately. A renal ultrasound scan will demonstrate a hydronephrosis and percutaneous placement of a nephrostomy tube will bypass the obstruction and allow the renal function to recover. Once the renal function is stable, the management of the cause of the obstruction can be planned.

Chronic renal failure

Renal damage from such causes as diabetic nephropathy, glomerulonephritis, polycystic renal disease or poor recovery from a treated obstructive uropathy can lead to permanent loss of renal function. The remaining renal tissue may then be inadequate for normal biochemical and fluid homoeostasis. A diet low in protein to reduce nitrogen products (urea) for excretion, along with fluid restriction will help limit the need for dialysis. Secondary effects of chronic renal failure, including anaemia, hypertension and osteoporo-

sis, must also be controlled with drugs such as erythropoietin (to stimulate erythropoiesis) and angiotensin-converting enzyme (ACE) inhibitors. Nephrotoxic drugs including gentamicin and non-steroidal anti-inflammatory drugs (NSAIDS) should also be avoided. With end-stage renal failure (ESRF) the renal function eventually becomes inadequate to maintain haemostasis and the patient requires dialysis or renal transplantation.

Dialysis

The principle of dialysis is to allow diffusion of water, electrolytes and waste products in the blood across a semi-permeable membrane into a solution that can then be discarded.

In peritoneal dialysis, the solution is run into the peritoneal cavity via an abdominally placed catheter. Diffusion takes place across the peritoneum, which acts as the membrane. The fluid is then drained out via the catheter and the process repeated until the biochemical status of the patient is satisfactory. This may take several hours and must be performed daily.

In haemodialysis, blood is circulated through filters. The blood flows across a semi-permeable membrane (the dialyser or filter), along with solutions that help remove toxins. Haemodialysis requires a blood flow of 400–500 ml/min and a standard intravenous line in an arm or leg cannot support that amount of flow. Therefore, in long-term haemodialysis, an arteriovenous fistula is surgically formed, for example between the radial artery and cephalic vein at the wrist. Dilated veins with fast-flowing blood open up in the arm and by direct puncture blood can be drawn off into the dialysis machine and then run back into an adjacent puncture site. Anticoagulation is required to prevent clotting during dialysis.

Transplantation

The natural response of the body to foreign tissue is to reject it, by way of an immune response. In kidney transplantation, the best immunologically matched kidney to the patient's own tissues is selected to reduce rejection and immunosuppressor drugs are used to 'damp down' the normal immune response.

The kidney donor's blood and tissue are matched as closely as possible with the recipient's blood ABO and major histocompatibility complex (MHC) antigens to reduce the risk of subsequent graft rejection.

The donor kidney is placed in the right or left iliac fossa and the renal vessels are anastomosed end-to-side to the external iliac vessels or end-to-end to the internal iliac vessels. The ureter is implanted directly into the bladder. Immunosuppression is achieved using a combination of drugs, including cyclosporin/tacrolimus, OKT3® (monoclonal antibody), azathioprine and prednisolone. Despite these precautions, acute rejection is frequently seen in the months following transplantation and the transplanted kidney occasionally has to be removed. Some patients also suffer from chronic rejection, where the initially good renal function deteriorates over several years until the patient develops chronic renal failure again and must return to dialysis.

Ureter

Reflux

If the anti-reflux valve mechanism at the VUJ is ineffective, urine will reflux up the ureter when the bladder contracts during voiding. When the bladder is empty and relaxes, the refluxed urine in the ureters refills the bladder, so giving an effective residual volume that can become infected and lead to recurrent urine infections. Refluxing urine can lead to pressure damage in the kidney and infected urine can lead to pyelonephritis, both of which may lead to renal scarring and renal tubular damage, particularly if it occurs in childhood. This condition is a developmental anomaly and is seen in children when the kidneys are still growing and are most susceptible to damage.

Reflux can be demonstrated by a MCUG. Most cases may be managed by prophylactic antibiotics to prevent the complications of infections and as the child grows the anti-reflux valve mechanism may improve. For those with severe or persistent reflux, a surgical operation to re-implant the ureter obliquely in the bladder wall or endoscopic injection of bulking agents into the area of the ureteric orifice can be employed. For children with severe reflux, renal damage can be irreversible and chronic renal failure may develop.

Hydronephrosis

This term is used to describe a dilated renal pelvis. It is also used to describe a dilated pelvis and ureter, although technically this is hydronephroureterosis. A hydronephrosis may be obstructive or non-obstructive.

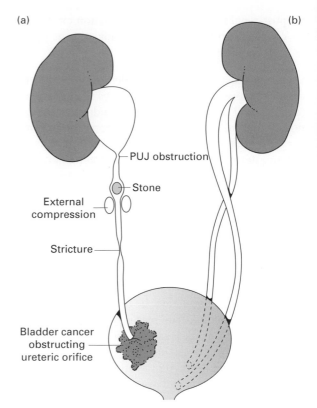

Figure 25.7 (a) Kidney showing sites of possible ureteric obstruction and (b) kidney with duplex ureters.

Obstructive hydronephrosis

A ureter may be obstructed in four different ways (Figure 25.7):

1. A mass within the lumen: a ureteric stone, blood clot or sloughed necrotic papilla may all get stuck within the ureter and cause obstruction. A tumour is a cause of 'mass within the lumen' and failure of normal ureteric peristalsis in the region of the PUJ leads to classical PUJ obstruction.
2. Narrowing of the wall: a stricture may result from previous surgery such as ureteroscopy or damage at open surgery (e.g. anterior resection). Fibrotic narrowing is seen as a result of chronic inflammatory conditions, such as renal tuberculosis and schistosomiasis.
3. Pressure from outside compressing the ureter: metastatic lymph nodes or retroperitoneal fibrosis (RPF) can result in ureteric obstruction.
4. A mass at the end of the ureter obstructing outflow of urine: a bladder carcinoma or prostate carcinoma infiltrating the trigone of the bladder

can occlude the ureteric orifice. In women, carcinoma of the cervix can cause a similar effect. A chronically distended bladder (due to benign prostatic hypertrophy (BPH) or urethral stricture) can cause backpressure and hydronephrosis.

Non-obstructive hydronephrosis

A dilated renal pelvis and ureter may be chronically distended rather than obstructed (e.g. VUR may produce a distended system). Following corrective surgery for a PUJ obstruction the hydronephrosis may seem unchanged, but prompt drainage will be demonstrated by renography. The congenital megaureter is another example of a dilated, but not obstructed ureter.

Investigation of hydronephrosis

Ultrasonography will confirm the presence of a dilated system and an IVU may reveal the level of the obstruction. Isotope renography, using MAG 3, gives a functional measure of renal excretion and drainage and is an accurate way of quantifying obstruction, but will not show the anatomical level of obstruction.

If an obstructive cause is suspected, a cystoscopy and retrograde ureteropyelogram (RGPG) will confirm the site of obstruction and often gives an indication as to the cause of the obstruction. If an RGPG fails, percutaneous nephrostomy and antegrade ureterography usually demonstrates the level and cause of obstruction reliably.

At the time of imaging it is possible to place an indwelling ureteric stent. This is a hollow plastic tube with a draining hole along its length and ends that curl up, hence the name double pigtail or double J® stent. This may be placed retrogradely or antegradely along the ureter from the renal pelvis to the bladder, effectively bypassing the obstruction. Further treatment will depend on the cause of the hydronephrosis.

Alternatively, in some circumstances, CT and MRI scanning may be used to diagnose the site and cause of an obstruction, particularly for conditions in and around the kidney.

Tumour

A TCC occasionally develops in the ureter or renal pelvis, and the tumour may cause haematuria and ureteric obstruction. Invasion can occur early because of the thin ureteric wall, resulting in lymph node metastases. Surgical treatment in the form of a nephroureterectomy is the usual treatment, but low-grade upper tract TCCs are increasingly being treated with endoscopic ablation and regular surveillance.

Stones

Ureteric colic due to a stone passing down the ureter is one of the commonest urological emergencies. The severe pain must be distinguished from the pain of biliary colic or a ruptured abdominal aortic aneurysm (AAA) and therefore a CT KUB scan or IVU is needed to confirm the diagnosis and establish the level the stone has reached. Pain relief using NSAIDS or opiates is usually effective.

Around 70% of ureteric stones of 5 mm or less in size will pass spontaneously. Passage of smaller stones may be facilitated by the use of alpha-blocker medication, which serves to relax the smooth muscle in the ureter. However, ureteric obstruction is not uncommon. Urgent relief of this obstruction is essential if the system becomes infected and this is achieved with percutaneous nephrostomy or retrograde placement of a ureteric stent. If the stone fails to progress, direct ureteroscopic manipulation and fragmentation (using a laser or lithoclast) is possible. Direct treatment of a ureteric stone by ESWL, although possible, has variable success.

Trauma

Injury to the ureter is most commonly the result of surgical intervention. Damage during ureteroscopy or bowel or gynaecological surgery is well recognized. Partial injures may be managed by ureteric stenting or the insertion of a nephrostomy tube, thus diverting urine. End-to-end re-anastomosis of the ureter is possible if little or no length has been lost. If the ureter is damaged close to the bladder, re-implantation is usually preferred. If the damage is higher with significant loss of ureter, a Boari flap, using a flap of bladder or direct anastomosis to the normal ureter on the other side (a transuretero-ureterostomy), will deal with the problem. The anastomosis should be stented with a ureteric stent until it has healed (Figure 25.8).

PUJ obstruction (PUJO)

Classical PUJO is due to abnormal ureteric peristalsis at the PUJ, or to external compression by vessel adjacent to the PUJ. This obstruction may be intermittent, precipitated by drinking large volumes of fluid. Surgery to widen the drainage through the PUJ and excise the redundant dilated portion of renal pelvis (pyeloplasty) is generally effective at relieving

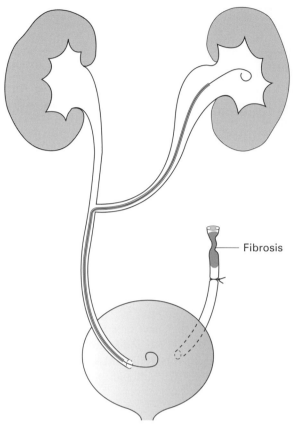

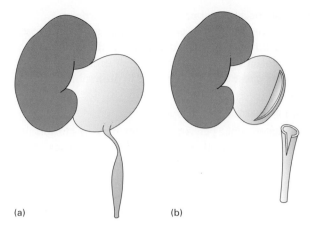

Figure 25.9 Anderson–Hynes dismembered pyeloplasty: (a) PUJ obstruction with hydronephrosis and (b) a contractile segment of ureter is excised and the ureter spatulated to anastomose to the trimmed renal pelvis.

Figure 25.8 Transuretero-ureterostomy with an indwelling double J® ureteric stent across the anastomosis from the bladder to the pelvis of the affected kidney.

the symptoms (Figure 25.9). Surgery can be carried out through a standard loin incision, or laparoscopically. Various minimally invasive endoscopic techniques are also used, but these tend to have lower success rates.

Bladder

Inflammation

Cystitis (inflammation of the bladder) may be caused by infection, mechanical trauma (e.g. stone or catheter), malignant disease (e.g. carcinoma *in situ* of the bladder), radiotherapy or intravesical chemotherapy. The symptoms are pain and frequency of voiding. An uncommon inflammatory condition is interstitial cystitis, which may form part of a painful bladder syndrome. In this condition, which is commoner in women, none of the above causes is demonstrated, but histologically the bladder biopsy shows an excess of mast cells, thought to release histamine, so causing inflammation. Treatment is

symptomatic, although agents such as intravesical dimethyl sulphoxide (DMSO), pentosan polysulphate (Elmiron) and regular cystodistension are used with some success.

The symptoms of cystitis are also seen in young women who have recently become sexually active. Some of the discomfort probably arises as a result of mild trauma to the urethra, giving the sensation of a constant urge to void ('honeymoon cystitis').

Stones

Bladder stones are seen most commonly in developing countries and this may be linked to diet and increased prevalence of UTI. In more affluent countries, most bladder stones develop as a result of urinary stasis, due to BOO, or in neurogenic bladders (e.g. following spinal injury).

Like all stones, those in the bladder may give rise to haematuria, urinary infections, pain and sepsis. Many stones can be fragmented and removed endoscopically, although large stones may have to be removed at open surgery (cystolithotomy). In men with outflow obstruction, it is often necessary to improve voiding and reduce subsequent urinary stasis, by performing a TURP.

Tumour

The commonest bladder cancer type is a transitional cell carcinoma (TCC). In countries where schistosomiasis is endemic, squamous carcinoma of the bladder is common. Adenocarcinoma is rare.

Transitional cell carcinoma

Classically, a TCC presents with painless haematuria, although urine infection is also commonly seen. Cystoscopy allows a biopsy to confirm the diagnosis and a resection biopsy of the base of the tumour will allow the pathologist to stage the tumour, by determining whether muscle invasion has occurred.

Treatment depends on the tumour stage and the general fitness of the patient. If the tumour is non-muscle invasive, simple endoscopic resection may be sufficient. This may be combined with adjuvant intravesical instillation of mitomycin C or epirubicin to reduce recurrence rates. Nevertheless, recurrence of new tumours in the bladder is common and so repeat check cystoscopies are necessary. The majority of superficial bladder cancers (>80%) will not progress to muscle invasion. However, they do have a tendency to recur over a period of many years. If a superficial bladder cancer is poorly differentiated and invasion of the lamina propria is demonstrated histologically (G3 pT1), the disease may be treated as though it were muscle invasive, as the disease tends to run a more aggressive course with an increased likelihood of progression to muscle-invasive disease.

If the tumour has invaded the muscle of the bladder wall (pT2), it is termed invasive. Local resection is unlikely to remove the entire tumour and the options for cure are radical radiotherapy or total removal of the bladder by surgery (cystectomy) and a urinary diversion procedure. The use of neoadjuvant chemotherapy has recently been shown to increase survival in patients undergoing radical cystectomy, though its use is limited by concurrent renal impairment and comorbidities. If staging by CT or MRI scans reveal the disease has spread to lymph glands or beyond, the tumour is less likely to be curable and may be managed symptomatically. Adjuvant chemotherapy may be used in an attempt to improve long-term survival following cystectomy.

Adenocarcinoma

Adenocarcinoma of the bladder and squamous carcinoma of the bladder are both treated by cystectomy, if they are not metastatic, as they are both resistant to radiotherapy.

Urine diversion

Urine may be diverted using segments of bowel anastomosed to the ureters. These techniques may be

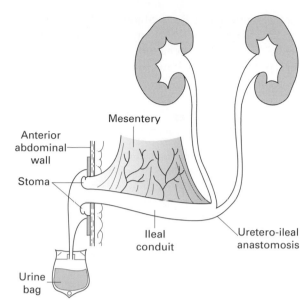

Figure 25.10 Ileal conduit urine diversion.

described as non-continent or continent diversions. In the UK, the most commonly performed non-continent urine diversion is an ileal conduit (Figure 25.10). A segment of small bowel is isolated, along with its blood supply. The divided ends of the remaining ileum are anastomosed to maintain bowel continuity. The cut ends of the ureters are implanted into one end of the ileal conduit and the other end brought out as a stoma (urostomy) on the right side of the abdomen. A stoma bag is then applied to collect the urine.

Continent urinary diversions include neobladder formation and Mitrofanoff formation. In a neobladder, bowel is used to create a new reservoir, or neobladder. The 'orthotopic bladder' can be anastomosed to the urethra and if the sphincter mechanism is preserved, controlled voiding in the normal way is usually possible. In a Mitrofanoff diversion the bowel urine reservoir can be drained onto the abdominal wall via a narrow lumen tube such as the appendix. Its closing pressure is such that the urine storage reservoir is continent and it is drained by the patient catheterizing the reservoir, via the stoma.

Trauma

For more details, see also Chapter 16.

Blunt abdominal trauma will produce the most dramatic effect if the bladder is full at the time. Rupture of the bladder frequently results and this will usually require surgical repair. Pelvic fractures may also rupture the bladder. Resuscitation of the patient and careful assessment of the bony injuries are required before the bladder is repaired. Catheterization, via a suprapubic cystotomy if necessary, will be required in the interim.

Functional abnormalities

Detrusor overactivity

An OAB may be seen in patients with intravesical inflammation (e.g. due to UTI or bladder stones) or as a result of neurological pathology causing overactivity of the detrusor muscle. The condition also occurs secondary to BOO. A third group has primary detrusor overactivity. They are neurologically intact, have a normal bladder capacity, but have symptoms of urine frequency, urgency and sometimes urge incontinence. A UDS demonstrates high detrusor pressure contractions at small bladder volumes.

Medical treatment aims to 'paralyse' the detrusor by blocking cholinergic receptors using anticholinergic drugs. Commonly used drugs include oxybutynin, tolterodine and trospium. As a result of generalized anticholinergic activity, side effects of these drugs are common and include dizziness, blurred vision and a dry mouth. Where medical treatment of OAB has failed, or if side effects are not tolerated, a patient may be considered for intradetrusor injections of botulinum A toxin. This has been shown to be efficacious in the short term; however, there are limited data regarding long-term outcome and treatment frequently needs to be repeated. Sacral nerve neuromodulation is also emerging as a potential treatment for cases refractory to drug therapy.

Occasionally, surgical treatment may be necessary if medical treatments fail or are not tolerated. Surgical treatment also aims to paralyse part of the detrusor muscle, as well as improve bladder compliance and capacity. This is achieved by cutting the bladder in half and then resuturing it with an interposing opened length of ileum in the opened bladder (clam ileocystoplasty). As a last resort, urinary diversion with an ileal conduit may be successful.

Detrusor underactivity and failure

Chronic retention of urine or the end stage of neurological diseases, such as diabetic neuropathy or multiple sclerosis, may result in the bladder becoming a flaccid, acontractile bag able to store urine, but unable to contract to expel it. Occasionally, long-term indwelling catheter drainage will allow the contracted bladder to regain some muscular tone. However, intermittent self-catheterization (ISC) is probably the best treatment, if this can be tolerated.

Bladder neck pathology

The internal or bladder neck sphincter is found only in men. Its primary function is to close during ejaculation to prevent the semen passing retrogradely into the bladder. The physiological function of this smooth muscle sphincter is usually compromised following TURP or bladder neck incision (BNI), leading to retrograde ejaculation.

The external sphincter mechanism is involved in maintaining continence. During normal micturition this sphincter relaxes as the detrusor muscle contracts. If this does not take place in a coordinated manner, for example following interruption of spinal micturition pathways after spinal cord injury, the sphincter remains closed, causing detrusor-sphincter dyssynergia (DSD). This can result in high-pressure chronic retention and irreversible obstructive nephropathy. Medical treatment aims to block the adrenergic receptors, using uroselective alpha-blockers (e.g. tamsulosin) to reduce sphincter tone. Surgical treatment consists of endoscopic division of the sphincter, but the patient must be warned about irreversible retrograde ejaculation, following division of the internal sphincter.

Spinal pathology

Spina bifida

Children born with a spinal defect often have neurological problems affecting the lower limbs, bladder and rectum. Many patients have neuropathic bladders and may require surgery because of severe voiding dysfunction. Options include management by an indwelling catheter, ISC or urinary diversion. Due to immobility and chronically poor voiding, renal stone formation and recurrent UTIs are common.

Spinal trauma

Traumatic spinal injury may result in paraplegia and an abnormally functioning bladder. Initially, during spinal shock, there is suppression of autonomic and somatic activity and the bladder becomes acontractile, areflexic and painlessly distended. It must therefore be drained, to prevent overdistension injury. As the neurological lesion stabilizes, reflex voiding may return, but this depends on the level of injury.

Detrusor hyper-reflexia and DSD may also be present. Self-catheterization, a permanent indwelling catheter or urinary diversion are all options. Renal stone disease is common due to immobility and urinary stasis.

Incontinence

The various causes of urinary incontinence have been described above.

Stress urinary incontinence (SUI) is a common problem seen by both urologists and gynaecologists. Risk factors for the condition include female sex, advancing age, childbirth and obesity. Initial treatment is aimed at strengthening the pelvic floor, reducing unnecessary intra-abdominal pressure and trying to elevate the prolapsed urethra. Physiotherapy, in the form of intensive pelvic floor training, to strengthen the pelvic floor structures, together with weight loss and cessation of smoking improve symptoms in at least half of patients. Contemporary surgical treatment options aim to support the urethra and/or elevate the bladder neck and include colposuspension and the use of tension-free mid-urethral slings. Potential complications of these procedures include voiding and sexual dysfunction. In frail patients, a vaginal pessary may be used to support the urethra and bladder neck.

Prostate gland

Inflammation

Prostatitis may be acute or chronic. Symptoms of perineal or rectal discomfort with non-specific urinary symptoms are common. Occasionally, the prostatitis is bacterial and is treated effectively with a fluoroquinolone antibiotic. More often the condition is abacterial and may be described as 'chronic prostatitis associated with chronic pelvic pain syndrome'. This form of prostatitis tends to run a chronic course and symptomatic treatment using NSAIDS and alpha-blockers may be helpful.

Tumour

Benign prostatic enlargement

Although BPE does not necessarily cause BOO, the two are frequently linked and it is common for elderly men with troublesome urinary symptoms to present to the doctor complaining about 'their prostate gland'. Conversely, a patient with classic symptoms of BOO may still have an obstructive prostate, even if the gland feels small on rectal examination.

Many patients reach retirement before they complain of troublesome LUTS, although on direct questioning they may admit to having had LUTS for some years beforehand. A full history and examination along with appropriate tests to confirm the diagnosis is essential. Diagnosis is usually confirmed following exclusion of other conditions (e.g. prostate cancer, urethral strictures) and when flow rate measurement has revealed an obstructed pattern, characteristic of the condition.

The following options are available for the management of BPE.

General supportive advice

A reduction of fluid intake, particularly in the evening, will reduce urine production at night. Voiding twice before going to bed may help to empty the bladder and reduce troublesome nocturia. Reassurance that the patient's symptoms are not due to prostate cancer is usually greeted with relief.

Medical treatment

Alpha-blockers –– The uroselective alpha-1-blockers (e.g. tamsulosin, alfuzosin) now form the mainstay of medical management of BPE. They work by relaxing the smooth muscle around the bladder neck and prostate and so help increase urine flow. They have a rapid onset in alleviating some of the symptoms, but do not cure BPE. The drugs are usually well tolerated, but side effects include lethargy and postural hypotension.

5-Alpha-reductase inhibitors –– These drugs block the enzyme 5-alpha-reductase, which converts testosterone to the active metabolite, dihydrotestosterone, which promotes BPE. Finasteride, taken orally, may take up to 4 months before any reduction in size of the prostate, or improvement in symptoms, is noted. A newer drug in this class is dutasteride, which is said to have a more rapid onset. The drugs are also well tolerated, but the prostate will regrow if treatment is stopped. Side effects include a reduced libido.

Surgical treatment

The commonest operation is TURP, in which the enlarged and obstructing adenoma is excised, using an endoscope and monopolar cutting diathermy loop. A laser can also be used to vaporize the tissue, and this technique may be appropriate in patients with comorbidities or on anticoagulant medication as blood loss may be lower than standard TURP; however, this is a relatively new technique and long-term outcome data are awaited. Bipolar diathermy is also emerging as a surgical technique which allows resection of the prostate gland using saline irrigation fluid, thus theoretically reducing the risk of perioperative complications. Open operations to remove the prostatic adenoma are less commonly performed, but may occasionally be required for very large adenomas. A BNI or transurethral incision of the prostate gland (TUIP) can be performed to release any bladder neck constriction, without removing any prostatic tissue. Several other methods exist to shrink the prostate, using different types of energy. These include thermotherapy and microwave therapy, where the prostate is heated to shrink it.

Cancer

There is a wide range of incidence of adenocarcinoma of the prostate worldwide, but in the West it is the commonest cancer diagnosed in men over 65 years. Symptoms from the primary tumour may be indistinguishable from BPE, hence the importance of palpating the prostate and measuring the PSA in men with LUTS.

To confirm the diagnosis a biopsy (ideally guided by a transrectal ultrasound scanner) is required. The PSA level may be normal in localized prostate cancer, but its level is important to monitor the response of the disease to treatment. It is invariably raised in metastatic prostate cancer.

The cancer most commonly metastasizes to bone and a bone scan is ideal for staging the disease. Both CT and MRI scanning provide important information regarding staging of prostate cancer. CT provides a satisfactory assessment of enlarged lymph nodes and MRI is used to confirm extension of the tumour beyond the capsule of the prostate.

If the tumour is confined to the prostate, curative treatment can be offered in the form of radical external beam radiotherapy, localized implantation of radioactive seeds (brachytherapy) or the surgical removal of the prostate gland and its capsule at open operation (radical prostatectomy). This technically demanding procedure can be performed via a standard open lower abdominal approach, a perineal approach or laparoscopically. It requires the urethra and bladder neck to be joined together when the gland has been removed. Side effects are significant and include erectile dysfunction (ED), urinary incontinence, bladder neck stricturing and damage to the rectum.

Metastatic prostate cancer is incurable, but significant improvements in survival as well as relief of local and systemic symptoms of the disease are seen with androgen deprivation. This may be achieved by bilateral orchidectomy or, more commonly, by the use of drugs. These include gonadotropin-releasing hormone (GnRH) agonists (e.g. Zoladex®), which block the release of gonadotropins from the pituitary gland and thereby inhibit production of testicular testosterone. These drugs are administered by monthly or 3-monthly depot injection. Antiandrogen tablets (e.g. bicalutamide, cyproterone acetate, flutamide) exist but may not represent a satisfactory monotherapy. However, GnRH agonists can be used in combination with antiandrogens to achieve maximum androgen blockade (MAB). Stilboestrol, which blocks the action of testosterone, is less widely used because of side effects, including thromboembolic events, but often gives a useful second-line response when luteinizing hormone-releasing hormone (LHRH) analogue treatment has failed. The use of chemotherapy, using docetaxel, for advanced prostate cancer is currently being investigated, as is the use of GnRH receptor antagonists.

A variable time after introducing hormonal treatment, the cancer will become refractory to this androgen deprivation and it is said to be hormone relapsed. Painful bone secondaries can then be treated by local radiotherapy or analgesics. Treatment is generally symptomatic, although changing the hormonal treatment can sometimes achieve a useful secondary response.

Asymptomatic prostate cancer is a common finding at autopsy in men over 75 years. Elderly or frail men diagnosed with the disease may be best treated conservatively with active monitoring of their disease and treatment of symptoms as they occur.

Testis and scrotum

Inflammation

Orchitis is an acute inflammatory reaction of the testis secondary to infection. Most cases are associated with a viral mumps infection; however, other viruses and bacteria can cause orchitis. Inflammation and swelling of the epididymis is relatively common and there may be associated orchitis – epididymo-orchitis. Usually, a specific organism is not identified, but the swelling and redness gradually resolve. This can be a painful and incapacitating condition, which requires bed rest, analgesics and antibiotic treatment. The symptoms usually develop more slowly than in testicular torsion and the men affected are usually older than the adolescents and young men affected by torsion. However, epididymo-orchitis can mimic a testicular tumour. If there is any doubt, an ultrasound scan may help to differentiate these conditions, but if the diagnosis is still in doubt, urgent scrotal exploration is necessary.

Fournier's gangrene is a rare necrotizing, inflammatory condition of the scrotum seen most commonly in elderly debilitated patients. The condition is also associated with diabetes and may occur following trauma or surgery. Initially a small black necrotic area develops in the scrotum. The inflammation spreads rapidly, due to synergism between aerobic and anaerobic organisms. The subcutaneous tissue becomes necrotic and gas-forming organisms may produce crepitus in the tissues. Urgent high-dose antibiotic treatment and radical surgical debridement of the affected tissues are required.

Swellings

These include:

- hydrocoele
- epididymal cyst
- tumour
- varicocoele
- inguinal hernia
- testicular torsion.

A hydrocoele lies anterior to the testis and will transilluminate. With a large hydrocoele, the testis itself may be difficult to palpate. An epididymal cyst may have multiple septa and lie posterior and superior to the testis, within the epididymis; it may transilluminate.

A hydrocoele can be drained percutaneously with a needle, but commonly recurs. Otherwise all these cystic swellings can be excised surgically, or treated conservatively if the symptoms are minimal. Although they are usually painless, once a patient has noticed them anxiety may make individuals conscious of them. If any doubt exists about whether the underlying testis is malignant, an ultrasound scan is a reliable way of excluding a testicular tumour.

A varicocoele results from the dilated pampiniform veins in the scrotum and cord. These veins can be ligated and divided in the inguinal canal, if they are symptomatic. Alternatively, embolization of the gonadal veins, using metallic coils, can be performed via the femoral vein.

In testicular torsion, the testis twists spontaneously on its spermatic cord, causing venous occlusion and subsequent arterial ischaemia. The majority of testes can be salvaged if scrotal exploration and untwisting of the cord is undertaken within 6 h. The peak age is 14 years, although a smaller peak also occurs in the neonatal period.

The hydatid of Morgagni is a small embryological remnant located at the upper pole of the testis, which can occasionally twist and cause pain. The symptoms can mimic those of true testicular torsion.

Tumours

A solid swelling of the testis is assumed to be malignant until proved otherwise. Often the swelling is painless, but trauma may produce a pain or haemorrhage into the tumour, which can produce a painful inflamed scrotum, mimicking epididymo-orchitis. Diagnosis is greatly helped by testicular ultrasound scanning and the presence of raised tumour markers (AFP, b-HCG).

Occasionally, the tumour spreads to para-aortic lymph nodes, lungs, liver and brain. These may present with backache, haemoptysis, jaundice or neurological events. Testicular tumours occur in relatively young men, late teens to early 30s. Teratoma tends to occur in the younger age range and seminoma in the slightly older group.

Treatment consists of a radical orchidectomy via a groin incision. If tumour markers return to normal following surgery, it is likely there are no metastases. A complete staging, using chest and abdominal CT scanning, is required. Metastatic disease requires cisplatin-based chemotherapy. Post-chemotherapy residual metastatic teratoma masses require surgical excision.

Seminoma is extremely radiosensitive and if the tumour is confined to the testis, abdominal lymph nodes may be irradiated to treat undetected micrometastases. Following orchidectomy, localized (stage 1) teratoma can be monitored by a surveillance programme (withholding adjuvant treatments), utilizing regular CT scanning and blood tests for tumour markers. In the good-prognosis group, only about 30% will relapse and require salvage chemotherapy, which is still curative in the majority of patients. With effective chemotherapy, over 90% of patients with a testicular tumour will be cured.

Rare testicular tumours include lymphoma in older men and rhabdomyosarcoma in infants.

Trauma

Direct trauma can cause testicular rupture, which requires surgical exploration and repair. Late presentation of trauma is not uncommon and a haematoma within the tunica vaginalis may form. This usually reabsorbs, but surgical exploration and drainage are occasionally necessary.

Fertility

Vasectomy is one of the commonest forms of contraception. Popularly regarded as a minor procedure, it is the urological procedure most likely to result in litigation. Postoperative haematoma or pain may be difficult to treat and sterility cannot be guaranteed until azoospermia has been confirmed on semen analysis. Even then, late recanalization of the vas is a rare but well-recognized complication.

Reversal of vasectomy may be attempted if the patient decides he wishes to have further children. Re-anastomosis of the vas is relatively straightforward. However, the longer it is since the vasectomy the greater the likelihood that sperm production and transport through the epididymis will be impaired.

Primary infertility is investigated initially with semen analysis to assess the number, motility and percentage of normal sperm. A hormonal screen is necessary to assess the hypothalamic-pituitary-testicular axis and testicular biopsy may be performed to assess spermatogenesis.

Penis and urethra

Inflammation

Inflammation of the foreskin and glans (balanitis) can result in a phimosis. In recurrent cases, this is best treated by circumcision. If the foreskin is drawn back over the glans, a paraphimosis results. Although this can usually be reduced, a dorsal slit may be necessary in the acute situation.

Stricture

Trauma to the urethra, by a catheter or surgical instrument, or inflammation from an infection such as *Neisseria gonorrhoeae* may produce fibrosis resulting in a urethral stricture. This may be divided under direct vision using an optical urethrotome, but recurrence is common. Urethroplasty using buccal mucosal grafts or penile foreskin allows the stricture to be excised and replaced with healthier tissue.

Tumour

The male distal urethra is lined mainly by transitional cells and in the female, squamous epithelium. Carcinomas can occur but they are rare.

Squamous carcinoma of the penis usually presents as an ulcerated lesion beneath the foreskin. The tumour may be in the coronal groove. Biopsy is essential for histological confirmation and staging is by CT scanning to assess the inguinal lymph nodes. A localized tumour can be treated by amputation (partial or complete), local excision or external beam radiotherapy. Very small, localized penile cancers can be treated successfully with topical 5-fluorouracil preparations. Although metastatic squamous carcinoma is usually incurable its rate of growth may be quite slow. Often the patient is elderly and frail, and careful surveillance may be the best option.

Trauma

A degloving injury to the penis results in the loss of skin from the penile shaft. The shaft can be buried with scrotal skin to allow healing and then removed, thereby preserving the scrotal skin covering.

Fracture of an erect penis involves rupture of one or both of the corpora cavernosa. These should be repaired at open operation.

Erectile dysfunction (ED)

Failure of normal erections occurs with advancing age and it is estimated that around 20% of men between 50 and 70 years of age have moderate or severe ED. The cause of this impotence may be psychogenic, but organic causes (such as diabetes, smoking and peripheral vascular disease) are more likely with increasing age. The mainstays of treatment are the phosphodiesterase type 5 (PDE 5) inhibitors, such as sildenafil, vardenafil and tadalafil. These drugs inhibit breakdown of cyclic guanosine monophosphate (cGMP), thereby enhancing the normal erectile response. They are effective in psychogenic and organic ED. Other modalities of treatment are occasionally necessary including intracavernosal prostaglandin E1 and intraurethral vasoactive drug therapy, and vacuum constriction devices. An uncommon side effect of drug therapy for ED is a prolonged erection lasting several hours (priapism), which may lead to ischaemic injury to the erectile tissue in the corporeal bodies. If priapism does occur, the blood must be drained from the corpora cavernosa by direct aspiration, or by surgical formation of a shunt with the corpus spongiosum, or a saphenous vein. Priapism may also occur as part of a sickle cell crisis or in a patient with leukaemia.

Aspects of general surgery and gynaecology that may cause urological problems

General surgery

Diverticular disease of the sigmoid colon may cause abscess formation that perforates into the bladder, producing a colovesical fistula. Symptoms include recurrent urine infections and air bubbles in the urine passed down from flatus in the colon (pneumaturia). It is uncommon for a carcinoma of either the bladder or colon to cause a similar fistula.

A leaking AAA is occasionally misdiagnosed as ureteric colic. Any patient over the age of 50 years with sudden onset of abdominal/loin pain must not be diagnosed as having a symptomatic renal stone until radiological confirmation has been obtained, or an AAA excluded by imaging.

Gynaecology

An ectopic pregnancy may cause lower abdominal pain and eventually an acute abdomen with shock. Establishing the date of a patient's last menstrual period is an important part of any history in a woman of childbearing age. Ovarian cysts may cause low abdominal pain and pelvic pain but these are easily identified by ultrasonography. A monthly cycle of lower abdominal pain and, more rarely, haematuria may result from endometriosis. Abdominal endometriosis can cause local fibrosis and ureteric obstruction.

Vaginal bleeding may present as 'haematuria'. A vaginal examination should always be performed at the time of cystoscopy to exclude a carcinoma of the cervix, or other pelvic mass. Locally advanced carcinoma of the cervix may present with hydronephrosis and renal failure due to local invasion, causing ureteric obstruction.

Following hysterectomy, unrecognized damage to a ureter may present as loin pain from an obstructive hydronephrosis, or a vaginal leakage of urine from a vesico-vaginal fistula.

Further reading

Bullock N, Sibley G, Whittaker R, Cox P. *Essential Urology*. Churchill Livingstone, 1989.

Lloyd-Davies W, Parkhouse H, Gow J, Davies D. *Colour Atlas of Urology*. 2nd edn. Wolfe Publishing, 1994.

Tanagho EA, McAninch JW. *Smith's General Urology*. 14th edn. Appleton & Lang, 1995.

Walsh P, Retik A, Vaughan E, Wein A (eds). *Campbell's Urology*. 7th edn. Saunders, 1998.

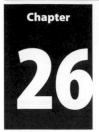

Chapter

26

Hernias

Andrew N. Kingsnorth

Landmarks in the history of surgical management

An appreciation of the history of hernia surgery may prevent us repeating the mistakes of the past and put in perspective the knowledge that has been accumulated in order to allow development of the successful techniques used today. The high prevalence of hernia, for which the lifetime risk is 27% for men and 3% for women, has resulted in this condition inheriting one of the longest traditions of surgical management.

- Hernia surgery has a 3500-year history (Figure 26.1)
- Castration was an essential part of the earliest operations for hernia, which carried with it an obvious stigma
- The Dark Ages until the sixteenth century halted further progress in effective treatment
- Femoral hernia was distinguished from inguinal hernia in the fourteenth century.

The great contribution of the surgical anatomists was between the years 1750 and 1865 and was called the age of dissection. The main contributors were Antonio Scarpa and Sir Astley Cooper and few major advances in our knowledge of the anatomy of the groin have been made since this time. The names of these great anatomists are Pieter, Camper, Antonio Scarpa, Percival Pott, Sir Astley Cooper, John Hunter, Thomas Morton, Germaine Cloquet, Franz Hesselbach, Friedrich Henle and Don Antonio Gimbernat.

Astley Cooper's seminal monograph was written in 1804 (Figure 26.2). Sir Astley Cooper (1768–1841) trained at St Thomas's Hospital, London and became a surgeon at Guy's Hospital and from 1813 to 1815 was Professor of Comparative Anatomy of the Royal College of Surgeons. Cooper published six magnifi-

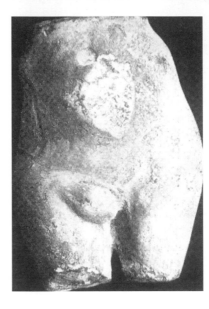

Figure 26.1 Greek terracotta illustrates general awareness of hernias around 900 BC.

cent books, two of which covered the subject of hernia, which were liberally illustrated by his own hand from dissections he had performed personally. Cooper was a charismatic lecturer and socialite and had an extensive surgical practice, which included being Sergeant Surgeon to King George IV. Cooper's recognition of the transversalis fascia positions him as one of the most important contributors to present-day surgery, which emphasizes this layer as being the first layer to be breached in groin hernias.

Franz Hesselbach was an anatomist at the University of Wurzburg who described the triangle now so important in laparoscopic surgery which originally defined the pathway of direct and external and supravesical hernias. The triangle as defined today is somewhat smaller.

As so often in surgery a new concept was needed before further progress could be made in herniology.

Fundamentals of Surgical Practice, Third Edition, ed. Andrew N. Kingsnorth and Douglas M. Bowley.
Published by Cambridge University Press. © Cambridge University Press 2011.

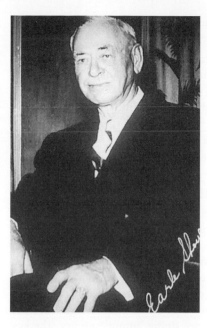

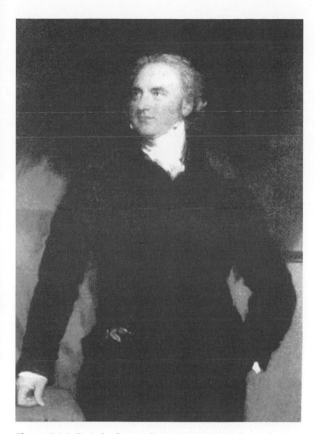

Figure 26.2 Sir Astley Paston Cooper (1768–1841). Surgical Anatomist, London, England.

Two pioneers – the American Henry Marcy (1889) and the Italian Eduardo Bassini (1884) – vie for priority for the critical breakthrough. Both appreciated the physiology of the inguinal canal and both correctly understood how each anatomic plane, transversalis fascia, transverse and oblique muscles, and the external oblique aponeurosis, contributed to the canal's stability. Bassini made another important advance when he subjected his technique to the scrutiny of the prospective follow-up. Bassini's 1890 paper is truly a quantum leap in surgery. He decided to open the inguinal canal and approach the posterior wall of the canal, which he achieved by reconstruction of the inguinal canal into the physiological condition, a canal with two openings, one abdominal, the other subcutaneous, and with two walls, one anterior and one posterior through the middle of which the spermatic cord would pass. Bassini dissected the indirect sac and closed it off flush with the parietal peritoneum. He then isolated and lifted up the spermatic cord and dissected the posterior wall of the canal, dividing the fascia transversalis down

to the pubic tubercle. He then sutured the dissected conjoint tendon consisting of the internal oblique, the transversus muscle and the 'vertical fascia of Cooper', the fascia transversalis, to the posterior rim of Poupart's ligament, including the lower lateral divided margin of the fascia transversalis. Bassini stresses that this suture line must be approximated without difficulty; hence the early dissection separating the external oblique from the internal oblique must be adequate and allow good development and mobilization of the conjoint tendon.

The Bassini operation re-emerged as the Shouldice repair in the 1950s (Figure 26.3). Earle Shouldice (1890–1965) also promulgated the benefits of early ambulation and opened the Shouldice clinic, a hospital dedicated to the repair of hernias of the abdominal wall. A huge experience accumulated with an annual throughput of 7000 herniorrhaphies per year enabled the surgeons at the Shouldice clinic to study the pathology in primary and recurrent hernias and to emphasize adjuncts to successful outcomes. Continuous monofilament wire was used in preference to other suture materials and the hernioplasty incorporated repair of the internal ring, the posterior wall of the inguinal canal and the femoral region. The cremaster muscle and fascia with vessels and genital branch of the genitofemoral nerve were removed and the posterior wall after division was repaired by a four-layer imbrication method using the ilio-pubic tract as its main anchor point. Until the introduction of mesh, the Shouldice operation became the gold standard for inguinal hernia repair.

- The surgical anatomy of the groin, on which modern hernia surgery is based, was defined between 1750 and 1865
- Bassini described his revolutionary operation in 1890
- The Shouldice clinic revived the Bassini operation in the latter half of the twentieth century.

Tension-free hernia repair

Irving Lichtenstein is the revolutionary thinker who introduced tension-free prosthetic repair of groin hernias into everyday, commonplace, outpatient practices. Lichtenstein pioneered the idea that, as well as being an office procedure under local anaesthetic, hernia surgery is special, that it must be performed by an experienced surgeon and cannot be relegated to the unsupervised trainee doing 'minor' surgery. The key feature of Lichtenstein's technique is the 'tensionless' operation. With his co-workers Shulman and Amid, he developed a simple prosthetic operation, which can be performed on outpatients. As a pioneer, Lichtenstein worked hard to promulgate his ideas but even so the first edition of his book *Hernia Repair Without Disability* written in 1970 sold rather poorly and never went beyond the first printing. Subsequent editions, however, required numerous reprints to meet demand paralleling the increase in popularity and worldwide success of the mesh-patch repair devised by Lichtenstein.

- Irving Lichtenstein had faith in his new operation in spite of opposition from the surgical establishment
- Mesh has contributed more to improvements in hernia surgery outcomes in the last 30 years than any other factor.

Laparoscopic repair

Laparoscopic repair has developed a place in the surgical armamentarium of inguinal hernia in the UK, representing about 15% of repairs. The use of the laparoscope has been extended to repair incisional, ventral, lumbar and paracolostomy hernias.

The first attempt to treat an inguinal hernia with the laparoscope was made by P. Fletcher of the University of the West Indies in 1979. He closed the neck of the hernia sac. The first report of the use of a clip (Michel) placed laparoscopically to close the neck of the sac was made by Ger in 1982, who reported a series of 13 patients: all the patients in this series were repaired through an open incision except the thirteenth patient, who was repaired under laparoscopic guidance with a special stapling device. The 3-year follow-up of that patient revealed him to be free of an identifiable recurrence. Ger continued his efforts to repair these hernias laparoscopically. He reported the closure of the neck of the hernia sac using a prototypical instrument called the 'Herniostat' in beagle dogs. The results in these models appeared to be promising. In that same article, he reported the potential benefits of the laparoscopic approach to groin hernia repair as: (1) creation of puncture wounds rather than formal incisions, (2) need for minimal dissection, (3) less danger of spermatic cord injury and less risk of ischaemic orchitis, (4) minimal risk of bladder injury, (5) decreased incidence of neuralgias, (6) possibility of an outpatient procedure, (7) ability to achieve the highest possible ligation of the hernial sac, (8) minimal postoperative discomfort and a faster recovery time, (9) ability to perform simultaneous diagnostic laparoscopy and (10) ability to diagnose and treat bilateral inguinal hernias. These potential advantages and advances in the laparoscopic repair of hernias continue to be the recognized goals that each method is attempting to achieve.

- Laparoscopic repair of an inguinal hernia was first performed in 1982
- Laparoscopic hernia repair requires greater skills than laparoscopic cholecystectomy or fundoplication
- The learning curve for laparoscopic hernia repair may be as high as 250 hernias, before recurrence rates reach an acceptable level.

Essential anatomy of the abdominal wall

The anatomy of the abdominal wall is well documented in several standard texts on anatomy, which contain accurate and detailed information that is readily available. The lined drawings in this chapter have been adapted from published reports for anatomists and surgeons with particular attention to applied surgical anatomy and anatomical variance of the normal. Pathological processes further disorganize the underlying anatomy and the surgeon who seeks to make a success of hernia repairs should fully understand these

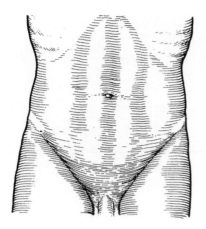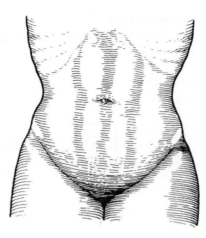

Figure 26.4 Topographical anatomy of the abdomen shows the distinctly different male and female characteristics.

anatomic variations. Today the surgeon should individualize the operation for the anatomy encountered.

Under normal circumstances the musculoaponeurotic layers of the abdominal wall are designed to retain the contents of the peritoneal cavity. There are certain limited areas, however, where the underlying anatomical structure is deficient and where hernias develop. This deficiency is most notable in the groin area in relation to the inguinal and femoral canals but there are several other sites, notably the umbilicus, epigastrium, lumbar triangle, obturator canal, sciatic foramina, perineum, pelvic sidewall and the spigelian line. The list is quite long and the clinician may or may not encounter one of the rarer types of abdominal wall hernias in a lifetime.

External anatomy – the surface markings

The abdominal wall, bounded by the lower margin of the thorax above, and by the pubes, the iliac crests and the inguinal ligaments below, is easily recognized in the upright man. Vertically down the centre of the abdomen the depression of the linea alba is obvious and is usually more apparent above the umbilicus. The umbilicus lies at the junction of the upper three-fifths and lower two-fifths of the linea alba. In the healthy young adult the rectus muscle is prominent on either side of the linea alba. The rectus muscle is particularly prominent inferolaterally to the umbilicus: this infra-umbilical rectus mound is of surgical importance. With ageing and obesity the lower abdomen sags but the infra-umbilical rectus mound remains obvious and visible to the subject, even into old age.

The outer margin of each rectus is indicated by a convex vertically directed furrow, the semilunar line

(linea semilunaris), which is most distinct in the upper abdomen where it commences at the tip of the ninth costal cartilage. At first it descends almost vertically, but inferior to the umbilicus it gently curves medially to terminate at the pubic tubercle. It is along this line that the internal oblique aponeurosis bands and splits to enclose the rectus muscle in the upper two-thirds of the abdomen. The broad furrow of the inferior semilunar line is also described as the Spigelian fascia and is the site of herniation. In the lower abdomen the configuration varies, a wider pelvis and greater pubic prominence being important female characteristics (Figure 26.4).

The surgeon must be aware of the elastic and connective tissue lines in the skin (Langer's lines) if optimum healing is to be obtained. Incisions made at right angles to Langer's lines gape and tend to splay out when they heal. The longitudinal contraction of the healing wound, particularly when the wound crosses a skin delve or body crease, can make healing very unsightly with contracture and for these reasons vertical incisions over the groin should be avoided. However, rapid abdominal access requires adequate vertical incisions and they continue to remain in everyday general surgical and gynaecological practice, particularly in emergency surgery.

The subcutaneous layer

Beneath the skin there is the subcutaneous areolar tissue and fascia. Superiorly over the lower chest and epigastrium this layer is generally thin and less organized than in the lower abdomen, where it becomes bilaminar – a superficial fatty stratum (Camper's fascia) and a deeper, stronger and more elastic layer (Scarpa's fascia). Scarpa's fascia is well developed in infancy, forming a distinct layer which must be separately incised when the superficial inguinal ring is approached in childhood herniotomy.

In the lower abdomen the deeper fascia (Scarpa's) is more membranous with much elastic tissue and almost devoid of fat. This fascia does not pass down uninterrupted to the thigh and perineum as the superficial fatty fascia does; instead, the deep fascia is attached to the inner half of the inguinal ligament, to the anterior fascia lata of the thigh and to the iliac crest laterally. Medially it forms a distinct structure containing much elastic tissue and descends, almost as a band, from the pubis to envelop the penis as the suspensory ligament. Internally it can be traced as a thin layer over the penis and scrotum. Behind the scrotum it becomes continuous with the deep layer of the superficial fascia of the perineum (Colles' fascia).

Superficial nerves

The most caudal of the abdominal wall nerves are derived from the first lumbar nerve; they are the iliohypogastric and ilio-inguinal nerves. The ilio-inguinal nerve is generally smaller than the iliohypogastric nerve – if one is large the other is smaller and vice versa. Occasionally the ilio-inguinal nerve is very small and may be absent. The anterior cutaneous branch of the iliohypogastric nerve emerges through the aponeurosis of the external oblique just above the superficial inguinal ring and innervates the skin in the suprapubic region. The ilio-inguinal nerve passes through the lower inguinal canal and becomes superficial by emerging from the superficial inguinal ring to supply the skin of the scrotum and a small area of the medial upper thigh.

The genitofemoral nerve arises from the first and second lumbar nerves and completes the innervation of the abdominal wall and groin areas. At first it passes obliquely forwards and downwards through the substance of the psoas major. It emerges from the muscle and crosses its anterior surface deep to the peritoneum, going behind, posterior to, the ureter. It divides a variable distance from the deep inguinal ring into a genital and a femoral branch. The genital branch, a mixed motor and sensory nerve, crosses the femoral vessels and enters the inguinal canal at or just medial to the deep ring. The nerve penetrates the fascia transversalis of the posterior wall of the inguinal ligament either through the deep ring or separately medially to the

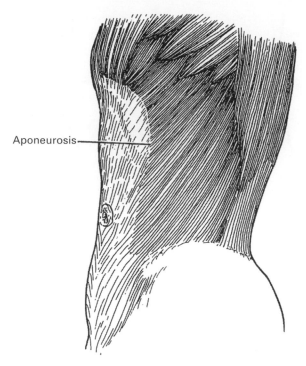

Figure 26.5 The external oblique muscle and its aponeurosis invests the abdomen.

deep ring. The nerve traverses the inguinal canal lying between the spermatic cord above and the upturned edge of the inguinal ligament inferiorly; the nerve is vulnerable to surgical trauma as it progresses along the floor of the canal (the gutter produced by the upturned internal edge of the inguinal ligament). The genital nerve supplies the motor function to the cremaster muscle and the sensory function to the skin of the scrotum. The femoral branch enters the femoral sheath lying lateral to the femoral artery and supplies the skin of the upper part of the femoral triangle.

The external oblique aponeurosis

The aponeurosis of the external oblique muscle fuses with the aponeurosis of the internal oblique in the anterior rectus sheath. This line of fusion is considerably medial to the semilunar line – the fusion line is oblique and somewhat semilunar, being more lateral above and more medial below. In fact, the external oblique aponeurosis contributes very little to the lower portion of the anterior rectus sheath. This latter point is of considerable importance in inguinal hernioplasty (Figure 26.5).

There is a defect in the external-oblique aponeurosis just above the pubis. This aperture – the superficial inguinal ring – is triangular in shape and in the male allows passage of the spermatic cord from the abdomen to the scrotum. In the female the round ligament of the uterus passes through this opening. The superficial inguinal ring is not a 'ring'; it is a triangular cleft with its long axis oblique in the same direction but not quite parallel to the inguinal ligament. The base of the triangle is formed by the crest of the pubis and the apex is lateral towards the anterior superior iliac spine. The superficial inguinal ring represents that interval between the aponeurosis of the external oblique which inserts into the pubic bone superiorly and, as the inguinal ligament, inserts into the pubic tubercle inferiorly. The aponeurotic margins of the ring are described as the superior and inferior crura. The spermatic cord, as it comes through the superficial ring, rests on the inferior crus, which is a continuation of the floor of the inguinal canal (the upturned internal margin of the inguinal ligament).

The crura of the superficial ring are joined together by intercrural fibres derived from the outer investing fascia of the external oblique aponeurosis. The size and strength of these intercrural fibres vary.

The external oblique aponeurosis in the region of the groin forms a free border known as the inguinal ligament, which is simply the lower margin of this aponeurosis; it is not a condensed thickened ligamentous structure. The ligament presents a rounded surface towards the thigh where the aponeurosis is rolled inwards back on itself to make a groove on its deep surface. Laterally the ligament is attached to the anterior superior iliac spine and medially to the pubic tubercle and via the lacunar and reflected inguinal ligaments to the iliopectineal line on the superior ramus of the pubis. The inguinal ligament is not straight; it is concave, with the concavity directed medially and upward towards the abdomen.

The medial attachment, or continuation, of the inguinal ligament as the lacunar (Gimbernat's) and the pectineal (Cooper's) ligament gives a fan-like expansion of the inguinal ligament at its medial end, which curves posteriorly to the iliopectineal ligament. This expansion has important surgical implications.

The lacunar ligament is a triangular continuation of the medial end of the inguinal ligament. Its apex is at the pubic tubercle, its superior margin continuous with the inguinal ligament, and its medial margin is attached to the iliopectineal line on the superior

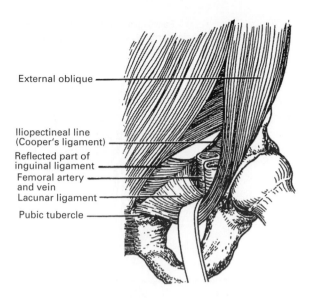

External oblique

Iliopectineal line
(Cooper's ligament)

Reflected part of
inguinal ligament

Femoral artery
and vein

Lacunar ligament

Pubic tubercle

Figure 26.6 The upper abdominal surface of the attachment of the inguinal ligament to the pubic tubercle is the floor of the inguinal canal.

ramus of the pubis. Its lateral crescentic edge is free and directed laterally, where it is an important rigid structure in the medial margin of the femoral canal. The ligament lies in an oblique plane, with its upper (abdominal) surface facing superomedially and being crossed by the spermatic cord, and its lower (femoral) surface looking anterolaterally. With the external oblique aponeurosis and the inguinal ligament, the superior surface forms a groove for the cord as it emerges from the inguinal canal (Figure 26.6).

The conjoint tendon

The conjoint tendon has a very variable structure and in 20% of subjects it does not exist as a discrete anatomic structure. It may be absent or only slightly developed, it may be replaced by a lateral extension of the tendon of origin of the rectus muscle, or it may extend laterally to the deep inguinal ring so that no interval is present between the lower border of the transversus and the inguinal ligament. A shutter mechanism for the conjoint tendon can only be demonstrated when the lateral side of the tendon, that is the transversus and internal oblique muscles, extend onto and are attached to the iliopectineal line. The extent of this insertion is very variable.

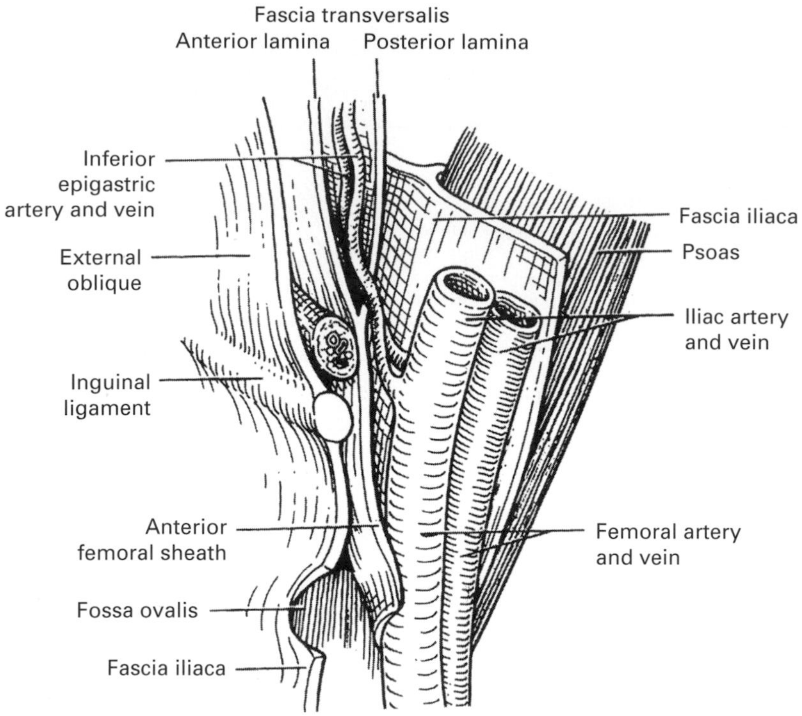

Figure 26.7 The bilaminar fascia transversalis in the groin.

The fascia transversalis – the space of Bogros

The fascia transversalis lies deep to the transverse abdominal muscle plane. It is continuous from side to side and extends from the rib cage above to the pelvis inferiorly.

In the upper abdominal wall the fascia transversalis is thin, but in the lower abdomen and especially in the inguinofemoral region the fascia is thicker and has specialized bands and folds within it. In the groin region, where the fascia transversalis is an important constituent of the posterior wall of the inguinal canal and where it forms the femoral sheath inferiorly to the inguinal ligament, the anatomy and function of the fascia transversalis are of particular importance to the surgeon. As originally described by Sir Astley Cooper in 1807, the fascia transversalis, in the groin, consists of two layers. The anterior strong layer covers the internal aspect of the transversalis muscle where it is intimately blended with the tendon of the transversus muscle. It then extends across the posterior wall of the inguinal canal medial to the deep ring aperture and is attached to the inner margin of the inguinal ligament. The deeper layer of fascia transversalis, a membranous layer, lies between the anterior substan-

tial layer of fascia transversalis and the peritoneum. The extraperitoneal fat lies behind this layer between it and the peritoneum (Figure 26.7). The deep epigastric vessels run between the two layers of fascia transversalis. Defects in it, congenital or acquired, are the aetiology of all groin hernias.

The peritoneum – the view from within

Hernia sacs are composed of peritoneum and they may contain intra-abdominal viscera. From within they consist of the peritoneum, then a loose layer of extraperitoneal fat, then the deep membranous lamina of fascia transversalis, then the vessels such as the epigastric vessels in the space of Bogros, then the stout anterior lamina of fascia transversalis, then the muscles and aponeuroses of the abdominal wall. The preperitoneal space lies in the abdominal cavity between the peritoneum internally and transversalis fascia externally. Within this space lies a variable quantity of adipose tissue, loose connective tissue and membranous tissue and other anatomical entities such as arteries, veins, nerves and various organs such as the kidneys and ureters. The clinically significant parts of the preperitoneal space include the space associated with the structural elements related

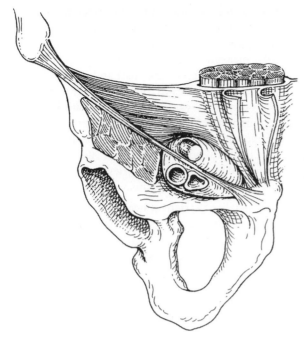

Figure 26.8 The myopectineal orifice of Fruchaud: the area of the groin closed by fascia transversalis with the inguinal canal above and femoral canal below the rigid inguinal canal.

and inferiorly the pecten of the pubis. The space is utilized in both the transabdominal preperitoneal and the totally extraperitoneal laparoscopic approaches to the repair of inguinal and femoral repairs. A thorough understanding of the limits of this myopectineal orifice is necessary to accomplish an effective repair of the inguinal floor with the laparoscopic approach.

Aetiology

The pathogenesis of groin hernia is multifactorial. Because indirect inguinal hernias are so common in infancy the first surgical speculation was that they were due to a developmental defect. Indirect inguinal hernia arises from incomplete obliteration of the processus vaginalis, the embryological out-pocketing of peritoneum that precedes testicular descent into the scrotum. The testes originate along the urogenital line in the retroperitoneum and migrate caudally during the second trimester of pregnancy to arrive at the internal inguinal ring at about 6 months of intrauterine life. During the last trimester they proceed through the abdominal wall via the inguinal canal and descend into the scrotum, the right slightly later than the left. The processus vaginalis then normally obliterates postnatally except for the portion surrounding and serving as a covering for the testes. Failure of this obliterative process results in congenital indirect inguinal hernia. Additional support for the congenital theory of indirect inguinal herniation is the finding at autopsy that 15–30% of adult males without clinically apparent inguinal hernias have a patent processus vaginalis at death.

Read made the crucial clinical observation which next advanced our understanding of the aetiology of inguinal hernia. In 1970 he noted, when using the preperitoneal approach to the inguinal region, that the rectus sheath is thinner and has a 'greasy' feel in those patients who turned out to have direct defects. This observation was confirmed by weighing samples of constant area; specimens from controls weighed significantly more than those from patients with indirect, pantaloon and direct hernias (in that order). Bilateral hernias were associated with more severe atrophy. Adjustment for age and muscle mass confirmed the validity of the primary observation. And, if surgical technical failure can be excluded, the logical treatment of recurrent herniation is prosthetic repair. This concept was enthusiastically promulgated by Irving Lichtenstein, one of the earliest protagonists of prosthetic

to the myopectoneal orifice of Fruchaud, the prevesical space of Retzius, the space of Bogros and retroperitoneal periurinary space. The myopectineal orifice of Fruchaud represents the potentially weak area in the abdominal wall, which permits inguinal and femoral hernias. The preperitoneal space that lies deep to the supra-vesical fossa and the medial inguinal fossa is the prevesical space of Retzius. The space of Retzius contains loose connective tissue and fat but more importantly vascular elements such as an abnormal obturator artery and vein. Bogros's space, which is a triangular area between the abdominal wall and peritoneum, can be entered by means of an incision through the roof and floor of the inguinal canal through which the posterior preperitoneal approach for hernia repair can be achieved. In the groin these muscles and aponeuroses are variously absent over the inguinal and crural canals. The myopectineal orifice of Fruchaud is divided into two parts by the inguinal ligament (Figure 26.8). This concept of one groin aperture is relevant for mesh repairs, whether anterior open operation or posterior laparoscopic operation. The boundaries of the myopectineal orifice of Fruchaud are superiorly the 'arch' of the transversus muscle, laterally the iliopsoas muscle, medially the rectus muscle repair for primary inguinal hernia. The aetiology of inguinal hernia is multifactorial:

- Genetic inheritance has a role
- Indirect hernias originate from a patent processus vaginalis
- A weakening of the transversalis fascia is the major factor contributing to the development of direct hernia, and also indirect hernia (*c.* 20% of males at autopsy have an intact transversalis fascia, a patent processus and no hernia)
- Smoking weakens collagen tissue, including the transversalis fascia.

Exertion and herniation

Manual work or strain is very rarely the sole cause of inguinal hernia. In a study of inguinal hernia and a single strenuous event, 7% of patients attributed their hernia to a single muscular strain. The anatomical and physiological basis for this is not well established but in a few studies, long-term heavy work seems to have an association with groin hernia. Mere occasional lifting, however, does not constitute a risk of developing of hernia. People with lung emphysema, aortic aneurysm, and collagen disorders are known to have higher risk of developing hernia. In all these conditions the primary problem is related to collagen biosynthesis. There is no clear evidence for prostatism, constipation and COPD as risk factors for developing hernia; however, they may exacerbate an existing hernia.

Economics

Economic evaluations of new and existing healthcare interventions are an essential input into decision-making. Healthcare systems around the world face steady increases in expenditure resulting from demographic change and improvements in medical technology. Increasingly, payors must choose which interventions will be provided and which will not be reimbursed from limited public or private funds. This creates difficult choices. In the UK the National Institute for Healthcare and Clinical Excellence (NICE) synthesizes evidence and reaches a judgement as to whether on balance the intervention can be recommended as a cost-effective use of NHS resources. In 2000 and 2004 NICE published recommendations for the use of laparoscopic hernia surgery and recommended its use in centres with the required expertise for primary, bilateral or recurrent inguinal hernia.

It is no longer sufficient to consider the clinical or therapeutic effects of healthcare interventions: purchasing choices will be predicated on studies which identify, measure and value what is given up when an intervention is used (the cost) and what is gained (improved patient health outcomes). This requires explicit economic evaluation of healthcare interventions. Purchasers have a fixed budget and are aware of the opportunity costs of interventions. Increasingly they are likely to require evidence of effectiveness and cost-effectiveness, and they may develop contracts and enforce protocols to ensure this.

- In a socialized system of healthcare (NHS) healthcare interventions must be cost-effective
- Laparoscopic repair for inguinal hernia is more expensive than open repair.

The type of economic evaluation depends upon the outcome measure chosen:

1. Cost minimization analysis is appropriate only when the outcomes of two or more interventions have been demonstrated to be equivalent, in which case the least costly alternative is the most efficient, and only cost analysis is required.
2. Cost-effectiveness analysis includes both costs and outcomes using a single outcome measure, usually a natural unit. This allows comparisons between treatments in a particular therapeutic area where effectiveness is unequal, but not between therapeutic areas where natural outcome measures differ.
3. Cost utility analysis combines multiple outcomes into a single measure of utility (e.g. a quality-adjusted life year, or QALY). This allows comparisons between alternatives in different therapeutic categories with different natural outcomes.
4. Cost-benefit analysis links costs and outcomes by expressing both in monetary units, forcing an explicit decision about whether an intervention is worth its cost. Various techniques have been used to attach monetary values to health outcomes, but the technique remains rare in health economics.

Economics of hernia repair

Hernia repair is an established and effective procedure and its relatively fixed cost and high volume amongst surgical procedures means that economic evaluation of the procedure itself has become a priority. Hernias create pain and discomfort for patients and limit ability to work or carry out other productive activities. While the increased risk of surgical procedures in elderly people means that repair of some small direct hernias may not be mandatory, there would seem to be clear clinical and economic arguments in favour of carrying out hernia repairs amongst the majority of the working population.

In selected patients with asymptomatic inguinal hernia, a wait-and-watch policy can be employed to avoid the risks of surgery (infection, chronic pain, recurrence) and anaesthesia-related problems. The risk of developing obstruction is small in asymptomatic inguinal hernias but it increases slowly over a period of time. In a randomized trial comparing watchful waiting and surgical repair, with 2 to 4.5 years follow-up, only one watchful-waiting patient (0.3%) experienced acute hernia incarceration without strangulation within 2 years; a second had acute incarceration with bowel obstruction at 4 years. This amounts to a frequency of 1.8 acute episodes per 1000 years of patient follow-up.

The experience from the Shouldice clinic in Canada and the results from the United States support the use of limited hospitalization for the repair of hernias.

- Hernia repair is common (20 million world wide, 100 000 in the UK annually)
- Hernia surgery is carried out most efficiently in dedicated units
- Ambulatory care is the most cost-effective means of care
- Local anaesthesia reduces complexity, time and money utilized (see below).

Return to normal activity and work

There is enormous variation in reported times for return to normal activity and work. For instance, in a socialized system of healthcare where patients' expectations and the insurance system still favour hospitalization, length of hospital stay after hernia surgery may be several days.

Advice concerning return to normal activity has been poorly managed by surgeons. Recent studies indicate that factors limiting a patient's return to activity and work are governed principally by the perceived amount of postoperative pain. Socioeconomic factors strongly influence this perception over and above the actual procedure performed or the anatomy involved.

In patients having National Insurance compared with patients having private insurance, the duration of postoperative pain and the days off work have been compared. The differences between the two groups is striking: the median duration of postoperative pain in the National Insurance group was 27 days, with 36.5 days off work. In the private insurance patients the duration of postoperative pain was 7.5 days and they went back to work after only 8.5 days. Personal motivation, therefore, appears to be the most important factor affecting clinical outcome and return to activities. Callesen from Copenhagen has demonstrated that well-defined recommendations and improved pain management can shorten convalescence. One hundred patients having elective herniorrhaphy under local anaesthetic and managed analgesia were recommended to have one day of convalescence for light/moderate work and 3 weeks for strenuous physical activity. The overall median absence from work was 6 days; the unemployed returning to activities in just one day, those in light/moderate work in 6 days and those in heavy jobs by 25 days. A more detailed prospective study of return to work after inguinal hernia repair has been undertaken by Jones and colleagues: data were collected by personal interviews, written surveys and medical record reviews in 235 patients, the main outcome measures being actual and expected return to work. Age, educational level, income level, occupation, symptoms of depression and the expected day of return to work (10 days) accounted for 61% of the variation in actual (12 days) return to work.

- Length of hospital stay is controlled overwhelmingly by the surgeon
- In the majority of cases local anaesthesia and a 1–2 hour recovery in hospital is sufficient
- Most patients can return to normal activities within 7–10 days of an uncomplicated, primary inguinal hernia repair.

Principles in hernia surgery

There are three principles which dictate the management of all abdominal wall hernia patients.

1. The patient must be adequately prepared for surgery. The mortality from hernia operations, particularly the mortality and morbidity of strangulated femoral hernias in older women, is almost entirely due to operating when the patient is in a less than optimal physiological condition. Hernias almost never require emergency surgery,

although they may require urgent surgery as soon as the patient is rendered fit. To operate before adequate rehydration and renal function is restored, or before the cardiorespiratory status is assessed and stabilized, is to court disaster. Even in the very elderly mortality can be reduced to a minimum; death is usually a result of complications of the strangulated hernia rather than associated diseases which should have been adequately treated before the urgent operation. For elective hernia repair the same golden principle applies – do not operate until the patient has been fully assessed and is in an optimum physiological state.

2. The contents must be reduced after inspection at open operation and following careful inspection for viability. If strangulation has occurred infarcted contents must be resected. The dangers of forcible reduction of contents into an inadequate cavity when there is 'lack of storage capacity of the abdominal cavity' or 'loss of domain' must be appreciated.

3. The defect must be repaired with a non-absorbable suture technique and then supplemented with a mesh hernioplasty. Each layer of the defect should be repaired discretely. The weak layers are then reinforced with mesh to restore the patient's anatomy so that it resembles the normal unoperated condition. The process of repair in aponeurosis is slow. Only tendinous/aponeurotic/fascial structures can be successfully sutured together: suturing red fleshy muscle to tendon or fascia will not contribute to permanent union of these structures.

Frequently, particularly with the repair of the larger incisional and ventral hernias, the reconstruction of the patient's anatomy is not feasible. The use of a prosthetic biomaterial is the only option for these individuals. When this is the case, the surgeon must ensure that a large overlap of the prosthetic is used so that the resulting repair will be sound and permanent.

Prosthetic biomaterials

The use of prosthetic biomaterials in the repair of hernias of the abdominal wall is now routine practice in many countries. In the USA and Europe over 90% of all inguinal and ventral hernias are repaired with a prosthetic material or device. In other parts of the world,

Table 26.1 The main indications for the use of prosthetic materials

Absorbable prosthetic materials	Temporary replacement of absent tissue (e.g. smaller infected wounds)
Collagen-based products	Form a 'neo-fascia' to repair defects in the abdominal wall
Flat prosthetic biomaterials	Differ in weight, porosity and thickness and utilized for fascial reinforcement
Dual-sided mesh products	The smooth surface is designed for use in the intra-peritoneal space

this is not the case. Limitations on the use of these products include a natural reluctance to place a biomaterial into a primary hernia or the cost of these products.

Incisional hernias will develop in approximately 10–15% of laparotomy incisions. The risk of herniation is increased by threefold if a postoperative wound infection occurs. Other factors that predispose to the development of a fascial defect include obesity, poor nutritional status, steroid usage, etc. While some of these may be avoided, those patients who are found to have such a hernia can present difficult management problems due to the high potential for recurrence. Without the use of a prosthetic biomaterial, the recurrence rate is as high as 51%. The use of a synthetic material will reduce this rate to 10–24%. The 'ideal' prosthetic product has yet to be found. There are at least 80 different products that can be used in the repair of inguinal, ventral, incisional and other hernias of the abdominal wall. In many of the products there is a paucity of published literature that verifies the claims that are made by the manufacturers. Surgeons recognize that the main purpose in the use of these materials will be the repair of a fascial defect in the abdominal wall. The main indications of use of the materials are listed in Table 26.1.

Synthetic prosthetic biomaterials can be divided into the absorbable and non-absorbable products. The absorbable biomaterials (polyglycolic or polyglactic acid) have been used to cover polypropylene prosthetics used to repair a fascial defect in an effort to protect the viscera from that product or as a temporary closure of the abdominal wall for intra-abdominal sepsis. While these materials may reduce adhesions, they do not prevent their development because of the inflammatory response that develops as a natural consequence of the use of these materials. Also, the fixation points (suture or tack) are a further source of adhesion formation.

Non-synthetic biomaterials are based either on the use of porcine tissues to produce a collagen matrix or on cadaveric skin. All of the products are not truly absorbable as they are intended to provide a scaffold for the native fibroblasts to incorporate natural collagen to repair a fascial defect.

Synthetic non-absorbable biomaterials are of many types, sizes and shapes. The use of these products is common in the repair of inguinal hernias. The current use of a prosthesis in the tension-free concept of a repair of the incisional hernias has gained widespread acceptance. The detailed description of the available prosthetic materials is beyond the scope of this chapter.

- Mesh utilization has become routine in countries where it is affordable
- Careful consideration should be given to the use of mesh in younger patients
- With meticulous technique mesh reduces recurrence rates by a factor of three in inguinal and incisional hernia
- Mesh design and mesh materials are undergoing continuous development
- A small proportion of patients may react adversely to prosthetic mesh.

Anaesthesia

Even though local anaesthesia with sedation (so called monitored anaesthesia care) is a more cost-effective anaesthetic technique for inguinal hernia repair, general and regional anaesthesia remain the most popular techniques in most district general hospitals. Interestingly, specialized hernia centres use local infiltration anaesthesia in more than 90% of these cases. The few audit data that exist indicate that on a national and regional scale, general anaesthesia is used in 60–70% of cases, regional anaesthesia in 10–20% and local infiltration anaesthesia in only 5–10% of cases.

General, regional or local anaesthesia is suitable for the repair of most hernias and the type of anaesthesia employed may depend on the preferences and skills of the surgical team rather than the wishes of the patient. In socialized systems of healthcare there are no effective incentives for the widespread adoption of cost-effective techniques and for this reason in Europe general anaesthesia and regional anaesthesia predominate. In contrast in the United States, where market forces prevail and the payor can demand that the less expensive local anaesthesia is utilized for herniorrhaphy, local anaesthesia is employed on a much larger scale.

Local anaesthesia for hernia repair does have particular advantages – organizational and economic as well as clinical. Local anaesthesia can be administered by the operator, thus no medical anaesthetist is required; the patient does require shared care during an operation performed under local anaesthetic and local practice and clinical governance guidelines will dictate whether the monitoring of the local anaesthetic with sedation is undertaken by a medical anaesthetist, a nurse anaesthetist, an operating department assistant or even in some healthcare environments no specialist monitor. Peripheral oxygen saturation must be monitored with a pulse oximeter, especially if intravenous sedation is being used. In addition intravenous access should be established in order that the complications of inadvertent intravascular injection of local anaesthetic agents, which may result in cerebral and cardiovascular side effects, can be counteracted. Blood pressure should be recorded on arrival in the operating theatre and after the injection of local anaesthetic, and preferably monitored throughout the procedure. This may be done by connecting the patient to a cardiac monitor supervised by the anaesthetic nurse throughout the operation and regularly recording pulse, blood pressure and respiratory rate. Emergency resuscitation equipment, including the requirements for endotracheal intubation, must be available in the event of severe respiratory depression needing intubation.

Modern general anaesthesia makes it possible for safe operations to be performed on patients who are to go home 2 h or so later. The need for tracheal intubation is no longer a contraindication to day surgery. The speed of recovery from general anaesthesia is paramount to facilitate full and rapid recovery to consciousness and a degree of physical performance commensurate with returning home by private car or taxi.

While the advantages and disadvantages of local or general anaesthesia must be considered for each and every patient, for open operations the patient's views should not be overruled by the surgeon's personal preference.

- The use of local anaesthesia in inguinal hernia surgery requires the acquisition of additional skills
- Patients having surgery under local anaesthesia should be carefully monitored
- A rate of 90% of patients having inguinal hernia repair under local anaesthesia is achievable.

Technique for local anaesthesia

The recommended local anaesthetic agent is a mixture of bupivacaine and lignocaine with the addition of adrenaline 1:200 000. The benefits of this mixture are the rapid onset of action of the lignocaine solution, the prolonged action of the bupivacaine and the possibility of reduced local haemorrhage with the addition of adrenaline. In practice 3 × 10 ml ampoules of bupivacaine 0.25% solution with adrenaline 1:200 000 are admixed with 3 × 10 ml ampoules of 1% lignocaine to produce 3 × 20 ml anaesthetic solutions. This 60 ml volume of local anaesthetic is suitable for most patients except the excessively lean or excessively obese patient, where the volume may be reduced or increased by up to 10 ml. The technique of application of the inguinal block can be achieved by a variety of techniques. If a preoperative inguinal block is applied, a 5 ml supplement of 1% lignocaine can be used intraoperatively should the need arise. Many experienced operators will use this supplementary local anaesthetic around the pubic tubercle before attempting dissection of the spermatic cord in this area. Amid from the Lichtenstein clinic has given an account of the step-by-step, infiltrate-as-you-go procedure of local anaesthesia for inguinal hernia repair. Care must be taken to avoid direct intravascular injection during the infiltration, which is a very rare event since the only major vein in the region is the femoral vein, which should be far from the wandering tip of the infiltrator's needle.

Although pre-anaesthetic drugs are unnecessary, patient morale is improved by giving midazolam intravenously just before the start of the procedure. In most patients the dose should be no more than 2 mg midazolam, except for young anxious patients where the dose required may be up to 4 mg, and in elderly patients with comorbid cardiorespiratory disease when sedation is contraindicated or unnecessary.

- A detailed knowledge of groin anatomy is required to achieve effective administration of local anaesthesia for hernia surgery
- Improved local anaesthetic agents have increased their effectiveness
- Surgical technique must be adapted to the local anaesthetic situation.

Complications of hernia in general

Complications include the following:

1. Rupture of the hernia – spontaneous or traumatic.

2. Involvement of the hernial sac in the disease process: (a) mesothelial hyperplasia; (b) carcinoma; (c) endometriosis and leiomyomatosis; (d) inflammation – peritonitis, acute appendicitis.
3. Incarceration, obstruction and strangulation. Reductio-en-masse.
4. Maydl's hernia and afferent loop strangulation. Strangulation of the appendix in a hernial sac. Richter's hernia. Littre's hernia.
5. Herniation of female genitalia. Pregnancy in a hernial sac.
6. Urinary tract complications, hernia of the bladder, the ureter and of a urinary ileal conduit.
7. Sliding hernia.
8. Testicular strangulation in: (a) infants; (b) adults with large giant inguinoscrotal hernias.

Incarceration, obstruction and strangulation

Incarceration is the state of an external hernia which cannot be reduced into the abdomen. Incarceration is important because it implies an increased risk of obstruction and strangulation. Incarceration is caused by (a) a tight hernial sac neck; (b) adhesions between the hernial contents and the sac lining – these adhesions are sometimes a manifestation of previous ischaemia and inflammation; (c) development of pathology in the incarcerated viscus, e.g. a carcinoma or diverticulitis in incarcerated colon; (d) impaction of faeces in an incarcerated colon.

Incarceration is an important finding. It should urge the surgeon to undertake operation sooner rather than later. If reduction of a hernia is performed it should be gentle; forcible reduction of an incarcerated hernia may precipitate reductio-en-masse (see below). If bowel with a compromised blood supply is reduced, stricturing and adhesions between gut loops will follow. This will lead to intestinal obstruction some weeks or months later. The best policy is to operate on incarcerated hernias and check the viability of the gut at operation.

Incarceration in an inguinal hernia is the commonest cause of acute intestinal obstruction in infants and children in the UK. In adults, postoperative adhesions account for 40% of cases of obstruction, external hernias for 30% and malignancy for 25% of cases. In tropical Africa, strangulated external hernia is the commonest cause of intestinal obstruction in all age groups.

Patients presenting with symptoms of intestinal obstruction should have all the potential hernial sites very carefully examined. The sites of obstruction are inguinal, femoral, umbilical, incisional, Spigelian, and obturator and perineal hernial orifices in that order. A partial enterocoele (Richter's hernia) is a particularly treacherous variety of hernia, especially in infancy. Partial enterocoele is a potentially lethal and easily overlooked complication of 'port site' hernia following laparoscopy.

Strangulation is the major life-threatening complication of abdominal hernias. In strangulation the blood supply to the hernial contents is compromised. At first there is angulation and distortion of the neck of the sac; this leads to lymphatic and venous engorgement. The herniated contents become edematous. Capillary vascular permeability develops. The arterial supply is occluded by the developing edema and now the scene is set for ischaemic changes in the bowel wall.

The gut mucosal defences are breached and intestinal bacteria multiply and penetrate through to infect the hernial sac contents. Necrobiosis and gangrene complete a sad and lethal cycle unless surgery or preternatural fistula formation saves the patient. Hypovolaemia and septic shock predicate vigorous resuscitation if surgery is to be successful.

Forty per cent of patients with femoral hernia are admitted as emergency cases with strangulation or incarceration, whereas only 3% of patients with direct inguinal hernias present with strangulation. A groin hernia is at its greatest risk of strangulation within 3 months of its onset. The general public, especially the elderly, should be aware of the potential dangers of a lump in the groin. The most easily missed of these lumps in the groin is a femoral hernia in an obese patient in whom the consequences of a missed diagnosis carry a high morbidity and mortality.

Obturator hernias are very prone to strangulation; however, their elective repair is rarely feasible and a high index of suspicion particularly in elderly, emaciated female patients with symptoms of intestinal obstruction is required. Clinical suspicion combined with preoperative ultrasonography or CT scan can correctly diagnose obturator hernia preoperatively and result in successful surgery.

- Incarceration should be treated urgently
- External hernias are one of the commonest causes of intestinal obstruction

- Strangulation should be treated as an emergency after adequate resuscitation
- Femoral and obturator hernias frequently present with strangulation and should be considered in a patient with an unidentified cause of intestinal obstruction.

Richter's hernia

Partial enterocele, the eponymous Richter's hernia, occurs when the antimesenteric circumference of the intestine becomes constricted in the neck of a hernial sac without causing complete intestinal luminal occlusion (Figure 26.9).

Richter's hernia is most frequently found in femoral or obturator hernias, although the condition has been described at other sites and there is an increasing incidence at laparoscope insertion sites, therefore awareness of this special type of hernia with its misleading clinical appearance is important.

According to localization and the mode of herniation and entrapment, the clinical picture and course can vary considerably. There are four main groups: (1) the obstructive group, in which early diagnosis and therapy leads to an excellent prognosis; (2) the danger group, in which symptomatology is vague and subsequent delay in surgery is responsible for a high death rate; (3) the postnecrotic group, in which local strangulation and perforation leads to formation of an enterocutaneous fistula; the fistula may close spontaneously ('the miracle cure') or remain chronic: and (4) the 'unlucky' perforation group, in which the postnecrotic abscess, as a result of unlucky anatomical constellations, accidentally finds its way into another compartment, resulting either in a large abscess with severe septic/toxic load or in peritonitis; both of these would lead to a high death rate.

Littre's hernia – hernia of Meckel's diverticulum

Meckel's diverticulum is the most common congenital anomaly of the gastrointestinal tract, arising as a result of incomplete obliteration of the vitello-intestinal duct. Approximately 4% of patients with Meckel's diverticulum develop complications, Littre's hernia being one of the least common. A Meckel's diverticulum may be a chance finding in an inguinal hernia. It has been described in incarcerated inguinal hernia in infants: in infants the diverticulum frequently becomes adherent

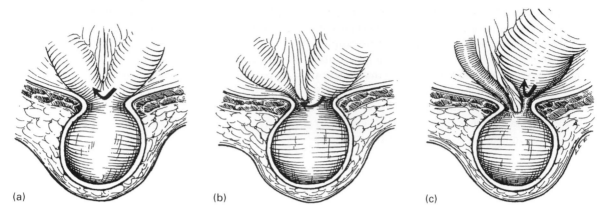

Figure 26.9 Richter's hernia (partial enterocoele). The antimesenteric circumference of the bowel is held by the rigid neck of the hernial sac.

to the sac and as a consequence the hernia becomes irreducible. This can be diagnosed when after taxis of a right inguinal hernia in an infant part of the hernia remains unreduced.

Groin hernias in children

Some 3% to 5% of full-term babies are born with clinically apparent inguinal hernias; in preterm babies this incidence is substantially increased up to 30%. Inguinal hernia is the commonest indication for surgery in early life. Approximately 20–25 live births per 1000 require operation for inguinal hernia, of which some 10% require emergency admission for incarceration and strangulation. The ratio of boys to girls is 9:1, which yields an incidence in male children of 4.2%.

Incarceration and strangulation

Ten per cent of children with inguinal hernias present as emergencies with incarceration or strangulation. Incarceration or strangulation has its highest frequency in the first 3 months of life; thereafter the incidence falls off so that incarceration is very rare after the sixth birthday. The incidence of incarceration is higher in premature and low-birthweight children. Incarceration or strangulation is 10 times more frequent in male than in female children. While incarceration is not infrequent, strangulation (an irreducible hernia containing viscera with a critically compromised blood supply) is very rare.

Treatment by sedation and gallows traction (Solomon position) is recommended initially. Eighty per cent of incarcerated hernias reduce spontaneously if the child is adequately sedated.

Prompt elective operation for inguinal hernia in infants is recommended, the probability of incarceration being 1:4 for hernias in male children diagnosed under 12 months of age.

- Groin hernia incarceration and strangulation are common in premature infants
- Resuscitation and preparation for surgery must take place in the environment of a paediatric unit
- Infant groin hernia is a specialist operation.

Clinical diagnosis of inguinal hernia in a child

A lump in the groin of a child is a common condition that presents to surgeons. In making a diagnosis, the sex and age of the patient and the history of the onset of the lump are critical determinants. Physical diagnosis usually only confirms what can be discovered by careful history-taking.

Sixty per cent of inguinal hernias are apparent within the first 3 months of life; the remainder are discovered in well-baby clinics or at school medical examinations. Few inguinal hernias are first noticed after 5 years of age.

Inguinal hernias may present at birth or at any date after that, and they are more frequent on the right side than the left side. Their early history often distinguishes them from other lumps. In the infant or child the lump is most often noticed by the mother. The lump is more prominent when the child screams or moves about vigorously, whereas it often disappears in the relaxed child; indeed when the child is brought to be examined in the clinic it may not be apparent. The mother's word alone is enough to make a diagnosis. The lump appears initially as a 'bulge' at the medial end of the groin. It increases in size and may progress down into the scrotum. Episodes of irreducibility are frequent.

The inguinal hernia in the male child should be distinguished from the hydrocoele. The symptoms are similar, except that with hydrocoele the mother will have noticed the swelling in the scrotum before there was a swelling in the groin. She may notice that the swelling is only in the scrotum.

On clinical examination the hernia extends from the superficial ring to the scrotum. The hydrocoele extends from the scrotum towards the superficial ring; it may not extend as far as the groin crease and external ring. The hernia is reducible and if it contains gut it will reduce with a gurgle. The hydrocoele is readily transilluminable.

- The diagnosis of groin hernia in an infant can be accepted on the basis of the history from the mother
- Hydrocoele and hernia should be distinguished
- Planned, elective surgery is the norm for infant hernia.

Burd and colleagues have suggested a strategy for the optimal management of metachronous hernias in children. A decision analysis tree was constructed with three approaches:

1. Observation and repair of a contralateral hernia only if it later becomes apparent
2. Routine contralateral groin exploration
3. Laparoscopy to evaluate the contralateral groin for a potential hernia.

The results indicated that observation was favoured over laparoscopy, and laparoscopy over routine exploration, with respect to preventing spermatic cord injury and preserving future fertility. Although observation was the favoured approach with respect to cost, laparoscopy was less expensive when the expected incidence of metachronous hernias was high. It was concluded that observation is the preferred approach to metachronous hernia repair because it results in the lowest incidence of injury and costs, and in most patients is associated with a minimal increase in anaesthesia-related morbidity and mortal-

ity. Laparoscopy may be advantageous for patients at high risk of development of a contralateral hernia.

The operation

In babies and young children, the inguinal canal has not yet developed its oblique adult anatomy. The superficial ring is directly anterior to the deep ring and the sac is indirect. There is no acquired deformity of the canal. In these cases the fascia transversalis is normal and a simple herniotomy is all that is necessary. Straightforward inguinal herniotomy should give a 100% cure rate.

Diagnosis of a lump in the groin in the adult

Although the distinction between femoral and inguinal hernias is difficult enough for practising surgeons, the clinical distinction between indirect and direct inguinal hernia is correct in little more than 50% of cases even in experienced hands. Even the position of fixed landmarks such as the midpoint of the inguinal ligament and the mid inguinal point cannot be accurately distinguished. Every groin lump should be carefully evaluated and hernias must be distinguished from other lesions.

Inguinal hernia – the adolescent and the adult

In the male adolescent or young adult the lump is most likely to be an indirect inguinal hernia. The story then is that when the lump first appeared there was acute, quite severe pain in the groin that passed off and after a day or two went away altogether. The pain may have been related to straining or lifting or playing some violent game. Overall, however, it has been estimated that only 7% of patients can attribute the presence of a hernia to a single muscular strain. At first the lump comes and goes, disappearing when the sufferer goes to bed at night and not being present in the morning until he gets out of bed and stands up. The lump comes in the groin and may descend down into the scrotum; this is the classic description of an indirect (oblique) inguinal hernia in the young adult. In the older man direct inguinal hernia is more likely.

A varicocoele cannot easily be confused with an inguinal hernia in the male. The varicocoele is invariably in the left inguinoscrotal line – it is like a mass of worms and disappears spontaneously if the subject lies down. It has no cough impulse.

Inguinal hernias are more common in adult males than adult females in a ratio of 10:1. However, inguinal hernias do occur in women; indeed, indirect inguinal hernias in women are as common as femoral hernias in women, a fact that is often forgotten in the differential diagnosis. Direct inguinal hernias are very rare in women.

- Direct and indirect inguinal hernias cannot be reliably distinguished
- Straining and coughing potentiate and are not the primary cause of groin hernia
- Beware the femoral hernia in a fat female with intestinal obstruction.

Femoral hernia

A femoral hernia accounts for approximately 5–10% of all groin hernias in adults. Most femoral hernias occur in women aged over 50 years. Atrophy and weight loss are common in patients with femoral hernias. The incidence of femoral hernias, male to female, is generally reported to be about 1:4. The different pelvic shape and additional fat in women render them more prone to femoral hernias than are men. Women with femoral hernias are usually multiparous – multiple pregnancy is said to predispose to femoral herniation. Femoral hernias are as common in men as in nulliparous women

Groin pain with a recent-onset irreducible groin lump is the presentation in 27%, a painless reducible groin lump occurs in 10%, a painful and reducible groin lump in 7%. Groin pain with no other symptoms and no complaint of a groin lump is the presentation in 3% of patients. Six per cent of patients present with recurrent obstructive symptoms. Missing the diagnosis of femoral hernia has dire consequences. Such patients are often frail and elderly with severe coexisting diseases and late hospitalization is one of the main causes of unfavourable outcome.

Other groin swellings

Other structures in the groin each contribute to the harvest of swellings, pains and discomforts patients complain of. These include:

1. Vascular disease. (a) Arterial – aneurysms of the iliac and femoral vessels; these may be complicated by distal embolization or vascular insufficiency, which will make the diagnosis easy. Femoral aneurysm as a complication of cardiac catheterization or transluminal angioplasty is a recent arrival in the diagnostic arena. (b) Venous – a saphenovarix could be confused with a femoral hernia. Its anatomical site is the same, but its characteristic blue colour, soft feel, fluid thrill, disappearance when the patient is laid flat and the giveaway associated varicose veins should prevent misdiagnosis. (c) Inguinal venous dilatation secondary to portosystemic shunting can result in a painful inguinal bulge that can even become incarcerated. Preoperative Doppler ultrasound in cirrhotic patients with suspected inguinal hernias is advised.

2. Lymphadenopathy. Chronic painless lymphadenopathy may occur in lymphoma and a spectrum of infective diseases. Acute painful lymphadenitis can be confused with a tiny strangulated femoral hernia. A lesion in the watershed area, the lower abdomen, inguinoscrotal or perineal region, the distal anal canal or the ipsilateral lower limb quickly resolves the argument.

3. Tumours. Lipomas are very common tumours. The common 'lipoma of the cord', which in reality is an extension of preperitoneal fat, is frequently associated with an indirect or direct inguinal hernia. Fawcett and Rooney examined 140 inguinal hernias in 129 patients to study the problem of lipoma. A fatty swelling was deemed significant if it was possible to separate it from the fat accompanying the testicular vessels. The fatty swelling was designated as being a lipoma if there was no connection with extraperitoneal fat and was designated as being a preperitoneal protrusion if it was continuous through the deep ring with extraperitoneal fat. Protrusions of extraperitoneal fat were found in 33% of patients and occurred in association with all varieties of hernia. There was a true lipoma of the cord in only one patient. It was concluded that the forces causing the hernia were also responsible for causing the protrusion of extraperitoneal fat. Read has commented that occasionally extraperitoneal protrusions of fat may be the only herniation and therefore inguinal hernia classifications need to include not only fatty hernias but sac-less, fatty protrusions. Lipomas also occur in the upper

thigh to cause confusion with femoral hernias. A lipoma is rarely tender; it is soft with scalloped edges and can be lifted 'free' of the subjacent fat.

4. Secondary tumours. A lymph node enlarged with metastatic tumour usually lies in a more superficial layer than a femoral hernia. Such lymph nodes are more mobile in every direction than a femoral hernia and are often multiple. A metastatic deposit of a tumour arising from the abdominal cavity such as adenocarcinoma can present as a rock-hard immobile mass that can be confused as either a primary incarcerated inguinal hernia or a postoperative fibrotic reaction following an inguinal hernia repair.

5. Genital anomalies. (a) Ectopic testis in the male – there is no testicle in the scrotum on the same side. Torsion of an ectopic testicle can be confused with a strangulated hernia. (b) Cyst of the canal of Nuck – these cysts extend towards, or into, the labium majorum and are transilluminable.

6. Obturator hernia. An obturator hernia, especially in a female, lies in the thigh lateral to the adductor longus muscle. Vaginal examination will resolve the diagnosis. Elective diagnosis is rarely entertained.

7. Rarities. (a) A cystic hygroma is a rare swelling; it is loculated and very soft. Usually the fluid can be pressed from one part of it to another. (b) A psoas abscess is a soft swelling frequently associated with backache. It loses its tension if the patient is laid flat. It is classically lateral to the femoral artery. (c) A hydrocoele of the femoral canal is a rarity reported from West Africa. In reality it is the end stage of an untreated strangulated femoral epiplocoele. The strangulated portion of omentum is slowly reabsorbed, the neck of the femoral sac remains occluded by viable omentum, while the distal sac becomes progressively more and more distended by protein-rich transudate.

Clinical examination

The groin should be examined with the patient standing erect and again with the patient lying flat. Hernias are sometimes only apparent when the patient stands up or only when the patient strains or coughs (Figure 26.10).

When the patient is examined a clinical decision should be made as to whether the lump is a hernia or not a hernia – this is the crucial initial decision

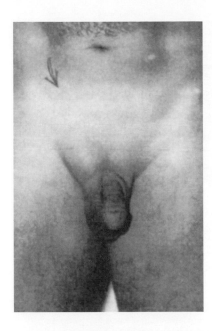

Figure 26.10 An inguinal hernia in the adult is above and medial to the inguinal ligament and pubic tubercle as the hernia emerges from the superficial inguinal ring.

to make. A hernia has a cough impulse, changes in size when the patient strains or lies down and may be reducible. The other lumps in the groin do not change their disposition when the patient stands or lies down.

Reducing the hernia and then using one finger or thumb to hold it reduced while the patient coughs is a useful test which will enable the inguinal canal or the femoral ring to be identified, almost with certainty. Scrotal hernias must be separated from other scrotal lumps – hydrocoele, varicocoele, testicular tumours, epididymal cysts, etc. If the hernia is reducible, the diagnosis is obvious. A cough impulse is a characteristic of hernias, but not of other scrotal masses.

The advent of sophisticated radiological investigation has enabled small and occult hernias to be more easily diagnosed. The chief utility of ultrasound is to enable scrotal and other swellings to be clearly differentiated.

- In the absence of a clinical hernia do not rely on radiological examination to make the diagnosis
- Radiological assessment helps identify the origin of unusual lumps in the groin and scrotum
- Expertise is required to interpret radiological images of the groin.

Anterior open repair of inguinal hernia in adults

The Shouldice operation is the gold standard for sutured repair. The most essential part of the Shouldice

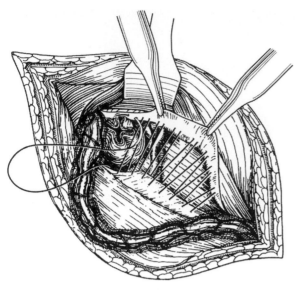

Figure 26.11 The second layer of suturing in the multi-layered Shouldice repair: the lower lateral flap of fascia transversalis is sutured to the undersurface of the upper medial flap along the 'white line' or 'arch'.

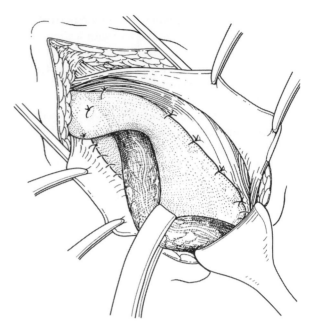

Figure 26.12 The completed Lichtenstein operation showing coverage of the posterior inguinal wall and overlap of 1–2 cm medially, laterally and superiorly.

operation is the repair of the fascia transversalis, which is divided along the length of the canal, beginning at the deep inguinal ring and continuing down to the pubic tubercle. The fascia transversalis is repaired in four layers and the deep ring is carefully reconstituted using a 'double breasting' technique (Figure 26.11).

The Lichtenstein technique

The true tension-free hernioplasty using mesh and no suture closure of the hernial defect was introduced in 1984 by Irving Lichtenstein in Los Angeles. Repair of the posterior wall with a suture line is abandoned, except for a simple imbrication suture for large sacs that aided flattening of the posterior wall before placement of the mesh. In the UK the Lichtenstein technique was first reported by Kingsnorth and colleagues, and subsequently by a private hernia clinic, The British Hernia Centre. Mesh repair is associated with three times fewer recurrences than non-mesh, in the repair of inguinal hernia. The incision, exposure, dissection of the canal and cord and the dealing with indirect hernial sacs is identical to that described for the Shouldice operation. A mesh (manufactured from polypropylene or polyester and having a weight of 40–80 g/m²) is pre-cut to 8 cm × 16 cm and is tailored to the individual patient's requirements. This will involve trimming

1–2 cm of the patch's width and the upper medial corner so that it will tuck itself between the external oblique and internal oblique muscles without wrinkles. After tailoring the mesh is sutured to the inguinal ligament and conjoint tendon and closed around the spermatic cord to recreate the internal ring (Figure 26.12).

Strangulated hernia

The use of mesh is not absolutely contraindicated if the amount of contamination is kept to a minimum and broad-spectrum antibiotics are used during and after the operation for several days. The Shouldice operative technique is recommended to treat a strangulated inguinal hernia, where there is gross contamination following bowel perforation due to necrosis. The additional risk of infection in this situation militates against the use of mesh, infection of which may cause morbidity.

Postoperative care

Immediate active mobilization is the key to rapid convalescence. The 'patient with a hernia' must not be allowed to become institutionalized into the 'postoperative patient'. If the operation has been performed under local anaesthesia, the patient should be helped to walk as soon as he is returned to the ward. If general anaesthesia has been used, the patient must be made to get up and walk as soon as he is conscious. There may be slight pain after surgery and a suitable mild analgesic should be prescribed. Analgesics with narcotic properties are never needed.

If social circumstances allow, patients should be discharged within a few hours of operation with minimal discomfort, for which mild analgesics are prescribed. Unrestricted activity is encouraged, and indeed most patients should resume normal activity in 2–10 days. 'Take it easy' is the wrong advice.

Integrity of the hernia repair depends on good surgical technique, rather than any supposedly deleterious, premature physical activity undertaken by the patient. Return to full activity does not increase recurrences and indeed caution will engender anxiety and perhaps justify the patient's decision to remain off work for up to 6 weeks. It is contradictory and counterproductive to warn against strenuous activity and is a recipe for long-term disability. Troublesome wound soreness is rare 7–10 days after the operation.

The recurrence rate after inguinal hernia repair is operator-dependent: the choice of operator is as important as the choice of operation

- Mobilization and return to activity must be actively encouraged by verbal and written information to patients and their carers
- Inadequate home support can compromise recovery
- Properly fixated mesh is stronger than innate tissues, allowing early return to normal activity.

Laparoscopic groin hernia repair

Laparoscopic repair involves placement of a preperitoneal prosthetic biomaterial. The repair follows the same principles as the open preperitoneal (Stoppa) repair. After reducing the hernia sac a large piece of mesh is placed in the preperitoneal space covering all potential hernia sites in the inguinal region (Figure 26.13). The mesh becomes sandwiched between the preperitoneal tissues and the abdominal wall and, provided it is large enough, is held there by intra-abdominal pressure until such time as it becomes incorporated by fibrous tissue.

The choice between the transabdominal preperitoneal (TAPP) and the totally extraperitoneal (TEP) repair is a matter of personal preference. There is

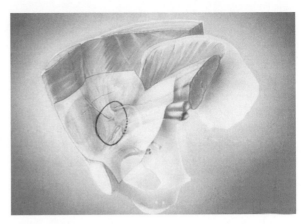

Figure 26.13 Mesh in the preperitoneal space overlying the myopectineal orifice.

no clinical difference between the conversions to open, the complications seen, or the recurrence rates between these two operations in experienced hands. The TEP may be the more expeditious and less costly procedure based upon operating room expenses.

Disadvantages of laparoscopic hernia repair

It is estimated that it may take as many as 250 laparoscopic hernia repairs before an inexperienced laparoscopic surgeon can bring the operating time for laparoscopic hernia repair into a range similar to that for open hernia repair. On the other hand, the surgeon who is experienced with other advanced laparoscopic operations will take approximately 30–50 cases to build an adequate experience and a decreased operative time. Since operating time is expensive this has significant cost implications. Added to this, laparoscopic hernia repair is already more costly than open repair, principally because of the use of disposable instruments. These costs, however, can be brought into a range similar to that of open repair by using reusable rather than disposable instruments and by suturing rather than stapling or tacking when indicated. A hidden cost, often not considered, is use of the laparoscopic equipment itself, which is currently less durable and more expensive than conventional instruments. These costs can be minimized by frequent use and extra care by nursing and medical staff during their use.

Laparoscopic hernia repair is technically more demanding than open anterior approaches. This, combined with a poor knowledge of the preperitoneal anatomy by many, will limit its use to surgeons with a special interest in laparoscopic or hernia surgery. Nevertheless, it has advantages in terms of reduced postoperative pain, lower wound morbidity, a more rapid return to normal activity and less chronic pain and numbness than open repair. The benefits that are realized to the individual patients can be expanded into the societal advantages because these patients are returned to the workforce more rapidly. Many surgeons are finding this technique more beneficial for the patients with bilateral and/or recurrent hernias. These advantages need to be balanced against increased costs and a high recurrence rate in the learning-curve period.

Femoral hernia

A femoral hernia is a variety of groin hernia – a defect in the fascia transversalis which occurs when the femoral sheath, a funnel of fascia transversalis enclosing the femoral vessels beneath the inguinal ligament, becomes dilated. A peritoneal sac enters the femoral funnel and then, as a plunger, causes it to dilate. Because the lacunar ligament medially and the pectineal ligament posteriorly are unyielding, strangulation is common at the neck of the sac.

The three open approaches

1. The low approach is recommended for the easily reducible uncomplicated femoral hernia especially in the thin patient, and in the frail ASA class 3 or 4 patient, when it can be undertaken electively using local anaesthesia.
2. The inguinal approach is best used when there is a concomitant primary inguinal hernia on the same side which can be repaired simultaneously.
3. The extraperitoneal approach is used when obstruction or strangulation is present, in patients who have undergone previous groin surgery, when inguinal and femoral hernias occur together, and in bilateral cases where both sides can be repaired simultaneously.

Open prosthetic repair

The use of prosthetic biomaterials is becoming the preferred method. This is especially true for recurrent repairs in which the recurrence rate is at least 25%. The concept of the plug-and-patch repair for femoral hernia is based upon the 'umbrella plug' and 'dart' repairs

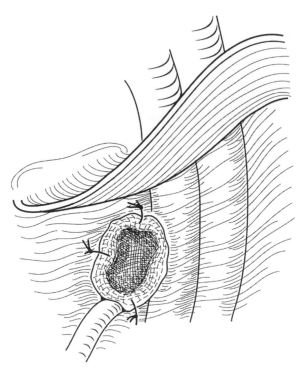

Figure 26.14 Insertion of a plug to repair a femoral hernia.

for inguinal hernia. The plug is fixed in position in the defect with non-absorbable sutures (Figure 26.14). This will prevent the migration of the plug.

Laparoscopic repair

The repair of femoral hernia with the laparoscopic placement of a preperitoneal mesh is identical to the transabdominal preperitoneal or the totally extraperitoneal inguinal operations. There is no difference in technique because the exposure of the myopectineal orifice by these two procedures will provide an excellent visualization of the femoral hernia.

Umbilical hernia in adults

Umbilical hernias in adults can be a cause of considerable morbidity and if complications supervene they can lead to death. Umbilical hernias are much less frequent in the adult population than inguinal hernias but rank second as a cause of external hernia causing strangulation in the UK. Of the patients with umbilical hernias, 90% are women, invariably women who are overweight and multiparous. Umbilical hernias have a high risk of incarceration. When these hernias incarcerate and strangulate, they frequently contain transverse colon and/or stomach. Strangulated umbilical hernias have a considerable morbidity dictated by the age of the patient and concomitant disease, atherosclerosis, obesity and diabetes mellitus.

Most patients with umbilical hernias complain of a painful protrusion at the umbilicus. This discomfort is indication enough for operation. In many patients, this protrusion may be asymptomatic but will be discovered by the primary physician or general practitioner on routine physical examination. Frequently, it is found in association with an inguinal hernia by the surgeon. Absolute indications for surgery include obstruction and strangulation. Irreducibility is not an absolute indication for surgery: many long-standing umbilical hernias have many adhesions in a loculated hernia and are thus irreducible. In larger hernias the overlying skin may become damaged and ulcerated. Skin complications may dictate the need for operation after the skin sepsis has been controlled. Surgery is advised for all umbilical hernias unless there are strong contraindications, which include obesity, chronic cardiovascular or respiratory disease or ascites (umbilical hernias can be manifestations of cirrhotic or malignant peritoneal effusions). In even these situations, however, the need for surgery may dictate that the procedure be performed after adequate preoperative preparation of the patient.

Umbilical hernias are an important complication of cirrhosis and ascites; the ascites should be controlled either medically or with a shunt before hernia repair is undertaken. Umbilical herniation is sometimes a consequence of chronic ambulatory peritoneal dialysis. In all patients who are to initiate CAPD, any hernia that is found prior to the insertion of the catheter must be repaired.

The overlapping fascial operation as described by Mayo can be used successfully in patients where there are no risk factors (Figure 26.15). However, the use of a prosthetic biomaterial for the repair of the larger defects (>4 cm) has been associated with a lowered rate of recurrence.

The use of the laparoscopic repair of these hernias has also been reported with acceptable results and may become a viable alternative to the repair of this hernia.

- Early diagnosis and repair represents optimal management for umbilical hernia
- A large incarcerated umbilical hernia in an obese patient represents a considerable operative risk
- An asymptomatic umbilical protrusion in a patient with ascites does not warrant surgical intervention.

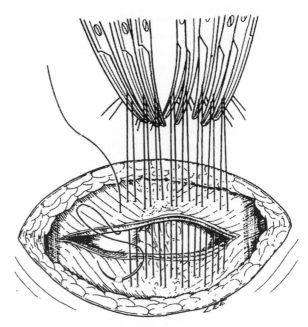

Figure 26.15 The first layer of sutures placed in the Mayo repair: the sutures are left lax and held in haemostats.

Incisional hernia

An incisional hernia is a bulge visible and palpable when the patient is standing and often requiring support or repair. Sixty per cent of patients with incisional hernias do not experience any symptoms; however, symptoms that predicate medical advice include difficulty in bending, cosmetic deformity, discomfort from the size of the hernia, persistent abdominal pain and episodic subacute intestinal obstruction. Incarceration persisting to acute intestinal obstruction and strangulation necessitate emergency surgery.

It is sometimes difficult to differentiate between a hernia and subcutaneous fat or small bowel in the hernia sac or in close proximity to a weakened anterior fascia. In most situations and particularly for massive complex incisional hernias a CT scan may be much more efficient and accurate in defining the defect and planning the preoperative preparation of the patient and the operation chosen.

Incidence

The overall incidence of incisional hernias is difficult to estimate, but at least 10–15% of abdominal operations are followed by incisional hernia. Certainly the reported incidence of this complication has fallen in the past 10 years, during which major sepsis has diminished, monofilament, non-absorbable sutures have been introduced and effective techniques of wound closure have been emphasized.

Long-term prospective studies of laparotomy wounds have revealed a high incidence of late wound failure in patients who have undergone laparotomy but who had sound wounds without herniation when examined at one year. More than half the incisional hernias first appeared more than one year after the initial operation. These 10-year results confirm that there is a continued attrition of the healed laparotomy wound, with incisional hernias developing up to and after 10 years.

Abdominal fascial closure of midline laparotomy wounds with a continuous, non-absorbable suture results in a significantly lower rate of incisional hernia than using either non-absorbable or interrupted techniques. The recent adoption of the laparoscopic techniques for the treatment of intra-abdominal pathology will undoubtedly decrease the occurrence of the midline incisional hernias.

Aetiological factors

The important causative factors include sepsis, steroid and other immunosuppressant therapy and inflammatory bowel disease. Obesity is an important risk factor both for the occurrence of the original incisional hernia and for the likelihood of recurrence of the hernia after repair. Less significant factors include age and sex, anaemia, malnutrition, hypoproteinaemia, diabetes, type of incision, postoperative intestinal obstruction and postoperative chest infection.

Midline incisions are at greater risk than paramedian incisions. Lower midline incisions seem to be at greater risk than upper midline incisions.

- Incisional hernias are common and are largely a consequence of faulty surgical techniques used in closure of laparotomy wounds
- All fit patients with incisional hernias should be offered surgery to improve quality of life and reduce complications
- All incisional hernias should be repaired with mesh
- Experienced surgeons should repair complex hernias.

Principles of open repair

The following principles should be followed:

1. Whenever possible the normal anatomy should be reconstituted. In midline hernias this means the linea alba must be firmly reconstructed; in more lateral hernias there should be layer-by-layer closure as far as possible. However, the use of suture alone with the repair of these hernias is associated with a high rate of recurrence. For this reason, the repair must be supplemented with mesh (see below).
2. Only tendinous/aponeurotic/fascial structures should be brought together. *In situ* darning over the defect without adequate mobilization and apposition of the aponeurotic defect gives a 100% recurrence rate.
3. The suture material must retain its strength for long enough to maintain tissue apposition and allow sound union of tissues to occur. A non-absorbable or slowly absorbable material must, therefore, be used.
4. The length of suture material is related to the geometry of the wound and to its healing. Using deep bites at not more than 0.5 cm intervals, the ratio of suture length to wound length must be 4:1 or more.
5. Repair of an incisional hernia inevitably involves returning viscera to the confines of the abdominal cavity with a resultant rise in intra-abdominal pressure. It is important to minimize this. Preoperative weight reduction is the first precaution. This, unfortunately, is generally not possible. Therefore the surgeon will usually be forced to repair these hernias with little consideration for the increase in the intra-abdominal pressure. In the majority of situations, this is not a clinical issue as few patients will experience an increase in the intra-abdominal pressure that is clinically significant.

A tension-free repair with prosthetic reinforcement is recommended, for which there are several different approaches:

1. The mesh is placed over the defect (onlay) and sutured in position (Figure 26.16).
2. The mesh is placed in the preperitoneal (and retro-muscular) space (Figure 26.17) so that it does not contact the bowel (sublay). Each rectus sheath is incised along its medial border and

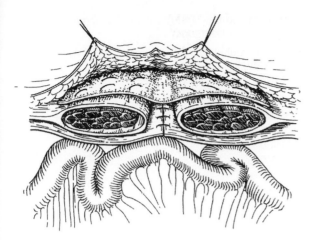

Figure 26.16 Incisional hernia repair using a mesh onlay.

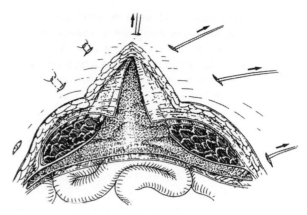

Figure 26.17 Incisional hernia repair using a mesh sublay with fixation by through-and-through sutures.

opened in the midline to expose the anterior and posterior aspects of the rectus muscle, which by blunt dissection is mobilized to its entire width along the length of the defect. The mesh is then placed posterior (retro-) to the rectus muscles, after first closing the posterior leaf of the sheath/peritoneum with monofilament nylon. The mesh is secured with interrupted absorbable sutures between the edges of the mesh and the underlying posterior rectus sheath/peritoneum. The layered closure is completed by approximation of the anterior rectus sheath over the prosthesis.

3. The mesh is placed between the unapproximated fascial edges (inlay). This exposes the bowel to the undersurface of the mesh and should only be used in the exceptional circumstance of inability to close the fascial layers without hernioplasty techniques (less than 5% of cases).

Whichever technique is employed, the mesh must overlap each margin of the aponeurotic defect by some 3–4 cm and must be well fixed to the aponeurosis.

Studies have shown a rate of recurrence that is consistently improved with the use of a synthetic biomaterial as an element to the open repair of incisional and ventral hernias. If there is any tissue loss, a defect greater than 4 cm or any risk factors prosthetic mesh reinforcement is mandatory.

Further reading

Aasvang E, Kehlet H. Surgical management of chronic pain after inguinal hernia repair. *Br J Surg* 2005;**92**:795–801.

Aufenacker TJ *et al.* The role of antibiotic prophylaxis in prevention of wound infection after Lichtenstein open mesh repair of primary inguinal hernia: a multi-centre double-blind randomized controlled trial. *Ann Surg* 2004;**240**:955–961.

Callesen T, Bech K, Kehlet H. The feasibility, safety and cost of infiltration anaesthesia for hernia repair. *Anaesthesia* 1998;**53**:35–35.

Davies N, Thomas M, McIlroy B, Kingsnorth AN. Early results with the Lichtenstein tension-free hernia repair. *Br J Surg* 1994;**81**:1478–1479.

Den Hartog D, Dur AhM, Tuinebreijer WE, Kreis RW. Open surgical procedures for incisional hernias. *Cochrane Database Syst Rev* 2008;**3**:CD006438.

Fitzgibbons RJ *et al.* Watchful waiting verses repair of inguinal hernia in minimally symptomatic men: a randomized clinical trial. *J Am Med Assoc* 2006;**295**: 285–292.

Gilbert AI. Medical/legal aspects of hernia surgery: personal risk. *Surg Clin N Amer* 1993;**73**:583–593.

Grevious MA, Cohen M, Jean Pierre F, Herrmann GE. The use of prosthetics in abdominal wall reconstruction. *Clin Plastic Surg* 2006;**33**:181–197.

Gullmo A. Herniography. *World J Surg* 1989;**13**:560–568.

Kingsnorth AN, LeBlanc KA. *Management of Abdominal Hernias*. 3rd edn. Arnold, 2003.

Kingsnorth AN, Bowley DMG, Porter C. A prospective study of 1000 hernias: results of the Plymouth Hernia Service. *Ann R Coll Surg Engl* 2003;**85**:18–22.

Korenkov M *et al.* Classification and surgical treatment of incisional hernia. Results of an expert's meeting. *Lang Arch Surg* 2001;**386**:65–73.

Lawrence K *et al.* An economic evaluation of laparoscopic versus open inguinal hernia repair. *J Publ Health Med* 1996;**18**:41–48.

Lichtenstein IL, Shulman AG, Amid PK, Montilier MM. The tension-free hernioplasty. *Am J Surg* 1989;**157**:188–193.

Miserez M *et al.* The European Hernia Society groin hernia classification: simple and easy to remember. *Hernia* 2007;**11**:113–116.

Robbins AW, Rutkow IM. The mesh-plug hernioplasty. *Surg Clin N Am* 1993;**73**:501–512.

Wantz GE. Ambulatory hernia surgery. *Br J Surg* 1989;**6**: 1228–1229.

Chapter 27

Fundamentals of vascular surgery

Donald J. Adam, Martin W. Claridge and Antonius B.M. Wilmink

Chronic lower limb ischaemia

Lower limb arterial disease is present in about 20% of the UK population aged over 60 years and is asymptomatic in 75%, causes symptoms of intermittent claudication in 4–5% and critical limb ischaemia in about 1%. All patients should be assessed for their cardiovascular risk factors, have a full vascular examination to assess co-existing carotid disease and aneurysmal disease, ankle:brachial pressure index (ABPI) measurement and imaging using Duplex ultrasound in the first instance and angiography if indicated (intra-arterial digital subtraction angiography, CT angiography, MR angiography).

Intermittent claudication (IC)

This is characterized by the gradual onset of pain in the calf muscles (infra-inguinal artery disease) and/or the thigh and buttocks (supra-inguinal artery disease) after walking a certain distance and disappears quickly with rest. The pain recurs if walking is resumed. Only about 1–2% of claudicants will progress to develop critical limb ischaemia per annum, but about 5% will die from other cardiovascular events such as myocardial infarction or stroke.

All patients with cardiovascular disease (where coronary, cerebrovascular or peripheral) should be commenced on best medical therapy to reduce cardiovascular risk (smoking cessation, exercise and dietary advice, diagnosis and treatment of diabetes, antiplatelets, statins, antihypertensives). In patients with IC, best medical therapy will also increase walking distance and improve their quality of life. Supervised exercise programmes have been shown to be beneficial especially in patients with infra-inguinal disease where collaterals may be encouraged to form. Cilostazol has been shown in several trials to improve claudication distance. Revascularization by surgery or endovascular techniques is rarely indicated in patients with IC due to infra-inguinal (femoro-popliteal) disease but may be worthwhile considering in patients with supra-inguinal (aorto-iliac disease) disease where the symptoms are often more severe, the response to best medical therapy and exercise is less satisfactory and the durability of endovascular or surgical intervention is superior compared to patients with infra-inguinal disease.

Critical limb ischaemia (CLI)

This is defined as persistently occurring ischaemic rest pain or night pain of greater than 2 weeks duration requiring analgesia, or tissue loss (ischaemic ulceration or gangrene). Whereas patients with IC often have a single level of arterial disease, most patients presenting with CLI will have multi-level arterial occlusive disease which makes revascularization more challenging. Best medical therapy should be commenced in all patients to reduce cardiovascular risk and increase the durability of any revascularization procedure.

Limb salvage treatment options include:

(a) endovascular intervention; principally in the form of angioplasty and/or stent placement for stenotic and occluded segments (Figure 27.1)
(b) endarterectomy of a localized atherosclerotic plaque such as the common femoral artery bifurcation and proximal profunda femoris usually completed with patch angioplasty
(c) bypass surgery using autologous vein (from lower or upper limb, either reversed or *in situ* with destruction of the venous valves using a valvulotome) or prosthetic (ePTFE or Dacron). Vein bypass is the conduit of choice for infra-inguinal occlusive disease

Fundamentals of Surgical Practice, Third Edition, ed. Andrew N. Kingsnorth and Douglas M. Bowley.
Published by Cambridge University Press. © Cambridge University Press 2011.

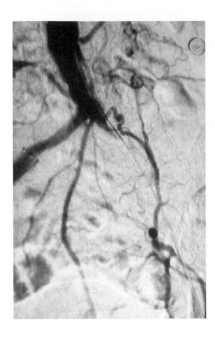

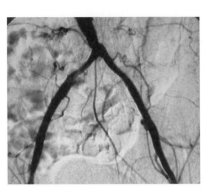

Figure 27.1 Left common and external iliac artery occlusion causing ischaemic rest pain. A stent has already been placed in the right iliac artery. Intra-arterial digital subtraction angiography before and after placement of a covered stent in the left iliac system.

(femoro-popliteal, femoro-tibial bypass) as it is associated with superior long-term patency compared to prosthetic grafts. Prosthetic grafts are used to treat aorto-iliac occlusive disease (aorto-femoral, ilio-femoral, fem-femoral cross-over, axillo-femoral bypass) as the grafts are of large calibre similar to the native vessels and associated with good long-term patency.

Major limb amputation (below the knee, above the knee) should be considered if:

(a) the patient has severe comorbidity and is unfit for surgery and has a pattern of arterial disease which is unsuitable for endovascular intervention

(b) the limb is unsalvageable

(c) the patient is systemically unwell with spreading gangrene or sepsis.

In many circumstances, revascularization is accompanied by minor amputation involving single or multiple digits or the forefoot (transmetatarsal amputation).

The optimal management of patients with critical lower limb ischaemia and a salvageable limb is controversial. In patients with severe limb ischaemia secondary to infra-inguinal disease, the BASIL trial has demonstrated that 'bypass-first' and 'angioplasty-first' strategies were associated with similar outcomes in terms of 30-day mortality, amputation-free survival

and all-cause mortality at 2 years, health-related quality of life out to 3 years and overall hospital costs. Bypass was associated with increased early morbidity, while angioplasty was associated with higher immediate failure rate and re-intervention within the first year. After 2 years, 'bypass-first' strategy was associated with a highly significant advantage in terms of all-cause mortality with a trend towards better amputation-free survival.

Acute limb ischaemia

Acute limb ischaemia (ALI) is limb-threatening ischaemia in a previously well-perfused limb which has an onset of less than 2 weeks duration. The underlying pathological process is acute occlusion of an artery or bypass graft secondary to:

(a) thrombosis of a pre-existing stenotic arterial segment (60%): acute plaque rupture, critical flow reduction, heart failure due to myocardial infarction, dehydration and hypovolaemia, and a pro-thrombotic tendency such as due to an undiagnosed malignancy may all be responsible; popliteal artery aneurysms may cause ALI by thrombosis and occlusion;

(b) thromboembolism (30%): more than 70% of peripheral embolic events are secondary to atrial fibrillation, and most of the remainder are

Table 27.1 Progression of symptoms of acute ischaemia with time

Time since onset	0–6 hours	6–12 hours	12 hours
Signs	Painful White foot Neurosensory deficit	Non-fixed mottling with blanching on digital pressure	Fixed mottling No blanching
Prognosis	Reversible	Partially reversible	Irreversible

secondary to mural wall thrombosis after myocardial infarction; the most frequent extra-cardiac cause of embolic arterial occlusion is a popliteal artery aneurysm and an abdominal aortic aneurysm may also present with acute limb ischaemia;

(c) or other causes such as arterial dissection, external compression, trauma (including iatrogenic injury) and popliteal entrapment or cystic adventitial disease in a young patient.

The classic clinical presentation is with pain (including pain of squeezing the calf, indicating severe muscle ischaemia), loss of function (paralysis and paraesthesia), pallor, pulselessness and perishingly cold to the touch. Examining for the presence of these signs in both the affected and unaffected limb is invaluable, as well as providing evidence of chronic limb ischaemia. When acute arterial occlusion occurs in the absence of previous disease, the signs and symptoms progress as the duration of ischaemia increases (Table 27.1). If arterial occlusion occurs in a limb with pre-existing chronic disease, then collateral vessels may exist and the limb may present with less severe ischaemia and progression to irreversible ischaemia may be slower.

History and cardiovascular examination should provide evidence for an embolic source, the presence of pre-existing atherosclerosis and any significant comorbidity that may require treatment. The presence of arterial pulses, as detected by palpation or with a hand-held Doppler, will help define the level of arterial occlusion: for example, acute bilateral lower limb ischaemia with bilateral absent femoral pulses and mottling to the waist occurs with a saddle embolus to the aortic bifurcation. Cardiac failure, extensive deep venous occlusion leading to phlegmasia cerulea dolens, acute neural entrapment and ergotism (fungus-derived drug poisoning causing acute

vasospasm) are all conditions that can present with similar symptoms and signs.

Immediate management

This group of patients usually have significant comorbidity. Resuscitation should be commenced immediately with correction of hypovolaemia or fluid overload, intravenous analgesia and oxygen. In the absence of contraindications, intravenous heparin is administered immediately to prevent thrombus propagation and maintain collateral circulation. Blood should be analysed for full blood count, urea and electrolytes and glucose. An ECG is performed to detect any cardiac arrhythmias or diagnose myocardial infarction. If an abdominal aortic aneurysm or popliteal artery aneurysm is suspected as a possible source of distal embolization then Duplex ultrasound should be performed.

If there is evidence of irreversible ischaemia, then palliative care may well be the appropriate course for the moribund patient. Otherwise, resuscitation should continue until the patient is stabilized before amputation is considered.

If there is evidence of reversible acute ischaemia, then intervention will be required. If ischaemia is incomplete then preoperative imaging (intra-arterial digital subtraction angiography, CT angiography or MR angiography) should be performed to assess the level and extent of the arterial occlusion and provide important information to guide appropriate intervention. In some circumstances, medical management with anticoagulation may be all that is required, such as the elderly patient with an upper limb embolus. If ischaemia is complete then the patient should proceed immediately to the operating theatre for exploration of the femoral artery with a view to performing thromboembolectomy and intraoperative angiography.

Surgical management

Preoperative preparation should include chest X-ray, ECG and group and save. The patient should be resuscitated and treatment of concurrent conditions should commence. An anaesthetist should always be present during the procedure. Local anaesthesia may be appropriate for the majority of cases where embolectomy is required, but general anaesthesia may be more appropriate for confused or obese patients and where extensive revascularization procedures or a fasciotomy may be required.

Table 27.2 Absolute and relative contraindications to thrombolysis

Absolute	Relative
Active bleeding	At any time
	Pregnancy, severe bleeding tendency, previous GI haemorrhage
	Within last 2 weeks
	Vascular or abdominal surgery
	Within last ten days
	Trauma (including CPR), puncture of non-compressible vessel
	Within 2 months
	Stroke, TIA, craniotomy

Arterial exploration (even if apparently successful) should be accompanied by completion angiography. This will help define any pre-existing aorto-iliac or infra-inguinal disease which may require treatment, particularly if thromboembolectomy has failed. Intraoperative thrombolysis may be attempted, an underlying stenosis may be amenable to angioplasty or stenting, and a persistent occlusion may require bypass grafting.

Successful revascularization will result in a large bolus of acidotic hyperkalaemic blood returning to the circulation as well as a systemic inflammatory reaction due to reperfusion, both of which may lead to significant organ dysfunction. The kidneys are also at risk from myoglobinuria. Continued resuscitation is usually required. Leg swelling may occur, necessitating fasciotomy.

Postoperatively, the patient should remain heparinized and subsequently be warfarinized to reduce the risk of recurrent embolic events.

Endovascular management

Peripheral arterial thrombolysis may be considered if ischaemia is incomplete as it usually takes several hours to dissolve the thrombus. Recombinant tissue plasminogen activator (t-PA) is delivered via a percutaneous catheter placed under local anaesthesia selectively in the occluded artery, thereby delivering a maximal dose of agent to the target lesion while minimizing the complications from systemic thrombolysis. The underlying lesion is usually identified after thrombolysis and can be treated by angioplasty, stenting or surgical reconstruction.

Active bleeding is the only absolute contraindication. All other contraindications should be viewed as relative, balancing their risk against that of the potential for limb salvage (Table 27.2).

Death, predominantly from myocardial infarction and stroke, occurs in 4–13% of cases. Major haemorrhage occurs in approximately 9%, stroke in 2%, minor haemorrhage in 40% and distal embolization in 4% of cases. A further 15% of patients will ultimately require amputation. A meta-analysis of randomized trials of thrombolysis and surgery for ALI demonstrated no difference in limb salvage rates or death at 30 days out to 1 year. Thrombolysis was associated with a significant increase in stroke, major haemorrhage and distal embolization at 30 days.

Abdominal aortic aneurysm

An aneurysm is an abnormal focal dilatation of an artery, vein or heart chamber. Most true aneurysms are degenerative but some may be infective in nature. Abdominal aortic aneurysm (AAA) is defined as a dilatation of the abdominal aorta greater than 3 cm in diameter. AAA is present in about 5% of men aged over 60 years and the male:female ratio is approximately 4:1. Aortic aneurysms are either asymptomatic and diagnosed incidentally, symptomatic but intact (abdominal and/or back pain, embolization or compression of adjacent structures) or ruptured (into the retroperitoneum, peritoneal cavity, inferior vena cava or duodenum). Ruptured AAA is associated with a community-based mortality rate of 80–90%. It is the thirteenth commonest cause of death in the UK, accounting for as many as 10 000 deaths per annum.

Management

(a) Asymptomatic AAA: abdominal ultrasound is the best method for identifying the presence of an AAA and assessing the diameter. CT angiography will provide more accurate information about the size and extent of the aneurysm, including its relation to the renal and visceral arteries and the iliac arteries, and whether the aneurysm is inflammatory in nature and suitable for endovascular repair (EVAR). CT will also identify other intra-abdominal pathology as well as potentially hazardous anatomical variants such as a retro-aortic left renal vein or horseshoe kidney. The likelihood of AAA rupture is directly related to the diameter of the aneurysm. The UK Small Aneurysm Trial demonstrated that, in patients with asymptomatic AAA less than 5.5 cm in diameter, the risks of open surgical repair were greater than the risk of rupture and that these aneurysms should be kept under surveillance. There is accumulating evidence that the diameter threshold for intervention should remain 5.5 cm if the aneurysm is also suitable for endovascular repair (EVAR) even though the early mortality risk is significantly lower than with open surgical repair. There are no robust natural history data on the risk of rupture of different-sized AAAs in fit patients. Therefore, the estimated annual rupture rates for aneurysms less than 5.5 cm, 5.5–5.9 cm, 6.0–6.6 cm, 7.0–7.9 cm and greater than 8 cm may be approximately <1%, 5%, 15%, 30% and 40%, respectively.

Patients with large AAA (>5.5 cm) should have their comorbidity (principally cardiac, respiratory and renal) assessed and management in order to optimize their fitness for intervention and reduce their cardiovascular risk: all patients should have best medical therapy regardless of the aneurysm diameter.

The UK Multi-centre Aneurysm Screening Study (MASS) demonstrated that, for men aged 65–74 years, an invitation to attend AAA screening reduced AAA-related mortality by almost 50%. Patients undergoing repair of screen-detected AAA also had lower operative mortality.

(b) Ruptured AAA: the classic triad of back pain/abdominal pain, hypotension and a pulsatile mass is present in less than half of the patients. A pulsatile mass may not be felt in obese individuals, or if the patient is profoundly hypotensive. A diagnosis of ureteric colic in patients over 60 years of age should be made only after an AAA has been excluded. Hypotensive resuscitation is of critical importance in the management of ruptured AAA. Fluid resuscitation can be harmful in the conscious patient, with increased blood pressure resulting in loss of the retroperitonal tamponade and vasoconstriction, causing a further, often refractory collapse as well as hypothermia and dilutional coagulopathy.

Transfer of an unstable patient to theatre should not be delayed by waiting for investigations to be performed. Blood is taken and red cell concentrate (10 units), fresh frozen plasma and pooled platelets are requested urgently from the transfusion service. ECG may diagnose a myocardial infarction which can present with epigastric pain and hypotension,

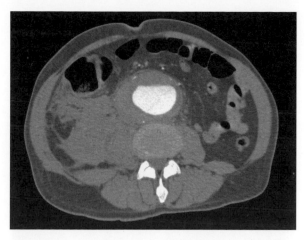

Figure 27.2 CT angiogram demonstrating ruptured AAA with right-sided retroperitoneal haematoma.

although acute ischaemic changes may be secondary to anaemia and hypovolaemia. In cases of clinical uncertainty, abdominal ultrasound will confirm the presence of an AAA and will give an estimate of size but is unreliable in identifying rupture. Abdominal contrast-enhanced CT angiography is useful in a stable patient when the diagnosis of ruptured AAA is in doubt and is indicated in stable patients who are being considered for emergency EVAR (Figure 27.2).

Open surgical repair

This involves general anaesthesia, laparotomy, aortic and iliac artery clamping, and replacement of the aneurysm with a prosthetic graft which is sutured to normal aorta proximally and aorta/iliac/femoral arteries distally. The average perioperative mortality rate for elective open surgical repair of asymptomatic infrarenal AAA in the UK is approximately 7%, with lower mortality rates achieved in higher-volume centres. Open surgical repair of juxtarenal AAA and suprarenal AAA is associated with significantly higher mortality and morbidity rates as the aortic clamp must be positioned on the more proximal aorta and this is associated with an obligatory period of renal and/or mesenteric ischaemia (and reperfusion) as well as lower limb ischaemia which occurs with infrarenal aortic clamping. Emergency open surgical repair for symptomatic intact AAA is associated with an approximate doubling of the mortality rate compared to elective surgery, and surgery for ruptured AAA is associated with a mortality rate of 40–50%.

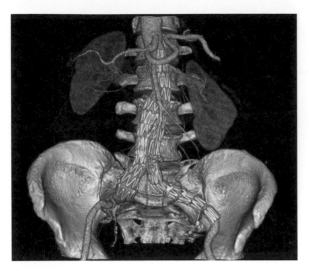

Figure 27.3 CT reconstruction of EVAR for an infrarenal aortic aneurysm.

Endovascular aneurysm repair (EVAR)

This involves general or locoregional anaesthesia, and insertion of a covered stent inside the AAA via the femoral arteries under radiological guidance. There must be an adequate length of normal aorta above the aneurysm and iliac arteries below the aneurysm for fixation and sealing of the covered stent which acts to exclude the aneurysm from the circulation (Figure 27.3). Laparotomy and aortic clamping are avoided. The UK EVAR1 trial demonstrated that, in patients with asymptomatic infrarenal AAA >5.5 cm who are suitable and fit for endovascular repair or open surgical repair, EVAR was associated with a significant reduction in 30-day mortality, hospital stay and AAA-related mortality out to 4 years, similar 4-year all-cause mortality, higher re-intervention rates, similar health-related quality of life and increased costs compared to open surgery. Patients with juxtarenal, suprarenal and thoraco-abdominal aortic aneurysms can also be treated in specialist centres using custom-designed fenestrated and branch EVAR grafts. Life-long stent-graft surveillance is currently required for all EVARs to detect impending graft failure and allow prophylactic re-intervention, which in the majority of cases can be performed using radiological techniques.

The UK EVAR2 trial demonstrated that, in patients with infrarenal AAA >5.5 cm who were considered unfit for open surgical repair, there was no difference in AAA-related mortality or all-cause mortal-ity at 4 years, similar health-related quality of life and increased costs for EVAR and best medical therapy compared to best medical therapy alone. The focus in this group of patients should be to improve their significant comorbidity where possible, so that they effectively become fit for EVAR or open surgical repair.

There is increasing evidence to demonstrate that there is a place for the use of EVAR in the treatment of acute symptomatic and ruptured AAA. This is because of the obvious theoretical advantages of avoiding a major emergency surgical procedure in a sick patient. The UK IMPROVE trial is currently under way, comparing EVAR with open surgical repair in patients with ruptured AAA.

Thoracic aortic aneurysms

The considerable majority (80%) of thoracic and thoraco-abdominal aortic aneurysms are degenerative in nature, 15% are related to a chronic aortic dissection and 5% are secondary to connective tissue diseases such as Marfan's syndrome, aortitis, infection or previous aortic surgery. Thoracic aneurysms are usually asymptomatic but may cause compression symptoms (dysphagia, recurrent pneumonia, dyspnoea, chest /back pain), embolize distally or rupture. For a 6 cm diameter thoracic aortic aneurysm, natural history studies demonstrate that conservative management is associated with a 14% annual risk of rupture, dissection or death. The prognosis of patients with thoraco-abdominal aortic aneurysms is particularly poor, with only 15–20% surviving 5 years.

Thoracic aneurysms may involve the ascending aorta, the aortic arch, the descending aorta or the descending thoracic and abdominal aorta to varying extents. The Crawford classification is used to describe thoraco-abdominal aneurysms: type I involves the descending thoracic and proximal abdominal aorta, sparing infra-renal aorta; type II, the entire descending thoracic and abdominal aorta to aortic bifurcation; type III, mid descending thoracic aorta and entire abdominal aorta; type IV, the entire abdominal aorta commencing at the level of the diaphragm.

Open surgical repair

This is a major undertaking and is only reserved for the fittest of patients with very large aneurysms. For every 100 AAA repairs performed in the UK, there will be 10 thoracic aortic aneurysm repairs and 1–2 thoraco-abdominal aortic aneurysm repairs. Open repair involves general anaesthesia with or without the use of a cardiopulmonary bypass circuit and hypothermia. A left thoracotomy (or thoracolaparotomy for thoraco-abdominal aneurysms) is used to expose the descending thoracic aortic aneurysm. A prosthetic graft is anastomosed to the normal proximal thoracic aorta and distally to either the thoracic aorta or abdominal aorta incorporating the coeliac axis, superior meseneteric and renal arteries, depending on the extent of the aneurysm. This type of procedure is associated with a considerable physiological insult with mortality rates of 15–30%, permanent renal failure in 10% and paraplegia in 10%. The patient invariably requires a prolonged stay in the ITU and hospital before discharge home.

Endovascular aneurysm repair (EVAR)

As with abdominal EVAR, thoracic and thoraco-abdominal aortic aneurysms can be repaired with covered stents inserted via the femoral or iliac arteries under radiological guidance (Figure 27.4). Normal aorta is required for proximal and distal fixation and seal and this can be accomplished by performing additional open surgical bypass procedures if required for more extensive aneurysms such as carotid-subclavian bypass or bypass grafting from the iliac arteries or infrarenal aorta to the visceral and renal arteries (hybrid open-endovascular repair) or by using custom-made fenestrated or branched aortic stent-grafts. Thoracic EVAR avoids the need for thoracotomy and cardiopulmonary bypass and is associated with a significant reduction in the risk of morbidity and mortality: approximately 3% mortality and 3% paraplegia for elective repair.

Popliteal artery aneurysms

These are the commonest peripheral artery aneurysm (80%). They are present in about 10–20% of patients with AAA. In 50% of patients with popliteal aneurysms there will be bilateral aneurysms and in 40% of patients there will be an associated AAA. Popliteal aneurysms are frequently asymptomatic but up to 50% will present with severe acute lower limb ischaemia secondary to either aneurysm thrombosis or distal microembolization which causes occlusion of the tibial vessels and often occurs without symptoms prior to presentation.

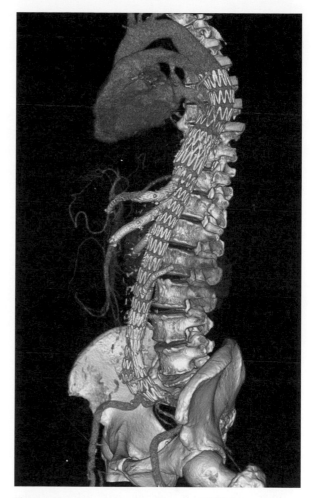

Figure 27.4 CT reconstruction of branched EVAR for type III thoraco-abdominal aortic aneurysm.

Rupture of a popliteal aneurysm is extremely uncommon. Elective popliteal artery aneurysm repair should be considered for aneurysms >2–3 cm in diameter especially if there is intraluminal thrombus. Surgery is currently the treatment of choice and involves either proximal and distal aneurysm ligation with surgical bypass, or interposition grafting. Covered stents may also be used but currently the outcomes are inferior to surgical repair with autologous vein.

Visceral arterial aneurysms

Visceral artery aneurysms are relatively rare. Splenic artery aneurysms are the commonest (60%) and, unlike other visceral aneurysms, are commoner in females (4:1). Hepatic artery aneurysms account for about 20% and are commoner in males. Coeliac and superior mesenteric artery aneurysms account for another 10%. Aneurysms may occur due to blunt abdominal trauma or inflammation (pancreatitis, septic embolization in intravenous drug abusers, or vasculitis). Increased blood flow combined with hormonal changes appears to explain why multiple pregnancies predispose to splenic artery aneurysm formation.

Rupture is the commonest mode of presentation and is associated with a mortality rate of 25%. Erosion may also occur into a major adjacent viscus. Ruptured aneurysms present with acute abdominal pain associated with severe intra-abdominal haemorrhage or with profuse gastrointestinal bleeding. Occasionally superior mesenteric artery aneurysms thrombose, causing acute mesenteric ischaemia. While intact splenic artery aneurysms are often asymptomatic, in up to 20% of patients they produce pain in the left upper quadrant and such a history may precede rupture. Intrahepatic hepatic artery aneurysms may rupture, causing haemobilia, biliary colic and obstructive jaundice.

Management

In cases of rupture or erosion, blood investigations will show evidence of bleeding as well as evidence of any underlying pathology such as pancreatitis or hepatic impairment. Visceral aneurysms are often saccular and tend to calcify with age so that signet ring calcification is visible on the plain abdominal X-ray in up to 70% of cases. Selective intra-arterial digital subtraction angiography of the coeliac and superior mesenteric arteries remains the most valuable investigation and should be performed in patients in whom the condition is suspected or when endoscopy fails to identify the source or cause of bleeding. Contrast-enhanced CT angiography will also identify the lesion.

Coil embolization of the bleeding vessel performed at the time of diagnostic arteriography is the treatment of choice in most specialist vascular units as it avoids major emergency surgery in a sick patient. Covered stents may also be used for hepatic and superior mesenteric aneurysms, thereby excluding the aneurysm while avoiding end-organ ischaemia. Splenic artery embolization rarely results in splenic ischaemia as the spleen remains perfused via the short gastric vessels. Open surgical repair is often hazardous and is reserved for those patients where coil embolization is contraindicated or fails.

Carotid artery disease

Approximately 75–80% of strokes are ischaemic in nature and about 50% of these ischaemic strokes are due to embolization from the carotid bifurcation. Embolization to the ipsilateral middle cerebral artery territory results in contralateral hemimotor and hemisensory signs and dysphasia if to the dominant hemisphere, while embolization to the ipsilateral ophthalmic and retinal artery leads to transient or permanent ipsilateral monocular blindness (amaurosis fugax). If the duration of the focal neurological deficit is less than 24 hours, then the event is called a transient ischaemic attack (TIA) and if more than 24 hours then it is called a stroke (CVA).

Management

Duplex ultrasound is the most widely used imaging technique for detecting carotid artery disease but MR angiography or CT angiography is usually required to confirm the severity of the carotid stenosis (especially if there is severe vessel calcification, a long stenosed segment, or near occlusion), the extent of the disease, the state of the contralateral carotid artery, vertebral arteries and circle of Willis and the presence of intracranial pathology (infarct, haemorrhage, space-occupying lesion).

Symptomatic carotid artery stenosis

Several major trials (ECST, NASCET) have demonstrated that in patients presenting with either a carotid territory TIA, amaurosis fugax or stroke with good recovery, and who have an internal carotid artery stenosis of 70–99% (carotid occlusions do not require intervention), carotid endarterectomy (CEA) combined with best medical therapy is associated with a highly significant reduction in stroke risk compared to best medical therapy alone.

In order to have the greatest impact on stroke prevention, CEA should be performed ideally within 48 hours of the index event but certainly within 2 weeks and with a perioperative mortality and stroke risk of less than 2–3%. Pooled data from large randomized trials have demonstrated that CEA within 2 weeks of the index event is associated with a 30% absolute risk reduction in stroke risk at 2 years. The type of anaesthesia used for surgery (local or general) and

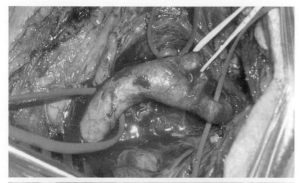

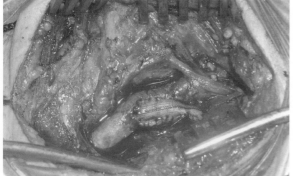

Figure 27.5 Carotid artery exposure and after CEA with prosthetic patch angioplasty.

carotid sinus nerve blockade have no influence on outcome, while routine carotid patching (either vein or prosthetic) is associated with a three-fold reduction in perioperative stroke risk, carotid thrombosis and late re-stenosis compared with routine primary closure (Figure 27.5).

The commonest causes of perioperative stroke are carotid thrombosis (which mandates emergency re-exploration) and intra-cerebral haemorrhage. Post-CEA hyperperfusion syndrome may occur in up to 3% of cases and is due to impaired cerebral autoregulation. Symptoms include severe frontal headaches, seizures and intracerebral haemorrhage and treatment is with aggressive control of blood pressure and any seizures.

Carotid stenting has been advocated as an alternative to CEA. It is performed under local anaesthesia via a percutaneous femoral artery puncture under radiological guidance. It avoids a neck incision and the risk of cranial nerve injury but to date randomized trials have reported an almost doubling of the risk of stroke and death compared to CEA in symptomatic patients.

Asymptomatic carotid stenosis

Several major trials have demonstrated that, in asymptomatic patients who have an internal carotid artery stenosis of 70–99%, CEA combined with best medical therapy is associated with a significant reduction in stroke risk compared to best medical therapy alone. A recent trial (ACST) demonstrated that, in asymptomatic patients less than 75 years old with a 70% or greater carotid stenosis, CEA and best medical therapy was associated with a 50% relative reduction in stroke risk compared with best medical therapy alone out to 5 years (6% CEA+BMT vs. 12% BMT alone).

Renovascular disease

A severe stenosis of the renal arteries will reduce the perfusion of the kidney, leading to hypertension (increased renin and angiotensin) or impaired renal function (renal parenchyma ischaemia and necrosis). Atherosclerosis is responsible for the considerable majority of renal artery stenotic disease although fibromuscular hyperplasia may be responsible in young and middle-aged women.

Renal revascularization may be indicated to control hypertension that is difficult to treat medically or to preserve renal function. Only rarely will revascularization lead to an improvement in renal function. The most commonly used approach to renal artery reconstruction is angioplasty and stenting with surgery (laparotomy with bypass or endarterectomy) reserved for those patients who cannot be managed with endovascular techniques. The ASTRAL trial demonstrated that, in patients with atherosclerotic renal artery stenosis, renal angioplasty/stenting and best medical therapy was not associated with a significant improvement in renal function, blood pressure, major cardiovascular events or mortality compared with best medical therapy alone.

Varicose veins

These are tortuous dilatations of the superficial veins, commonly affecting the lower limbs. The majority of varicose veins (VV) are primary or idiopathic and are thought to be due to a structural vein wall defect which predisposes the vein to progressive dilatation with increased venous pressure and secondary valvular incompetence; and a minority of cases may be secondary to an underlying cause such as pelvic mass (pregnancy, fibroids, ovarian tumour), previous deep venous thrombosis (DVT), arteriovenous fistula or congenital absence of venous valves. When standing the venous pressure at the ankle is about 100 mmHg. When walking, competent venous valves and the calf muscle pump act to propel venous blood up the leg and prevent backflow such that the pressure at the ankle is less than about 25 mmHg. Failure of these mechanisms (valves and calf pump) leads to high pressure in the superficial system at rest as well as when walking and this leads to the symptoms and signs of VV and chronic venous insufficiency (CVI). VV are classified as: truncal varices affecting the main trunk and major tributaries of the great and small saphenous veins, which are usually greater than 4 mm in diameter and lie subcutaneously; reticular varices, which are usually less than 4 mm in diameter and lie deep in the dermis; and telangiectasias, which are usually less than 1 mm in diameter and lie superficially in the dermis.

Patients will present with cosmetic issues, symptoms (heaviness and aching) or complications which include: thrombophlebitis with painful inflamed and thrombosed VV; haemorrhage into subcutaneous tissue or externally due to chronic venous hypertension; varicose eczema with itching, scaling and a rash especially around ankles; ankle and calf oedema; haemosiderin pigmentation and lipodermatosclerosis due to chronic venous hypertension which leads to leakage of red blood cells from capillaries into the subcutaneous tissues, degradation of the haemoglobin into brown haemosiderin deposits, and subsequent scarring and fibrosis of the skin and subcutaneous tissues; chronic venous ulceration (CVU). VV are not a risk factor for DVT in young healthy people but may indicate co-existing deep venous disease in elderly people which may be a risk factor for DVT. Duplex ultrasound is the principal investigation for lower limb venous disease. It can determine the presence, severity and precise anatomy of any superficial and/or deep venous disease. Co-existing arterial occlusive disease may be present and so ABPI and arterial duplex are indicated in the absence of palpable pedal pulses.

Management

In the first instance, patients should be reassured and advised about weight loss, avoiding constricting clothing, regular walking (calf muscle contraction increases venous return) and avoiding prolonged standing.

Conservative treatment with graduated elastic compression hosiery may be indicated in those with mild symptoms, the elderly, unfit and pregnant patients, and when there is significant deep venous insufficiency and intervention is not possible.

The aim of intervention for varicose veins is abolition of superficial venous reflux. This can be performed using one of the following:

(a) Conventional superficial venous surgery. The incompetent connections between deep and superficial veins are exposed and interrupted (flush saphenofemoral and/or saphenopopliteal ligation) and the varices are removed. It is common practice to strip the great saphenous vein from the groin to just below the knee to reduce the risk of recurrence. The small saphenous vein is not normally stripped. The procedure usually requires general anaesthesia, incisions and some recovery before returning to normal activities. Major complications are uncommon but minor morbidity may occur in up to 20% of patients. Complications include major venous or arterial injury (very rare), haematoma, wound infection, temporary or permanent nerve injury (saphenous, sural, popliteal or common peroneal) and venous thromboembolism (although rare, some surgeons give prophylactic subcutaneous low molecular weight heparin before or during surgery).

(b) Ultrasound-guided foam sclerotherapy. Foam sclerosant is injected into the truncal superficial veins and tributaries under direct vision using duplex ultrasound guidance. The foam causes intense venospasm and displaces blood from the vein thus increasing the time and surface area of contact between the sclerosant and the venous endothelium. The procedure is performed under local anaesthesia in the out-patient setting, requires no incisions and the patient can return immediately to normal activities.

(c) Endovenous catheter-based intervention. A catheter is placed into the refluxing truncal superficial vein percutaneously under duplex ultrasound guidance and thermal energy (radiofrequency ablation, RFA) or laser energy (endovenous laser treatment, EVLT) is delivered via the catheter to damage the vein and abolish reflux. These procedures have similar advantages to ultrasound-guided foam sclerotherapy but are more expensive.

Chronic venous insufficiency and ulceration

Failure of the superficial and/or deep venous valves, poor calf muscle pump and venous obstruction lead to high lower limb venous pressure at rest and when walking and this leads to chronic venous hypertension and insufficiency (CVI) with irreversible damage to the lower leg skin and subcutaneous tissues (haemosiderin pigmentation, lipodermatosclerosis and ultimately chronic venous ulceration). CVI affects 5–10% of the adult population and chronic venous ulceration affects 2–3% of people aged over 65 years. The majority (>70%) of leg ulcers are venous and another 15–20% are mixed arterial and venous in aetiology.

Careful history (including previous episodes of ulceration, venous thromboembolism, any surgery; comorbidity; musculoskeletal conditions; medications and allergies, and symptoms of intermittent claudication or critical limb ischaemia), examination (including ulcer characteristics, peripheral pulses, gait, ankle movements) and additional investigations (including ABPI, venous and arterial duplex ultrasound, standard haematology and biochemistry, glucose, rheumatoid serology and thyroid function) should clarify the aetiology of the ulcer and guide management.

Management

Elasticated, multilayer, graduated compression bandaging is the first-line treatment and is very effective at healing the majority of chronic venous leg ulcers. The four-layer system is commonly with 30–40 mmHg compression at the ankle reducing to 15–20 mmHg at the knee. Significant arterial disease must be excluded by history, palpation of the pulses and ABPI measurement before applying compression. If the ABPI is <0.8 or there is a good history of ischaemia then full compression should be avoided until further investigations (toe pressures, arterial duplex or angiography) have been performed with a view to revascularization if indicated. Once the ulcer has healed with bandaging, the patient should wear graduated compression hosiery to reduce the risk of ulcer recurrence. There is also evidence to suggest that, in patients with

chronic venous ulceration due to superficial venous reflux alone, superficial venous surgery and compression bandaging is associated with reduced ulcer recurrence (but not ulcer healing rates) compared with bandaging alone. There is little evidence for any other form of intervention other than compression in patients with chronic venous ulceration who have combined superficial and deep venous reflux.

Venous thromboembolism

Venous thromboembolism (VTE) may present as deep-vein thrombosis (DVT) alone or in combination with pulmonary embolism (PE) or occasionally as PE with no detectable DVT. VTE is responsible for considerable morbidity and mortality, both in hospital and in the community. The principal late complication of DVT is the post-thrombotic syndrome. Destruction of the valves or residual obstruction of the deep veins of the leg causes deep venous insufficiency which is manifest as swelling, venous claudication and the skin changes of chronic venous insufficiency.

VTE is principally due to the interaction of three factors – reduced or static venous blood flow, injury to the vein wall and a hypercoagulable state (Virchow's triad). DVT can occur in any part of the venous system but most commonly originates in the soleal veins of the calf and can extend into the popliteal, superficial femoral or iliac veins or inferior vena cava. As the thrombus forms it either propagates proximally to become free-floating and non-occlusive (and more likely to embolize) or attaches to the vein wall and occludes the vein (and is unlikely to embolize).

Primary DVT

This occurs due to a primary hypercoagulable state (or thrombophilia) where there is a specific abnormality of the coagulation system which results in increased risk of thrombosis (such as antithrombin III deficiency, protein C deficiency, protein S deficiency, antiphospholipid syndrome, and activated protein C resistance). The patient is usually young (<45 years old), there is no obvious precipitating cause, there may be a family history, thrombosis may occur in unusual sites (such as mesenteric, renal and cerebral veins) or there may be a history of recurrent DVTs. Activated protein C resistance (APCR) is the commonest risk factor for VTE, characterized by the inability of activated protein C to degrade an altered form of coagulation factor Va (factor V Leiden).

Secondary DVT

Most DVTs have a precipitating cause or event consistent with Virchow's triad. Patient risk factors include previous VTE, age greater than 40 years, prolonged surgery; trauma; sepsis; malignancy and chemotherapy; inflammatory bowel disease and other chronic inflammatory conditions; immobility due to recent surgery, obesity, stroke and paralysis, cardiac failure, diabetes and pregnancy. After surgery, there is increased activation of the coagulation system and a hypofibrinolytic state for at least 10 days. In addition to the above, risk factors for postoperative VTE include thrombophilia (primary or secondary), cardiovascular complications, major joint replacement, peripheral vascular reconstruction, and surgery for cancer and inflammatory bowel disease. Secondary thrombophilia also occurs in association with liver dysfunction, disseminated intravascular coagulopathy and chronic renal failure.

Phlegmasia and venous gangrene

Phlegmasia caerulea dolens occurs when the thrombotic process extends from the major veins into the capillaries and venules resulting in secondary arterial insufficiency. The resultant increased capillary hydrostatic pressure leads to interstitial oedema which may be so massive that the patient develops hypovolaemic shock. The increase in the interstitial pressure compresses the capillaries and further compromises capillary flow. It usually occurs in the presence of a massive iliofemoral DVT and is usually found in patients with advanced malignant disease. It is characterized by a severe 'bursting' pain, cyanosis and extreme swelling of the entire limb, and in 50% of patients venous gangrene develops affecting the toes and foot initially. It is associated with considerable morbidity and mortality. Although the appearances of the limb may be alarming, it is a mistake to embark on early amputation (unless there is compartment syndrome with impending muscle necrosis) since tissue loss can often be minimized by aggressive medical treatment. Phlegmasia alba dolens occurs due to thrombotic occlusion of the microcirculation initially and is characterized by a swollen, painful, pale or erythematous limb. The natural history is similar to phlegmasia caerulea dolens.

Upper limb DVT

The condition appears to present earlier than is the case with lower limb DVT and the diagnosis is usually clinically obvious with sudden onset of heaviness, swelling and cyanosis of the arm accompanied by engorgement of the collateral veins of the upper arm, shoulder and chest wall. It may occur due to chronic thoracic outlet compression as a consequence of ligamentous or bony abnormality, indwelling catheters in the great veins of the upper limb or neck, or malignancy, or it may occur spontaneously in an otherwise healthy young person after physical activity (so-called 'effort syndrome').

Pulmonary embolism

Lower limb DVT is responsible for more than 90% of PE, but is clinically apparent at the time of the PE in only 10% of patients. Symptomatic PE is associated with acute-onset dyspnoea, pleuritic chest pain and haemoptysis. Clinical signs include a low-grade pyrexia, cyanosis, tachycardia, hypotension, tachypnoea and a raised jugular venous pulse. As the symptoms and signs may be subtle and non-specific, VTE should always be suspected in a patient who is in a high-risk situation. Massive PE may present as cardiovascular collapse and cardiac arrest.

Management

Clinical diagnosis of VTE is very inaccurate. Nevertheless, a careful history should be taken (including family history, previous events, recent trauma, surgery, immobility, pregnancy, malignant disease or air travel; symptoms of calf pain and swelling, usually unilateral), and examination should be performed (signs include pitting oedema, tenderness, erythema, increased temperature, and dilated collateral superficial veins; severe swelling and cyanosis in cases of phlegmasia caerulea dolens; severes swelling and pallor in cases of phlegmasia alba dolens; and venous gangrene). Venous duplex ultrasonography is the first-line diagnostic method in patients with suspected lower limb DVT. It is non-invasive, avoids ionizing radiation and contrast media and is very accurate in assessing the presence of DVT in the superficial femoral and popliteal veins. The method relies on the ability to visualize luminal thrombus, interference with venous flow or non-compressibility of the vein. Venography may be useful, in addition to duplex ultrasound, in patients with upper limb DVT. D-dimer (a fibrin degradation product) is a useful screening blood test in patients with suspected VTE as a negative test essentially excludes VTE. A positive value must be considered in the light of other clinical evidence.

In suspected PE, a plain chest X-ray is rarely diagnostic but may help to exclude alternative pathology as a cause of the patient's symptoms and signs. Features suggestive of PE include atelectasis, prominent hilar markings, pleural effusion, oligaemic lung fields, elevated hemidiaphragm and cardiomegaly. ECG features suggestive of PE include signs of right heart strain and/or ischaemia. Arterial blood gas analysis may demonstrate hypoxia and hypocarbia. Echocardiography may demonstrate intracardiac clot or signs of right ventricular dysfunction (such as right ventricular and pulmonary artery dilatation, right ventricular wall dyskinesia, tricuspid regurgitation). CT pulmonary angiography is the current investigation of choice for diagnosing PE.

Where there is clinical suspicion of VTE and in the absence of contraindications, full anticoagulation with heparin should commence pending definitive diagnosis. If possible, a thrombophilia screen should be performed before commencing heparin in certain clinical situations (such as VTE before 45 years of age, if there is no apparent precipitating factor, history of recurrent VTE or thrombophlebitis, family history of VTE or thrombophilia, venous thrombosis in an unusual site, warfarin or heparin-induced skin necrosis). The treatment of DVT has three principal aims – prevent clot propagation, reduce the risk of PE, and enhance resolution of the clot to minimize the post-thrombotic syndrome. In uncomplicated DVT (for example, DVT confined to the calf veins in a fully mobile patient with reversible risk factors), then the patient is managed as an out-patient with mobilization, an elastic stocking and intermittent subcutaneous low molecular weight heparin followed by warfarin therapy. In complicated DVT (where the DVT is more extensive or recurrent; PE may have occurred; there are irreversible risk factors; heparin is contraindicated), then further treatment may be indicated. For example, patients with phlegmasia or venous gangrene will initially require anticoagulation, high limb elevation and fluid resuscitation for hypovolaemic shock, which will improve limb perfusion. Catheter-directed intra-clot thrombolysis (with or without mechanical assistance) results in more rapid thrombus clearance compared with anticoagulation alone and may reduce

the incidence of PE and post-phlebitic syndrome in patients with extensive ilio-femoral-popliteal DVT. In patients with phlegmasia, this may be combined with intra-arterial thrombolysis in an attempt to clear the thrombosed microcirculation. Surgical venous thrombectomy is rarely performed in the UK and has largely been replaced by endovenous techniques. In cases of upper limb DVT, treatment includes elevation and anticoagulation, with some advocating early catheter-directed intra-clot thrombolysis. In most cases, once the thrombus has been cleared, an underlying anatomical cause of thoracic outlet compression will become apparent. The patient should be maintained on heparin therapy pending thoracic outlet decompression.

Inferior vena caval filters

These are designed to trap emboli and prevent PE. The devices are made of titanium or nickel titanium alloy and are usually placed in the infra-renal IVC percutaneously under local anaesthesia via the common femoral or internal jugular veins. Some filters are designed to be temporary and can be removed percutaneously. Absolute indications for insertion of an IVC filter are recurrent PE despite effective anticoagulation, complications of VTE or anticoagulation which prevent further anticoagulation, and where anticoagulation is contraindicated due to an increased risk of bleeding.

VTE prophylaxis

Without thromboembolic prophylaxis, the risk of DVT is 25% for major general and cardiovascular surgery, and 40–80% for major hip and knee surgery. Prophylaxis in low-risk groups (minor surgery or trauma, major surgery in patients <40 years old, and minor medical illness) consists of leg elevation and early mobilization. Prophylaxis in moderate-risk groups (major trauma, burns or medical illness, major surgery in patients >40 years, minor surgery in patients with additional risk factors, and patients with inflammatory bowel disease) consists of leg elevation, early mobilization, graduated thromboembolic deterrent (TED) compression stockings and subcutaneous low molecular weight heparin (LMWH) once daily. Prophylaxis in high-risk groups (major cancer, pelvic and lower limb joint surgery, those undergoing surgery or suffering illness associated with previous VTE or thrombophilia) consists of leg elevation, early mobilization, TED stockings, subcutaneous LMWH, and mechanical calf compression. In some areas of surgery, particularly where the surgeon wishes to avoid intraoperative anticoagulation, mechanical compression is a useful option for the medium- and high-risk groups.

Lymphoedema

This is abnormal limb swelling due to accumulation of increased amounts of protein-rich interstitial fluid due to defective lymphatic drainage (aplasia, hyoplasia, hyperplasia or fibrosis).

Primary lymphoedema is an inherited developmental abnormality of the lymphatic system. The causes are most commonly classified according to the age of onset: lymphoedema congenita is present at or within 2 years of birth, is commoner in males, more likely to be bilateral and involve the whole leg; lymphoedema praecox develops between the ages of 2 and 35 years, is commoner in females, is three times more likely to be unilateral than bilateral, and usually only extends to the knee; lymphoedema tarda develops after 35 years of age and is often associated with obesity and lymph nodes are replaced by fibro-fatty tissue.

Secondary lymphoedema is the commonest form and occurs due to lymphatic obstruction by tumour, bacterial infection causing lymphangitis and lymphadenitis, infestation by filariasis, and injury secondary to trauma, surgery or radiotherapy.

Unlike other forms of oedema, lymphoedema characteristically involves the foot, with infilling of the submalleolar depressions of the ankle, a 'buffalo hump' on the dorsum of the foot, 'square' toes and the skin on the dorsum of the foot cannot be pinched due to subcutaneous fibrosis. In the early stages, lymphoedema occurs with dependency and will pit easily but, left untreated, fibrosis, dermal thickening and hyperkeratosis occur which prevent pitting. Ulceration is uncommon.

Management

Duplex ultrasound may be useful to exclude any concomitant venous disease but, in general, lymphoedema is a clinical diagnosis and investigations are not usually required. The aims of treatment are to reduce limb swelling (by elevation at rest, manual lymphatic drainage, intermittent pneumatic compression, graduated compression hosiery with 50 mmHg pressure at the ankle), reduce risk of infection (well-fitting shoes, good skin hygiene, early or possibly long-term antibiotic therapy for cellulitis, and treatment of fungal infections) and improve function. Surgery is rarely indicated and includes reduction procedures or bypass procedures.

Vascular trauma

Blunt vessel injury

Direct crush injury or stretching can cause vessel injury. The commonest presentations are motor-vehicle accidents causing transection of the descending thoracic aorta immediately distal to the left subclavian origin; and tibial plateau fractures, posterior knee dislocations or misadventure during knee replacement surgery causing popliteal injury, thrombosis with lower limb ischaemia, or false aneurysm formation.

Penetrating vessel injury

Stab wounds cause injury which is limited to the tract of the wound. Knowledge of the weapon used will assist in determining which organs may have been injured.

Missile injuries cause direct trauma to the vessel as well as indirect trauma adjacent to the missile tract due to the shock wave and cavitatory effect which results in a larger area of injury as well as drawing debris such as clothing into the wound. Higher-velocity missiles cause greater direct and indirect injury and so a greater area of debridement is required. Missile injury may cause intimal injury with thrombosis and/or embolization (which can lead to stroke in carotid injury); a lateral tear with thrombosis, or false aneurysm formation and subsequent risk of delayed haemorrhage, thrombosis, embolization or compression of adjacent structures (airway, brachial plexus), or haemorrhage externally or into a body cavity; or complete transaction with haematoma formation and vessel thrombosis, or haemorrhage externally or into a body cavity. As well as the primary injury, sepsis can lead to delayed secondary haemorrhage at the site of injury.

Simultaneous arterial and venous injury can lead to arteriovenous fistula formation, which presents with a machinery murmur on auscultation or a thrill, but if large can lead to distal ischaemia due to a steal phenomenon or high-output cardiac failure.

Management

Unstable patients should be resuscitated according to the standard trauma protocols. A urinary catheter should be inserted (if safe to do so), and wide-bore venous cannulae should be placed avoiding the upper limbs in cervical or mediastinal trauma or the lower limbs in lower limb trauma. Every attempt should be made to avoid or correct hypothermia. If the patient is awake and passing urine then so-called hypotensive resuscitation (or permissive hypotension) is advised with only small volumes of fluid resuscitation to maintain haemodynamic stability, thereby avoiding disruption of the haemostatic thrombus, coagulopathy and hypothermia which are associated with large volumes of fluid resuscitation. If the patient fails to respond adequately to resuscitation or deteriorates then transfer to the operating theatre is indicated for urgent surgical intervention.

The history and nature of the injury and careful clinical examination are important. Absent pulses, a bruit or thrill, an expanding haematoma and external or internal haemorrhage are strong indicators of arterial injury but more subtle signs include a history of hypotension, a small non-expanding haematoma, anaemia and any associated injuries in the vicinity of major arteries (such as a brachial plexus injury). Erect chest X-ray may demonstrate a haemothorax, widened mediastinum or cardiac tamponade. Intra-arterial digital subtraction angiography (either pre- or intraoperatively) and more recently CT angiography may be useful in cases of clinical uncertainty and is vital where endovascular intervention is being considered, but it should not delay surgical intervention if the patient is unstable.

External haemorrhage requires application of direct digital pressure or temporary inflation of a sphygmomanometer cuff proximal to the extremity bleeding followed by exploration in the operating theatre. Urgent surgical exploration is indicated if there is evidence of free haemorrhage (tense distended abdomen or a large volume of blood in the chest drain). Antibiotic prophylaxis should be administered in the operating theatre and the patient should be prepared and draped to allow both proximal and distal vascular control, and harvest of the long saphenous vein from an injured lower limb if required.

Vascular repair first requires debridement back to healthy vessel to reduce the risk of thrombosis. The two ends of the vessel are then back-bled and an embolectomy catheter is passed proximally and distally to remove thrombus which will have propagated to the next patent collateral. The proximal and distal vessel is usually instilled with heparinized saline and the vessel is occluded for repair. Lateral tears in large arteries may be repaired by simple transverse sutures. If there is a risk of narrowing, however, then careful proximal and distal mobilization of the vessel may allow tension-free primary anastomosis (with spatulation of the vessel ends for anastomosis of small-calibre vessels to reduce stenosis, and interrupted sutures in children to allow vessel growth). If primary anastomosis is not possible due to tension, then interposition grafting can be performed. Reversed long saphenous vein is the conduit of choice in the extremities or in contaminated fields, but prosthetic grafts may be used for large vessel repair (carotid, aorta, iliac, common femoral arteries) or extra-anatomical bypass of aorto-iliac injuries in a contaminated field (axillo-femoral, femoro-femoral bypass grafting). Alternatively, vein patch angioplasty may be considered provided the vessel is otherwise healthy. Intraoperative completion angiography should be performed before ensuring there is soft tissue cover of the vessel repair.

Endovascular techniques include occlusion of non-critical bleeding vessels or false aneurysms (using coils, plugs or glue to induce thrombosis), temporary balloon-occlusion of injured vessels that are not directly accessible allowing time for surgical exposure, and the use of covered stents across a lateral tear thereby avoiding open surgical intervention. Endovascular treatment may be definitive or provide a bridge to surgery once the patient has been stabilized.

Further reading

ASTRAL trial investigators. Revascularisation versus medical therapy for renal artery stenosis. *N Engl J Med* 2009;**361**:1953–1962.

BASIL trial participants. Bypass versus angioplasty in severe ischaemia of the leg (BASIL): multi-centre, randomised controlled trial. *Lancet* 2005;**366**:1925–1934.

EVAR trial participants. Endovascular aneurysm repair versus open repair in patients with abdominal aortic aneurysm (EVAR trial 1): randomised controlled trial. *Lancet* 2005;**365**:2179–2186.

EVAR trial participants. Endovascular aneurysm repair and outcome in patients unfit for open repair of abdominal aortic aneurysm (EVAR trial 2): randomised controlled trial. *Lancet* 2005;**365**:2187–2192.

MASS trial participants. Screening men for abdominal aortic aneurysm: 10 year mortality and cost effectiveness results from the randomized Multicentre Aneurysm Screening Study. *BMJ* 2009;**338**:b2307.

MRC Asymptomatic Carotid Surgery Trial (ACST) Collaborative Group. Prevention of fatal and disabling strokes by successful carotid endarterectomy in patients without neurological symptoms: randomized controlled trial. *Lancet* 2004;**363**:1491–1502.

North American Symptomatic Carotid Endarterectomy Trial Collaborators. Beneficial effect of carotid endarterectomy in symptomatic patients with high-grade carotid stenosis. *N Engl J Med* 1991;**325**: 445–453.

Randomised trial of endarterectomy for recently symptomatic carotid stenosis: final results of the MRC European Carotid Surgery Trial (ECST). *Lancet* 1998; **351**:1379–1387.

UK Small Aneurysm Trial Participants. Mortality results for randomised controlled trial of early elective surgery or ultrasonographic surveillance for small abdominal aortic aneurysms. *Lancet* 1998;**352**:1649–1655.

Chapter 28

Fundamentals of orthopaedics

Jon Clasper

Introduction

The aim of this chapter is to introduce the reader to orthopaedic surgery. Core training in orthopaedics has four key topics, all concerned with trauma rather than elective surgery. This chapter will cover the topics:

1. Simple fractures and dislocations
2. Soft tissue injuries, including open fractures and compartment syndrome
3. Ankle fractures
4. Proximal femoral fractures in the elderly.

Fracture healing

Fracture healing is a complex physiological process, and unlike other tissues that heal by the formation of connective scar tissue of poor quality, bone is regenerated and the pre-fracture properties are usually restored.

Fractures can heal by:

- primary direct bone healing
- secondary (callus formation) bone healing.

The vast majority of fractures heal by secondary bone healing, which proceeds in five distinct stages:

- stage 1: tissue damage and haematoma formation
- stage 2: inflammation and cellular proliferation
- stage 3: callus formation
- stage 4: consolidation
- stage 5: remodelling.

Tissue damage and haematoma formation

Bleeding occurs from the medullary cavity, the periosteum, as well as adjacent soft tissue and muscle. This results in the formation of a haematoma within and around the fracture site. The disruption of the Haversian systems leads to death of the osteocytes at the fracture surface.

Inflammation and cellular proliferation

Within hours, the fibrin mesh within the haematoma forms a framework for the influx of various cells (platelets, neutrophils, lymphocytes, monocytes, macrophages and mast cells).

The haematoma organizes over the next week into granulation tissue. The inflammatory cells and platelets release a variety of cytokines which activate cell migration, proliferation, and differentiation of mesenchymal stem cells. Angiogenesis occurs as the haematoma organizes and osteoclasts resorb the dead bone ends. Inflammatory mediators increase vascular permeability, causing an exudate of plasma and promoting phagocytosis of necrotic material.

Callus formation

Callus is a physiological reaction to inter-fragmentary movement. The initial haematoma matures into granulation tissue at the fracture gap. Soft callus or cartilage then forms and finally the soft callus is replaced by endochondral ossification to become hard callus or woven bone. The chondrocytes become hypertrophic, calcify and die. Angiogenesis occurs and osteoblasts lay down bone matrix on the collagen scaffold left by the chondrocytes.

Osteoblasts beneath the periosteum deposit a subperiosteal layer of woven bone at the fracture site. This woven bone forms the framework of the bridging external callus. External callus forms on the outside of the fractured bone to bridge the gap. Internal callus forms more slowly from the medullary canal. Finally, the cortical continuity is restored.

Fundamentals of Surgical Practice, Third Edition, ed. Andrew N. Kingsnorth and Douglas M. Bowley.
Published by Cambridge University Press. © Cambridge University Press 2011.

Consolidation

Consolidation is the conversion of woven bone into lamellar bone. Woven bone can be considered as 'temporary' callus. The collagen fibres that run through the osseous matrix are arranged in an irregular network. Lamellar bone, on the other hand, is the permanent bone of the mature trabeculae and the shafts of long bone. Lamellar bone is laid down in orderly layers and the osteocytes are distributed evenly between the layers. The fibres in each layer run in parallel, but at a different angle to adjacent layers. This configuration increases the bone's strength.

Lamellar bone cannot be deposited in fibrous tissue and cannot therefore bridge a moving gap spanned only by fibrous tissue. The solid framework on which lamellar bone is normally deposited is the woven bone of callus which has formed a temporary scaffold. The woven bone is finally removed by osteoclasts when the lamellar bone has acquired an adequate thickness.

Remodelling

Remodelling can continue for many months after the fracture has clinically healed; eventually the temporary woven bone is replaced by lamellar bone and there is reconstitution of the medullary canal and restoration of the bone shape. In remodelling, osteoclastic and osteoblastic activity occurs in synergy to regain the shape of the bone based on the stresses to which the bone is exposed.

In children, the remodelling is so effective that even completely displaced fractures may heal and remodel without trace. However, axial rotation deformity should not normally be accepted as it will persist. In adults, there is very little correction of angulation or axial rotation. Therefore both should be corrected to an acceptable position before the fracture heals.

Primary bone healing

If the fracture is anatomically reduced and movement is eliminated primary bone healing can occur. Osteoclasts tunnel across the fracture line, and establish a 'cutting cone' across the fracture. Osteoblasts follow and lay down bone matrix and re-establish continuity between Haversian systems. Vessel ingrowth is absent and the bone filling the interfragmentary gap appears without the intermediate formation of cartilage or granulation tissue.

For primary bone healing to occur, interfragmentary strain must be minimal and the fracture gap between the bone ends should be <200 μm. This requires full anatomical reduction with intrafragmentary compression using a lag screw or compression plate to prevent motion.

Primary bone healing is essentially the same biological process as occurs in normal bone turnover and late remodelling. This can therefore be a slow process and any internal fixation device implanted must be maintained until this healing process is complete.

Implications for fracture fixation

The principles of fracture management should take into consideration the mechanisms of fracture healing. In fractures of long bones, accurate reduction of axes and rotation are important. Whenever possible, the blood supply at the fracture site should not be compromised.

If secondary fracture healing is the goal, movement of the fracture along the axes is beneficial for the formation of soft callus. However the movement should be small (ideally amplitude 0.2–1.0 mm and fracture gap <2 mm). Higher strain amplitudes may inhibit osteoblastic activity and delay fracture healing. In the later stages the formation of hard callus is compromised by vigorous mechanical stimulation. Therefore motion should be limited in the final phase of consolidation. Ideally this increase in fracture site stiffness is a biological response from formation of hard callus.

If fracture fragments are rigidly fixed but the fracture gap is greater than 200 μm, then neither secondary bone healing nor primary (direct) healing can occur and the fracture is at risk of developing into nonunion and ultimately the implant failing.

With intra-articular fractures, where absolute stability and accurate reduction are required, primary fracture healing is desirable and can be achieved with lag screw fixation.

Principles of fracture immobilization/ stabilization

The vast majority of fractures will be immobilized in some manner to:

- relieve pain, by reducing or eliminating movement of the bone ends
- optimize use by placing the limb in a functional position

- aid healing by reducing the fracture gap
- facilitate recovery by eliminating deformity.

A number of methods are available but in general the principles of reduction and stabilization can be summarized as:

- If the position of the fracture is acceptable and stable, simple measures are usually sufficient. These include plaster of Paris and other splints, slings and other orthotics.
- If the position of the fracture is unacceptable then reduction is required. This may simply be reducing a toe under local anaesthetic in the emergency department, to complex surgery under anaesthetic.
- If closed reduction is possible by manipulation and the position is stable after reduction (many wrist fractures) then simple measures are again used. If, however, closed reduction is possible but the position is unstable then other methods are considered. This is the most common reason for reduction and K-wire fixation of wrist fractures. With the tibia and femur, closed reduction is usually possible, but this is usually supplemented by intramedullary fixation, both to stabilize the fracture and also to allow earlier mobilization.
- If a closed reduction is not possible, and the position is unacceptable, then open reduction of the fracture is carried out. Having opened the fracture site to reduce it, internal fixation with a plate and/or screws is usually carried out. This is the situation with many articular fractures, and again facilitates early movement of the joint.

Open fractures

An open fracture refers to a break in the skin and underlying soft tissue which communicates directly with the fracture and its haematoma. The term can also be used when a fracture is in communication within a body cavity, e.g. pelvic fractures through the bowel or vagina. In the UK, the annual incidence of open long-bone fractures is 11.5 per 100 000, with 40% occurring in the lower limb. Any wound occurring on the same limb segment as a fracture should be assumed to be an open fracture until proven otherwise.

Soft tissue injuries related to an open fracture have these important consequences:

- contamination of the fracture site by exposure to the external environment

- crushing, stripping, and devascularization resulting in soft tissue compromise and increased susceptibility to infection
- destruction of the soft tissue envelope affects the options for fracture fixation; there is also a loss of function from damage to muscle, tendon, nerve, vascular or ligamentous structures.

The extent of the associated soft tissue injury is one of the major determinants of the infection risk after a civilian open fracture. Gustilo and Anderson (1976) have reported a grading of wounds, which remains a universally accepted classification of the wound associated with an open fracture.

Type I: An open fracture with a wound less than 1 cm long and clean.
Type II: An open fracture with a laceration more than one centimetre long without extensive soft tissue damage, flaps, or avulsions.
Type III: Either an open segmental fracture, an open fracture with extensive soft tissue damage, or a traumatic amputation.
Type III fractures are further sub-divided:
Type IIIA: Adequate soft tissue cover of the bone despite extensive laceration.
Type IIIB: Extensive soft tissue loss, with periosteal stripping, and exposed bone. Usually associated with massive contamination.
Type IIIC: Open fracture with vascular injury that needs repair.

For Gustilo type I fractures an infection rate of 1% or less can be expected, and for type II fractures a rate of approximately 3% has been reported. For type IIIA fractures an infection rate of 17% has been reported, and for type IIIB 26%. Type IIIC fractures have a variable infection rate, depending on the soft tissue injury and delays in revascularization.

Management in the emergency department

Approximately one-third of patients with open fractures have multiple injuries. Patients should be assessed along ATLS protocols with appropriate management of life-threatening conditions. Clinical evaluation of the limb should involve:

- addressing wound haemorrhage with direct pressure using a sterile dressing

- a full neurovascular assessment of the injured limb; if necessary, Doppler ultrasound can be used to assess distal pulses; the location of the pulse should be marked for future examination. Consider early referral to a vascular surgeon, if vascular injury is suspected
- assessing skin and soft tissue damage; if possible photograph the wound, and then cover the wound with a sterile dressing
- following adequate analgesia, reducing the fracture if possible and placing in a splint; if the fracture is manipulated in the emergency department, ensure that the neurovascular status is rechecked and documented in the medical notes
- getting senior help early.

Principles of surgery for open fractures

The aim of fracture management is to produce a united fracture with intact soft tissues and normal function. The essential features of management are:

- antibiotic prophylaxis
- wound debridement +/− fasciotomy
- early stabilization of the fracture
- early wound cover.

In fractures with significant soft tissue damage, this will require a multidisciplinary approach, and early communication with a plastic surgical unit is advised. The traditional dictum is that the initial debridement should occur within 6 hours of injury. However, recently it has been reported that delays up to 24 hours did not increase infection rates.

Antibiotic prophylaxis

Antibiotics should be commenced promptly as delays increase the risk of infection. Each hospital will have its own protocols or guidelines, but a general guide is:

For type I and II open fractures, *Staphylococcus aureus*, streptococci and aerobic Gram-negative bacilli are the most common infecting organisms and can be covered with a first- or second-generation cephalosporin or alternatively with a quinolone (e.g. ciprofloxacin). As the predominant organisms are staphylococcus and streptococci many hospitals will use a combination of a penicillin and flucloxacillin.

For type III open fractures, better coverage for Gram-negative organisms should be considered, and the addition of an aminoglycoside to the cephalosporin may be appropriate.

For severe injuries with soil contamination and tissue damage with areas of ischaemia, a penicillin should be added to provide coverage against anaerobes, particularly *Clostridia* species.

Tetanus prophylaxis

If the patient has not been vaccinated or had a booster injection in the last 10 years, then they will require 0.5 ml intramuscular tetanus toxoid. In addition 250 IU of tetanus immunoglobulin (75 IU for patients less than 5 yrs old, 125 U for ages from 5 to 10 years) should be administered. Consider giving tetanus immunoglobulin in all patients with grossly contaminated open fractures.

Debridement

The aim of debridement is to remove foreign material and non-viable tissue, in order to leave a clean healthy bed for soft tissue reconstruction. As open fractures are frequently high-energy injuries with severe tissue damage, the most experienced surgeon available should perform the debridement. The principles of debridement are:

- Wound excision – skin is generally very resistant to trauma and has a good capacity to heal. Therefore the wound edges should be excised with care and only enough to leave healthy skin edges.
- Wound extension – the zone of soft tissue injury will often extend far beyond the wound. Therefore the wound will need to be extended proximally and distally to enable full examination of the injured tissue. As part of this a formal fasciotomy may be required (see below).
- Removal of non-viable tissue – devitalized tissue, especially muscle, will provide a focus for infection and needs to be excised.

When assessing damaged tissue, look for the four Cs:

- Colour: dead muscle is often dark and discoloured
- Consistency: non-viable tissue has a mushy consistency
- Contractility: dead muscle will not contract when crushed with forceps or touched with a diathermy probe
- Capillary bleeding: non-viable bone fragments (i.e. without significant soft tissue connection) should be removed.

- Wound washout – an essential feature of wound debridement is copious wound irrigation. A minimum of 6 litres of saline is recommended.

Fasciotomy and compartment syndrome

A compartment syndrome occurs when the pressure within a fixed fascial compartment rises to the point that it impedes capillary circulation and muscle ischaemia occurs. This in turn will lead to an increase in pressure, worsening the situation. If unrelieved, muscle necrosis will occur, although pulses will usually remain present throughout.

The cardinal symptom of a compartment syndrome is excessive pain. The compartment is tense, and any further pressure worsens the pain, as does passive stretching of the muscles within the compartment such as extending the toes.

Compartment syndrome can occur in almost any muscle compartment, but is most common in the lower leg.

Diagnosis is clinical, when the condition is suspected, although pressure monitoring can be used if the condition is anticipated or suspected and accurate clinical examination is not possible, such as with a head-injured patient, or an anaesthetic limb.

Treatment is emergency decompression of the compartment by full-length, longitudinal incisions through the fascia, when the muscle will be seen to bulge out.

Upper arm

This has two compartments, the flexor, containing the biceps and related muscles, and extensor, containing the triceps. Both can be decompressed by longitudinal incisions, which may be possible through an open wound.

If exposure of the vessels is also required, the incision can be placed medially. A lateral incision can be used to avoid exposing the artery, but if external fixation is also required, closure of a lateral wound may be compromised.

Forearm

Although the forearm also has a flexor and extensor compartment, release of individual muscle may be required at the time of fasciotomy, and can be carried out through a single curved volar incision. If fasciotomy is required, consideration should also be given to releasing the carpal tunnel.

Carpal tunnel

This is formed by the transverse carpal ligament of the wrist forming a roof over the carpal bones of the wrist. The flexor tendons of the fingers pass through it, along with the median nerve, and it is compression of this against the roof of the tunnel that results in the symptoms of paraesthesia in the median nerve distribution.

Although it can occur with trauma, the majority of cases are idiopathic and associated with nocturnal symptoms which are relieved by shaking or hanging the hand down. Carpal tunnel syndrome is the most common nerve entrapment seen.

Diagnosis is made from the history, and in addition percussion over the nerve in the canal will reproduce the symptoms (Tinel's sign), or palmar-flexing the wrist. Neurophysiological tests are also invaluable.

Treatment is by surgically dividing the transverse carpal ligament and is very successful, with minimal complications. This can be carried out under local anaesthetic although it will take place under general anaesthetic if it is part of a forearm decompression.

Thigh

The thigh contains three compartments, flexor, extensor and a medial adductor compartment. In most situations release of the anterior and posterior compartments, through a single lateral incision, may be sufficient, but penetrating injuries to the thigh may require release of the medial compartment, particularly when associated with a vascular injury. This will require a separate incision.

Lower leg

There are four compartments, anterior and lateral, and superficial and deep posterior compartments. Failure to release the deep posterior compartment is the most common error in lower limb fasciotomy, and occurs when the soleus muscle is released from the posterior aspect of the tibia, which fails to release the whole compartment. The posterior tibial artery is located between the two posterior compartments, and this can be used as a landmark during surgery. A two-incision technique should be used in the lower limb, decompressing the posterior compartments through an incision just posterior to the medial border of the tibia. An incision too posterior will damage the perforators and may compromise soft tissue closure.

Fracture stabilization

Early fracture stability is required to prevent further soft tissue damage and reduce the risk of infection. Traditionally, the external fixator has been the method of choice as it allows management of the fracture without placing metalwork within the zone of injury and it does not require further exposure of the damaged soft tissue. However, pin site infection is a problem, with infection rates of 25% in type IIIA and 50% in type IIIB reported.

In low energy type I fractures and selected type IIIB fractures of the tibia and femur, an intramedullary nail can be placed with no significant increase in infection. A meta-analysis of fixation methods in open tibial fractures showed that use of an intramedullary nail significantly reduced the incidence of superficial infection and the reoperation rate compared with external fixation. There was no difference in deep infection or non-union rates.

Wound coverage

Small uncontaminated type I wounds may be primarily sutured after the initial debridement or just left to heal. However, in general it is advisable to dress the wound with sterile gauze and consider wound closure at 48 hours.

A number of reconstructive options are available and form the 'reconstructive ladder', which ranges from delayed primary closure to free tissue transfer. Whichever option is used, soft tissue coverage within 3–5 days of injury has been reported to reduce the risk of osteomyelitis and deep infection.

Pathological fractures

Pathological fractures occur in bone which is abnormal, and, in general, less injury is required to break the bone, with some even occurring spontaneously. They occur in two peaks, in adolescents and in the over 50s.

Osteoporosis is the most common pathological process that predisposes to fracture, and is associated with a reduction in the amount of bone present, which results in bone fragility. Unlike osteomalacia where there is deficient mineralization of bone, the bone present in osteoporosis is of normal composition.

The most common cause is age-related, and particularly affects postmenopausal females due to oestrogen deficiency. Endocrine causes such as Cushings

syndrome, thyrotoxicosis and pituitary insufficiency, as well as prescribed corticosteroids, can also cause it.

As well as treating the specific fractures, the cause of the osteoporosis should be sought. Elderly patients who sustain an osteoporotic fracture should be considered for screening and/or treatment as there is a very high risk of further fractures, which carry significant risks of both mortality and morbidity, as well as place a considerable financial burden on society.

Tumours, both benign and malignant, are also a frequent cause of pathological fracture. The most common tumour in bone is a secondary metastasis, and this is usually from a breast, lung or prostate primary. Less commonly the primary is renal or thyroid in origin.

The management of the patient depends on the underlying diagnosis. In children with benign lesions such as primary bone cysts, treatment is usually conservative, the fracture will heal, and the cyst may also fill in.

If the patient has a known primary and the fracture is through a metastatic lesion then stabilization is usually required to relieve pain, and allow mobilization, and this is particularly important if the patient has a relatively prolonged life expectancy. In general intramedullary fixation is preferred, but with all fractures there is a need to image the entire bone, as other lesions may influence the choice of implant.

Intramedullary fixation would not normally be indicated for a primary tumour (or an isolated secondary, particularly from a renal primary) to avoid disseminating the tumour. Resection of the tumour and stabilization may be indicated, but this will usually be carried out in specialist centres after staging of the disease.

Specific injuries

Clavicle fractures

Incidence – this is one of the most common sites, accounting for 5% of all fractures. In males it is most common in the under 20s with a decreasing frequency with each subsequent decade. In women there are two peaks, in the young and the 70s.

Aetiology – they are commonly due to road traffic accidents or sport. In the older female it may occur following a simple fall.

Management – treatment is usually conservative with a broad arm sling and mobilization as comfort allows. There is currently some controversy surrounding the treatment of displaced midshaft fractures associated with >2 cm overlap or displacement, which may benefit from plate fixation. Lateral 1/3 fractures can also be associated with significant displacement and many authors recommend primary internal fixation.

Complications – non-union is one of the most common complications and is associated with midshaft fractures with overlap, and displaced lateral 1/3 fractures. Symptomatic non-unions are treated by internal fixation with a plate and supplemental bone graft.

Proximal humerus

Incidence – this is predominantly a fracture of older patients, and this and hip, vertebral body and distal radius fractures are the most common osteoporotic fractures. Of the three limb sites proximal humerus is the least common site.

Aetiology – these are commonly the result of a simple fall; in younger patients they are associated with significant trauma such as traffic accidents.

Management – commonly the fractures are classified based on the four major bony segments – the anatomical neck, separating the articular surface from the rest, the separate lesser and greater tuberosities and the surgical neck, separating the humeral shaft.

Treatment is often based on age and degree of displacement, but also needs to be based on surgeon experience. Most proximal humeral fractures can be managed non-operatively in a sling followed by relatively early mobilization, but controversy remains for the more displaced three- and four-part fractures, particularly in the older patient. These have a very high rate of avascular necrosis, although even when this occurs the outcome is not universally poor. In addition although ORIF and hemiarthroplasty allow early mobilization and a potentially better functional result, there is no guarantee this will occur.

Complications – these are common and often related to the method of treatment. Avascular necrosis is most common with four-part fractures, and if these have been treated by ORIF, this can result in collapse of the humeral head and penetration of the joint by screws. Malunion is also common, particularly after conservative treatment,

but good function can still result. Many of the complications are treated by salvage hemiarthroplasty, but this may not alleviate the symptoms.

Humeral shaft fractures

Incidence – there is a small peak in the 20s but in general these are fractures of the elderly, with an increasing incidence with increasing age. Five to eight per cent may be pathological fractures, usually from a breast or prostate primary.

Aetiology – it is usually an isolated fracture due to a simple fall in an elderly patient. In the younger patient the cause is often sporting or a motor accident and this may be associated with polytrauma and/or an open fracture.

Management – the majority will heal with conservative measures, predominantly by an early functional brace after an initial period of a U slab for comfort. In general hanging casts should be avoided, due to the risk of non-union. Open fractures and polytrauma are indications for internal fixation, with either a plate or intramedullary device.

Complications – radial nerve palsy can occur in up to 10%, which is the most common nerve palsy associated with long bone fractures; 90% of the palsies will heal without any specific treatment. Non-union is also a common complication, again occurring in approximately 10%, and is commonly associated with mid-shaft transverse fractures. Satisfactory healing can be obtained with compression plating with bone graft.

Distal humeral fractures

Incidence – these account for about 30% of fractures around the elbow occurring in a bimodal age distribution, in males around 20 and elderly females.

Aetiology – the bimodal age distribution is due to the mechanism of injury: in younger patients it is usually high-energy mechanisms such as motor-vehicle accidents, falls from heights and sport. In the older patients the fracture occurs in osteoporotic bone often as a result of a simple fall.

Management – unfortunately the majority of these injuries are complex fractures, with involvement of the articular surface, and complex separation of the joint from the humeral shaft. There are three treatment options:

(1) Conservative with early mobilization. This 'bag of bones' technique was the standard method of treatment prior to the advances in internal fixation in the 1960s and '70s and still has an occasional place today.

(2) Internal fixation, usually with two plates. This is a difficult procedure due to poor access to the fracture and small, often osteoporotic bone fragments. It is important that stable fixation is achieved to allow early movement and as a result a formal olecranon osteotomy, to improve access, and specially designed implants are utilized.

(3) Total early replacement. This is indicated in the elderly patient with a low fracture, where a stable reduction may not be obtained, particularly if there is pre-existing disease such as rheumatoid arthritis.

Complications – these are relatively common and are usually related to the implant, with loss of reduction, prominent metal and non-union occurring. The ulnar nerve is at risk, but should have been identified and protected during the procedure.

Olecranon fractures

Incidence – these account for approximately 10% of fractures around the elbow in adults, ranging from simple avulsion fractures to complex fracture dislocations.

Aetiology – the simple fractures are commonly seen in the more elderly and usually result from an indirect mechanism such as a fall onto the outstretched hand, the fracture probably resulting from the sudden contraction of the triceps against a fixed elbow. In the younger patient direct trauma is a more common cause, particularly road traffic accidents and may be complex injuries with dislocation of the radial head.

Management – treatment is usually operative, but in the older patient with a minimally displaced avulsion type, non-operative treatment is appropriate. Although these are articular fractures, the more important functions of the proximal ulna are stability of the elbow joint, and as part of the extensor mechanism. If the patient has a stable

elbow joint that can move through a functional range of motion, and can extend against gravity or light resistance, initial rest in a sling followed by early mobilization is entirely appropriate.

For the simple two-part fractures a tension band technique can be used with two K wires together with a figure-of-8 wire. This implant resists the distraction forces applied across the fracture site by the triceps, and results in compressive forces across the articular side of the fracture.

For more complex fracture dislocations, or when multiple fragments are present, internal fixation with a plate and screws is required. Unlike distal humeral fractures, prosthetic replacement of the elbow is not indicated for proximal ulnar fractures.

Complications – these are relatively common and are related to the implant rather than the fracture, with prominent wires being the most common.

Radial head fractures

Incidence – these are the most common fractures around the elbow and can occur at most ages. They may be isolated or part of a complex injury involving dislocation and fractures of the coronoid process of the ulna.

Aetiology – they commonly result from a fall on the outstretched hand.

Management – isolated injuries have been classified into (Mason) type I minimally displaced, type II which are displaced, but only involve part of the radial head, and type III which are multifragmentary and involve the whole head.

Treatment of type I fractures is conservative, with early mobilization. In the acute situation if the elbow is particularly painful it can be aspirated under sterile conditions and a long-acting local anaesthetic instilled. The treatment of type II and III fractures is more controversial. With type II injuries the debate centres on the need for open reduction and screw fixation. The main indication is a block to motion, particularly flexion and supination. In the absence of a block, early motion can result in a good functional result and should be considered, as an alternative to fixation. Operative fixation can still result in permanent loss of motion as well as complications due to the implant.

In general type III fractures are not amenable to fixation, and the debate centres on the need for replacement versus excision, although some clinicians will still treat these by early mobilization. When associated with a complex injury involving elbow dislocation or an injury to the intra-osseous ligament radial head excision is contraindicated and replacement is indicated, but should be combined with fixation of any significant coronoid fracture and the medial ligament if possible.

Complications – pain and loss of motion are common, and may improve with removal of the implant and/or late excision of the radial head.

Forearm fractures

Incidence – fractures of the shaft of the radius and/or ulna are uncommon when compared to those around the elbow or wrist.

Aetiology – fractures involving both bones are commonly isolated injuries and are usually due to a fall on the outstretched hand. A fracture of a single bone, usually the ulna, can result from a direct blow, the so-called nightstick injury. However, unless there is a definite history of a direct blow, an injury to the adjacent joint should be suspected. These include the eponymous Monteggia fracture, with a radial head dislocation in association with a (usually proximal) ulna fracture, or a Galeazzi fracture with disruption of the distal radio-ulnar joint in association with a distal radius fracture.

Management – the majority of these injuries should be managed by open reduction and fixation, usually by plates. Due to the mechanically complex nature of forearm rotation, even small degrees of malunion can result in quite profound loss of rotation. In addition prolonged treatment in plaster may be required as these fractures can be slow to heal. Normally two strong plates will be used, preferably with compression across the fracture site to reduce the risk of delayed or malunion.

Complications – as noted above, delayed and malunion can occur particularly if there is instability at the fracture site, or loss of reduction. Non-union can also occur, particularly of the ulna, and this may occasionally require revision plating and bone graft.

Wrist fractures

Incidence – fractures of the distal radius are one of the most common fractures seen, and have been estimated to account for 20% of all new attendances at fracture clinics.

Aetiology – the fact that nearly 80% are reported to occur in females, with an average age of 64, demonstrates that this is an osteoporotic fracture, and usually results from a simple fall. In men they are seen at a younger age and arc usually due to higher-energy mechanisms such as sporting injuries or falls from a significant height.

Management – there is considerable debate about the correct management of these injuries, centred on what degree of displacement can be accepted, before functional impairment occurs.

Extra-articular fractures with less than 10 degrees of dorsal angulation and no significant shortening or loss of radial inclination can be managed non-operatively. Traditionally plaster has been applied for 6 weeks, but early mobilization is felt to be of benefit, and commonly 3 weeks in plaster are advised. Some fractures, particularly impacted fractures, can be managed in a removable splint.

For significantly displaced fractures reduction is required, and, if stable, these injuries can again be managed in plaster, although weekly radiographs may be required for the first 2–3 weeks. The management of unstable fractures is again controversial, with some clinicians advocating K-wire fixation, and others open reduction and plate fixation. Bone graft or bone substitutes may be required if impaction results in a defect when the fracture is reduced.

Partial articular fractures usually involve the palmar aspect (volar Bartons) and are unstable. These can be difficult to reduce and stabilize and a volar buttress plate is usually indicated.

With high-energy multifragmentary fractures associated with instability, external fixation can be used, but with the development of better locking plate systems, external fixation is now less commonly used.

Complications – these are frequent, and the most common complications result from loss of reduction and malunion, but function may be good despite considerable deformity. If function is restricted, corrective osteotomies can be considered. Tendon rupture, particularly extensor pollicus longus can also occur.

Chronic regional pain syndrome can also occur and may be difficult to manage, particularly if associated with malunion, which may also be a contributing factor to the pain and loss of function.

Scaphoid fractures

Incidence – the scaphoid is the most commonly fractured carpal bone, often occurring in young adults.

Aetiology – it often results from a fall on the outstretched hand, commonly during sport or a fall from a (motor)cycle.

Management – depends on the degree of displacement. Minimally displaced fractures are commonly managed in a cast for 6–12 weeks, and radiological evidence of healing should be obtained before the patient is mobilized. Some surgeons advocate early internal fixation even for the minimally displaced fractures.

More displaced fractures are usually treated by closed reduction and percutaneous compression screw, or by open reduction and internal fixation. Some fractures are associated with collapse of the fracture site, particularly if there have been delays, and these are usually managed with a bone graft to restore length and alignment.

Complications – avascular necrosis is relatively common and affects the proximal pole with collapse. This is due to the blood supply from the radial artery entering the distal pole; this is then disturbed with displaced fractures across the waist of the bone. Treatment is related to symptoms and degree of collapse, and may be conservative or operative including open reduction and a vascularized bone graft.

Non-union is also common, occurring in 5–10%, particularly with displaced fractures treated conservatively. Symptomatic non-unions are treated with internal fixation and bone-grafting. The management of asymptomatic non-union is controversial.

Pelvic fractures

Incidence – fractures of the pelvis are relatively common.

Aetiology – these can be broadly divided into stable injuries, commonly occurring in elderly patients following a simple fall, and often resulting in pubic rami fractures, and complex injuries, usually occurring in younger patients after significant trauma, such as traffic accidents and commonly resulting in both haemodynamic and mechanical instability.

Management – the key to the management of pelvic fractures is the haemodynamic status and stability of the patient. A classification based on mechanism of injury can give a guide to stability, prognosis and resuscitation requirements:

Lateral compression – these are the most common, accounting for 50–60%. They are usually due to a side impact, commonly a road traffic accident or a pedestrian struck on the side by a vehicle. They have been associated with a mortality rate of 13%, but this is usually due to associated abdominal or head injuries. Radiographs usually show overlap of the pubic rami and little specific treatment is required.

Antero-posterior compression – this is also relatively common, accounting for up to 30%, and occurs in motorcyclists or pedestrians struck from the front. This results in opening up of the pelvis (open book). The most severe injuries are associated with mortality rates up to 50%, usually from haemorrhage from the pelvis. Treatment involves aggressive resuscitation together with reducing the pelvis. In the acute situation this can be achieved with a pelvic binder or sheet placed around the level of the trochanters, and definitively by external or internal fixation.

Vertical sheer – these are less common and as the name suggests involve a vertical element which can result in significant instability that cannot be adequately managed with a binder or other splints. They commonly result from a fall or a motorcycle accident and can be associated with a significant mortality.

Management again involves resuscitation and obtaining pelvic stability.

With both open book and vertical shear fractures, the aim of the binder or external fixation is to reduce the pelvic volume, to both reduce the space to bleed into as well as to allow tamponade. In most situations this will control the venous bleeding, but approximately 10% will involve arterial bleeding and pelvic packing or embolization may be required.

Complications – although the elderly patients appear to have sustained insignificant injuries, it is associated with a high 1-year mortality due to immobility of the patients' medical comorbidities.

Fractures in younger patients are also associated with significant mortality, as noted above, but this is due to the fracture itself, or other injuries sustained in the accident.

Proximal femoral fractures

Incidence – although commonly referred to as 'neck of femur' fractures many do not involve the femoral neck. They are one of the most common osteoporotic fractures, increasing in frequency with increasing age. They can be classified as:

- intracapsular fractures (femoral neck fractures)
- extracapsular fractures: intertrochanteric or subtrochanteric.

The majority of the fractures are treated operatively to allow early mobilization of the patient, to minimize the risk of the complications associated with prolonged immobilization such as chest infection, pressure sores and deep-vein thrombosis. The specific techniques vary but are largely determined by the blood supply to the hip.

The femoral head is supplied by endosteal branches, branches that run with the capsule, and by vessels in the ligamentum teres in the hip joint.

All displaced fractures will disrupt the endosteal supply, and given the variable nature of the supply by the ligamentum teres, the viability of the femoral head is related to capsular attachment. When the fracture is outside the capsular the femoral head maintains a blood supply and therefore these fractures can be managed by reduction and fixation. When the fracture is inside the capsule, the blood supply is disrupted and avascular necrosis may occur.

Management – given this then the fractures are usually managed as follows:

Intracapsular fractures – replacement of the femoral head should be considered. This will not usually involve replacement of the acetabular and therefore hemiarthoplasty, as opposed to total hip replacement, is carried out. This may be cemented or uncemented depending on patient factors, especially comorbidities, as well as surgeons' preferences.

In younger patients, particularly with a short history (6–12 hours or less since injury) especially with minimal displacement an attempt can be made to preserve the head. Reduction of the fracture is carried out and fixation by screws.

In some patients there will be pre-existing hip disease such as osteoarthritis. In these patients a primary total hip replacement should be considered, although this is associated with a higher complication rate.

Extracapsular fractures: intertrochanteric – these are usually treated by reduction of the fracture under image intensifier, and fixation with a sliding screw device. This allows compression of the fracture site, resulting in stability and rapid healing.

Subtrochanteric – compression of the fracture cannot usually be achieved and a stable and strong implant is required. This is commonly achieved with an intra-medullary device such as a nail.

Complications – these are significant injuries in the elderly patient and are associated with a 30% 6–12-month mortality. Even in survivors there is considerable morbidity, with the majority losing some degree of mobility and/or independence. Following these injuries patients often require long-term nursing or rest home placement.

Femoral shaft fractures

Incidence – although frequently seen, these are less common than either proximal femoral fractures or tibial shaft fractures.

Aetiology – in general a significant amount of violence is required to break the femur, and in younger adults they are frequently due to traffic accidents and are commonly associated with other injuries. In more elderly patients they may result from simple falls.

In toddlers and young children, non-accidental injury should be considered, particularly if the history is not consistent with the injury. However, pathological conditions of the bone can occur and should also be considered.

Management – in adults the vast majority of femoral fractures are managed operatively, due to the prolonged treatment of traction that would be required if the patient were treated in skeletal traction. In developing countries skeletal traction, via a proximal tibial pin, is a viable option, but in the more elderly patient can be associated with significant morbidity from chest or urinary tract infections or pressure areas.

The most common method of operative fixation is by a locked intramedullary nail, although plate fixation is occasionally performed. External fixation is less commonly used, even with open fractures.

Complications – general complications are related to comorbidities in older patients, and associated injuries in younger patients.

Specific complications are less common than with tibial or humeral shaft fractures, due to the larger implants resulting in less implant failure, and a better blood supply resulting in a lower non-union rate.

Patella fractures

Incidence – these are uncommon fractures in adults, quoted as 1% of all fractures. Unlike most fractures, they appear to be more common in middle age.

Aetiology – they can result from direct injury such as contact with a dashboard, when they are often multi-fragmentary fractures. They also occur with indirect violence, such as a fall from height, resulting in tensile forces on the front of the patella and three-point bending, resulting in a transverse fracture.

Management – this depends on the fracture pattern, displacement and function of the extensor mechanism of the knee. Undisplaced, or minimally displaced fractures, associated with a good straight leg raise test (minimal extensor lag) are managed non-operatively in a plaster cylinder or brace. Displaced transverse fractures are managed using a tension band technique as described for olecranon fractures.

Management of multifragmentary fractures is more complicated. Restoration of the extensor mechanism is paramount and multiple wires and or screws may be used, often in combination with a tension band device. This can result in an incongruous joint, and significant anterior knee pain, and so for mulifragmentary fractures involving the upper lower pole, partial patellectomy can be considered. Total patellectomy has been described, but is rarely used, and can cause significant weakness.

Complications – These are relatively common, and can be significant. Due to the subcutaneous nature of the bone the hardware is prominent and commonly requires removal. Anterior knee pain is common and can be debilitating, and infection and wound healing problems are not uncommon.

Tibial plateau fractures

Incidence – these have been reported to have a similar incidence to patella fractures, at around 1%, and can occur in all age groups.

Aetiology – the level of violence required is related to the age of the patient. In young adults they are often due to high-energy mechanisms such as motor-vehicle accidents, and are often complex injuries. In the elderly they are usually associated with low-energy mechanisms, and, although less complex injuries, can still be difficult to manage, especially if associated with significant osteoporosis, and/or pre-existing degenerative joint disease.

Management – undisplaced or minimally displaced fractures are usually managed non-operatively, although minimally invasive techniques such as percutaneous screws can be used, occasionally with arthroscopic assistance. More displaced fractures are usually treated by open reduction and buttress plates, often with bone graft.

With high-energy injuries, external fixation can be used, and in elderly patients with significant injuries the displacement may be accepted with a view to later total knee replacement if required. Acute management by knee replacement, however, is not commonly used.

Complications – there are few specific complications, although debate centres on the incidence and symptoms from late degenerative arthritis. Infection, although uncommon, can be a devastating complication.

Tibial shaft fractures

Incidence – the tibia is the most commonly fractured long bone, approximately 10 times more common than humeral shaft fractures, and 20 times more common than femoral shaft fractures.

Aetiology – in some series traffic accidents are the most common cause, with sporting injuries a close second. The fractures are less common in the elderly and may occur following a simple fall. Many of the fractures are open, particularly from the higher-energy injury mechanisms.

Management – this depends on the displacement, associated injuries, and whether the fracture is open. Minimally or undisplaced closed fractures can be managed in plaster, and even displaced fractures can be reduced and held in a plaster. When the fracture is open, or difficult to control in plaster, and in polytrauma, operative fixation is indicated. Closed reduction and intramedullary fixation with a nail is the most common method, although plate fixation, particularly by a minimally invasive approach, is becoming more common. External fixation is indicated for the more severe open fractures.

Complications – unfortunately these are relatively common. Healing is slow, often requiring 12 weeks in plaster, and non-union can occur, particularly with open fractures. This can be a complex problem requiring bone transport, particularly with open fractures, with associated bone loss. Infection is also common, and some of these injuries result in late amputation for failed salvage.

Distal tibial – pilon fractures

Incidence – these have a similar incidence to tibial plateau fractures, although their relative incidence will depend on the population being described.

Aetiology – pilon fractures are usually caused by higher-energy mechanisms than ankle fractures, and usually result from axial loading rather than just rotational injuries. They form a spectrum from severe loading from high-speed vehicle crashes and falls from heights to skiing injuries and the outcome is related to the energy involved.

Management – these are severe injuries, and require skilled management. Frequently there is an associated significant soft tissue injury with swelling and skin blisters.

For lower-energy injuries open reduction and internal fixation are commonly performed, with the joint reduced and fixed with screws and plate fixation to the shaft, often with bone grafting to any defect caused by impaction. Although the aims for higher-energy injuries are the same open reduction through compromised skin can result in significant complications. A number of alternatives are available, including minimally invasive techniques including percutaneous screws and small incisions and sliding low-contact plates above the periosteum.

External fixation is also used widely, including fine-wire techniques, and both external fixation and skeletal traction may be used initially, with internal fixation delayed until the soft tissues have improved.

Complications – due to the higher-energy and soft tissue problems associated with these injuries, complications are common. Wound breakdown and infection can occur, and both malunion and late arthrosis are common. Ultimately late amputation may be required.

Ankle fractures

Incidence – ankle fractures are among the most common of all fractures.

Aetiology – unlike pilon fractures, ankle fractures are typically the result of lower-energy, rotational injury mechanisms. These may be due to sporting injuries or simply low-energy injuries at home or in the garden.

Two main classifications have been described – Lauge-Hansen and Weber. With the Lauge-Hansen classification four patterns are described: supination-external rotation, supination-adduction, pronation-abduction, and pronation-external rotation.

The supination-external rotation pattern is the most common injury pattern and accounts for 40–75% of all ankle fractures. A supination-external rotation injury includes: a spiral oblique fibula fracture at or just above the ankle mortise (see Weber B below), rupture of the deep deltoid ligament or transverse avulsion fracture of the medial malleolus, and a posterior malleolar fracture may also occur.

A supination-adduction pattern includes: a low avulsion fracture of the lateral malleolus or lateral ligament injury, and a vertical shear fracture of the medial malleolus.

The pronation-abduction injury is commonly associated with instability of the syndesmosis and includes: tension failure of the deep deltoid ligament or transverse avulsion fracture of the medial malleolus and a transverse fibula fracture at or above the ankle mortise, typically with lateral comminution because of the bending forces applied to the fibula.

A pronation-external rotation pattern includes: tension failure of the deep deltoid ligament or transverse avulsion fracture of the medial malleolus, a spiral oblique fibula fracture above the ankle mortise (Weber C – see below); and possibly a posterior malleolus fracture. This pattern is also commonly associated with instability of the syndesmosis.

Weber – this classification is based on the level of the fibula fracture, and is a guide to treatment rather than based on mechanism of injury.

Weber A fractures occur below the syndesmosis, possibly as an avulsion following an inversion injury.

Weber B fractures occur at the syndesmosis and are commonly oblique on the lateral radiograph. They can be considered as stable or unstable dependent on the integrity of the medial deltoid ligament. This can be determined by clinical examination at the time of presentation, with significant pain and swelling medially. It can also been seen on plain radiographs.

Weber C fractures occur above the syndesmosis, which is often injured with diastasis of the tibia and fibula. This may require operative stabilization.

Management – this depends on the degree of displacement and stability at the fracture site. Minimally displaced fractures (particularly Weber A and Weber B) with an intact deltoid ligament are managed non-operatively, without plaster immobilization if symptoms are minimal. Potentially unstable fractures can also be managed in plaster if a satisfactory reduction can be maintained, although weekly radiographs are recommended initially.

If closed reduction cannot be achieved or maintained, and for very unstable injuries, internal fixation with a plate and/or screws is recommended.

Complications – inadequate or loss of reduction can occur and may require revision surgery, and wound infection and breakdown can occur; particularly with more severe soft tissue injuries, or in diabetics. Diabetics may also require up to 3 months immobilization in plaster, as opposed to 6 weeks or less for most other patients.

Dislocations

Glenohumeral joint

The glenohumeral joint is the most commonly dislocated joint in the body, and in a Swedish study was esti-

mated to affect 1.7% of the population at some time in their life. Its ease of dislocation is due to its inherent instability, the price paid for the considerable range of movement. Although dislocations can affect all age groups, they are most common in young males, usually due to sporting injuries.

There are a number of features which increase stability, which include the labrum, a circumferential fibrocartilage structure which increases the concavity of the glenoid. Damage to this is very common following dislocations and predisposes to recurrent instability.

The majority (usually quoted as 95%) of acute dislocations are anterior and are associated with detachment of the antero-inferior labrum (Bankart lesion), and an impaction injury to the humeral head (Hill-Sachs lesion).

A number of methods are described to reduce the dislocation, but most rely on traction of the arm, rotation and pressure on the humeral. Following reduction the arm is rested and then gently mobilized. There is little evidence that any specific period of immobilization is beneficial, although immobilization in an external rotation brace has been shown to reduce the recurrence rate.

The risk of redislocation is related to the age at first dislocation, with those under 20 years having a reported recurrence rate of 80–90% in some series, and up to 50% require surgery to treat the recurrent instability. Much of the risk is due to the individual continuing to play sport.

In the older patient, the recurrence risk is much smaller, but recovery may be prolonged. There is also a lower rate of Bankart lesions, but there is a higher risk of associated rotator cuff tears and early MRI scan is commonly required.

Posterior dislocation can also be due to trauma and sport, but is also associated with epilepsy and electric shock. The recurrence rate seems to be smaller but this may be due to the age and initial cause of the dislocation.

Acromio-clavicular joint

This is also a relatively commonly dislocated joint, usually due to a direct blow to the outer aspect of the top of the shoulder. It is most commonly seen in young males due to a sporting injury, or a fall from a cycle/motorcycle.

When viewed standing up the patient has a very prominent lateral end of clavicle due to inferior displacement of the arm due to gravity. The dislocation is usually reducible, and will often reduce spontaneously if the patient lies down.

Classifications are described usually based on the degree of displacement, which is often considered as part of a spectrum of injury.

Minimally displaced injuries are managed conservatively with a supporting sling and early mobilization, while the most displaced injuries are commonly treated by reduction and stabilization. Debate continues on the intermediate injuries as to whether conservative or operative treatment is appropriate.

Persisting displacement associated with functional problems is treated by late reconstruction.

Elbow dislocation

This is the most commonly dislocated joint in young children and the third most common, after the glenohumeral joint and fingers, in adults.

It is usually due to a fall on the outstretched hand, and the forearm is displaced posteriorly relative to the distal humerus, and may be due to a rotational injury rather than a direct force applied to the front of the joint.

Reduction is usually easy with traction on a slightly flexed arm with anterior and inferior pressure applied to the olecranon.

If a stable reduction is possible, early mobilization is recommended, but immobilization may be required for unstable injuries. Operative treatment may be required for fracture dislocations, or instability that persists when the elbow is flexed to 90 degrees.

Hip dislocation

Due to its inherent stability, from both bony architecture and strong ligaments within a thick capsule, hip dislocation is a relatively uncommon injury and is usually due to high-energy mechanisms.

The most common cause is a motor-vehicle accident, and is usually posterior from a blow to the knee when the hip is flexed. Due to the high-energy nature, other injuries are common, and in addition associated fractures of the acetabulum, femoral neck, or even femoral head occur. On examination the hip is flexed and internally rotated, and acutely painful when moved.

Closed reduction is attempted with the patient prone and in-line traction applied to the flexed hip. Open reduction may be required, both for irreducible injuries as well as for unstable injuries due to fractures of the acetabulum.

A post-reduction CT is obtained, particularly with any associated fracture, and if reduction is satisfactory and stable the patient can be mobilized, with restricted weight-bearing initially. Unlike the glenohumeral joint, chronic instability is unusual, but avascular necrosis of the femoral head can occur.

Patella dislocation

This is not an uncommon injury, although because many spontaneously reduce and the diagnosis is not made, the true incidence is unknown.

It is more common in females and affects the second and third decades. The dislocation usually occurs with a low-energy twisting injury, and the patella most commonly dislocates laterally.

The diagnosis is usually straightforward if the dislocation persists, and reduction is possible by gently extending the knee.

Recurrent dislocations can occur, and may require surgical stabilization. However, the most common cause of morbidity is due to articular damage, or even an osteochondral fracture which can result in chronic anterior knee pain.

Imaging in orthopaedics

Plain radiographs

The majority of fractures are diagnosed by plain radiographs, which were the earliest images available following the discovery of X-rays by Roentgen at the end of the nineteenth century. In general X-rays are generated in a tube, and pass through the area being imaged and into a receptor. In conventional radiography the receptor is a film cassette and the X-rays are converted to visible light which exposes (darkens) the film, such that the more light that reaches the cassette, the darker the image. Structures such as bone which impede the passage of X-rays are seen as white on the film.

Digital radiography is beginning to replace standard radiography. With digital radiography, the cassette and film are replaced with a plate several times more sensitive. A laser reader extracts the image, and the data are managed by an image processor. Work stations replace the conventional viewing boxes, and the digital image can be easily manipulated.

Computed tomography (CT)

This also utilizes X-rays, with the source and the detectors placed opposite each other in a gantry. The gantry rotates around the patients, and the detectors are connected electronically to a computer, allowing continuous image transmission. This allows a complete axial image, or slice, to be generated. With appropriate software three-dimensional images can be created from multiple axial slices, as well as slices in the sagittal or coronal plane. One of the main disadvantages is the X-ray dose that may be required, and in addition, axial fractures, such as some cervical spine injuries, may be missed if the fracture line is between slices. This can be eliminated with the use of newer-technology spiral or helical CT, when the gantry does not just rotate around the patient, but the patient also moves within the scanner. In addition to improving accuracy, this also shortens the time required for scanning.

Magnetic resonance imaging

This is indicated when soft tissue rather than bony detail is required, and uses completely different technology to X-rays.

MRI uses the magnetic properties of hydrogen atoms, which usually exist as H^+, with an unpaired proton. If a strong magnetic field is applied to the body some of the protons will align themselves with the field, but will spin around the axis of the field, known as precession, similar to the wobble of a spinning top. The precession differs depending on the tissue the H^+ is part of. In addition the alignment of the proton can be disturbed by applying a radiofrequency pulse. As the protons return to their original alignment an electromagnetic signal is given out which can be detected and used to formulate an image.

Unlike X-ray-based imaging which measures the density of tissue, reflected by the ease with which the X-rays pass through, MRI can differentiate between different tissues, which makes it ideal for soft-tissue imaging. As well as anatomy it can also demonstrate pathology due to the different properties within the tissues.

Ultrasound

This uses high-frequency sound waves, rather than any radiation. The hand-held probe not only emits the waves, but also detects any that are reflected back, from structures such as bone. Because of the dynamic nature of the investigation, it is useful for motion such as the imaging of the achilles, patella tendon or the rotator cuff. The machines are portable and relatively cheap so are suitable for smaller out-patient departments, although the accuracy is dependent on the skill and experience of the operator, and there is a learning curve.

Nuclear medicine

This is also commonly used within orthopaedics. An isotope is given to the patient, which then accumulates in the body, where it can be detected with an appropriate 'camera'.

The most commonly used isotope is technetium-99, which is given intravenously and is rapidly taken up by bone. It can be detected by a gamma camera and will show areas of new bone formation as high activity, or hot spots. It is a very sensitive test, but not particularly specific as high activity could represent bony metastases, infection or healing fractures.

Fundamentals of plastic surgery

Tania C.S. Cubison

Introduction

The term plastic surgery is derived from the Greek word '*plastikos*' which translates as 'to form or mould'. Although often associated with skin conditions, plastic surgery is not limited to the skin. Modern plastic surgery includes a wide variety of subspecialty areas, many of which are far away from the 'nip and tuck' image commonly portrayed by the media. The British Association has recently changed its name from the British Association of Plastic Surgeons to the British Association of Plastic, Reconstructive and Aesthetic Surgeons (BAPRAS) to highlight the role of the modern plastic surgeon as a reconstructive surgeon as well as an aesthetic surgeon. As with all surgical specialties, there are a number of subspecialty areas of interest for plastic surgeons including hand or breast surgery, burns, craniofacial, cleft lip and palate, head and neck surgery, skin cancer and aesthetic (cosmetic) surgery. The theme of soft tissue reconstruction underlies all these areas and is the fundamental core of the plastic surgery specialty.

To mould the skin a surgeon needs to understand a number of basic principles that have changed little since the writings of Sir Harold Gillies in 1920 (Table 29.1). The careful handling of tissues, replacement of like with like, replacing the landmarks, and the understanding of the relationship between beauty and blood supply are vital.

In 1957, Millard expanded on Gillies's theories and outlined the plastic surgeons' creed:

Know the ideal beautiful normal; diagnose what is present, what is diseased, destroyed, displaced, or distorted, and what is in excess. Then, guided by the normal in your mind's eye, utilize what you have to make what you want – and when possible go for even better than what would have been.

These fundamental techniques allow plastic surgeons to achieve both functional and aesthetically pleasing results in many anatomical areas.

Soft tissue reconstruction

The blood supply of the skin

The detailed blood supply of the skin has been thoroughly investigated; in all parts of the body an area of skin is supplied by a dominant vessel, and the zone of tissue supplied by that vessel is termed an angiosome. Between the angiosomes are connecting vessels that allow some blood flow and open up when the flow is limited in the main vessel. These vessels are termed choke vessels and are responsible for the extra bleeding from the skin edges when extending a wound that surgeons often describe as the 'lateral incisional artery of sod'! The choke vessels also allow larger areas of tissue to be incorporated into flaps for transfer, especially after delay. The term delay in plastic surgery describes a procedure where the area of tissue is isolated from its primary blood supply by either dividing the tissue or obstructing its vessel. This encourages the dilatation of the surrounding choke vessels and increases the volume of tissue that can be reliably transferred.

Options to achieve soft tissue cover

One of the main contributions of plastic surgery is the provision of soft tissue cover, especially skin, to a wound where direct closure is either not possible or would be functionally or cosmetically unsatisfactory.

To achieve this soft tissue must be moved from another anatomical location and provided with adequate blood supply. Tissue can be moved in two major forms, either as a graft or as a flap.

Fundamentals of Surgical Practice, Third Edition, ed. Andrew N. Kingsnorth and Douglas M. Bowley.
Published by Cambridge University Press. © Cambridge University Press 2011.

Table 29.1 The principles of plastic surgery; Gillies and Millard 1957

Plastic surgery is a constant battle between blood supply and beauty
Observation is the basis of surgical diagnosis
Diagnose before you treat
Make a plan and a pattern for this plan
Make a record – sketches and photographs
The lifeboat – another flap or skin graft
A good style will get you through – dexterity and gentleness
Replace what is normal in normal position and retain it there
Treat the primary defect first – borrow from Peter to pay Paul only when Peter can afford it
Losses must be replaced in kind
Do something positive – start with a landmark or two pieces that definitely fit
Never throw anything away – a preserved piece may be used later
Never let routine methods be your master
Consult other specialists
Speed in surgery consists of not doing the same thing twice
The after-care is as important as the planning
Never do today what can honourably be put off till tomorrow – when in doubt, don't
Time, although the plastic surgeon's most trenchant critic, is also his greatest ally

Graft

A graft is an isolated piece of tissue that is removed from the patient or donor and has no integral blood supply. It is then placed into a vascularized bed and takes its nutrition by diffusion before revascularization occurs if the conditions are favourable (see below). The most commonly used graft is a skin graft, but grafts can also be made of other tissues such as tendon, nerve, bone or cartilage.

Flap

A flap is a vascularized piece of tissue that either remains attached to its blood supply during the transfer or is temporarily disconnected and then reattached by microvascular anastomosis to a new blood supply during the same procedure.

The classification of flaps can be complex but there are a few simple rules. A flap disconnected and then reattached by microsurgery is termed a free flap. A flap connected only by its blood supply is a pedicled flap. Flaps from other anatomical areas are referred to as distant flaps and flaps from the same area are local flaps. Flaps are also described by their type of blood supply, as either random or axial pattern flaps. A random-pattern flap is a piece of tissue that does not have a predetermined blood vessel with it, and relies upon the width of its base to incorporate adequate blood supply. This means that the volume of tissue that

can be moved is dependent on its base width to length ratio. In the head and neck the high vascularity means that long flaps with narrow bases are safe to plan. However, in the lower limb the blood supply is less, so that only 1:1 flaps are safe on a random-pattern blood supply.

The majority of currently used flaps are axial pattern, where there is a known vessel incorporated within the flap. The vessel is either a well-recognized anatomically described vessel or is identified during the planning of the flap using a Doppler ultrasound or exploratory incision. The volume of tissue that can form an axial-pattern flap is far larger than that of random-pattern flaps and allows the current plastic surgeon a wide number of options for immediate soft tissue reconstruction.

The reconstructive ladder

The reconstructive ladder describes the sequence of methods of wound closure (Figure 29.1). This starts with healing by secondary intention and finishes with the most complex free tissue transfer. It was initially described as a ladder, suggesting that all the methods should be attempted in sequence. However, the ladder relates to the thought process to ensure simpler methods are considered first and in practice it has been termed the reconstructive elevator, which allows the surgeon to go directly to the most appropriate level for the particular wound having considered the risks and benefits of each technique.

Primary closure and healing by secondary intention

Many wounds can be treated with primary closure, sometimes assisted by careful undermining. However, it is important to remember that closure under tension is only a temporary solution, as the subsequent ischaemia will often result in poor healing and later wound breakdown. Methods that spread tension over a wider area can be helpful but aggressive suture technique or mechanical closure devices should be used with caution.

The natural process of wound healing involves the production of granulation tissue with collagen synthesized from fibroblasts, which then causes contraction in the wound bed to aid in the closure of the defect. This can be beneficial in some situations such as the closure of a pressure sore or abdominal dehiscence,

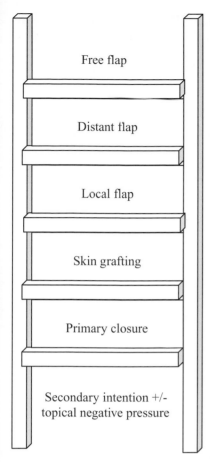

Figure 29.1 The reconstructive ladder, starting with the most simple procedures and building up to the most complex.

ulates the production of granulation in the wound, which may allow the application of a split skin graft as a later procedure. However, it is not a substitute for adequate wound preparation and it should be applied after all necrotic tissue and gross contamination are removed. The mechanisms of action are thought to include mechanical wound contraction, removal of exudate, interstitial fluid and bacteria, increasing the rate of angiogenesis and increased formation of granulation tissue.

There are a number of commercial systems now available with different wound interface dressings. The wound is covered with a porous primary dressing then a bulky layer of either foam sponge or gauze is applied and a suction drain tube is incorporated within or on top of this. The negative pressure (suction) is provided by a pump and the exudate is collected in a removable canister. The level of pressure used varies from 50 mmHg to 125 mmHg, either continuously or intermittently. Higher pressures are suitable for acute wounds, although if TNP is being used to secure a skin graft or skin substitute a lower setting is recommended (75 mmHg). Often the higher pressures are painful, especially in a chronic wound, and there is little evidence to show that the higher pressures are any more effective in these patients.

but in areas where the full thickness wound crosses a joint the excess contraction produced can flex joints and cause the severe deformity sometimes seen after neglected burn injury. The process of granulation and angiogenesis can be stimulated by the addition of topical negative pressure to the wound, and this modality would usually be considered with the secondary healing component of the reconstructive ladder.

The role of negative pressure

Topical negative pressure (TNP) dressings are used extensively to optimize healing conditions in difficult wounds. In some situations such as pressure sores TNP may provide the definitive treatment with the expectation of eventual healing after a considerable period of treatment. In other patients TNP may be used to optimize the wound environment and manage exudate prior to definitive wound management. TNP stim-

Indications for negative pressure
Definitive management of pressure sores
Production of granulation to produce a graftable surface
Wound management in high exudate chronic wounds
Wound stabilization after skin graft or skin substitute
Temporary safe wound cover for open fractures (short term only)
Maintain moist environment and prevent wound edge retraction in open abdomen

Skin grafting

Split skin graft

A split skin graft (SSG) consists of the epidermis, basement membrane and a variable thickness of dermis. It is harvested using a special knife (Figure 29.2) or a mechanical dermatome (Figure 29.3). As the remaining dermal layer contains adnexal elements, the keratinocytes lining these glands and follicles will divide and migrate, allowing re-epithelialization to occur. The

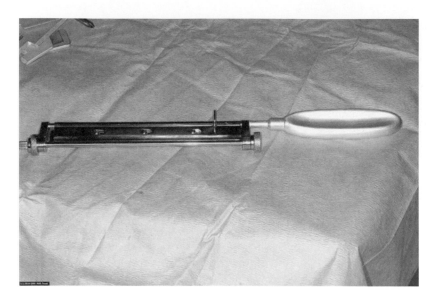

Figure 29.2 Watson skin knife.

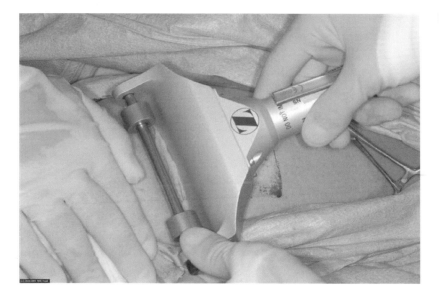

Figure 29.3 Mechanical dermatome.

donor site will therefore heal spontaneously with simple dressings. The thicker the split skin graft the more dermis is removed to form part of the graft and the less dermis and dermal elements remain. A thick split skin graft donor site will take longer to heal and is more likely to leave an unfavourable scar. Thin split skin graft donor sites heal quickly and the donor site can be re-cropped if there is a shortage of skin, e.g. in major burns.

There are a large number of potential donor sites for split skin grafting and large pieces of skin can be harvested. A thin split skin graft has less bulk of tissue associated with it and the diffusion distance is less, therefore a thin SSG is more likely to take on a poorly vascularized bed than a thicker graft.

However, it is the dermal elements of the skin that provide the cushioning and support for the skin and the lack of dermis in a thin graft results in a high level of contracture as the graft matures; a thin SSG is also less durable than a thick SSG. To increase the area that a skin graft can cover a process of meshing is used. This can be done using a meshing-machine that provides a series of cuts that allow the graft to expand in a pre-defined ratio (Figure 29.4). A 2:1 mesh pattern allows

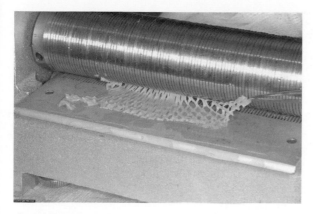

Figure 29.4 The 2:1 Brennan mesher.

the skin to expand to cover twice the area of the original piece of skin. As the graft takes, the epidemal cells divide and migrate to fill in the spaces left within the mesh pattern. Wider expansions have larger areas to heal in this way and comparatively smaller amounts of available dermis. The resulting scar from wider meshing is therefore less satisfactory with more contraction and poor cosmesis.

Full-thickness graft

A full-thickness graft (FTG or Wolfe graft) consists of epidermis and the full thickness of dermis. It is cut with a scalpel and the donor site will not heal unless closed or covered with SSG as all the dermal adnexal elements have been transferred to the new site. There are a limited number of FTG donor sites that can be closed primarily and these include the pre- and post-auricular, clavicular, upper arm and groin. The colour match is important with FTG and where possible the graft should be harvested from the same anatomical region. Skin from behind the ear is a good colour match with the nose, whereas a groin FTG will appear very yellow if applied to the face. Although a large piece of FTG can sometimes be harvested, in routine practice FTG is indicated for small defects. The bulk of dermis requires good early nutrition and the FTG will only take properly if the bed is well vascularized and conditions are optimal. The thicker dermis of a FTG results in a more durable surface and less shrinkage once matured.

Principles of graft take

Graft take requires revascularization and maturation; the process of graft take is similar in all tissues but is described here for the skin. The first phase is adhe-

sion; the graft sticks to its new bed by fibrin adherence during the first hours after its placement. It is supplied with essential nutrients by inhibition (drinking) from the tissue fluid surrounding it. Over the first 3 days new tiny blood vessels start to bridge the gap, growing into the transplanted tissue, and these attach to the existing vascular structure of the graft by a process called innosculation (kissing). It is likely that new endothelium grows into the graft relining the previous vascular channels. Fibroblasts then move into the gap and the grafted tissue and lay down fibrin that is converted to fibrous tissue. Over the next few weeks lymphatic channels also develop into the grafted tissue and eventually there is some nerve growth into the skin graft but this takes a number of months.

To ensure good graft take a number of practical issues need to be considered. The blood supply of the bed must be adequate for the type of graft. If the bed is poorly vascularized, especially if there is exposed bone or metalwork, then a graft will not take and a different method of skin cover such as a flap may be required. Alternatively the vascularity of a potential bed can be improved by a period of negative pressure therapy to encourage a layer of granulation tissue which will then support a skin graft as a delayed procedure.

Good fluid balance and maintenance of blood count and oxygen saturation are essential. The oxygen carriage and nutrient levels of the blood must be adequate to support the graft during the early inhibition phase, therefore comorbid conditions can significantly reduce graft take as the keratinocytes struggle to survive long enough for revascularization to occur. Protein and vitamin C levels, iron stores and certain trace elements such as zinc, copper and selenium have been shown to cause problems with graft take if they are abnormally low.

Smoking, which causes vasoconstriction in the smallest vessels for up to 1 hour after each cigarette, should be avoided and not replaced with high-dose nicotine substitutes as these have a similar effect.

Mechanical factors can also reduce graft take; a collection of fluid such as haematoma prevents close approximation and reduces new vessel growth and any shearing between the graft and its bed easily disrupts the new vessels, preventing their successful ingrowth. Careful wound preparation is essential; ensuring good haemostasis and removing any non-viable tissue before the graft is applied. Stabilizing methods such as tie-overs are commonly used over grafts (especially full-thickness grafts) to reduce shear and reduce

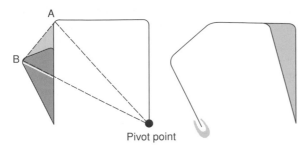

Figure 29.5 The transposition flap.

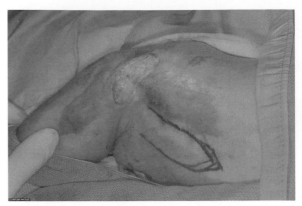

Figure 29.6 Planning an axial transposition flap of normal tissue for resurfacing the axilla.

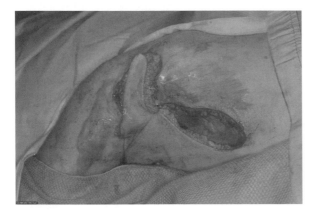

Figure 29.7 The transposition flap raised and transposed. The donor site is closed primarily in this case.

haematoma formation although they do not actively apply pressure to the bed for more than the first few minutes. Negative pressure dressings are also used over skin grafts especially in difficult areas such as in the axilla, and these appear to have a positive mechanical effect. Certain bacteria are known to destroy skin grafts even when they have apparently taken well and these must be actively treated. Many bacteria have a detrimental effect to graft take and common organisms such as *Streptococcus pyogenes* Groups A, C or G and *Staphylococcus aureus* can have a devastating effect. Other pathogens such as *Pseudomonas aeruginosa* often colonize skin grafts but can sometimes be managed by simple methods such as regular dressings.

Flap coverage

Local flaps

Small local flaps are most commonly performed on the face where there is excellent blood supply and maximal need for cosmesis and in the hand where their sensate

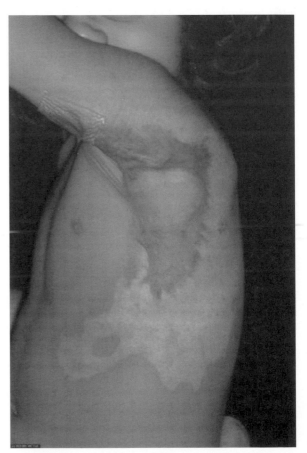

Figure 29.8 Axillary transposition flap; postoperative result.

nature is important. In other areas, larger local flaps may be used for non-graftable defects. Local flaps are described either by their shape or by the movement that they undertake to fill the defect.

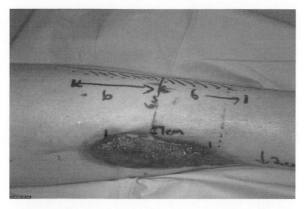

Figure 29.9 Planning a bipedicle flap for an exposed tibia.

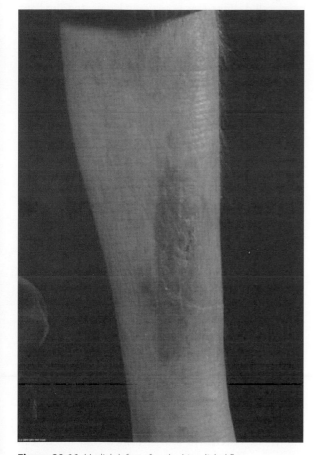

Figure 29.11 Medial defect after the bipedicled flap.

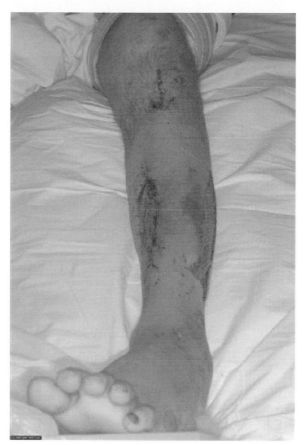

Figure 29.10 The flap at 2 weeks with a skin grafted donor site.

Transposition flaps

The flap of tissue is lifted and moved sideways into a prepared triangulated defect. The pivot point is on the furthest corner and limits the movement of the flap. A classic transposition flap needs to be planned longer than the apparent length of the wound to allow it to reach the far side of the defect. The pivot point of the flap is the furthest corner and this determines the zone of greatest tension (Figure 29.5). The donor site where the flap is taken from is either closed directly (if planned to utilize an area of skin excess) or a split skin graft is applied to the donor defect. The length to breadth ratio needs to be considered in view of the local blood supply and a vessel is often incorporated within the flap to improve its blood supply. In regions such as the lower limb the deep fascia is incorporated into the flap. Long flaps can be planned with an axial vessel and transposed into areas such as the axilla (Figures 29.6–29.8). A very simple technique is the bi-pedicled flap, which involves releasing a strip of skin that remains attached at both ends and moving the central part into the wound. The resulting donor defect is then skin grafted. The width to

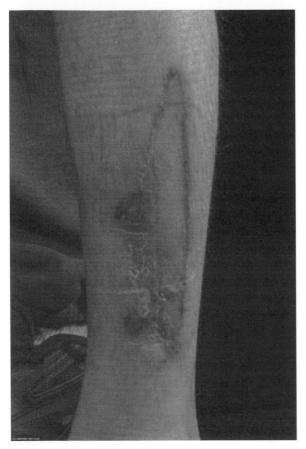

Figure 29.12 V–Y advancement. It is the skin on each side of the V that is actually advanced.

commonly used to lengthen a tight scar by recruiting lateral excess tissue, but is also used to change the alignment of unsatisfactory scars and to release special three-dimensional areas such as the medial canthus. The Z-plasty as classically described has two flaps which are transposed into the defect (Figure 29.17). The basic Z-plasty can be adapted into a running Z-plasty, double opposing z-plasties (jumping man) and four-flap Z-plasty and with adjustment to its angles and geometry can be adapted to a wide variety of sites with different degrees of lengthening and contour. A basic Z-plasty can be used to extend a tight band of scar. The central incision is made through the scar tissue along the line of maximal tension and two limbs are planned at 60-degree angles. If the Z-plasty has been well designed, as scar tissue is released the flaps will transpose themselves into their new positions. If the flaps do not fall into the new positions easily with minimal undermining they may need to be put back where they came from.

Rotation flaps

Rotation flaps rotate around a pivot point. They are usually planned as very large areas of tissue that allow direct closure of the donor defect by stretching the flap and then taking up the tension away from the defect to allow a tension-free closure of the wound. The defect is triangulated and the flap planned. The edge of the flap is four or five times the length of the base of the defect triangle. A backcut may be required or the excision of a small triangle of skin (Burow's triangle – Figure 29.18). The pivot point of a rotation flap is the furthest corner. Rotation flaps are commonly used in the scalp and for closing pressure sores on the buttocks.

Many described flaps move with a combination of transposition and rotation. Examples include the hatchet flap.

Advancement flaps

The tissue is released and stretched into the defect; either the releasing incision can be on the sides of the flap (H flap on forehead – Figure 29.19) or the skin of the flap can be incised all around and the flap advanced on the subcutaneous tissue or simply the vascular pedicle.

The V to Y or Y to V flaps are a variation on advancement flaps and are used to import tissue from

base ratio does need to be considered especially when there is no axial vessel in the flap. Although a useful technique for covering areas such as the exposed tibial fracture it never moves quite as well as expected (Figures 29.9–29.12).

The rhomboid flap or its descendant 'square flap into a round hole' is an example of the classic transposition flap with direct closure of the donor site (Figure 29.13).

A bilobed flap is a double transposition flap that allows excess tissue to be used that is at some distance from the initial defect, and allows closure of the donor site without a skin graft (Figures 29.14–29.16).

The Z-plasty is a very versatile two-flap transposition-type flap and has a wide variety of uses. Although easy to perform, it can be difficult to plan and without effective planning it can produce very unsatisfactory results. The Z-plasty is most

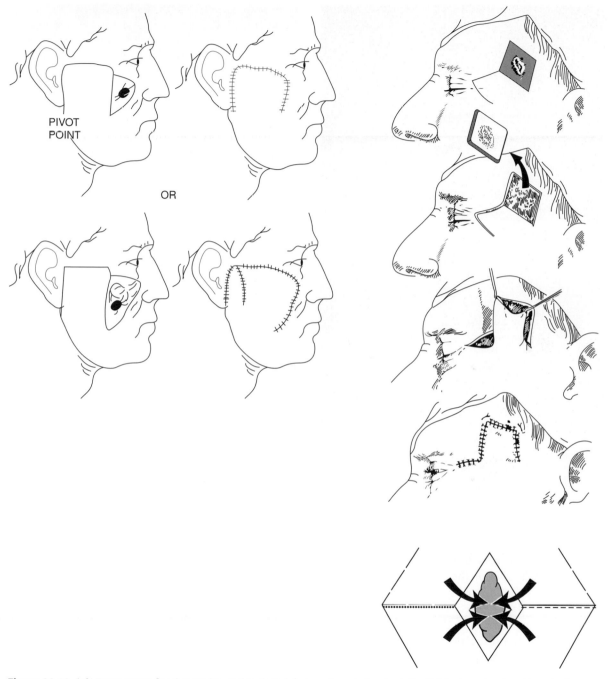

PIVOT
POINT

OR

Figure 29.13 (left) Transposition flap that can be used to close defects on the anterior cheek. Small defects can be closed by a single transposition flap that follows the skin lines. Large defects can be closed by a double transposition flap that uses a flap of postauricular skin to close the cheek flap donor site. (right) The rhomboid flap, using local excess tissue.

an area of excess to an area of deficit (Figure 29.20). They are classically designed to fill defects or release contracture. A running Y to V sequence of flaps is very useful in linear scarring (Figure 29.21).

Perforator flaps

With increasing awareness of the blood supply of the skin and using a hand-held Doppler ultrasound probe it is possible to identify the perforating vessels to the

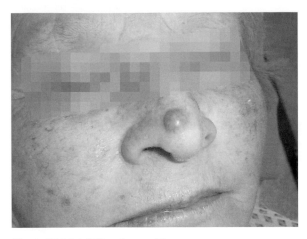

Figure 29.14 A BCC on the nasal tip.

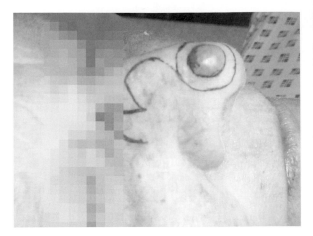

Figure 29.15 The bilobed flap marked out to move the excess tissue around the bridge of the nose to fill a defect on the tip where there is no excess skin.

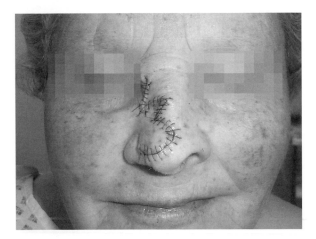

Figure 29.16 The bilobed flap completed, with primary closure of the superior defect.

skin. These can then be used to plan the design of a flap very specifically for the patient and the wound. Propeller flaps are a special type of rotated perforator flap where the flap is raised with only the perforating vessels attaching the flap to the patient. The tissue is then rotated up to 180 degrees into the defect and if the vessels are prepared very carefully there remains sufficient flow to allow flap survival (Figures 29.22–29.26). These flaps are particularly useful in the distal lower limb where traditional methods of reconstruction are very limited (Figures 29.27–29.30).

Distant flaps

These flaps import tissue from outside the local area to the site of tissue loss. The most commonly used distant flaps in modern plastic surgery are the pedicled latissimus dorsi flap or pedicled transverse rectus abdominus myocutaneous (TRAM) flap for breast reconstruction, and in hand surgery the cross finger flap. Staged techniques used very often in the past have now been replaced with free tissue transfer techniques. However, it is sometimes necessary to bury a hand in the groin or swing a deltopectoral flap to the head and neck (Figure 29.31), or even waltz a tube pedicle (Figure 29.32). These traditional techniques used distant flaps from another anatomical region which were inset into the defect while still attached to the original site and then, after a number of weeks when an adequate blood supply had developed, the pedicle of the flap was divided and the flap finally inset.

Free flaps

The skill of small vessel anastomosis has revolutionized the art of plastic surgery over the last 50 years. In 1968, John Cobbett moved a toe from the foot of a patient to reconstruct a lost thumb, and the free groin flap, free omentum and free scalp flap were all reported in 1973. By the mid 1980s microsurgery was no longer experimental and by the 1990s microsurgery had become mainstream. By 2009, the reconstructive surgeon could choose from a large number of well-described flaps including a number of different tissue types, or prefabricate the combination that is required using complex planning and surgical techniques to tailor the reconstruction.

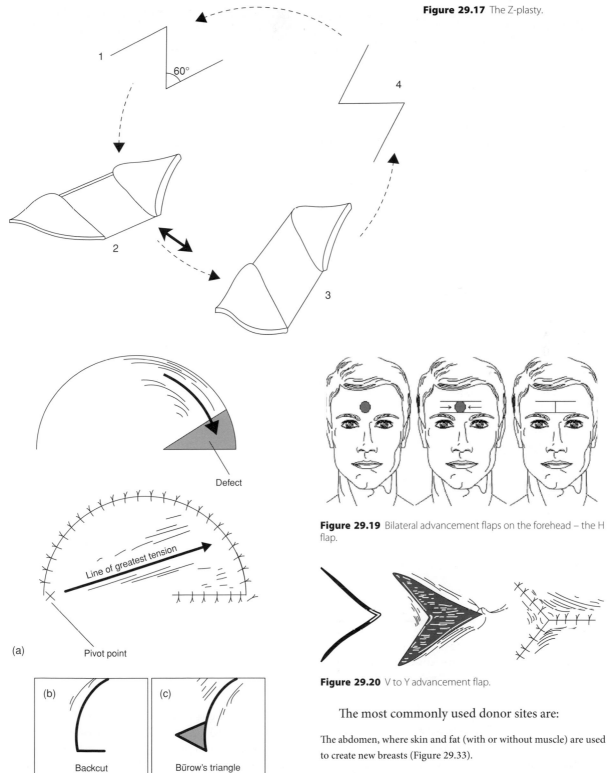

Figure 29.17 The Z-plasty.

Defect

Line of greatest tension

Pivot point

(a)

(b) Backcut

(c) Būrow's triangle

Figure 29.18 The rotation flap.

Figure 29.19 Bilateral advancement flaps on the forehead – the H flap.

Figure 29.20 V to Y advancement flap.

The most commonly used donor sites are:

The abdomen, where skin and fat (with or without muscle) are used to create new breasts (Figure 29.33).

The thigh, where skin, fascia and fat (with or without muscle) can be taken as the antero-lateral thigh (ALT) flap. Fasciocutaneous flaps

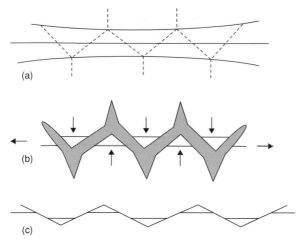

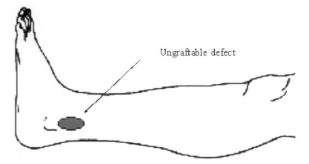

Figure 29.22 The principle of a propeller flap. The initial defect.

Figure 29.21 Running Y to V flaps, each tongue of tissue is advanced into the incision ahead of it so that the wider parts of each triangle provide the extra tissue for elongation of the scar.

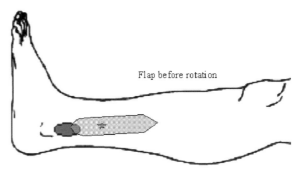

Figure 29.24 The flap is marked and an exploratory incision is performed to identify the perforator.

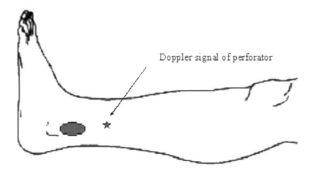

Figure 29.23 A suitable perforator is identified by hand-held Doppler ultrasound and marked.

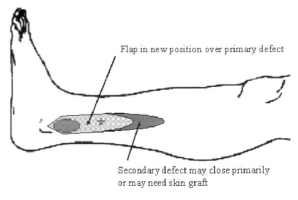

Figure 29.26 The secondary defect is grafted or closed primarily.

Muscle flaps are reliable, robust and reasonably predictable to raise; they are usually covered by a split skin graft. Examples are the latissimus dorsi muscle flap, gracillis muscle flap and rectus abdominus muscle flap.

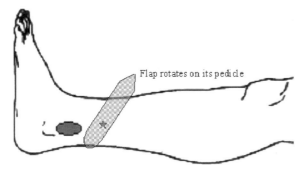

Figure 29.25 The flap is rotated around the skeletalized vessels.

like these are very good cosmetically and have minimal donor-site morbidity. However, they can be a challenge to raise as long intramuscular courses of the supplying vessels are not unusual and muscle damage during the harvest can result in significant postoperative morbidity.

Vascularized bone is taken as a free fibular flap or deep circumflex iliac artery (DCIA) flap which incorporates a piece of the pelvis. This is most commonly performed for mandibular reconstruction in head and neck reconstruction. Other tissue types such as omentum and jejunum are also used as free tissue transfer in specialized situations.

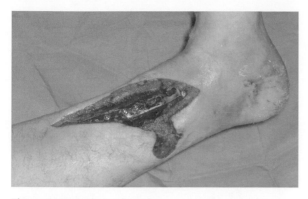

Figure 29.27 Defect on lower leg.

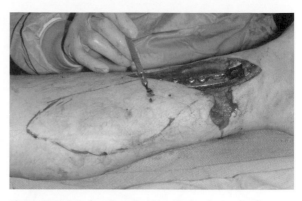

Figure 29.28 Perforating vessel identified and propeller flap marked.

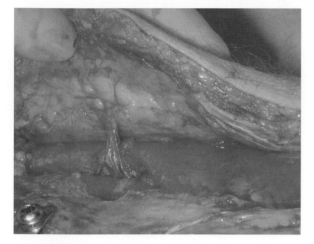

Figure 29.29 Perforating vessel skeletalized.

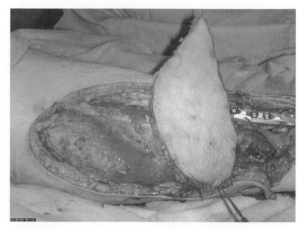

Figure 29.30 Propeller flap, rotated on its vessels.

Burns

Aetiology

A burn is a wound caused by heat, chemicals or electricity. The main groups of heat injury are flame, flash, contact and scald. The term scald refers to a burn from a wet heat source such as fluid or steam.

In heat injury the intensity of the heat source and the duration of contact time determine the depth of burn. In chemical injury, pH, concentration and contact time determine the depth, and in electrical injury the voltage and type of current are the key factors.

Epidemiology

In the UK 0.5% of the population (275,000) suffer a burn injury each year. Fifty per cent of those injured have only minor inconvenience to their daily lives and 10% require admission to hospital. One per cent of burn patients have a serious burn injury that may make them critically ill.

Although some patients sustain a purely accidental burn injury, the majority are associated with carelessness or risk-taking behaviour, commonly alcohol or drugs are involved and pre-existing psychiatric problems are common in the burn population.

Physiology

Jackson described a model of burn injury (Figure 29.34) with a central area of coagulative necrosis, surrounded by a zone of stasis and a surrounding zone of hyperaemia. In a burn over 25% of the body surface, the area of hyperaemia can be the whole body.

The size of the central area of necrosis is determined by the initial injury and is dead tissue. The

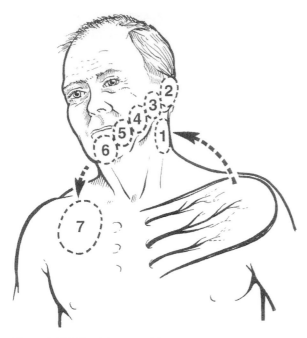

Figure 29.31 The deltopectoral flap.

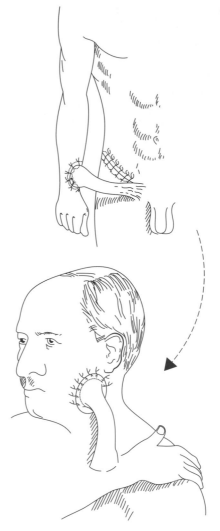

Figure 29.32 The tube pedicle flap.

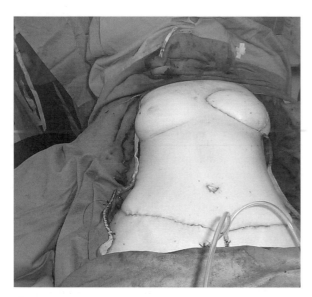

Figure 29.33 Transverse rectus abdominus musculocutaneous flap breast reconstruction.

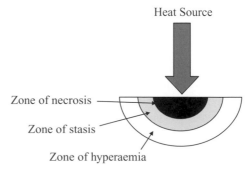

Jackson's Burn Model

Figure 29.34 Jackson's zones of the burn wound.

zone of stasis is an area of circulatory compromise with intermittent ischaemia but the cells may survive if the area is cooled quickly and the patient well resuscitated. However, prolonged vasoconstriction due to poor resuscitation, low temperature or the use of certain inotropes can result in the progression of the zone of stasis into a larger zone of necrosis. There can be considerable fluctuation in the capillary flow in the zone of stasis over the first 48 h after burn injury and this makes assessment of burn depth inaccurate. The outer zone of hyperaemia is involved in the inflammatory response but the skin will return to normal after the hyperdynamic vascular response has died down. Ischaemic and necrotic tissues produce inflammatory mediators, resulting in both local and systemic responses to the burn injury. Early excision of the zone of necrosis reduces the production of these mediators and is the physiological reason behind the current doctrine of early total burn excision.

At a local level the mediators cause vasodilatation resulting in capillary leak and tissue oedema. In larger burns there is a whole-body systemic response. Abnormal capillary exchange occurs due to vasodilatation, increased capillary permeability and breakdown or uncoiling of the intracellular matrix. This affects many parts of the Starling equation (see box below) with vasodilatation causing increased capillary hydrostatic pressure, separation of the endothelial cells allowing protein leak, increase of colloidal osmotic pressure of the interstitial space and reduction of the hydrostatic pressure of the interstitial space due to its physical expansion. All these factors result in the net movement of fluid out of the intravascular compartment and into the interstitial space, causing hypovolaemia and effective protein loss.

There are also other systemic changes associated with a major burn.

The hypermetabolic response to the burn injury is caused by secretion of stress hormones (cortisol, catecholamines and glucagon) and the suppression of anabolic hormones (anabolic steroids, insulin and growth hormone). This catabolic state is associated with tachycardia, hyperthermia and loss of muscle protein (wasting). Immunosuppression, bacterial translocation in the gut and acute inflammatory response syndrome are also common. In children there is significant growth disruption with changes in bone, muscle and fat deposition that can last for a number of years after a large burn. Although these children do start to grow again after 2 or 3 years they do not typically catch up this lost growth.

Healing of the superficial or partial-thickness burn occurs due to re-epithelialization of the wound surface by the epithelial cells of the hair follicles and other skin appendages. The deeper the burn injury the fewer are the skin appendages that remain and the longer is the time taken for a confluent epidermis to form. If the skin is sealed within 14 days there is minimal scar formation. However, especially in children if the burn wounds take over 30 days to heal the risk of aggressive (hypertrophic) scarring is very high. If burns are deep partial or full thickness it is therefore necessary to remove the necrotic tissue and replace with a split skin graft as soon as practical to reduce the risk of severe scarring.

> **Starling's hypothesis**
>
> The net fluid movement is the difference between the forces moving fluid out (hydrostatic pressure in the capillary pushes fluid out and the colloidal osmotic pressure pulls the fluid out) and the forces moving fluid in (hydrostatic pressure in the interstitial space pushing fluid back in and plasma colloid osmotic pressure pulling fluid in).

Initial management

First aid

The first aid for the burn is active cooling with cool (not ice-cold) running water for 15 minutes; this is vital to stop the burn progressing further and may still be effective up to 2 or 3 hours after the incident. If the burn still feels warm to touch, actively cool the area. Chemical burns require irrigation for longer periods to return to a safe pH (between 6 and 9).

Resuscitation

The initial management of a patient with burn injury should be the same as the primary management of the patient with any general trauma. All trauma patients should be treated using the principles of the Advanced Trauma and Life Support Course (ATLS®). It is vital that the patient is not just seen to have a burn, and all focus then changed to the management of the burn, because there is often other associated trauma that also needs to be assessed and treated. In the early stages other injuries may be a much greater risk to the patient's life than the burn injury, even if the burn is major.

Burn injury is managed following the principles of the EMSB Course (Emergency Management of Severe Burns) which itself incorporates much of the ATLS guidance.

A = Airway with C spine control

B = Breathing with oxygen

C = Circulation with haemorrhage control

D = Disability with pupil assessment

E = Exposure within warm environment

F = Fluids with analgesia

A = Airway with cervical spine control

Although the patient may have an isolated burn injury it is also important to remember that they may have sustained other injuries including cervical spine damage when sustaining their burn or in escaping from the burn situation; for example, jumping out of a window or being thrown by an electric current.

Airway compromise can be associated with peri-oral swelling as well as laryngeal swelling and both can develop over a number of hours following a burn injury. It is important that the airway is continually reassessed and, if there are signs of significant swelling or risk factors in the history to suggest significant risk of inhalation injury, the airway should be secured early. Life-threatening airway obstruction can develop quickly and emergency intubation can be very difficult even in experienced hands. Do not cut down the endotracheal tube as the swelling of lips can be very extensive. Surgical airways are very occasionally needed. However, if airway swelling is anticipated and an appropriate anaesthetist involved early, emergency tracheostomy is seldom required.

Risk factors for inhalation injury/airway swelling
Flame burn in an enclosed space
Singeing of nostril and eyebrow hair
Soot in or around nostrils and/or mouth
Peri-oral burns
Intraoral burns
Change in voice
Cough +/− sooty sputum
Wheeze – late
Stridor – very late

B = Breathing with oxygen

All burns should receive high-flow oxygen via a non-rebreathing mask. High levels of oxygenation are important to prevent ischaemia in the zone of stasis around the established burn injury, and to wash out toxic gases such as carbon monoxide and cyanide that may have been inhaled. The treatment of inhalation injury is principally supportive with airway management, respiratory support and mechanical measures being used in a similar manner to that with general ITU patients with SIRS (systemic inflammatory response syndrome). Bronchoscopy, irrigation with a variety of medications and regular physiotherapy are all important.

C = Circulation with haemorrhage control

Although major burns can be associated with hypo-volaemic shock, if a patient presents shocked within an hour of burn injury there is another cause until proved otherwise. This may be a ruptured spleen or closed pelvic fracture. These other injuries are far more likely to be immediately life-threatening and it is vital that a full ATLS® survey is carried out to ensure that there is no active bleeding. Two large-bore cannulae should be inserted through unburned skin (if possible), and blood samples should be obtained for full blood count, urea and electrolytes and blood cross-match.

D = Disability and pupil reaction

The basic neurological status of the patient is assessed using the AVPU score (A = alert, V = responds to voice, P = responds to pain, U = unconscious), and the pupil reactions are recorded.

E = Exposure within a warm environment

The patient should be undressed and the burn assessed for depth and surface area, while the environment is kept very warm to prevent the development of hypothermia. Hypothermia is very serious in burn patients and has a correlation with poor outcome (as demonstrated with other ITU patients). Jewellery should be removed before it can cause problems as swelling develops.

F = Fluids and analgesia

To combat the loss of effective circulating body fluid due to the physiological mechanisms above it is necessary to aggressively resuscitate patients with larger burns. The assessment of burn size is covered below. Children with more than 10% total body surface area (TBSA) burns and adults with over 15% TBSA burns should be formally resuscitated. Elderly patients with moderate-sized burns (5–15% TBSA) should be carefully monitored as significant physiological and fluid balance changes can easily destabilize their cardiac function.

Fluid resuscitation is carried out guided by formulae. The most common current formula is the Parkland crystalloid formula. Some burn units still use the more traditional Muir and Barclay formula that resuscitates with colloid (originally plasma, now human albumin

% Total Body Surface Area Burn (TBSA)

Be clear and accurate, and do not include erythema

(Lund and Browder)

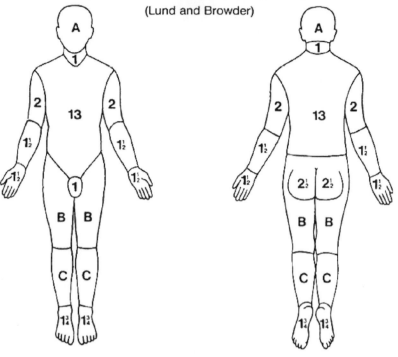

Figure 29.35 The adult Lund and Browder chart.

AREA	Age 0	1	5	10	15	Adult
A = ½ of head	9.5	8.5	6.5	5.5	4.5	3.5
B = ½ one thigh	2.75	3.25	4	4.5	4.5	4.75
C = ½ one lower leg	2.5	2.5	2.75	3	3.25	3.5

solution). Remember to use the correct fluid for the formula used as the volumes needed are very different for crystalloid and colloid formulae. Catheterization is required to allow accurate measurement of the urine output as this is the main method to monitor the effectiveness of resuscitation. The target should be 0.5 to 1 ml per kg in the adult and 1–2 ml per kg in children. Patients with high-voltage electrical injury are at risk of developing haemachromogens in the blood due to breakdown products from ischaemic muscles and myoglobinuria may develop. These damage the renal tubule and may cause acute renal failure. Any sign of darkening of the urine should be investigated and urine volumes of 1–2 ml/kg per %TBSA should be achieved to wash out the pigments. Analgesia should be provided using IV opiates titrated to the needs of the patient; intramuscular routes should be avoided due to patchy absorption and risk of late release after adequate resuscitation.

> 2–4 ml × weight (kg) × %TBSA
> Given as Hartmann's solution
> Half in the first 8 hours following the burn and the remainder in the next 16 hours

Assessment

The severity of a burn is described using size and depth. Burn size is related to the overall surface area of the patient and expressed as a percentage of the total body surface area or %TBSA burn. Small burns are also described in square centimetres. The %TBSA relates to the area of actual epithelial loss and does not include erythema (transient redness of the skin where the epithelium does not separate with rubbing). There are various methods of establishing the %TBSA of a burn with different degrees of accuracy. The most accurate commonly used method is to shade the burn area onto a Lund and Browder chart (Figure 29.35).

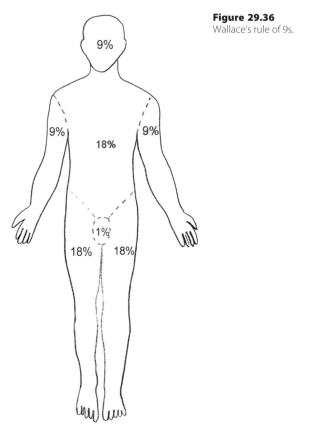

Figure 29.36
Wallace's rule of 9s.

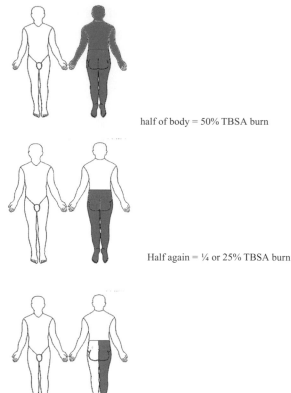

half of body = 50% TBSA burn

Half again = ¼ or 25% TBSA burn

Half Again = 1/8 or 12.5% TBSA bu

Figure 29.37 Serial halving.

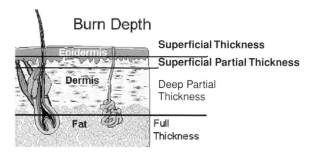

Burn Depth

Figure 29.38 The depth of burn injury.

These charts are specially designed for burn size assessment and are produced for adults and various paediatric ages as the comparative sizes of parts of the body change with growth of a child. The numerical values for each anatomical area can then be added together. In larger burns always double check the %TBSA burn by also adding up the percentage of unburned skin: if the combined figure is not 100% there has been a mathematical error in the calculations. Addition error is the most common reason for poor percentage assessment.

Other methods to calculate the burn percentage include Wallace's rule of 9s (Figure 29.36) and serial halving (Figure 29.37) and for smaller or patchy burns the most useful method is the approximation that the patient's own hand (fingertips to wrist crease) is 1%TBSA. Children have different proportions and different charts are needed; this is discussed in the paediatric burns section below.

Burns are classified in the UK by their depth related to the layers of skin involved in necrosis (Figure 29.38). The most superficial burns are simply epidermal loss and these appear as severe sunburn with desquamation of the most superficial layer. Partial-thickness burns are those where there is partial damage of the dermis and these are divided into superficial partial and deep partial. The superficial partial-thickness burns are characterized by blister formation, and when these blisters are removed the underlying surface is wet and pink with good capillary return after blanching on digital pressure (Figure 29.39). The patient is able to feel touch and exposure of the burn surface to the air

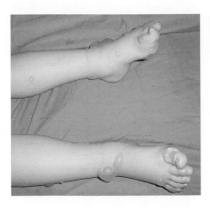

Figure 29.39 A superficial partial-thickness scald to the feet.

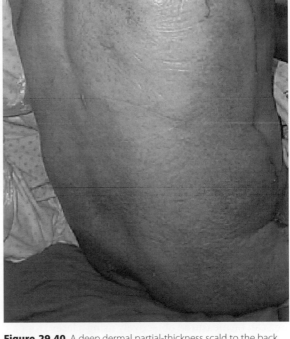

Figure 29.40 A deep dermal partial-thickness scald to the back.

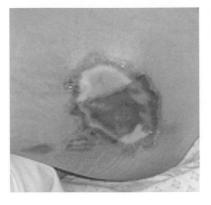

Figure 29.41 A full-thickness flame burn to the buttock.

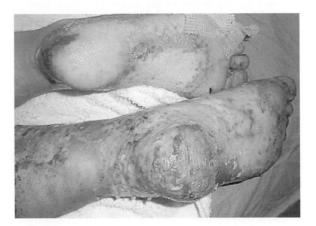

Figure 29.42 A full-thickness scald to the feet.

is painful. The use of a pin/needle to assess pain in burns is unnecessary as it adds nothing to the assessment and is distressing to the patient. Deep partial burns are less likely to have intact blisters on presentation, the underlying surface is white or fixed stained (dark red that does not blanch with pressure) and the patient is less concerned about the exposure of the area (Figure 29.40). These burns are less painful to touch. Full-thickness burns are burns involving the complete skin structure and the necrosis extends into the underlying soft tissue. The appearance of full-thickness burn injury depends on the mechanism of injury. Full-thickness flame burns appear white, brown or sooty with a dry leathery texture and sometimes a luminescent quality showing the coagulated veins underneath (Figure 29.41). Full-thickness scald injury is a soft creamy white often with a flaky surface, and a damp appearance (Figure 29.42).

In the USA burns are described using degrees, with first degree relating to simple erythema, and second degree a dermal burn. Although the term third-degree burn (a full thickness injury involving all layers of the skin) is universally used, terminology for deeper burns is confusing, with fourth, fifth and sixth degree being referred to in some texts.

Although the differentiation between truly superficial burn and full-thickness burn is easily recognized clinically, the depth of a partial-thickness burn can be difficult to assess especially within the first 48 h when the circulatory fluctuations are still occurring. The most accurate time to assess the depth of burn is

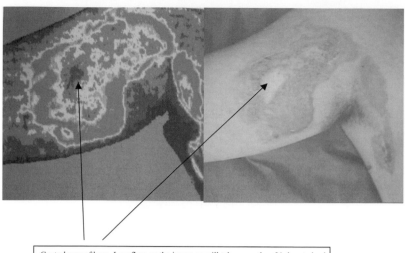

Central area of burn. Low flow on the image so will take more than 21 days to heal

Figure 29.43 Laser Doppler imaging scan and the clinical photograph demonstrating the healing potential of the burn, which relates to the depth of injury.

after 48 h and this is traditionally the time of the first dressing change. The blood supply within the burn area can be measured objectively using a laser Doppler imager (LDI) and this provides good correlation with healing time, which therefore provides an indirect measure of the depth of the burn. However, due to the blood flow variations this method is only accurate between 48 h and 5 days after the burn injury. The scan provides a coloured image that relates to the healing potential of the burn wound. A high-flow image (red) represents a healing potential of less than 14 days and a low-flow image (blue) represents a healing potential of over 21 days (Figure 29.43).

Wound management

The burn wound should be cleaned with soap and water to reduce contamination and allow proper assessment. Any loose epithelial elements are removed and blisters de-roofed (except on palms and soles). If the patient is to be transferred to the burns service, the area should be covered with cling film and then a secondary cover of cotton wool or gamgee used to keep the patient warm in transfer. Small superficial burns can be managed with non-adherent dressings in the community. Topical creams such as silver sulphasalasine can be used in the deeper burn but only if specialist opinion has not been requested, as these substances significantly change the appearance of the burn depth and can make management decisions difficult. After the depth assessment has been made topical antimi-

crobial agents are helpful and these are used in preference to systemic antibiotics.

Paediatric burns

Paediatric burn patients differ from adults in a number of ways. In adults one-third of all burns are scalds; in children two-thirds are scalds, and in children most burns happen in the home. Burns occur in young children/toddlers and also with risk-taking behaviours in the young male teenager. Children are different, with thinner skin and different body proportions than adults. Water at 60°C causes full-thickness injury in adult skin after approximately 20 seconds, but will cause a similar injury after 5 seconds in an older child and in less than 1 second in an infant. Children have a higher surface to body weight ratio; this means that for a given body weight they have greater evaporative water loss and greater heat loss as well as a higher metabolic rate. Wallace's rule of 9s varies with age group. In an infant the head represents 18% of the total body surface as compared with 9% in the adult and each leg is 14% (18% in adults). As the child develops the body grows disproportionately with the head reducing in percentage terms by 1% each year and the legs increasing by 0.5% on each leg, until adult proportions are reached by approximately age 10 years. Lund and Browder charts are also available in different ages to ensure accurate mapping of the younger child. The different body shape also has effects on the surface-to-volume ratio which leads to increases in fluid requirement; children shiver less, which affects temperature regulation, they are prone to hyponatraemia and hypo-glycaemia, and have a very small total blood volume. Even a small scald in children can result in toxic shock syndrome, the response to a toxin produced by some *Staphylcocci* and which can produce a very rapid deterioration and cardiovascular collapse. Intensive care treatment is sometimes required. Fluid resuscitation is indicated in children with a %TBSA greater than 10% and is given as 3–4 ml per kg per % burn over 24 h with half given in the first 8 h. Maintenance fluid is also given to paediatric patients. This can be given as Hartmann's or as another crystalloid such as dextrose/saline.

Paediatric maintenance fluid for 24 h
100 mg/kg for the first 10 kg
+50 mg/kg for each kg between 10 and 20 kg
+20 mg/kg for each kg between 20 and 30 kg

The psychology of children's burns is very complex. Every injured child needs to be carefully assessed. Why did it happen? There is often real or perceived responsibility for the situation if not the actual injury. Blame may be laid, and often this has a far-reaching impact on family dynamics. There is a wide spectrum from actual deliberate non-accidental injury (NAI) to neglect and lack of comprehension of risk. Burned children should always be assessed by the paediatric team and referral to the burns network made early to ensure all the necessary child-protection issues are explored and managed appropriately. Always consider NAI until proved otherwise. Watch out for delayed presentation and conflicting histories and remember to compare the history to the child's size and developmental milestones. Classic patterns of injury such as the round lesions of cigarette burns should immediately arouse suspicion, and the child should be carefully examined for bruises, bite marks and other signs of other injury. You are required to act if you suspect NAI. Arrange to admit the child under paediatrics or burns to watch the family interaction and ensure the child is in a place of safety while the situation is investigated.

Referral

All significant-sized burns, full-thickness injury and burns of special areas such as faces and hands should be referred to the burns network. The guidelines for referral are shown below.

Guidelines for referral to burns network
Airway burns, or potential smoke inhalation
Burns over 10% TBSA in adults
Burns over 5% TBSA in children
Full-thickness burns large enough to require grafting
Burns of special areas (face, hands, feet, perineum)
Chemical burns
Electrical burns
Circumferential burns of limbs or chest
Burns at extremes of age
Patients with polytrauma or comorbidity
Any suspicion of non-accidental injury

Total burn care

Regional burn networks now provide burn care in the UK with multidisciplinary team management to defined standards of care. The most serious injuries are managed in the burn centre, with burns units and facilities providing more local care for the less complex burn patients. The burn team approach reflects the range of integrated needs that burn patients and their family have during the acute burn management, and which continues into rehabilitation and secondary surgery if this is needed. The team is led by the burns surgeon. In the UK burns surgeons are plastic surgeons and anaesthetists provide critical care, perioperative management and specialized pain management. Specialized nursing staff play a major part in the holistic management of burn patients with significant input from physiotherapy, occupational therapy and psychological therapy. Other vital members of the team include a pharmacist, microbiologist, dietician, social worker and play therapist.

Surgery in burn care

Emergency surgery

Airway management is the first priority, with surgical tracheostomy being required in some cases. This is rarely performed as an emergency as the majority of burns patients are successfully intubated as part of their pre-transfer preparation.

Circumferential deep burns to either the trunk or extremities can prevent expansion; as hyperaemia develops and resuscitation progresses there may also be significant swelling. In the trunk this can reduce ventilation and acute division of the burn eschar (escharotomy) may be needed as an emergency. The chest should be released with mid-axial incisions joined under the rib margin and across the clavicles forming a breast plate that can move freely, allowing the thorax to expand properly. Chest escharotomy may occasionally be necessary in an emergency before the patient reaches the burns centre. However, escharotomy can result in significant bleeding and does result in permanent scarring, so should be performed by burns surgeons wherever possible. In the limbs, critical ischaemia takes longer to develop but the need for escharotomy should be regularly reassessed and patients should be transferred urgently to the burn centre where this can be performed if necessary. Limb escharotomy, especially if delayed, will release a significant amount of lactic acid and other mediators into the general circulation. This can have a marked effect on blood pressure and it is important that the anaesthetist is prepared for this.

Superficial and partial-thickness burns

Superficial and partial thickness burn injury does not involve all the depth of the dermis and therefore an appropriate wound-healing environment is vital to allow rapid healing to occur from the adnexal elements as the epidermal cells divide and migrate over the wound surface. Traditional dressing routines require alternate day painful dressings and are potentially distressing for patients and staff. Modern developments in wound care and analgesics have significantly improved this and products such as Biobrane® are now routinely applied to moderate-sized superficial and superficial partial-thickness injury. Biobrane® is a nylon fabric mesh with a layer of porcine collagen on one side and a thin film of silicone on the other. The collagen adheres to the prepared wound surface by fibrin adherence and remains *in situ* until the wound heals under the dressing and it separates. The patient usually requires a general anaesthetic to apply the Biobrane®. However, once in place and adherent, subsequent dressings are considerably less painful and only minimal over-dressings are required. This product is particularly beneficial in hand burns and larger areas of superficial injury, providing good pain control and early mobilization.

Full-thickness burns

Full-thickness burns require replacement of all layers of the skin. The non-viable tissue is excised and the healthy wound bed resurfaced. Skin cover can be autologous (patient's own skin), allogenic (donated skin from the transplant programme) or xenograft (other species' skin, usually pig skin). Only the patient's own autologous tissue will potentially form a permanent multi-layer epidermis, with both allograft and xenograft separating after a few weeks.

In the majority of cases primary cover is achieved with autologous split skin graft. However, in large area burns or if the patient is too unwell, it may be necessary to simply excise the burnt skin during the first procedure and cover with a temporary skin. This is usually allograft (cadaveric skin) but biological dressing such as Biobrane® can also be used as a temporary cover.

Definitive skin cover can also be achieved using a dermal regeneration template such as Integra®; this provides a biological scaffold for the production of a neodermis as proliferating cells migrate into the collagen matrix. After the scaffold has been vascularized it can then sustain a split skin graft. The use of a dermal replacement allows the split skin graft to be very thin without the significant contraction that occurs with thin split skin graft alone. The donor sites therefore heal more quickly and it is possible to re-harvest earlier.

In major burns the most common approach is early total burn excision (in the first few days post burn), then immediate autograft of the anterior neck so that an elective tracheostomy can be performed a week later if required. Neck grafts are usually meshed at 2:1 to achieve good take rates; 2:1 gives better cosmesis than the wider mesh while still allowing the exudate and any bleeding to escape from under the graft. The next priority is to cover as wide an area as possible with the patient's own skin. To achieve this wide meshing is performed (4:1) of the remaining available autograft and this is then covered by donated allograft (meshed at 2:1) which is applied over the autograft, to protect it and optimize healing in the exposed areas between the mesh pattern. This is called sandwich grafting. When there is insufficient autograft to cover all the excised burn then the meshed allograft is applied directly to the wound and this will adhere for a few weeks before it is usually rejected. When the donor sites are healed enough to allow re-harvesting the cadaveric allograft is removed and further sandwich grafting performed. Hands and face should be resurfaced with sheet graft and this may need to be delayed until donor sites are available.

Although the acute phase of burn care may involve multiple surgical procedures, this is the beginning of the long journey of rehabilitation and secondary reconstruction that, in the major burn, may continue for much of the patient's life. As scars mature

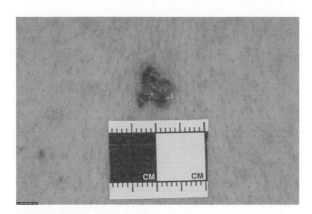

Figure 29.44 A malignant melanoma.

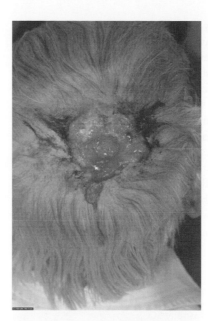

Figure 29.45 A squamous cell carcinoma.

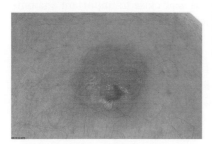

Figure 29.46 A well-differentiated squamous cell carcinoma.

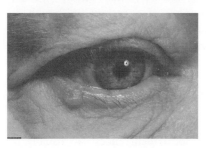

Figure 29.48 A BCC on the lower eyelid.

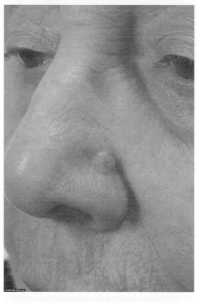

Figure 29.47 A BCC on the nose.

and patients age scar release and resurfacing may be required and the balance between function and cosmesis continues to direct the selection and timing of further surgery.

Skin cancer

Skin cancer is the most common form of cancer in the current UK population; often caused by sun damage it is most common in white-skinned races. There are three main types of skin malignancy; these are malignant melanoma (MM) (Figure 29.44), squamous cell carcinoma (SCC) (Figures 29.45 and 29.46) and basal cell carcinoma (BCC) (Figures 29.47, 29.48 and 29.14). Malignant melanoma is by far the most aggressive form of skin tumour; it commonly metastasizes and is frequently fatal. At the other end of the spectrum

is the basal cell carcinoma; this is usually less aggressive, rarely metastasizes, and is only very occasionally fatal.

Basal cell carcinoma (basal cell epithelioma, basaloma, rodent ulcer)

Epidemiology and aetiology

Basal cell carcinoma (BCC) is the commonest cancer in the West and in Australia (BCC:SCC 3:1). It occurs almost exclusively in the fair-skinned patient although it can occur in dark-skinned races in chronic wounds and albinos. Ninety-five per cent of BCCs occur over the age of 40 years, and they are twice as common in males as in females, although females are three times more likely to have BCC on the legs. The majority of BCCs occur in the head and neck region, with the nose being the commonest site in the head and neck. Risk factors for BCC development are related to either host or environment. They typically occur in association with high levels of sun exposure over a long time-frame, but can be associated with syndromes such as Gorlin's syndrome or Bazex's syndrome and are very common after immunosuppression for transplants.

BCC risk factors
UV light
Chronic wounds (usually SCC)
Chemicals (polycyclic hydrocabons – creosote, fuel oil, pitch, arsenicals and nitrogen mustard)
Immunosuppression (transplants , HIV)
Familial forms (Gorlins, Bazex)
Malignant change in sebaceous naevus of Jadassohn
Xeroderma pigmentosum

Pathology

BCCs arise from the pluripotential cells of the stratum germinatum, most often where there are many pilosebaceous follicles. They are almost all on hair-bearing skin, not palms or soles. They do not occur on mucosal surfaces. They are a slow-growing tumour because only the outer layers actively divide. Histologically BCC may be classified into nodular, ulcerating, superficial, morpheaic (or sclerosing) and pigmented. A multi-centric type of BCC is also described, although whether this is truly a different form is controversial. The lesions may also be described based on their differentiation, with undifferentiated tumours being more aggressive.

Management

The management of basal cell carcinomas is either excisional or ablative. The surgical option is usually full-thickness excision, although Mohs micrographic surgery can sometimes be used in order to ensure clear margins. Ablative options are electro-desiccation, curettage, cryosurgery, carbon dioxide laser ablation and also topical chemotherapy or radiotherapy.

The main advantage of surgical excision of BCC is that histological confirmation both of diagnosis and of completeness of excision is possible. With ablative methods neither diagnosis nor completeness of excision can be given. However, all these methods are totally acceptable and do produce good tumour clearance. Surgical excision margins are controversial. Although the majority of people would recommend a 5 mm margin for a tumour with an indistinct edge, a 3 mm margin is probably adequate for nodular tumours with a clearer edge clinically.

Mohs micrographic surgery is used when there is a concern that the edge of the tumour is very indistinct or the lesion is very close to important anatomical structures such as the eye where it is important to minimize the amount of tissue that is removed. In this situation serial sections are taken and individually analysed until the tumour is cleared. When the tumour is fully removed reconstruction can then take place. Mohs surgery can be done as a single sitting with the patients, often under local anaesthetic, returning to the operating theatre on a frequent basis during the day. Alternatively this can be done on a number of occasions. Although an accurate technique, it can be fairly stressful for the patient and is time-consuming for both surgeon and histopathologist.

If lesions are incompletely excised then there is a potential for local recurrence and often further excision is recommended if a lesion is incomplete. However, it may be more appropriate to watch and wait, as early local recurrences can usually be treated with further surgical excision, and many of these elderly patients will die from other pathology before there is any local recurrence from a low-grade tumour.

Long-term follow-up of BCC is rarely carried out as they are unlikely to have either recurrence or metastatic spread, although very aggressive tumours in difficult locations can occasionally metastasize and these clearly need to be watched carefully.

Following surgical excision the defects are commonly treated with simple skin grafts as this allows good monitoring of the tumour bed for recurrence. However, often a more cosmetically pleasing result can be obtained with a local flap, although it is important to balance the risk of a local flap covering early recurrence and making any recurrent lesions more difficult to manage.

Table 29.2 SCC risk factors

UV light
Bowens disease and actinic keratoses
Chronic wounds (Marjolins ulcer), old burns, osteomyelitis sinus, venous ulcers
Granulomatous infections
Hydradenitis superativa
Industrial carcinogens and oils
Immunosuppression (transplants , HIV)
Xeroderma pigmentosum
Leukoplakia

Squamous cell carcinoma (squamous epithelioma)

Epidemiology and aetiology

SCC is common in light-skinned races and occurs from late middle age onwards .They are more common in males than in females in a ratio of 2:1. The lesions appear most commonly on the sun-exposed surfaces: the dorsum of the hand, scalp and face, and on mucosal surfaces such as the lips. The aetiology of SCC is related to irritation; this is usually ultraviolet light but can also be mechanical, infection and due to exposure to carcinogens (Table 29.2).

Pathology

SCCs are malignant epidermal tumours whose cells show maturation towards keratin formation. Histology shows dermal invasion of atypical malpighian or spindle cells; tumours show variable degrees of cellular atypia and differentiation with the well-differentiated tumours having a much better prognosis. Clinically they often have inverted edges with keratotic appearances. Well-differentiated tumours can also develop keratin horns although the less well-differentiated lesions may be flat and ulcerated. Tumours have a high propensity for metastatic spread via lymph nodes.

Treatment

The main treatment is with primary excision. The recommended excision margin for the majority of lesions is 5 mm. The secondary spread to local lymph nodes is managed with therapeutic lymph node dissection and radiotherapy is used for regional /metastatic disease.

Prognosis

Metastatic potential is worse in larger, deeper tumours; a lesion >2 cm is twice as likely to locally recur and three times more likely to metastasize; tumours over 4 mm thick have a greater than 45% chance of metastatic spread. Poorly differentiated tumours and perineural involvement correlate with higher distant spread and host immunosuppression is also a high-risk factor.

Malignant melanoma

Malignant melanoma (MM) is a tumour derived from the melanocytes in the base layer of the epidermis and is usually a pigmented condition. After malignant transformation it becomes invasive by penetrating into and beyond the dermis. The incidence of MM in developed countries has increased by 50% in the past 20 years and is 10 times higher in white populations. There are certain risk factors for development of malignant melanoma; some people have a genetic predisposition for MM such as the association with atypical dysplastic naevi. There is also an association with sunburn and excessive sunlight, particularly in childhood. Lentigo maligna is a premalignant condition that becomes the invasive lentigo maligna melanoma in 30–50% of cases.

The most common type of MM is the superficial spreading melanoma (50–70% of all MM). Nodular melanoma makes up 10–20% of MM, with acral lentiginous melanoma (palms, soles and subungal) representing 2–8% of MMs in white races but up to 60% in dark skin types. Amelanotic melanomas are less common but can be aggressive. A small number of identified melanomas are secondary deposits and a primary tumour is not always found. That exposure to sunlight is not an absolute prerequisite for MM can be noted in the occurrence of MM of the anal canal and other parts of the gastrointestinal tract.

The depth of cutaneous MM is assessed using the Breslow thickness. This is a measurement of the thickness of the tumour from the granulating layer of the epidermis to the deepest part of the melanoma; the Breslow thickness is directly related to survival.

Diagnosis

Major signs of MM and the likelihood that a lesion is a melanoma are changes in size, shape and colour, with minor signs being a diameter greater than 5 mm, inflammation, itching, crusting or bleeding.

Management

Excision biopsy of a suspicious lesion should usually be carried out with a 2 mm margin.

Table 29.3 Staging (AJCC/UICC)

Stage	Description	T	N	M	Prognosis – 5 yr survival (approx.)
1A	<1.0 mm no ulceration	pT1a	0	0	<95%
1B	<1.0 mm with ulceration	pT1b	0	0	95%
	1.01–2.0 mm no ulceration	pT2a	0	0	90%
2A	1.01–2.0 mm with ulceration	pT2b	0	0	75%
	2.01–4.0 mm with no ulceration	pT3a			80%
2B	2.01–4.0 mm with ulceration	pT3b	0	0	65%
	>4.0 mm with no ulceration	pT4a			70%
2C	>4.0 mm with ulceration	pT4b	0	0	50%
3A	One occult metastatic node	Any pT	1a	0	65%
3B	One palpable metastatic node	Any pT	1b	0	55%
	Two to 4 occult metastatic nodes		2a		45%
3C	Two to 4 palpable metastatic nodes	Any pT	2b	0	30%
	Five or more nodes		3		25%
4	Skin, subcutaneous or distant lymph nodes	Any pT	Any	1	20%
	Lung			2	<10%
	All other sites or any site with raised LDH			3	<10%

Incisional biopsies are sometimes acceptable particularly if the diagnosis is uncertain and the lesion is large and if the area is more of a field change such as a change within an area of lentigo or a subungal melanoma. It is unwise, however, to carry out shave biopsy or curettage as the primary treatment because this means that the Breslow thickness of the tumour cannot be determined and this has implications for prognosis. Check for other lesions, lymphadenopathy and hepatomegaly. Prophylactic excision of other moles with no suspicious features is not recommended.

Once the diagnosis of melanoma has been confirmed then a wider excision should be performed and the extent of this excision will depend on the Breslow thickness. If the Breslow thickness is less than 1 mm then a 1 cm excision margin is recommended. Thicker lesions should be excised with a 2 cm margin. All tissue superficial to the deep fascia should be removed and the area reconstructed with either a skin graft or a local flap, although it is to be remembered that if local flaps are used recurrent lesions are difficult to identify in the early stages.

If a patient with a melanoma has palpable lymph nodes these should be assessed by a fine-needle aspiration and/or open biopsy, although any open biopsy should be planned carefully so as not to compromise a subsequent block dissection.

Patients who have histologically positive lymph nodes should have chest X-ray and liver function tests performed and also an ultra-sound, CT scan and MRI of their abdomen and pelvis. If these investigations show that the disease is simply in one lymph node area then a block dissection should be carried out. It is not currently recommended that prophylactic lymph node dissection should be carried out for malignant melanoma as this does not confer any survival benefit.

Sentinel node biopsy is a technique that aims to identify which lymph node is most likely to be the first draining node from the area where the tumour is situated. This is identified by a combination of coloured dye and radioactive injection around the tumour site and the identification with a gamma camera and visually to identify the central node in the lymph basin so this can be removed for histological examination. This will allow identification of lymph node spread to be carried out and may help determine which patients would benefit from a block dissection. However, it is not clear that sentinel node biopsy in malignant melanoma actually improves the prognosis for the individual patient.

If there is local or regional recurrence within a limb then it is possible to treat the limb with isolated limb perfusion, or isolated limb infusion. These techniques have a high complication rate and although effective treatment for local recurrence do not necessarily have a major impact on the overall survival.

Adjuvant therapy for malignant melanoma is indicated in certain patients; radiotherapy has been used successfully, particularly with metastatic brain disease; single-agent or combination chemotherapy has been extensively investigated but there is little evidence for survival benefit in patients with disseminated disease. There are, however, a number of trials under way for different chemotherapy regimes and also immunotherapy. Adjuvant treatment for melanoma therefore should only be carried out by a multidisciplinary team fully aware of the latest research and the majority of patients should be managed in centres where recruitment into a number of trials is available.

Follow-up and prognosis

All patients should self-examine as many recurrences are not found by doctors in clinics but by the patients repeatedly self-examining. *In situ* melanoma should only need one follow-up appointment after complete excision. Invasive MM should be followed up 3 monthly for 3 years then discharged if less than 1.0 mm Breslow thickness. Tumours over 1.0 mm thick require a further 2 years of 6 month reviews, discharging at the 5-year point. At each visit the patient should be checked for local recurrence, new lesions and clinical lymphadenopathy; no routine imaging is needed although photographs can be useful in certain cases.

Prognosis of MM is determined by the depth of invasion of the primary lesion, the presence of ulceration and the involvement of regional lymph nodes. Prognosis is better in females but worse with lesions on the trunk. Five-year survival figures for malignant melanoma relate to the clinical staging of the disease, with superficial tumours having up to a 95% survival rate at 5 years and metastatic tumours less than 10% 5-year survival (see Table 29.3).

Chapter

30

Surgical care of the paediatric patient

Paul K.H. Tam

Introduction

Paediatric surgery has developed as a specialty based on the facts that infants and children are different from adults. They differ in their anatomy, physiology and psychology. Unlike adults, children are growing organisms. Children also differ in the diseases they encounter: congenital anomalies (Figure 30.1) are common whereas malignancies are less common, and degenerative diseases are rare.

Paediatric surgery is a broad specialty that is defined by age rather than by organ systems. There are two levels of specialization: specialist paediatric surgery and general paediatric surgery.

Specialist paediatric surgery consists of:

- neonatal surgery from birth to postconceptional age of 44 weeks
- surgery of major or complex conditions in infants and older children, including neoplasms, hepatobiliary diseases, specialized gastrointestinal conditions, thoracic anomalies, major trauma, etc.
- paediatric urology.

General paediatric surgery encompasses relatively common and less demanding disorders, including elective conditions such as inguinal hernia and emergency conditions such as appendicitis in older children.

The outcome of infants and children requiring surgery has improved enormously in recent years as a result of a better understanding of the physiology of children, improvement of surgical techniques, advances in paediatric anaesthesia and intensive care and the adoption of a multidisciplinary approach. Attention to the psychological needs of children, involvement of the family in the management process and more effective postoperative

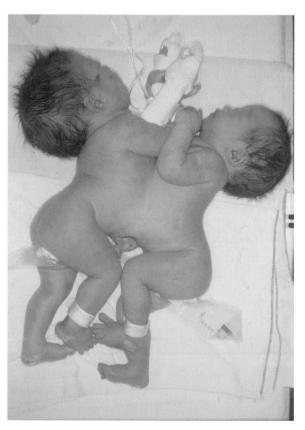

Figure 30.1 Conjoint twin: a challenging congenital anomaly.

pain relief enhance the quality of care for these children. Advances in basic science (e.g. genetics, stem cell biology and immunology), new technologies (e.g. minimal invasive surgery, robotics, extracorporeal membrane oxygenation, tissue engineering, fetal surgery) and evidence-based medicine (randomized controlled trials) will bring further improvements in future.

Fundamentals of Surgical Practice, Third Edition, ed. Andrew N. Kingsnorth and Douglas M. Bowley.
Published by Cambridge University Press. © Cambridge University Press 2011.

Table 30.1 Maintenance fluid requirements (ml/kg per day)

Day 1	40
Day 2	60
Day 3	80
Day 4	100
Day 5	120
Day 10	150
Infants	100
Pre-school	80
Adolescent	60

Table 30.2 Normal values

Age	Pulse rate (min)	Blood pressure (mmHg)	Urine output (ml/kg per day)
Infant	160	80	100
Pre-school	120	90	60
Adolescent	100	100	30

Physiology of infants and young children

Children are not 'small adults'. The differences between children and adults are greatest immediately after birth as the infant adapts to extra-uterine life: these are further accentuated in preterm babies.

Temperature

The infant is vulnerable to hypothermia because of the high surface area to body weight ratio and the small amount of subcutaneous fat. This is aggravated in the operating theatre when the viscera are exposed to a low ambient temperature. Increased heat production is needed to maintain body temperature resulting in increased oxygen consumption and metabolic acidosis. Meticulous care to preserve body heat must therefore be taken before, during and after operation to prevent the development of hypothermia.

Fluid and electrolytes

The total amount of fluid and electrolytes required by a child daily is determined by the maintenance requirements and replacement needs of abnormal losses. The maintenance fluid requirement is age- and weight-dependent (Table 30.1). It can also be conveniently summarized in the 4–2–1 rule for infants and children after the first week of life: 4 ml/kg per h for the first 10 kg of body weight, 2 ml/kg per h for the second 10 kg of body weight and 1 ml/kg per h thereafter. The maintenance requirements of sodium, potassium and chloride are 2–4 mmol/kg per day. Infants and small children become dehydrated easily because of a high surface area to body weight ratio and immature regulating mechanisms. Surgical conditions often incur abnormal losses, e.g. water loss from exposed bowel

in gastroschisis and loss of gastric contents (fluid and electrolytes) in intestinal obstruction, etc. An intravenous line and nasogastric tube are the best first steps in the management of a child with a surgical problem. Infants become hypoglycaemic easily, hence the need for dextrose in the intravenous fluid for any significant period of fasting. A useful solution is 0.18% saline in 10% dextrose (neonates) or 5% dextrose (children). Potassium is added as required.

Severe electrolyte disturbances can lead to acid-base imbalance, as can poor tissue perfusion, respiratory distress, etc. In addition to acid-base correction, the cause of the imbalance needs to be identified and treated.

Changes in circulatory volume are reflected in the vital signs and urine output (Table 30.2). Tachycardia, cool extremities, hypotension and oliguria (<1 ml/kg per h) indicate shock and demand vigorous fluid resuscitation. The blood volume of infants and young children is approximately 80 ml/kg, whereas that of older children approaches the adult value of 70 ml/kg. Because of the infants' low body weights, blood loss which would be considered inconsequential in adults represents a substantial proportion of the infant's circulating blood volume, e.g. 20 ml represents 20% of the blood volume of a preterm infant. Paediatric surgeons take meticulous care to minimize intraoperative blood loss.

Nutrition

Infants and young children have a relatively higher metabolic rate and energy requirements than adults. In addition to maintenance needs, the child requires nutrition for growth. Enteral feeding is the preferred method of providing fluid, calories (carbohydrate, protein and fat), minerals and vitamins but may not be possible in critically ill or postoperative patients having paralytic ileus. Refinements in parenteral nutrition have undoubtedly been a major factor in the improved outcome of major surgery for infants and children. As a rule, parenteral nutrition should be considered in neonates when there is a delay of >4 days before adequate enteral feeding can be established. Long-term parenteral nutrition in infants carries the same risks as in adults (metabolic complications, sepsis, venous access problems, etc.) but infants appear to be particularly prone to develop cholestasis, which can lead to liver failure.

Respiration

The respiratory rates are 40 breaths/min in infants, 30/min in pre-school children and 20/min in adolescents.

The mechanisms controlling respiration are inadequately developed in infants. Preterm infants are particularly at risk of developing apnoea and need close monitoring for at least 24 hours after even relatively minor surgical procedures such as inguinal hernia repair. The presence of hyaline membrane disease in low birth weight babies demands expert neonatal care. Abdominal distension, shock and sepsis can compromise the fragile respiratory status of a neonate, and trigger the need for mechanical ventilation.

Sepsis

Infants are predisposed to septic complications because of their immature defence system. Neonatal sepsis may not always be accompanied by fever or leukocytosis and may present with non-specific features, e.g. lethargy, intolerance of feeds. Neonatal sepsis needs to be treated empirically and rapidly once cultures have been taken and before results are available. Once septicaemia becomes established, shock, disseminated intravascular coagulation and multiple system organ failure may follow.

Endocrine and metabolic response to surgery

Surgery represents a major stress, the metabolic effects of which are more pronounced in infants than in adults. In response to surgery, there is an increase in plasma concentrations of adrenaline, noradrenaline, insulin, glucagon, glucose, lactate, pyruvate and alanine. The response is directly proportional to the severity of surgical stress. Cortisol and prolactin levels are also increased postoperatively. Cytokines, which mediate the host response to injury, are also implicated. Plasma levels of interleukin-6 and interleukin-8 are increased postoperatively and the increase is exaggerated when postoperative complications arise.

The metabolic complications induced by operative stress may be sufficient to upset the delicate metabolic balance in a sick surgical infant with limited body reserves and immature defence mechanisms. As a result, for similar surgical procedures, infants have a higher morbidity and mortality than adults. To minimize the metabolic consequences in children undergoing surgery, much emphasis is now placed on the need for correction of metabolic abnormalities preoperatively.

Transfer to specialist centres

Sick infants and young children requiring specialist surgery should be transferred to centres with adequate facilities and expertise. There are few conditions under which a sick infant will benefit from being 'rushed to theatre' in a hospital without proper paediatric anaesthetic, intensive care and surgical support.

Upon recognition of a paediatric surgical condition, the child should be resuscitated, kept in a warm, humidified environment and well hydrated. Measures to prevent respiratory complications should be undertaken including orogastric drainage to minimize the risk of aspiration. Good communication with the referring centre is essential. For very sick patients, a doctor should accompany the patient during transfer. Results of simple investigations such as complete blood picture, serum biochemistry, blood grouping and plain radiographs, when available, should be transferred with the patient.

Increasingly congenital anomalies are diagnosed by antenatal ultrasound examination. This allows parental counselling, and referral to specialist centres for delivery and planned surgical treatment. Fetal surgery is seldom indicated, and should only be performed in highly specialized centres for a few carefully selected life-threatening conditions.

Surgical techniques

Most incisions should be placed along the skin crease to improve healing. The 'squareness' of the abdomen of infants and young children means that laparotomy can usually be accomplished with a transverse incision. For thoracotomy, ribs should be spared and not removed. Haemostasis must be meticulous because children have a small blood volume, hence diathermy is used liberally. Instead of non-absorbable sutures, the fascia is repaired with slowly absorbable synthetic sutures. Skin is approximated with absorbable sub-cuticular sutures or adhesive tapes. Intestinal anas-tomosis is often accomplished with a single layer of interrupted, mucosa-inverting (or extramucosal), absorbable sutures.

Postoperative pain-relief is achieved by a com-bination of oral analgesics, local wound anaesthesia (0.25% bupivacaine), regional/spinal/epidural anaes-thesia, and patient/parent/nurse-controlled analgesia with intravenous morphine infusion (see the chapter on postoperative management).

Minimal invasive techniques are increasingly adopted in paediatric surgery. With advances in the miniaturization of instruments and improved endosurgical experiences, most procedures that pre-viously required open surgery can now be performed with a laparoscopic or thoracoscopic approach. The laparoscopic/thoracoscopic approach gives better access to deep cavities and improves visualization of internal organs as a result of magnification and better illumination. Operations that range from appendicectomy, pyloromyotomy and herniotomy to fundoplication, splenectomy, pyeloplasty and even repair of oesophageal atresia can be achieved endoscopically using ports of 2–5 mm in diameter. Short-segment Hirschsprung's disease can be treated by one-stage transanal pullthrough with or without laparoscopy assistance, without a laparotomy incision or colostomy. Robotic surgery has also been described and may be increasingly applicable for complex recon-structive procedures. The minimal invasive approach results in improved cosmesis, reduced postoperative pain, decreased adhesion formation and shorter hospital stay.

Head, face and airway

External angular dermoid

This is typically a pea-sized subcutaneous swelling above the lateral end of the eyebrow. Excision is curative.

Dermoid cyst

A dermoid cyst in the scalp is not uncommon. Com-munication with the dura has been recorded rarely and where present is usually associated with midline lesions. Treatment is with excision.

Preauricular sinus

Preauricular sinus is an ectodermal inclusion related to aberrant development of the auditory tubercles. It is prone to infection and may be bilateral. The tract with a pin-sized external opening anterior to the helix leading to the auricular cartilage has to be completely excised during the quiescent phase to prevent recurrence.

Haemangioma

Haemangioma can occur in any part of the body. There are many forms of haemangiomas but the commonest is juvenile or strawberry capillary haemangioma (with or without cavernous components). The lesion, usu-ally undetected in the first few days or weeks of life, appears as a red spot which grows in size at an alarm-ing rate in the next few months. The majority resolve spontaneously between 1 and 4 years of age. First there is the arrest of growth and subsequently the appear-ance of pale areas. Intervention is only rarely indicated in the presence of complications, e.g. platelet trap-ping (Kasabach-Merritt syndrome), congestive heart failure or interference with important functions such as acquisition of visual-cortical circuitry in the case of a haemangioma blocking the eye. Short-course high-dose steroid therapy is sometimes effective. Vin-cristine, propanolol and alpha interferon therapy are newer alternative therapeutic options. Lesions persist-ing into adolescence may require excision.

In contrast to haemangiomas, vascular malforma-tions do not involute and may require excision with or without preoperative embolization.

Ranula

A ranula is a cyst of the floor of the mouth. Small lesions are excised and large ones marsupialized.

Tongue tie

A tight frenulum which impedes speech development or causes feeding problems should be divided.

Cleft lip and palate

Cleft lip and palate affects 1 in 500 births, singly or in combination. The defect may be unilateral or bilat-eral. A complete cleft lip and palate is a severe anomaly affecting appearance, speech, feeding, breathing, hear-ing, etc. Antenatal diagnosis by ultrasound examin-ation is possible and allows parental counselling. In the

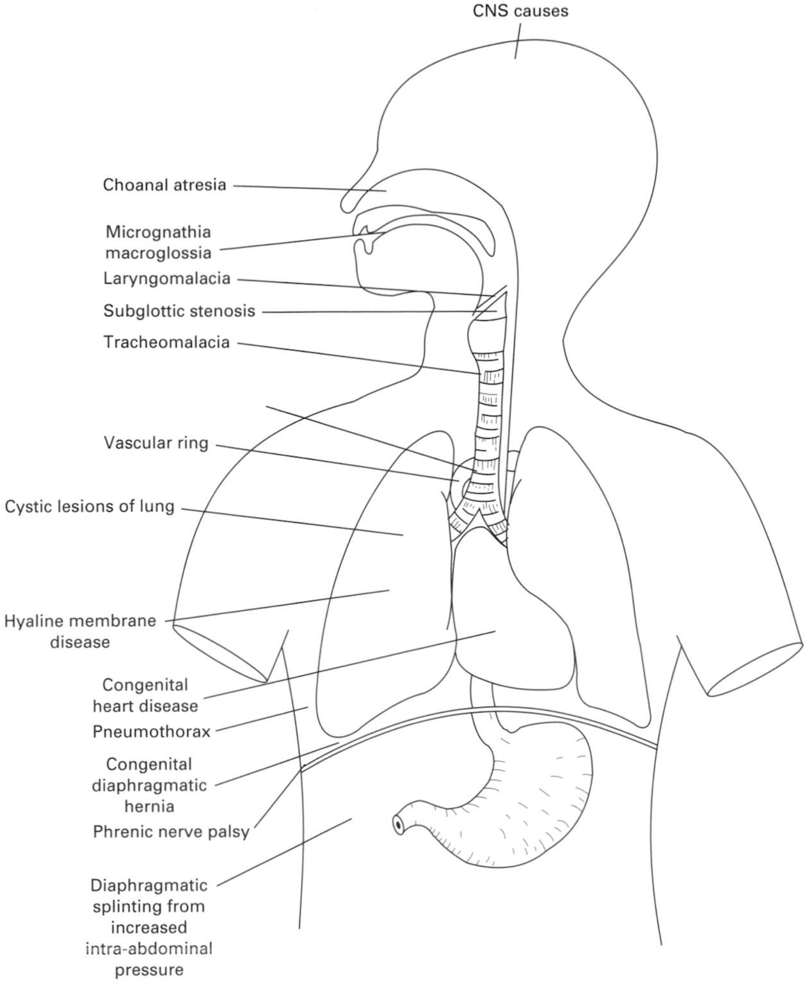

Figure 30.2 Major causes of respiratory distress in the newborn.

Labels on figure:
- CNS causes
- Choanal atresia
- Micrognathia macroglossia
- Laryngomalacia
- Subglottic stenosis
- Tracheomalacia
- Vascular ring
- Cystic lesions of lung
- Hyaline membrane disease
- Congenital heart disease
- Pneumothorax
- Congenital diaphragmatic hernia
- Phrenic nerve palsy
- Diaphragmatic splinting from increased intra-abdominal pressure

newborn period, attention is paid to airway patency (e.g. Pierre Robin syndrome – see below) and ability to feed (special feeding regimens). Management is long-term and multidisciplinary involving the surgeon, orthodontist, speech therapist and supporting staff. Cleft lip is generally repaired at the age of 3 months (10 weeks of life, 10 grams of haemoglobin and 10 pounds of weight) for optimal wound healing and safe anaesthesia. Cleft palate is repaired at 9 months of age for better speech function. Secondary revision of the lip, nose or both is often necessary in later life.

Respiratory distress of the newborn (Figure 30.2)

A baby in respiratory distress should first be resuscitated and then the underlying cause is determined.

There may be disorders of the airway, chest or other parts of the body (see below). Airway diseases often present with stridor which may be inspiratory (pharyngeal, glottic), expiratory (bronchial) or biphasic (subglottic, tracheal).

Airway disorders

Choanal atresia causes respiratory distress because neonates are obligatory nasal breathers. A nasal catheter cannot be passed into the pharynx. Treatment is by perforation of membrane or excision of bone.

Pierre-Robin syndrome is characterized by micrognathia, glossoptosis and cleft palate. Initial treatment consists of positioning of the baby to prevent the tongue from falling back; breathing improves with growth of the mandible.

Laryngomalacia is the most common cause of new-born stridor and is caused by supraglottic prolapse ('a floppy larynx') during inspiration. Treatment is supportive as most infants will improve with age.

Tracheomalacia is collapse of the trachea and may be primary or secondary (e.g. association with oesophageal atresia/tracheoesophageal fistula). Most will resolve with growth. Resistant cases may require aortopexy or stenting.

Subglottic stenosis can be congenital or acquired (post-intubation). Treatment is conservative or surgical (laser, excision).

Tracheal stenosis may require stenting or tracheoplasty.

Foreign bodies

Foreign bodies that are aspirated into the airway cause respiratory symptoms and require removal by ventilating rigid bronchoscopy under general anaesthesia.

Foreign bodies that are impacted in the oesophagus, e.g. bones, coins, need to be removed endoscopically. Blunt objects that have passed into the stomach can usually be observed. Button batteries are, however, more risky as leakage can cause perforation or poisoning.

Caustic ingestion can result in varying degrees of oesophageal and gastric injury. Management is guided by a diagnostic upper endoscopy within the first 48 hours. Mild injuries respond to symptomatic treatment. Severe corrosive oesophagitis may be complicated by oesophageal stricture, perforation or aspiration pneumonia. Oesophageal stricture is treated with dilatation; resistant and extensive strictures may eventually require oesophageal replacement.

Bezoars – collections of hair (trichbezoar) or vegetable matter (phytobezoar) – are typically found in the stomachs of children with psychiatric illnesses and require surgical removal.

Neck

Neck masses can be solid or cystic. The common causes of lateral neck masses are lymphadenopathy, branchial cyst, thyroid swelling, salivary gland swelling, laryngocoele, hamartoma (lymphangioma, haemangioma) and neoplasms (teratoma, neurogenic/mesenchymal tumours). The differential diagnoses of median neck masses include thyroglossal cyst, thyroid swelling, ectopic thyroid and submental lymph node. Lipomas, fibromas, pilomatrixoma, naevus, dermoids and sebaceous cysts can occur in any part of the body.

Thyroglossal cyst

A thyroglossal cyst is a midline neck lesion with a tract originating from the foramen caecum and therefore moves upwards on protrusion of the tongue. The cyst can be situated above, at or below the hyoid level, but the tract is invariably embedded in the inner surface of the central part of the hyoid bone. A 1 cm segment of hyoid must be excised together with the cyst and the tract followed to the foramen caecum to prevent recurrence (Sistrunk's operation).

An ectopic thyroid can mimic a thyroglossal cyst (or rarely even a tongue lesion – lingual thyroid) and may be the only functional thyroid tissue of the patient. In such a case, ultrasound or thyroid scan is advisable. Treatment may be either suppressive thyroxine therapy or autotransplantation.

Thyroid diseases

Thyroid enlargement in children is uncommon and is most often due to simple goitre. Other causes of diffuse thyroid swelling are chronic lymphocytic thyroiditis (Hashimoto's), subacute viral thyroiditis (de Quervain's), acute suppurative thyroiditis and Graves' disease (thyrotoxic). Congenital hypothyroidism may be detected in neonatal screening. Thyroid nodules may be caused by cyst, adenoma, carcinoma and ectopic thyroid.

Thyroid carcinoma is rare in children and may be associated with previous irradiation or alkylating agents. It affects girls more commonly. Most patients have papillary thyroid carcinoma. Medullary thyroid carcinoma is usually familial, may be associated with RET mutations, and can be part of multiple endocrine neoplasia (MEN) 2 syndromes. Total thyroidectomy (+/− modified neck dissection for regional metastasis) and thyroxine therapy is usually recommended.

Branchial sinus and branchial cyst

A branchial sinus is usually a remnant of the second branchial cleft with an external opening anterior to the sternomastoid muscle in the lower neck. The condition may be familial and may be complicated by infection. The tract, which courses upward along the carotid sheath between the external and internal carotid arteries towards the tonsillar fossa, needs to be completely excised, sometimes requiring two incisions. The treatment for a branchial cyst which is situated laterally at the upper neck is similar.

Cervical lymphadenopathy

Hyperplastic lympadenopathy associated with viral illnesses usually resolves on observation. Acute suppurative lympadenitis is treated with antibiotics; progression to pyogenic abscess requires aspiration or drainage. Chronic lymphadenopathy caused by atypical mycobacteria is managed by surgical excision. Lymphoma, leukaemia and metastatic neoplasms can present with enlarged cervical lymph nodes which should be biopsied for diagnosis.

Cystic hygroma

Cystic hygroma is a lymphangioma (a lymphatic hamartoma) most commonly occurring in the neck (75%), sometimes in the axilla (20%) and other parts of the body (5%). The mass is composed of multiple lymphatic channels and cystic spaces which may or may not be communicating, and is often multiloculated. Unlike haemangiomas, lymphangiomas do not resolve spontaneously. Enlargement, which may be precipitated by infection, bleeding or trauma, can result in airway obstruction or dysphagia. For uncomplicated cases, sclerotherapy with OK-432 (picibanil) may induce partial or complete response, especially in unilocular and macrocystic lesions. Surgery is indicated for complications and when sclerotherapy fails. Complete excision is difficult to achieve because of the multicystic nature and possible extension to the mediastinum, oral cavity and vital structures. Postoperative residual disease and recurrence are common.

Torticollis

Torticollis, which is the result of a shortened fibrosed sternomastoid, is often associated with a 'sternomastoid tumour' or haematoma. It results in rotation and tilting of the head. The condition is benign and the majority respond to physiotherapy. Very rarely, surgical division of the muscle contracture is required.

Chest

Chest wall deformity

The commonest chest wall deformity is pectus excavatum, or funnel chest, which is characterized by a sharp posterior curvature of the sternal body. Boys are more often affected. Symptoms are mostly cosmetic and psychological. Some have exercise intolerance or chest pain. Investigation may show cardiopulmonary dysfunctions (arrhythmia, mitral valve prolapse). For surgical treatment, the minimally invasive Nuss procedure, which involves elevation of the sternum by a bar without resection or division of costal cartilages, is becoming increasingly popular.

Breast conditions

Mastitis in the newborn period is most often caused by *Staphylococcus* and responds to antibiotics. A small breast abscess can be aspirated.

Gynaecomastia occurs in pubertal boys; most is physiological and results from hormonal imbalance. The majority will regress after reassurance. Severe cases may be treated medically (tamoxifen) or surgically (subareolar mastectomy). Rarely gynaecomastia is due to an underlying cause (Klinefelter's syndrome, hormonal/liver disorders, drug-induced).

Breast growth in adolescent girls may be asymmetric. Most breast masses in prepubertal girls are benign (fibroadenoma); phylloidal tumours and cancer are rare.

Congenital diaphragmatic hernia

This occurs in 1 in 4000 live births or 1 in 2000 births if stillbirths are included. The defect is usually left-sided (85–90%) and affects the foramen of Bochdalek, which is situated in the posterolateral aspect of the diaphragm. The parasternal (anteromedial) foramen of Morgagni is rarely affected. The size of the defect varies from a small opening with a good muscle rim to a near-complete absence of diaphragm (diaphragmatic agenesis). A left-sided hernia usually contains small bowel, stomach, spleen, colon and occasionally the left lobe of the liver. In right-sided hernias, the right lobe of the liver and intestines are the usual contents. Herniation of the intestine results in its non-rotation. Associated anomalies, especially cardiac anomalies, are present in 20–40% of cases and affect the outcome adversely. Gastro-oesophageal reflux is also common. CDH can also be associated with chromosomal abnormalities or syndrome, e.g. Fryns syndrome (CDH, facial and distal limb abnormalities).

Embryology and pathophysiology

The diaphragm is derived from: (1) the septum transversum (anterior central), (2) pleuroperitoneal membranes (posterolateral), (3) oesophageal mesentery and (4) intercostal muscles. Diaphragmatic hernia is believed to arise from a failure of closure of the pleuroperitoneal canal/delayed fusion of the muscle components.

Lung development occurs in stages: (1) embryonic (3–6 weeks of gestation): foregut diverticulum; (2) pseudoglandular (7–16 weeks): bronchial branching; (3) canalicular (16–24 weeks): acini (crude air sacs), capillaries; (4) saccular (24 weeks – term): alveoli, surfactant synthesis; (5) alveolar (term – 2 years): alveolar maturation and multiplication.

Fetal diaphragmatic herniation results in pulmonary hypoplasia and pulmonary hypertension: the earlier it occurs, the greater is the functional loss. Development of the ipsilateral lung is most affected but the contralateral lung can also be involved as a result of the mediastinal shift and compression. The abnormal pulmonary arterioles have hypertrophied muscular walls: postnatally these vessels constrict in response to hypoxaemia. As a result, the infant's respiratory status may deteriorate after an initial 'honeymoon' period due to a vicious circle of hypoxaemia and pulmonary hypertension.

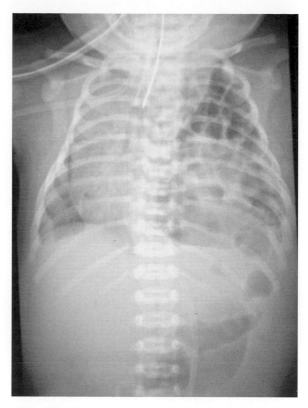

Figure 30.3 Chest X-ray in congenital diaphragmatic hernia (left-sided) showing bowel loops in left hemithorax and mediastinal shift to the right.

Diagnosis

Increasingly, the condition is discovered during antenatal ultrasound examination. Diagnosis before 24 weeks' gestation, liver herniation into the chest and a low lung-to-head ratio are associated with severe pulmonary hypoplasia and a high mortality. The typical presentation of a left-sided diaphragmatic hernia is respiratory distress (cyanosis, dyspnoea) within the first few hours of life, apparent dextrocardia and a scaphoid abdomen. In the ipsilateral chest, air entry is reduced and bowel sounds may be present. Infants who remain asymptomatic for >12 hours after birth have good pulmonary reserve and a good prognosis. Plain radiography (Figure 30.3) showing air-filled bowel loops on the chest and mediastinal shift is usually diagnostic. Differential diagnosis includes diaphragmatic eventration and cystic lesions of the lung.

Management

An orogastric tube should be inserted for gastrointestinal decompression. Face-mask resuscitation is con-traindicated as gas pushed into the gastrointestinal tract in the chest aggravates compression of the lungs. The infant may be given oxygen supplementation via nasal cannula but more often endotracheal intubation and mechanical ventilation are necessary. Care must be taken to avoid barotrauma from excessive pressures. Vital signs, oxygen saturation and arterial blood gases are closely monitored.

Operative repair is only undertaken after a period of stabilization. The systemic circulation is maintained by appropriate fluid and inotropic therapy. Adequate arterial oxygenation should be achieved with low-pressure ventilation (conventional or high-frequency oscillatory ventilation) and moderate 'permissive hypercapnia'. Pulmonary hypertension is treated with inhaled nitric oxide. Infants who are resistant to conventional therapies may benefit from support of extracorporeal membrane oxygenation (ECMO). The effectiveness of new therapies such as surfactant replacement and liquid (perfluorocarbon) ventilation has yet to be proven. Fetoscopic tracheal occlusion has been attempted to encourage the severely hypoplastic lung to grow in utero, but clinical trials have so far not shown survival benefit for fetal surgery for severe congenital diaphragmatic hernia.

Surgical repair of diaphragmatic hernia is usually carried out transabdominally via a left subcostal incision, or alternatively thoracoscopically. The visceral contents are reduced and the defect is closed primarily. For very large defects, muscle flaps or synthetic patches (e.g. Gortex) may be necessary. The chest is not routinely drained.

The overall hospital survival rate has improved to about 60–70% but there remains a substantial hidden mortality due to stillbirths and infants who die before surgery. Long-term follow-up reveals significant pulmonary and extrapulmonary morbidity such as neurodevelopmental and growth problems, gastro-oesophageal reflux and sensorineural hearing loss.

Diaphragmatic eventration

This may be congenital or acquired as a result of phrenic nerve palsy (often due to birth injury). The patient may be asymptomatic or have a varying degree of respiratory distress. Diagnosis is made by chest X-ray with fluoroscopy or ultrasonography. Symptomatic patients may benefit from placation of the diaphragm.

Cystic lesions of the lung

Cystic lesions can be congenital or acquired, the latter often occurring as a complication of staphylococcal pneumonia. Congenital causes include congenital cystic adenomatoid malformation (CCAM), bronchopulmonary sequestration (typically associated with an anomalous arterial supply often from the descending aorta), lobar emphysema and bronchogenic cyst. The congenital lesions are increasingly diagnosed on routine antenatal ultrasound screening. The condition may be asymptomatic but is more often associated with chest infection or respiratory distress. Diagnosis is made with chest X-ray and CT scan. While acquired lesions may respond to expectant treatment (antibiotics, etc.), congenital cystic lesions require excision.

Pleural conditions

Pneumothorax may be traumatic or spontaneous. Spontaneous pneumothorax most commonly occurs in teenage boys; it is prone to recurrence and may be caused by pulmonary blebs. Tension pneumothorax,

Table 30.3 Mediastinal masses

	Cystic	Solid
Anterior mediastinum	Teratoma Lymphangioma Thymic cyst	Teratoma Lymphoma Thymic hyperplasia, thymoma
	Pericardiac cyst	Thyroid goitre
Middle mediastinum	Bronchogenic cyst	Lymphoma
Posterior mediastinum	Bronchogenic cyst	Pulmonary sequestration
	Oesophageal duplication	Neural tumours

with a valve-like air leak, may be life-threatening. Initial management of pneumothorax is chest drainage. Recurrent pneumothorax is treated by thoracoscopic sealing of air leak or chemical pleurodesis (using tetracycline).

Empyema thoracis is most commonly a complication of pneumonia (pneumococcal or staphylococcal). Treatment consists of antibiotics and chest drainage with or without intrapleural fibrinolytic (streptokinase or urokinase) or thoracoscopic debridement. Resistant cases require open decortication and even partial lung resection when a bronchopleural fistula has developed.

Chylothorax may result from malformation of the thoracic duct, trauma, operative injury, infection or neoplasm. Most cases will resolve after repeated thoracocentesis, chest drainage and a period of fat-free or medium-chain triglyceride-only diet, or total parenteral nutrition.

Mediastinal masses

Mediastinal masses can be either cystic or solid (Table 30.3). A mediastinal mass is often discovered incidentally but may also be associated with:

- chest infection
- airway obstruction
- swallowing difficulties
- superior vena caval syndrome
- neurological symptoms such as spinal cord compression, Horner's syndrome, etc., depending on the location and nature of the lesion.

Surgical excision is often needed for diagnosis and treatment.

Thymic hyperplasia is the most common anterior mediastinal mass seen in infants; it can be diagnosed by the characteristic 'sail' sign on chest X-ray

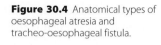
Figure 30.4 Anatomical types of oesophageal atresia and tracheo-oesophageal fistula.

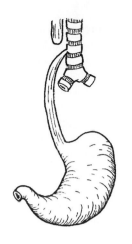
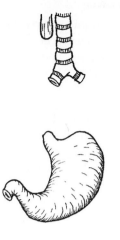
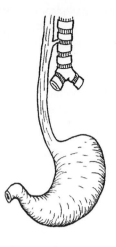

Proximal oesophageal atresia, distal tracheo-oesophageal fistula

Pure oesophageal atresia

H-type tracheo-oesophageal fistula

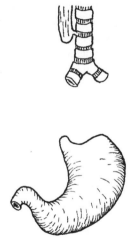
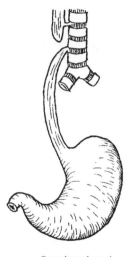

Oesophageal atresia, proximal tracheo-oesophageal fistula

Oesophageal atresia, double tracheo-oesophageal fistula

and requires no treatment. Bronchogenic cysts and gastrointestinal duplication (enterogenous) cysts often present in infancy and early childhood and require excision. Occasionally an enterogenous cyst may have an intraspinous component (neurenteric cyst) which may give rise to neurological symptoms and requires MRI evaluation and excision via laminectomy. A teratoma normally has both cystic and solid components and can be benign or malignant. A lymphangioma may be either entirely in the chest or more often an extension from a cystic hygroma in the neck. Neural tumours may be benign (neurofibroma, ganglioneuroma) or malignant (neuroblastoma).

Oesophageal atresia and/or tracheo-oesophageal fistula

This is one of the most challenging conditions in neonatal surgery. It affects 1 in 2500 live births. The anatomical variations (Figure 30.4) in order of frequency are:

- proximal oesophageal atresia with distal tracheo-oesophageal fistula (85%)
- pure oesophageal atresia without a fistula (10%)
- H-type tracheo-oesophageal fistula without atresia (4%)

- oesophageal atresia with proximal tracheo-oesphageal fistula (0.5%)
- oesophageal atresia with proximal and distal tracheo-oesophageal fistulae (0.5%).

There is a high incidence of associated anomalies (50%), the best known of which is the VACTERL association:

- *v*ertebral anomaly (e.g. hemivertebra, thirteenth rib)
- *a*norectal anomaly
- *c*ardiac anomaly
- *t*racheo-oesophageal fistula and o*e*sophageal atresia
- *r*enal and *l*imb anomalies (e.g. radial aplasia).

The CHARGE syndrome describes:

- *c*oloboma (cleft eyelid)
- *h*eart anomaly
- choanal *a*tresia
- *r*etarded growth and development
- *g*enital hypoplasia
- *e*ar anomaly with deafness.

The survival rate of this once fatal condition is now much improved but mortality remains substantial in infants with major congenital cardiac anomalies and low birth weight.

Diagnosis

There is often maternal polyhydramnios. Pure oesophageal atresia may be diagnosed antenatally – the stomach is small due to a lack of swallowed amniotic fluid. A newborn infant with oesophageal atresia has frothy salivation and develops cyanosis and choking if feeds are given. An orogastric tube cannot be passed >10 cm from the gum margin – this can be confirmed by plain radiography which shows a coiled-up tube in a blind oesophageal pouch in the neck and upper chest. Abdominal X-ray shows gas in the stomach and intestines in the common type of oesophageal atresia with distal tracheo-oesophageal atresia, but an absence of gas in pure oesophageal atresia without fistula. CT scan of the thorax can be used to assess the gap between the proximal and distal ends of the oesophagus before operation. Preoperative cardiac assessment should be undertaken.

Management

Aspiration pneumonia should be prevented by constant oropharyngeal suction – the use of a Replogle tube (sump mechanism) minimizes tissue trauma. In patients with tracheo-oesophageal fistula, the major risk is reflux of gastric acid via the fistula into the tracheo-bronchial tree. The tracheo-oesophageal fistula is divided and repaired via right thoracotomy (fourth intercostal space, extrapleural approach) or thoracoscopically. Primary anastomosis of the oesophageal segments is attempted. In the presence of a wide gap, this may be facilitated by mobilization of the upper pouch and techniques such as circular myotomy and postoperative mechanical ventilation with paralysis for several days. Pure oesophageal atresia is characterized by a long gap between the proximal and distal oesophagus. It can be managed initially with gastrostomy and oropharyngeal suction. Delayed primary anastomosis can be undertaken a few weeks later to allow time for the oesophagus to grow. Where anastomosis is not possible, a cervical oesophagostomy is performed and the oesophagus is later substituted by an intestinal segment (most often the stomach or colon).

Complications include:

- anastomotic leak
- anastomotic stricture
- recurrent tracheo-oesophageal fistula
- tracheomalacia
- gastro-oesophageal reflux
- incoordination of swallowing, etc.

The child may develop repeated chest infection and failure to thrive. Long-term follow-up is necessary to anticipate and avert these problems.

Abdomen

Gastrointestinal tract

Achalasia

Failure of lower oesophageal sphincter (LES) relaxation results in dysphagia, regurgitation and respiratory complications. Contrast oesophagram shows a smooth tapering of the gastro-oesophageal junction ('bird's beak') with a dilated proximal oesophagus. Oesophageal manometry reveals elevation of resting LES pressure; the LES fails to relax on swallowing and the oesophageal body is aperistaltic. Upper endoscopy shows an atonic, dilated oesophagus and a

LES which appears tightly closed but allows advancement of the endoscope. Pharmacotherapy (calcium channel blockers or nitrates), endoscopic botulinum injection and pneumatic dilatation have limited usefulness as long-term treatment for children. Cardiomyotomy (Heller's) combined with an antireflux procedure (open or laparoscopic) is recommended.

Gastro-oesophageal reflux

Gastro-oesophageal reflux is common in infants. In the majority, it resolves with simple measures. Persistent reflux, however, is harmful. Gastric acid (and sometimes bile) refluxes into the oesophagus when one or more of the protective mechanisms becomes defective. The protective mechanisms are:

- a high-pressure zone in the lower oesophagus
- an intra-abdominal segment of the oesophagus
- the acuteness of the gastro-oesophageal angle (angle of His)
- mucosal folds at the gastro-oesophageal junction.

The commonest complication is reflux oesophagitis, which causes upper gastrointestinal bleeding and may develop into a stricture. Barrett's oesophagus (columnar metaplasia) predisposes to malignancy. Acid reflux into the tracheobronchial tree results in respiratory complications.

Diagnosis

Non-bilious vomiting is the commonest symptom. Other oesophageal symptoms include feeding problems, pain/heartburn, bleeding and dysphagia. Respiratory symptoms include aspiration pneumonia, apnoea, bronchospasm, near-miss sudden infant death syndromes, etc. Rarely, there may be seizure-like events and dystonic posturing (Sandifer syndrome).

The gold standard for diagnosis is 24-hour oesophageal pH monitoring. Upper gastrointestinal endoscopy allows evaluation of oesophagitis and Barrett's oesophagus. Contrast studies have a low sensitivity but are occasionally performed to identify anatomical abnormalities such as hiatus hernia, oesophageal stricture, malrotation or delayed gastric emptying. The latter is often better assessed by radioisotope scintigraphy ('milk scan').

Management

Uncomplicated gastro-oesophageal reflux is usually managed by a combination of upright posturing, small frequent feeds, milk thickeners, antacids (e.g.

alginates), H_2-receptor antagonists/proton pump inhibitors and prokinetic agents (e.g. metoclopramide). Surgery is indicated for failure of medical treatment (persistence of failure to thrive) and for severe complications (near-miss sudden infant death syndrome, oesophageal stricture and unresponsive oesophagitis). Patients with underlying pathological conditions, e.g. neurological deficits, oesophageal atresia, etc. may respond poorly to medical treatment.

The commonest form of antireflux surgery is Nissen's fundoplication. The procedure is effective but may be associated with dumping, retching, gas-bloat and recurrences. Alternative procedures with partial wraps, e.g. Thal procedure, cause less gas-bloat but may be less effective. Surgery can be accomplished by a laparotomy but increasingly it is performed laparoscopically. Concomitant gastrostomy may be performed for children with neurological deficit who have feeding problems. Oesophageal strictures need to be dilated, preferably by balloon dilators. Persistent strictures may require resection.

Neonatal gastric perforation

This is a rare condition, possibly due to mechanical disruption but may also be related to stressful clinical settings resembling necrotizing enterocolitis (see below). There is an acute onset of abdominal distension which may be accompanied by respiratory distress and vomiting. Pneumoperitoneum is evident. At laparotomy, the defect, often in the greater curvature, is excised and repaired.

Gastric volvulus

This is also rare: the stomach may rotate around the axis connecting the cardia and pylorus (organo-axial), or less commonly the axis connecting the midpoints of the curvatures (mesenterico-axial). Typically there is acute epigastric distension and pain, unproductive attempts at vomiting and failure of passage of a nasogastric tube. Emergency laparotomy is necessary for derotation and fixation of the stomach.

Pyloric atresia

Atresia, web or membrane can affect the pylorus, resulting in non-bilious vomiting. Pyloric atresia may be associated with epidermolysis bullosa or may occur as part of a familial multiple intestinal atresia. A single enlarged gastric bubble without distal bowel gas is evident on plain radiograph. Gastroduodenostomy is curative.

Peptic ulcer

Children with peptic ulcer can present with pain, bleeding, perforation or obstruction. Primary peptic ulcer is usually associated with *Helicobacter pylori*, and its eradication is curative. Secondary peptic ulcer usually occurs in children with severe stress and injuries and initial treatment is acid reduction.

Hypertrophic pyloric stenosis

Infantile hypertrophic pyloric stenosis is the commonest surgical cause of non-bilious vomiting in Caucasian infants outside the newborn period. Hypertrophy of the pyloric muscle (mainly the circular muscle layer) narrows the pyloric lumen and results in gastric outlet obstruction. The pathogenesis remains unknown. Defective innervation involving fibres which contain neuropeptides and nitric oxide synthase has been reported.

Pyloric stenosis occurs in 3 in 1000 Caucasian births; it is less common in Asians and Blacks. The male:female ratio is about 4:1. Firstborns are more often affected (40–60% of all cases). With an affected father, there is a 5% risk for the son and 2.5% risk for the daughter of developing pyloric stenosis. With an affected mother, the risks rise to 20% and 7%, respectively. Overall there is an 18-fold increase in incidence in first-degree relatives compared to the general population. A sex-modified, polygenic inheritance has been suggested with susceptible loci identified in chromosomes 11, 12 (neuronal nitric oxide synthase gene), 16 and X. Association with Smith-Lemli-Opitz syndrome, chromosomal disorders, joint hypermobility, other anomalies and early exposure to macrolide (e.g. erythromycin) has been described.

Diagnosis

Typically, a previously well baby develops non-bilious, projectile vomiting at the age of 3–4 weeks. Occasionally symptoms occur as early as the newborn period and as late as several months of age. Delayed recognition, rare nowadays, can result in dehydration and starvation changes – constipation, 'starvation diarrhoea', passage of greenish 'hungry stool', failure to thrive, weight loss and lethargy. Occasionally haematemesis occurs as a result of oesophagitis/gastritis. Jaundice due to hepatic glucuronyl transferase deficiency occurs in 2% of cases and resolves after surgery. The hydration and nutritional status of the infant should be assessed on examination. There is often a 'worried' facies. Gastric peristalsis is often visible. The definitive sign of pyloric stenosis is a palpable olive-shaped mass, the so-called 'tumour', in the right upper quadrant. Detection is facilitated by a small feed with dextrose water and improves with the examiner's experience.

When a pyloric 'tumour' is felt, further studies for diagnosis are not required. For equivocal cases, provided the expertise is available, ultrasonography is the investigation of choice. The usual criteria for diagnosis are:

- a pyloric muscle thickness of 4 mm or more
- an anteroposterior diameter of 15 mm or more
- an elongated pyloric canal of 19 mm or more.

Alternatively, a contrast study may be used to confirm the diagnosis or to evaluate possible alternative causes of vomiting such as malrotation and gastro-oesophageal reflux.

Loss of gastric juice results in hypochloraemic alkalosis (serum bicarbonate 26 mmol/l, chloride <106 mmol/l). Sodium and potassium are also depleted. 'Paradoxical aciduria' occurs in severe alkalosis.

Management

The infant must be adequately rehydrated and the biochemical abnormalities are corrected before operation. Intravenous fluid and electrolytes are given (usually a combination of dextrose, saline and potassium supplements); alkalosis will be reversed with sufficient hydration and repletion of chloride and sodium deficits. Nasogastric decompression and irrigation are undertaken preoperatively.

Ramstedt's pyloromyotomy is the standard operation (Figure 30.5). In the open procedure, an umbilical fold or right upper quadrant transverse incision is made. The pyloric 'olive' is delivered out of the wound and is held between the thumb (duodenal end) and finger (antral end). An incision is made along the length of the mass anterosuperiorly and the hypertrophied muscle is split either by using a pyloric spreader or by twisting the blunt end of a scalpel holder until the submucosa bulges out. Myotomy is complete when the divided muscle blocks can be moved in opposite directions. Mucosal integrity is confirmed by air insufflation into the stomach: the commonest site of perforation is the duodenal fornix. Laparoscopic pyloromyotomy is associated with faster recovery and better cosmesis. Feeding can be started several hours after surgery and most patients can be discharged from hospital

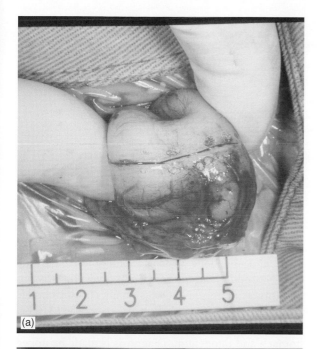

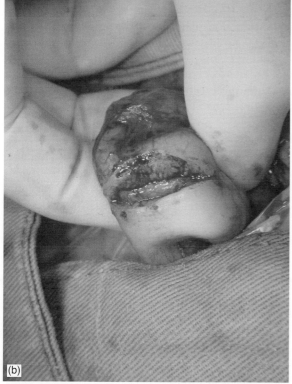

Figure 30.5 Hypertrophic pyloric stenosis (a) incision on 'olive', (b) completed pyloromyotomy.

within 2 postoperative days. Complications, including duodenal perforation, incomplete myotomy, bleeding, wound dehiscence, wound infection and incisional hernia, are mostly avoidable. Rarely, medical treatment with atropine may be used for patients unsuitable for surgery,

Duodenal atresia and annular pancreas

Duodenal atresia occurs in about 1 in 10 000 live births. Obstruction may be complete (atresia) or incomplete (stenosis, diaphragm, 'windsock' web) and most commonly occurs near the ampulla of Vater. The pathogenesis is thought to be due to a failure of recanalization following a solid core phase during early embryonic development. Associated malformations are common (50%) and include Down's syndrome (30%), cardiac anomalies (20%), malrotation (20%) and oesophageal atresia.

Annular pancreas is believed to arise from the failure of rotation of the ventral anlage to fuse with the larger dorsal anlage. There is often an associated duodenal atresia.

Congenital duodenal obstruction may be detected on antenatal sonographic screening. Vomiting is often bilious as 80% are postampullary lesions. Classically, there is a 'double-bubble' on the plain abdominal radiograph showing the distended stomach and the first part of the duodenum. Distal gas is absent in duodenal atresia but present in stenosis. Treatment is by duodeno-duodenostomy. Postoperative feeding may be delayed because of dysmotility of the dilated proximal duodenal segment and requires a period of parenteral nutrition (or transanastomotic tube feeding). Tapering of megaduodenum is sometimes practised.

Neonatal intestinal obstruction

Features of neonatal intestinal obstruction (Table 30.4) are:

- bilious vomiting, which in a newborn is abnormal and has to be considered as indicative of intestinal obstruction until it is proved otherwise
- abdominal distension (the degree of which depends on the level of obstruction)
- constipation/failure to pass meconium.

Plain abdominal radiography is a useful investigation of intestinal obstruction in neonates for whom air is an excellent contrast. It is, however, difficult to distinguish between large and small bowel in neonates on plain radiographs because of the lack of haustra in

Table 30.4 Causes of neonatal intestinal obstruction

	Intraluminal	Intramural	Extramural
Organic obstruction			
Duodenum		Duodenal atresia	Annular pancreas
			Ladd's band (Malrotation)
Small intestine	Meconium ileus	Jejunal and ileal atresia	Midgut volvulus
		Duplications	complicating malrotation
			Meconium peritonitis
			Hernia
Large intestine	Meconium plug	Colonic atresia	
		Anorectal anomaly	
Functional obstruction			
Hirschsprung's disease (intestinal aganglionosis)			
Necrotizing enterocolitis			
Medial causes: sepsis, prematurity, hypothyroidism, hypoglycaemia			

the infant colon. In addition the sigmoid colon can be very redundant in infants and young children and may not be restricted only to the left lower quadrant. All infants with intestinal obstruction will require initial resuscitation with intravenous fluid therapy and gastric decompression. These general points will not be repeated and only specific points of treatment for individual conditions are presented.

Malrotation

The incidence of symptomatic malrotation is 1 in 6000 live births; the incidence in the general population is 0.2% as the majority are asymptomatic.

During the 4th–10th weeks of normal embryological development, the midgut grows faster than the coelomic cavity and herniates into the umbilical cord, rotating 90° anticlockwise. In the next 2 weeks, the midgut returns to the abdomen undergoing a further 180° anticlockwise turn. The 270° rotation results in the retroperitoneal fixation of the duodenojejunal junction in the left upper quadrant and the ileocaecal junction in the right lower quadrant. This gives a wide root of mesentery. Malrotation results in a narrow pedicle of mesentery, predisposing to midgut volvulus. Ladd's bands, which arise from the posterior parietal peritoneum to the abnormally situated ascending colon, may compress the duodenum, leading to obstruction. Non-rotation invariably exists in exomphalos, gastroschisis and diaphragmatic hernia.

Diagnosis

The commonest symptom is bilious vomiting. When midgut volvulus supervenes, there may be rectal passage of blood, acute abdominal distension, peritonitis,

shock and metabolic acidosis. Sometimes the symptoms are milder and intermittent, suggesting twisting and untwisting episodes. Occasionally, chronic duodenal obstruction is the only feature.

Plain abdominal radiograph may show a dilated stomach and duodenum. Diagnosis is made by upper gastrointestinal contrast study showing the duodenojejunal junction to the right of the midline. The duodenum may be dilated and have a corkscrew appearance. A barium enema may demonstrate an abnormally high and mobile caecum but this test is less reliable than a barium meal. Ultrasonography reveals the superior mesenteric artery to the right of the vein.

Management

Malrotation should be treated surgically (Ladd's procedure) as early as possible after diagnosis as midgut volvulus is a life-threatening possible complication. All abnormal adhesions are divided. The duodenum is 'straightened'. The intestines are replaced with the duodenum and small intestines on the right and the caecum and colon on the left of the abdomen. If the appendix is not removed, the family should be made aware of its abnormal position to avoid diagnostic difficulties of appendicitis in future. When there is volvulus: the bowel is untwisted. Obviously infarcted bowel is resected but massive resection results in short gut syndrome.

Jejunal and ileal atresia

Jejunoileal atresia occurs in 1:1000 live births and is classified into:

- stenosis
- type I atresia (membrane/web)

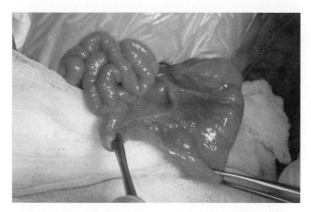

Figure 30.6 Type IIIa ileal atresia showing blind, dilated proximal segment, and a V-shaped gap in mesentery.

- type II atresia (blind ends joined by a fibrous cord)
- type IIIa atresia (disconnected blind ends) (Figure 30.6)
- type IIIb atresia (apple-peel or Christmas tree deformity in which the distal bowel coils round a solitary supplying vessel which arises from the ileocolic or right colic vessel)
- type IV atresia (multiple atresias).

Jejunoileal atresia usually results from an intrauterine mesenteric vascular accident leading to localized intestinal ischaemia, infarction and resorption. Some cases of multiple atresias are familial and probably have a non-vascular pathogenesis. Extra-abdominal associated anomalies are uncommon.

Diagnosis

Proximal small bowel atresia may be suspected from antenatal ultrasonography (dilated bowel segments). The neonate presents with bilious vomiting. There may be abdominal distension depending on the level of obstruction. Failure of passage of meconium may be a feature but this is not invariable as the causative intrauterine mesenteric ischaemia may occur after intestinal contents have passed into the distal bowel. Plain abdominal radiographs are usually diagnostic, showing dilated loops of proximal bowel with fluid levels and absent distal bowel gas.

Distal ileal atresia may be difficult to differentiate from, and in some instances may coexist with, other causes of low intestinal obstruction, e.g. meconium ileus, Hirschsprung's disease, etc. A contrast enema shows disused microcolon in ileal atresia and meco-

nium ileus, and a transitional zone in Hirschsprung's disease.

Management

Surgical treatment involves resection of atretic bowel and primary anastomosis (end-to-end or end-to-back). It is essential to check for patency of distal bowel by intraluminal saline infusion as multiple atresias may exist. The outcome of treatment of isolated intestinal atresia is highly satisfactory.

Gastrointestinal duplications

Duplications are rare congenital anomalies which may occur anywhere along the alimentary tract; 80% are located within the abdomen, most commonly at the ileocaecal region. Most duplications are cystic and are non-communicating; some are tubular and may or may not communicate with the adjacent bowel. Typically, duplications are situated on the mesenteric aspect of the bowel as opposed to the antimesenteric location of Meckel's diverticulum. All duplications have a muscle wall and are intimately attached to at least one point of the alimentary tract with which they share a common blood supply. The inside of duplications is lined with gastrointestinal epithelium, occasionally ectopic gastric mucosa. The pathogenesis is unknown. For those associated with vertebral anomalies, the most popular explanation is an abnormal splitting of the notochord.

Diagnosis

The majority of duplications present in early childhood. Presentations include:

- asymptomatic masses
- space-occupying effect
- haemorrhage
- infection
- perforation
- intussusception.

Diagnosis may be made by imaging studies, e.g. ultrasonography, CT, etc. Especially for foregut lesions, exclusion of associated vertebral anomalies is advisable.

Management

The preferred treatment is complete surgical excision. Rarely, this may not be possible because of the location, extent and size of the duplication and alternative approaches such as mucosal stripping or internal drainage into normal bowel may have to be adopted.

Meconium ileus

Meconium ileus is the commonest intraluminal cause of neonatal intestinal obstruction in Caucasians and is nearly always associated with cystic fibrosis (95–100%). Cystic fibrosis is transmitted as an autosomal recessive trait and represents the commonest inherited disease in Caucasians (carrier rate 5%, incidence 1 in 2000 births). Meconium ileus occurs in 10% of neonates with cystic fibrosis. Abnormal exocrine secretions result in thickened meconium obstructing the terminal ileum. The distal ileum is inspissated with pellets of hard meconium, proximal to which the meconium is putty-like. There is microcolon because of disuse.

Diagnosis

Half of the neonates present with uncomplicated intestinal obstruction while the remainder present with complications associated with volvulus (twisting of dilated bowel segment) and its sequelae, including perforations, meconium peritonitis and atresia. Neonates with simple meconium ileus develop bilious vomiting, abdominal distension and failure to pass meconium in the first 48 hours. The presentation, in complicated cases, is more acute and more severe. Bowel loops distended with meconium or giant cystic collections may be palpable.

Abdominal radiographs reveal dilated loops of bowel. There are no fluid levels as meconium is viscid, giving a soap bubble or 'ground glass' appearance instead in the right lower quadrant. If meconium ileus has been complicated by intrauterine perforation, calcification may be apparent.

Management

For uncomplicated meconium ileus, a contrast enema may be both diagnostic and therapeutic. Gastrografin is the most commonly used medium for non-operative treatment. Reflux of the hyperosmolar gastrografin (1800 mOsm/l) into the terminal ileum results in shifting of fluid into the intraluminal compartment, disimpacting the meconium. A wetting agent (Tween 80) may be added. To avoid drastic fluid depletion, a 1:3 dilution of gastrografin is more commonly used and attention to intravenous fluid therapy must be meticulous. A 50% success rate is recorded for uncomplicated cases.

For complicated meconium ileus, and failed non-operative treatment of simple cases, there are a number of surgical options. Non-viable bowel needs to be resected – the ends can be exteriorized or anastomosed primarily. As a variation, one end may be exteriorized, with the other end joined to its side (Bishop–Koop anastomosis), thus giving external access to irrigate and disimpact thick meconium. If the bowel is viable and distension is not severe, enterotomy, irrigation and primary closure can be performed. A variation involves a T tube may be inserted for subsequent irrigation.

The diagnosis of cystic fibrosis should be confirmed by a sweat test. Genetic screening of Δ F508, which accounts for 70% of mutations, is advisable. Comprehensive management of cystic fibrosis, including respiratory care, should be implemented.

Meconium peritonitis

Meconium peritonitis results from gut perforation in the last 6 months of the intrauterine period after meconium has formed. The peritoneal reaction gives rise to adhesions and radiologically is characterized by intra-abdominal calcifications. The gut perforation is usually secondary to an underlying pathology, e.g. intestinal atresia, meconium ileus, etc., but occasionally a primary cause cannot be found. At birth, the perforations may or may not have been sealed off. Surgical treatment consists of laparotomy, identification of possible gut perforation and treatment of underlying pathology.

Necrotizing enterocolitis

Necrotizing enterocolitis (NEC) is the most common and most lethal neonatal abdominal condition requiring emergency surgery. NEC classically affects sick, low birth weight infants. The incidence varies between 1% and 6% of admissions to a neonatal unit and increases with decreasing birth weights. NEC is characterized by pneumatosis intestinalis (intramural gas) and may progress to transmural necrosis. The terminal ileum is the most frequently affected site, followed by the colon and other segments of the small bowel. In 10–20%, there is extensive involvement of the intestine, resulting in high mortality.

Risk factors for the development of NEC include low birth weight, perinatal stress (hypoxia, polycythaemia, exchange transfusion and umbilical catheterization) and formula feeding. The pathogenesis is unclear but probably involves an immature intestinal barrier and bacterial proliferation. Perinatal stress such as hypoxia in a premature infant causes a redistribution of blood flow to vital organs (heart and brain) resulting in intestinal ischaemia. The ensuing mucosal injury allows translocation of bacteria. Intramural proliferation of bacteria is aided by nutrient from enteral feeds. Immature gut immunity and inappropriate inflammatory response aggravate the injury.

There is often clustering of cases. Some premature infants develop localized intestinal perforation (usually in the terminal ileum) with or without NEC in the remaining intestine.

Diagnosis

Early NEC presents with systemic features (lethargy, apnoea, etc.), poor feeding, vomiting, abdominal distension and blood in stool. On progression to definite NEC, these clinical features deteriorate and pneumatosis intestinalis becomes radiologically apparent. Portal vein gas is associated with a poor prognosis. Septicaemic shock, disseminated intravascular coagulopathy (thrombocytopenia, metabolic acidosis, etc.), peritonitis and pneumoperitoneum indicate advanced disease.

Management

The cornerstones of management of NEC are:

- early diagnosis
- correction of predisposing factors
- cessation of feeding
- orogastric decompression
- intravenous fluid and electrolyte therapy
- intravenous antibiotics
- close clinical, biochemical and radiological monitoring.

About 30% of cases fail to respond to such measures and require surgery. The main indications for surgery are bowel perforation and gangrene. The timing of surgery is critical. Operating too early will fail to select out potential responders to conservative treatment and will not allow sufficient demarcation of necrotic and viable bowel segments in those requiring resection. Operating too late may result in irreversible septicaemia and multiorgan failure.

At laparotomy, non-viable bowel is resected. The bowel ends are usually exteriorized but primary anastomosis can be done for good-risk patients. Patients with multiple segments of dubious intestinal viability may benefit from a second-look laparotomy 24–48 hours after conservative surgery. Very sick, premature infants with bowel perforation may benefit from initial peritoneal drainage: laparotomy is undertaken when haemodynamic and respiratory stability is restored. Pan-intestinal necrosis is associated with high mortality and morbidity; survivors often need prolonged parenteral nutrition. Intestinal strictures can complicate successful medical or surgical treatment and require contrast studies for diagnosis and bowel resection for treatment.

Intussusception

Intussusception, the invagination of a segment of bowel (intussusceptum) into the distal bowel (intussuscipiens), is a common and important cause of intestinal obstruction in infants and young children. Although intussusception can occur at any age, the peak incidence is at 5–9 months and over 80% occur before the age of 2 years. Males are more often affected (60–70%).

The majority of cases (90%) are idiopathic. The commonest (>90%) site of involvement is the ileocaecal region: ileocolic intussusception usually begins several centimetres proximal to the ileocaecal valve and advances into varying lengths of the colon, occasionally presenting at the rectum. Ileo-ileal and jejuno-jejunal intussusception may be secondary to a pathological lead point or previous surgery. In Africa, there is an increased incidence of colo-colic intussusception which tends to affect older children. The risk of intussusception lies in delayed diagnosis and treatment, which can result in bowel strangulation and perforation.

In primary idiopathic intussusception, lymphoid hyperplasia in the terminal ileum is thought to provide a lead point. A preceding viral illness, often related to adenovirus and rotavirus, is aetiologically implicated in 30–50% of cases. A weaning diet, loss of maternal immunity and differences in diameters of an infant's ileum and caecum have also been speculated to contribute to its pathogenesis.

Secondary intussusception (2–12%) should be suspected in those with atypical presentations, older children, ileo-ileal intussusception and recurrent intussusception. The common pathological lead points are Meckel's diverticulum, polyp, neoplasm, especially lymphoma, duplication, appendiceal stump, intramucosal haematoma (e.g. Henoch-Schönlein purpura) and intraluminal lesions (e.g. inspissated stool in cystic fibrosis, ascaris).

Postoperative intussusception occurs rarely; most often following certain intra-abdominal or retroperitoneal procedures. The small bowel is most commonly involved and diagnosis is seldom made before operative treatment because of atypical presentation.

Most intussusceptions are acute. Occasionally, chronic intussusception occurs in the older child and may be associated with pathological lead points.

Diagnosis

The classic presentation of intussusception is abdominal pain (85%), vomiting (85%) and rectal bleeding/passage of red currant jelly (50%): the complete triad is only found in 30% of cases. Typically, a previously healthy baby develops screaming episodes of abdominal colic, each of which lasts for a few minutes. The colic is often accompanied by circumoral pallor and drawing up of the legs. The child is initially well in between attacks but becomes restless as the frequency of attacks increases. Food is refused and this is followed by bilious vomiting. Rectal passage of blood and mucus (from venous congestion of intussusception) results in 'red currant jelly' stool. If the condition remains unrecognized, dehydration and septicaemia set in. The child becomes lethargic and paradoxically quiet. Coma and convulsions may be mistaken for meningitis.

On examination, a sausage-shaped mass is palpable in 60% of cases, most often in the right hypochondrium. There may be a sense of emptiness in the right iliac fossa (Dance's sign). Rectal examination confirms the presence of blood and rarely reveals the apex in an intussusception. Shock, abdominal distension, peritonitis and hyperpyrexia are signs of advanced disease.

For diagnosis, a high index of suspicion is necessary. A plain abdominal radiograph may reveal absence of gas in the colon and a soft tissue mass in the right iliac fossa/hypochondrium. Ultrasonography is highly sensitive and specific, showing a 'target' sign in the transverse section (Figure 30.7a) and a 'pseudokidney' sign in longitudinal section (Figure 30.7b). Rarely, a pathological lead point may be identified. Barium enema typically demonstrates a mass and the 'coiled spring' sign (Figure 30.7c).

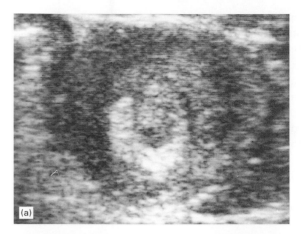

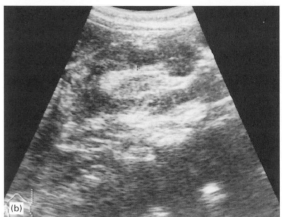

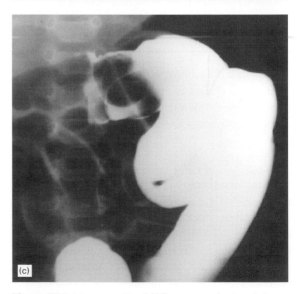

Figure 30.7 Intussusception. (a) Ultrasonography: target sign; (b) ultrasonography: pseudokidney sign; (c) barium enema: coiled spring sign.

Management

Intussusception is potentially lethal but most deaths are preventable. The key points for successful management in intussusception are:

- early diagnosis
- adequate resuscitation
- effective reduction.

Resuscitation begins with intravenous fluid therapy. Advanced cases require antibiotics and nasogastric aspiration. Reduction of intussusception may be non-operative or operative. The child should always be prepared for surgery as non-operative reduction may fail or result in perforation. Blood is cross-matched. The operating theatre is made available and the anaesthetist is informed. Non-operative reduction should generally be attempted for most cases of acute intussusception. The contraindications are perforation, peritonitis indicating bowel necrosis and profound shock. If a pathological lead point is present, non-operative reduction is usually unsuccessful. A long history (>48 hours), radiological evidence of small bowel obstruction and extremes of age are associated with lower success rates but are not absolute contraindications to non-operative reduction.

Non-operative reduction can be hydrostatic or pneumatic. The child is sedated with morphia, diazepam or, rarely, general anaesthesia. Traditionally, hydrostatic reduction is achieved with a barium enema. Barium is introduced via a rectal balloon catheter with the buttocks strapped. The hydrostatic pressure should not exceed the equivalent of 1 mH$_2$O for a maximum of 10 min. The procedure is monitored fluoroscopically. Reduction is indicated by a free flow of barium into the terminal ileum, expulsion of faeces and gas with the barium and resolution of symptoms and signs. Alternatively, hydrostatic reduction can be carried out using Hartmann's solution or saline under ultrasonographic guidance, which avoids the risk of irradiation. Successful reduction rates vary between 50% and 90%. Pneumatic reduction is performed with manometric and fluoroscopic control. If perforation complicates reduction, air or saline is less damaging to the peritoneum than contrast.

Surgery is indicated for failed or complicated reduction. Operative reduction can be done openly or laparoscopically. If viability of the reduced bowel is doubtful, warm packs are applied. Bowel resection is carried out for irreducible intussusception, gangrenous bowel and pathological lead points.

The mortality rate of intussusception should nowadays be <1%. Recurrent intussusception occurs in 5–10% of cases after non-operative reduction but less often after operative reduction. First recurrences can be treated by non-operative reduction. Second recurrences should be managed operatively. Multiple recurrences suggest the presence of pathological lead points. Adhesive intestinal obstruction is a late complication (3–6%) of operative reduction.

Acute appendicitis

Acute appendicitis affects all ages and is discussed in detail in the chapter on upper gastrointestinal surgery. The specific points relevant to the paediatric age group are presented here. Older children are more often affected; while pre-school children account for just 5% of childhood appendicitis, they often have advanced appendicitis at diagnosis. Neonatal appendicitis is rare, and underlying conditions such as Hirschsprung's disease and necrotizing enterocolitis should be excluded.

Diagnosis

The commonest triad of symptoms is vomiting, abdominal pain and fever but a normal temperature does not exclude appendicitis and may be present in 80% of affected pre-school children. The diagnosis is particularly difficult in the young child because of inability to communicate, atypical presentation and other associated illness – diarrhoea, upper respiratory tract infection, otitis media, etc. may coexist with or precede appendicitis. Physical examination reveals right lower quadrant tenderness, muscle spasm and involuntary guarding. Rovsing's sign is positive when palpation of the left lower abdomen elicits pain at McBurney's point. Pain is elicited by extension of the right thigh (psoas sign) or passive internal rotation of the flexed right thigh (obturator sign).

Investigations are needed only when the clinical picture is atypical. Leukocytosis is present in 80% of cases. Abdominal radiograph may show a faecolith, sentinel bowel loops (due to localized ileus) and lordosis away from the right side. Ultrasonography may reveal an enlarged, noncompressible appendix, and exclude tubo-ovarian pathology in adolescent girls. Computed tomography may be helpful but is not recommended as a routine in children because of irradiation.

Diffential diagnosis

Causes of acute abdominal pain in childhood are:

- surgical conditions:

    appendicitis

    intussusception

    mesenteric adenitis

    peptic ulceration/gastritis

    constipation

    Meckel's diverticulum

    malrotation/volvulus

    adhesive intestinal obstruction

    ovarian cyst

    rare miscellaneous conditions (primary peritonitis, pancreatitis, cholangitis/ choledochal cyst, inflammatory bowel disease, mesenteric/duplication cyst, etc.);

- medical conditions:

    pneumonia

    urinary tract infection

    gastroenteritis

    parasitic infestation

    rare miscellaneous conditions (Yersinia infection, Henoch-Schönlein purpura, haemolytic uraemic syndrome, blood dyscrasias, e.g. leukaemia, sickle cell crisis, diabetes mellitus, meconium ileus equivalent, etc.);

- acute non-specific abdominal pain.

Acute appendicitis and acute non-specific abdominal pain (ANSAP) each account for about one-third of hospital admissions for this complaint. ANSAP is a diagnosis made only after a period of 'active observation' including repeated reassessment, during which there will be gradual improvement in symptoms and signs.

Management

There is often a delay in seeking a surgical opinion by both parents and general practitioners. The delay in diagnosis, and possibly the thin-walled paediatric appendix, results in a greater risk of perforation (30–45%). Perforation is associated with a greater morbidity. Diagnosis is facilitated by an increased clinical awareness, and, if in doubt, repeated reassessment. Intravenous fluid and antibiotics are given preoperatively. Appendicectomy is performed

Table 30.5 Causes of gastrointestinal bleeding

Systemic disease (coagulopathy, septicaemia)
Swallowed blood
Oesophagitis
Oesophageal varices
Mallory-Weiss tear
Peptic ulcer (gastritis, duodenal ulcer)
Necrotizing enterocolitis
Midgut volvulus
Intussusception
Meckel's diverticulum
Duplication
Vascular malformation
Inflammatory bowel disease
Colitis: allergic (milk), infectious, Hirschsprung's
Polyp
Anal fissure

via a grid-iron incision or laparoscopically. Antibiotics should be continued postoperatively in perforated cases. The commonest postoperative complications are wound infection, intra-abdominal abscess and small bowel obstruction. Appendicular mass is treated non-operatively with antibiotics and interval appendicectomy 3–6 months later.

Meckel's diverticulum

The vitelline (omphalomesenteric) duct which connects the midgut to the yolk sac normally regresses at 5–7 weeks gestation. Meckel's diverticulum is the most common vitelline duct remnant. It occurs in 2% of the population, is twice as common in males as in females, is about 2 inches long and within 2 feet of the terminal ileum, contains two types of ectopic mucosa (gastric and pancreatic) and if symptomatic often becomes so by 2 years of age ('rule of 2s').

Clinical presentation is related to complications: gastrointestinal bleeding (Table 30.5), diverticulitis (abdominal pain, fever), intussusception and intestinal obstruction (volvulus, internal herniation). A technetium 99 m isotope scan is diagnostic in 80–90% of cases. Symptomatic Meckel's diverticulum should be resected with its base using an open or laparoscopic technique.

Short bowel syndrome

The extensive loss of functioning intestine results in inadequate nutrient absorption to sustain life and growth. The common surgical causes of short bowel syndrome include necrotizing enterocolitis, volvulus, intestinal atresia, gastroschisis and total intestinal aganglionosis. The normal small intestine length for a full-term infant is 200–250 cm. After massive bowel resection (more than two-thirds), the patient becomes parenteral nutrition-dependent to varying degrees. Adaptation occurs over time and is more likely to succeed in patients whose remnant intestine is longer and consists of the ileum rather than jejunum, especially if the ileocaecal valve is intact. Medical therapy consists of enteral feeding (elemental formulas) supplemented by parenteral nutrition/fluids, suppression of gastric hypersecretion with H_2 receptor antagonist or proton pump inhibitor and slowing of intestinal transit with loperamide; the use of octreotide and parenteral fish oil has also been advocated. A variety of surgical procedures to slow intestinal transit and increase intestinal length have been described; the most promising technique is serial transverse enteroplasty (STEP). Prolonged total parenteral nutrition is associated with significant morbidity due to central venous line related problems, hepatic dysfunction and sepsis. Small bowel transplantation is a clinical option but is associated with high morbidity and mortality due to severe immune rejection and its treatment.

Hirschsprung's disease

Hirschsprung's disease is characterized by an absence of intrinsic nerve cells in the rectum (congenital rectal aganglionosis), which extends proximally for varying lengths. The majority (70%) have short-segment aganglionosis (rectal/rectosigmoid); 30% have long-segment aganglionosis. Total colonic aganglionosis occurs in 10% and rarely innervation is absent from the entire small bowel.

The distal aganglionic bowel segment fails to relax, resulting in functional intestinal obstruction. The proximal normoganglionic bowel becomes secondarily dilated and hypertrophied, giving a paradoxical abnormal appearance (congenital megacolon). The intervening hypoganglionic bowel tapers into a transitional zone.

During normal embryonic development, neural crest cells migrate via the vagi into the oesophagus and colonize the entire alimentary tract in a craniocaudal direction. Hirschsprung's disease results from perturbation of migration, proliferation, differentiation or survival of the enteric neuroblasts. The pathogenesis remains elusive but several genes including RET and endothelin B receptor are implicated.

Hirschsprung's disease affects 1 in 5000 births. There is a 4–8% incidence of familial involvement, especially with long-segment cases. A male preponderance (4:1) exists in short-segment cases. There is a known association with chromosome anomalies such as Down's syndrome, deletions of chromosome 10 and 13 and malformation syndromes such as Waardenburg syndrome (pigmentary disorder), Ondine's curse (central hypoventilation), etc.

The most dreaded complication of Hirschsprung's disease is enterocolitis, which occurs in 20–58% of cases and can be rapidly fatal. Another serious complication is bowel perforation, which may be a result of enterocolitis or obstruction. Early diagnosis and treatment of Hirschsprung's disease is therefore important.

Diagnosis

Functional intestinal obstruction in Hirschsprung's disease can be acute, recurrent or chronic. The majority can be diagnosed in the neonatal period. Typically, the infant presents with bilious vomiting, delayed passage of meconium (>24 hours) and abdominal distension. Examination reveals a tight anus and an empty rectum. In Hirschsprung's disease, withdrawal of the finger or instrument (e.g. thermometer) from the rectum is often accompanied by an explosive passage of flatus or meconium. Older children present with chronic constipation dating back to early infancy, abdominal distension and malnutrition. Acquired megacolon or idiopathic chronic constipation is distinguished by the finding of a dilated rectum which is impacted with faeces down to the anal verge.

Diagnosis of Hirschsprung's disease is established by the histological finding of aganglionosis in a rectal biopsy specimen. Suction rectal biopsy is often adequate in infants; open biopsy is only occasionally necessary. Acetylcholinesterase staining is helpful in demonstrating abnormal proliferation of nerve fibres in lamina propria and hypertrophy of nerve trunks which accompany the aganglionosis. Ancillary investigations include contrast enema (demonstration of a transitional zone) and anorectal manometry (failure of anal sphincter relaxation in response to rectal distension).

Management

Functional obstruction can usually be relieved by daily bowel washout. Definitive surgery consists of resection of aganglionic bowel and pullthrough of histologically proven normoganglionic bowel. Most infants with short-segment aganglionosis can be treated by primary transanal endorectal pullthrough at 1 month of age. Patients with intractable obstruction, fulminant enterocolitis and total colonic aganglionosis

Table 30.6 International Classification (Krickenbeck) of anorectal anomalies

Major clinical groups	Rare/regional variants
Perineal (cutaneous) fistula	Pouch clon

Rectourethral fistula
    Prostatic
    Bulbar
	Rectal atresia/stenosis
	Rectovaginal fistula
	H fistula

Rectovesical fistula	Others
Vestibular fistula Cloaca No Fistula Anal stenosis	

require initial bowel diversion and staged definitive surgery 3–6 months later. There are different approaches of pullthrough – rectorectal (Duhamel), endorectal (Soave) and abdominoperineal (Swenson, State-Rehbein). Frozen section examination of biopsy samples obtained intraoperatively is essential to ensure that normoganglionic colon is used for anastomosis.

Hirschsprung-like disease

Some patients have bowel dysmotility despite the presence of ganglion cells on rectal biopsy. The best-described condition is intestinal neuronal dysplasia, which is characterized by hyperplasia of the submucous and myenteric plexuses and giant ganglia. The treatment is in the first instance conservative. Other conditions include hypoganglionosis, immature ganglia, internal anal sphincter achalasia, smooth muscle disorders and the generally fatal megacystis-microcolon-intestinal hypoperistalsis syndrome.

Meconium plug syndrome

Occasionally, a meconium plug in the rectum may cause intraluminal intestinal obstruction. This readily resolves after an enema with the passage of a tenacious strip of meconium. Hirschsprung's disease and cystic fibrosis have to be excluded before such a diagnosis is established.

Anorectal anomaly

Anorectal anomaly, or imperforate anus, occurs in 1 in 4000 births. Boys are slightly more affected than girls. There is a wide spectrum of anomalies and these are classified according to the relationship of the terminal bowel to the puborectalis muscle and presence/absence of a fistula to the urinary tract/vagina (Table 30.6). Low imperforate anus (perineal fistula, or where bowel terminates within 1 cm of skin level

with no fistula) is suitable for perineal procedures without colostomy. Intermediate, high and complex anomalies require colostomy and total surgical reconstruction.

Boys tend to have more high than low lesions, the commonest defect being rectourethral fistula. In girls, the commonest anomaly is vestibular fistula, which may be anal or rectal, requiring different treatments.

Associated anomalies are common, especially with high lesions. VACTERL association is discussed above. The commonest associated anomaly is urological: 60% in high and 20% in low lesions. Sacral agenesis involving two or more vertebrae is associated with poor bowel control; some may also develop neurogenic bladder.

Diagnosis

Careful inspection of the perineum should be an integral part of neonatal examination. Occasionally the diagnosis of anorectal anomaly may be delayed because of adequate bowel decompression through a perineal/vestibular fistulous opening and failure to recognize the correct position of the anus. Rarely, in rectal atresia, there is a normal anal opening and the diagnosis is suspected on failure of attempts to pass a rectal thermometer. An abnormal skin tag (the so-called 'bucket handle' deformity) or a 'covered' anus with bulging meconium suggests a low lesion. In boys, meconium-stained urine denotes high anomaly.

An invertogram (a plain radiograph with the baby held upside down) or a lateral radiograph with the baby prone and buttocks elevated is done after the first 24 hours of life (to allow adequate passage of bowel gas). A rectal gas shadow above the coccyx suggests a high lesion. Ultrasonography, fistulogram, CT and MRI may also be used to define the level of anomaly; MRI additionally assesses pelvic musculature.

Management

For low imperforate anus, anoplasty is satisfactory. For all other lesions, a colostomy is recommended. Definitive surgery is undertaken at 1 month of age. The commonly performed procedure is posterior sagittal anorectoplasty (PSARP): the fistula to the urethra/vestibule/vagina is repaired and the rectum is brought to the perineum through the sphincter complex. The sphincter complex is then reconstructed. Laparoscopic anorectoplasty is preferred in some centres. Patients with persistent faecal incontinence or intractable constipation after surgery require intensive bowel management, sometimes with the aid of an ante-grade continence enema (ACE) procedure using the appendix as a conduit.

Inflammatory bowel disease

In children, Crohn's disease (CD) is more common than ulcerative colitis (UC); some are indeterminate colitis. CD can occur at any age, though most often after 10 years; 5% present before 10 years. Clinical features include abdominal pain, weight loss, growth failure, fever, diarrhoea, rectal bleeding and anaemia; perianal disease (fissures, fistula, abscess, skin tags) and extraintestinal manifestations (arthritis, conjunctivitis, erythema nodosum) are especially common in children with CD. Investigations are similar to those in adults. The mainstay of treatment is elemental nutrition, 5-aminosalicylate and corticosteroid. Additional therapies include immunosuppressant (azathiaprine), TNF-α antibody (infliximab – especially for fistulas), antibiotic for sepsis; surgery is rarely indicated, e.g. for complications, and should always aim at bowel preservation.

UC is more aggressive in children than in adults. The risk of colon cancer is estimated as 1–3% 10 years after onset of UC, increasing 1% after every year. Medical treatment (see CD) aims to alleviate symptoms, restore growth and avoid disease complications. Emergency operations for toxic megacolon, colitis and bleeding are rare; restorative proctocolectomy is the preferred form of definitive surgery.

Acquired anorectal disorders

Anal fissure is the most common cause of minor rectal bleeding in infants and toddlers, and is associated with constipation and painful defaecation. The tear in the anal mucosa is typically located in the posterior mid-line. Chronic fissure is sometimes associated with a sentinel skin tag at 12 o'clock position. Treatment consists of stool softener, sitz bath and local anaesthetic gel application. Occasionally a chronic fissure requires topical nitroglycerin, botox injection or lateral sphincterotomy. Rarely, Crohn's disease and immuno-deficiency can present with laterally located anal fissures.

Rectal polyp causes painless rectal bleeding in school-aged children. The juvenile polyp is a hamartoma and sometimes autoamputates. A rectal polyp which persists can be removed endoscopically with a diathermy snare. More than one polyp may be found in up to 25 % of patients upon colonoscopic examination.

The condition is benign and should be distinguished from diffuse adenomatous polyposis in Peutz-Jeghers syndrome and familial polyposis coli.

Perianal abscess occurs commonly in infants and is treated by antibiotics (small) or incision and drainage (large). Approximately one-third of abscesses develop into a fistula-in-ano. Fistulas in infants may be treated conservatively; those which persist after 1 year are treated by fistulectomy. Crohn's disease should be considered in older children with multiple fistulas.

Rectal prolapse usually occurs in the toilet-training age group and is often associated with constipation. The prolapse usually involves the mucosa only and responds to conservative treatment. Persistent prolapse may require hypertonic saline injection or Thiersch procedure using a strong nylon suture. The possibility of cystic fibrosis should be considered.

Liver, pancreas and spleen

Biliary atresia

Biliary atresia is an important surgical cause of conjugated hyperbilirubinaemia. It is characterized by an obliteration of the extrahepatic bile ducts which represents the end-result of an inflammatory destructive process. Unrelieved, progressive intrahepatic damage will occur, leading to the histological findings of cholestasis, portal tract proliferation and inflammation with giant cell infiltration. Cirrhosis and liver failure are the eventual outcome.

Biliary atresia affects 1 in 10 000 births. Associated anomalies occur in 5% (biliary atresia splenic malformation syndrome), most commonly polysplenia, situs inversus, preduodenal vein, absent inferior vena cava, malrotation and congenital heart disease. Biliary atresia is classified into:

- type 1: atresia of common bile duct (5%)
- type 2: atresia of common hepatic duct (2%)
- type 3: atresia of most or the entire extrahepatic ducts including porta hepatis (>90%).

Type 1 biliary atresia has been termed correctable type and a biliary-enteric anastomosis for drainage is possible. The basis of surgical treatment (Kasai's operation) is that in the early course of the disease, the fibrous remnant at the porta hepatitis contains patent bile ductules and adequate bile drainage may be obtained by portoenterostomy. Success depends on early diagnosis and timely operation (before 60–75 days).

Table 30.7 Causes of neonatal jaundice

Unconjugated hyperbilirubinaemia
  Physiological jaundice of newborn
  Rh, ABO incompatibility
  Breast feeding
  Haemolytic disease

Conjugated hyperbilirubinaemia
  Anatomical:
    Extrahepatic: biliary atresia, choledochal cyst, spontaneous
      bile duct perforation, inspissated bile syndrome
    Intrahepatic: bile duct hypoplasia (Alagille's syndrome)
  Infectious: neonatal hepatitis; idiopathic giant-cell hepatitis;
    B, A or non-A, non-B hepatitis
  Systemic: septicaemia, cytomegalovirus, rubella,
    toxoplasmosis, syphilis
  Metabolic: α_1-antitrypsin deficiency, galactosaemia, cystic
    fibrosis
  Endocrine: hypothyroidism, hypopituitarism
  Iatrogenic: parenteral nutrition-induced cholestasis

Diagnosis

The infant presents with deepening jaundice, darkening urine and clay-coloured stool. Serial liver function tests reveal persistent or increasing levels of conjugated bilirubin as well as enzyme derangement. Other causes of jaundice (Table 30.7) are excluded.

Ultrasonography may show an absent or contracted gallbladder. A radioisotope (HIDA) scan typically shows absence of excretion into the gastrointestinal tract. Liver biopsy may help differentiate conditions such as Alagille's syndrome, neonatal hepatitis. The gold standard for diagnosis, however, is examination at laparotomy/laparoscopy (the gallbladder is either atretic or if patent only contains mucus and no bile) and operative cholangiogram.

Management

Kasai's operation is the first-choice treatment for most patients. The fibrous remnant is excised up to the level of the porta hepatis (proximal to the posterior surface of the bifurcation of portal vein) and portoenterostomy is performed with a Roux-en-Y jejunal loop. Results are best with timely surgery and in patients with large bile ductules in the fibrous remnant. Postoperative steroid and intravenous antibiotic therapies are believed to improve the operative outcome.

Clearance of jaundice can be accomplished in 50–70% of treated infants. There are ongoing risks of cholangitis, portal hypertension and liver failure – it is estimated that 50–60% of patients will require liver transplantation in the long term. Patients who present late (>100 days) and with signs of cirrhosis may be treated primarily by liver transplantation.

Choledochal cyst

Choledochal cyst is congenital cystic dilatation of the biliary tree, affecting 1 in 100 000 births in the West (but estimated to be at least 10 times more frequent in Japan and China). The aetiology is believed to relate to reflux of pancreatic enzymes associated with either anomalous junction of the pancreatic and common bile ducts (long common channel) or distal common bile duct stenosis. It is classified into:

- type I: cystic or fusiform dilatation of common bile duct (commonest type)
- type II: diverticulum of bile duct
- type III: choledochocoele
- type IV: intrahepatic and extrahepatic cysts
- type V: intrahepatic cysts only (Caroli's disease).

Diagnosis

Most cases present in childhood but diagnosis may also be made antenatally and in adulthood. Jaundice, pain and mass are the commonest clinical features but presentation with the complete triad is infrequent. Occasionally, patients may present with vomiting, failure to thrive and complications including cyst perforation, cholangitis, gallstones, pancreatitis, portal hypertension, cirrhosis and malignancy.

In addition to abnormal liver function tests, the plasma amylase level may be elevated. Ultrasonography is frequently diagnostic. CT, MRI and endoscopic retrograde cholangiopancreatography (ERCP) may be used selectively for better anatomical delineation.

Management

Treatment consists of excision of the cyst and hepaticoenterostomy with a Roux-en-Y loop. Simple drainage procedures are unsatisfactory because of long-term risk of malignancy and anastomotic stricture.

Pancreas

Acute pancreatitis is a rare but known cause of abdominal pain in childhood. The causes are: idiopathic, hereditary (e.g. associated with SPINK1 gene), viral, traumatic, developmental (pancreatic divisum, pancreatic biliary malunion including choledochal cyst), gallstones, drug-induced, and metabolic (e.g. cystic fibrosis). Diagnosis and management are similar to those in adults.

Persistent hyperinsulinaemic hypoglycaemia of infancy (PHHI) is a rare disorder caused by hyperactive islet cells which may be diffuse or focal (nesidioblastosis). Upon biochemical diagnosis, intravenous glucose is given. Insulin secretion is controlled medically with diazoxide and somatostatin analogue. Positive emission tomography is useful for localization of lesions: focal lesions are resected (partial pancreatectomy) whereas diffuse disease is treated with 95% pancreatectomy.

Spleen

Most splenic traumas are managed non-operatively. The main indication for splenectomy in children is haematological (e.g. congenital spherocytosis). Post-splenectomy sepsis is a known risk; triple vaccination (pneumococcus, meningococcus and H influenzae) and antibiotic prophylaxis (oral penicillin) are advised.

Abdominal masses

Abdominal masses may be a presenting or associated clinical feature of a variety of conditions, most of which are discussed in other sections:

- gastrointestinal system: faecal impaction, duplication cyst, appendix mass, intussusception, hypertrophic pyloric stenosis, Crohn's disease, etc.
- urinary system: distended bladder, hydronephrosis (pelviureteric junction obstruction, advanced vesicoureteric reflux, posterior urethral valve, etc.), polycystic/multicystic kidney, Wilms' tumour
- genital system: ovarian mass (cyst), uterus (haematocolpos)
- liver, spleen, pancreas: hepatosplenomegaly (blood dyscrasia, neoplasm), choledochal cyst, pancreatic pseudocyst
- other solid tumours: neuroblastoma, rhabdomyosarcoma, teratoma, lymphoma, etc.
- other cysts: mesenteric cyst, omental cyst.

It is important to determine the age, sex, presence of associated symptoms, duration of symptoms, rate of growth, size, location, solid or cystic nature and other signs so that appropriate investigations are carried out for diagnosis.

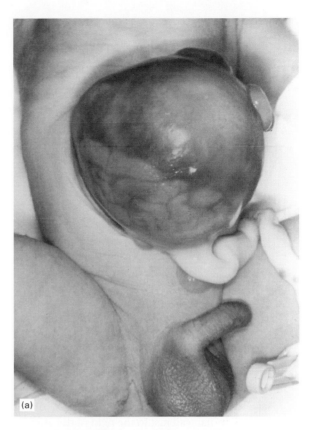

(a)

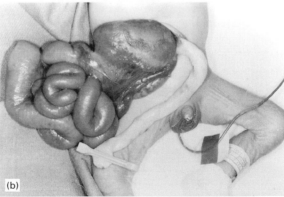

(b)

Figure 30.8 (a) Gastroschisis , (b) exomphalos.

Abdominal wall

Gastroschisis and exomphalos (omphalocoele)

Gastroschisis (Figure 30.8a) and exomphalos (or omphalocoele) (Figure 30.8b) are two distinct types of major congenital abdominal wall defects (Table 30.8), each accounting for about 1 in 5000 births. In recent years the incidence of gastroschisis appears to be increasing.

589

Table 30.8 Abdominal wall defects

	Exomphalos (omphalocoele)	Gastroschisis
Location	Umbilical ring	Right side of umbilical cord
Defect size	Large	Small
Sac	Present	Absent
Contents	Liver, bowel, etc.	Bowel
Bowel appearance	Normal	Matted; inflamed thickened wall
Non-rotation	Present	Present
Atresia	No additional risk	Additional risk
Function	Normal	Prolonged ileus
Abdominal cavity	Small	Small
Associated anomalies	Common (30–70%)	Uncommon (except bowel atresia 10–15%)
Syndromes	Common: Beckwith-Wiedemann, Trisomy 13–16, 16–18, 21, lower midline syndrome, pentalogy of Cantrell	None

Gastroschisis is a small full-thickness defect of the anterior abdominal wall just to the right of the umbilicus. The aetiology is unknown but is believed to be either an in utero rupture of a small exomphalos or a localized infarction related to abnormal involution of the right umbilical vein. Unlike exomphalos, there is no peritoneal sac in gastroschisis and the eviscerated bowel is exposed to the damaging effects of amniotic fluid in the intrauterine period. The bowel becomes matted and foreshortened and its walls are inflamed, thickened and covered with fibrin. Prolonged ileus can be expected. There is invariable non-rotation and frequently bowel atresia (10–15%) as a result of intrauterine mesenteric occlusion at the tight hernia ring. Other viscera are seldom involved and extra-abdominal associated anomalies are rare.

Exomphalos is a central defect involving the umbilical ring and its neighbouring abdominal wall. It is likely to be a persistence of the anatomical arrangement in the early embryological period (weeks 3–12) during which the rapidly elongating midgut resides in the extracoelomic yolk sac. The size of the defect varies. Small defects (2–4 cm) sometimes called hernia of the umbilical cord can be considered as a separate entity from exomphalos as they have fewer associated anomalies and an excellent prognosis. Large

exomphalos has a poorer prognosis. The umbilical cord inserts onto a peritoneal sac which often contains nearly the entire gastrointestinal tract as well as the liver, spleen, etc. The sac is intact in 90% of cases and therefore, unlike in gastroschisis, the bowel is relatively unaffected. Associated anomalies are common (30–70%), involving the cardiovascular (most frequent), gastrointestinal, genitourinary, musculoskeletal, central nervous and respiratory systems. There is association with a number of chromosomal abnormalities (trisomy 13–15, trisomy 16–18, trisomy 21) and syndromes (Beckwith-Wiedemann syndrome characterized by exomphalos, gigantism, macroglossia, visceromegaly and hypoglycaemia due to islet cell hyperplasia). Extension of the defect in the upper midline is classically known as pentalogy of Cantrell (abdominal wall, sternal, anterior diaphragmatic, pericardial and cardiac effects). In the lower midline, exomphalos may coexist with bladder or cloacal extrophy.

Diagnosis

Increasingly, gastroschisis and exomphalos are recognized antenatally by ultrasonography. An elevated maternal serum alpha-fetoprotein is also seen in gastroschisis and ruptured exomphalos. Amniocentesis for chromosomal analysis may be considered for large exomphalos.

Management

The child should be delivered in a centre with paediatric surgical expertise; vaginal delivery is adequate. The infant is often preterm. The defect and its eviscerated contents are covered with sterile plastic sheet/bag or moist packs to prevent heat and water loss. An orogastric tube is inserted to prevent aspiration and distension of the gastrointestinal tract due to air swallowing. Intravenous fluid and antibiotics are given.

Surgery is carried out as soon as possible, preferably with primary fascial repair. This is facilitated by good paralysis, decompression of the gastrointestinal tract and, if necessary, manual stretching of the abdominal wall at operation to enlarge the small abdominal cavity. Excessively tight closure, however, may result in diaphragmatic splinting and caval compression, compromising respiration and circulation, respectively. If fascial closure is not possible, either a prosthetic sheet is used, or the fascial defect is left with skin cover to form a ventral hernia for repair at an older age.

Defects which cannot be repaired primarily are managed by staged repair. A strong prosthetic (e.g. silastic) sheet is sutured to the edge of the abdominal wall defect in the form of a chimney or 'silo' to provide temporary cover for the viscera. Alternatively, pre-made silastic silo with a wire-ring covered base can be used without anaesthesia. The top of the silo is hung from the ceiling of the incubator to encourage gradual return of viscera into the abdominal cavity. Over a period of 5–10 days, the size of the silo is gradually reduced by rolling in or suturing the top of the silo. At the second-stage operation, the silo is removed and closure of fascia and skin is achieved.

A period of postoperative ventilation and paralysis is often necessary. For gastroschisis, there is often a delay in return of normal gastrointestinal function, requiring total parenteral nutrition for support.

For massive exomphalos with an intact sac or infants with life-threatening medical conditions, non-operative management may be adopted. Epithelialization is encouraged by daily topical application of escharizing agents such as silver sulfadiazine.

Umbilical and midline abdominal hernias

Umbilical hernia is common in the newborn period and results from a delay in the closure of the umbilical ring. The intestinal contents are easily reducible and complications are extremely rare. The majority will resolve spontaneously. Surgery (repair of fascial defect with a periumbilical incision) is indicated only in the minority of cases which persist after the age of 4 years. Hernias with a diameter greater than 2 cm are less likely to close spontaneously. Umbilical hernia related to increased intra-abdominal pressure, e.g. ascites, is a separate clinical entity and management is directed at the underlying cause.

Hernias in the midline of the abdominal wall excluding the umbilicus represent abnormal defects in the fascia and are most commonly located near the umbilicus: paraumbilical hernia, supraumbilical hernia. They may also be located anywhere along the midline between the xiphisternum and the umbilicus: epigastric hernia. Usually, an extraperitoneal pad of fat (or occasionally the omentum) protrudes through a small defect, presenting as a pea-sized swelling which is best felt by rolling the fingers along the midline of the abdominal wall. There may be a history of abdominal pain. Surgical repair is indicated. The site of hernia must be marked preoperatively as the hernia may be

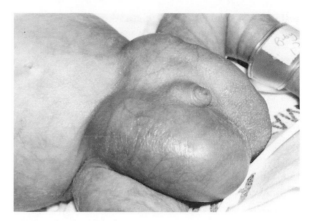

Figure 30.9 Bilateral inguinal hernia in a preterm infant.

difficult to locate when the child is anaesthetized and in a reclined position.

Divarication of recti occurs commonly in infants and requires no treatment.

Umbilical granuloma

Umbilical granuloma often results from low-grade infection of the stump of the umbilical cord after delivery and usually clears up on regular dressing. Healing may be expedited by topical application of silver nitrate. Rarely, a persistent granuloma may need local excision.

Occasionally umbilical discharge becomes persistent. The presence of mucosa in the umbilicus and gastrointestinal or urinary contents in the discharge may point to an underlying pathology: a patent vitellointestinal duct or urachal remnant, for which exploration and excision are indicated.

Groin and scrotum

Inguinal hernia and hydrocoele

Inguinal hernia

Inguinal hernia (Figure 30.9) and hydrocoele are common groin and scrotal conditions in infants and children. They differ from the same conditions in adults in both their aetiology and treatment.

Childhood inguinal hernia and hydrocoele are congenital anomalies resulting from a persistence of processus vaginalis. As the testis descends from its retroperitoneal position to beyond the internal ring, it carries with it an anteromedial diverticulum of peritoneum (the processus vaginalis). The process of obliteration of the processus vaginalis begins at 32 weeks gestation and may continue for the first 2 years of life. A widely patent processus vaginalis which allows the passage of visceral contents results in an indirect inguinal hernia. A narrowly patent processus vaginalis which allows the passage of peritoneal fluid results in a communicating hydrocoele. An inguinal hernia does not regress whereas most infantile hydrocoeles will resolve spontaneously upon completion of obliteration of the processus vaginalis. Occasionally, the fluid collection may persist after closure of the processus vaginalis, resulting in a hydrocoele of cord (hydrocoele of canal of Nuck in females) or a non-communicating hydrocoele.

The incidence of inguinal hernia in term neonates has been estimated to be 1–5%. Preterm infants have an even higher incidence (10%). Boys are more commonly affected – the male:female ratio is 8:1. Right-sided hernias are commoner than left-sided hernias. Bilateral occurrence is common: 10% in children and 40% in infants with hernia.

Conditions associated with a higher incidence of inguinal hernia include cryptorchidism, raised intra-abdominal pressure, connective tissue disorder (Marfan syndrome, Ehlers-Danlos syndrome) and testicular feminization.

Diagnosis

The commonest presentation is a swelling in the groin, with or without extension into the scrotum (labia majora in females). The swelling appears on straining and is reducible. When the swelling is not obvious on examination, a thickening of the cord or the 'silk-glove' sign may be found instead. The usual contents of a hernia are intestine (giving rise to a gurgling sensation on reduction), or ovaries and fallopian tubes in females.

There is a high risk of incarceration (10% in children, 30% in infants): the hernia becomes irreducible and tender. Unrelieved, intestinal obstruction, strangulation and gonadal ischaemia (compression of testicular vessels in the inguinal canal in males, incarceration of ovaries in females) may result. Urgent reduction is necessary for an incarcerated hernia to avoid complications. Upon sedation, the hernia either spontaneously reduces or is manually reduced. To avoid recurrent incarceration, elective surgery is undertaken 24 hours after reduction when the oedema of the hernia sac has settled. A hernia which is persistently irreducible or shows signs of strangulation requires emergency exploration after resuscitation.

Management

Inguinal hernia repair (herniotomy) is one of the most frequently performed operations in childhood. To avoid incarceration, early elective surgery should be arranged once the diagnosis of inguinal hernia is made.

Unlike the case in adults, there is no need to repair the posterior wall of the inguinal hernia. For open herniotomy, a groin crease incision is made. In infants, the inguinal canal is short and need not be opened; in older children, the external oblique aponeurosis is incised. After careful dissection to avoid damage of the vas and testicular vessels, the sac is removed at its neck and transfixed. At the end of the procedure, the testes must be retracted back into the scrotum to avoid the complication of iatrogenic high testes. Laparoscopic hernia repair is equally safe and effective, may be associated with less postoperative pain, better cosmesis and is advantageous for bilateral hernia.

A preterm infant presents a higher risk of anaesthesia and postoperative apnoea. Herniotomy is done when the infant is medically fit for discharge from the special care baby unit. Monitoring for apnoeic attacks is undertaken for 24 hours postoperatively.

Complications of herniotomy include recurrence, scrotal haematoma, testicular atrophy, high testes and wound infection; complication rates are higher for preterm infants and emergency surgery.

There is controversy as to whether contralateral groin exploration should be undertaken for unilateral hernia because of the possibility of unrecognized/metachronous bilateral hernia. The conventional approach is not to explore because not all patent processus vaginalis (30% contralateral patency) will become symptomatic inguinal hernias (10% contralateral hernia). Laparoscopic hernia repair obviates this uncertainty as the contralateral inguinal ring can be examined and, if desired, repaired at the same operation.

Hydrocoeles

Although a hydrocoele may fluctuate in size due to gravitation of peritoneal fluid during the day, the swelling does not disappear completely like a reducible hernia. Rarely an acute tense hydrocoele may present – however, unlike an incarcerated hernia, a hydrocoele is not tender. A hydrocoele transilluminates brilliantly (Figure 30.10). However, a hernia in an infant may also transilluminate because of the thin bowel wall.

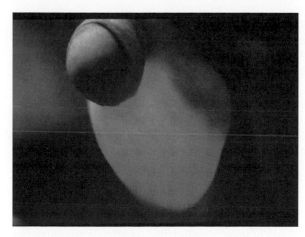

Figure 30.10 Transillumination sign in hydrocoele.

Most infantile hydrocoeles will resolve and can be safely observed until the age of 1 year. High ligation of processus vaginalis, similar to herniotomy, is performed for persistent hydrocoele.

Direct inguinal hernia and femoral hernia are rare in childhood and the diagnosis is often missed pre- and intraoperatively.

Inguino-scrotal emergencies

Causes of an acute scrotum in childhood are:

* testicular torsion
* torsion of testicular appendage
* epididymo-orchitis
* idiopathic scrotal oedema
* incarcerated inguinal hernia
* acute tense hydrocoele
* Henoch-Schönlein purpura
* acute leukaemia
* testicular tumour
* testicular trauma.

Testicular torsion

Testicular torsion is one of the commonest and most important causes of acute scrotum and there are two types:

* extravaginal (neonatal) (Figure 30.11a)
* intravaginal (adolescent) (Figure 30.11b).

Extravaginal testicular torsion occurs in the perinatal period and is characterized by a twist of the whole spermatic cord above the testis and tunica vaginalis. Intravaginal testicular torsion occurs from infancy to young adulthood, peaking in adolescence, and is characterized by a twist of the testis inside the tunica. Normally, the tunica envelopes only the anterior two-thirds of the testis, leaving the posterior surface of the testis fixed to the posterior scrotal wall. Abnormal complete enclosure of the testis by the tunica results in the testis being freely suspended within the space

Figure 30.11 Testicular torsion: (a) extravaginal (neonatal); (b) intravaginal (adolescent).

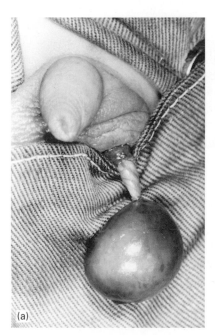

(a)

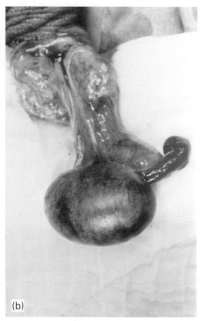

(b)

('bell-clapper' deformity). Contraction of the cremaster muscle may initiate intravaginal torsion of the spermatic cord. Alternatively, intravaginal torsion of the mesorchium of the testis may occur. The testis is often in a transverse lie.

Diagnosis

Neonatal testicular torsion may be relatively painless and presents as a firm discoloured scrotal swelling which does not transilluminate. Intravaginal testicular torsion causes acute scrotal pain which may be associated with lower abdominal pain, nausea and vomiting. The left testis is twice as commonly involved as the right. There may be a history of similar, milder complaint, suggesting previous twisting and untwisting of the testis. The testis is tender, swollen and often elevated. The contralateral testis may have a transverse lie.

Testicular torsion is an emergency as delay in diagnosis and treatment will result in testicular infarction: necrosis occurs within 6 hours of the onset of symptoms and few testes will survive >24 hours of torsion. The commonest differential diagnoses are torsion of testicular appendages and epididymo-orchitis (see above). Doppler ultrasound and radioisotope scan demonstrating reduced testicular blood flow in testicular torsion have been advocated for use in doubtful cases but these should only be attempted if the expertise is available and the tests can be performed without delay. Prompt scrotal exploration is the safest approach for any child with the slightest doubt in testicular torsion.

Management

The treatment of testicular torsion is to untwist the testis. Bilateral fixation of the testes with non-absorbable sutures is performed since the contralateral testis may have the same anatomic abnormality which predisposes to torsion. Viability of the testis may be assessed by the colour and bleeding on incision of the tunica albuginea. The testis in neonatal torsion is seldom viable. Retention of a non-viable testis may result in persistent symptoms and possible abscess formation and subsequently subfertility through an autoimmune reaction. After removal of a necrotic testis, prosthetic insertion may be considered for psychological reasons.

Torsion of testicular appendages

Torsion of the appendix testis or appendix epididymis (remnants of Mullerian and mesonephric ducts, or hydatids of Morgagni) gives rise to acute scrotal pain which is usually less severe compared to testicular torsion. The peak incidence is at the age of 10 years. In the early stage, there may be a 'blue-dot' sign – discolouration at the upper pole of the testis where a tender pea-sized swelling can be felt separate from a normal testis. Later on, oedema spreads to obscure these localized findings. Treatment may be conservative (analgesics) if the diagnosis is certain but more often exploration and excision of the testicular appendage is performed, leading to speedy recovery.

Epididymo-orchitis

Most commonly epididymo-orchitis occurs in young adults and is related to sexually transmitted infection. In pre-school children, epididymo-orchitis (infective or chemical) is often related to urinary tract pathology. Viral orchitis, e.g. mumps and epididymo-orchitis secondary to blood-borne infection, are rare.

The presentation is gradual scrotal pain. The scrotal swelling and tenderness may be bilateral and mainly involves the epididymis. The testis is usually normal. Urine microscopy may be helpful. As emphasized, exploration is required for doubtful cases to exclude testicular torsion. Antibiotic treatment is usually effective. Ultrasonography of the urinary tract and micturating cystourethrogram should be performed in children with epididymo-orchitis unrelated to sexually transmitted infection to exclude urinary tract abnormalities.

Acute idiopathic scrotal oedema

Acute idiopathic scrotal oedema can present with sudden painless oedema of the scrotal skin (unilateral or bilateral) with or without extension to the neighbouring skin, e.g. perineum, lower abdomen. The child is otherwise healthy and asymptomatic. An allergic or infective cause has been postulated but not proven. There is no tenderness and the testis is normal on palpation. Treatment is reassurance as the oedema resolves spontaneously within 2–3 days.

Undescended testes (cryptorchidism)

The testes is not found in the scrotum in 4–5% of boys at birth; and 1–2% at 3 months of age. Intra-abdominal descent of the testis from the posterior abdominal wall occurs in the first 28 weeks of gestation. Further descent along the inguinal canal into

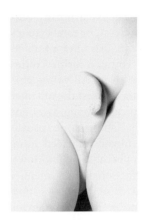

Figure 30.12 Empty scrotum.

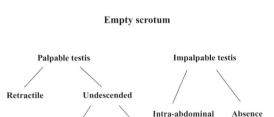

the scrotum occurs in the last 12 weeks of gestation and may continue for another 3 months postnatally. Cryptorchidism may result from an arrest of descent along the normal pathway or rarely an aberrant descent into an ectopic position, e.g. perineal or femoral. The commonest location of an undescended testis is the superficial inguinal pouch (just above and lateral to the external inguinal ring), which is not considered as ectopic. Other positions of arrested descent are 'canalicular' or, less commonly, intra-abdominal.

Diagnosis

Undescended testes must be differentiated from retractile testes (Figure 30.12). Retractile testes result from an overactive cremasteric reflex and can be coaxed into the scrotum. Most retractile testes will descend spontaneously with age and do not require treatment. A small number of patients have testes in the scrotum at birth but the testes ascend at an older age, possibly as a result of failure of the spermatic cord to elongate normally postnatally (the ascending testes or acquired undescended testes).

Twenty per cent of undescended testes are impalpable, which can be due to absence of testes, intra-abdominal testes or canalicular testes. Testicular absence usually results from intrauterine torsion (vanishing testes) rather than agenesis. Unilateral congenital testicular absence or mono-orchidism is commoner (1 in 25 cases of undescended testes) than bilateral absence or anorchidism (1 in 20 000). For bilateral impalpable testes, XY karyotyping and a human chorionic gonadotrophin (HCG) stimulation test to demonstrate the presence of testosterone-secreting tissue should be performed. To locate impalpable testes, ultrasound and MRI (better accuracy, especially with contrast enhancement to show testicular veins) are non-invasive tests; the gold standard, however, is laparoscopy.

Management

Orchidopexy is indicated mainly because of:

1. Subfertility: impaired germ-cell development (reduction of spermatogonia, abnormalities of seminiferous tubules) is evident by the age of 1 year because of damage caused by the higher temperature in the undescended position (35–37°C) compared to the scrotal position (33°C). Hormonal function is not affected.
2. Risk of malignancy: approximately 10% of testicular tumours arise in undescended testes. Undescended testes have 10–40 times higher risk of malignancy than normal; the risk is increased further by six-fold in intra-abdominal testes. Scrotal placement of an undescended testis allows early detection of malignant changes in later life. There is no proof, but some suggestion, that early orchidopexy may lower the risk of malignancy.
3. Psycho-cosmetic reasons: an empty scrotum may be detrimental to the psycho-social development of a child or young adult.

Additional reasons for surgery are the need to treat concomitant hernia and increased risks of torsion and trauma.

Orchidopexy is now recommended between 6 months and 1 year of age if the expertise is available. For the inexperienced surgeon, the advantage of early orchidopexy has to be balanced against the risk of testicular vessel damage in a young infant. Orchidopexy is carried out via a groin incision. The gubernaculum is divided. The patent processus vaginalis, which is often present, is isolated, divided and ligated. The testicular pedicle is mobilized sufficiently to allow tension-free transfer of the testis to the scrotum. The testis is fixed in the dartos pouch.

For high undescended testes, pre- or perioperative localization (e.g. laparoscopy) is indicated as some procedures for high undescended testes depend on an intact collateral blood supply to the testes, which may be disturbed by unplanned exploration. The following surgical options are available:

- Staged orchidopexy: at the initial operation, the testis is fixed to the pubis, and, together with the cord, is encased in a silastic sheet. A second operation is undertaken 8–16 months later.
- Testicular vessel division (Fowler-Stephen's procedure): a high undescended testis is often associated with a long-loop vas which provides collateral circulation to the testis, allowing the testicular vessel to be divided high above the testis in one- or two-stage orchidopexy. This is the most popular procedure and can be done laparoscopically.
- Microvascular orchidopexy: with the available expertise, transfer of testes to the scrotum can be achieved by anastomosis of the testicular and inferior epigastric vessels.
- Orchidectomy +/− prosthesis for post-pubertal man with a unilateral intra-abdominal testis and a normal contralateral testis.

Varicocoele

Varicocele represents a dilatation of the testicular veins in the pampiniform plexus and occurs predominantly in the left hemiscrotum, probably related to the drainage of the left spermatic vein into the left renal vein at a 90° angle. It usually presents in an adolescent as a 'bag of worms', which decreases as he lies supine. There is a risk of subfertility. Surgical treatment consists of high ligation/clipping of the spermatic vein via a groin incision or preferably laparoscopically. For a young child with a varicocoele, the possibility of an underlying neoplasm such as Wilms' tumour should be considered.

Paediatric urology

Urinary tract infection in infants and children is most often caused by urinary stasis, which can result

from vesicoureteric reflux, obstructive uropathy, neuropathy/dysfunction of urinary tract, or rarely stones; ascending infection can occur in girls after a bubble-bath because of the short urethra. A urine culture is obtained and antibiotics are given. All young children should be investigated after the first documented episode of urinary sepsis with ultrasonography and micturating cystourethrogram. Radioisotope (usually technetium 99) imaging has mostly replaced intravenous urography in children because of the lower ionization risk and better functional assessment: a DMSA (dimercaptosuccinic acid) scan assesses functional renal parenchyma, and a MAG3 (mercaptoacetyl triglycerine) or DTPA (diethylenetriamine-pentaacetic acid) scan assesses drainage.

Hydronephrosis can be caused by severe reflux nephropathy or urinary obstruction due to pelviureteric junction (PUJ) obstruction, primary obstructive megaureter, ureterocoele or posterior urethral valve.

Multicystic dysplastic kidney

This condition is distinguished from polycystic kidney disease, which is a rare genetic disorder. Multicystic dysplasia is usually unilateral and may be detected by ultrasonography both ante- and postnatally. The cysts are unconnected and there is no functioning renal parenchyma. Many multicystic dysplastic kidneys will atrophy with age and may not require treatment. Nephrectomy is carried out for persistent and symptomatic (urinary infection) lesions. The risk of late malignancy is considered very unlikely.

Pelviureteric junction obstruction

Pelviureteric junction (PUJ) obstruction is a common congenital anomaly which results in hydronephrosis without hydroureter. There is typically a narrow segment at the pelviureteric junction with disorganized musculature and fibrosis and often an aberrant artery crossing it anteriorly. Rarely, it can be caused by a kink, band, valve or polyp. It is commoner in boys and on the left side; 5% are bilateral.

Diagnosis

The condition is increasingly detected antenatally by ultrasonography (1:100 pregnancies, although only 1 in 1000 have persistent uropathy). An abdominal mass in infants is often renal in origin (50%), and 40% can be attributed to hydronephrosis secondary to PUJ obstruction. Loin pain (known as Dietl's crisis when intermittent and associated with vomiting, followed by diuresis and resolution of symptoms) and urinary infection are common symptoms. Occasionally haematuria, hypertension or stone occurs. In addition to anatomic diagnosis by ultrasonography, renal function and degree of obstruction should be assessed by a dynamic radioisotope renal scan (MAG3 or DTPA).

Management

Antenatal pelvic dilatation ≤12 mm (anteroposterior diameter) is considered mild; and ≥20 mm severe. An infant with mild asymptomatic PUJ obstruction can be observed; an infant with significant antenatal hydronephrosis is given antibiotic prophylaxis until a micturating cystourethrogram is performed as 30% have vesicoureteric reflux.

Surgery is indicated when the hydronephrosis is symptomatic, complicated or shows deteriorating renal function on periodic isotope renography (≤35% differential renal function). The standard procedure is dismembered pyeloplasty (Anderson-Hynes), which can be performed by the open or laparoscopic approach. For bilateral PUJ obstruction, the side that is symptomatic or has a better function is corrected first. For kidneys with <10% of overall renal function, nephrectomy is performed instead.

Duplex system and ureterocoele

Duplications of the upper urinary tract occur in 0.8% of the population. Females are more often affected (60–70%); 40% are bilateral.

The ureteric bud arises from the mesonephric duct at the fifth week of gestation and grows towards the developing kidney (metanephros) to form the collecting tubules, renal pelvis and ureter. Abnormal division of the ureteric bud results in varying degrees of duplications. Incomplete duplications, e.g. bifid ureters, are more frequent than complete duplications and are often asymptomatic. The upper pole ureter has a more medial and caudal orifice (ectopic) than that of the lower ureter (Weigert-Meyer law). The upper pole ureter is associated with ectopic insertion and ureterocoele whereas the lower pole ureter is associated with vesicoureteric reflux and PUJ obstruction.

The commonest entity requiring treatment consists of a poorly functioning upper kidney moiety drained by an ectopic ureter. The ureter may open into a ureterocoele in the bladder, or rarely outside the bladder (urethra, vagina, vestibule), in which case the child typically wets in between normal voids. Urinary infection is more commonly the presenting symptom. Investigations include ultrasonography +/− MR urography, micturating cystourethrography, radioisotope scan (DMSA, MAG3) and cystoscopy.

Upper pole nephroureterectomy is performed for a non-functioning moiety. Symptomatic refluxing or obstructing ureteric duplications draining functioning renal units are treated as in nonduplicated systems; common sheath reimplantation avoids ischaemic injury as the duplicated ureters share a common blood supply.

Ureterocoele is cystic dilatation of the lower end of the ureter and can be intravesical or extravesical. Most often it is associated with an ectopic ureter from the upper moiety of a duplex system; rarely, it is orthotopic from a single ureter. It commonly obstructs the upper pole ureter, but a prolapsing ureterocoele can cause obstruction to the urethra. The common presentations are antenatal detection and urinary tract infection. A small ectopic ureterocoele may collapse after upper pole nephroureterectomy, but a large obstructing ureterocoele requires decompression by endoscopic incision. Occasionally, cyst excision, ureteric reimplantation and bladder base reconstruction are needed.

Vesicoureteric reflux

Vesicoureteric reflux (VUR) is found in 1% of children, and is a common cause of urinary infection (20–50%). There is a female preponderance (85%) and a familial tendency (30% incidence in siblings of affected patients, suggesting an autosomal dominant inheritance with variable penetrance). The oblique course of an intravesical, submucosal ureteral segment normally functions as a valve, failure of which (e.g. a short ureteral tunnel) results in reflux. Vesicoureteric reflux is only harmful when complicated by infection. Repeated urinary infection is associated with renal scarring, loss of renal function and eventually hypertension and renal failure.

Diagnosis

Vesicoureteric reflux is diagnosed by micturating cystourethrography and the severity is graded as:

- grade I: partial filling of an undilated ureter
- grade II: total filling of an undilated upper tract
- grade III: dilated calyces

- grade IV: blunted fornices
- grade V: massive hydronephrosis and tortuous ureter.

A radioisotope (DMSA) renogram delineates the degree of renal scarring and loss of function.

Management

Treatment of vesicoureteric reflux may be medical or surgical. For mild grades of reflux, prophylactic antibiotics are often adequate in preventing urinary infection and allow spontaneous resolution of reflux, which usually completes by the age of 4 years (grade I, 90%; grade II, 75%; grade III, 50%; grade IV, 25%; grade V, 0–5%). Surgery is considered for children with severe reflux or failure of medical treatment, e.g. breakthrough urinary infections, progressive renal scarring, drug intolerance or non-compliance, and associated anomalies. Endoscopic treatment is the preferred surgical option for moderate VUR. The biodegradable paste Deflux is injected subureterally, resulting in a submucosal 'volcanic' bulge and a slit-like ureteric orifice. The outpatient/day procedure has an 80–90% success rate. Ureteric reimplantation is reserved for extreme/unresponsive VUR or those requiring surgery for concomitant anomalies; the most popular method is submucosal, transtrigonal (Cohen) and this can be performed by the open or pneumovesical technique.

Vesicoureteric junction obstruction

Occasionally, the lower end of the ureter is stenosed, resulting in urinary infection and megaureter. This should be excised and the ureter (which may need tapering) reimplanted.

Posterior urethral valve

Posterior urethral valve (PUV) is the most common life-threatening urological anomaly in male infants. The common form of posterior urethral valve originates from the inferior margin of the verumontanum that extends anteriorly and distally as two leaflets; rarely, it presents as a perforated diaphragm. There are varying degrees of bladder outlet obstruction. Vesicoureteric reflux is present in 50% of PUV patients; 15% of PUV patients have unilateral VUR associated with renal dysplasia – VURD (valve, unilateral reflux, dysplasia) syndrome – which acts as a 'pop-off', avoiding pressure and damage to the contralateral kidney. Rupture of calyx may lead to urinary ascites or urin-

oma and similarly acts as a pop-off. Fetal urine is a main component of amniotic fluid which is required for lung development; severe oligohydramnios can lead to pulmonary hypoplasia.

Antenatal ultrasound may reveal hydronephrosis (bilateral, or unilateral – VURD), megaureter, distended thick-walled bladder, dilated posterior urethra, oligohydramnios and renal dysplasia. The neonate may present with urosepsis (fever, failure to thrive, vomiting, dehydration), urinary retention (suprapubic mass), abdominal distension (urinary ascites), renal failure (metabolic acidosis, hyperkalaemia) and rarely respiratory distress. The sick infant should be stabilized initially with appropriate fluid and electrolyte management, antibiotics and bladder catheterization with a fine feeding tube. Older children can present with voiding dysfunction such as wetting, poor stream, acute urinary retention, etc.

Postnatal imaging begins with ultrasonography. A micturating cystourethrogram typically shows a dilated posterior urethra with abrupt distal narrowing. Ablation of the valve can usually be achieved endoscopically. Long-term sequelae include vesicoureteric reflux, 'valve bladder' (progressive upper tract dilation despite adequate PUV ablation, an insensitive and non-compliant bladder), bladder dysfunction and incontinence, and renal failure.

Wetting

Most children achieve day and night urinary continence by 5 years of age. Urinary incontinence may be continuous, intermittent (daytime and/or nocturnal), urge or stress. The causes are anatomic, neurogenic, functional, enuresis and others (urinary infection, polyuria).

Anatomic incontinence may result from ectopic ureter, bladder obstruction (posterior urethral valve, urethral stricture, meatal stenosis), or bladder extrophy.

Neurogenic incontinence arises from disturbed innervation of the bladder: neural tube defect, spinal trauma and tumours. The patient has failure of voluntary bladder control and incomplete bladder emptying. There may be bowel incontinence and other neurological sequelae. Complications include urinary infection, stones and renal failure. Evaluation is achieved by urodynamic studies. Clean intermittent catheterization is the mainstay treatment; this may be achieved per urethra or via a conduit (appendix implanted into the bladder – the Metrofanoff procedure). Bladder augmentation, urinary diversion and artificial urinary sphincters may be selectively applicable.

Functional incontinence may manifest as urge syndrome (frequent voiding and a small bladder) or fractional voiding (infrequent, incomplete voiding and a large bladder). A child with functional incontinence or enuresis frequently has constipation; successful treatment of constipation often leads to resolution of urinary symptoms. Specific treatment of urinary incontinence may be guided by urodynamic diagnosis:

1. Detrusor overactivity: desmopressin (antidiuretic hormone analogue) + oxybutinin (antimuscarinic) + urotherapy.
2. Bladder neck dysfunction: desmopressin + alpha blocker (relaxation of bladder neck) +/− oxybutinin (detrusor overactivity present).
3. Dysfunctional voiding: desmopressin + urotherapy +/− oxybutinin (detrusor overactivity present).

Enuresis is identified with nocturnal incontinence: the child is capable of voluntary bladder emptying but is unaware when wetting occurs at night. Primary nocturnal enuresis (PNE), defined as wetting ≥ 2 times per week for ≥ 3 months in a child ≥ 5 years, affects 15–20% of 5-year-old children. The natural course is spontaneous resolution, at a rate of 15% of patients per year. Even though enuresis causes no physical harm, adverse psychological consequences may be sustained. The pathophysiology of PNE is unclear but may be related to nocturnal polyuria, impaired sleep arousal response and bladder dysfunction. The diagnosis of PNE is achieved by exclusion, starting with a good history including psychological evaluation, and proper physical examination. The child has never been dry in primary enuresis, whereas in secondary enuresis the child has been dry for ≥ 6 months. Primary enuresis is essentially monosymptomatic; workup for other causes of wetting is necessary when enuresis is polysymptomatic. The parents are reassured by counselling on the epidemiology and natural history of enuresis. Behavioural therapy (reduced fluid intake before bedtime, retraining to achieve a good urinary habit, prevention of constipation) is enhanced with a star chart and alarms, leading to 60–80% success. Medical treatment may be necessary in resistant/recurrent cases. Desmopressin is effective in 60–70% of cases but relapse is common on cessation of treatment.

Imipramine (a tricyclic antidepressant) has anticholinergic and central effects, and gives 10–50% response.

Hypospadias

Hypospadias is characterized by a proximal location of the urethral meatus ventrally. There is a spectrum of severity: glandular, coronal, subcoronal, midshaft, penoscrotal and perineal. Except for very mild hypospadias, there is often an associated chordee, a ventral curvature of the penis, which is exacerbated on erection. The foreskin has an abnormal appearance of a dorsal hood. Some degree of torsion of the axis of the penis often exists.

Hypospadias affects 1 in 300 boys. There is a familial tendency: 8% of fathers and 14% of brothers of patients are affected. Associated anomalies include undescended testes (9%), hernia-hydrocoele (9%) and upper urinary tract anomalies (2–3%).

Management

It is important to recognize the condition as circumcision is absolutely contraindicated: the dorsal hood of foreskin is a valuable piece of tissue for reconstruction. Uncorrected, the penile curvature and abnormal urination and semen delivery could lead to major psychological and sexual sequelae and infertility. The goal of surgery is to straighten the penis, provide a urethra which opens at its tip and achieve a normal appearance. A variety of techniques have been employed. Most are repaired at around the age of 1 year. A single-stage operation is performed except for very severe hypospadias. If chordee is present, this is excised completely. For proper placement of the new urethral opening, a short distance may be covered by meatal advancement and glanuloplasty. In moderate and severe hypospadias, a neourethra has to be fashioned, usually from penile skin, which commonly is meatal-based or pedicled from the dorsal hood, or by tubularizing the urethral plate. Complications include meatal stenosis, urethrocutaneous fistula, stricture, diverticulum, etc. Bladder or buccal mucosa grafts may be needed for secondary procedures.

Phimosis

True phimosis affects only 1% of boys and is usually the result of a chronic inflammatory process, balanitis xerotica obliterans (BXO) (Figure 30.13). BXO is probably a form of lichen sclerosis, which leads to a scarred

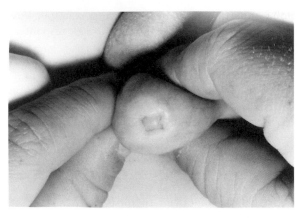

Figure 30.13 Phimosis resulting from BXO.

and non-retractile foreskin. Circumcision is indicated for true phimosis.

Non-retractility of foreskin in early life is, however, normal (physiological phimosis) as the epithelial layers of the glans and foreskin are fused at birth. This probably protects the infant from ammoniacal excoriation and hence neonatal circumcision has no medical grounds. This procedure is commonly performed in the USA for reasons of 'hygiene', 'perhaps lowering the risk of urinary infection', 'social habit', etc. The other major non-medical reason for circumcision is religion, notably for Jews and Muslims. Natural separation of foreskin usually occurs so that by the age of 4 years the foreskin becomes retractile in 90% of boys. Prior to this, sometimes anxious parents may discover pea-sized swellings underneath the foreskin. These are collections of smegma, are harmless and will resolve when foreskin separation is complete.

Balano-prostitis may also be a concern and repeated attacks after the age of 4 years constitute a relative indication for intervention.

Rarely, a foreskin with a narrow preputial ring which has been retracted cannot be pulled forward, resulting in acute, painful swelling, i.e. paraphimosis. This needs to be reduced manually with sedation. A dorsal slit under anaesthesia is sometimes required. When the inflammation has settled, elective circumcision is arranged.

Circumcision is usually performed as a day-case procedure under general anaesthesia. Complications include bleeding, infection, meatal stenosis, fistula formation, excessive/inadequate skin removal, etc. It is important that penile abnormalities, e.g. hypospadias, buried penis, webbed penis, etc., are excluded before circumcision.

Alternatives to circumcision include topical steroid treatment, separation of preputial adhesion under general or local anaesthesia and preputioplasty.

Buried penis

In buried penis, the shaft is retracted into the subcutaneous tissue and obscured by preputial skin. It may be concealed (poor penile skin attachment, prepubic obesity), webbed (penoscrotal fusion) or trapped (scarring following excessive removal of shaft skin at neonatal circumcision). Most concealed penis improve with age with redistribution of prepubic fat. Surgical correction for functional, cosmetic and psychological reasons is achieved by degloving of the penile shaft and fixation of penile skin to subcutaneous tissue and fascia at the base of the penile shaft.

Ambiguous genitalia

Disorders of sex development (DSD) are congenital conditions in which development of chromosomal, gonadal or anatomic sex is atypical. The ambiguous genitalia phenotype may be a result of abnormal chromosomes, gonads or sex steroid synthesis and action. DSD patients may be classified as:

1. Overvirilized 46XX female ('female pseudohermaphroditism'): congenital adrenal hyperplasia, often due to 21-hydroxylase deficiency.
2. Undervirilized 46XY male ('male pseudohermaphroditism'): testosterone biosynthesis deficit, 5α-reductase deficiency and partial androgen insensitivity.
3. Abnormal gonadal development: mixed gonadal dysgenesis (45X/46XY), ovotesticular dysgenesis (46XX, 'true hermaphroditism') and testicular dysgenesis.

Gender is assigned on an individual basis and only after expert evaluation at a centre with an experienced multidisciplinary team and discussion with the patient's family. Diagnostic procedures include examination of external genitalis, palpation for gonads, karyotyping, biochemical and hormonal studies, imaging (ultrasound, genitography), gonadal examination and biopsy (inguinal, laparoscopic). Management includes psychosocial care, hormonal therapy and surgery. Streak and dysgenetic gonads are associated with risks of malignancy; streak gonads and any gonad inappropriate to the sex of rearing should be removed, and any retained testes should be placed in a palpable position for easier surveillance. A child assigned as a female will have reduction clitoroplasty, reconstruction of vagina and labioplasty. A child reared as a male will have urethral and penile reconstruction; Mullerian remnants and symptomatic prostatic utricle may be removed laparoscopically.

Trauma

Most paediatric injuries result from blunt trauma caused by falls, vehicle accidents, etc.; penetrating injuries are less common but in some countries firearms cause significant morbidity. The basic principles of early management of paediatric trauma are similar to those for adult trauma (Advanced Trauma Life Support; ATLS) including prompt assessment and attention to airway, breathing and circulation. Children are prone to multiple injuries; those with multiple or complex injuries should be treated in paediatric trauma centres.

Spleen and liver are the most and second most commonly injured solid organs in blunt abdominal trauma. Typically there is upper quadrant tenderness and pain that may radiate to the shoulder. Haemoperitoneum may manifest as abdominal distension, umbilical bruising and even scrotal bruising (if processus vaginalis is patent). Ultrasonography is a helpful screening procedure, but the gold standard of diagnosis is contrast-enhanced CT scan. Over 90% of cases can be managed successfully with the non-operative approach: close monitoring and bed rest for 2–5 days and activity restriction for 3–6 weeks. Surgery is only indicated in severe continued blood loss (e.g. persistent low blood pressure, blood replacement >40 ml/kg in the first 24 hours) or concomitant hollow viscus injuries. Splenic salvage procedures are attempted instead of splenectomy because of the risk of post-splenectomy sepsis, and these include segmental resection, splenorrhaphy (suture, topical haemostatic agent, mesh) and splenectomy with autotransplantation. Most liver lacerations requiring laparotomy can be managed by suture repair. For the exsanguinating unstable patient, a 'damage control' strategy is adopted: abbreviated laparotomy with packing, resuscitation and planned reoperation. Excessive intra-abdominal pressure may result in abdominal compartment syndrome manifesting as respiratory insufficiency and haemodynamic com-

promise from inferior vena cava compression, and requires temporary patch abdominoplasty.

Most renal injuries respond to non-operative management. Bowel injuries may result from direct impact to the abdomen. Small bowel and duodenum are common sites. Perforations and avulsions are treated by laparotomy, repair or resection. Intramural haematoma may respond to bowel rest and parenteral nutrition. Seat-belt or bicycle handlebar injury typically involves the duodenum and pancreas.

The majority of chest injuries are blunt injuries. As a child's chest wall is pliable, severe intrathoracic injuries may occur without overt external damage or rib fracture. Pneumothorax, haemothorax and lung contusions are the common manifestations; their mangement has been described elsewhere.

Birth injuries may occur during difficult labours and often affect large or premature babies. These are classified into head, nerve, bone and visceral injuries. Head trauma may result in extracranial haematoma (cephalhaematoma), skull fracture or intracranial haematoma (subdural, subarachnoid, epidural). Injuries to the nerves include brachial plexus, which may be upper (Erb's palsy), lower (Klumpke's palsy) or combined; facial nerve; and phrenic nerve. Fractures most commonly occur in the clavicle, humerus and femur. Liver, spleen and adrenals are the abdominal organs most vulnerable to birth trauma.

Non-accidental injury is intentional injury of the child by parents, guardians or acquaintances and often occurs in the first year of life. The pattern of offence is often repetitive. Inappropriate history and physical findings should raise suspicion; all suspected cases should be reported to the relevant authorities. The shaken baby syndrome results from violent shaking leading to subdural haematoma. Munchausen by proxy is an unusual form of child abuse whereby an illness is simulated or produced by a parent and the child is presented repeatedly to unsuspecting institutions for multiple medical procedures.

Burns may be due to thermal, chemical or electrical injuries; in children, over 80% are caused by hot liquid accidents (scald). In estimating burn area, the adult 'rule of nines' is adjusted as follows: the infant's head is 18%, and each leg 14%; for each year after the first, the head decreases by 1%, and each leg increases by 0.5% of total body surface area. The burn depth, airway and respiratory system (inhalation injury, acute respiratory distress syndrome), circulation and extremities (compartment syndrome) are assessed. Fluid loss is replaced according to the Parkland formula: 4 ml/kg per % burn in the first 24 hours (half in the first 8 hours, the rest in the next 16 hours). Sepsis is a major complication which can lead to multiorgan failure. Wound care consists of cleansing, debridement, sterile dressing and topical therapy (silver sulfadiazine); decompression escharotomy, excision and skin grafting are carried out as appropriate. The child requires pain management, nutritional care and in the long term rehabilitation measures (e.g. pressure garment for hypertrophic scar).

Paediatric solid tumours

Management of malignant neoplasm is one of the great success stories of paediatric surgery. Overall survival rate has improved from <20% in the 1950s to 75% now predominantly because of better multimodal therapy involving chemotherapy, surgery and radiotherapy. The availability of new and potent drugs, a better understanding of tumour behaviour and the formation of large multicentre cancer study groups have allowed the evolution of more effective treatment protocols.

Neuroblastoma

Neuroblastoma is the most common extracranial solid malignancy in children, comprising 10% of all childhood cancer and affecting 10 per million children. It remains a serious clinical problem, accounting for 15% of deaths due to malignancy in children. Neuroblastoma arises from the neural crest, most commonly in the adrenal medulla (50%), but also anywhere along the sympathetic ganglion chain in the abdomen and pelvis (25%), thorax (20%) and neck (5%). The clinical behaviour of neuroblastoma is unique and heterogeneous: most tumours grow aggressively and metastasize; on the other hand, some tumours regress spontaneously by undergoing differentiation and/or apoptosis. The majority (70%) have advanced disease at presentation; infants, however, have good prognosis.

The tumour is usually vascular, nodular and locally invasive. The typical histological features are small round blue cells with scanty cytoplasm arranged in rosettes with fine nerve fibres in the centres. The spectrum of cell differentiation can range from immature neuroblasts (anaplastic neuroblastoma) to mature ganglion and Schwann cells (benign ganglioneuroma). Associated anomalies include Hirschsprung's disease (neurocristopathy), Klippel-Feil syndrome, Beckwith-Wiedemann syndrome, di George syndrome, Ondine's curse (congenital central hypoventilation) and trisomy 18.

Diagnosis

The age of presentation is infancy (30%), 1–4 years (50%) and older children (20%); a small number are detected antenatally. The commonest presentation of abdominal neuroblastoma is a palpable abdominal mass. The child often has non-specific symptoms such as anorexia, weight loss and fever; sometimes these are related to metastasis (e.g. bone pain due to bone metastasis). Skin metastasis ('blueberry muffin baby') is a manifestation of stage IV S tumour. Rarely, excessive catecholamine or vasoactive intestinal peptide production leads to hypertension or diarrhoea respectively. Some patients present with opsomyoclonus (dancing eye syndrome) or periorbital bruising ('racoon' or 'panda' eyes denoting orbital metastasis). Thoracic lesions may give rise to respiratory symptoms; cervical tumours may cause Horner's syndrome; pelvic tumours are associated with urinary and bowel dysfunction; paraspinal tumours often have dumb-bell extensions into the spinal canal resulting in neurological symptoms.

Elevated urinary levels of catecholamine metabolites, vanillylmandelic acid (VMA) or homovanillic acid (HVA) are found in 90% of neuroblastomas. A plain radiograph may show calcification. Ultrasonography, CT and MRI provide useful anatomical information. Metastasis is evaluated by bone marrow aspiration, skeletal survey and more recently ^{131}I scan using MIBG (m-iodobenzylguanidine), which is taken up by neuroectodermal tumours. Biopsy (percutaneous, laparoscopic or open) is taken both to confirm the diagnosis and to assess tumour biology to guide treatment.

Tumour behaviour is related to age, stage, histology and biology; age >2 years, advanced stage, unfavourable histology and aggressive biology are associated with worse outcome.

Biochemical markers for tumour biology include lactate dehydrogenase (LDH), neuron-specific enolase (NSE) and ferritin; high serum levels are associated with advanced staging and worse outcome. Molecular markers of poor outcome include multiple copies of N-myc oncogene, diploidy, 1p deletion, 11q deletion, 17q gain and 6p22 risk allele.

Shimada pathological classification describes favourable and unfavourable histology. Stroma-rich tumours have a favourable prognosis, unless a nodular

Table 30.9 International Neuroblastoma Staging System

1. Localized tumour with complete gross excision, with or without microscopic residual disease; negative lymph nodes
2A. Localized tumour with incomplete gross excision; negative lymph nodes
2B. Localized tumour with or without complete gross excision, with positive ipsilateral regional lymph nodes positive for tumour
3. Localized unilateral tumour infiltrating across the midline, with or without regional lymph node involvement; or unilateral tumour with contralateral regional lymph node involvement; or midline tumour with bilateral infiltration or lymph node involvement
4. Tumour with dissemination to distant lymph nodes, bone, bone marrow, liver, skin and/or other organs (except as defined for stage 4S)
4S. Localized primary tumour (as defined for stage 1 or 2), with dissemination limited to skin, liver and/or bone marrow (limited to infants < 1 year of age)

pattern is present. Stroma-poor tumours that are associated with older age, undifferentiation and a mitosis-karyorrhexis index (MKI) <100/5000 cells have an unfavourable prognosis.

The International Neuroblastoma Staging System (Table 30.9) is used. Advanced staging, except stage IV S, is associated with poorer outcome.

Management

Management is multimodal (chemotherapy, surgery and radiotherapy) and protocol-driven. Stage I and II tumours are excised and chemotherapy +/− radiotherapy is given for stage II. Stage III and IV tumours are best treated by preoperative chemotherapy to reduce tumour size and vascularity, followed by delayed excision. Treatment of stage IV S disease is individualized; in some, tumours will mature and disappear without specific treatment; in others, the primary tumour is excised. Occasionally respiratory distress may develop from a rapidly enlarging liver, requiring low-dose irradiation, hepatic artery embolization or insertion of a temporary silastic patch in the abdominal wall. Chemotherapy usually consists of a combination of alkylating agent (cyclophosphamide, cisplantin), topoisomerase inhibitor (topotecan), vinca alkaloid (vincristine) and anthracycline (doxorubicin). The role of surgery is biopsy, vascular access and excision. Locally advanced neuroblastoma frequently surrounds major vessels but rarely invades the tunica media, allowing excision in the subadventitial plane following preoperative

chemotherapy. Radiotherapy is used for local tumour control or rarely in the form of total body irradiation as conditioning for bone marrow transplantation following megachemotherapy.

Overall survival rate is 40–60%; survival in stage I, II and IV S is >90%, stage III >70% and stage IV 30–50%. Advanced stage, age >2 years, unfavourable histology and aggressive biology are poor prognostic factors.

Neonatal screening programmes based on urinary catecholamine studies for early detection of neuroblastoma have failed to provide survival benefits.

New strategies for treatment of advanced diseases include megachemotherapy with total body radiation and bone marrow transplantation, immunotherapy, target therapy with monoclonal antibody antiganglioside GD2, retinoids to induce differentiation, and gene therapy.

Wilms' tumour

Wilms' tumour is the second most common extracranial and the most common intra-abdominal malignant solid tumour in children, with an incidence of 7 per million. Wilms' tumour, or nephroblastoma, is a large and heterogeneous renal embryonoma which is usually confined within a pseudocapsule but can invade neighbouring tissues, especially the renal vein. Histologically, there is a mixture of primitive blastemal, stromal and epithelial cells. Anaplasia, a variant in Wilms' tumour, is associated with aggressive biological behaviour. Rhabdoid (metastasis to brain) and clear cell (metastasis to bone) sarcomas of the kidney are now considered to be unrelated to Wilms' tumour and respond poorly to treatment. Blastemal cell clusters (nephrogenic rests) may be found within normal parts of the kidney and may be transformed into normal or Wilms' tumour elements; rarely diffuse nephrogenic rests affect both kidneys (nephroblastomatosis).

Associated anomalies occur in 10% of patients: WAGR syndrome (**W**ilms' tumour, **a**niridia, **g**enitourinary anomalies and mental **r**etardation), Denys-Drash syndrome (intersex, nephropathy), Beckwith-Wiedemann syndrome, hemihypertrophy, etc. About 2% of patients have a family history. Genetic alterations are found in chromosomes 11p13 (WT1 gene, 50%), 11p15 (WT2, Beckwith-Wiedemann syndrome), 17q (FWT1, familial), 19q (FWT2, familial), 16q and 1p 36.

Diagnosis

The majority present before the age of 5 years, usually as an asymptomatic abdominal mass. There may be non-specific constitutional symptoms such as abdominal pain, malaise, weight loss, anaemia, hypertension and occasionally haematuria. Rarely, a left varicocoele arises from tumour occlusion of the left renal vein. Investigations should include ultrasonography, chest and abdominal X-rays and CT scan with intravenous contrast.

Management

Treatment is multimodal and depends on staging and histology. The National Wilms' Tumour Study Staging System (NWTS-3) is:

- stage I: tumour limited to kidney, completely excised
- stage II: tumour extends beyond kidney, completely excised
- stage III: residual tumour with abdomen
- stage IV: haematogenous metastasis
- stage V: bilateral renal tumour.

Treatment for stages I and II is surgical resection and chemotherapy and for stages III, IV and unfavourable histology (any stage) radiotherapy is added. Some protocols advocate primary nephrectomy while others prefer preoperative chemotherapy followed by secondary nephrectomy; postoperative chemotherapy is given in both protocols. Treatment of stage V is individualized and typically consists of primary chemotherapy, followed by nephron-sparing surgery (partial nephrectomy); bilateral nephrectomy will necessitate subsequent transplantation. The duration and intensity of chemotherapy increase with advancing stages. The most commonly used chemotherapeutic agents are vincristine and actinomycin D. Advanced stage, unfavourable histology and age >2 years are poor prognostic indicators. The overall survival rate of Wilms' tumour now approaches 90%.

Congenital mesoblastic nephroma was initially regarded as a variant of Wilms' tumour, but now has been identified as a separate entity. It is the most common renal neoplasm detected in the antenatal and neonatal periods. It is a low-grade spindle cell tumour that rarely metastasizes. Surgical resection results in virtually 100% survival.

Soft tissue sarcoma

Soft tissue sarcomas account for 7% of all childhood tumours. They are classified into rhabdomyosarcomas, which originate from striated muscle and are more common, and the heterogeneous non-rhabdomyosarcoma soft tissue sarcoma.

Rhabdomyosarcoma is the third most common solid tumour (after neuroblastoma and Wilms' tumour) in childhood. It arises from embryonic tissue capable of muscular differentiation and can occur in any part of the body except the brain and bone. Rhabdomyosarcoma is a small round blue cell tumour, characterized by positive staining with antibodies against actin and myosin. There are two major histological subtypes. Embryonal (55%) rhabdomyosarcoma is the most common subtype and has an intermediate prognosis; the botryoid (5%) variant seen in cavitary structures (e.g. vagina) as a 'cluster of grapes' and the spindle cell variant have the best prognosis. The other major subtype, alveolar (20%) rhabdomyosarcoma, has a poor prognosis. Undifferentiated (20%) tumours also have a poor prognosis. Pleomorphic tumours are rare and have an intermediate prognosis.

There are two peak age incidences, at 2–5 years and 12–18 years, with a slight male preponderance. Familial tendency and association with neurofibromatosis, Li Fraumeni syndrome, Beckwith-Wiedemann syndrome and p53 mutation have been described.

Clinical features relate to the location of the tumour. Head and neck (35%) rhabdomyosarcomas often present with a swelling or bleeding from an orifice (ear, nose or proptosis of the eye); parameningeal tumours can give rise to meningeal symptoms and cranial nerve palsy; histology is commonly embryonal. Genitourinary (25%) rhabdomyosarcomas are mostly embryonal tumours and can be divided into bladder-prostate and other tumours; tumours of the prostate and bladder base present with bladder outlet obstruction, haematuria or constipation, and have a poorer prognosis; paratesticular tumours present with a painless scrotal mass, and/or inguinal swelling (regional lymph node involvement); those with a spindle cell variant have excellent prognosis; vaginal tumours present in infants and young children with vaginal bleeding, discharge or mass, rarely spread, are often botryoid and have excellent prognosis; uterine tumours occur in older girls and have a worse prognosis. Rhabdomyosarcomas of the extremities (20%) present as a mass, often in the lower limbs, and frequently with regional lymph node involvement; they are mostly alveolar and aggressive. Trunk rhabdomyosarcomas present as a paraspinal, retroperitoneal, pelvic, chest or abdominal wall mass and are usually alveolar tumours with poor prognosis. Lung and bone are common metastatic sites.

Diagnosis is made by biopsy after imaging studies (ultrasound, CT, MRI) and work-up for metastasis. Treatment is multimodal (surgery, chemotherapy, radiotherapy) and depends on staging (stage I: localized disease, completely resected, no lymph node involvement; stage II: localized or regional disease with grossly total resection but with microscopic residues; stage III: incomplete resection; stage IV: distant metastasis). Biopsy should be carefully planned, e.g. a longitudinal rather than a horizontal incision is used for extremity rhabdomyosarcoma as subsequently the muscle and biopsy tract need to be resected en bloc. Surgery is site-specific: the principle is to achieve complete excision of the primary tumour with healthy margins while preserving function and cosmesis; advances in chemotherapy have minimized mutilating surgery. Overall survival is 70%. Prognosis is dependent on stage (I, 90%; II, 80%; III, 70%; IV, 30%), pathology (embryonal type is favourable, alveolar and undifferentiated are unfavourable) and location (orbit and genital organs have a favourable prognosis).

Nonrhabdomyosarcomatous soft tissue sarcomas are heterogeneous (e.g. primitive neuroectodermal tumour (PNET), synovial sarcoma, fibrosarcoma, etc.), and individually relatively rare. They can occur in any part of the body. Unlike rhabdomyosarcoma, which is highly chemosensitive, the mainstay of treatment for this group of tumours is complete surgical resection with or without adjuvant radiotherapy to prevent local recurrence.

Other tumours

Gonadal tumours

Ovarian mass has an incidence of 2.5 per 100 000; it can be non-neoplastic (30%), benign neoplastic (50%) or malignant (20%).

Ovarian cysts are often discovered incidentally, are benign and follicular, and can be observed. Surgery is indicated when they are symptomatic, complex, increasing in size or size >5 cm, complicated (torsion, rupture or haemorrhage) or suggestive of malig-

nancy or hormone overactivity. Benign tumour is usually a mature cystic teratoma which appears complex on ultrasonography/CT and may show teeth or hair. Surgery consists of cyst removal with ovarian preservation by laparotomy or laparoscopy.

Malignant tumours may be germ cell, stromal or epithelial. Germ cell tumours may be gonadal or extragonadal (aberrant migration of primitive germ cells); these may arise from primordial germ cells (dysgerminoma), embryonic totipotent cells (teratoma, embryonal carcinoma) or extraembryonic totipotent cells (yolk sac tumour, choriocarcinoma) and account for two-thirds of paediatric ovarian malignancies. Sex stromal tumours may originate from granulosa-theca or Sertoli-Leydig cells and secrete hormones. Dysgerminoma and granulosa-theca cell tumours may present with precocious puberty; Sertoli-Leydig cell tumours may be masculinizing. Serum markers are helpful for diagnosis and follow-up monitoring: α-fetoprotein (malignant teratoma, embryonal carcinoma, yolk sac tumour and Sertoli-Leydig tumour), human chorionic gonadotrophin (HCG) (choriocarcinoma and dysgerminoma). Epithelial tumours are serous or mucinous and have an indolent course; CA-125 is a useful biomarker. Malignant tumours require multimodal treatment (surgery, chemotherapy, radiotherapy).

Testicular tumour has a bimodal age distribution: in prepubertal boys (peak incidence at 2–4 years) and post-pubertal men. The difference in pathology and metastatic potential allows a different treatment approach in the two age groups: younger patients may be considered more often for testes-sparing procedures. Testicular tumours represent 1% of all paediatric solid tumours. The risk of malignancy is 1% in inguinal testes and 5% in intra-abdominal testes. Testicular tumours may be germ cell, stromal or gonadoblastoma. Germ cell tumours may be seminoma, teratoma, yolk sac or mixed. Stromal tumours originate from Leydig, Sertoli or granulosa cells, or epidermoid cyst. Teratoma and yolk sac tumours are the most common prepubertal testicular tumours; teratoma is often benign in children; yolk sac tumour is malignant. Mixed germ cell tumour (malignant) is the most common adolescent tumour; teratoma is potentially malignant in adolescents; seminoma is malignant and predominantly affects adolescents. Epidermoid cyst, Sertoli and Leydig cell tumours affect both age groups and are usually benign in children. A nontender, solid scrotal mass is the usual

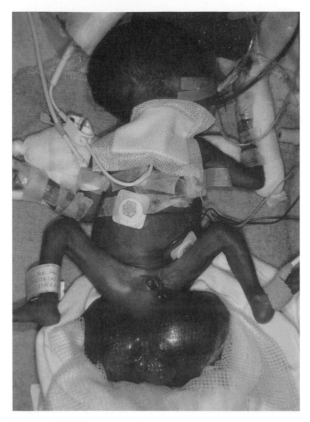

Figure 30.14 Sacrococcygeal teratoma.

coccyx and can be classified into types I (exterior only) (50%), II (exterior and intrapelvic) (35%), III (exterior, intrapelvic and intrabdominal) (10%) and IV (intrapelvic only) (10%). Most sacrococcygeal teratomas are benign: malignancy is rare in type I tumour, but occurs in 6–20% of type II–IV tumours; incompletely excised tumour is associated with a significant risk of malignant change. Sacrococcygeal teratoma may be detected antenatally and may cause perinatal complications and death (e.g. fetal hydrops due to vascular steal syndrome as a result of blood shunting away from the placenta). The most common presentation is a large sacral mass (partly solid, partly cystic) at birth. The anus is often displaced anteriorly. An intrapelvic extension may be palpable behind the rectum. Diagnosis of type IV tumour (intrapelvic only) is often delayed until the child presents with pressure symptoms on the rectum and bladder. Investigations include ultrasonography, X-ray (bone, teeth), CT scan, MRI and serum α-fetoprotein. Treatment is by excision, which should always include the coccyx. Long-term follow-up for bowel and bladder dysfunction and malignant recurrence (α-fetoprotein) is recommended.

Malignant liver tumours are more common than benign liver tumours. Liver malignancies account for 1% of all paediatric malignancies and are the third most common intra-abdominal cancer. The most common primary hepatic malignancies are hepatoblastoma (60%) and hepatocellular carcinoma (30%); sarcoma and lymphoma are less common. Liver may also be the site of metastasis of other primary tumours.

Hepatoblastoma has an incidence of 1 per million and predominantly affects infants and young children (>75% occur in children <2 years of age). The risk factors are Beckwith-Weidermann syndrome, familial adenomatous polyposis, hemihypertrophy and low birth weight. It is an embryonal tumour and is composed of cells resembling the developing fetal and embryonic liver; antenatal diagnosis has been reported. The prognosis is excellent (85% survival).

Hepatocellular carcinoma occurs in older children, often complicating underlying liver disease such as hepatitis B and cirrhosis. The prognosis is poor (20% survival).

Males are more commonly affected in both hepatoblastoma and hepatocellular carcinoma. Clinical presentation is an asymptomatic abdominal mass for hepatoblastoma, and pain and non-specific symptoms such as anorexia and weight loss for hepatocellular carcinoma. Serum α-fetoprotein is elevated in both

presentation; a history of trauma may have alerted the boy but is not causal. There may be an associated hydrocoele. Serum α-fetoprotein is elevated in yolk sac tumour; HCG is raised in choriocarcinoma, malignant teratoma and mixed germ cell tumour, and sometimes in seminoma. The standard initial surgical treatment for malignant testicular tumour is inguinal orchidectomy with early control of the vessels. Prepubertal tumours without an elevated HCG level may be considered for testes-preserving surgery: the lesion is excised via an inguinal incision with testicular vessel occlusion, and examined by frozen section; orchidectomy is performed if the frozen section suggests malignancy. For malignancies, postoperative platinum-based chemotherapy is given and, where appropriate, retroperitoneal lymph node dissection.

Teratoma is composed of tissues from all three embryonal germ layers. Sacrococcygeal teratoma (Figure 30.14) is the most common teratoma in children, with an incidence of 1 in 40 000 live births and a female preponderance (3:1). It arises at the tip of the (hepatoblastoma is associated with a higher level), and HCG in some hepatoblastomas. Diagnosis is achieved with imaging studies including ultrasonography, CT scan with contrast enhancement or MRI, and biopsy. Hepatic resection is the main form of treatment. Children are noted for their excellent capacity for hepatic regeneration, allowing resection of up to 80% of the liver. Hepatoblastoma is chemosensitive; pre- and postoperative chemotherapy is often effective. Inoperable hepatocellular carcinoma may be palliated by transarterial oily chemoembolization (TOCE). Liver transplantation is an option for unresectable primary lesions confined to the liver. Occasionally a liver tumour may be complicated by rupture, requiring emergency embolization or surgery to control bleeding.

Benign liver tumours include vascular tumours (haemangioma, haemangioendothelioma, haemangioblastoma), mesenchymal hamartoma, focal nodular hyperplasia, hepatocellular adenoma, teratoma and inflammatory pseudotumour.

Lymphoma (Hodgkin and non-Hodgkin) is a common malignancy in childhood but the majority are treated effectively by chemotherapy and radiotherapy. The role of surgery is limited to diagnostic biopsy (the most accessible suspected lesion), vascular access and treatment of complications, e.g. intussusception due to Burkitt's lymphoma.

Gastrointestinal tumours are uncommon in children and may be lymphoma, gastrointestinal stromal tumour (GIST) (commonest in the stomach) or carcinoid tumour (appendix); epithelial cancer is rare. GIST and carcinoid are treated by surgical resection. GIST expresses KIT protein; tyrosine kinase inhibitor (imatinib) is effective as adjuvant therapy.

Further reading

Grosfeld JL, Coran AG, O'Neill JA Jr, Fonkalsrud EW, Caldamone AA (eds). *Pediatric Surgery*. 6th edn. Mosby, 2006.

Majid AA, Kingsnorth AN (eds). *Advanced Surgical Practice*. Greenwich Medical Media, 2003.

Puri P, Hollwarth M (eds). *Pediatric Surgery: Diagnosis and Management*. Springer, 2009.

Spitz L. Esophageal atresia. Lessons I have learned in a 40-year experience. *J Pediatr Surg* 2006;**41**:1635–1640.

Spitz L, Coran AG (ed). *Rob & Smith's Operative Surgery: Paediatric Surgery*. 6th edn. Hodder Arnold, 2006.

Wong KKY, Tam PKH. Recent advances in minimal access surgery for infants and children. *Curr Pediatr Rev* 2006; **2**:177–186.

Chapter

31

Fundamentals of organ transplantation

Matthew Bowles

Introduction

On 3 December 1967 a patient with end-stage cardiac disease received a heart transplant from a deceased donor who had recently sustained a severe head injury. The operation took place in South Africa and the recipient lived for 3 weeks after the operation. This was not the first 'successful' human organ transplant – kidney transplantation was already established, but this particular event captured the public imagination worldwide.

This clinical achievement marked the turning point from organ transplantation being just a technical dream (100 years ago a French surgeon called Carrel described a technique to anastomose blood vessels), to being the treatment of choice for many types of organ failure, with demand for organs for transplantation far outstripping supply.

Transplantation is a fascinating and exciting area in which to work: the patients are often very sick, the surgery may be very technically challenging, there are many ethical issues to debate and the specialty involves a large multidisciplinary team, bringing together surgeons, physicians, radiologists, pathologists, immunologists, transplant coordinators, intensivists and pharmacists, not to mention an extremely well-informed group of patients.

Types of transplantation

Transplantation involves the transfer of part of the body to another location in the same individual, or to another individual. We tend to think of it in terms of kidney, liver and heart transplants, but its scope is much wider (Table 31.1).

Organ transplantation – This term describes the transplant of a vascularized organ, in which the blood supply to the organ is directly from the recipient's circulation. Such organs include kidney, liver, heart, lungs, pancreas and small bowel. On some occasions multi-organ transplants are carried out, e.g. heart/lung or liver/small bowel.

Tissue transplantation – Here there are no vascular anastomoses performed as part of the transplant, and the graft obtains its oxygen and nutrition without such a vascularized supply. Examples are cornea, skin and bone transplants.

'Composite' transplants are grafts that are vascularized, but the tissue transplanted is not a single organ; examples are limb and face transplants.

Cell transplants – Here individual cells are transplanted, suspended in a suitable medium. The most common example is blood transfusion, although this is not usually regarded under the umbrella of transplantation. The next most common is bone marrow transplantation, and others include islet cell and hepatocyte transplantation.

Organs, such as heart, kidney and liver, need to be removed (retrieved) from the donor whilst the organs are still (or until very recently) perfused with oxygenated blood. Tissues such as skin, bone and corneas can be taken up to 24 hours (and possibly longer) after cessation of the circulation of the deceased donor.

Transplantation within an individual (auto-transplantation), such as skin grafting and the use of free flaps in plastic surgery, is not part of the remit of this chapter, which will focus on organ transplantation, as described above.

Definitions (Table 31.2)

The transplanted organ, tissue or cell is called a 'graft'. The individual from whom the graft comes is called a 'donor' and the individual into whom the graft is

Fundamentals of Surgical Practice, Third Edition, ed. Andrew N. Kingsnorth and Douglas M. Bowley.
Published by Cambridge University Press. © Cambridge University Press 2011.

Table 31.1 Types of transplants

Organs – heart, lung, liver, kidney, pancreas, small bowel
Tissues – skin, bone, cornea
Cells – bone marrow, hepatocytes, pancreatic islets

Table 31.2 Types of graft

Autograft – transplant within same individual
Isograft – between genetically identical individuals – identical twins
Allograft – between genetically different individuals of same species
Xenograft – between different species

transplanted is called the 'recipient'. The most common form of transplantation is between one individual and another; this is called an 'allograft'. An 'isograft' is a transplant between genetically identical individuals such as identical twins. An 'autograft' is a transplant within one individual, most commonly skin grafting but also applicable, for example, to resiting a kidney during complex aortic aneurysm surgery. A 'xenograft' is a transplant between species; there has been considerable scientific interest in this in recent years but, irrespective of the ethical issues, it remains experimental at present due to problems controlling the immune responses and ensuring prevention of transfer of diseases from animal species into humans.

Indications and outcomes

Indications for organ transplantation

An all-embracing description of the indications for organ transplantation could be 'end-stage organ disease with poor prognosis', although there are exceptions to this. Examples of end-stage organ disease are cardiomyopathy, cystic fibrosis, glomerulonephritis, cirrhosis and diabetes respectively for heart, lung, kidney, liver and pancreatic transplantation.

However, other factors have to be taken into account, such as the availability, morbidity and mortality of non-transplant methods of organ support or replacement. So for renal failure, it has long been accepted that both clinically and economically a kidney transplant is better than long-term haemodialysis (the financial costs involved in a renal transplant procedure are about the same as those of one year's dialysis). However, for small bowel failure, the overall advantages of small bowel transplantation over long-term home total parenteral nutrition are not so clearly established.

One of the great challenges of transplantation is that it is probably the only branch of medicine in which activity is not limited by finance or facilities. The number of transplants that are performed is restricted primarily by the number of organs that become available from cadaveric donors. Increasing use of living donors has relieved this situation somewhat, but there remains a large imbalance between organ supply and demand.

However, one must be careful not to talk of an 'organ shortage' as this may be interpreted as a need for more people to die and donate their organs, a situation to which nobody aspires.

Malignant disease presents a challenging alternative to the 'end-stage organ disease' indication. Some presentations of hepato-cellular carcinoma (HCC), a primary tumour of the liver, are best treated by liver transplantation. However, because of the imbalance between supply and demand of transplant organs, one of the criteria for liver transplantation in the UK is that the chance of survival of the patient should be at least 50% at 5 years after the transplant.

Thus patients with an HCC and an expected survival of less than 50% at 5 years post transplant are turned down for liver transplantation. If this criterion was applied to cancer surgery in general, many patients would not receive operations which are currently performed with 'curative intent'. Within the rest of upper gastrointestinal surgery, it would exclude from surgery most patients with oesophageal, gastric or pancreatic cancer.

Outcomes of organ transplantation

Survival after organ transplantation is measured in two ways: graft survival, which is the time from transplantation until failure of the graft; and patient survival, which is how long the patient lives following transplantation. For an individual patient these two may be the same if the patient dies as a result of graft failure, or dies from an unrelated cause with a fully functioning graft. However, patient survival may be longer than graft survival if, for example, the patient goes back on dialysis after renal graft failure or receives a retransplant, etc.

The 1- and 5-year patient and graft survival rates for different transplants in the USA are shown in Table 31.3. One-year patient survival is greater than 80% in all cases, and greater than 90% for kidney transplantation. Patient survival at 5 years is greater than 70% for all apart from lung transplant recipients. Given that the life expectancy of most of these patients would

Table 31.3 Patient and graft survival rates following transplantation

Transplant type	Survival type	Survival (%)	
		1 year	5 years
Kidney – cadaveric donor	Graft	90	68
	Patient	95	81
Kidney – living donor	Graft	96	81
	Patient	98	91
Liver – cadaveric donor	Graft	82	68
	Patient	87	73
Liver – living donor	Graft	85	71
	Patient	90	77
Heart	Graft	87	73
	Patient	88	74
Lung	Graft	82	50
	Patient	84	53

Data from: http://www.ustransplant.org/annual_reports/current/survival_rates.htm.

Table 31.4 History

1902 – Carrel describes technique of vascular anastomosis
1945 – Medawar describes immunology of rejection
1954 – First kidney transplant between identical twins
1960 – Calne describes use of Azathioprine
1963 – First liver transplant
1967 – First heart transplant
1980 – Cyclosporin introduced
1990 – Tacrolimus introduced

have been extremely limited without transplantation, this table demonstrates the overall success of transplantation as a form of treatment.

History of transplantation

Understanding many aspects of transplantation is helped by an appreciation of the history of the evolution of the specialty (Table 31.4).

The first transplants

The first successful human transplants were carried out in the 1950s between identical twins – isografts. This was possible if a patient with end-stage renal failure had an identical twin who was healthy, had two well-functioning kidneys and was willing to donate one of their kidneys to their twin. These transplants were successful because there were no immunological consequences to overcome. Many of these types of transplants were carried out in the 1950s, particularly in the USA.

Of course this therapeutic option was clearly unavailable for the vast majority of patients with renal failure. With the introduction of immunosuppressive agents – steroids and then azathioprine – attention turned to transplanting organs from donors unrelated to the recipient. The only available source of organs was from patients who had died suddenly in hospital and for whom resuscitation attempts had been unsuccess-ful or not attempted. With the consent of relatives, the recently deceased cadaver was taken immediately to the operating theatre and the kidneys were removed, perfusing them immediately via the renal arteries with cold perfusion solution. The kidneys were then transplanted as soon as possible.

A degree of success was achieved with these transplants from deceased donors. They demonstrate two concepts within transplantation. The first is the nature of the cadaveric donor, in this case so called 'non-heart-beating' to distinguish from 'heart-beating', which will be described in the following paragraphs. The second is the concept of 'warm ischaemia', which describes the period from cessation of the heart beat to perfusion of the kidneys with cold perfusion solution.

The concept of brainstem death (BSD)

In 1976, the Conference of Medical Royal Colleges in the UK published a Statement in the British Medical Journal and the Lancet on the Diagnosis of Brain Death (Conference of Medical Royal Colleges and their Faculties in the United Kingdom 1976). It is an eloquent and precisely written article which speaks for itself:

With the development of intensive care techniques and their wide availability in the United Kingdom it has become common-place for hospitals to have deeply comatose and unresponsive patients with severe brain damage who are maintained on artificial respiration by means of mechanical ventilators.

This state has been recognized for many years and it has been the concern of the medical profession to establish diagnostic criteria of such rigour that on fulfilment the mechanical ventilator can be switched off, in the secure knowledge that there is no possible chance of recovery.

It is agreed that permanent functional death of the brainstem constitutes brain death and that once this has occurred further artificial support is fruitless and should be withdrawn. It is good medical practice to recognize when brain death has occurred and to act accordingly, sparing relatives from the further emotional trauma of sterile hope.

The Statement went on to describe the conditions for considering the diagnosis of brainstem death (BSD) and then set out the tests for confirming BSD (see below). These were a development of the 1968 Harvard criteria (Report of the Ad Hoc Committee of Harvard Medical School 1968) but EEG testing was not included in these UK guidelines. These guidelines were subsequently adopted by the Courts in the UK as part of the law for the diagnosis of death.

It cannot be over-emphasized that the principal purpose of these BSD guidelines was to enable ITUs to withdraw treatment in a timely fashion, but to allow a potentially more dignified death. Transplantation was mentioned only once in the Statement: the Transplant Advisory Panel was one of several groups which gave advice to the Conference of Medical Royal Colleges.

Heart-beating organ donation

The Statement meant that patients fulfilling the BSD criteria could be declared dead, and a death certificate issued, even though they were on a ventilator with their heart still beating and many organs still functioning satisfactorily. Decisions about when and how to withdraw treatment could then be made; organ donation for transplantation was a by-product of this practice.

As a result of the establishment of these BSD criteria, the concept of 'heart-beating' organ donation was introduced. Once declared dead, a patient, now a heart-beating cadaver on mechanical ventilation, could be transferred to the operating theatre where an organ retrieval operation could be carried out in an unhurried fashion.

This resulted in two major advances. First, there was time for planning. Once the patient had been declared dead they could be maintained on the ventilator while organ retrieval team(s) could travel from transplant centres. Second, the organs remained perfused and oxygenated until the time of cold perfusion (see below), thus keeping the 'warm ischaemic time' to an absolute minimum. This low warm ischaemic time resulted in much improved graft function compared to the longer warm ischaemic times of non-heart-beating donation in the pre-BSD testing era.

Table 31.5 Ischaemia (applicable to both deceased and living donation)

Warm ischaemic time in donor – time from cessation of perfusion of organs with warm, oxygenated blood in donor to perfusion with cold perfusion solution.
Cold ischaemic time – time from perfusion with cold perfusion solution to removal of organ from cold (4°C) storage immediately prior to implantation (organ starting to be warmed by surroundings)
Warm ischaemic time in recipient – time from removal of organ from cold (4°C) to reperfusion of organ with recipient's warm, oxygenated blood.

Warm and cold ischaemia

In order to function, all organs need oxygen, and they function optimally at 37°C. If an organ is deprived of oxygen then it becomes ischaemic. The length of time that an organ can endure ischaemia varies, related to the metabolic rate of the cells within the organ. If the organ's temperature is reduced, the metabolic rate is reduced and the organ can tolerate ischaemia for much longer periods of time. This gives rise to the principles of warm ischaemia, which is lack of oxygen at 37°C, and is very harmful, and cold ischaemia, which is lack of oxygen at 4°C, which is usually much better tolerated by the organ.

There are two periods of warm ischaemia in transplantation (Table 31.5). The first occurs during organ retrieval and is the time from cessation of perfusion of organs with warm, oxygenated blood to perfusion with cold perfusion solution. Then follows a period of cold ischaemia, which is the time from perfusion with cold perfusion solution to removal of the organ from cold (4°C) storage immediately prior to implantation. The second period of warm ischaemia occurs during implantation of the graft and is the time from removal of the organ from storage at 4°C to reperfusion of the organ with the recipient's warm, oxygenated blood.

Organ procurement

The process of cadaveric, heart-beating, organ donation

The process through which deceased, heart-beating organ donation takes place in the United Kingdom and many other counties represents a considerable feat of organization, cooperation and coordination within a national framework. The typical series of events is as follows (subject to significant variations):

A patient sustains a massive head injury or sub-arachnoid haemorrhage but survives long enough to be intubated and ventilated and then managed on an intensive care unit.

After a variable period of neurosurgical investigation and treatment it becomes apparent that the patient has an unrecoverable brain injury and has no brain-stem function, as confirmed by the absence of all brain-stem reflexes.

Brainstem death testing

Certain conditions must be fulfilled before BSD testing can be carried out. These are:

(a) There should be no doubt that the patient's condition is due to irremediable brain damage of known aetiology.
(b) The patient is deeply unconscious and the possibility that this is due to drugs, hypothermia or circulatory/metabolic/endocrine causes has been excluded.
(c) The patient is being maintained on the ventilator because spontaneous respiration has been inadequate or has ceased altogether and drugs have been excluded as a cause of this.

The brainstem death tests are:

- Fixed, unresponsive pupils
- Absent corneal reflexes
- Absent vestibulo-ocular reflexes, tested by injecting ice-cold water into each external auditory meatus in turn
- Absent motor responses within the cranial nerve distribution
- Absent gag reflex and absent response to bronchial stimulation
- No respiratory effort when, following disconnection from the ventilator, the pCO_2 has risen above 6.7 kPa, whilst hypoxia is prevented by delivering 100% oxygen via a tracheal catheter.

The brainstem death tests described above are performed according to the 1998 guidelines (http://www.dh.gov.uk/dr_consum_dh/groups/dh_digitalassets/@dh/@en/documents/digitalasset/dh_4035462.pdf). They are carried out on two separate occasions by two doctors (usually intensivists or neurosurgeons who must not be members of the transplant teams), both of whom have been registered for 5 years or more and at least one of whom is a consultant. Doctor A performs the tests alone at time 1 and then Doctor B alone at Time 2, and there is no lower limit to the interval between times 1 and 2. However, it is common practice for both doctors to be present for both sets of tests, which are usually at least half an hour apart. Death can be declared after the second set of tests is complete, although the time of certification of death is then given as the time that the first set of tests were completed.

Decisions regarding organ donation

Once death has been certified, a decision is made either to withdraw treatment or to take the patient for organ donation. This is obviously discussed in detail with the next-of-kin and family, and discussions may well have started prior to BSD testing, often very soon after the concept of BSD testing is first raised with the family.

This discussion is obviously very difficult. It is vital to separate the issue of brainstem death and its testing from that of subsequent management, i.e. withdrawal of treatment and/or organ donation. Withdrawal of treatment on the ITU will involve some or all of extubation, giving air rather than oxygen and stopping inotropic support, etc. Organ donation will involve the deceased patient being taken to the operating theatre still heart-beating on a ventilator, an operation lasting several hours, finishing with the exsanguination of the cadaver at the time of organ perfusion (see below).

The discussion may be helped if the family know that the patient carried an organ donor card (introduced in the UK in 1971) or was on the NHS Organ Donor Register (established in 1994; it now has over 16 million registrants); ITU staff will routinely check this register prior to discussion because it may help to be able to tell the family that the patient was registered even if the family were not aware, as it may make them feel that the decision had already been made by the patient.

The role of the transplant coordinator

If the decision is made that the deceased patient could be an organ donor, then the local donor transplant coordinator will be called (and they may well have been called earlier to help with the discussions about potential organ donation). They will continue the discussions with the family, give a full explanation of the process of organ donation, assess the patient and then 'offer' organs to transplant centres.

Another important aspect to the discussions with the coordinator is the need for virological testing of the potential donor. In order to prevent transmission of viral infection to a transplant recipient, the donor is tested for HIV and hepatitis B and C. Organs from HIV-positive donors are 'never' used, but those from hepatitis B/C-positive donors are sometimes used in similarly infected recipients. Previously unknown positivity may have significant implications for the donor's family, so careful consent must be taken for such pre-donation testing.

Depending on the location of the hospital (the 'donor' hospital) where the potential organ donor is there will be a designated retrieval centre for each organ. The donor coordinator contacts the recipient coordinators in each of these centres; this can be very time-intensive if all organs are being offered, i.e. heart, lungs, liver, pancreas and kidneys.

The clinicians at the transplant centres will make judgements based on information about the donor (past history, current physiological state and virological status) as to whether or not 'their' particular organ is suitable for transplantation and therefore worth retrieving. If so, a retrieval team will be sent out to the donor hospital in as timely a fashion as possible. Over the years the term 'retrieval' has replaced 'harvest'.

Organ retrieval operation

Between the retrieval of an organ from a donor and its implantation into a recipient, the organ will not have any oxygen supply. In order to keep damage to a minimum, it is kept at 4°C. During retrieval, as an organ loses its blood supply the object is to cool it as rapidly as possible so that warm ischaemia is kept to a minimum. For the abdominal organs this is achieved by cannulating the distal aorta with a large-bore cannula and then simultaneously clamping the aorta at the level of the diaphragm, infusing perfusion fluid rapidly through the aortic cannula and dividing the inferior vena cava to exsanguinate the cadaver. At the same time cold cardioplegia solution is infused via the ascending aorta into the coronary arteries in order to cool and arrest the heart.

Cooling organs *in situ* via the aorta in the cadaver is not as effective as cooling them directly by perfusion into the organ's artery on the 'backtable' – usually a theatre trolley draped with sterile theatre drapes. For this reason it is desirable to remove the organs from the donor as soon as possible after cross-clamping and per-

fusion. To achieve this without damaging the organs, a considerable amount of dissection and mobilization is required prior to cross-clamping of the aorta at the diaphragm, and all teams must be sure they are all ready prior to cross-clamping.

It should be clear from the above that the organ retrieval operation is lengthy and demanding as a surgical technique, particularly as it usually involves coordination between more than one surgical team from different transplant centres, all working in an unfamiliar hospital, often during the night.

The final part of the retrieval operation involves the removal of lymph nodes (usually ileo-colic) and the spleen for cross-matching purposes (see below) for the renal transplants and also removal of the iliac arteries and veins which may be needed for reconstruction of the graft or recipient vasculature.

Living donation

Going back to the history of developments in transplantation, having demonstrated that the immunological consequences of human allografting could be controlled to a certain extent, attention turned back to the use of living donors who were not identical twins. These living donors were family members. The recipients required immunosuppression (unlike the identical twins) but the advantage of living donation was the short warm ischaemic time that could be achieved, essentially just a few minutes from clamping the renal vessels in the donor to perfusing the kidney with cold solution once removed from the donor.

In those countries which do/did not recognize the concept of BSD, living related donation has been the cornerstone of transplantation for many years; Japan is a prime example of this, although recently BSD legislation has been passed.

Deceased non-heart-beating donation

The demand for transplantable organs has always outstripped the supply and the transplant community is continually looking for ways to maximize the potential for organ donation (Table 31.6). The advent of BSD testing led to a shift towards heart-beating donation, because it is much more controlled than retrieving organs from patients who have not been resuscitated from a cardiac arrest, because the warm ischaemic times can be kept much lower and because as a consequence the outcomes for the recipients are better.

Table 31.6 Types of organ donors

Deceased
Heart beating / brainstem dead / donation after brain death (DBD)
Non-heart-beating (NHBD) / donation after cardiac death (DCD)
Living
Related
Unrelated – e.g. spouse or altruistic donation
Domino

However, over the last 10–20 years for kidneys and 5–10 years for livers, there has been a revival of interest in using organs from patients who have suffered cardiac arrest, so called 'non-heartbeating donors' – NHBD. The most common method of donation for these patients is that they are on the ITU and deemed as having no chance of recovery, but for one reason or another they do not fulfil BSD criteria and therefore cannot be certified as dead whilst still on the ventilator and maintaining a cardiac output. In this situation ventilation and inotropic support are withdrawn, the ITU staff wait until the heart stops beating, wait for 5 minutes to ensure that it does not start again, certify death based on the lack of heart beat and then the patient/cadaver is taken to the operating theatre where the organ retrieval team(s) is standing by.

The organ retrieval operation is then carried out as speedily as possible, particularly until the moment of aortic perfusion with cold fluid, in order to keep the warm ischaemic time to a minimum, although it is inevitably much longer (minutes rather than seconds) than the warm ischaemic time of a heart-beating organ retrieval operation.

Numbers of organ donors in United Kingdom

In the year 2008–2009 there were 899 deceased organ donors in the UK (Table 31.7). Of these 611 (two-thirds) were heart-beating donors and 288 (one-third) non-heart-beating. There were a total of 2559 organ transplant operations performed from these donors, representing just less than three grafts from each deceased donor – two kidneys and the liver being the most common combination.

In the same period there were 954 living donors and the same number of transplants from living donors, the vast majority being kidney transplants plus 27 living donor liver transplants.

Table 31.7 Organ transplant activity in the UK: figures for 2008–2009

Organ donors	
Deceased organ donors	899
Heart-beating	611
Non-heart-beating	288
Living organ donors	954
Total organ donors	1853
Transplants	
From deceased donors	
Kidney	1403
Liver	644
Lung	143
Heart	129
Pancreas	54
Combined kidney/pancreas	152
Others	34
Total	2559
From living donors	
Kidney	927
Liver	27
Total	954
Overall total organ transplants	3513

Data from: http://organdonation.nhs.uk/ukt/statistics/latest_statistics/latest_statistics.jsp.

In addition to the above deceased donor numbers, there were approximately 2000 corneas-only deceased donors.

However, in the same period there were 7877 patients waiting for a transplant in the UK, with some waiting many years and some dying on the waiting list. In 2008, in response to the ever-increasing imbalance between the supply of organs and the demand, the Department of Health Organ Donation Taskforce committed to achieving a 50% increase in organ donation numbers over 5 years (http://www.dh.gov.uk/dr_consum_dh/groups/dh_digitalassets/@dh/@en/documents/digitalasset/dh_082120.pdf).

Principles of implantation

The principles of implantation of any vascularized organ are very similar: they require an arterial supply, venous drainage and then connection of any other structures, e.g. ureter, bile duct, pancreatic duct and bronchus respectively for kidney, liver, pancreas and lung transplants. The heart requires anastomosis of two sets of vessels but no ductular structures.

The first stage of the recipient operation involves preparation of the site of graft implantation. This may either be 'orthotopic' – where the diseased organ is removed and replaced by the graft – e.g. heart, liver and lung transplants, or 'heterotopic' – where the diseased organ(s) is left *in situ* and the graft is placed in a non-anatomical position – e.g. kidney and pancreas transplants.

Explantation of the diseased organ prior to orthotopic transplantation can be very challenging technically, particularly if the patient has had previous surgery to the organ. This is often considerably more demanding than the implantation of the graft.

Once the vessels to be used for anastomosis to the graft vessels have been prepared, the organ is removed from its storage at 4°C and usually covered with a swab soaked in cold saline as it is implanted. The order of arterial and venous anastomoses varies and is not important whilst all vessels are clamped. The venous clamps are removed first, allowing low-pressure backflow of blood into the organ, and it begins to warm. Bleeding from the venous anastomosis or the surface of the organ is dealt with and then the arterial clamps are released. This usually results in dramatic 'pinking up' of the organ, and beating in the case of the heart. Arterial anastomotic bleeding is dealt with as appropriate. The organ is usually left to 'settle in' a bit before the duct/ureter, etc. is anastomosed to the recipient.

Kidney

Kidney grafts are usually placed in the right or left iliac fossa, using a curved oblique incision. The peritoneum is not opened and space for the graft is created extra-peritoneally, by pushing the peritoneum upwards, thus exposing the external iliac vessels. The renal artery and vein of the graft are anastomosed onto these external iliac vessels. The graft ureter can then be cut quite short and implanted into the dome of the bladder, by one of a variety of techniques designed to reduce vesico-ureteric reflux. A 'double-J' stent is usually placed through the ureteric anastomosis and can be removed at cystoscopy some weeks after transplantation.

The advantages of this technique of heterotopic kidney transplantation are that access is much easier than it would be to the orthotopic position, and the native, failed kidneys can be left *in situ*. The blood supply to the ureter would be fairly precarious if its full length was used, and this technique necessitates only a short length of ureter. Additionally, post-transplant biopsy of the kidney is relatively straightforward when the graft is easily palpable in the iliac fossa.

The native kidneys are rarely removed, and if so not usually at the same time as the transplant. The most common reason for native nephrectomy is probably polycystic disease, when the kidneys cause pain and discomfort as a result of their large size.

Pancreas

There have been a variety of techniques described for implantation of the pancreas and, as for the kidney, the pancreas is always transplanted in a heterotopic position with the native pancreas being left *in situ*. The venous outflow of the pancreas is relatively straightforward in that the entire organ drains into the portal vein. However, the arterial inflow is more complicated, coming from both splenic and superior mesenteric arteries, so these have to be joined prior to implantation, sometimes with a 'Y' graft using the common iliac artery bifurcation retrieved from the donor.

The pancreas is often implanted in one of the iliac fossae, like the kidney, with vascular anastomoses to the iliac vessels. The pancreas is retrieved with a short segment of the duodenum, stapled off at both ends, to which it is intimately attached and into which drains the pancreatic duct. One way of draining the pancreatic duct is to attach the duodenal segment to the bladder. One of the advantages of this is that urinary amylase can be used as a measure of graft function. However, a more physiological method of pancreatic drainage is achieved by attaching the duodenal graft to a Roux loop of small bowel, so that the pancreatic enzymes end up in the small bowel. The pancreas is not transplanted for its exocrine function, but instead for its endocrine function in patients with unstable diabetes.

Liver

The liver is transplanted in an orthotopic position, the native liver being removed as part of the transplant operation. In end-stage liver disease the combination of hepatomegaly, cirrhosis with severe portal hypertension, deranged clotting and thrombocytopaenia make liver explantation a very technically and anaesthetically demanding operation. A temporary porto-caval shunt is often fashioned to help reduce the portal hypertension and thus blood loss.

Liver implantation is complicated by the presence of the dual blood supply to the liver – arterial and portal. Additionally, if the graft is to be truly orthotopic then the inferior vena cava (IVC) has to be clamped above and below the liver; this may only be tolerated haemodynamically if veno-venous bypass from the iliac to the axillary or jugular veins is employed. To avoid this, a partially heterotopic variant of liver transplantation, called the piggy-back technique, is often used: the native liver is 'filleted' off the retro-hepatic IVC and then the supra-hepatic IVC of the graft is anastomosed to the hepatic veins of the patient. So for a short segment there are two IVCs in parallel, one 'piggy-backed' onto the other.

The common bile duct of the graft is usually anastomosed to the common bile duct of the recipient. However, there are circumstances where this is not possible or desirable and in these cases the graft bile duct is anastomosed by a hepatico-jejunostomy to a Roux loop of jejunum. The graft gallbladder is removed in order to avoid any complications related to it.

Heart

Anastomosis of the outflow of the heart is done at the level of the great vessels: aorta and pulmonary artery. The inflow anastomoses are carried out at the level of the atria: the back walls of the atria are left in place in the transplant recipient and atrial to atrial anastomoses are performed.

Lung

The lung is implanted orthotopically with the graft pulmonary vessels and bronchus all being anastomosed with their corresponding structures in the recipient.

Variations on 'standard' transplantation techniques

In renal transplantation, there may be occasions when both of a deceased donor's kidneys are used for one recipient. This may be when the donor is very small or is a child and the recipient requires more renal function than can be provided by one of the kidneys alone. Similarly, if the donor kidneys are 'marginal' in that they are not particularly good organs, then both may be transplanted into one recipient to ensure adequate overall renal function.

In liver transplantation, a very good donor liver may be 'split' into two grafts. Usually the left lateral segment of the liver (about 20–30% of the liver) is used for a paediatric recipient and the remaining liver is used for an adult recipient. The splitting operation in itself is quite complex and requires several hours work on the backtable in the operating theatre.

Table 31.8 Immunology

MHC – major histocompatibility complex – group of genes found close to each other on chromosome 6
HLA – human leucocyte antigen – the locus for the MHC on chromosome 6
APC – antigen-presenting cell – take up antigen and present it to T lymphocytes
CD – clusters of differentiation – surface markers which define cell types
TCR – T cell receptor

Auxiliary transplantation describes the use of a graft to temporarily maintain organ function when there is the hope/expectation that the diseased organ will recover function sufficiently for the auxiliary graft to be removed eventually. This form of transplantation is very occasionally employed in liver and heart transplantation.

Domino transplantation occurs when an organ is removed from the transplant recipient which is suitable for use as a graft in another patient. The classic example is in cystic fibrosis, when the traditional operation was a heart/double lung en-bloc operation; the recipient's heart was removed when in fact it worked pretty well, and so could be used to transplant another heart-only patient. The other example is in liver transplantation, in rare forms of amyloid disease, when the diseased liver is quite able to give another patient a good 10 years or so of improved quality of life.

Transplant immunology

One of the fundamental attributes of the immune system is the ability to distinguish self from non-self (Table 31.8). Under normal circumstances an immune response will only be triggered when an individual comes into contact with non-self antigens. A transplanted organ contains an abundance of such non-self antigens and rejection of the transplant is the end result of the immune response directed against them.

The major histocompatibility complex

The major histocompatibility complex (MHC) is a large group of genes found in close proximity to each other. In humans this region is called the human leucocyte antigen (HLA) locus and is located on chromosome 6.

The MHC encodes for cell membrane proteins which are of two types: MHC class 1 molecules and MHC class 2 molecules. MHC class 1 molecules are found on all nucleated cells and platelets; MHC class 2 molecules are principally found on antigen-presenting cells (APCs) – these are a functionally defined group of cells which are able to take up antigen and present it to T lymphocytes. This group includes B lymphocytes, macrophages and dendritic cells.

There are several groups of MHC class 1 and MHC class 2 molecules, each encoded by a single gene locus. The HLA-A, -B and -C loci encode MHC class 1 molecules and the HLA-DP, -DQ and -DR loci encode MHC class 2 molecules.

At each locus (e.g. HLA-A) the genes are highly polymorphic, with a defined range of between 5 and 30 possible genes. Each individual has two genes at each locus, one from each parent. This gives rise to the way we describe an individual in terms of their HLA type.

The set of genes inherited from one parent reside on one chromosome and are called a haplotype; every individual has two haplotypes, one from each parent. The chance of two unrelated individuals having exactly the same combination of MHC class 1 and 2 genes is extremely low, but for siblings, because haplotypes are inherited en bloc, the chance is 25%.

The clusters of differentiation (CD) nomenclature

In contrast to MHC molecules, which are widely different between individuals (but are the same on all the cells on which they are expressed within any one individual), the CD system of nomenclature describes other cell surface markers which vary widely between different cell populations within an individual but which are exactly the same on the equivalent cell population from all individuals in the species (and are often well conserved between species).

The CD system of nomenclature defines functionally different cell populations. CD3 is part of the T cell receptor (TCR) and is present on all T lymphocytes. CD4 and CD8 are mutually exclusive mature T cell markers which broadly define the cells as having either collaborative 'helper' functions (Th) or cytotoxic potential (Tc) respectively, although CD4+ and CD8+ cell populations can contain both Th and Tc cells.

Rejection

The major immunological problem in clinical transplantation is acute graft rejection, which usually occurs within a few days or weeks of transplantation. The rejection response is equivalent to the cell-mediated (rather than antibody mediated) immune response to any non-self antigen; we are used to thinking about cell-mediated immunity in terms of the response to antigen from another species, e.g. viral etc. In transplantation, the non-self antigen is from another individual of the same species.

The acute rejection process can broadly be divided into two phases. There is an induction phase, in which recognition of the non-self antigens of the graft initiates a cascade of immune events that leads to an effector phase, during which damage to the transplanted tissue takes place.

Antigen presentation and recognition

Recognition of alloantigen takes place by two pathways: indirect and direct recognition.

Indirect recognition

Indirect recognition is the mechanism through which many non-transplantation antigens, for example bacteria, are handled. It involves processing of the antigen by an antigen-presenting cell (APC), which then presents the antigen to T lymphocytes. In the case of transplantation, antigen is in the form of alloantigenic peptide shed from the graft; this peptide material is internalized by an APC, processed by the APC and associated with the APCs class 2 MHC molecules and then expressed on the cell surface of the APC as part of a foreign antigen/self MHC complex.

The peptide/MHC class 2 complex on the APC cell surface is then recognized by a T lymphocyte using the T cell receptors (TCRs) on the surface of the T cell. The CD4 molecule acts as a co-receptor for the TCR complex; CD4 molecules cluster on the T cell surface at the T cell/APC interface and help the two cells to bind together.

One of the principal differences between CD4+ and CD8+ T cells is that MHC class 2 molecules on APCs exclusively associate with the CD4 molecule and MHC class 1 molecules exclusively associate with the CD8 molecule (see below).

The binding of the APC and CD4+ T cell in this way results in the first step towards full activation of the CD4+ cell, which can then interact with, or help, a variety of other cells which mediate damage to cells bearing foreign antigens.

Direct recognition

Transplanted tissue differs from the vast majority of non-self antigens in that the cells of the graft themselves express human class 1 MHC molecules.

Recipient T cells are able to recognize directly non-self MHC molecules on graft cells, either alone or as peptide/MHC complexes. This recognition pathway is called direct recognition. This form of allo-recognition is by CD8+ T cells; it results in their differentiation into cytotoxic T lymphocytes (CTL), which are harmful to the MHC class 1-bearing cell.

Virtually all graft cells express MHC class 1 molecules on their surface and this partly explains the aggressive nature of allo-responses: rather than a few host cells recognizing and processing foreign antigen, the majority of the cells of the transplanted tissue present antigen either as graft MHC molecules or, much more commonly, as MHC molecules in association with a wide variety of graft MHC-derived peptides.

Direct recognition is the predominant process in allo-recognition, but more recently it has been accepted that the indirect pathway of allo-recognition can also be important. The direct pathway is important in the early acute rejection of MHC mis-matched grafts and less so in chronic rejection. The indirect pathway becomes more important with increasing time from transplantation.

HLA matching

The vigour of the rejection response is therefore linked to the disparity between the graft and host MHC molecules. In renal transplantation this gives rise to the clinical practice of HLA matching of prospective recipients to an organ donor prior to transplantation. The recipient with the HLA profile closest to that of the donor is selected for transplantation.

An important consideration is that HLA identity between donor and recipient, such as may occur in living related transplantation, does not preclude rejection because there will still be minor (as opposed to major) histocompatibility differences. True immunological identity only occurs between phenotypically identical twins.

Adhesion molecules

Central to all cell/cell interactions are the group of cell surface molecules known as adhesion molecules. Each adhesion molecule has a specified distribution amongst the cells of the immune system (and other cells of the body) and a ligand or ligands which are also distributed on a variety of cell types. Adhesion molecules serve two functions.

1. They enhance cell/cell binding and therefore play a key role in cell migration and localization, for example in lymphocyte/endothelial cell interactions.
2. They have important roles in intercellular signalling.

Second or co-stimulatory signal

The recognition of the complex of MHC class 1 or 2 with peptide by the TCR and its associated CD8 or CD4 molecules respectively, as described above, and the subsequent binding of these two complexes result in a signal within the T cell which is the first step towards its activation. Adhesion molecule interactions between the MHC-bearing cell and the T cell are responsible for a second, or co-stimulatory, signal. This leads to full T cell activation.

The role of activated T lymphocytes

The differentiation of alloantigen primed CD8+ T cells into activated CTLs results in their being able to inflict damage directly on graft cells; the cytotoxic mechanisms are described below. This CD8+ differentiation is enhanced by help from activated CD4+ T cells. In addition, activated CD4+ T cells provide help for the differentiation of B lymphocytes into alloantigen-specific antibody-producing plasma cells: this occurs when the APC in contact with the CD4+ cell is a B cell. Activated CD4+ cells may also more directly damage the graft through a delayed type hypersensitivity reaction.

Cytokines

Cytokines are a group of molecules which are produced and released by a variety of cells and which have diverse effects on other cells, usually in a paracrine fashion. The interleukins (IL) are a series of cytokines; others include tumour necrosis factor (TNF) and interferon (IFN). They are of great importance in the immune system and thus in transplant rejection. They form the link between the induction and effector phases of the rejection process. One of the crucial roles is that of IL2 released from CD4+ cells to help activation of CD8+ cells into CTLs.

Graft damage

The effector mechanisms of graft destruction can be both antigen-specific, accomplished by CTLs, and antigen-non-specific, caused by inflammatory cells or their secretory products.

CTLs have cytoplasmic granules which contain perforin and granzymes; these are released by the CTL into the junction between the CTL and the MHC class 1-bearing target cell and result in the death of the target cell by apoptosis. Activated CD4+ cells may inflict graft damage themselves by releasing cytokines. Another form of cell-mediated cytotoxicity is natural killer cell damage, by cell lysis.

Steps in the rejection process

The chain of events leading to the rejection of the transplanted organ described above can be summarized as follows:

Induction phase

1. Non-specific infiltration of the graft by inflammatory cells of the recipient results in graft antigens being expressed on the surface of APCs in association with MHC molecules.
2. Initial contact between APCs and T cells is established by non-cognate (non-specific) adhesion between their surface adhesion molecules, thus allowing presentation of alloantigen by APCs to T cells.
3. Recognition of the alloantigen occurs by means of the cognate interaction between MHC/peptide and TCR/CD4 or CD8 complexes. This results in an initial activation signal within the T cell.
4. The second, non-cognate, interaction between adhesion molecules results in the essential co-stimulatory signal necessary for full T cell activation.

Effector phase

5. The activated T cells release cytokines which in turn induce the activation of a number of other cell types.
6. These cells possess a number of effector mechanisms which result in tissue destruction.

Graft-versus-host disease

In some forms of transplantation there are enough lymphocytes carried in the transplant (so called 'passenger' lymphocytes) for them to mount a type of rejection reaction against the transplant recipient. This is called 'graft-versus-host disease' (GVHD) and is the main immunological consequence of bone marrow

Table 31.9 Immunosuppressive agents used in transplantation

Steroids
Azathioprine
Cyclosporin A
Tacrolimus
Mycophenolate mofetil
Sirolimus
Polyclonal antibodies – ALG
OKT3
Anti-IL2R monoclonal antibodies

transplantation, although it may also occur following small bowel, lung and liver transplantation.

Immunosuppression

The aim of immunosuppression is to interrupt the immune events described in the preceding sections and thus attempt to prevent the rejection process from inflicting damage on the transplanted tissue, or GVHD doing the same to host tissue. Immunosuppressive agents (Table 31.9) can broadly be divided into pharmacological immunosuppressants and biological immunosuppressants. The former are what we would consider as 'normal' drugs produced by chemical processes; the latter are biologically produced antibodies.

Pharmacological immunosuppression

Prednisolone

The corticosteroid prednisolone has been the cornerstone of post-transplantation immunosuppressive protocols for many years. Prednisolone principally acts on monocytes/macrophages: there is inhibition of cytokine release by activated monocytes/macrophages which deprives T cells of an important stimulus to their proliferation. This all occurs relatively early in the overall rejection response.

In addition to the actions mediated by inhibition of monocyte/macrophage activity, steroids also inhibit neutrophils. This results in more non-specific anti-inflammatory and immunosuppressant actions.

Steroid immunosuppression chiefly affects cell-mediated rather than humoral immunity and is used not only for induction and maintenance therapy following transplantation but also, in high doses, for treatment of rejection episodes. Steroids are of little use in hyperacute and chronic rejection, which are both chiefly antibody-mediated.

Side effects are common, especially if the maintenance dose of prednisolone is high. Side effects include infections, poor wound healing, diabetes and masking of the clinical signs of sepsis. When used in high doses (typically 1000 mg intravenously daily for 3 days), steroid-induced psychological changes may also occur.

Calcineurin inhibitors – cyclosporin and tacrolimus

The introduction of cyclosporin A (CsA) in the 1980s and then tacrolimus in the 1990s revolutionized the outcomes of clinical organ transplantation. They are both calcineurin inhibitors (CNI) and act specifically on T lymphocytes. They inhibit the calcium-dependent pathway between receptors on the T cell surface and transcription of genes encoding cytokines (particularly IL-2) in the nucleus.

The inhibition of IL-2 and other cytokine production by $CD4^+$ cells results in blockade of the help required for the various effector mechanisms which result in graft damage. CsA and tacrolimus have no direct effects on events occurring after T cell gene activation.

As both drugs act only on T lymphocytes, one of their principal side effects is immunosuppression, leading to infection, which tends to be viral and fungal rather than bacterial. Cytomegalovirus (CMV) is a particularly problematic post-transplant viral infection.

Clinical effects

The inclusion of a CNI in immunosuppressive protocols, most frequently in combination with steroids and azathioprine, reduced the incidence and severity of rejection in most types of clinical organ transplantation. At the same time it allowed reduced doses of steroids to be used, with resultant diminution in steroid toxicity. This is an important principle in immunosuppressive regimens: use of several drugs allows smaller doses of each to be used, with less toxicity.

Toxicity

Infective complications

Immunosuppressive protocols in which a CNI is the major component significantly reduce the incidence of opportunistic infection compared to the high-dose steroid regimens, but such infection remains a major problem following transplantation.

Compared to the general population, there is an unusual spectrum of infectious disease in transplant patients. As described above, CNIs, azathioprine and steroids predominantly exert their effects via inhibition of T lymphocyte and macrophage function while having limited influence on B lymphocyte and plasma cell function. Thus cell-mediated immune responses are suppressed whereas antibody-mediated immunity is relatively spared. For these reasons, viral infections are the greatest cause of infectious disease morbidity and mortality in transplant recipients and bacterial infections are numerically less important. Cytomegalovirus (CMV) is the single most important pathogen in such patients.

The CMV antibody status of the organ donor is routinely tested prior to transplantation. The risk of subsequent CMV infection is increased if an organ from a CMV-seropositive donor is transplanted into a CMV-seronegative recipient. In this situation the recipient is usually considered for antiviral prophylaxis, with gancyclovir for example.

Other important opportunistic infections include fungal infections such as aspergillosis and pneumocystis pneumonia, and tuberculosis, which occurs in transplanted patients at a rate 100 times that of the general population.

Nephrotoxicity

Nephrotoxicity is a major problem associated with CsA and tacrolimus therapy and results from a combination of haemodynamic and histological changes. The therapeutic window for CNIs, particularly in respect of nephrotoxicity, is narrow, and therefore monitoring of CNI blood levels is required in both the short and long term following transplantation.

Other side effects

Other side effects of CNIs include neurological problems such as tremors and fitting, particularly in association with low serum magnesium levels, hypertension, diabetes and hyperlipidaemia. Cardiovascular morbidity and mortality are therefore very important long-term sequelae of CNI immunosuppression. In addition, all immunosuppressants result in an increased risk of neoplastic disease.

Sirolimus

Cyclosporin and tacrolimus are structurally distinct but have very similar mechanisms of action. Sirolimus is very similar in structure to tacrolimus but acts further down the immune activation pathway, by inhibiting lymphocyte proliferation. It is a relatively recent addition to the immunosuppressive armamentarium and is very effective in this action and also has some anti-neoplastic activity. In addition, it is not significantly nephrotoxic, a great advantage over the CNIs. However, it has profound detrimental effects on wound healing, which limits its widespread routine use.

Azathioprine and mycophenolate mofetil

Azathioprine was the first drug to be used in combination with steroids as long-term post-transplant immunosuppression. Mycophenolate mofetil (MMF) has a similar mechanism of action and has been in clinical use since the mid-1990s. Both drugs act by preventing cell proliferation at a DNA level. This is a non-cell-specific effect, but principally affects rapidly dividing cells, such as those in the early stages of allo-recognition and rejection.

MMF has been shown to be more effective than azathioprine in the prevention of acute graft rejection. Its major advantage in clinical practice is its lack of nephrotoxicity, so it is often used to replace the CNI if renal function is becoming a problem.

Azathioprine and MMF have several side effects, the most important of these being myelosuppression: the peripheral leucocyte count is a reasonably sensitive and consistent measure of such toxicity. Diarrhoea is often a problem with MMF, but may be transient and can usually be managed by introducing MMF at a low dose and then gradually increasing the dose over a period of weeks/months.

Biological immunosuppression

Another approach to immunosuppression is to use antibodies which are reactive against a specific part of the rejection cascade. These have been available, in one form or another, since the 1970s.

Polyclonal antibodies

Anti-lymphocyte globulin (ALG) is a polyconal antibody preparation that has been used for both the prevention and treatment of rejection for many years. The principle behind its production is as follows: an animal from another species, usually horse or rabbit, is immunized with human lymphocytes; after a certain time the serum from these immunized animals contains anti-human antibodies. The term 'polyclonal' refers to the fact that the antibodies produced by the immunized animal are derived from multiple B cell clones, each with its own specificity for a particular human lymphocyte surface marker, of which there are many.

The animal serum is then purified to form the ALG preparation.

Mechanisms of action/uses

Administration of ALG results in a rapid decrease in the circulating lymphocyte count. This contrasts with azathioprine and MMF, which cause a pan-leucocytopenia. ALG also depletes lymphocytes from lymph nodes. As a result it significantly interferes with the rejection response. ALG is used as prophylactic immunosuppression at the time of organ transplantation in combination with other immunosuppressants. It is usually given over a 1 to 2 week course. It allows some steroid sparing and also means that the dose of CNI can be reduced in the immediate post-transplant period when, particularly in the renal transplantation, the combination of acute tubular necrosis (as a result of graft ischaemia) and CNI nephrotoxicity can be difficult to manage. The CNI can then be introduced/increased at the end of the ALG course when the graft should be stabilizing.

ALG is also used as a treatment of acute rejection, usually if the organ dysfunction has not improved following the usual treatment with high-dose steroids (steroid-resistant rejection).

Clinical toxicity

The administration of horse or rabbit immunoglobulin is associated with a significant number of immunological side effects. Anaphylaxis is rare but fever and chills occur in 20–25% of patients at the time of the first and sometimes subsequent intravenous injections. Skin rashes affect about 15% of recipients. 'Serum sickness', due to immune complex formation and deposition in the kidneys and joints, is relatively rare.

Monoclonal antibodies

One of the drawbacks of polyclonal antibodies is that even in purified immunoglobulin preparations such as ALG, only about 2% of the immunoglobulins are active against human lymphocytes, with the majority being ordinary horse or rabbit immunoglobulins, which are not reactive against any human antigen, let alone human lymphocytes.

The concept and development of monoclonal antibodies (MAb) represented a great advance in biological science; they are much more specifically targeted than polyclonal preparations and their dose can be precisely known. There are many monoclonal antibodies in regular clinical use.

For many years the only widely used MAb in clinical organ transplantation was orthoclone OKT3 (OKT3). It is a mouse MAb directed against the human T cell receptor (TCR) present on all T lymphocytes. Just as ALG results in a profound fall in total lymphocyte counts, a single dose of OKT3 rapidly depletes the peripheral circulation of all its T lymphocytes. As with ALG, this prevents its use for more than a 1 to 2 week course. It has been used for treatment of steroid-resistant rejection but its role has been limited due to its profound immunosuppression and a variety of other side effects.

Over the last decade or so MAbs to the interleukin-2 receptor (IL-2R) have come into clinical use. They are used for immunosuppressive induction in the first week or two after transplantation and, like ALG, allow reduction in the doses of other immunosuppressants. Their side-effect profile is much less severe than ALG or OKT3 and for this reason their use has become fairly widespread.

Postoperative care

Depending on the organ transplanted and the institution, immediate postoperative care of the transplant patient takes place on the intensive care unit, high-dependency unit or in a designated area on the transplant ward. As with all major surgery, particular attention is paid to fluid balance and maintenance of cardiovascular stability. Of critical importance is the patency of the vascular anastomoses, so there is usually a tendency to over-hydrate rather than under-hydrate the patient.

Standard blood tests are done on a daily basis initially. In addition, trough levels of CNI and/or MMF immunosuppressants are measured regularly, in order to guide the dosing of these drugs. Doppler ultrasound examination of the graft vasculature is usually performed on the first post-op day and then at intervals afterwards, depending on the organ, the institution and any abnormalities seen on the previous scan.

Responsibility for post-op care is often shared between medical and surgical teams. Again, this varies between organs and institutions, but in many cases the physicians (cardiologists, nephrologists, hepatologists, etc.) take primary responsibility for fluid balance, medications, immunosuppression and antimicrobial prophylaxis, whilst the surgeons concern themselves primarily with graft imaging, surgical drains, wound care, etc. The most important principle here is to main-

tain close communication and cooperation between the teams.

Complications of transplantation

In general terms, the early complications of transplantation tend to be those arising as a result of surgical or technical problems, whereas the later complications are often related to immunological responses and the immunosuppressive medications that patients have to take.

'Technical' or 'surgical' complications

Bleeding – intra- or postoperative

Bleeding from one of the vascular anastomoses is quite a common occurrence immediately after the anastomosis has been formed, and may require several further sutures to control. Surgical drain(s) are usually placed to aid detection of postoperative bleeding, but this is relatively rare; when it does occur it is often from small cut vessels on the surface of the organ, probably cut during the post-perfusion dissection in the donor, or from the explant dissection in the recipient. Significant postoperative bleeding may require a return to the operating theatre. Even if the bleeding appears to have stopped without surgery, it is often sensible to wash out any haematoma as it may easily become infected in an immunosuppressed patient.

Pseudoaneurysm formation can occur when there is infection adjacent to a vascular anastomosis. This represents a risk of bleeding and is usually dealt with by interventional radiology, either embolizing the pseudoaneurysm or stenting its origin.

Thrombosis – arterial or venous

While postoperative bleeding is a nuisance and may set back a patient's recovery by some time, vascular thrombosis, arterial or venous, is usually a catastrophe for the graft and almost invariably leads to graft failure and removal of the graft as it becomes necrotic. Such thrombosis may be asymptomatic but is picked up on biochemical testing and ultrasound examination of the graft. If diagnosed promptly, such thrombosis may be salvageable by immediate re-exploration of the graft.

Vascular stenosis

This may occur as a technical complication, where the anastomosis is too tight, or kinked. Percutaneous angioplasty is often used to dilate up the stenosis.

Bile/urine leak

Leaking of blood from vascular anastomoses is relatively easy to identify intraoperatively, but it is harder to spot leaks of urine or bile from the ureteric or biliary anastomoses and these may only become apparent in the surgical drain postoperatively.

The ureteric anastomosis is usually stented at the time of transplantation, but in the case of biliary leaks the initial management is to place a biliary tent across the leak at ERCP.

Biliary/ureteric stricture/stenosis

As for vascular stenoses, such strictures may be technical in origin, but may also be the result of ischaemia of the ureter/bile duct, which may have an immunological cause rather than being purely vascular. The stricture may respond to dilatation and/or stenting, but ultimately further surgery may be required.

Immunological complications

Rejection of the graft is the end result of the immune response to the transplant and may occur despite immunosuppression.

Hyperacute rejection is a particular problem in kidney transplantation. It is an antibody-mediated immune response. It is prevented by (a) matching donor and recipient blood group, (b) matching donor and recipient HLA typing ('tissue typing'), ideally with no A, B or DR mis-matches, and finally (c) running a cross-match prior to transplantation between the recipient's serum and donor lymphocytes. If the cross-match is negative, then the transplant can go ahead.

Acute rejection: this is the most clinically relevant type of rejection and is cell-mediated. It typically occurs several days to several weeks after transplantation. The host immune system attacks the cells of the graft with resultant cell injury and loss of function. Clinically it results in a rising creatinine level after kidney transplantation and a rising AST/ALT after liver transplantation. There are other causes of rising biochemical markers, so frequently a percutaneous core biopsy of the graft is obtained prior to commencing treatment for rejection. Pathology laboratories in transplant centres will be used to processing and reporting such biopsies on a same-day basis, to allow the timely start of treatment. Treatment is

Table 31.10 Clinically significant toxicities of principal immunosuppressants and

Steroids
Poor wound healing
Infection
Diabetes
Psychosis
Calcineurin inhibitors (cyclosporin and tacrolimus)
Viral infection
Hypertension
Diabetes
Renal impairment
Hyperlipidaemia
Neurological
Mycophenolate mofetil
Marrow suppression
Diarrhoea
Sirolimus
Poor wound healing
Anti-lymphocyte globulin
Skin rash
'Serum sickness'
OKT3
Profound lymphocytosis
Anti-IL2R monoclonal antibodies
Few

usually in the form of 'pulsed' intravenous steroids, typically three daily doses of 1000 mg of methylprednisolone. Treatment is monitored by a fall back to normal values of the relevant biochemical marker.

By reducing the incidence of acute rejection, the introduction of cyclosporin in the 1980s improved the results of kidney transplantation and then tacrolimus had a similar impact on liver transplantation in the 1990s.

Chronic rejection: this is a much more insidious process than acute rejection and tends to be a chronic fibrotic process, often involving gradual occlusion of arterioles within the graft. The immunological processes are less clear than in hyperacute and acute rejection and treatment is less straightforward, with less scope for reversibility than with acute rejection.

Complications of immunosuppression

The principal clinically important complications of immunosuppression have been described above, and are summarized in Table 31.10.

In addition to these, there is a general tendency of all immunosuppression to inhibit the immune response to neoplasia and therefore all transplant recipients are at higher risk than the general population of developing cancer. Skin cancer (of all types) is the most common problem, particularly if the patient is exposed to excess sunlight.

Post-transplant lymphoproliferative disease (PTLD) is a disorder of the lymphatic system which presents with multiply enlarged lymph nodes in patients on immunosuppression. It is frequently associated with Epstein-Barr virus. It is not strictly a malignant process and may regress with reduction in the dose of immunosuppressants and anti-viral treatment.

Ethical considerations

The legal body through which all organ transplantation in the UK is currently regulated is the Human Tissue Authority (http://www.hta.gov.uk), which was established in 2005. In turn, the HTA is bound by two laws: the Human Tissue Act (2004) and the European Union Tissue and Cells Directives.

The practice of transplantation requires legislation because of its nature – removing organ(s) from one individual and transplanting them into another. Many ethical dilemmas are raised by transplantation, which can be one of the attractions of working in this field. Among these dilemmas are the following:

Opting in or opting out of organ donation

The current system in the UK for gaining consent for organ donation from a deceased potential donor is based on 'opting in' – consent is obtained from a donor card, donor register and/or next-of-kin. No presumption of willingness to be a donor is made. In 'opting out' the assumption is that all individuals are potential donors at the time of death unless they specifically indicated unwillingness to be a donor during life. Would a system of opting out produce more organ donation in the UK?

Use of marginal grafts

How do we choose recipients for 'marginal' grafts, i.e. grafts that are not as good as we would like? Poor-risk patients will do badly with a marginal graft, whereas a good-risk patient will probably manage. However, should we give our good-risk patients poor-risk transplants? To what extent should patients have a say in whether or not they wish to be transplanted with a particular organ?

Living donation

Based on the 'first do no harm' principle, can surgeons justify performing living donation operations? A healthy individual is subjected to an operation which carries a mortality of about one in 2000 for kidney retrieval and one in a few hundred for liver retrieval. Who should decide on the acceptable level of risk for such procedures?

Payment for organs

Should money ever be involved in encouraging organ donation, whether it be a financial incentive to put your name on the Organ Donor Register, a payment to hospitals which have had a patient become an organ donor, or direct payment to be a living organ donor?

Further reading

Barnard CN. Human cardiac transplantation: An evaluation of the first two operations performed at the Groote Schuur Hospital, Cape Town. *Am J Cardiol* 1968;**22**:584–596.

Carrel A. La technique operatoire des anastomoses vasculaires et la transplantation des visceres. *Lyon Med* 1902;**98**:859–864.

Conference of Medical Royal Colleges and their Faculties in the United Kingdom. Diagnosis of brain death. *Br Med J* 1976;**2**:1187–1188.

Report of the Ad Hoc Committee of Harvard Medical School to examine the definition of brain death. *J Am Med Assoc* 1968;**205**:337.

Index

Note: page numbers in *italics* refer to figures and tables